PROFESSIONAL PARAMEDIC

FOUNDATIONS OF
PARAMEDIC CARE

▷▷▷▷▷▷▷▷▷▷▷▷▷▷▷▷▷▷▷▷▷▷▷▷▷▷▷▷▷▷▷▷▷▷▷▷

VOLUME I

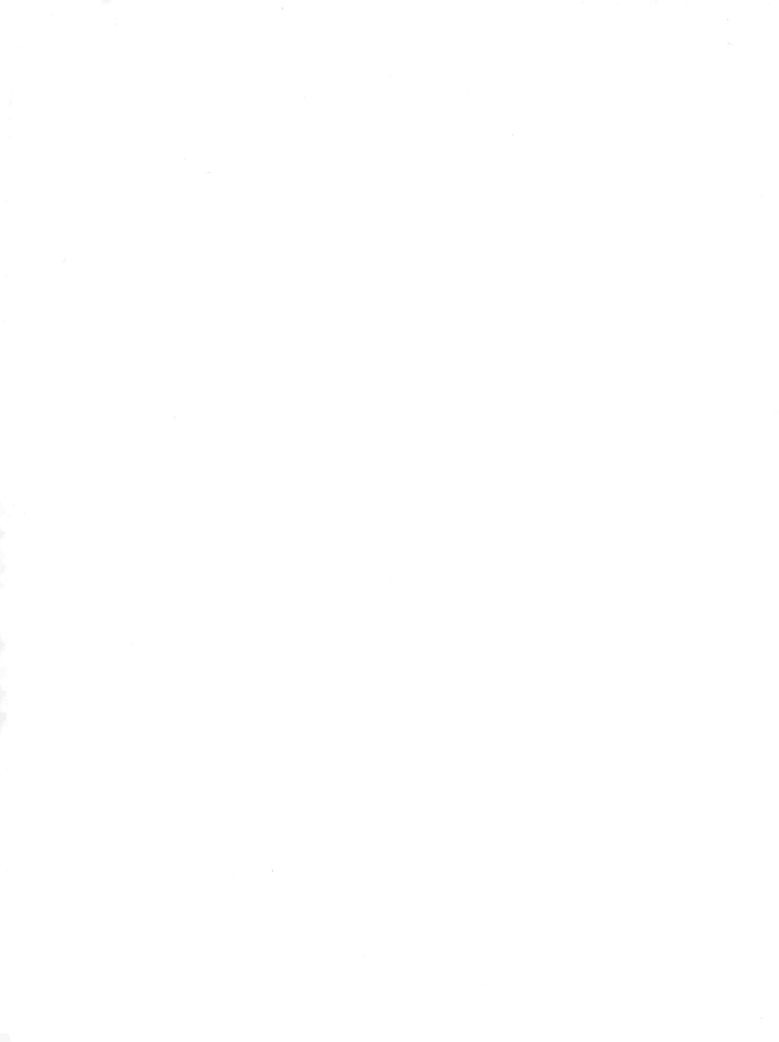

PROFESSIONAL PARAMEDIC

FOUNDATIONS OF
PARAMEDIC CARE

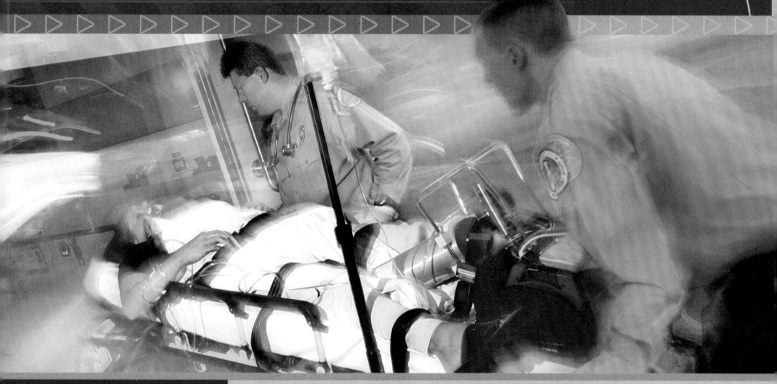

VOLUME I

RICHARD BEEBE | JEFFREY MYERS, DO

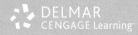

DELMAR
CENGAGE Learning

Australia · Brazil · Japan · Korea · Mexico · Singapore · Spain · United Kingdom · United States

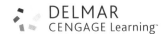

Professional Paramedic: Foundations of Paramedic Care
Richard Beebe and Jeffrey Myers, DO

Vice President, Career and Professional
    Editorial: Dave Garza

Director of Learning Solutions: Sandy Clark

Product Development Manager:
    Janet Maker

Managing Editor: Larry Main

Senior Product Manager: Jennifer A. Starr

Editorial Assistant: Amy Wetsel

Vice President, Career and Professional
    Marketing: Jennifer Baker

Executive Marketing Manager:
    Deborah S. Yarnell

Senior Marketing Manager: Erin Coffin

Marketing Coordinator: Shanna Gibbs

Production Director: Wendy Troeger

Production Manager: Mark Bernard

Senior Content Project Manager:
    Jennifer Hanley

Art Director: Benj Gleeksman

Technology Project Manager:
    Christopher Catalina

For product information and technology assistance, contact us at
Cengage Learning Customer & Sales Support, 1-800-354-9706

For permission to use material from this text or product, submit all requests online at **www.cengage.com/permissions**. Further permissions questions can be emailed to **permissionrequest@cengage.com**

Library of Congress Control Number: 2009924715
ISBN-13: 978-1-4283-2345-2
ISBN-10: 1-4283-2345-7

Delmar
5 Maxwell Drive
Clifton Park, NY 12065-2919
USA

Cengage Learning is a leading provider of customized learning solutions with office locations around the globe, including Singapore, the United Kingdom, Australia, Mexico, Brazil, and Japan. Locate your local office at: **international.cengage.com/region.**

Cengage Learning products are represented in Canada by Nelson Education, Ltd.

To learn more about Delmar, visit **www.cengage.com/delmar.**

Purchase any of our products at your local college store or at our preferred online store **www.ichapters.com.**

NOTICE TO THE READER
Publisher does not warrant or guarantee any of the products described herein or perform any independent analysis in connection with any of the product information contained herein. Publisher does not assume, and expressly disclaims, any obligation to obtain and include information other than that provided to it by the manufacturer. The reader is expressly warned to consider and adopt all safety precautions that might be indicated by the activities described herein and to avoid all potential hazards. By following the instructions contained herein, the reader willingly assumes all risks in connection with such instructions. The publisher makes no representations or warranties of any kind, including but not limited to, the warranties of fitness for particular purpose or merchantability, nor are any such representations implied with respect to the material set forth herein, and the publisher takes no responsibility with respect to such material. The publisher shall not be liable for any special, consequential, or exemplary damages resulting, in whole or in part, from the readers' use of, or reliance upon, this material.

Printed in the United States of America
1 2 3 4 5 XX 11 10 09

DEDICATION

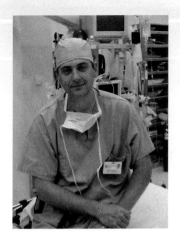

Dedicated to the memory of John Pryor: Paramedic, surgeon, father, husband, brother, and son.

On Christmas Day, 2008, while serving his country in Iraq, Dr. Pryor was tragically killed in the line of duty. Dr. Pryor felt compelled to join the U.S. Army Reserve after witnessing the effects of September 11, 2001, from the rubble pile at Ground Zero. As a member of the U.S. Forward Army Surgical Unit, Dr. Pryor volunteered for not one, but two tours of duty in Iraq, believing that he needed to be there to help others, especially his fellow soldiers. Dr. Pryor's history as a volunteer in medical service started at age 17 with the Clifton Park-Halfmoon Volunteer Ambulance Corp., where he became an Emergency Medical Technician and later a Paramedic. These early beginnings in EMS may have led Dr. Pryor to a career as a widely respected trauma surgeon in Philadelphia.

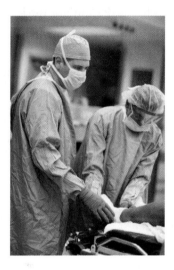

Dr. Pryor often wrote eloquently about his view of the human condition, whether he observed it in war-torn Iraq or the streets of Philadelphia. In one letter he wrote to the family of a mortally wounded Marine, he described his struggle to save the soldier. He expressed that he, his fellow physicians, and especially the Paramedics and EMTs who had the honor of serving with the dead Marine "more than anyone else, know he was a true American hero."

The life of service, love for others, and spirit of devotion of Dr. John Pryor is an example for us all. We, his fellow Paramedics, more than almost anyone else, know he was a true American hero.

TABLE OF CONTENTS

10. BASIC HUMAN PHYSIOLOGY   156

11. PRINCIPLES OF PATHOPHYSIOLOGY   174

SECTION V: PRINCIPLES OF CLINICAL PRACTICE

27. INTRAVENOUS ACCESS   552

28. BLOOD PRODUCTS AND TRANSFUSION   598

29. INTRODUCTION TO PHARMACOLOGY   612

30. PHARMACOLOGICAL INTERVENTIONS FOR CARDIOPULMONARY EMERGENCIES   636

31. PHARMACOLOGICAL THERAPEUTICS FOR MEDICAL EMERGENCIES   682

32. PRINCIPLES OF ELECTROCARDIOGRAPHY   718

33. THE MONITORING ECG   734

34. DIAGONOSTIC ECG— THE 12-LEAD   754

FOREWORD

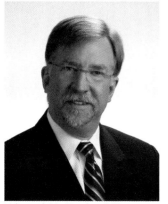

Edward M. Racht, MD

EMS is a practice of medicine....

In medicine, there is an art and a science to everything. The science is *what* we need to do to improve our patient's condition. In its purest form, *what* we do is based on rigorous scientific scrutiny and all the available evidence applicable to the conditions we treat. The art of medicine is *how* we apply the science to our patients in a way that maximizes the potential for an improved outcome. Ironically, the science is often much easier to master than the art. This is perhaps no more pronounced than in the ever-changing, often unpredictable world of EMS.

One thing is very clear: A good practitioner must be accomplished at both the art and the science of medicine.

This is a fascinating time to work in emergency health care. EMS is undergoing tremendous evolution. Not only do we know more about the conditions we treat, but more and more of our clinical practices are now based on sound scientific evidence that applies specifically to our patient population. In the early days of EMS, we adapted evidence from inpatient studies or the laboratory environment and applied it to what we did in the field. While that was certainly appropriate for much of what we did, the challenges of the field and the unique environment of medical care outside the hospital created the need for very targeted research in out-of-hospital medicine. Fortunately, we have more academic initiatives focused on the field than ever before in our brief history. The more we study, the more we learn.

We also understand much more about the seemingly insignificant details that can have a dramatic impact on patient outcomes. Paying attention to those details and focusing on what's truly important in the field practice of medicine is another characteristic of the EMS evolution. For example, there are major changes in the way we attempt to resuscitate our patients. A very consistent, focused attention to perfusion is at the core of everything we do during resuscitation attempts. While many would say we've always believed that to be true, the fact is we didn't always focus on those details during patient care. During those critical moments of assessing and repairing altered physiology and broken anatomy, paying attention to details can often mean the difference between life and death.

As we learn more about the amazing science of the human body and how it behaves when it's "broken," we appreciate that the best approach to management of illness and injury requires more than just memorizing facts. It requires us to put together everything we know, use all our available resources, and develop a plan of action that incorporates clinical care, different modes of transport, and different receiving facilities that have different capabilities. EMS, as a unique practice of medicine, is charged with making complex decisions in short periods of time, often with only limited data. The educational toolbox you hold in your hand will follow you throughout your career and guide you in making the tough calls.

Our role in the Big Picture of Medicine is also evolving. The devastating and unfortunate events of September 11th and the emerging challenges of terrorism, intentional violence, and newer, unpredictable threats have forever focused the American public's attention on the importance of emergency medical care. EMS providers must have the knowledge and ability to deal with an entire spectrum of out-of-hospital problems, ranging from the simple to the unimaginable. Because of the potential for rapidly changing scenarios, we as Paramedics must now know where to go to get the right information and how to rapidly access data we need to make our decisions. Our ability to rapidly deploy our resources throughout a community has also highlighted the value of using EMS providers and systems to disseminate emergency medications and immunizations in the event of a need for rapid public health interventions.

As economic conditions change, our society is retooling healthcare delivery and our patients are using EMS in different ways than they have historically. While that creates some new stresses on EMS, it's a vitally important part of our EMS culture. We are the safety net for many communities suffering from inadequate healthcare resources. Regardless of the number of facilities, patients still get sick and hurt. We should be very proud of our collective ability to care for our fellow human beings regardless of their ability to afford it or our community's ability to provide it. It's who we are.

The newly promulgated Educational Standards are the result of thousands of hours of work from the most accomplished EMS educators, clinicians, and administrators in the profession. The standards provide us with a new approach to delivering the tools that perfect the out-of-hospital delivery of medical care. Rich Beebe, Jeff Myers, and their colleagues have done a spectacular job of presenting the latest evidence in a very comprehensible manner.

As you embark on your educational journey to master the art and science of field medicine, you will continuously discover the valuable educational approach of the *Professional Paramedic Series*. Volume I provides a solid foundation in the knowledge and clinical skills a Paramedic needs to expertly assess and treat patients. In Volumes II and III, the clinical material is presented in a unique way that facilitates the development of critical thinking skills (remember the art?). These volumes use an interrupted case format that narrows a patient's chief concern into a paramedical diagnosis. Volume III also discusses the wide range of operational issues faced by the Paramedic and presents students with the many niches within EMS. In addition, the accompanying student resources and instructor curriculum provide additional cases and avenues to test student knowledge, further refine critical thinking skills, and enhance the teaching and learning experience. Throughout the learning process, students will not only understand what's important, they will also learn how to think their way into the diagnosis and develop an approach that has the best opportunity to improve a patient's condition. *That* is critical thinking.

Enjoy. Enjoy this part of your journey. Enjoy taking care of people when they need you the most. Enjoy learning about the fascinating intricacies of the human body, and enjoy the impact you will have on people's lives every day.

Always remember how important your knowledge, skills, and compassion are for those at the other end of the 9-1-1 call.

Edward M. Racht, MD

PREFACE

THE INTENT OF THIS BOOK

You are about to embark on an exciting career as a Paramedic! Within these pages we will present to you the knowledge, skills, and practical advice needed to become a skilled and proficient Paramedic.

With a focus on future Paramedics *and* the Paramedics of today, the *Professional Paramedic Series* was designed as a comprehensive resource for Paramedic students during their education and as a source for life-long learning. This series seeks to prepare aspiring Paramedic students in community colleges, universities, and other educational programs by not only providing the knowledge needed to become a Paramedic, but also developing the ability to think critically and decisively when seconds count. Beyond the basic foundation of information and skills, this series helps the Paramedic student reach a higher level of understanding. For this reason, the series is also an essential source for recertification and continuing education for practicing Paramedics.

In January 2009, the new National EMS Education Standards were released to the EMS community, setting an academic standard for all Paramedic education programs. This series was specifically developed with the National EMS Education Standards in mind, yet can also be used in Paramedic programs that have not yet transitioned to the new standards. Each of the three volumes, as a series, meet *and exceed* these new education standards by not only teaching the essential information and skills, but also by preparing each student in how to *think* like a Paramedic. As Paramedics who started in the streets and who continue to practice in the streets, we support the vision of the National EMS Education Standards, and have created this aptly named *Professional Paramedic Series*.

WHY WE WROTE THIS BOOK

As educators, we *challenge* our learners—the students of this series—to be the best Paramedics they can be. While there are other Paramedic textbooks available, we felt that the evolving nature of the Paramedic field demanded a fresh approach. We wanted our textbook to challenge Paramedic students to think about the application of medical knowledge to field practice. This approach changed the focus of a Paramedic textbook from being the center of a Paramedic's education to one in which it serves as an authoritative resource that implores the student to explore the current state of the science.

As part of our vision in writing this series, we wanted to recognize the practice of *paramedicine*. What is paramedicine? Paramedicine is a unique practice of emergency medicine that happens in the out-of-hospital setting. First described in the *EMS Agenda for the Future* in 1996, paramedicine is the result of the growth of EMS over almost one half of a century. It encompasses the complete roles and responsibilities of the Paramedic within the domains of health care, public health, and public safety systems. We offer this series as a guide to prehospital emergency medical care and the practice of paramedicine, providing learners with a reference for the often complex, at times ambiguous, and always challenging field of emergency medicine.

We understand that often the best Paramedics are those who start with a natural curiosity about emergency medicine and inquisitiveness about how that medical knowledge could be practically applied in the streets. These students know it is important to be *street smart* as well as *book smart*. This book seeks to help answer their questions through a conversation with the student.

THE *PROFESSIONAL PARAMEDIC SERIES*

This series is designed to follow a logical progression of learning, in which information and skills are presented first in Volume I, followed by the application of those skills in emergency situations in Volume II, and trauma and special response considerations in Volume III. The framework of each book is practical in approach: introducing principles, skills, and terminology; presenting a typical case; walking through critical response steps; and again reviewing key concepts to ensure understanding for successful application on the job.

The series is inclusive of all of the content areas listed in the National EMS Education Standards and contains material on most of the critical and emergent disorders listed in the EMS core content, as well as many of the lower acuity conditions. This coverage helps ensure the student prepares for the National Registry or state Paramedic certification examinations. More importantly, the series helps prepare the Paramedic student for professional Paramedic practice.

VOLUME I: FOUNDATIONS OF PARAMEDIC CARE
ISBN: 978-114283-2345-2

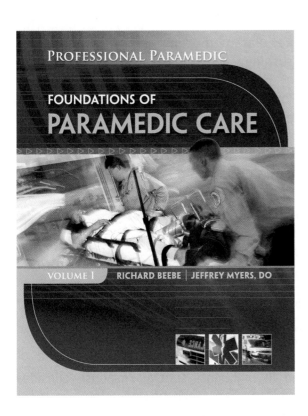

To be able to make a diagnosis, the Paramedic must be well grounded in the basics of medicine including anatomy and physiology as well as pathophysiology. *Volume I: Foundations of Paramedic Care* begins with the basics. This first volume in the series introduces the fundamental information and skills needed for success, as well as the necessary tools to begin developing a professional approach to emergency medicine and Paramedic care.

This volume is divided into six sections.

SECTION I: FRAMEWORK FOR PARAMEDIC PRACTICE

All things must be built on a solid foundation, and the practice of EMS is no different. What do Paramedics do, why do they do it, and how did the field develop? How are EMS systems put together and why? How do we remain safe at what we do? What is research, how do I read it, and why is it important during my daily practice in the street? The four chapters in this section answer these questions and examine these subjects in depth. As the field of paramedicine becomes more evidence based, understanding research and how it applies to our practice becomes more important.

SECTION II: ETHICS AND LAW IN EMS

The public as a whole—and each individual patient and family—entrusts Paramedics with their lives and expects them to provide appropriate care. Some situations pose a dilemma for the Parame-dic, whether it is with a patient, family member, partner, supervisor, or medical director. A strong sense of ethics, displayed by following accepted ethical and legal practices, helps Paramedics maintain the trust and privilege that is placed in them by society.

SECTION III: EMS AND PUBLIC HEALTH

Since September 11, 2001, the EMS community has recognized that there is a strong link between EMS and public health. In some areas of the United States, Paramedics are utilized to augment the public health system, whether as part of a response team to a public health emergency or to assist with day-to-day public health activities in areas of need. These chapters provide a foundation in the field of public health and illness and injury prevention. This allows the Paramedic to fulfill these important roles in the healthcare system.

SECTION IV: SCIENTIFIC PRINCIPLES

The four chapters in this section provide a basic foundation in lifespan development, physiology, pathophysiology, and medical terminology. These areas again help lay a solid foundation for the Paramedic to build upon in the later technical and clinical chapters.

SECTION V: PRINCIPLES OF CLINICAL PRACTICE

Communication with and assessment of the patient is essential to every encounter. Through this process, the Paramedic gains the information needed to form a differential diagnosis and develop an appropriate treatment plan for the patient. These seven chapters provide the Paramedic with the base skills to obtain an effective history and perform a thorough physical examination.

SECTION VI: CLINICAL ESSENTIALS

The final section of this volume includes the essential material regarding airway management, monitoring devices, intravenous access, pharmacology, ECG monitoring, and acquisition that forms the basis for our assessment and treatment. This section provides the foundational material nece-ssary to progress into the clinical chapters in Volume II.

VOLUME II: MEDICAL EMERGENCIES, MATERNAL HEALTH & PEDIATRICS
ISBN: 978-1-4283-2351-3

As Paramedic students, you must learn to apply the skills introduced in the first volume within Volume II of the series. Through introduction of an *interrupted case* approach, this book walks you through a wide range of emergency response situations, from cardiac emergencies to various diseases and disorders, from gynecological concerns to neonatal resuscitation, from the chronically ill to the victims of domestic violence and sexual assault. Each chapter walks you through a typical emergency that a Paramedic might encounter in the field—each case associated with the subject of the chapter-presenting critical information that leads you to develop a Paramedic's diagnosis from the information provided.

It should be understood that each case represents only one potential patient presentation. To that end, we have included additional cases in the accompanying *Study Guide*. It is the responsibility of the student and the instructor to explore these other cases, and other real world examples, to fully appreciate other potential patient presentations. Even so, this cannot possibly cover the entire universe of potential patient presentations. This fact makes Paramedic emergency care exciting and refreshing. These cases are intended to reinforce the commonalities of presentation for the different disorders and syndromes that will permit the Paramedic to make a diagnosis, regardless of the individual patient-specific conditions.

Volume II is divided into four sections:

- **Section I:** Medical Emergencies
- **Section II:** Maternal Health
- **Section III:** Pediatric Medicine
- **Section IV:** Special Patients

PROFESSIONAL PARAMEDIC

MEDICAL EMERGENCIES, MATERNAL HEALTH & PEDIATRICS

VOLUME II   RICHARD BEEBE | JEFFREY MYERS, DO

VOLUME III: TRAUMA CARE AND EMS OPERATIONS
ISBN: 978-1-4283-2348-3

Volume III highlights special response considerations and a broad range of operational medical topics needed to prepare readers with the complete spectrum of knowledge required to succeed as a Paramedic. These aspects of Paramedic practice help to make paramedicine unique and help make paramedicine a profession.

Volume III is divided into four sections:

- **Section I:** Trauma Care
- **Section II:** Environmental Medicine
- **Section III:** EMS Operations
- **Section IV:** Emergency Incident Management

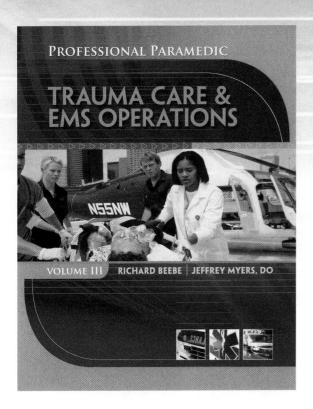

PROFESSIONAL PARAMEDIC

TRAUMA CARE &
EMS OPERATIONS

VOLUME III   RICHARD BEEBE | JEFFREY MYERS, DO

and instructor within the classroom. By portraying realistic emergency situations that a Paramedic is likely to encounter on the job, the book introduces the student to the material in a meaningful manner. This presentation also encourages the decision-making process involved in making a field diagnosis, and outlines a plan of treatment that meets the standard of care within the scope of practice for the patient—for prehospital care and transport to the hospital. Each case is designed to encourage a Paramedic thought process, relates to the subject under discussion within the chapter, and includes follow-up *Case Study Questions* at the end of the chapter.

▶ CASE STUDY QUESTIONS:

Please refer to the Case Study at the beginning of the chapter and answer the questions below.

1. What should be included in the radio report to the medical control physician?
2. How important was the first-due report given by the first member of the public safety team on-scene?

FEATURES

Along with an appealing design, this series has many features intended to motivate the student to read and learn the content and skills presented in each volume.

COMPREHENSIVE COVERAGE

The complex depth and comprehensive breadth of information required for a working knowledge of Paramedic practice, for Paramedic certification, and, ultimately, for success on the job are all provided in an engaging and reader-friendly manner. Students will be properly prepared for these challenges with evidence-based information presented within the content that meets and exceeds National EMS Education Standards.

KEY CONCEPTS

Presented in the beginning of each chapter, the key concepts set learning goals for students and prepare readers for both the didactic and psychomotor skills presented in the chapter.

CASE STUDIES

The case studies included in each chapter facilitate the *conversation*—both the internal dialogue within the student and the dialogue between the student

CHEATED METHOD

This method follows the standard medical intelligence of a Paramedic (sometimes called "medic think"), and encourages students to engage in the critical thinking process needed for a proper field diagnosis and treatment—Chief concern, History, Examination, Assessment, Treatment, Evaluation, and Disposition.

PROFESSIONAL PARAMEDIC

Integrated throughout the book, this advice highlights the professional attitudes that signify the difference between a competent Paramedic and a proficient Paramedic—one fellow Paramedics respect and look to as a leader.

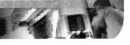

PROFESSIONAL PARAMEDIC

The professional Paramedic does not blame the patient for the disease. For example, tobacco smoking is now known to be a risk factor for lung diseases such as emphysema and cancer. However, tobacco smoking was encouraged by the U.S. government in World War II and tobacco companies advertised that tobacco was an aid to digestion.

STREET SMART

Street Smart tips, lessons learned by the authors while in practice in the field, focus on practical information that can help new Paramedic students perform in less-than-ideal or unusual situations.

CULTURAL/REGIONAL DIFFERENCES

Important considerations are pointed out for responding to patients of different cultural backgrounds. This prepares students for the diverse patient population that the Paramedic will encounter in emergency situations. Understanding these cultural/regional differences increases the Paramedic's effectiveness in the field.

STEP-BY-STEP SKILLS

Photos and descriptions are combined to present critical information on the fundamental skills of Paramedic practice. Each skill is included at the end of the chapter to avoid interrupting the flow of learning, and is referenced in the applicable discussion within the chapter.

CONCLUSION AND KEY POINTS

Critical points in the chapter are covered and provide a basis of review for the student. While the *Conclusion* provides an overall summary of the chapter's main theme, the *Key Points* provide a bulleted list of important information that is helpful for study or review.

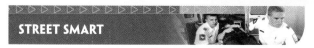

Skill 23-5 King Airway Placement

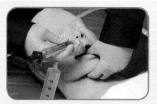
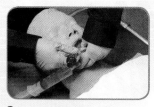
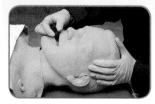
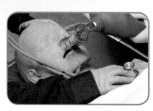
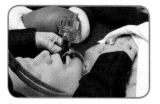
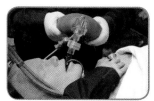

1 Grasp tongue and jaw, lifting toward ceiling. Place tip of tube toward oropharynx, approaching from the patient's right.

2 Rotate the airway counterclockwise as it is advanced.

3 Advance until the orogastric port is at the level of the teeth.

4 Inflate balloon, bag-ventilate the patient, and auscultate breath sounds.

5 Slowly withdraw while listening until breath sounds are the loudest.

6 Confirm placement and secure airway.

REVIEW QUESTIONS

Review Questions at the end of each chapter are helpful for evaluating student knowledge of the concepts presented in the chapter. Review Questions are followed by *Case Study Questions* that encourage students to apply critical thinking skills to the case studies that are presented at the beginning of each chapter.

REFERENCES AND AN EVIDENCE-BASED APPROACH

The content each student learns must be substantiated by science and medicine. Each chapter is thoroughly researched and includes documentation of references that support the content presented in the chapter.

REFERENCES:

1. Kelly CG. The ways and whys of documentation. Good documentation is more than what's on a PCS form. *Emerg Med Serv.* 2007;36(7):30.
2. Perkins TJ. Tell me a story. The importance of good documentation. *Emerg Med Serv.* 2007;36(9):30, 32–33.
3. Krentz MJ, Wainscott MP. Medical accountability. *Emerg Med Clin North Am.* 1990;8(1):17–32.

THE *PROFESSIONAL PARAMEDIC SERIES* CURRICULUM PLAN

We are proud to present a robust curriculum plan for the Paramedic student and instructor. As part of this plan, we offer resources that work hand-in-hand with each volume in the series, serving to further enhance both the teaching and the learning experience. For the students, resources are available that will help them review important concepts through practical application, develop and practice critical thinking skills, and guide them toward further research and discovery. For the instructors, we offer tools that will help them efficiently prepare for classroom instruction, manage and track student progress of didactic and skill requirements, keep informed of new advances in the EMS field, and overall, engage students in learning both in and out of the classroom.

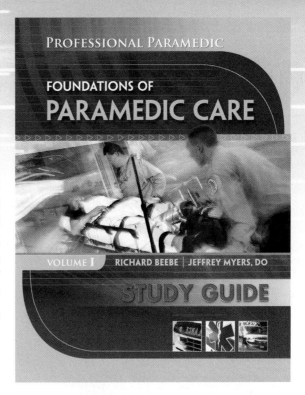

FOR THE STUDENT

STUDY GUIDES

Volume I Study Guide, ISBN: 978-1-4283-2346-9
Volume II Study Guide, ISBN: 978-1-4283-2352-0
Volume III Study Guide, ISBN: 978-1-4283-2349-0

Bridging the gap between knowledge and application, one *Study Guide* accompanies each volume to offer learners additional case studies for each chapter, along with multiple types of practice questions and activities required for comprehension of the material.

ONLINE COMPANIONS

Students are provided with FREE access to our website with an *Online Companion* to accompany each volume. This website invites students to further study and explore the concepts presented in each volume. The website includes articles and up-to-date information on the EMS field, related links to important industry organizations and resources, information related to national guidelines, illustrated glossaries, and bonus content. Each Online Companion is uniquely designed to the corresponding volume in the series, and contains information relevant to the topics covered within that volume.

Visit www.cengage.com/community/ems to access these Online Companions!

FOR THE INSTRUCTOR

INSTRUCTOR RESOURCES (CD-ROM)

Volume I Instructor Resources,
ISBN: 978-1-4283-2347-6
Volume II Instructor Resources,
ISBN: 978-1-4283-2353-7
Volume III Instructor Resources,
ISBN: 978-1-4283-2350-6

The Instructor Resources for each volume are designed to help instructors effectively prepare students to become well-rounded, street-smart Paramedics within the guidelines of the new National EMS Educational Standards. The *Instructor Resources on CD-ROM* includes tools that help instructors and administrators prepare their Paramedic program in a timely and efficient manner. Each CD-ROM includes the following features:

■ **Administration:** This section includes information on setting up the program, as well as practical advice for transitioning your program to the new National EMS Educational Standards. In addition, it includes the following tools:
  ● **Equipment Checklist:** The checklist provides a resource for instructors to ensure that they have the necessary tools for classroom

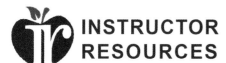

INSTRUCTOR RESOURCES

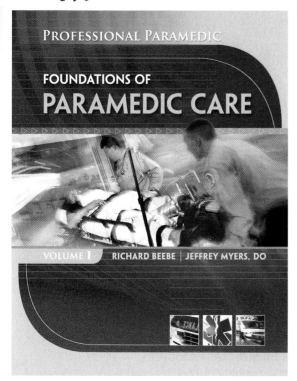

PROFESSIONAL PARAMEDIC

FOUNDATIONS OF
PARAMEDIC CARE

VOLUME I   RICHARD BEEBE | JEFFREY MYERS, DO

instruction and for setting up and running skill sequences.

● **Concept Maps:** Highlighting the decision-making process, these *Concept Maps* offer a way for instructors to help students conceptualize ideas in the classroom and develop the critical thinking skills necessary for determining a field diagnosis. Each Concept Map, utilizing a typical emergency scenario, walks students through the critical thinking steps used during an EMS response.

● **Correlation to National EMS Education Standards and D.O.T Paramedic Curriculum:** These guides map out Paramedic content and provide students with the volume, chapter, and pages where this content is covered in the *Professional Paramedic Series*.

■ **Lesson Plans:** Including an outline of each chapter, with correlations to the accompanying PowerPoint presentations, skill sheets, and helpful teaching tips, these *Lesson Plans* provide a helpful guide for classroom instruction. These plans are provided in Word format so that instructors may revise them according to local practice variations and regional/state medical protocols.

■ **PowerPoint Presentations:** Correlated to the accompanying Lesson Plans, these presentations combine key points with photos, graphics, and video to serve as a basis for either interactive classroom instruction or as augmentation of an asynchronous distance learning program.

■ **Computerized Test Banks:** Containing over 1,000 questions and covering the content in each chapter, these *Test Banks* in ExamView format allow instructors to manage test administration in the classroom. Instructors may create or edit tests based on existing questions, edit questions, and add or delete questions to fit local practice variations and regional/state medical protocols—all in this user-friendly program.

■ **Teaching Sheets:** Highlighting the Paramedic skills necessary for Paramedic practice, these *Teaching Sheets* provide a baseline for skills learning. Each Teaching Sheet provides a breakdown of the critical principles for the skill, and is included in Word format to allow instructors to add specifics based on their local requirements and/or regional/state protocols and procedures.

■ **Clinical Logs:** Based on the Teaching Sheets, these *Clinical Logs* provide forms for tracking student accomplishment of prehospital (field) and in-hospital (clinical) skills. These forms, complete with a signature page, are provided in Word format to allow instructors to edit them in order to meet local requirements.

■ **Research and Discovery—Instructor Reference Guide:** Paramedicine, like medicine, has an ever-changing body of knowledge. To remain current, the Paramedic must be a life-long learner. In addition to the listing of references that appears at the end of chapters in each volume in the series, this *Instructor Reference Guide* provides additional resources—including articles, websites, organizations, and other reference materials—to find information on specific topics. This ensures that instructors remain informed of current practices in the EMS field.

ONLINE COMPANIONS

Linked to the student Online Companions, these resources provide instructors FREE access to bonus content, including podcasts, articles on new information and technology, links to EMS community websites, information related to national guidelines, and additional classroom materials. Each Online Companion is uniquely designed to the corresponding volume in the series, and contains information relevant to the topics covered within that volume.

WEB TUTOR ON WEBCT AND BLACKBOARD

Providing a content-rich, Web-based teaching and learning aid, this tool helps to emphasize and clarify complex concepts, provides a forum for discussion, and offers a venue for tracking course syllabus and other program-related activities.

WebTutor on Blackboard Course allows instructors to quickly and easily jump-start their on-line course development. Whether you want to Web-enable your class or put an entire course on-line, WebTutor delivers!

ABOUT THE AUTHORS

RICHARD BEEBE, MSEd, BSN, RN, NREMT-P

Richard Beebe started his EMS career in 1974 as an Explorer Scout with the Moyers Corners Volunteer Fire Department in upstate New York. Since obtaining his Emergency Medical Technician certification in 1975, Mr. Beebe has continuously maintained his certification and his practice. During his career Mr. Beebe has served in fire/EMS, commercial EMS, volunteer EMS, and as a municipal Paramedic. During that time, he has served as a volunteer crew chief, a squad captain, and Paramedic supervisor. Mr. Beebe currently serves as a civilian Paramedic for the Guilderland Police Department, outside of Albany, New York.

Mr. Beebe has also been a critical care nurse since 1985, having practiced for 10 years in both the Emergency Department and the Intensive Care Unit. During these years, Mr. Beebe developed his knowledge of medicine and—perhaps, more importantly—an appreciation of the potential impact that prehospital advanced life support could have on patient morbidity and mortality.

Consistent with that belief, Mr. Beebe became a Paramedic in 1988 and, in hopes of advancing the practice of his fellow Paramedics, started his career as a Paramedic Educator.

During his tenure as a Paramedic Educator, Mr. Beebe has served in the capacity as lecturer, instructor-coordinator, and Paramedic program director. He continues to speak at local, regional, state, and national conferences on topics of importance to both the EMT and the Paramedic.

Mr. Beebe is presently a clinical assistant professor at the State University of New York at Cobleskill and Paramedic program director for Bassett Healthcare's Center for Rural Emergency Medical Services Education.

Mr. Beebe has been published in several journals, including the *Journal of Emergency Medical Services* and *Fire-Engineering,* as well as being a co-author for Delmar's *Fundamentals of Basic Emergency Care,* now in its third edition.

Mr. Beebe has contributed to the previous editions of the National Standard Curriculum for Paramedic, Intermediate, and Basic; to the national EMS Education Agenda for the Future; to the national EMS Scope of Practice; and served as content leader for the National EMS Education Standards. Mr. Beebe is also a charter member of the National Association of EMS Educators.

JEFF MYERS, DO, EdM, NREMT-P, FAAEM

Dr. Myers has been involved in EMS for over 20 years, including 12 years in the prehospital environment and 18 years as an EMS educator. Dr. Myers began his EMS journey in 1988 in upstate New York by volunteering for his college ambulance (RPI Ambulance) and a local community ambulance (North Greenbush Ambulance Association). He began teaching in 1990 for the Rensselaer County Ambulance and Rescue Association, eventually becoming a state Certified Instructor Coordinator. Dr. Myers ran the EMT-Basic original course in Rensselaer County for three years before leaving to attend medical school. During the early 1990s, he also served as a Rensselaer County Deputy County EMS Coordinator for four years, responding to multi-ambulance and multi-agency incidents. His field experience includes volunteer, commercial, and combination paid-volunteer agencies as a Paramedic in upstate New York and in southern Maine.

Dr. Myers attended medical school at the University of New England College of Osteopathic Medicine in Biddeford, Maine. While in medical school, he continued to teach ACLS and BCLS classes through the local hospital.

Dr. Myers then moved to Buffalo, New York, completing his residency in Emergency Medicine at SUNY-Buffalo in 2004. In his final year of residency, he served as Chief Resident. He stayed at SUNY-Buffalo for a two-year EMS Fellowship through the Erie County Medical Center and completed a Masters in Education at the University of Buffalo. He is board certified in Emergency Medicine and a Fellow of the American Academy of Emergency Medicine.

He is currently on faculty at SUNY-Buffalo as a clinical assistant professor and serves as the associate system EMS medical director and EMS fellowship director at the Erie County Medical Center. Dr. Myers is an active member of the Specialized Medical Assistance Response Team, western New York's physician response team, which is called upon to augment local EMS during MCIs, and special situations, for example patient entrapment and providing tactical medical support. He is the assistant medical director for Rural Metro Medical Services of Western New York, based out of Buffalo, New York. Dr. Myers has several publications in peer-reviewed journals and is an author for Delmar Cengage Learning, writing *Automated Defibrillation for Professional and Lay Rescuers* and *Principles of Pathophysiology and Emergency Care*. He also produced and directed the *Techniques in Airway Management* DVD series. Dr. Myers has spoken at several regional and national conferences on a variety of topics. For more information on topics or to provide feedback on the textbook, please check out Dr. Myers' website at http://ems-ed.photoemsdoc.com.

ACKNOWLEDGMENTS

As with all of our projects, the *Professional Paramedic Series* would not have been possible without the support, guidance, and participation of the contributors, reviewers, and advisory board members. We owe these individuals our sincere thanks.

CONTRIBUTORS

During the development of *Volume I: Foundations of Paramedic Care*, we were honored to have the following contributors participate in researching, writing, editing, and reviewing materials to ensure a comprehensive and accurate Paramedic guide:

Anthony Billittier, IV, MD, Commissioner of Health, Erie County, New York; Assistant Professor Emergency Medicine, Department of Emergency Medicine, School of Medicine and Biomedical Sciences; Assistant Professor, Department of Social and Preventative Medicine, School of Public Health and Health Professions, State University of New York at Buffalo

Jonnathan Busko, MD, MPH, EMT-P, Emergency Physician, Eastern Main Medical Center, Bangor, Maine

Steve Carson, BS, PA, CCEMT-P, Physician Assistant, Army National Guard, Afghanistan

Deborah Kufs, MS, RN, EMT-P, Interim Director, Paramedic Program, Hudson Valley Community College, Troy, New York

Jeffrey Thompson, MD, Attending Physician, Professional Emergency Services and Clinical Instructor of Emergency Medicine, State University of New York at Buffalo, Buffalo, New York

Brett Williams, MD, Florida Emergency Physicians, Orlando, Florida

For the development of the art program in this volume—the countless hours spent in preparation, set up, and shooting of the photography appearing in this book, as well as the extensive research, persistence, and acquisition of those "hard to find" photos and graphics—we express our gratitude to the following individuals:

Jon Behrens, AAS, EMT-P, Paramedic Instructor, State University of New York at Cobleskill

Chris Lenaghan, Photographer, CML Media Services

Abigail Reip, Photo Acquisition and Permission Coordinator

Liana Dypka, Art Manuscript Development

REVIEWERS

To the reviewers, who provided an honest evaluation of the content in the book and continual guidance throughout development of this volume, we express our appreciation:

Melissa Alexander-Shook, Director of EMS Academy, University of New Mexico, New Mexico

Steve Kanarian, Paramedic Instructor, Rockland Community College, New York

Mike McLaughlin, Director of Health Occupations, Kirkwood Community College, Iowa

M. Jane Pollock, Extension Education Training Specialist, Emergency Medicine, East Carolina University, North Carolina

Don Royder, Emergency Medical Services Program Coordinator, Texas Engineering Extension Service, Emergency Services Training Institute, Texas

EMS ADVISORY BOARD

We offer special thanks to our Advisory Board Members, who take time out of their schedules to advise us on our training materials, the status of the EMS field, and to work with us as partners in striving to meet the needs of the students and instructors of today—and those of the future:

Scott Bourn, National Director of Clinical Programs, National Resource Center, American Medical Response, Colorado

Deb Cason, Associate Professor, University of Texas Southwestern Medical Center, Texas

Don Collins, Captain, Massport Fire-Rescue, Logan International Airport, Boston

Stephen Dean, Director, Corporate Training, Paramedic Plus, Oklahoma

Joe Grafft, President, Customized Safety Training

Art Hsieh, Chief Executive Officer and Director of Education, San Francisco Paramedic Association, California

Mike Kennamer, Director of Workforce Development, Northeast Alabama Community College, Alabama

Guy Piefer, Paramedic Program Coordinator, Borough of Manhattan Community College, City of Yonkers Fire Department, New York

Ed Racht, Vice President of Medical Affairs and Chief Medical Officer, Piedmont Newnan Hospital, Georgia

Karla Rickards, EMS Training Coordinator, Unified Fire Authority, Salt Lake County

John Rinard, Training Coordinator, TEEX, Texas A&M University

John Sinclair, Fire Chief, Kittitas Valley Fire Rescue Emergency Manager, City of Ellensburg, Washington; Immediate Past Chair and International Director, International Association of Fire Chiefs, Emergency Medical Services Section

Mike Ward, Director of Emergency Health Services, George Washington Medical Center, Washington, DC

FROM THE AUTHORS

BEEBE

First, I would like to acknowledge my friends and family, and particularly my wife Laura, whose support has sustained me over the 10 years that it took to write this book. Thank you for your love.

I would also like to thank the professionals at Delmar/Cengage Learning who have helped support this idea from its onset and continue to encourage me to greater accomplishments. I would like to thank Sandy, Benj, Erin, and particularly Jennifer, the backbone of this excellent team.

Finally, I would like to thank my students who, each and every year, challenge me to be the best Paramedic and educator that I can be and who, even to this day, continue to inspire me. In the 30-plus years I have been involved in EMS and EMS education, I have truly seen EMS in general—and Paramedics in particular—evolve into a caring profession that we all can be proud of.

MYERS

Thanks and love to my family. This textbook (and all my life's projects) would not be possible without their support.

DELMAR/CENGAGE LEARNING TEAM

For the team that always finds a way, every day, to turn an idea into a reality, we thank these extraordinary people for their hard work, dedication, support, and creativity:

Janet Maker, Product Development Manager
Jennifer Starr, Senior Product Manager
Amy Wetsel, Editorial Assistant
Jennifer Hanley, Senior Content Project Manager
Erin Coffin, Senior Marketing Manager
Shanna Gibbs, Marketing Coordinator

CLOSING THOUGHTS

In this time when the importance of quality improvement is understood and appreciated, we encourage students and instructors alike to communicate with us. Via these conversations, all parties can improve their understandings. We are all enriched through this communication.

Richard W.O. Beebe
Bassettmedic@gmail.com

Jeffrey W. Myers
http://ems-ed.
photoemsdoc.com

SECTION 1

FRAMEWORK FOR PARAMEDIC PRACTICE

All things must be built on a solid foundation, and the practice of EMS is no different. What does a Paramedic do, why do they do it, and how did the field develop? How are EMS systems put together and why? How do we remain safe at what we do? What is research, how do I read it and why is it important during my daily practice in the street? The four chapters in this section answer these questions and examine these subjects in depth. As the field of paramedicine becomes more evidence based, understanding research and how it applies to our practice becomes more important.

- **Chapter 1:** Roles and Responsibilities of the Professional Paramedic
- **Chapter 2:** Introduction to Emergency Medical Service Systems
- **Chapter 3:** Workforce Safety and Wellness
- **Chapter 4:** Research and EMS

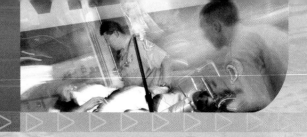

CHAPTER 1

ROLES AND RESPONSIBILITIES OF THE PROFESSIONAL PARAMEDIC

KEY CONCEPTS:

Upon completion of this chapter, it is expected that the reader will understand these following concepts:

- The profession of paramedicine combines aspects of public health, public safety, and health care
- Standards and scope of practice define the Paramedic's knowledge, skills, and attitudes
- The Paramedic's role is as a healer, clinician, and teacher
- Quality assurance, Quality improvement, and continuing education enhance both the Paramedic's individual practice and that of the profession as a whole
- The Paramedic is a physician extender through stewardship, leadership, and followership

▶ CASE STUDY:

Traffic was slowed around the accident site. As the two teens drove slowly by, each looked at the Paramedics who were providing and directing care of the victims. The first teen stated, "They sure looked like they knew what they were doing." The second teen added, "I wonder what else they do."

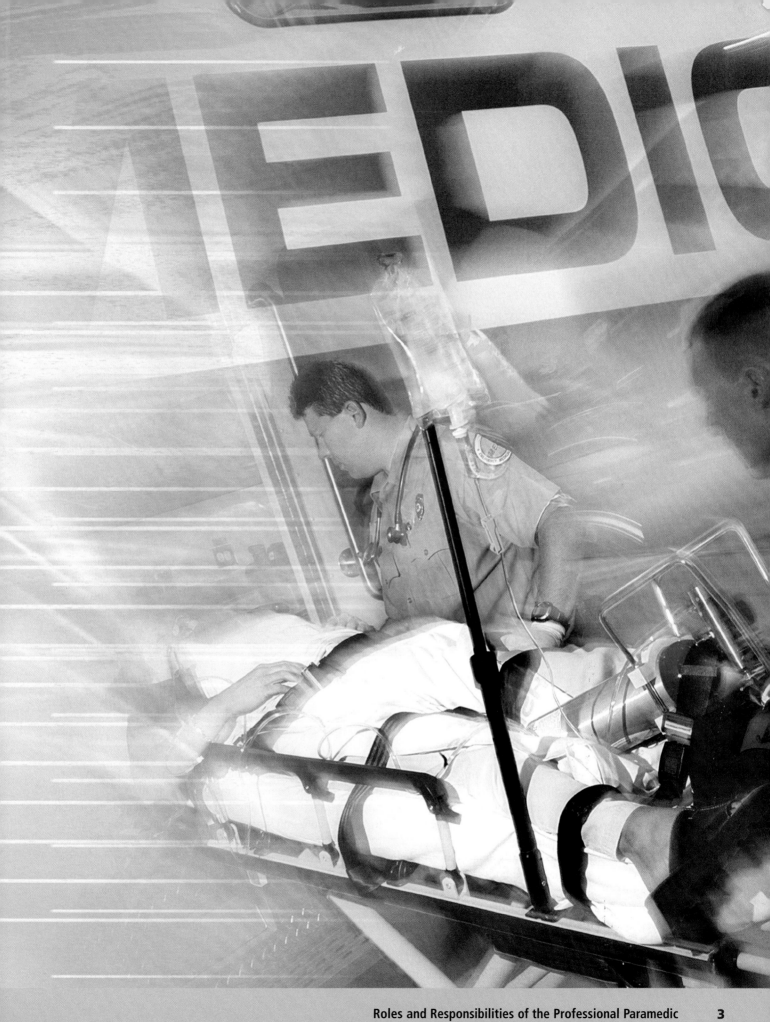

OVERVIEW

Although paramedicine is a relatively young profession compared to many others, it has found its footing as a unique part of the healthcare system. The Paramedic's role has evolved from simply responding to emergencies to now practicing an expanded scope of practice as a physician extender. In this way, the Paramedic has proved to be a vital part of the public health and safety team. This chapter not only examines the origins of paramedicine but also how national education standards and accreditation of educational programs coupled with professional organizations have helped to validate paramedicine as a profession. The chapter also examines the Paramedic's core values and his or her role as healer, clinician, and teacher. As the Paramedic's scope of practice and community responsibilities continue to develop, quality assurance, quality improvement, and continuing educational programs need to be established. The Paramedic's independent and interdependent role as a physician extender relies on leadership and stewardship.

What Is Paramedicine?

Paramedicine is a special subset of medicine that Paramedics provide in the out-of-hospital setting. Paramedics, as allied healthcare professionals, practice paramedicine under often austere conditions and with a minimum of equipment. Paramedic practice is both independent as well as interdependent. The universe of independent Paramedic practice includes disaster planning, response readiness, scene management, and emergency vehicle operations. Collaboratively, Paramedics work interdependently with emergency physicians to bring the highest level of medical care outside of the hospital.

While Paramedics traditionally have provided emergency care as part of the emergency response system, Paramedics also provide care during transportation between medical facilities. Interfacility patient care often involves a high level of medical complexity and requires education above that of the entry-level Paramedic.

Paramedicine is positioned at the intersection of health care, public health, and public safety. Owing its existence to each, the Paramedic is cross-trained in each of these areas. As a result, a synergy occurs among the knowledge from these three areas and the result is paramedicine, a unique body of knowledge which is exclusive of its origins.

More than a vocation, paramedicine involves extensive educational preparation, typically at a collegiate level, to attain the specialized knowledge necessary to become a Paramedic. Paramedic education is usually attained in an educational program that is accredited by a body which includes professional Paramedics.

Paramedicine is also an applied science. To attain proficiency at patient care skills and apply the knowledge gained to care of patients, Paramedic students learn and work under the watchful eye of preceptors. Upon completion of a program of study, Paramedics complete professional certification examinations and become licensed to practice paramedicine. All Paramedics understand the importance and the necessity of giving back to their profession through teaching Paramedic students.

The practice of paramedicine, like the practice of medicine, is constantly evolving. Professional Paramedics incorporate and apply new information and technologies in their practice. Through programs of competency assurance and professional development, offered in continuing education programs, the Paramedic stays current with the profession.

The Paramedic's professional identity revolves around the voluntary assumption of certain roles and responsibilities and a code of ethics. Once Paramedic status is attained, that person is a Paramedic and, regardless of other roles the person may have in a lifetime, will always see himself as a Paramedic.

The practice of medicine is an art, not a trade; a calling, not a business; a calling in which your heart will be exercised equally with your head.

—William Osler, MD

The professional Paramedic has many roles, the first of which is as a healer. Healing is an attempt to mollify the effects of disease. In many instances the Paramedic is unable to effect a cure and strives instead to relieve pain and suffering. Healing is a process of helping people physically, mentally, and spiritually endure their illness. As one of the healing professions, when the practicing Paramedic demonstrates empathy, respect, and a genuine interest in the patient, the Paramedic is seen as a compassionate caregiver—a healer. This ability to help the patient in distress to heal while providing medical care could be seen as the art of paramedicine.

While Paramedics rarely cure a disease, the practice of paramedicine is also based, in part, on the science of medicine.[1,2] The science of medicine focuses on cure and medical research is continually improving the treatment of patients with diseases. In turn, the medical treatments that Paramedics provide are based, to the extent possible, on medical research. A professional Paramedic always keeps abreast of the medical science which has an impact on the practice.

Paramedics are also stewards. As a shared practice that originates in medicine, Paramedics are responsible for maintaining the ideals of medicine and to practice in a manner that would bring honor to themselves and their physician colleagues. The right to practice paramedicine is given to Paramedics by physicians who understand the importance of collaborative practice.

As members of the healthcare team Paramedics are also leaders. Paramedics are not leaders by virtue of their position but by their ability to affect the behavior of other members of the team to accomplish the goal of patient care. As a leader, the Paramedic may have to take on the role of teacher or patient advocate, but in every instance the patient's welfare is foremost in the Paramedic's mind.[3]

As the leader, the Paramedic also understands the importance of followership. A Paramedic's adherence to the physician's orders, as well as those of other authority figures, is an example of followership. Followership is not offered begrudgingly but instead willingly, with an understanding of the importance of teamwork for patient care.

PROFESSIONAL PARAMEDIC

The role of patient advocate encompasses all of the Paramedic's other roles and responsibilities.

Hallmarks of a Profession

In the past, Paramedics were considered auxiliary healthcare providers, unlicensed care providers who received the majority of their training "on the job" (OJT) and were not considered to be healthcare professionals. Classic examples of healthcare professionals are physicians, nurses, and physician assistants. These groups are considered professional because they meet certain criteria to be considered a profession. Paramedics have not yet met those criteria. However, the field of paramedicine is in the process of professionalization.

Some of the criteria for consideration as a healthcare professional were discussed in the fourth report of the Pew Health Professions Commission entitled, "Recreating Health Professional Practice for a New Century."[4] The section entitled, "Professional Characteristics of Allied Healthcare Providers" describes what is needed for a group to be considered an allied healthcare provider.

To be considered an allied healthcare provider, Paramedics would first need extensive educational preparation. This type

Table 1-1 Qualities of a Profession

- Extensive educational preparation
- Accreditation of educational programs
- Mentoring
- Certification
- Licensing
- Professional development
- Professional societies
- Code of ethics—professional boundaries

of education is typically provided in a college or university environment in accredited educational programs. During their education, Paramedic students would need professional models, or mentors to guide them along in their educational development. Upon successful completion of the original education, the Paramedic's rite of passage into the profession would be certification and licensure. Once in the field, the practicing professional Paramedics would be expected to maintain their education through competency assurance and professional development.[5] Paramedics would also be expected to contribute to the profession through active participation with fellow Paramedics in an association or society. Central to these professional associations or societies is a code of ethics which helps define the profession. Many qualities are common in all professions (Table 1-1).

Currently Paramedics are required to obtain extensive educational preparation to acquire a unique body of knowledge. An increasing number of Paramedic programs are being offered in accredited programs provided at postsecondary schools where Paramedic students also learn from experienced preceptors during an internship. Plus, there is a growing trend toward licensing Paramedics. These efforts, and others, will help to shape and develop the Paramedic profession.

CULTURAL/REGIONAL DIFFERENCES

No national exam serves as a culminating point for entry into the profession of paramedicine as does the NCLEX for professional nursing. A tapestry of county, regional, and state requirements often create difficulties in transferring from one geographical area to another.

To assist current and aspiring healthcare professionals, the Pew Health Commission listed what were felt to be the 21 competencies that healthcare professionals needed to aspire to in the twenty-first century. Some of these are especially germane to Paramedics (Table 1-2).

Table 1-2 Partial List of the 21 Competencies for Healthcare Professionals for the Twenty-First Century from the Pew Health Commission

- Embrace a personal ethic of social responsibility and service
- Exhibit ethical behavior in all professional activities
- Provide evidence-based clinically competent care
- Integrate population-based care in services into practice
- Improve access to healthcare for those with unmet health needs
- Provide culturally sensitive care to a diverse society
- Use communication and information technology effectively and appropriately
- Work in an interdisciplinary team
- Practice leadership
- Contribute to continuous improvement of the healthcare system
- Continue to learn and help others learn

Education Systems

Key to a profession is the educational preparation required to enter that profession. In the past, the DOT National Standard Curriculum has served as the basis for EMS education. Since the creation and adoption of the first EMT-A National Standard Curriculum (NSC) in 1969, the DOT NSC has served as both curriculum and a scope of practice in that EMS lacked any other unifying documents. The document which will replace the NSC is the National EMS Education Standards. The standards, together with the national core content and national scope of practice, identify the Paramedic's knowledge, skills, and attitudes.

The National EMS Education Standards (NEMSES) provide the foundation for that final terminal objective of every EMS education program—the graduation of a competent entry-level Paramedic.[6]

Commission on Accreditation of Allied Health Education Programs

To ensure that Paramedic education programs adhere to these educational standards, the Commission on the Accreditation of Allied Health Education Programs (CAAHEP) charges the Committee on Accreditation of Educational Programs for the EMS Professions (CoAEMSP) to investigate and report to CAAHEP.

Accreditation of a Paramedic program is evidence of a satisfactory report from the CoAEMSP having been furnished to CAAHEP. At present, CAAHEP accredits over 2,000 educational programs in 19 healthcare professions.

Beginning in 2012, the National Registry of Emergency Medical Technicians will only permit those individuals who have completed their education in an accredited Paramedic education program to seat for the Paramedic national certification examination.

National Registry of Emergency Medical Technicians

The culmination of a Paramedic education should be certification. A certification is a formal process in which an outside organization, often an organization that represents the profession or the professional association, verifies through written and/or practical examination the competency of an individual who wishes to enter the profession. This process seeks to ensure that the individual possesses the minimum level of knowledge and skill required to practice that profession.

The **National Registry of Emergency Medical Technicians (NREMT)** presently provides a certification process of practical testing and written examinations for the certification of Paramedics. Successful completion of the National Registry testing demonstrates that the Paramedic has demonstrated a minimally acceptable level of proficiency in the core elements.

The National Registry was initiated by recommendation of the American Medical Association's (AMA) Committee on Highway Traffic Safety, chaired by Dr. Oscar Hampton Jr. The committee included notable EMS authorities such as Dr. J.D. "Deke" Farrington, author of the influential article "Death in the Ditch." The National Registry of EMT was formed in June 1970 and—under the leadership of its first executive director, Rocco V. Morando—proceeded to meet its mission "to certify and register EMS professionals throughout their careers by a valid and uniform process to assess the knowledge and skills for competent practice."

National Association of Emergency Medical Technicians

The EMS profession is relatively young compared to other healthcare professions. While EMS has roots in the past, the emergence of EMS as a profession has occurred in less than four decades. Nevertheless, EMS has strived to meet its ideals and become recognized as a profession.

One of the other attributes of a profession is a professional organization or society that speaks on behalf of the members. The **National Association of EMT (NAEMT)** is a professional organization, founded in 1975, whose mission is to represent the views and opinions of all prehospital care providers. As the voice of the profession, it has been leading efforts to help professionalize EMS. Through its leadership, the NAEMT has been influential with the advancement of EMS as an allied healthcare profession. The NAEMT has liaisons with at least 28 federal agencies and professional organizations with interests in EMS. That list of collaborating organizations includes the American College of Emergency Physicians (ACEP), the National Association of EMS Physicians (NAEMSP), the Advocates for EMS, the National Registry of EMT (NREMT), the International Association of Firefighters (IAFF), the International Association of Fire Chiefs (IAFC), the Emergency Nurses Association (ENA), the American Red Cross (ARC), EMS for Children (EMSC), the Federal Emergency Management Agency (FEMA), the National Rural Health Association (NRHA), and the Commission on the Accreditation of Ambulance Services (CAAS), to name a few.

National Institute of Medicine Report

The landmark National Institute of Medicine Reports entitled "EMS at the Crossroads" and "Hospital Based Emergency Care: At the Breaking Point," released in 2006, spoke of the dysfunctional and fragmented emergency services in the United States.[7] These reports encouraged standardization of emergency services through processes such as national accreditation of the Paramedic programs, national certification of Paramedics, and organized efforts at improving the delivery of patient care through cooperation with other healthcare professions.

Core Values

The clinical care provided by Paramedics, guided by evidence-based science, is dictated by protocols, guidelines, and algorithms. But the human side of paramedicine—that aspect of EMS which makes it part of the patient care realm—is dictated by another set of rules, the core values of a Paramedic professional. Paramedics must possess these core values, which complement and enhance their clinical skills and medical knowledge. Otherwise, Paramedics will be ineffectual as patient care providers.

The key professional attribute and the first core value of a Paramedic is caring. Caring is an expression of concern toward the patient by the Paramedic and is foundational to the Paramedic–patient relationship. To practice caring, some Paramedics have been taught to use the PEARLS model advanced by the American Academy on Physician and Patient. The letters in the **PEARLS** mnemonic stand for *partnership, empathy, apology, respect, legitimization,* and *support*. These are the qualities that provide for a strong Paramedic–patient relationship.

While in the past most patients willingly accepted a physician's advice without question, patients today are less tolerant of this paternalistic approach. Patients now want to be knowledgeable about their choices and to be involved in their healthcare decisions. They want to **partner** with their healthcare provider. Paramedics who involve patients in their own care, in a partnership, are demonstrating an acceptance of the patient's wishes to be involved and in control. Paramedics who involve patients in decisions about their own care empower the patients to take more responsibility for their own health. This Paramedic–patient cooperation tends to improve the patient's overall satisfaction with the care provided by the Paramedic.

Another key to quality patient care is **empathy**. Empathy is an emotional understanding of the patient's feelings; to be able to understand what it is like to walk in the other person's shoes. Some refer to empathy as a good bedside manner. Paramedics can demonstrate their empathy through both action and words.

Like the teachable moment—that point in time when the student is most susceptible to learning—empathy is best expressed when the provider recognizes the presence of strong emotion and then responds to the patient in a supportive manner. To be supportive, all the Paramedic need do is imagine the feeling the patient is experiencing, be it anger or fear or hopelessness, and then acknowledge those feelings to the patient in a simple statement such as, "This must be difficult for you." This simple offer of respect and support will be appreciated by the patient.

Sympathy is the quality of suffering with the patient. While empathy is a quality to be practiced, sympathy can interfere with the patient–provider relationship. Sympathy is lending an emotional quality to the relationship that is neither wholesome nor professional and which can lead to burnout. The Paramedic should strive to understand the patient's feelings (empathize) but not take on the patient's feelings (sympathy).

Caring implies emotional vulnerability on the part of both the patient, who confides in the Paramedic, and the Paramedic, who is trying his best to provide care, often under trying circumstances. To be truly caring, the Paramedic must be willing to also share his mistakes with the patient and **apologize** if necessary.

While the thought of apologizing for an error may seem abrasive or unwise to some, physicians and Paramedics are increasingly accepting of the need to apologize. Simply stated, no matter how skillful or knowledgeable the Paramedic, mistakes will be made. The Institute of Medicine (IOM) 1999 report estimated that between 44,000 and 98,000 patients will die while in the hospital from mistakes.[8] Mistakes are a part of the practice of paramedicine and each mistake represents an opportunity for improvement. The Paramedic's acceptance of the mistakes and willingness to apologize will be important to the patient's satisfaction with care.[9] Whenever a professional standard of care is breached, or the outcome is unwanted or unexpected, a caring Paramedic admits the error and demonstrates caring when he apologizes.

The first step whenever an error is encountered is to investigate why the error occurred. If there is no immediate explanation forthcoming, then the Paramedic should explain to the patient that an error occurred and, if appropriate, explain that "I will find out why" and get back to the patient later with an answer.

If the decision is made to apologize, the Paramedic should choose an appropriate time and place—perhaps after patient care has been turned over at the emergency department—and explain the situation, stating that an error has been made. A skillful Paramedic listens to the family's response and answers their questions thoughtfully and after a moment's reflection.

Fundamental to the Paramedic–patient relationship is **respect** for the patient. Respect is based upon a nonjudgmental attitude toward the patient, regardless of the personal circumstances. While many Paramedics are aware of prejudices about race or religion, the problem of economic prejudice is less recognized. Regardless of the social status or economic position that a patient holds at any one moment, the Paramedic should respect the patient as a person in need of help and worthy of care.

On occasion some Paramedics have difficulty understanding the patient's concerns, and may even cite "9-1-1 abuse" when speaking about these patients. Regardless of the Paramedic's attitude, these patients have a concern that prompted them to call for emergency medical services. The caring Paramedic listens and seeks to understand the patient and the patient's concern, regardless of how seemingly insignificant the problem. This process of **legitimization** supports the patient and demonstrates caring. A patient who is put at ease is more cooperative with care and has a more positive regard for the Paramedic.

Finally, the Paramedic demonstrates caring and compassion by offering the patient **support** and acting as a patient advocate. Being a patient advocate is important in a chaotic world where people are "lost in the process" and "treated like a number."

The secret of the care of the patient is in caring for the patient.

—Dr. Francis Weld Peabody—
Harvard Medical School—1925

Another key to quality patient care is the attribute of **integrity**. Professional integrity, described in more detail in Chapter 5 on ethics, involves an unabashed truthfulness with the patient which serves as a foundation for the patient–provider relationship.

Inherent within interpersonal communications is the concept of **diplomacy**. A thoughtful consideration of the words spoken, to ensure that the message spoken does not have an unintended meaning, improves interpersonal understanding and, ultimately, patient care.

While the science of emergency medical care can be learned from a book, the art of emergency medical service—combining the previously stated qualities in an effective manner—is best learned by practice in the field with a master Paramedic. A professional mentor can help with the process of socialization needed to create a professional Paramedic. A novice Paramedic subjected to intense socialization at the hands of seasoned professionals within a healthy EMS culture can quickly mature into a professional Paramedic.

Roles of a Paramedic

A Paramedic assumes many roles during the course of a career. The primary roles are those of healer, clinician, and patient advocate. As the Paramedic's practice evolves, the Paramedic may become involved as a researcher or a teacher. These changing roles keep a Paramedic engaged with the profession and continuously striving to improve his practice.

Healer

The Paramedic's primary role is that of healer. A healer is a person who supports another during illness. From the old English "Haelan" meaning to make whole, sound, and well, the Paramedic, as a healer, supports the patient, both physically and spiritually, through an illness or injury.

The role of the healer revolves around showing compassion. Dr. Bernard Lown, noted cardiologist and Nobel Peace Prize winner, states in his book *The Lost Art of Healing* that healing involves two aspects: preserving the personhood of an individual and providing comfort measures.

By its nature, illness is an attack upon an individual's sense of person, the individual's personhood. Illness threatens the patient's quality of life and perhaps even the patient's life itself. Moreover, illness is something that the patient has limited ability to prevent and little control over once it occurs. As a result of illness, the patient may feel helpless. This sense of helplessness leads to suffering.

To help reduce suffering, the Paramedic need only show compassion. Compassion is an awareness of another's suffering. In some cases it only takes the Paramedic's concerned presence (presencing) to help alleviate the suffering. The importance of presencing is exemplified by the common feeling often voiced by others that no one wants to die alone. By merely being there and showing compassion, the Paramedic helps to support the patient and, specifically, helps the patient validate himself and his sense of personhood.

Illness also brings pain. The Paramedic, as healer, can provide a range of comfort measures to the bedside. In some cases that comfort measure is in the form of pharmaceutical pain management. But in almost every case the Paramedic's therapeutic use of touch helps to relieve the patient's pain and provides comfort. Therapeutic touch has long been recognized by nursing as an effective treatment for pain. Therapeutic touch involves one-on-one attention and human touch.

Clinician

A clinic is a place dedicated to the diagnosis and care of a patient. A clinician is the person who works in that place. It could be said that the Paramedic's clinic is the back of an ambulance, a place where the Paramedic assesses and diagnoses a patient's ailment.

A Paramedic's diagnosis is a broad diagnosis made after an assessment. During the assessment the Paramedic ascertains a **symptom complex**. This symptom complex is simply a list of abnormal conditions found by the Paramedic during the history of the present illness and the physical examination. The Paramedic then, in turn, takes the symptom complex, compares it to his knowledge of disease, and matches it to a known **symptom pattern** associated with a disease to arrive at a diagnosis.

With only crude medical instruments and a limited time for history taking, the **Paramedic's diagnosis**, sometimes called a field diagnosis, must be broad and comprehensive. Typically a Paramedic makes a diagnosis of a syndrome, a group of signs and symptoms that signifies a specific disease, or of a primary disorder of homeostasis, such as hypoxia.

As a clinician, the Paramedic's first responsibility is to treat disorders of homeostasis which threaten the patient's survival. The brain's survival is paramount. The three essential conditions for the brain's survival are adequate oxygen, glucose, and perfusion. If the brain lacks any of these three conditions, then the patient has a fundamental disorder of cerebral function and manifests an altered mental status.

The approach to the assessment and treatment of these disorders is exemplified by the mnemonic ABC. The patient is assessed for hypoxia, hypoperfusion, and hypoglycemia. While this description is technically accurate, it is a gross simplification of a process which is expanded upon and discussed throughout this series.

The Paramedic, as clinician, keeps one invaluable rule foremost in the mind when treating the patient. That rule, simply stated, is "do no harm." While some harm will always come from a treatment or drug (e.g., the pain of a needle), the harm is outweighed by the benefit that the treatment or drug will have for the patient. The rule "do no harm" is intended to cause Paramedics to pause and consider every treatment intervention before proceeding.

The decision to treat in the field is multifactorial. In some instances it is more prudent to withhold certain treatments until arrival at the hospital where more experienced physicians can make the judgment about which treatments to initiate. At other times, delaying treatment in the field can be detrimental to the patient. The concept of "do no harm" is further discussed in Chapter 5 on ethics.

The Paramedic, as clinician, understands that medicine is a practice, meaning the science of medicine must be matched to the patient to try to obtain a maximum benefit for the patient. In some instances that match is not perfect. Learning the right time to perform specific procedures or administer particular medication is often a function of trial and error. It takes practice.

The Paramedic, as clinician, understands that the practice of medicine is first and foremost about the patient. The Paramedic understands that while the technology to treat the patient is becoming truly amazing, the priority remains to treat the patient as a person. The Paramedic understands that the love of technology and the science of medicine (philotechnia) comes second to caring for the person (philanthropia).

Expanded Scope of Practice

The traditional role of a Paramedic has been in the out-of-hospital setting responding to medical emergencies. But as necessity has required, the Paramedic's role has expanded in some limited situations and the Paramedic's scope of practice has expanded as well.

Driven by the increasing specialization of hospitals (i.e., trauma centers), interventional cardiology centers, stroke centers, children's hospitals, and so on, and accelerated by the nursing shortage, more Paramedics are becoming involved in specialty care transport (SCT). Paramedics who perform SCT have training above that of the typical Paramedic. The flight medic is an example of a specially trained Paramedic who performs SCT.[10]

In some other circumstances, such as rural communities, or under special conditions such as an epidemic, it may be appropriate to give Paramedics an **expanded scope of practice** to supplement existing healthcare resources.[11]

The American College of Emergency Physicians, in a position paper on expanded scope of practice, specifies several conditions that must be met before Paramedics can perform an expanded scope of practice.[12] ACEP maintains that all expanded scope of practice must be closely monitored, with intimate physician involvement and a rigorous quality assurance process that has standards and mechanisms for remediation. ACEP, in its position paper, further states that such expanded scope of practice must fulfill a community need, usually based on an assessment and plan of action, and that the practice is legally permissible.

Self-Evaluation and Continuous Quality Improvement

The Paramedic, as clinician, is always trying to improve the practice of paramedicine. This is best accomplished by critical self-evaluation and planned action. For example, an often quoted goal of EMS is the patient's satisfaction. Patient satisfaction may result from many factors including the provision of high-quality emergency medical care, timeliness of response, or respect for the patient's rights. An EMS system objective would be an eight-minute response in 90% of calls for EMS. It might also be in response to a patient demand for a timely response. If that objective is met then, to some extent, patient satisfaction with EMS should be higher.

While an EMS system may periodically look at certain practice parameters, a superior EMS system is always in a process of review and re-engineering, trying to refine the process and improve the delivery of EMS. This approach is called **continuous quality improvement (CQI)** and involves a process that can be summarized as plan-do-check-act (PDCA). This PDCA cycle is different than simply verifying compliance with established standards, or **quality assurance (QA)**, because it has an action component.

Any system of self-analysis, whether it is QA/CQI or others, is dependent on the data collected. These information systems can be real-time (i.e., direct observation of skills or performances in the field), but are often done retrospectively, after the fact, by a **chart audit**. For a chart audit to be reliable and dependable, it is important that Paramedics accurately and completely describe the care given. As the saying goes, "If it wasn't written down then it didn't happen."

Continuing Medical Education

Another responsibility of a professional Paramedic as clinician is to stay current with the state of the art. This is best accomplished through continuing medical education which culminates in periodic recertification. Paramedics also have a responsibility to re-register every two or three years. The re-registration is intended to ensure the public that the Paramedics that serve them have remained competent as Paramedics.

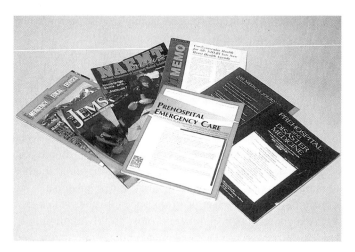

Figure 1-1 EMS journals are a means to obtain information about the state of the art.

However, the Paramedic understands the necessity of not only maintaining minimal skills and an adequate knowledge base, or **competency assurance**, but the need to continue to remain current with the state of the art. Paramedics are expected to keep abreast of new developments in the field of medicine as they pertain to EMS through involvement in **professional development**.

Attendance at state and national EMS conferences as well as attending regional workshops help ensure that the Paramedic is continuing to develop and provide high-quality emergency medical care. Alternatively, Paramedics often turn to their medical directors for guidance and education on new technologies. Another way to keep up with the profession is reading EMS trade journals (Figure 1-1). The best EMS trade journals have research that is peer-reviewed or articles that are refereed.

Whenever research has been **peer reviewed**, that means the article or research was critically appraised by experts in the field for validity. To be valid, the research has to objectively support its conclusion. In other words, the research must not be personal opinion, contain exaggerated statements, or make unjustifiable claims.

However, articles are not peer reviewed per se but rather are **refereed**. Typically an editor will distribute an article to a panel of expert Paramedics, in this case, and these expert Paramedics offer input. They edit the article and act as referees. Then the article is returned to the author and the author is allowed to revise the article before re-submission. Often the comments offered by these referees cite current research or best practices.

The commitment made by all Paramedics when they attain that first certification is to remain current with the profession through **life-long learning**.

Researcher

EMS practice in years past was based upon either in-hospital practice, which sometimes did not fit into the prehospital environment, or anecdotal experience. This approach has led to a great deal of concern regarding the effectiveness of EMS by some. To counter these claims, Paramedics have turned to an **evidence-based** approach to the practice. Changes in practice are now driven by research and the practice is becoming more **reliable** and **valid** in the process.

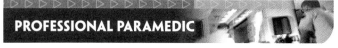

PROFESSIONAL PARAMEDIC

The professional Paramedic is interested in research because it offers the opportunity to improve the efficiency of paramedicine.

Teacher

Paramedics, in an effort to reduce injury and illness, have started to educate the public. These opportunities to educate the public sometimes occur during an emergency call, on a one-to-one basis, or in public education programs.

To be effective, this education must occur when the person, or the public, is ready to learn. This is called the **teachable moment**. For example, a campaign to wear seat belts may have more impact immediately following a fatal motor vehicle collision involving teenaged drivers. At that moment the public is sensitive to preventable death from motor vehicle collisions.

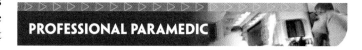

PROFESSIONAL PARAMEDIC

A newer role for the Paramedic is that of health educator.

Public Education

Public education is one means of garnering public support while simultaneously providing the public with the information they need about injury and illness prevention. A model public education system called **PIER** was developed by the National Highway Traffic Safety Administration (NHTSA).[13] PIER stands for public information, education, and relations, and incorporates the three aspects of public education.

The first aspect, public information, pertains to information regarding people and events that the media traditionally communicates to the public. Many EMS agencies have a **public information officer (PIO)** whose responsibility is to interface with the news media and to provide public information. The PIO must be cautious about not revealing restricted personal health information (PHI), a violation of the Health Insurance Portability and Accountability Act (HIPAA) regulations, while simultaneously providing the

Table 1-3 Public Education Activities

Public Information
• Press conferences
• Newspaper announcements about weekly EMS activity
• Annual reports to government boards or councils
Public Education
• CPR classes
• Life-saving classes
• Pediatric drowning education
• Elderly fall prevention classes
Public Relations
• Open house
• Blood pressure clinics

news media the information that it is entitled to due to the freedom of the press.

The second aspect of PIER is public education. All education is an attempt to change behaviors. Public education, from an EMS perspective, is an attempt to change the public's behavior toward medical emergencies. Examples of public education programs include CPR classes for citizens or public access defibrillation (PAD) for school officials.

The final aspect of PIER is public relations. Public relations is less an effort to educate the public (though there can be overlap) as it is to garner the public's support of Paramedics. The public's opinion of Paramedics can be directly translated to support for new programs or support of public funding. The Paramedic is involved in a number of public education activities (Table 1-3).

Patient Advocate

Finally, the professional Paramedic is a **patient advocate**. Being a patient advocate means that the Paramedic defends and supports the patient's rights to health care. Whenever a Paramedic acts to help a patient obtain needed health care he is acting in the advocacy role. A Paramedic is also acting in an advocacy role when she supports, through constructive argument, the need for equipment that will improve patient care. Some would see reporting child abuse as a Paramedic acting in an advocacy role as well.

Paramedics as Physician Extenders

While physicians are educated in medical schools, it is the state, through licensing legislation, that authorizes the physicians to practice medicine. Most states have state statutes, called a medical practice act, that define medical practice.

Many of these medical practice acts have a reference to **physician extenders**, allied health professionals who work under the license granted to the physician. Paramedics, as physician extenders, are among those allied healthcare professionals who are permitted to perform limited medical procedures while under the supervision of a licensed physician.

Stewardship

Because Paramedics work under the physician's license, paramedicine is a **shared practice** with physicians. However, often a physician is not present when the Paramedic is taking care of the patient. Nevertheless the Paramedic is still representing the physician and the responsibilities of medicine.

Therefore, in the absence of the physician, the Paramedic shares the physician's responsibilities, including veracity, fidelity, beneficence, avoidance of malfeasance, and justice. These concepts are discussed in Chapter 5 on ethics. Whenever a Paramedic upholds noble traditions of medicine the Paramedic is acting in the role of a steward. **Stewardship** is a weighty responsibility for the Paramedic. A Paramedic's failure to properly conduct himself, as a physician would, often leads to conflict between the Paramedic and physician and loss of medical privileges.

Leadership

As the highest level of out-of-hospital EMS provider, Paramedics are often thrust into the leadership role by virtue of their education. This traditional form of top-down management (vertical leadership) was common in the immediate post-World War II business world. It can be visualized as a pyramid with a distinctive chain of command.

However, enlightened Paramedics as leaders seek to "flatten the pyramid" and work toward linking, or networking, with the members of a public safety team. This **horizontal leadership** style demonstrates that the Paramedic values the contributions of every team member. Horizontal leadership emphasizes an "out and back" line of communication instead of an "up and down" line of communication and can be visualized more like a wagon wheel.

In an information intensive era, horizontal leadership is an effective technique for knowledge management. Nevertheless, there still needs to be a nexus for control. Traditionally the Paramedic assumes that role, offering common direction and a strong vision to fellow EMS team members as well as other public safety partners.

The Paramedic, as leader, needs to have a sense of direction and a strong personal vision of paramedicine. He must also constantly reflect upon the values common to a professional Paramedic (ethics) and work to incorporate those values into daily practice.

Besides being a model of ethical behavior, the Paramedic as a leader is also a coach. As coach the Paramedic teaches others, or trains the team, to work together to reach a common goal.

The qualities of a good leader can be summed up in the 5 "C's": competence, command presence, choreography, communications, and conflict resolution. Competence goes beyond merely being technically proficient at skills and instead means having **operational competence**. Operational competence includes knowing how the various team members interact, knowing an organization's policies and procedures, and possessing situational awareness.

The Paramedic, as leader, has situational awareness. He can read the scene and can detect both opportunity and threat. These opportunities include teaching moments, times for the team members to learn, without risk to either the team's or the patient's safety. This skill cannot be easily learned from books but rather is a result of witnessing master medics function in the field.

Another quality of a good leader is **command presence**. Command presence can be defined as that ability to present oneself as the person of authority. The Paramedic's authority flows, in part, from the respect that the team has for the medical director and the Paramedic's role as the medical director's steward.

Outwardly, the Paramedic's appearance can demonstrate confidence, a key command trait. A clean pressed uniform and the "tools of the trade," such as a stethoscope, give the Paramedic the appearance of a medical professional. A professional appearance, along with a professional attitude, can substantially improve one's command presence.

Confidence can also be manifest in one's behaviors. The confident Paramedic walks purposefully toward the patient with an eye toward the patient as well as the surrounding environmental, i.e., situational awareness. Confidence is further demonstrated in purposeful speech with a low tone. Instead of yelling into the scene, instructions are pointedly given to individuals by looking toward that individual and speaking an unambiguous message in a directive manner.

The next quality of a Paramedic leader is the ability to organize the team's efforts in order to deliver appropriate interventions in a timely manner. This skill could be described as **choreography**. While algorithms are helpful with organizing patient care, acting almost like a pre-plan, on-scene conditions and other variables make it imperative that the Paramedic take an active role in leading the team down the treatment pathway.

To be truly effective, the Paramedic, as leader, must also be a strong communicator. A key to success in teamwork is possessing excellent communication skills. The Paramedic must be articulate with both patients and family, speaking to them in terms that they understand while still being able to be conversant with fellow healthcare professionals, most notably the emergency physician, in terms that they will understand.

It is inevitable that disputes about patient care will occur among team members. Without the authority given in a traditional chain of command, the Paramedic must be masterful at conflict resolution in order to maintain order and control. In high stress situations (i.e., those with a high life hazard), it may be necessary for the Paramedic to assert authority, issue a command, and offer to review the call later with the team. In those cases it is important for the Paramedic to institute an "after action review" and allow all parties to express their viewpoints and vent their emotions. But if time permits, and it is not disruptive to patient care, the Paramedic may elect to listen to the suggestions of other team members offered in civil discourse. During these teachable moments learning can occur for all involved, including the Paramedic leader.

Followership

Consistent with the concept of leadership is **followership**. Followership is a willingness to follow a leader's direction and to support the mission, putting aside personal ambitions. Every leader is a follower at some level. Inherent in the definition of paramedicine is the willing submission to medical command. But followership is more than submission.

A Paramedic, as follower, understands the mission (patient care) and is dedicated to that mission. The Paramedic, as follower, understands the team's need for compliance (team play) in order to achieve the team's common goals. The good follower puts the needs of the team and the patient above one's own needs.

A Paramedic, as follower, makes timely recommendations to the leader. That includes respectfully disagreeing with the leader when need be, if that is what is in the best interests of the team and/or the patient.

A Paramedic, as follower, sets the example for others by understanding the leader, anticipating the orders of the leader, and complying with those orders. Perhaps more importantly the Paramedic, as follower, knows when to take appropriate action when no orders are forthcoming.

Finally, the Paramedic, as follower, keeps the information flowing to the leader and does not horde vital information. Through clear communications, all members of the team can provide the highest quality of care.

CONCLUSION

Paramedicine is a pattern of thinking and behaviors, that outward manifestation of thinking, that is consistently applied in varying situations until a practice has been achieved. The art of paramedicine is the ability to apply that practice while maintaining focus, using one's wits and creative abilities.

KEY POINTS:

- Paramedic practice is both independent, encompassing specialized prehospital practices, and interdependent, through a working relationship with emergency physicians.

- The Paramedic is cross-trained in health care, public health, and public safety.

- The National EMS Education Standards, together with the national core content and national scope of practice, identify a paramedic's knowledge, skills, and attitudes.

- Professional organizations or societies, such as the National Association of EMT (NAEMT), provide a voice for the profession and have been leading efforts to professionalize EMS.

- The landmark National Institute of Medicine Reports entitled "EMS at the Crossroads," and "Hospital Based Emergency Care: At the Breaking Point," released in 2006, encouraged changes in the delivery of patient care.

- Caring is an expression of concern toward the patient and is foundational to the Paramedic–patient relationship.

- A Paramedic may assume the role of healer, clinician, and patient advocate.

- During the assessment, the Paramedic ascertains a symptom complex.

- The Paramedic, as clinician, keeps one rule in mind when treating the patient: do no harm.

- Roles and responsibilities describe a Paramedic's scope of practice.

- A superior EMS system is always in a process of review and re-engineering through continuous quality improvement (CQI) and quality assurance (QA).

- Involvement in professional development provides the Paramedic with competence assurance, and allows the Paramedic to remain current with the state of the art as a life-long learner.

- Changes in EMS are now driven by research, and the process has become more reliable and valid to the Paramedic practice.

- In an effort to reduce injury and illness, the Paramedic has become a health educator.

- The professional Paramedic is also a patient advocate.

- As a physician extender, the Paramedic is authorized to practice under the license granted to the physician.

- The Paramedic serves as a model of ethical behavior.

- A Paramedic leader is a strong communicator and has the ability to organize a team's efforts to deliver appropriate intervention in a timely manner.

- The Paramedic, as a follower, is willing to follow a leader's direction and support the mission.

REVIEW QUESTIONS:

1. How has the Paramedic's role changed since the inception of the profession?

2. What professional organizations or societies serve as a voice for the Paramedic profession? How have they helped to advance EMS?

3. Using the mnemonic PEARLS, explain how caring is the Paramedic's first core value.

4. Why is it important for the Paramedic to take part in continuing education?

5. How does the rule "do no harm" relate to a Paramedic's scope of practice?

6. Describe how a Paramedic develops a Paramedic field diagnosis.

7. How do continuous quality improvement (CQI), quality assurance (QA), and research improve the practice of paramedicine

8. What is the relationship between stewardship and the Paramedic as a physician extender?

9. What leadership qualities should the Paramedic exhibit?

10. How is being a good follower as important as being a good leader?

CASE STUDY QUESTIONS:

Please refer to the Case Study at the beginning of the chapter and answer the questions below:

1. How would you counsel high school students who are interested in EMS?

2. What could you say to someone who says, "I want to be a Paramedic but I only want to take care of trauma patients"?

3. Discuss the importance of a science and mathematics curriculum as the basis for Paramedic study.

REFERENCES:

1. Fan E, MacDonald RD, Adhikari NK, Scales DC, Wax RS, Stewart TE, et al. Outcomes of interfacility critical care adult patient transport: a systematic review. *Crit Care*. 2006;10(1):R6.

2. Svenson JE, O'Connor JE, Lindsay MB. Is air transport faster? A comparison of air versus ground transport times for interfacility transfers in a regional referral system. *Air Med J*. 2006;25(4):170–172.

3. American Academy of Pediatrics. Committee on Pediatric Emergency Medicine. American College of Critical Care Medicine. Society of Critical Care Medicine.

4. Minarik PA. A vision for health professions regulation in the new millennium: recommendations from the Pew Health Professions Commission. *Clin Nurse Spec*. 1999;13(6):306–309.

5. Bartlett WD. Paramedic education and the development of professional status: a prognosis. *Paramed Int*. 1979;4(1): 36–39.

6. http://www.nemses.org

7. National Academies Press. *Hospital-Based Emergency Care: At the Breaking Point (Future of Emergency Care)*. Washington, DC: National Academies Press; 2007.

8. Leape LL. Institute of Medicine medical error figures are not exaggerated. *Jama*. 2000;284(1):95–97.

9. Brennan TA, Leape LL, Laird NM, Hebert L, Localio AR, Lawthers AG, et al. Incidence of adverse events and negligence in hospitalized patients. Results of the Harvard Medical Practice Study I. *N Engl J Med*. 1991;324(6):370–376.

10. Gryniuk J. The role of the certified flight Paramedic (CFP) as a critical care provider and the required education. *Prehosp Emerg Care*. 2001;5(3):290–292.

11. Hatley T, Ma OJ, Weaver N, Strong D. Flight Paramedic scope of practice: current level and breadth. *J Emerg Med*. 1998;16(5):731–735.

12. American College of Emergency Physicians. Expanded roles of EMS Personnel. Revised April 2008. Available at: **http://www .acep.org/practres.aspx?id=29444.** Accessed May 4, 2009.

13. Thoma T, Vaca F. National Highway Traffic Safety Administration (NHTSA) notes. PIER: public information, education, and relations for EMS injury prevention modules. *Ann Emerg Med*. 2004;43(4):521–524.

INTRODUCTION TO EMERGENCY MEDICAL SERVICE SYSTEMS

KEY CONCEPTS:

Upon completion of this chapter, it is expected that the reader will understand these following concepts:

- The paradigm in EMS has shifted from ambulance transport to advanced prehospital care
- Emergency Medical Services are incorporated into all levels of public life: local, state, and national
- The EMS Agenda for the Future has redefined both the scope of practice and educational standards

▶ CASE STUDY:

The Paramedics were at the squad building and the group of them stared at the invitation. The local Emergency Physician's Advocacy Group had invited a Paramedic to their next meeting to speak on the history of paramedicine, its scope of practice, its educational requirements, and its role in the local healthcare system. Who would go and represent them to their physician colleagues and what would they say, everyone asked. One thing was for sure, they wanted to put their best foot forward.

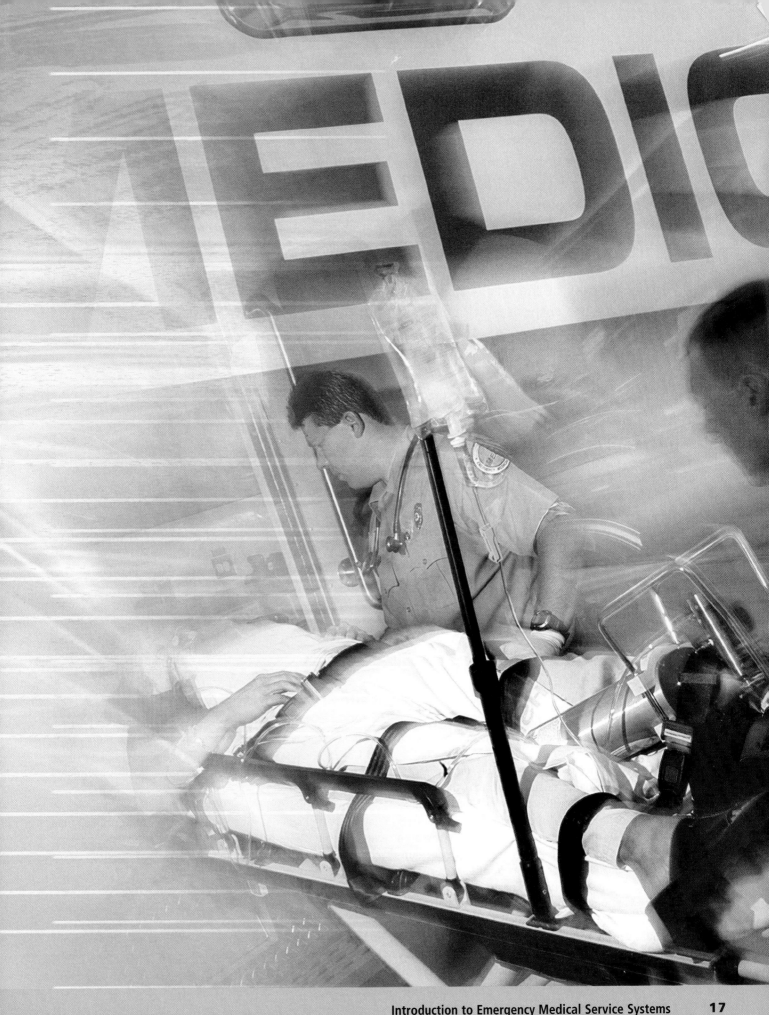

OVERVIEW

What started out as the simple idea of transporting the sick or wounded to medical care has evolved into an integral component of our healthcare system in the United States. Its development—one that originated out of necessity—now plays a vital role in an ever-expanding system of health care. This chapter will not only outline the history and progression of EMS but also identify what defines EMS practices. The evolution of EMS in the healthcare system prompted the development of an EMS Agenda for the Future that establishes a clear vision for the future of EMS. This vision has been implemented by means of national core content, a defined scope of practice, and educational standards. With knowledge of how the EMS system is constructed and an understanding of the origin of its various components, a Paramedic can better appreciate the responsibility and function they have in the healthcare system.

The Evolution of EMS

While medicine has been in existence since the beginning of recorded time, **Emergency Medical Services (EMS)** is a relative newcomer to the field of medicine. Modern EMS, with its specially trained EMS providers and a systems approach, is generally considered to have started in the late 1960s and early 1970s.[1–3] From these early beginnings EMS, and specifically Paramedics, have rapidly developed into one of the newest allied healthcare professions.

A constant throughout the development of EMS is the close working relationship of EMS with other parts of the healthcare system, particularly the emergency department. Therefore, to understand the evolution of EMS it is important to first review the history of American health care.

Historical Evolution of American Health Care

Before the 1800s, health care was largely delivered by physicians who traveled by mule to the homes of the sick and injured. In its day that level of health care was satisfactory for the fledgling republic.

As cities grew during the 1800s, largely due to a dramatic influx of European and Asian immigrants, the demand for more public healthcare facilities escalated. Forward thinking physicians helped develop large urban hospitals to meet that demand. These hospitals (e.g., Massachusetts General in Boston and Bellevue in New York City) could care for hundreds of patients, and allowed economies of scale (savings made from bulk purchases), which in turn made health care affordable to vast legions of poor and underserved persons.

The physician in the 1800s, armed with only limited experience and even more limited education—or no formal education at all—dealt largely with infectious diseases. Many of these infectious disease outbreaks occurred because of overcrowding in inadequate housing and almost nonexistent sanitation systems.[4,5]

Revolution in the Laboratory

During the early and mid-1900s, discoveries in the laboratories brought about a revolution in medicine. Scientists used microscopes to identify the sources of many infectious diseases and developed crude but effective treatments—using the scientific method—to treat these diseases. Word of these medical breakthroughs was widely disseminated via journals such as the *New England Journal of Medicine*. The field of medicine began to change.

Almost overnight, county and state medical societies were created and physicians gathered to discuss new developments in medicine in a climate of openness that fostered more medical research and established the beginning of modern medicine.

Public Health Care Emerges

As great strides were being made against infectious disease, the delivery of health care also changed. For example, in 1906 St. Luke's Hospital in New York City opened its first private pavilion. This change marked the beginning of a healthcare system.[6,7]

Prior to that time there was no perceived advantage to having patients cared for in the hospital setting rather than in the home where patients could receive equally good care. However, after the turn of the century—with the advent of hospital laboratories equipped with powerful microscopes as well as expansive pharmacies filled with new cures—the hospital setting provided distinct advantages. These resources empowered the physicians to encourage patients to be admitted into the hospital. Soon hospital admission for illness, predominantly infectious diseases, became a public expectation.

Evolution of Medicine

Following World War II and the successful introduction of modern antibiotics, the incidence of infectious diseases was waning. For example, smallpox was being eradicated due to the use of a new vaccine. Soon chronic diseases, such as cancer, stroke, and heart disease, were replacing infection as the leading killers. As a result, medicine began to concentrate less on infectious diseases and more on chronic diseases. Also during this time the development of medical sciences (biology, pharmacy, etc.) blossomed and the biotechnology industry—the marriage of medical science and technology—emerged in the health care industry.

At the same time, the growth of widespread employer-provided health insurance permitted an increasing segment of the U.S. population to afford medical care. With the widespread availability of health insurance the healthcare industry was then firmly established.

Also beginning in the 1980s, medicine began to integrate information technologies such as computers, and other biomedical devices, into healthcare. The advancement of pharmaceutical research had also taken on revolutionary new directions, including the development of new bioengineered drugs.

Partially as a result of the significant advances in medical science, healthcare costs have skyrocketed. For this reason the federal government, in part because of Medicaid and Medicare health programs, has taken a greater role in healthcare policymaking in an effort to curb rising healthcare costs.

Public Health Movement

Paralleling the advances in medicine, and the development of healthcare systems, was the public health movement. The public health movement started in the early 1800s as a result of the smallpox, yellow fever, and cholera epidemics that ravaged the larger cities.[8,9]

During that time, quarantines and in-house confinement were the only effective means of preventing the further spread of disease. As a result of widespread illness, business and the manufacturing industries suffered and productivity was affected.

In order to temper the effect of illness and sick call outs on business a few wealthy patrons hired graduate nurses to care for the sick and the poor in Boston, Cincinnati, and Washington, DC. These nurses, referred to as community nurses, worked tirelessly in the ghettos and tenements of major cities trying to improve sanitation and decrease morbidity and mortality as a result of infectious disease.

Similar to modern-day Paramedics, these public health nurses would leave the safety of the hospital to go to workers' homes and worksites. Some community nurses established clinics to advance sanitary practices in the home and improve maternal–child health, as infant mortality was particularly high in the inner cities. Lillian Wald, RN (Figure 2-1), an early social work pioneer, is credited with starting the Henry

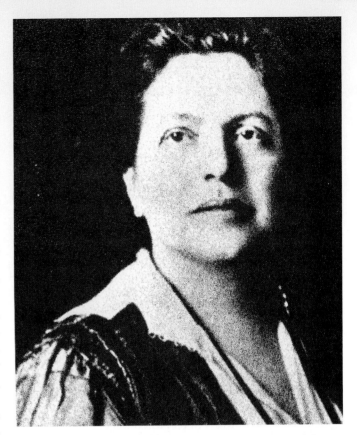

Figure 2-1 Lillian Wald, RN, a pioneer in public health. (Photo courtesy of American Nurses Association)

Street Settlement in New York City, a social services shelter, in 1793 and coining the term "Public Health Nurse."[10]

Public Health Service

The federal **Public Health Service** actually evolved out of the need for health care for the maritime fleet. The Public Health Service roots can be traced to the creation of the Marine Hospital Service in 1798. At that time, sailors paid 20 cents a month to fund the Marine Hospital Service. The service provided them with medical care if they should get sick away from home and while in a distant port of call. As the public health movement grew, and pressure mounted on the federal government to provide service to the poor, the Marine Hospital Service became the federal Public Health Service.

The federal Public Health Service is a key portion of the Department of Health and Human Services today. With 5,700 commissioned health services officers and 51,000 civilian employees, all led by the Surgeon General, the current United States Public Health Service provides support to county and state Public Health Departments as well as health care to medically underserved areas.

The United States Public Health Service (PHS) consists of eight agencies, including the National Institute for Health (NIH), the Food and Drug Administration (FDA), the Agency for Toxic Substances and Disease Registry (ATSDR), and the Centers for Disease Control and Prevention (CDCP).

Current challenges to public health, including Lyme disease, West Nile virus, SARS, Avian flu, and swine flu, to name a few, have placed a renewed emphasis on public health medicine.

The mission of EMS is now seen as being more in step with the Public Health Service than previously thought. Relationships between Paramedics and the Public Health Service's physicians, nurses, scientists, and sanitarians are growing and evolving; especially in light of the threats of pandemic flu and natural disasters.

The History of Emergency Medical Service

The transportation of the sick and injured has seen many developments over the past millennium. The earliest examples may be seen in the Roman Empire. Romans would use chariots to move battle-injured soldiers from the battle field in the time of Caesar (100 A.D.). This innovation was followed by the first hammock-wagon, a wagon designed specifically for transporting the sick and injured, and a forerunner of the modern ambulance, but the hammock-wagon was not created until about 900 A.D. In their day these crude carriages and horse litters would carry one invalid patient to medical care at a distant physician, at a monastery, for example, but the long transfer over rough roads often proved to be more dangerous to the wounded patient than the original battlefield wound.

During the Spanish crusade of Ferdinand and Isabella against the Moors in the late fifteenth century, the use of *ambulancias*, or mobile military hospitals, came into being. These facilities, which were located closer to the battlefront, helped provide more immediate care to the wounded. As a result, this more timely medical intervention improved the chances for a soldier's survival from battle wounds.

However, credit for the concept of the modern ambulance is generally given to Dominique-Jean Larrey of Baudean, France. A surgeon, Larrey got a great deal of his training treating victims of the French Revolution during his stay at the Hotel Dieu, the premier French hospital in Paris. Larrey, pressed into military service by the Prussians, was disturbed by the then-common practice of waiting for the battle to end before rescuing the wounded. Larrey went about creating a light carriage that could swoop into a battle, scoop up the wounded, and then rapidly transport them to the waiting surgeons at the "ambulance." Those light two-wheeled carriages that carried an attendant as well as a driver were called *les ambulance volantes,* or flying ambulances.

The American Civil War utilized what could be described as weapons of mass destruction, such as rapid fire or repeating rifles and devastatingly accurate cannon fire. These improved weapons caused greater casualties and put greater demands on battle surgeons. While casualties were greater, medical attention to these combat casualties improved and resulted in many advances in field care of wounded soldiers. And to respond to the mass casualties sustained during these military engagements, army surgeon Major Jonathan Letterman completely reorganized the military field medical service, called the Letterman plan, into what was to be the forerunner of the modern trauma system.

The Letterman plan called for "an act to establish a uniform system of ambulances in the Armies of the United States," and was ratified by the United States Congress in 1864. The act declared that ambulances were a special corp. that needed personnel, in distinctive special uniforms, who drove specially marked wagons, and answered to the head of the medical department of the army, a physician, and not the battlefield commander (Figure 2-2).

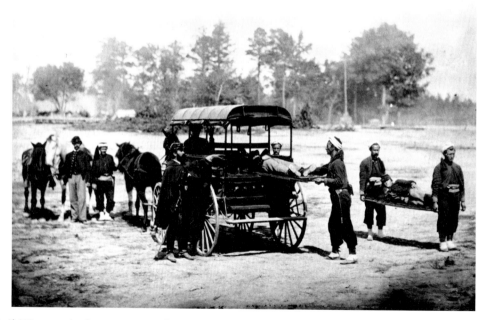

Figure 2-2 Civil War ambulance accepting patients. (Courtesy of the Library of Congress, Selected Civil War Photographs, Photo No. LC-B8171-7636)

As a result of the shear number of casualties and the horrible carnage of war there was a public outcry to control warfare. In 1864, a convention was held in Geneva, Switzerland, to "civilize" warfare. The result was the Geneva Treaty. Among its many precepts, the Geneva Treaty established the neutrality of all ambulance workers who wore the "Red Cross"—an icon created by the reversed colors of the Swiss flag created in honor of the Swiss, who hosted the convention. In 1882 the United States Congress ratified the Geneva Convention accords.

In keeping with the accords of the Geneva Treaty, and with the help of Clara Barton (Figure 2-3), the American Red Cross was formed and chartered by the Congress in 1881 "to provide volunteer aid in time of war to the sick and wounded of the armed forces."[11,12]

The American Red Cross differs from its European counterparts because it was active during peacetime as well as during war, responding during peacetime with disaster relief and humanitarian aid. Since the American Red Cross is not a government agency, it offers neutral humanitarian service to victims of war.

Around the same time as the appearance of the American Red Cross, hospital-based civilian ambulance services started to appear in the United States. The first hospital-based ambulance, the ambulance of the Commercial Hospital of Cincinnati (later Cincinnati General), was started in 1865, followed by Bellevue Hospital ambulance in 1869. By 1891 Bellevue Hospital's ambulance had responded to 4,392 calls. Shortly thereafter, hospitals throughout New York City provided ambulances staffed with an ambulance driver and a surgeon in accordance with a plan advanced by Dr. Dalton. These ambulances responded to medical emergencies throughout the City of New York.

The practice of prehospital care rapidly advanced as new technologies were created to deal with the unique environment encountered in the civilian world as well as on the battlefield. For example, the outbreak of World War I and the invention of the motorized ambulance coincided, improving both the quality and the speed of ambulance transportation. Another example is the splint created by Sir Hugh Owen-Thomas. Dr. Thomas invented an external fixation and traction splint, called the Thomas half-ring, which reduced the number of fatalities resulting from a traumatic fractured femur from roughly 80% to less than 20%.

The combination of advances such as the Thomas half-ring splint, rudimentary first aid treatments to stop bleeding, and the introduction of motorized ambulances substantially reduced battlefield mortality during World War I. These battlefield advances, which were also adopted for the civilian population, led to improved survival from trauma in general during the same time.

Emergence of Civilian EMS

After World War I, citizens started to see the importance of an organized emergency medical service and subsequently the first volunteer rescue squad was formed in Roanoke, Virginia. The Roanoke Rescue Squad, lead by Stanley Wise (Figure 2-4), started to provide emergency medical service to the citizens of Roanoke in 1921.

After early successes with this model, community-based rescue squads began to spring up across the country. Many of these "independent" rescue squads (i.e., not hospital-based or commercial ambulance services) sprang from local volunteer fire departments and heralded an era of volunteer ambulances.

Changing Paradigms

Before World War II, the ambulance was chiefly seen as an expedient means to get a patient to a hospital. Following the successes of army "para-medical" personnel during World War II and the advent of a new treatment for cardiac arrest called "cardiopulmonary resuscitation" or CPR, it became apparent that the ambulance driver might be able to provide more than just a fast ride.

In 1958, Dr. Peter Safar demonstrated the safety and efficiency of mouth-to-mouth ventilation, using trained Baltimore firefighters, on anesthetized medical residents. This idea of non-medical personnel performing medical procedures was revolutionary in its day. The introduction of the lifesaving CPR technique quickly intrigued the public.[13–16]

The "can do" attitude in America led organizations such as the American Red Cross and the American Heart Association to conduct mass CPR and first aid training for the public in firehouses and rescue squad buildings across the country. By 1960, firefighters in major cities like Columbus,

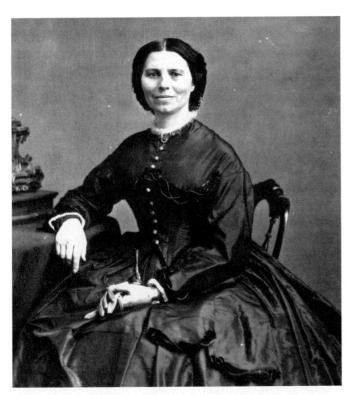

Figure 2-3 Clara Barton, founder of the American Red Cross. (Courtesy of the National Archives, Photo No. 111-B-4246, Brady Collection)

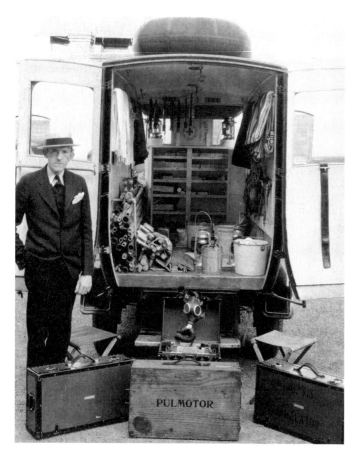

Figure 2-4 Julian Stanley Wise, founder of the first volunteer rescue squad. (Courtesy of the Julian Stanley Wise Foundation)

Los Angeles, Seattle, and Miami, to name a few, were trained to provide CPR.

Also in 1960, Asmund S. Laerdal, a Norwegian dollmaker, created the first "resusci-annie," a manikin for CPR practice. With an acceptable simulator/manikin, the American Red Cross and the American Heart Association began to train the public in vast numbers. CPR training, along with American Red Cross advanced first aid training, became the standard for ambulance drivers.

The White Paper

As America prospered, and medical care improved, it was becoming increasingly apparent that prehospital care, particularly for motor vehicle trauma, was not keeping pace with the medical community. In 1960 President John F. Kennedy made the statement that "Traffic accidents constitute one of the greatest, perhaps the greatest, of the nation's public health problems."[17]

At that time, the majority of ambulance service was provided by a variety of tow truck operators, hospital supply companies, and funeral homes. To illustrate the point, in the 1950s and 1960s over 50% of ambulances in the United States were owned and operated by some 12,000 morticians. Funeral hearses were often used as ambulances as they were the only public conveyance that could transport a patient horizontally on a stretcher.

From 1965 to 1966, two reports on highway safety were produced. One, by the National Academy of Sciences, entitled "Accidental Death and Disability: The Neglected Disease of Modern Society," discussed shortfalls in the nation's EMS system.[18–20] The other, the report of the President's Commission on Highway Safety, entitled "Health, Medical Care and Transportation of the Injured," also echoed the problems EMS was experiencing.[21]

In 1966, President Lyndon B. Johnson signed into law the National Highway Safety Act. This act provided for federal funds as well as other improvements in highway safety.[22] The Highway Safety Act, among its many provisions, created an EMS program within the Department of Transportation (DOT) and is seen as the first federal commitment to EMS.

Following the passage of the Highway Safety Act there was a flurry of activity in emergency medicine. For example, The American College of Emergency Physicians was formed in 1968, a group consisting of physicians who specialized in emergency medicine. These early physicians, pioneers in emergency medicine, provided medical oversight and control to the growing EMS community.

In support of the EMS community the federal DOT produced the first **Emergency Medical Technician-Ambulance** curriculum in 1969, a national standard curriculum for the training of ambulance drivers/attendants in new skills and life-saving techniques.

While the EMT curriculum was developed to deal with vehicular trauma, cardiologists were dealing with another threat to Americans: the heart attack. Physicians, like Dr. Barnard Lown, noted that when certain drugs, such as lidocaine, were given during a heart attack there was a decrease in the incidence of sudden cardiac death (SCD).

Another cardiologist, Dr. Paul M. Zoll (Figure 2-5), also theorized that an electrical current passed through the heart could terminate the lethal dysrhythmia called ventricular fibrillation. And in 1956 Dr. Zoll delivered the first external, 750-volt, alternating current countershock to a fibrillating heart, which effectively stopped the dysrhythmia. Shortly thereafter defibrillators, now battery-powered direct current (DC) defibrillators, were placed in service in many hospitals and emergency departments.

Prehospital Coronary Care

Dr. J. "Frank" Pantridge, of Belfast, Ireland, noted that 90% of young or middle-aged men who died from heart attacks did so

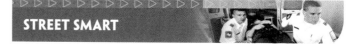

STREET SMART

The defibrillators, some weighing over 100 pounds, were placed on top of mobile carts which had a tendency to roll over, or "crash," when pushed through the halls of the hospital; hence the term "crash carts."[23–25]

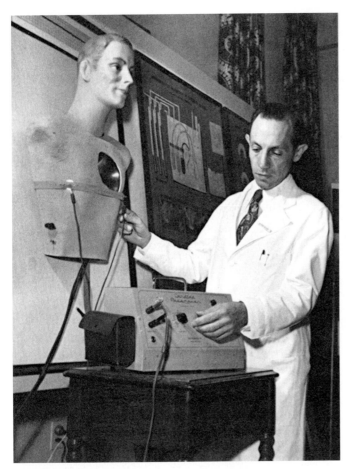

Figure 2-5 Dr. Zoll, inventor of the external cardiac defibrillator. (Photo: Paul Showstark. Paul M. Zoll, MD, 1954. Courtesy of Beth Israel Deaconess Medical Center Archives)

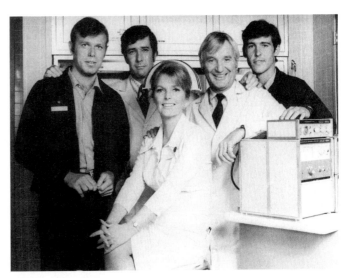

Figure 2-6 Emergency Paramedics Jon Gage and Roy DeSoto. (Courtesy of Everett Collection, Inc.)

due to ventricular fibrillation. These deaths usually occurred within one hour of onset of initial symptoms. Realizing the potential of rapid defibrillation in the field to reverse sudden cardiac death, Dr. Pantridge placed the "heart-shockers" into ambulances and staffed those ambulances with trained coronary care nurses.

The patient survival rates from sudden cardiac death were remarkable and Dr. Pantridge reported his success in the British medical journal *Lancet* in 1967. After reading of his success with prehospital defibrillation, the American College of Cardiology invited Dr. Pantridge to speak at its annual convention the following year.[26]

After learning of Dr. Pantridge's success, physicians at Ohio State University started their own version of the mobile coronary care unit which they dubbed the "heartmobile." The heartmobile continued to operate through Ohio State University until July 1971 until it became a part of the Columbus Division of Fire as Squad 52.

Emergency Hits TV Screens

Robert A. Cindar was interested in emergency medical services, and particularly the advent of the Paramedic. Following

his success with creating the television show *Adam-12*, Mr. Cindar approached then Captain James Page of the Los Angeles Fire Department and asked him if he would be the technical advisor for a new "reality" television program to be called *Emergency*. The show was to be loosely based on the new Paramedic program. Subsequently, the crew of the television Squad 51 of the L.A. County Fire Department began to roll. These fire department Paramedics, or fire-medics, responded to all variety of emergencies, from fires to special and technical rescue to every imaginable medical emergency, always rendering expert medical care in the field. An entire generation of future Paramedics was raised watching the emergency medical care provided by Firefighter/Paramedics Gage and DeSoto (Figure 2-6).

EMS Act of 1973

In 1973 Congress passed the EMS Act, Public Law 93-154, an amendment to the Public Health Service Act of 1944, which offered technical assistance to regions and municipalities.[27] The **EMS Act of 1973** delineated the 15 aspects of an EMS system that needed improvement including education (both public as well as provider), improved communications (including public access), and system evaluation but offered little money to help make those improvements.

Federal EMS Efforts in the 1980s

The 1981 Omnibus Budget Reconciliation Act took monies previously earmarked for EMS and placed them under a broader rubric of preventive health money. The federal government provided the states with large "block" grants to fund various programs including EMS. While the intention was to continue to fund EMS, the effect was to turn control of EMS funding over to the states. The states then choose how to spend the allocated monies. Some states did not support funding for EMS to the same level as the federal government had.

1500 B.C. Roman Wars

- Evidence of first treatment protocols.
- Romans and Greeks used chariots to remove wounded from the battlefield.

1797 The Napoleonic Wars

- Baron Dominique-Jean Larrey, Napoleon Bonaparte's chief surgeon, constructed a horse-drawn carriage called the *ambulance volante* or "flying ambulance."

1860s The U.S. Civil War

- The first ambulance service in the United States was developed by U.S. Army surgeon Jonathan Letterman, who reorganized the Army Medical Corp to include ambulances, similar to Baron Dominique-Jean Larrey's flying ambulances.
- Clara Barton was a volunteer on the Civil War battlefields and saw the mayhem first hand. Returning from the Franco–Prussian War, where she witnessed the good work of the Red Cross on the battlefield, she founded the American Red Cross.

1865–1950 U.S. Ambulance Service

- (1865) Cincinnati established the first civilian ambulance service.
- (1869) New York City established an ambulance service with hospital interns riding in horse-drawn carriages designed specifically for the sick and injured.
- (1901) At the Pan American Expo in Buffalo, NY, the first electric-powered ambulance was demonstrated and used to transport people to the on-site hospital.
- (1910) One of the first ambulances, called the "Invalid's Car," ran out of Iowa Methodist Hospital, Des Moines, Iowa, staffed with a nurse and resident from the hospital.
- (1928) The Roanoke Life Saving and First Aid Squad was the first volunteer rescue squad in the United States.

1910–1940s The World Wars

- An unmodified French fighter aircraft was used for air medical transport during the retreat of the Serbian army from Albania.
- "Combat medics" cared for the wounded in the field with advanced procedures including intravenous solutions, crude antibiotics, and intraosseous (bone) needles.
- Improved systems for trauma care were established including field hospitals and forward first-aid stations.
- Mechanized ambulances with the characteristic Red Cross emblem on the side were used and the era of the ambulance driver had arrived.

1950s Out of Hospital Medical Advances

- American Red Cross took the lead in providing basic medical training, making classes such as Standard and Advanced First Aid the standard of care for rescue squad members.
- Cardiopulmonary resuscitation (CPR) was taught to civilians for the first time in the late 1950s and early 1960s.
- (1958) Mouth-to-mouth ventilation was demonstrated by Dr. Peter Safar using volunteers from the Baltimore Fire Department, who agreed to be paralyzed.
- (1958) Dr. Joseph K. "Deke" Farrington, known as the Father of EMS, and Dr. Sam Banks started a trauma training course for the Chicago Fire Department in what was to become the prototype of the EMT-Ambulance course.

1950–1970 Korean and Vietnam Wars

- Mobile Army Surgical Hospitals (MASH) were developed during the Korean and Vietnam conflicts in an attempt to save the most seriously injured patients through a transportation-dependent method of triaging.
- Transportation of wounded soldiers by helicopter to medical units, used first during the Korean War, was the genesis of modern aeromedical transportation.
- The HU-1 (Huey) helicopter used during the Vietnam War had a large patient compartment to allow emergency care to begin while in flight.

1960s Development of an EMS System

- (1966) The National Academy of Sciences produced a white paper, "Accidental Death and Disability: The Neglected Disease of Modern Society" for President Kennedy. It stated that, to that date, more Americans had died on American Highways than in all of the U.S. wars.
- (1966) The National Highway Safety Act of 1966 encouraged states to begin organized EMS programs.
- (1967–1968) The first paramedic services were established in Miami, Florida, using telemetry units designed by Dr. Eugene Nagel and Dr. John Hirchmann.
- (1968) St. Vincent's Hospital in New York City established the first coronary care unit in the United States, and Columbus, Ohio established mobile coronary units staffed with cardiology fellows from OSU. Both soon replace physicians with advanced trained EMTs.
- (1969) The first nationally recognized EMT course was held in Wausau, Wisconsin. Dr. J. "Deke" Farrington was the course medical director.
- (1969) Dr. Leonard Cobb, Harborview Medical Center, and Seattle Fire Department established the Medic One paramedic program.

1970s The Star of Life and Voice of EMS

- (1970) The National Registry of EMTs (NREMT), a national EMS certification organization that maintains a registry of certifications, was established.
- (1971) "Emergency!" debuted on television, putting a public face on EMTs and Paramedics providing expert medical care on the scene of an accident. The show increased public awareness of EMS and possibly influenced government funding of EMS.
- (1973) Star of Life was adopted as the national EMS symbol, representing the six points of the complete EMS system: detection, reporting, response, on-scene care, care in transit, and transfer to definitive care. The central staff with a serpent wrapped around it represents medicine and healing.
- (1973) U.S. Congress passed the Emergency Medical Services Systems Act (PL93-144), which identified 15 essential components of an EMS system and allocated federal funding for individual EMS regions to address these components.
- (1975) National Association of EMTs (NAEMT) was formed to represent the needs of all EMTs to the public and government.
- (1979) American Ambulance Association (AAA), a representative organization for the ambulance service industry and legislation affecting EMS, was founded.

Figure 2-7 EMS Timeline.

1970s–Present Iraq War

- With an advanced skill set, the 68W healthcare specialist (a.k.a. Army medic) is prepared to treat combat casualties as well as civilian combatants.
- Development and deployment of special blood-stopping dressings, one-handed tourniquets, and special surgical procedures for extremity injuries and burns.

1980s–2000 Agenda for the Future—Education and Federal Funding

- (1981) The Omnibus Budget Reconciliation Act of 1981 consolidated EMS funding into state preventative health and health services block grants. Funding under the EMSS Act is eliminated.
- (1984) Medical Priority Dispatching began in Salt Lake City, Utah.
- (1984) EMS for Children (EMS-C) program, under the Public Health Act, was established, providing funds for enhancing the EMS system to better serve pediatric patients.
- (1985) The National Research Council published "Injury in America: A Continuing Public Health Problem," describing deficiencies in the progress in addressing the problems of accidental death and disability.
- (1986) The Comprehensive Omnibus Budget Reconciliation Act (COBRA) prevented patient "dumping," or transferring patients incapable of paying for services.
- (1988) The National Highway Traffic Safety Administration initiated the Statewide EMS Technical Assessment program based on ten key components of EMS systems.
- (1990) The Trauma Care Systems and Development Act of 1990 provided funding to states for trauma system planning, implementation and evaluation, encouraging development of inclusive trauma systems.
- (1993) The Institute of Medicine published "Emergency Medical Services for Children," pointing out deficiencies in the healthcare system's ability to address the emergency medical needs of pediatric patients.
- (1996) "The EMS Agenda for the Future" was released, outlining 14 essential attributes for future EMS development.
- (2006) The controversial report, "The Future of Emergency Care: Emergency Medical Services at the Crossroads" was released by the Institute of Medicine.

Figure 2-7 *(continued)*

EMS Agenda for the Future

As shown in Figure 2-7, EMS has developed out of a long and rich history. In 1995, the National Association of State Emergency Medical Services Directors (NAEMSD) and the National Association of EMS Physicians (NAEMSP), with assistance from the National Highway Traffic Safety Administration (NHTSA), met to reflect upon the previous 25 years of EMS practice experience and to establish their vision for the future of EMS. Their intention was to guide EMS toward its own destiny. The product of those meetings was called the **EMS Agenda for the Future** (Table 2-1).

The EMS Agenda for the Future suggests that EMS will be more intimately intertwined with public health, as well as public safety, and continue to evolve along with health care. The EMS Agenda suggested that public expectations and demands of EMS will remain high. These expectations will be fueled in part by increasing media attention by the press, television, and Internet as well as consumer demand.

To meet those expectations, Paramedics and emergency physicians are going to need to make better decisions regarding what care provides the best patient outcomes in the most cost effective manner. The standard of care that was formerly provided may not be the best care that can be offered. In that case, the public is going to demand performance improvement and cost efficiency.

In other words, EMS practice is going to have to become more evidence-based (i.e., supported by the medical research). In situations where the evidence is lacking, EMS should review their experience and reflect upon those practices that have led to the most desirable outcomes and strive to replicate them. These practices are the so-called **best practices**.

Table 2-1 Statement from the EMS Agenda for the Future

Emergency Medical Services (EMS) of the future will be community-based health management that is fully integrated with the overall healthcare system. It will have the ability to identify and modify illness and injury risks, provide acute illness and injury care and follow-up, and contribute to the treatment of chronic conditions and community health monitoring. This new entity will be developed from redistribution of existing healthcare resources and will be integrated with other healthcare providers and public health and public safety agencies. It will improve community health and result in more appropriate use of acute healthcare resources. EMS will remain the public's emergency medical safety net.[28]

EMS agencies should also strive to improve their operational preparedness. Proactive EMS agencies will look to the leaders in the EMS industry and use their operational practices as benchmarks. These benchmarks will rapidly become the standard of care and public officials will measure their EMS systems operations against the EMS standard of care.

To survive in a world of ever tightening fiscal constraints, and in order to remain the public's "safety net," EMS will have to demonstrate its efficiency and effectiveness and its willingness to adapt to improved medical technology.

The EMS Agenda for the Future describes the attributes of an effective and efficient EMS system. The EMS Agenda for the Future was reviewed by 500 EMS organizations and individuals, who came to consensus about EMS excellence. The panel that created the EMS Agenda for the Future listed 14 attributes of EMS (Table 2-2) and noted that EMS needs to continue to develop those 14 attributes if it is to reach its greatest potential.

Table 2-2 Attributes of an EMS System According to the EMS Agenda for the Future

1. Integration of Health Services
2. EMS Research
3. Legislation and Regulation
4. System Finance
5. Human Resources
6. Medical Direction
7. Education Systems
8. Public Education
9. Prevention
10. Public Access
11. Communication Systems
12 Clinical Care
13. Information Systems
14. Evaluation

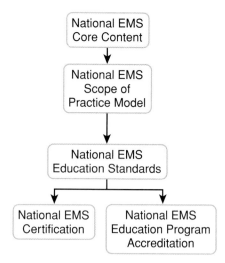

Figure 2-8 The five essential elements of the EMS educational system. (Courtesy of National Highway Traffic Safety Administration)

National EMS Education Agenda for the Future

In 1996 the National Highway Traffic Safety Administration convened a meeting of over 30 EMS organizations with the intent of implementing the educational portions of the EMS Agenda for the Future. The results of that meeting became known as the national **EMS Education Agenda for the Future**.[29] The Education Agenda set out to describe how all EMS providers, including Paramedics, would be prepared for service in EMS by following a systems approach. The National EMS Education Agenda, a systems approach, established five components that incorporated the essential elements of an educational system and how these elements interacted in a system (Figure 2-8).

The first component was the **National EMS Core Content**. The core content defines the entire universe of disorders, diseases, syndromes, and skills that an EMS provider might encounter and for which he would be expected to provide emergency care (i.e., the domain of EMS practice). Naturally, EMS physicians had a lead role in defining the domain of EMS practice. To the extent possible, the core content tried to include those practices that had strong evidence to support them or those that appeared in the 2004 practice analysis conducted by the National Registry of EMT.

The second component of the EMS Education Agenda for the Future was the **National EMS Scope of Practice (NEMSSOP)** model.[30] The **scope of practice** defines and divides EMS into four groupings. The National EMS Scope of Practice, created under the leadership of the National Association of State EMS Officials (NASEMSO), formerly known as the National Association of EMS State Directors (NAEMSD), clearly defines four levels of EMS providers. More importantly, it identifies the knowledge and skills required for each level (i.e., what is the scope of practice for that level within the domain of EMS practice).

One advantage of a national SOP is that there is a standardization of EMS providers of four levels. The four levels of EMS providers described in the NEMSSOP include the emergency medical responder (formerly the certified first responder), the emergency medical technician (formerly the emergency medical technician–basic), the advanced emergency medical technician (formerly the advanced emergency medical technician–intermediate), and the Paramedic (formerly the emergency medical technician–Paramedic).

The **emergency medical responder (EMR)** is an EMS provider who is expected to render lifesaving care with minimal equipment. This person may be the lone provider on scene for an extended period of time. For example, a member of the emergency response team at a plant or a security officer at a shopping mall, would be an emergency medical responder.

The **emergency medical technician (EMT)–Basic** is part of a team that responds to the emergency scene, typically aboard an ambulance, and is trained to provide initial care on scene as well as medical care to the patient while in transit to the hospital.

The **advanced emergency medical technician (AEMT)** is an EMT with additional skills. These additional skills are skills or medications that have been shown to positively impact patient survival (i.e., evidence-based practices). These skills include the administration of a limited number of drugs as well as, among other things, supraglottic airway devices.

The highest level of EMS provider is the **Paramedic**. The Paramedic's medical education includes advanced assessment and diagnosis of syndromes and disorders and the treatment thereof. In many states a Paramedic can obtain an associate's degree or higher.

Each level of EMS provider has knowledge and skills that are clearly delineated. If an EMS provider was to perform a procedure that was not within one's scope of practice then that individual could be accused of practicing medicine without a license.

Education Standards

In the past, the scope of practice for many EMS providers was defined by the **National Standard Curriculum (NSC)** for EMS. A seminal document, created with the assistance of the NHTSA in the 1970s, the NSC quickly became the only available source of information about the domain of prehospital emergency care (i.e., the scope of practice).[31,32]

With a definition of both the core content of EMS and the scope of practice of EMS establishing the domain of EMS, the National Association of EMS Educators (NAEMSE) set out to replace the NSC with the broader **National EMS Education Standards**. These National EMS Education Standards serve as the basis for EMS instruction and provide direction for EMS educators regarding both the core content and the scope of practice.

Accreditation

National EMS Education Program Accreditation, like other educational program accreditations, assures students who enter an EMS education program that the education they are about to receive meets national standards. Perhaps more importantly, accreditation helps assure the public, who depends on the graduates of those educational programs, that the graduates will be competent providers.

Presently the Commission on Accreditation of Allied Health Education Programs (CAAHEP) accredits Paramedic education programs. CAAHEP grants accreditation after receiving a favorable report from the Committee on Accreditation of Educational Programs for EMS Professions (CoAEMSP). CoAEMSP site visitors visit the program and review the facilities, faculty, and courses of a Paramedic program to determine if they meet the national accreditation standards and then issue their report either recommending for or against accreditation. For most healthcare professions, graduation from an accredited school or program is a minimum requirement for entry to certification examinations. Eventually this will become the standard for Paramedic education as well.

Licensure and Certification

All states, as a matter of state rights, license individuals for practice in that state. Licensure permits an individual to practice a trade or a profession. Generally that license is issued after demonstration of satisfactory completion of a course of education, usually called a certification. By definition, a license precludes other non-licensed individuals from practicing in the profession or trade. If a non-licensed person was to practice, then that person could be accused of "practicing without a license," which might involve criminal and/or civil penalties.

In some cases the state not only licenses but also certifies those individuals, through written and practical testing, before they are licensed. This has been cause for some confusion about the difference between licensure and certification. Simply stated, any time a state gives an individual exclusive rights to perform a function or profession it is a license. The use of the term "certification" in this regard is a semantic difference. The National Registry of EMT has a well written legal opinion on the matter on its website.[33, 34]

In a growing number of states the certification of the **National Registry of Emergency Medical Technicians (NREMT)** is accepted as proof positive that the individual being licensed is minimally competent to provide that level of care. Presently, the majority of states accept National Registry certification for licensure.

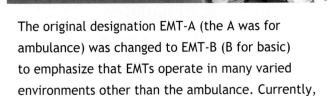

STREET SMART

The original designation EMT-A (the A was for ambulance) was changed to EMT-B (B for basic) to emphasize that EMTs operate in many varied environments other than the ambulance. Currently, the letter B has been eliminated altogether.

Mission of the EMS System

The fundamental mission of EMS has been to respond to a medical emergency, provide on-scene care, and transport patients to the closest appropriate medical facility. This mission is exemplified in the **star of life**, the symbol of EMS as represented by the six points; detection, reporting, response, on-scene care, care in transit, and transfer to definitive care.[35]

To be effective, the EMS system must provide a coordinated response of health and safety resources in a timely manner and be successful in mitigating the effects of illness and injury. To attain this goal, EMS must have both horizontal linkage with other public safety agencies and vertical linkage with the rest of the healthcare system.

Through complementary relationships (i.e., horizontal linkage) with other emergency services, such as law enforcement and/or the fire service, EMS can realize efficiencies through rapid response and treatment.

Take, for example, a citizen who experiences a cardiac arrest. If a law enforcement officer (LEO) in a quick response system (QRS) were to arrive on-scene within minutes of the cardiac arrest, the officer could apply an automated external defibrillator (AED). Following the instructions of the AED, and the lessons learned during CPR training, lifesaving care could be initiated. (LEO is used to categorize that large group of professionals that are involved in law enforcement, including but not limited to constables, Sheriff's deputies, police officers, state troopers, border patrol officers, agents and investigators from the Federal Bureau of Investigation, Drug Enforcement Agency, and so on.) Immediately afterward a **basic life support (BLS)** engine company from the fire service would arrive to support the LEO effort and provide additional skills and equipment, such as suction and oxygen. An advanced life support (ALS) ambulance would then arrive. The Paramedic would assume care of the patient, provide additional skills and equipment (such as intubation and ventilation), and transport the patient to the emergency department for stabilization. Once stabilized in the emergency department, the patient would be transferred to a coronary care unit (CCU) for further treatment and evaluation by a team of cardiologists. The patient's entry into this critical care pathway is an example of horizontal linkage between EMS and the rest of the healthcare team.

This ideal system illustrates one example of the effectiveness that can be realized from an integrated approach to emergency response by all public safety agencies.

Legislation and Regulation

EMS at its core is a public service. As such, the public has certain expectations of performance. To ensure that EMS is available, states have enacted legislation that provides for the existence of EMS and regulates its functions.[36-38]

In many states this enabling legislation describes the various levels of providers and, more importantly, links the practice of those providers with the state medical practice act and physician oversight. Furthermore, these statutes typically empower either the state health department or the state department of state with responsibility for EMS system oversight.

At a larger, macro level, local, state, and federal government have an interest in EMS. EMS responds to and mitigates the consequences of a disaster as part of the larger government response. For that purpose, government often funds EMS disaster preparedness through grants and other mechanisms.

A further discussion of other medical–legal responsibilities is contained in Chapter 6 on the law and EMS.

Public Access

When a citizen is suddenly confronted with a potentially life-threatening emergency, the person turns to EMS for help. To get that help, the citizen can use a variety of telecommunications devices but by far the most common means is to call on a telephone.

Previously the citizen had to memorize a seven-digit number for that jurisdiction. This often led to confusion and mistakes, some that were fatal. The obvious answer was to have a universal number for emergencies. Britain has had a universal number, 9-9-9, since 1937. However, the United States did not see a universal number, 9-1-1, until 1967.[39-42] When that famous 9-1-1 call was made from Haleyville, Alabama, in 1967, the era of modern telecommunications was ushered in.

Early 9-1-1 service provided the public immediate access to the local **public safety access point (PSAP)**, as well as automatic number identification (ANI), so that a "call-back" could be performed if necessary. Since that time, basic 9-1-1 has been improved. Enhanced 9-1-1 is now in use. Not only does it provide rapid access to emergency services, but

computer-assisted dispatch (CAD) technology identifies the caller's location as well.

With the growing number of mobile cellular telephones which cannot utilize the 9-1-1 technology, the early advantages of 9-1-1 location identification may have been lost. The Federal Communications Commission (FCC) is now working with the telecommunications industry and has undertaken a special wireless project that permits identification of a cellular telephone's location within 125 meters. Telecommunications professionals, represented by the National Emergency Number Association, have been working to improve the public's access to EMS.

Communication Systems

A typical EMS communication starts at the public safety access point (PSAP) when the professional telecommunicator, or dispatcher, answers the call and starts the emergency medical dispatch process. It ends when the Paramedic presents the patient over the radio to the medical control physician.

An overview of emergency communications underscores its importance. The emergency communications centers alert the public of impending natural disasters or terrorist attacks. From the simple color-coded terrorist alert used in the Homeland Security Advisory System to the Emergency Alert System (EAS) that predates the Homeland Security Advisory System, emergency communications professionals have been alerting the public to potential danger for years. Keeping up the tradition of watchfulness over our communities, telecommunicators can now alert drivers of a child abduction, via Amber alert, or dangerous persons with a special "be on the lookout (BOLO)" alerts via public signs and television announcements using the Emergency Notification System (ENS).

As technology improves, emergency communications takes advantage of these advances and incorporates them into the emergency communications system. There is a further discussion of emergency communications, both process and technology, in Chapter 18 on communications.

Architecture of EMS Systems

The wide variety of EMS system configurations speaks to the ingenuity of EMS officials and system administrators whose planning reflects the community's capability to provide EMS.

Contemporary EMS depends on a number of configurations of emergency responders—some fire-based, some municipal, some volunteer, some proprietary, and some a combination of these—to ensure EMS is provided to the community.

System Configurations

The predominant means of delivering EMS in the United States is via **fire-based EMS**.[43,44] The combination of trained personnel, lifesaving equipment, emergency vehicles, and strategically located stations make the fire service an ideal platform for the delivery of EMS.

The fire service has a long tradition of rescue and first aid. During World War II, in a time before self-contained breathing apparatus, many early fire services carried heavy E&J or Emerson Resuscitators for use in reviving firefighters and fire victims overcome by smoke and fumes. Eventually, the fire service started getting requests for "resuscitator" runs. Despite the availability of this equipment, medical calls remained infrequent until a few visionary physicians saw the potential of fire-based EMS.

Leaders in fire-based EMS—such as Dr. "Deke" Farrington of Chicago, Dr. Nagal of Miami, and Dr. Cobb of Seattle—saw the advantages in fire-based EMS and encouraged the fire service to get involved in EMS. Today, many major cities operate fire-based EMS services. For example, the Fire Department of New York (FDNY) operates the largest fire-based EMS service in the United States and had 1.2 million ambulance "jobs" or trips in 2007.

The International Association of Fire Chiefs (IAFC) and the International Association of Fire Fighters (IAFF) has supported the development of fire-based EMS and has made EMS a major priority for the Fire Service (Figure 2-9).

Hospital-based EMS is another common EMS system design. When the large urban hospitals—such as the Commercial Hospital in Cincinnati or Bellevue in New York City—were started it became clear that these hospitals needed ambulance service to bring invalid patients to the hospital. In some cases proprietors of local livery stables dedicated a specially outfitted carriage for the hospital to provide special transportation. That tradition continues today in many large cities. New York City, for example, still has a large number of ambulances that respond from the "voluntary" hospitals.

In still other cases, groups of physicians established ambulance services, such as the Physicians and Surgeons Ambulance Service (P&S) of Columbia University.

Commercial ambulance services, or for-profit EMS, have long provided interfacility medical transportation as well as emergency medical services to patients. Many of these commercial ambulance services originated from the funeral homes that previously provided the service.

Today, commercial ambulance services provide EMS to vast areas. Some companies (e.g., Rural-Metro and American Medical Response) are so large that the company's stock is sold in the market on the stock exchange.

Following the example of the Roanoke Volunteer Rescue Squad in 1920, rescue squads sprang up across America. These **community-based EMS** squads were independent of local fire departments and largely staffed with volunteers. Pressured by a lack of volunteers today, many of these community-based ambulances have turned to paid crews. However, the fact that these community-based ambulance services remain not-for-profit differentiates them from commercial ambulance services.

Some citizens believe that the government should provide EMS as part of its responsibilities for public safety. In those communities, a **municipal EMS service** was established as the third of three public safety departments (the other two public safety services being law enforcement and the fire service). In some cases small cities and villages would cross-train police officers as Paramedics to provide service and efficiency.

The military is decidedly the largest provider of emergency medical care (i.e., **military emergency medicine**) and

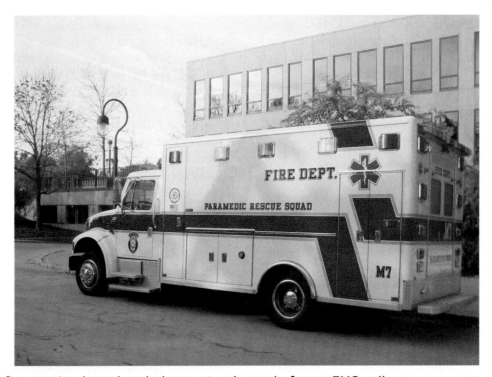

Figure 2-9 A fire service-based ambulance stands ready for an EMS call. (Image copyright 2009, Jenny Woodworth. Used under license from Shutterstock)

has been providing EMS for a longer period of time than any other EMS system. The healthcare specialist and corpsmen of today's military care for some 1.37 million active service men and women alone.

Modern EMS in the armed forces can be traced back to surgeon Jonathan Letterman's efforts to establish a system of ambulances in 1864. In many respects the lessons that the military has learned while providing emergency medical care on the battlefield have been translated to emergency medical care in the civilian sector.

Resource Management

Resource management involves placing vehicles and personnel in a position to provide the most expeditious response to an emergency. Some communities require, through contract or regulation, a minimal response time. While there is not a national standard response time, many EMS services have accepted a 6- to 10-minute response time. This time is consistent with cardiac arrest studies that indicate the greatest likelihood of return of spontaneous circulation (ROSC) is within 6 to 10 minutes of cardiac arrest.[45–50]

Traditionally EMS was stationed in standing facilities and many EMS services still utilize this **fixed-post staffing** method of resource distribution. Using squad buildings, ambulance bays, or fire stations, ambulances respond from these centrally located stations to calls for emergency medical service.

Some EMS services have gone to a dynamic posting method called **system status management (SSM)** or event-driven deployment. Instead of posting in fixed locations, such as a fire house, the ambulances or emergency response vehicles are "on-the-road" moving to new locations, or posts, that optimize response times. The decision of where to post these resources is typically made after an analysis of historical data of call volume and knowledge of geography and traffic conditions.

Still other systems, trying to combine fixed-post staffing with system status management, provide **peak-load staffing**. During predictable hours of high demand, additional ambulances are placed in-service at strategic locations.

Specialization

Unique environments, certain occupations, and special circumstances require specially trained Paramedics. Over a dozen subspecialties have been created in EMS. The following are short descriptions of some of the notable subspecialties.

A growing subspecialty in EMS is the area of **Specialty Care Transport (SCT)**. Called to transport sick and injured patients from outlying clinics and critical access hospitals to **tertiary care** centers, such as trauma centers and cardiac centers, for example, these Paramedics perform critical care interfacility transportation.

Many consider the **flight Paramedic** as the most highly trained level of EMS provider.[51–53] Flight Paramedics transport critically ill patients in either **fixed-wing aircraft**

or rotor aircraft from scenes or other facilities to definitive care. Upon completion of advanced EMS education, with emphasis on critical care medicine and flight medicine, flight Paramedics may test to become certified flight Paramedics.

Frontier/rural Paramedics and woodlands search and rescue teams are tasked with providing patient care in wilderness areas. The **Wilderness EMT (WEMT)** has special training that fosters critical thinking as well as creativity in an environment where supplies may be limited and patient transport to definitive care prolonged.

Paramedics who provide EMS in a rural setting often have different circumstances and more difficult obstacles to overcome than their counterparts in the city. To prepare for these emergencies many Paramedics take the **FarMedic®** course, which is specifically directed to the farm emergency. The FarMedic® course teaches how to care for a patient under an overturned tractor (Figure 2-10) and a number of other rural emergencies.

Another area of EMS specialization is medical support for special weapons and tactics (SWAT) teams. Despite careful planning and preparation, casualties do occur in these highly charged operations. **Tactical EMS (TEMS)** providers are trained on how to provide care to the wounded while in hostile surroundings as well as maintain the health of the SWAT team members on prolonged operations.

Information Systems

In the age of computers EMS began to incorporate information systems into patient care. From electronic patient care reports that are capable of being transmitted prior to the arrival of the ambulance to integrated information systems that permit inter and intra-agency communications, EMS systems are embracing information technology.

Some new challenges have also been presented with this new technology. Patient confidentiality, a fundamental tenet of patient care, is at greater risk for inadvertent disclosure. Recent federal legislation, the **Health Insurance Portability and Accountability Act (HIPAA)**, has placed conditions upon all healthcare providers that protect patient privacy during claims processing, data analysis, utilization review, quality assurance, and practice management.[54–59]

There is further discussion of information systems in Chapter 19 on documentation.

Integration of Health Services

EMS does not operate independently but is a link between the public and the rest of the healthcare continuum. EMS can be seen as one of the doors to health care, a system within a system. The seamless transition of care from the streets to the hospital ensures the continuation of quality medical care.

A number of healthcare "stakeholders" depend on EMS. Social service workers depend on the assistance of Paramedics to report child abuse, domestic violence, and elder abuse. Trauma surgeons depend on Paramedics to

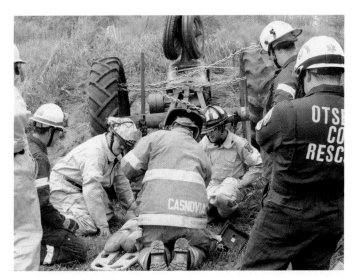

Figure 2-10 Disentangling a patient under an overturned tractor. (Courtesy of Chris Randall/Michigan Rural Rescue, Inc.)

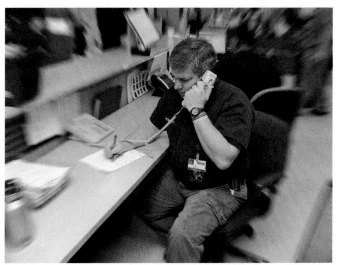

Figure 2-11 Radio communications permit the physician to have direct access and control of the Paramedic in the field.

expeditiously transport trauma patients to definitive care at the trauma center. Cardiologists have an interest in the provision of advanced life support and stabilization of cardiac patients in the field, including the identification of high-risk patients using 12-lead ECG.[60–63]

Medical Direction

In 1989, the American College of Emergency Physicians (ACEP) published a position paper, "The Principles of EMS Systems," which called for strong physician involvement in prehospital medicine as well as the active participation of physicians in EMS.[64]

Terms such as **medical oversight** and **medical command** illustrate the direct control that a physician has over a Paramedic's practice.

Medical oversight is present whenever a physician is involved in the quality assurance/quality improvement process and provides direction, either in the form of protocols or education, to Paramedics. This medical oversight is often retrospective and may be remedial in nature.

Medical command implies a more immediate and direct involvement in patient care. The physician's authority can be exercised either on-scene or over-the-air at the time of an emergency, referred to as **on-line medical control**. Physicians can give medical direction via the base radio and exercise medical command (Figure 2-11).

More commonly, the physician's authority is exerted through a written set of instructions, called protocols. The **protocols** can be used by the Paramedic in specific situations in the absence of the physician.[65–67] These preauthorized medical orders, or **standing orders**, are often given to Paramedics in a flowchart format called an **algorithm**. An algorithm is a logic tree that simply states: if this, then do that; if not this, then do this other thing. Algorithms can be useful during an emergency when time is of the essence.

Finance Systems

The means of financing EMS systems is typically driven by community capabilities. For example, a fire-based EMS system may be supported, in part or in whole, from property taxes, whereas a volunteer EMS rescue squad may receive its funds from taxes collected in a special district similar to a fire district. Other volunteer ambulances or fire districts may depend on community generosity by seeking donations.

The majority of EMS—be it commercial, hospital-based, or any other configuration—is funded by billing a fee-for-service. In a fee-for-service system, the patient is billed a charge that is customary for such a service in the area. Payment for ambulance service may come from the patient but is usually paid by the patient's health insurance.

One of the largest payers for EMS is Medicare. Medicare reimbursement is paid according to a schedule established by the Centers for Medicaid and Medicare Services (CMS) which is part of the federal Department of Health and Human Services.

Grants for special projects or research are also available to EMS services from government agencies or groups (e.g., the Centers for Disease Control and Prevention (CDC), the Maternal and Child Health Bureau, or the EMS for Children program).

One of the difficulties facing EMS is the inconsistency in funding. Driven by patient transportation, as opposed to the emergency medical care provided, payments have been erratic and undependable. The CMS has attempted to modify the federal Medicare rules to account for not just transportation but emergency medical care as well.

Some health insurance organizations have tried to eliminate payments by limiting the definition of a medical emergency to these conditions, listed in a discharge diagnosis, that without immediate care and treatment would result in harm to the patient's health. Any medical condition that does not fall under this definition and could have been treated later and at less expense to the insurance company is thus not a covered condition. This limited retrospective view of an emergency fails to take into account the patient's fears and anxiety when suddenly faced with an unknown illness or injury.

Many health insurance carriers have adopted a more flexible and a reasonable approach to defining an emergency. These organizations use the **prudent layperson standard** to establish medical necessity. The prudent layperson standard simply places the proverbial "average person" in the situation and asks if that average person would reasonably think, under those conditions, that this problem was an emergency.[68–72] This approach allows for the inclusion of human factors such as fear and anxiety.

National Healthcare Systems

Medical care in the majority of the world is a government-operated enterprise, a social welfare system of sorts which ensures the health and well-being of the citizens within its borders.

Health care in the United States is more of a medley of private payment and public funds, private physicians, and government-run treatment centers. This unique blend of different approaches to healthcare delivery has resulted in a healthcare system that provides numerous opportunities, as well as remarkable inefficiencies.

Previously the majority of health care was provided on a **fee for service** basis, or pay as you go, with a certain amount of medical care provided gratis to the poor or uninsured. However, the pressures of modern economics have generally encouraged all healthcare providers to embrace the concept of **managed health care**.

Managed health care is a system where there is a purchaser of services, such as a large corporation or the government. The purchaser in turn obtains health insurance for its workers via private sources, such as Blue Cross/Blue Shield, or governmental sources, such as state-run Medicaid or federal Medicare programs.

These insurers then gather groups of healthcare providers—physicians as well as allied healthcare providers—and obtain a reduced rate in exchange for a guaranteed client base. These savings could only be possible because of the economies of scale. The managed healthcare insurance plan then mandates that patients seek treatment from this preferred medical group, in essence managing the care that the patient will receive by providing medical care for the lowest price.

A multiplicity of managed care arrangements exist. However, generally managed care can be broken down into three basic configurations.

The first and earliest system is the **health maintenance organization (HMO)**. The HMO provides payments to healthcare providers at a negotiated annual per capita rate. These rates are based on practice history of the insured patients and helps to prevent fluctuations in payments, thus making expenses, costs, and budgets more predictable.

The next configuration is the **preferred provider organization (PPO)**, a modified fee-for-service schedule, that permits patients to choose their healthcare provider from amongst a roster. Although there is increased flexibility for the patient with the PPO, some limitations still exist in terms of the patient's choice of provider if not on the roster.

The last configuration is called **point of service (POS)**. POS has qualities of both an HMO and a PPO. In a POS program the patient is allowed to choose a healthcare provider from amongst a list of preferred care providers (PCP) but may elect to see another "out of system" provider, without a referral, at a substantially higher copayment and/or deductible, similar to a fee-for-service arrangement. The employer, in turn, gets the advantages of cost savings whenever the patient/employee participates in the managed care program. The POS is gaining increasing popularity with patients and employers alike.

CONCLUSION

From its early beginnings, when hearses were used as ambulances and the patient might be lucky enough to have an ambulance driver with basic first aid training, EMS has evolved into a highly complex system of emergency responders who provide the public with an emergency medical safety net and who work as part of the larger healthcare system.

KEY POINTS:

- Emergency Medical Services (EMS) became recognized as part of the public health services in the late 1960s.

- The historical evolution of American health care began with physicians making house calls to treat the sick and injured.

- Following World War II, medicine began to concentrate less on infectious diseases and more on chronic diseases, such as cancer, stroke, and heart disease.

- Health insurance made it more affordable to receive health care. However, technology has significantly increased costs. To curb rising costs, the federal government has taken a greater role in healthcare policymaking.

- Public health was advanced by nurses who sought to improve sanitation and decrease morbidity and mortality as a result of infectious diseases.

- The Public Health Service is a key portion of the Department of Health and Human Services overseen by the Surgeon General.

- Deriving from once crude horse-drawn carriages used as far back as Roman times, the concept of the ambulance developed from the trials of several wars.

- While the tools of war became more devastating, the field care of soldiers improved. During the American Civil War the military field medical service was reorganized and became the forerunner of the modern trauma system.

- Stemming from the Geneva Convention in 1864 the American Red Cross, founded by Clara Barton, was created to provide aid in a time of war to the sick and wounded of the armed forces.

- Hospital-based civilian ambulance services began to appear in the United States during the 1860s.

- The emergence of civilian EMS came from the first volunteer rescue squad in Virginia, 1921. Many of these "independent," or non-hospital-based services, developed from local volunteer fire departments.

- A paradigm shift occurred as ambulances were seen as more than just fast rides but rather as a way to deliver faster medical care to the patient.

- The White Paper addressed public health concerns regarding traffic accidents and led to the development of stronger educational programs for emergency care providers.

- New drug therapies and defibrillators developed as a result of research in sudden cardiac death.

- Television helped demonstrate the role of emergency services to the public.

- The EMS Act of 1973 amended the Public Health Service Act of 1944 and outlined needed improvements in the EMS system.

- The National EMS Education Agenda for the Future established a core content, scope of practice, educational standards, accreditation, and certification.

- National EMS Core Content listed the knowledge and skills necessary for the provision of emergency care.

- The National EMS Scope of Practice delineated the four levels of EMS providers.

- Replacing the National Standard Curriculum, the National EMS Education Standards serve as the basis for EMS instruction and provide direction for EMS educators.

- EMS Education Program Accreditation assures students that their education meets national standards.

- A license is issued by a state, giving the license holder the right to perform a function.

- Completion of a specific educational program leads to certification.

- The EMS system provides a coordinated response of resources with other public safety agencies. The EMS system also constitutes a vital link with the rest of the healthcare system by providing rapid response and emergency treatment.

- Expectations of performance for each provider are maintained through the state medical practice act and physician oversight.

- The 9-1-1 system created a public safety access point (PSAP) to provide immediate public assistance.

- A wide variety of EMS system configurations provide EMS to communities ranging from urban to rural.

- Resource management involves placing vehicles and personnel in a position to provide the most expeditious response to an emergency.

- Subspecialties exist in EMS. Some include training as a Specialty Care Transport (SCT), Flight Paramedic, Wilderness EMT, or Tactical EMS.

- EMS systems use information technology to incorporate information systems into patient care.

- A key component to an EMS system is medical oversight and command performed by emergency physicians.

- In a fee-for-service billing system, the patient is billed for service but the cost is usually covered by the patient's health insurance. Most EMS systems are funded this way with Medicare being the largest payer.

- A health maintenance organization (HMO) provides payment to a specified group of healthcare providers at a negotiated annual rate in turn for health care for employees.

- The preferred provider organization (PPO) is similar to a HMO but permits patients to choose their healthcare provider from among a roster.

- A point of service (POS) configuration contains qualities of both an HMO and PPO by allowing patients to choose a healthcare provider or see another "out of system" provider without referral.

▶ REVIEW QUESTIONS:

1. Name the key developments in the evolution of American health care.
2. What effect do wars have on the advancement of public health?
3. What is the role of the public health nurse?
4. What departments in government are overseen by the U.S. Surgeon General?
5. Who was Clara Barton? What agency was derived from her interventions?
6. Describe the paradigm shift from ambulances as transportation to ambulances delivering fast medical care.
7. In what way did the White Papers address public health concerns?

8. What is the EMS Agenda for the Future?
9. How does the National EMS Scope of Practice model define the different practice levels of EMS providers?
10. Explain the importance of educational standards and accreditation.
11. What is medical oversight of the Paramedic?
12. How do protocols assist the Paramedic?

CASE STUDY QUESTIONS:

Please refer to the Case Study at the beginning of the chapter and answer the questions below:

1. Respond to the statement: The role of EMS is still to transport the sick or injured to medical care.
2. After your presentation, a physician asks for clarification of the role of ER physicians in local prehospital care. How would you respond?
3. In what ways is EMS meeting the goals set out by the EMS Agenda for the Future?
4. What opportunities exist to strengthen the relationship between EMS and physicians?

REFERENCES:

1. Bencze B. From the history of ambulance and rescue squad services. *Orv Hetil.* 1976;117(42):2557–2559.
2. Donchin Y. On the history of the ambulance. *Harefuah.* 2001;140(7):658–660.
3. Pal E. The history of ambulance services. *Orv Hetil.* 1978;119(13):802–805.
4. English PC. Diphtheria and theories of infectious disease: centennial appreciation of the critical role of diphtheria in the history of medicine. *Pediatrics.* 1985;76(1):1–9.
5. Kass EH. A brief perspective on the early history of American infectious disease epidemiology. *Yale J Biol Med.* 1987;60(4):341–348.
6. Jahiel RI. Healthcare system of the United States and its priorities: history and implications for other countries. *Croat Med J.* 1998;39(3):316–331.
7. Kearney PR, Engh CA. History of the American healthcare system: its cost control programs and incremental reform. *Orthopedics.* 1997;20(3):236–247; quiz 248–249.
8. Lloyd S. The Ottawa typhoid epidemics of 1911 and 1912: a case study of disease as a catalyst for urban reform. *Urban Hist Rev.* 1979;8(1):66–89.
9. White CR. Yellow fever; history of the disease in the eighteenth and nineteenth century. *J Kans Med Soc.* 1959;60(8):298–302 passim.
10. Reed AS. Looking back. A tribute to my great aunt, Marguerite Wales: author, leader, consultant, public health nurse, and director of Henry Street Visiting Nurse Service. *Home Healthc Nurse.* 2007;25(4):235–239.
11. The American Red Cross charter section 2, paragraph 1.
12. Evans GD. Clara Barton: teacher, nurse, Civil War heroine, founder of the American Red Cross. *Int Hist Nurs J.* 2003;7(3):75–82.
13. Berry D. The history of cardiopulmonary resuscitation. *Circulation.* 2007;115(5):f20.
14. Cooper JA, Cooper JD, et al. Cardiopulmonary resuscitation: history, current practice, and future direction. *Circulation.* 2006;114(25):2839–2849.
15. DeBard ML. The history of cardiopulmonary resuscitation. *Ann Emerg Med.* 1980;9(5):273–275.
16. Vrtis MC. Cost/benefit analysis of cardiopulmonary resuscitation: a history of CPR—Part I. *Nurs Manage.* 1992;23(4):50–54.
17. **http://www.jfklink.com/speeches/jfk/publicpapers/1961/jfk338_61.html**
18. National Academy of Sciences. Accidental death and disability: the neglected disease of modern society. National Academy Press; 1966.
19. Howard JM. Historical background to accidental death and disability: the neglected disease of modern society. *Prehosp Emerg Care.* 2000:4(4):285–289.
20. Gaston SR. Accidental death and disability: the neglected disease of modern society. A progress report. *J Trauma.* 1971;11(3):195–206.

21. National Highway Traffic Safety Administration. *The National EMS Scope of Practice Model*. Washington, DC: U.S. Department of Transportation/National Highway Traffic Safety Administration; 2005.

22. Guide to Federal Records in the National Archives of the United States. Compiled by Robert B. Matchette et al. (September 9, 1966). Washington, DC: National Archives and Records Administration (80 Stat. 718 and 80 Stat. 731).

23. Benhamou-Jantelet G, Heron L, et al. Emergency crash cart and its use in an academic medical center. *Soins*. April 2007;(714):35.

24. Clarke RH, Phillips OC, et al. Hospital designs crash cart for each nursing station. *Mod Hosp*. March 1965;104:126.

25. Nussbaum GB, Fisher JG. A crash cart that works. *Am J Nurs*. 1978;78(1):45–48.

26. Pantridge JF, Geddes JS. Cardiac arrest after myocardial infarction. *Lancet*. 1966;1(7441):807–808.

27. Public Law 93-154–Nov. 16, 1973. Title XII–Emergency Medical Services Systems. 58 Stat. 682; 86 Stat. 137.

28. National Highway Transportation Safety Administration. EMS agenda for the future. 1996. Available from: **http://www.nhtsa .gov/people/injury/ems/agenda/emsman.html**

29. National Highway Transportation Safety Administration. EMS education agenda for the future: a systems approach. 2000. Available from: **http://www.nhtsa.gov/people/injury/ems/ FinalEducationAgenda.pdf**

30. **http://www.nasemsd.org/documents/FINALEMSSept2006_ PMS314.pdf**

31. **http://www.health.state.ny.us/nysdoh/ems/original/intro/ intro.pdf**

32. Salzman JG, Page DI, et al. Paramedic student adherence to the national standard curriculum recommendations. *Prehosp Emerg Care*. 2007;11(4):448–452.

33. **http://www.nremt.org/nremt/about/Legal_Opinion.asp**

34. Cannon GM, Jr., Menegazzi JJ, et al. A comparison of paramedic didactic training hours and NREMT-P examination performance. *Prehosp Emerg Care*. 1998;2(2):141–144.

35. Alberts ME. The star of life. *J Iowa Med Soc*. 1972;62(8):431.

36. Doyle OJ. Federal EMS legislation. *JEMS*. 1997; 22(9):26–27, 30.

37. Lipsky J. The need for EMS legislation. *J Iowa Med Soc*. 1978;68(3):85–86.

38. McKenna W. Understanding EMS legislation. *Emerg Med Serv*. 1988;17(5):52–55.

39. Davenport J. Anatomy of a 911 call. *Northwest Dent*. 2005;84(4):37–38.

40. Isler C. Dial 911 for the coronary ambulance. *RN*. 1969;32(8):48–51.

41. Kimball KF. 911—the emergency number. *Nebr State Med J*. 1971;56(2):68–70.

42. McSwain NE, Jr. The effectiveness of 911. *Ann Emerg Med*. 1992;21(10):1242–1243.

43. Greiff SJ. Fire-based EMS: the trend of the future? *Emerg Med Serv*. 1999;28(6):43, 45–46, 48 passim.

44. Davis J. Fire-based EMS. *Emerg Med Serv*. 2000;29(1):12, 14, 16; author reply 93, 101.

45. Krep H, Bottiger BW, et al. Time course of circulatory and metabolic recovery of cat brain after cardiac arrest assessed by perfusion- and diffusion-weighted imaging and MR-spectroscopy. *Resuscitation*. 2003;58(3):337–348.

46. Matot I, Shleifer A, et al. In-hospital cardiac arrest: is outcome related to the time of arrest? *Resuscitation*. 2006;71(1):56–64.

47. Morley PT. Improved cardiac arrest outcomes: as time goes by? *Crit Care*. 2007;11(3):130.

48. Ornato JP, Gonzalez ER, et al. Arterial pH in out-of-hospital cardiac arrest: response time as a determinant of acidosis. *Am J Emerg Med*. 1985;3(6):498–502.

49. Schoerkhuber W, Kittler H, et al. Time course of serum neuron-specific enolase. A predictor of neurological outcome in patients resuscitated from cardiac arrest. *Stroke*. 1999;30(8):1598–1603.

50. Vukmir RB. Survival from prehospital cardiac arrest is critically dependent upon response time. *Resuscitation*. 2006;69(2): 229–334.

51. NFPA. The role of the flight paramedic in the prehospital environment. NFPA (National Flight Paramedics Association) position paper. *Air Med J*. 1993;12(6):203–204.

52. Gryniuk J. The role of the certified flight paramedic (CFP) as a critical care provider and the required education. *Prehosp Emerg Care*. 2001;5(3):290–292.

53. Hatley T, Ma OJ, et al. Flight Paramedic scope of practice: current level and breadth. *J Emerg Med*. 1998;16(5):731–735.

54. Bacon GV. Legislative activity: HIPAA and recommendations to protect individual privacy. *J Law Med Ethics*. 1997;25(4):316–319.

55. Burkhartsmeier G. HIPAA: where are we now? *MLO Med Lab Obs*. 2007;39(6):28.

56. Gaines R. HIPAA: privacy and public good. *Update*. 2003;18(4):9–13.

57. Hansen, E. HIPAA (Health Insurance Portability and Accountability Act) rules: federal and state enforcement. *Med Interface*. 1997;10(8):96–98, 101–102.

58. Kumekawa J. HIPAA: how our healthcare world has changed. *Online J Issues Nurs*. 2005;10(2):1.

59. Schoppmann MJ, Sanders DL. HIPAA compliance: the law, reality, and recommendations. *J Am Coll Radiol*. 2004;1(10): 728–733.

60. Collins D. The prehospital 12-lead EKG: starting outside the emergency department. *J Emerg Nurs*. 1997;23(1):48–50.

61. Cummins RO, Eisenberg MS. From pain to reperfusion: what role for the prehospital 12-lead ECG? *Ann Emerg Med*. 1990;19(11):1343–1346.

62. Davis DP, Graydon C, et al. The positive predictive value of paramedic versus emergency physician interpretation of the prehospital 12-lead electrocardiogram. *Prehosp Emerg Care*. 2007;11(4):399–402.

63. Greiff SJ. Taking it to the street: advanced monitoring and 12-lead EKGs in prehospital care. *Emerg Med Serv*. 1998;27(9):47–48, 54–55.

64. John A, Brennan E. *Principles of EMS Systems* (3rd ed.). American College of Emergency Physicians; Boston, MA: Jones and Bartlett, 2005.

65. Myers MB, Norwood SH. Standing orders for trauma care. *J Emerg Nurs*. 1994;20(2):111–117.

66. O'Connor R. Paramedic standing orders. *Del Med J*. 1993;65(7):465–466.

67. Schedler P. Standing trauma orders should also be cost-effective. *J Emerg Nurs*. 1994;20(5):346–347.

68. American College of Emergency Physicians. Definition of emergency medicine. *Ann Emerg Med*. 1994;24(3):553–554.

69. Kucera WR. Narrow definition of "emergency" can spell "litigation." *Hosp Med Staff*. 1978;7(9):21–27.

70. Li J, Galvin HK, et al. The "prudent layperson" definition of an emergency medical condition. *Am J Emerg Med*. 2002;20(1):10–13.

71. Mitchell TA. Nonurgent emergency department visits—whose definition? *Ann Emerg Med*. 1994;24(5):961–963.

72. Schneider SM, Hamilton GC, et al. Definition of emergency medicine. *Acad Emerg Med*. 1998;5(4):348–351.

WORKFORCE SAFETY AND WELLNESS

KEY CONCEPTS:

Upon completion of this chapter, it is expected that the reader will understand these following concepts:

- Paramedic wellness defined as more than absence of disease
- The body's responses to both positive and negative stresses
- Stress management techniques for managing acute stress and chronic stress
- Safety tips and stress management prevention strategies

▶ CASE STUDY:

"I can't believe that I pulled my back on that last call," said the young Paramedic. "Now what am I supposed to do? We're expecting our first baby and I've got the house payment and car payment. I can't be out of work and I need the overtime!"

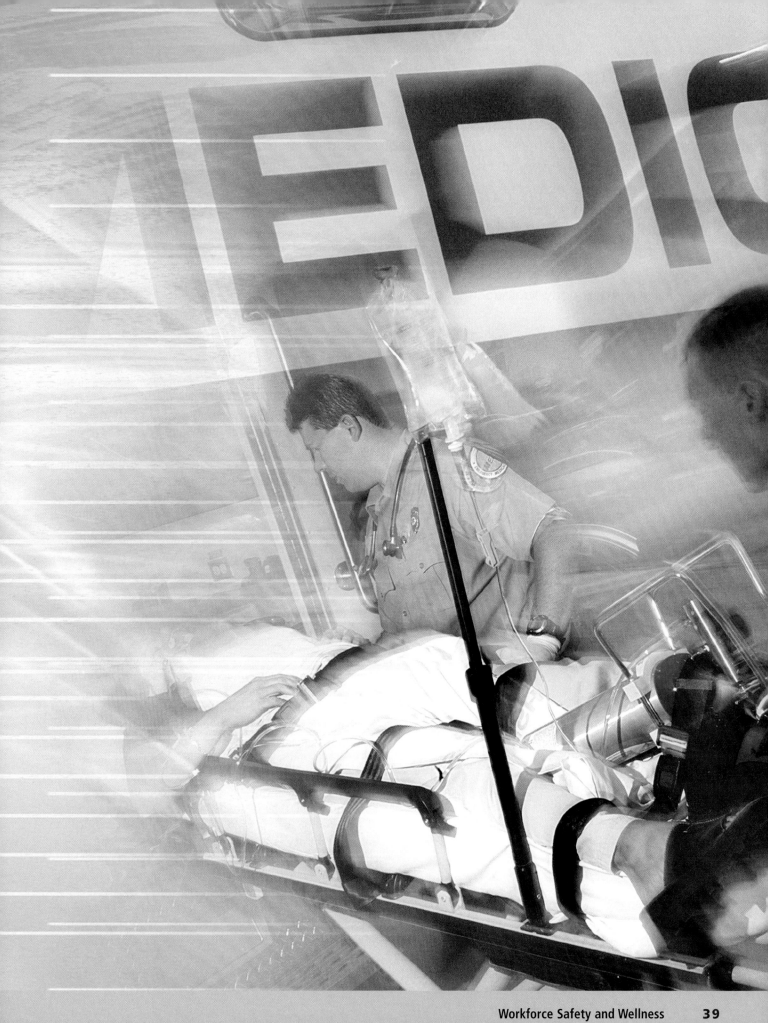

OVERVIEW

The health and wellness of the Paramedic goes beyond simply avoiding illness. It involves the social, spiritual, intellectual, emotional, and physical well-being as a part of a well-balanced lifestyle. The Paramedic encounters stress each day. This stress can have a harmful physiological effect on the body. It is important for the Paramedic to have built-in mechanisms for stress management and be familiar with the methods of crisis intervention to help prevent stress related illness.

The Paramedic has many responsibilities, but perhaps the most important is personal safety. Focusing on the Paramedic's response to emergencies and scene hazards, awareness is what can keep the Paramedic, his team, and the public safe. Safety is more than body substance isolation.

Wellness

The concept of wellness could be thought of as merely the absence of illness. However, this simplistic approach fails to take into account the complexity of human existence. Wellness is a multidimensional concept which includes all aspects of a person—social, spiritual, intellectual, and emotional—as well as physical well-being (Figure 3-1).

One definition of **wellness**, advanced by DePaul University, is that wellness is an active process of becoming aware of, and making choices toward, a more successful existence. This definition, intrinsically, implies that wellness is more than an absence of illness, which could be thought of as the lowest level of wellness. Paramedics who are aware of the practice of wellness are more likely to not experience illness and to lead more productive lives.

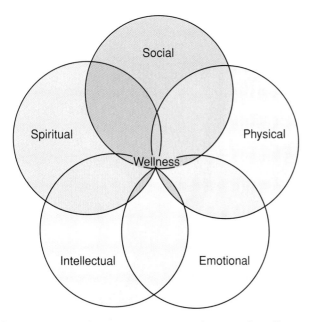

Figure 3-1 The interconnectedness of wellness.

Benefits of Wellness

The benefits of wellness include a heightened sense of purpose, an inner tranquility, as well as a physical being capable of greater feats. Physical health is the most outward sign of wellness. Physically, the healthy body is more resistant to injury (such as back injuries), as well as to illness. The body, as a machine, functions better with a lower resting heart rate and blood pressure, more respiratory reserve, and generally has a better cardiovascular capacity when it is healthy. Risk factors for all of the major diseases—cardiovascular disease, diabetes, and cancer—are reduced in healthy people.

Methods Used to Achieve Wellness

Nutrition

The components of physical health include a proper diet, one that provides the necessary nutrients, in the quantities sufficient for life. A balanced intake of carbohydrates for quick energy, fats and proteins for body maintenance, as well as essential vitamins and minerals, can help the body maintain optimal functionality. These nutrients can be obtained from the major food groups illustrated in the Department of Agriculture's Food Pyramid (Figure 3-2). Foods, taken in the quantities indicated, can sustain a body and provide it with the materials and resources it needs to withstand the stresses encountered in emergency services.

Food should always be eaten in moderation, with attention paid to the type of foods being eaten. Excess amounts of fatty foods, for example, or excessive intake can lead to obesity. **Obesity** is a growing health crisis, second only to cigarette smoking as the leading cause of preventable death.[1,2] Obesity can lead to a host of associated complications including diabetes and cardiovascular disease.[3–6]

Medically speaking, a person is obese when his body mass index is 30 or greater.[7] A common layperson definition of morbid obesity is 100 pounds over ideal weight. Over 60% of American men are obese by definition and therefore have an increased chance of illness, injury, and premature death.

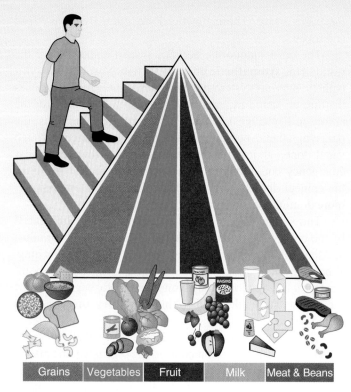

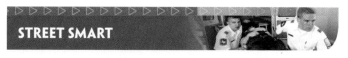

| Grains | Vegetables | Fruit | Milk | Meat & Beans |

Figure 3-2 United States Department of Agriculture's Food Pyramid with a new emphasis on exercise. (Courtesy of United States Department of Agriculture)

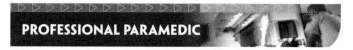

STREET SMART

Specialized bariatric equipment is available to help transport patients with obesity. The Paramedic should know how to obtain this equipment and use it to prevent personal injury.

Exercise

Exercise is also essential to physical health. A combination of aerobic exercise (e.g., walking or jogging), as well as strength training is considered optimal for maintaining

PROFESSIONAL PARAMEDIC

Some Paramedic employers contract with chiropractors, personal trainers, or health educators with a specialty in injury prevention to conduct assessments and teaching sessions in an effort to reduce back injuries.

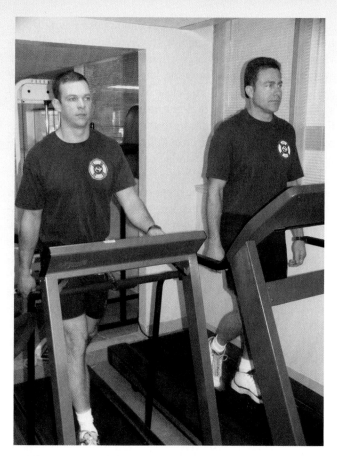

Figure 3-3 Physical fitness is essential to longevity in EMS.

health. Whether using free-weights (**isometric**) or resistance exercises (**isotonic**), strength training can lead to increased muscle strength and flexibility (Figure 3-3). This in turn can help reduce the incidence or the severity of on-the-job injuries, particularly back injuries.

Stress

Stress is a function of daily living, a result of the interaction between the person and the environment. During the course of a day, the human body is constantly being bombarded by stimuli. The body reacts to this stimuli accordingly. The amount of stimulation results in a certain level of stress in the body. If the stress is manageable (i.e., tolerable within the limits of a person's physical, psychological, emotional/ spiritual, and intellectual capacity to respond to the stimuli), then it is a positive form of stress or **eustress**. Eustress can lead to improved health as well as a sense of fulfillment or accomplishment.

Alternatively, overwhelming stimuli can lead to unhealthy stress, which in turn can have a negative impact on the person. This is called **distress**. Distress is the result of the body's maladaptive reaction to stress. The stimulus causes the body to react in a self-protective manner. This "survival instinct," awareness of and the ability to respond to one's surroundings, is immediate and uncontrollable.

When distress occurs, the body undergoes a reaction controlled by the autonomic nervous system. The autonomic nervous system can affect organ function throughout the body. Walter Cannon coined the term "**fight or flight**" to describe the generally adaptive response of the autonomic nervous system to stress. "Fight or flight" describes the body's instinctive response to a potential life threat. This primitive stress response may have been critical to the survival of primeval man, but can be unhealthy today.

Modern man faces a host of new behavioral and emotional **stressors** beyond the mere physiologic stressors faced by early man. Modern stressors include psychosocial pressures from family, coworkers complaints, and supervisors' demands. In addition, intellectual pressures to perform to perhaps unrealistic expectations, as well as new physiological stressors that include noise pollution from sirens wailing, can lead to distress. Distress can be caused by any stimulus that creates a maladaptive response from the autonomic nervous system.

Hans Selye, an endocrinologist, observing the impact of stress upon physiology, advanced his theory of the "general adaptation syndrome." In his theory he suggested that all human experience creates stress, but it is how the person responds to that stress that determines if it is eustress or distress.[8–10] Selye believed that the power of the body to resist distress, over a prolonged period of time, was limited and that the body would eventually become exhausted and typically manifest in mental or physical illness.

Symptoms of Stress

The manifestations of a Paramedic's pending exhaustion from stress can be divided into psychological, cognitive, behavioral, and physiological signs and symptoms.

For some people, the psychological signs of distress include an unreasonable irritability at seemingly minor annoyances, uncharacteristic angry outbursts, open or covert hostility, and a general restlessness. For other people, distress is manifested by depression, withdrawal, self-deprecation, as well as reduced self-esteem. The Paramedic may also manifest stress by having uncharacteristic bouts of forgetfulness, reduced creativity, shortened attention span, and disorganized thought.

The person under extreme stress may demonstrate uncharacteristic changes in behavior such as increased smoking, aggressive behavior (e.g., road rage), increased alcohol or drug use, over-eating, and a general carelessness about and withdrawal from activities of daily living. All of these may be signs of impending stress-induced crisis.

Walter Cannon referred to the symptoms of stress as a "fight or flight syndrome" and all of the manifestations of stress, system by system, are all attributable to a heightened autonomic nervous system state. The autonomic nervous system's function can be roughly divided into two portions. The first portion, the **parasympathetic nervous system**, is responsible for the involuntary vegetative functions including digestion, heart rate, and the like, largely controlled by the vagus nerve. These functions are summarized as "feed and breed."

The other autonomic nervous system responses are the result of the **sympathetic nervous system**. Normally the sympathetic nervous system includes those emergency responses that are at "stand-by," ready to provide the person with the ability to flee (flight) or fight. Under normal conditions, the parasympathetic nervous system takes dominance, through vagal tone, and maintains homeostasis. However, under emergency conditions in which there is sufficient stimulus, the epinephrine-based sympathetic nervous system assumes more dominant control of the organs' functions.[11,12]

The sympathetic nervous system is greatly influenced by the brain's cognition, that ability to comprehend stimulus, and thought, the ability to comprehend a stimulus's meaning. When repeatedly overstimulated, perhaps by constant bombardment by stress-inducing stimuli, the body begins to show the fatigue, a prelude to illness in many cases, in a condition called **strain**.

The chief neurotransmitter in the sympathetic nervous system is epinephrine. Epinephrine has organ-specific effects that alter that organ's function. For example, epinephrine attaches to beta-receptors in the heart to make it contract more forcefully (inotropy) and more quickly (chronotrophy). Simultaneously, epinephrine also attaches to alpha-receptors in the peripheral vasculature, leading to increased peripheral vascular resistance (PVR).

The stimulation of both receptors, alpha and beta, by epinephrine released during a stimulus response causes the heart to beat faster and harder against a greater resistance (PVR). The heart's increased workload leads to cardiovascular complications if the stress is prolonged.

Stress can also cause abnormal contraction of skeletal muscles, contractions beyond their functional needs, leading to muscle spasms, spinal column misalignment and resultant backache, contraction of facial muscles leading to headache, jaw clenching, nocturnal teeth-grinding (bruxism), and neck pain. Internally, the immune system, set on high alert for potential bacterial invasion, eventually fatigues. T-lymphocyte counts drop, resulting in immunosuppression and, paradoxically, more infections. The signs and symptoms of overstress, or distress, include persistent tachycardia, palpitations, hypertension, chest pressure, and chronic pain.

Physical disorders associated with chronic high stress include, from head to toe, migraine and tension headaches, cardiovascular disorders, respiratory disease, ulcers, and colitis, as well as hypertension and cancer.

Emotional and behavioral disorders are also associated with stress. These include anxiety, with associated panic attacks, depression, alcoholism, and conduct disorders. These emotions, behaviors, and somatic complaints should alert fellow Paramedics that the person is under stress and may or may not be coping well emotionally.[13]

The human psyche is not immune to the effects of chronic stress either. The psychological defense mechanisms against stress include projection, denial, and conversion, among many others. When the individual's coping mechanisms fail to provide the relief needed, the individual may resort to maladaptive coping mechanisms. Examples of these maladaptive coping mechanisms include substance abuse, alcoholism, smoking, and the use of other addictive substances.

The Crisis Process

A person is in crisis when he has experienced a threatening event but no longer has the capacity to respond, due to mental and/or physical exhaustion. The crisis process is somewhat analogous to the transition from compensated to decompensated shock. Anxiety, panic, and, in some cases, terror sets in and the patient may become profoundly depressed or start to manifest frank psychiatric symptoms.

Like the shock syndrome, the crisis process is reversible, provided a crisis intervention is provided in time. The goals of crisis intervention start with stopping the acute process. Depending on the situation, this may be accomplished simply by removing the person from the source of the stimulus. Once removed, the downward spiral of emotions must be stopped and the person's thoughts and/or feelings can stabilize. In other cases it will take psychotropic medications and/or acute crisis intervention to stop the crisis. With the acute symptoms managed, the goal of crisis management is to return the person back to independent functioning.

One example of a crisis intervention approach used for emergency services personnel is the **SAFE-R** model (Table 3-1). The letters in the SAFE-R model each stand for a step in the process. Stimulation reduction (S) is the first goal of crisis intervention using the SAFE-R model. Next, the facilitator would then acknowledge (A) the crisis and, using carefully chosen probing questions, facilitate (F) an understanding of the situation.

After gaining the person's attention, using empathy and therapeutic communications, the facilitator would explain (E) the basic concepts of stress. The universality of stress would be emphasized and the facilitator would offer some plans for coping with the current situation. Finally, the facilitator would discuss a plan to return or restore (R) the person back to independent function.

While the SAFE-R technique appears easy, as the saying goes, the devil lies in the details. Crisis interventions are best left to personnel trained in critical incident stress management.

Stress Management

Stress management is a process of coping with chronic stress in an effort to recover from its effects. In some instances, the individual can take action to eliminate the source of the stress. This activity would constitute **stress reduction**. A job change or even divorce can be examples of stress reduction. If the source of the stress cannot be eliminated, then some action must be taken to reframe the brain's interpretation of the stimulus so that it is non-threatening. This technique, called **cognitive restructuring**, provides hope for recovery for some people with fatigue, strain, or stress.

To understand the benefits of stress management, Paramedics need to first learn to recognize the early warning signs of stress, both immediate and long-term. Examples of the effects of long-term stress include recurrent headaches and unremitting fatigue. Part of managing stress is recognizing events that trigger stress and attempt to either eliminate them or respond to them differently.

There are several effective models for stress management, both short-term and long-term. For short-term stress some EMS responders use controlled breathing or isotonic exercise. Long-term methods of stress management are discussed shortly. In every case, Paramedics need to become aware of their warning signs of impending stress and plan how they are going to respond to those stressors.

While stress management is focused on the individual, in this case the Paramedic, there are organizational benefits to stress management training. In a cost–benefit analysis, the loss of time in stress management training is outweighed by loss in sick leave, worker's compensation, associated medical costs, and employee turnover. Paramedics who learn how to manage their stress tend to have increased morale, decreased conflict with fellow workers and supervisors, reduced errors, and enhanced performance while on-the-job.

Paramedics can learn a number of stress management techniques that will help mitigate the long-term effects of stress.[14-17] The majority of these techniques can be done quietly, on-the-job, and without additional equipment. One technique, autogenic training, stems from the practice of autohypnosis first advanced by Vogt in 1900. A form of "self-regulation" akin to biofeedback, autogenic training was developed in 1932 by Johannes Schultz as a means to train the autonomic nervous system. Other stress management techniques that emphasize the power of the mind–body connection include progressive muscle relaxation and diaphragmatic breathing. Some Paramedics have been trained in the use of mental imaging, which is useful for immediate stress relief, as well as meditation. Meditation has long been known as a technique for stress reduction.

Specific Stressful Situations

Acute Traumatic Stress

Witnessing horrific and disturbing events can generate intense fear and a sense of helplessness in Paramedics. Unchecked, these feelings can lead to **acute traumatic stress**. Acute traumatic stress is an unexpected and sudden stressful event which is unlike the stress of day-to-day EMS and understandably requires a different approach.

Table 3-1 SAFE-R Model

S	Stimulation reduction
A	Acknowledge the crisis
F	Facilitate
E	Explain
R	Return or restore

Like medicine, the most effective critical stress management is prevention-oriented. Planning for the ability to provide humane relief during a major incident provides the best opportunity to reduce acute stress.

When possible, a predeployment briefing that explains the situation, and potential stressors that the Paramedic is about to encounter, can go far toward decreasing the shock and subsequent acute traumatic stress. For example, search and rescue predeployment briefings should include a discussion of the possibility of the operation changing from one of rescue to a recovery operation. Tempering the hopes of concerned rescuers can help to reduce the impact of a poor outcome, thereby protecting rescuers, without diminishing the prospect of a rescue.

Clear delegation of authority and the assignment of specific tasks can help to eliminate some of the confusion and helplessness that Paramedics will experience when confronted with a horrific situation. With proper guidance, command, and control, Paramedics can persevere against incredible adversity.

Incident command also needs to consider the mental and physical limitations of the emergency service responders under their command. Rotations to out-of-service in order to take a rest break, eat some food, drink fluids, and use lavatories, all part of **rehabilitation**, can help responders handle stress more effectively. It is also useful to have trained counselors who are observing for signs of stress and can provide immediate interventions in the case of an acute stress reaction.

Whenever possible, the media should be restricted from the rehabilitation area. Reporters tend to use inflammatory or untactful language in their questions in order to achieve a desired effect or to prompt a response. Unfortunately, ill-chosen or less than tactful words can have devastating effects upon emergency services responders.

Demobilization is another opportunity to mitigate the effects of the acute stressors and to decrease the incidence of acute traumatic stress reactions. Debriefings, or "after action

reports," should be used to emphasize the successes on-scene. Disagreements regarding specific aspects of scene development should be reserved until later. During a debriefing, first-line responders should be monitored, possibly including an exit physical examination. These post-event physicals can reveal signs of stress including sustained tachycardia, persistent headaches, and hypertension.

After a major incident all responders should be encouraged to get rest, moderate their intake of alcohol, and reduce their caffeine intake. Responders should also be encouraged to engage in self-affirming activities such as spending time with family and friends or getting involved in a favorite sport.

Defusings

On occasion, and because of the nature of the incident or based upon an observation of emergency services responders, it may necessary to order a **defusing**. A defusing is an immediate intervention intended to avert acute stress reactions among the responders. Usually initiated within eight hours, a **critical-incident response team (CIRT)** is called in to meet with the affected personnel, typically front-line responders.

The purpose of a defusing is to quickly explore the event and then educate responders about the effects of stress. The lesson includes a discussion of signs and symptoms of acute stress reaction as well as means of managing stress. If done correctly, a defusing can either eliminate the need for further critical incident stress debriefings or enhance the productivity of future critical incident stress debriefings. Crew leaders, educated in debriefing techniques, can support their fellow crew members (Figure 3-4).

Several criteria can establish the need for a **critical incident stress debriefing (CISD)**.[18–20] Perhaps the most common reason for a CISD is an extraordinary event-related occurrence. Examples of responder-related extraordinarily stressful events include a line-of-duty death, serious injury of a coworker while on-the-job, and post-event suicide of a fellow responder. Examples of event-related extraordinarily stressful events include the traumatic death of a child or children; prolonged rescues, especially those that turn into a body recovery operation; and prolonged hostage situations.[21–24] Dr. Jeffrey Mitchell, a leader in critical incident stress management, has identified 10 critical incidents with high potential for stress (Table 3-2).[25]

A CISD can be triggered by a request for CISD, often from either an affected responder or an enlightened incident commander. It can also be triggered by indirect personnel, such as family members, who observe behavioral changes in the responder. Concerned coworkers, who are still witnessing signals of distress, such as constant ruminating after three weeks, can also request a CISD.

A CISD is a private meeting, where only the CIRT and responders are invited. Typically, rank holds no privilege and conditions are established from the outset. This encourages open dialogue among the CISD's participants. With all

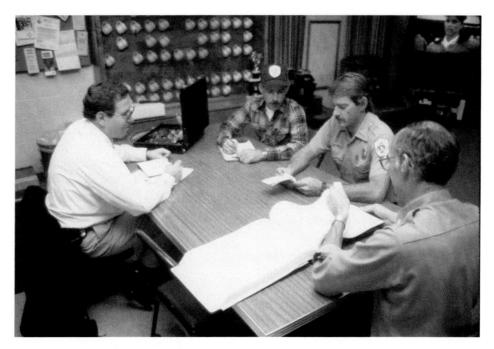

Figure 3-4 Defusing session led by a Paramedic.

Table 3-2 High Potential Critical Incidents

1. Line of duty death
2. Suicide of a colleague
3. Serious work-related injury
4. Multi-casualty incident
5. High threat incident (terrorism)
6. Severe traumatic injury to children
7. Close relationship with victim
8. Excessive media exposure
9. Prolonged operations
10. Overwhelming events (disasters)

responders and the CIRT assembled in one room, the CIRT leader begins by making introductions. A typical CIRT has a mental health practitioner as well as emergency responders who are trained in critical incident stress debriefings. Once the introductions are completed, the leader starts the process of divining the facts, asking for thoughts and reactions, all in a nonconfrontational atmosphere.

Timing is important to a CISD. If responders are still experiencing acute stress they will have a limited number of communication channels to handle incoming information. They will not be able to tolerate the ambiguity that may occur during the discussion.

The objective of every CISD, and the next step in the process, is education. Responders are first taught about typical or "normal" reactions to stress, asked to reflect upon these symptoms, then taught about means to manage the stress that naturally accompanies any incident.

Following a CISD, a member of the CIRT may have identified a responder manifesting symptomology consistent with acute stress reaction who might benefit from professional psychiatric services. These psychiatric interventions, provided immediately after the event, can potentially prevent long-term disability such as post-traumatic stress disorder.

Post-Traumatic Stress Disorder

If symptoms of acute stress disorder do not resolve within a four-week period, then **post-traumatic stress disorder (PTSD)** must be considered.[26,27] The essential feature in post-traumatic stress disorder, per the American Psychiatric Association's (APA) *Diagnostic and Statistical Manual, fourth edition* (DSM-IV), is the development of "characteristic symptoms following exposure to an extreme traumatic stress involving direct personal experience of an event that involves actual or threatened death or serious injury, or other threat to one's physical integrity; or witnessing an event that involves death, injury or a threat to the physical integrity of another person."

Symptoms of PTSD include persistent intrusive recollections of the event and flashbacks. Chronic absenteeism may represent the Paramedic's attempts to avoid anything associated with the psychological trauma. Paramedics who have experienced a violation of a key psychological assumption, such as safe return from duty, might have tendencies toward PTSD.

Personal Injury Prevention

Many individuals get involved with emergency services because of the excitement and danger of a rescue, never really thinking that they themselves might actually get hurt. To the

Paramedic, nothing may be more stressful than personal injury. Despite their best efforts to mitigate hazards, injuries do occur. In many situations, these injuries could have been lessened, or eliminated altogether, with proper preplanning and a safety-conscious attitude on the part of Paramedics.

The problem of emergency responder death and injury may have been brought to the forefront by a 1973 publication entitled *America Burning*. *America Burning,* a presidential white paper, brought to light the indifference to safety in the fire service.[28] Subsequently, all emergency responders have experienced an increased emphasis on safety, primarily through increased regulations and standards (Table 3-3). Paramedics, both in and out of the fire service, must be aware of the standards and regulations that affect them.

Regulations are mandatory and carry the weight of law, whereas guidelines and standards are voluntary and only offer directions for safe practice. Other recognized sources of standards include the American National Standards Institute (ANSI) and the American Society of Testing and Materials (ASTM). However, when specific injuries increase in certain areas lawmakers frequently turn to standards and guidelines for direction.

Back Injury

The prevalence of back injury among Paramedics is high and potentially preventable.[29-31] A reduction in the incidence of back injury can be realized if Paramedics adhere to a few basic back safety rules. In many cases, back injury occurs because of improper lifting and carrying.

A Paramedic should lift only those loads that can be carried safely. Many EMS agencies have guidelines regarding safe lifting, often tied to a functional job description, and mandate that additional rescuers be called for heavy lifting. When lifting any object—stretchers to jump kits—Paramedics should bend their knees, stoop down, and lift with their legs. Keeping the object close to the body and in-line helps to reduce the chance of a back injury. Part of back safety is back health. Exercise, discussed earlier, helps to maintain the strength and flexibility of the back and reduces the chance of injury.

Table 3-3 Sample of Safety Regulations and Standards Applicable to Paramedics

- Safety Regulations within the Code of Federal Regulations (CFR)
- Confined Space Rescue 29 CFR 1910.146
- Hazardous Materials Response 29 CFR 1910.120
- Bloodborne Pathogens 29 CFR 1910.1030
- National Fire Protection Association Standards
- Fire Department Infection Control NFPA 1581
- Hazardous Materials Awareness Competencies NFPA 472
- Centers for Disease Control and Prevention (CDC)
- Guidelines for Exposure to Tuberculosis
- Guidelines for Hepatitis B Exposure

Risk Management

Progressive EMS agencies have developed a plan for **risk management**, a plan that emphasizes safety and whose goal is to reduce Paramedic injury in an effort to promote a culture of safety in their organization.

In those agencies, either a **risk manager** or a safety committee identifies known hazards and then tries to mitigate those hazards. These activities are consistent with requirements under the general duty clause contained within the Occupational Safety and Health Administration's (OSHA) regulations.

Through a study of the frequency of injury, the severity of injuries, and the economic impact of those injuries (including workers' compensation claims), the risk management team identifies trends and implements change (e.g., new regulations, procedures, or protocols). The risk management team would then perform an audit and reassess the success of the change. This plan-do-check-act approach, the PDCA cycle, is a form of continuous quality improvement and is the same model used in business.

Safety

The saying goes "safety starts at home." Every Paramedic has a responsibility to help maintain the safety of both the station and the emergency response vehicle (ERV).

Of immediate concern in the station is the problem of fire and life safety. EMS stations should serve as models of a safe building for the community. Sprinklers should be placed in all living areas and fire extinguishers, as well as fire alarms, should be readily available. In addition, fire escape routes should be posted and clearly visible and fire drills should be routinely practiced.

Another concern is falls that occur while on the premises. Wet floors and snow-covered walkways present a clear and present danger. Precautions should be taken to eliminate or mitigate the danger if possible.

Vehicle Safety

Paramedics depend on their emergency response vehicle (ERV) for protection during an emergency response. A combination of lights, reflective surfaces, and sirens help to increase the visibility of EMS while on-scene. Therefore, these safety devices should be regularly checked to be sure they are in working order. However, a greater danger may exist from mechanical failure. High speed driving, sudden stopping, and multiple drivers driving in all kinds of conditions combine to put an extraordinary stress on ERVs.

To prevent mechanical failure, and ensure a timely response, EMS agencies should have a program of **preventative maintenance (PM)** for their ERV. As opposed to a traditional "wait until it breaks then fix it" approach, a preventative maintenance program forestalls the incidence of failure, thereby decreasing the incidence of injury and potential litigation.

Emergency Response

Paramedics are at greatest risk of personal injury during the initial response to the scene of an emergency. Despite safe vehicle operation, collisions with other vehicles on the road do occur. Every **emergency vehicle operator (EVO)** should practice caution when advancing upon intersections. Many EMS agencies require all ERV to come to a complete stop, when opposed by the red light, before proceeding.

When passing other vehicles, while running lights and sirens, the EVO should expect the unexpected and be prepared to drive evasively in order to avoid collision. Most states require emergency vehicles to pass on the left. Passing on the right runs the risk of having confused drivers suddenly turn into the path of the ERV.

Paramedics should be on a heightened state of alert when multiple emergency vehicles are on the road. Unsuspecting motor vehicle operators, seeing one emergency vehicle pass, may pull out into the path of the next emergency vehicle. Police escorts are discouraged in many EMS systems for this reason.

If more than one emergency vehicle is traveling the same route it may be prudent to change siren modes. There is a better chance that the motorists will hear two distinctly different sounds and recognize that there is a second emergency vehicle. While a safe following distance increases the safety of the chase vehicle, the wisdom of having two ERV responding lights and sirens must be questioned. If it is plausible, the chase vehicle should turn off its lights and siren, allowing the first ERV to be the first responder to arrive on-scene.

A defensive driving attitude, or due regard for others on the road, can help to limit the number of motor vehicle collisions. A number of emergency vehicle operator courses and accident reduction programs are available to Paramedics. Some insurance companies offer a reduction in premiums (personal and corporate) for participation in these programs.

Scene Hazards

Personal safety is the primary concern of Paramedics upon arrival on the scene of an emergency. The responsibility for scene safety is both an individual responsibility as well as a collective responsibility of the team. At larger incidents a **safety officer** may be assigned to maintain safety. However, at a small incident (e.g., a typical call for an emergency), overall responsibility falls to the officer-in-charge.

When approaching the scene of a motor vehicle collision, the driver and the Paramedic should slow the vehicle and take a moment to get a "windshield survey" of the scene. Obvious hazards, such as a patient lying in the roadway or smoke and fire, should be reportedly immediately as part of the "first due" report. It is safe practice to call out, by radio, or note somewhere in the cab of the ERV the license plate numbers of the vehicle being approached. Some EMS agencies are not allowed to approach vehicles that are reported stolen until law enforcement officers arrive.

If the emergency responder is the first emergency vehicle on-scene then the vehicle should be placed in such a manner so as to protect the patient and the responders. Typically, the ERV is staggered, out-of-line, from the vehicle ahead so that a safety zone is created.

The ERV is now acting as a warning device, with its lights flashing, and as a physical barrier. To improve its functionality as a barrier, the tires should be turned sharply, away from the pathway to the vehicle ahead.

If the scene is already protected by another emergency responder, then most EMS agencies have a policy of parking beyond the scene, parking in the direction of the most likely destination hospital, and toward the route of intended exodus. Parking in front of the scene helps reduce the exposure of the second emergency vehicle to collision.

Before approaching an unknown vehicle, headlights should be turned on high and any available takedown lights or spotlights aimed toward the vehicle ahead. This lighting helps to illuminate the interior of the vehicle as well as create a safe working zone.

Some EMS systems require that the Paramedic radio the license plate of the vehicle before it is approached. If the plate comes back on a stolen vehicle the Paramedic is to wait for the arrival of law enforcement.

After selecting only the minimal equipment required for an initial response, the Paramedic would approach the rear of the vehicle. Carrying additional equipment, such as ECG monitors and so forth, is unnecessary and presents an additional burden if the Paramedic has to flee suddenly. The Paramedic should choose to either approach the vehicle from the passenger side or to go around the back of the ERV and approach the vehicle from the driver's side. The Paramedic should avoid walking in front of the ERV headlights, back-lighting his position and announcing his presence to the driver. Surprise is an important safety technique.

With flashlight in hand, and carried away from the body, the Paramedic would examine the inside of the vehicle for weapons as well as for the number of patients and then position him- or herself behind the B-post of the vehicle. From this venue the Paramedic can continue to inspect the interior of the vehicle's occupant compartment for evidence of damage as well as weapons before proceeding with patient care.

A Paramedic approaches a house call much differently than a road call for a motor vehicle collision. While houses vary, from the apartment in a high-rise development to the bungalow on a beach, the basic safety principles remain the same for all and need only be modified to the conditions on-scene. A current controversy in EMS concerns the style of uniforms. Some EMS agencies advocate the button-down style of uniform that presents a clean image and portrays a military bearing to the wearer. Other Paramedics argue that these uniforms make Paramedics look like law enforcement officers, especially to the distorted eyesight of a confused or intoxicated patient (Figure 3-5). Patients could respond inappropriately, even violently, to this misperception.

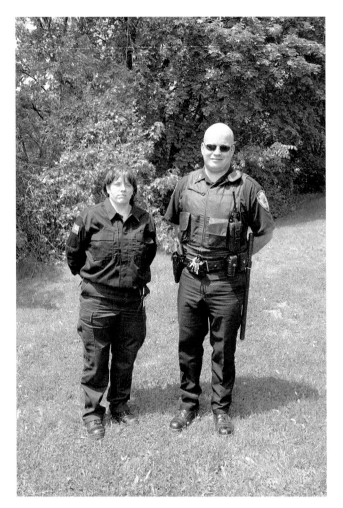

Figure 3-5 Similarities between law enforcement officer uniforms and EMS uniforms.

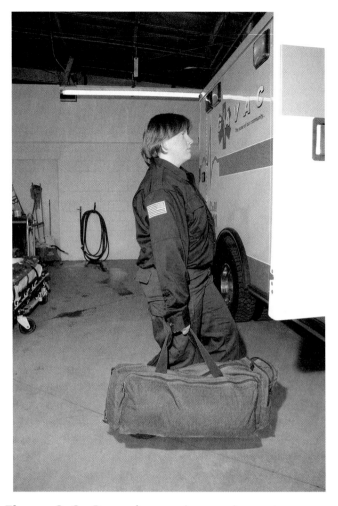

Figure 3-6 Properly carrying equipment can ensure the Paramedic's safety.

An alternative EMS appearance, dubbed the soft look, consists of polo-style shirts. These shirts, without the badges of authority, are argued to be safer.

The use of personal **body armor** while performing EMS is another controversy in EMS. Some argue that body armor is necessary to protect Paramedics. Citing gun ownership statistics, body armor advocates believe that body armor is part of personal protective equipment (PPE). In opposition, other Paramedics believe that wearing body armor will encourage Paramedics to enter scenes that they would otherwise not have entered, under the false assumption that the body armor will protect them. Opponents of body armor argue that Paramedics do not have a duty to enter into unsafe scenes.

Like their approach to a motor vehicle collision, Paramedics should slow their approach to a house call until both the driver and the Paramedic can get a windshield survey. Emergency lights should be extinguished well before arrival, so as to not alert the occupants of the impending approach of emergency responders. The ERV should be slowed to a near stop at a 45-degree angle from the scene. From this vantage,

the Paramedic can take a moment to look and listen for evidence of scene violence.

If there is no evidence of scene violence, the Paramedic should park the ERV either diagonal across the end of a driveway, or backed into the scene. This position permits a hasty retreat if need be.

Carrying only the minimum equipment needed, the Paramedic should approach the house from an oblique angle if possible, cutting across the lawn if necessary. Potential attackers assume the Paramedic will approach the house from the sidewalk or other walkways. If a flashlight is needed to illuminate the pathway, then it should be carried away from the body and care should be taken to not backlight the Paramedic.

Equipment bags should be slung over the shoulder, or carried by hand, where they can be slipped off and dropped in front of pursuers. If the equipment bag is slung over the neck, attackers can grab the strap and drag the Paramedic to the ground. Paramedics must be sure to properly carry their equipment bag (Figure 3-6).

If possible, the EVO should remain in the vehicle, with the ERV running and the mobile radio on, while the Paramedic approaches the house. This permits the EVO to contact LEO if assistance is needed and to more quickly depart the scene.

If the residence is an apartment complex or similar structure with an elevator, then the Paramedic should consider using the fire service functions. Upon arrival at the intended floor, the elevator alarm should be silenced and the elevator locked. One Paramedic should approach the apartment door while another Paramedic surveys the scene for stairwells, fire escapes, and other emergency exits. Once safe entry is made into the apartment, the elevator can be released for regular service.

The Paramedic should verify the address, then approach the door from the door handle side; this cuts down on the Paramedic's angle of exposure. Using the door's jam as a barrier, the Paramedic would position himself perpendicular to the wall and loudly announce his presence, using the butt of a flashlight or similar object to knock on the door while shouting out, "Ambulance!" or "Fire department!" These terms are generally understood by most citizens and cannot be confused with "police" or other terms.

Entering the residence, many Paramedics suspend the EMS equipment bag and carry it in front of them, providing a barrier to attacking dogs and/or an obstacle to pursuers. Paramedics should request that all dogs be locked in another room, regardless of pleas from the family or innocent appearances. Even small, apparently harmless dogs can attack if they sense that the Paramedic is hurting their master.

Whenever possible, two responders should enter the scene together. One responder acts as the contact medic. The contact medic makes contact with the patient and begins patient care. This second responder acts in the role of the "cover medic." The cover medic watches the scene for hazards. The cover medic always keeps the "big picture" in mind, watching both the patient and the other people on scene. The cover medic should ensure that the doorway to the exit is never blocked. If possible, the cover medic should be stationed in the path to the doorway, to ensure that it remains open. Often the cover medic carries the radio in case additional aid is needed.

The cover medic should also do a quick scan of the scene to identify **deadly weapons** and **dangerous instruments**. Deadly, or lethal, weapons are those objects that are, by design, intended to inflict death or disability (e.g., a pistol or a knife; Figure 3-7a). The definition of a dangerous instrument is more amorphous. A dangerous instrument is any object that could be used, under the right circumstances, to produce serious injury or even death. An example of a dangerous instrument would be a box cutter or broken beer bottle (Figure 3-7b), both of which could produce serious lacerations.

If a cover medic is not available then the Paramedic must perform a scene survey alone. The Paramedic should avoid tunnel-vision and, borrowing a term from the fire service,

perform a scene size-up before proceeding. Some Paramedics, once they are inside the door, immediately step to the side, with their back to the wall, and start asking family members simple questions. Taking advantage of the moment, these Paramedics perform a quick sweep of the room for deadly weapons and dangerous instruments.[32–35]

Domestic violence calls are some of the most dangerous calls for LEO and Paramedics alike. When arriving on the scene with a potential for domestic violence, the Paramedic is well advised to wait for the arrival of LEO before entering. If Paramedics have inadvertently entered into the scene of probable domestic violence, they should consider the severity of the patient's injuries versus their personal safety, keeping their safety foremost in their minds. If the scene is unsafe, and the Paramedic can get the patient into the relative safety of the ERV, they should attempt to do so. If the scene is unsafe, the Paramedic should immediately withdraw and call for assistance.

If Paramedics are attacked or feel they are about to be attacked they should immediately withdraw from the scene. Some Paramedics will throw the clipboard into the hands of a potential attacker, to confuse the attacker and to allow them more time to escape.

The first goal for Paramedics during a hasty retreat is to get two or more objects called **cover** between themselves and their would-be attackers. Cover is any object that cannot be penetrated by a projectile, from bullets to frying pans. Examples of cover include telephone poles and even fire hydrants. The tires and engine block of the ERV also make good cover; however, Paramedics are reminded that a bullet tends to follow the plane of the ground after it ricochets and can travel under an ERV.

If cover is not immediately available then the Paramedic will have to settle for **concealment**. Concealment is created by any object that blocks the pursuer's vision of the Paramedic. However, concealment does not offer protection and should be abandoned in favor of cover and retreat as soon as possible.

Special Operations

Special operations, such as confined space rescue, vehicle rescue, and water rescue, require special protective apparel as well as training in its proper use. For example, a Paramedic inside a vehicle should have, from head to toe, a helmet or bump cap with strap, ear protection, eye protection, a fire-retardant turnout coat, leather or firefighter-grade gloves, overalls or bunker pants, and boots.

Infection Control

The ever-present danger on the scene of every EMS call is infection. Paramedics have a good chance of preventing an infection for themselves provided they have up-to-date immunizations and use proper barrier protection. Immunizations considered standard in most EMS agencies include tetanus, diptheria, polio, and MMR (measles, mumps, and rubella).

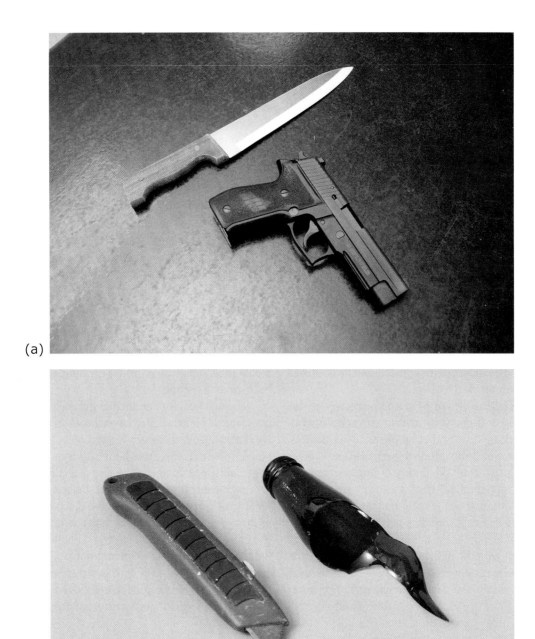

Figure 3-7 Deadly weapons versus dangerous instruments.

Other common immunizations include the vaccination series for hepatitis B, offered free to Paramedics as part of the OSHA regulations regarding bloodborne pathogens, and (in the future) smallpox vaccination. Many Paramedics also receive vaccination for influenza, not only to protect themselves, but to protect their infant and elderly patients who do not recover as easily from these contagions. While, at present, there are no immunizations against tuberculosis (Tb) or human immunodeficiency virus (HIV), many Paramedics obtain periodic testing, in order to obtain life-prolonging chemotherapy in the event they are infected.

On-scene of a medical emergency, Paramedics utilize a **dress-up philosophy**, meaning Paramedics add barrier devices for protection as the situation warrants. Practicing **body substance isolation**, Paramedics frequently don gloves before approaching the patient. In many cases, the patient's chief complaint determines what additional barrier device is worn. Paramedics should be aware of commonly used barrier protection for certain situations (Table 3-4). The list is not comprehensive nor should Paramedics limit themselves to the listed devices if conditions warrant more protection.

Table 3-4 Barrier Devices Used in Selected Activities

Task	Disposable		Protective	
	Gloves	Gown	Mask	Eyewear
Bleeding control Spurting blood	Yes	Yes	Yes	Yes
Bleeding control Minimal blood	Yes	No	No	No
Emergency childbirth	Yes	Yes	Yes	Yes
Intravenous line insertion	Yes	No	No	No
Endotracheal intubation	Yes	No	Yes	Yes
Suctioning	Yes	No	No	No
Measuring blood pressures	No	No	No	No

Appropriate use of Body Substance Isolation (BSI) is recommended any time open skin or mucosa may be exposed to body fluids.[36–40]

Source: This table is taken from the New York State Department of Health, Bureau of Emergency Medical Services, Recommendations for Body Substance Isolation.

Infectious Disease Exposure

Whenever blood or bodily fluids from a patient are spilled, splashed, or dripped onto or injected into a Paramedic, an **exposure** to a potentially infectious material may have occurred. The prevention of exposure to blood and bodily fluid is paramount and all efforts to provide equipment with built-in safety devices and for the proper disposal of sharps and other potentially infected materials should be given priority.

Barrier devices, such as eye protection and gowns, should also be readily available and used in anticipation of a blood or bodily fluid exposure (Figure 3-8).

Whenever a potential exposure has occurred, the exposed area should be immediately blotted clear of visible blood or fluids, then thoroughly washed with soap and water. If soap and water is not immediately available, the Paramedic should use a gelled alcohol cleanser, then (as soon as possible) use soap and water to cleanse the area.

Blood or bodily fluids inadvertently splashed into the eyes, nose, or mouth should be flushed away, using clean water. The Centers for Disease Control and Prevention (CDC) reports that there is no scientific evidence to support the practice of applying antibiotics or squeezing fluid from the wound to reduce or prevent the transmission of disease.

Following agency guidelines, and after caring for the patient, the Paramedic should immediately report the exposure and seek medical treatment. Treatment may include obtaining a blood sample from both the Paramedic and the source patient, assuming the patient grants permission as well as post-exposure chemotherapy.

Factors that combine to determine the risk of exposure to hepatitis B (HBV), hepatitis C (HCV), and human immunodeficiency virus (HIV) is a function of the number of infected persons in the community, the type and number of blood or

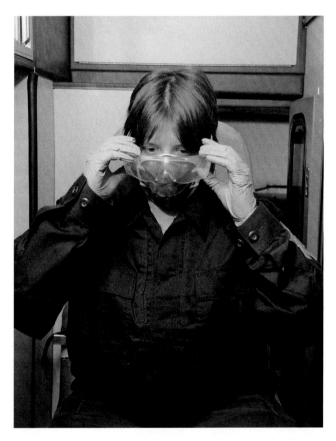

Figure 3-8 Preparing for an intubation by first donning personal protective equipment.

fluid contacts, and the chance of the Paramedic being infected from a single blood contact with an infected patient.

A great deal of concern is expressed about exposure to HIV, but the CDC reports that the risk of HIV infection, even after needlestick with HIV-infected blood, is 0.3% (1 in 300).

The risk for a splash of HIV-infected blood into the eye, nose, or mouth is less than 1 in 1,000.[41-43]

Following a call where potentially infectious material has been present, the equipment and the ERV should be decontaminated. Decontamination of the emergency response vehicle diminishes the potential for disease transmission and should be done as soon as practical. Moist blood should be immediately blotted with a disposable towel at the time of the spill, using a gloved hand. The towel should then be disposed of in a red biohazard waste container. More thorough cleaning should occur after the call.

Using heavy-duty utility gloves, kitchen-type, the Paramedic should mix a 1:100 solution of bleach and water (1/4 cup of bleach to a gallon of tap water) and wipe down any contaminated surfaces. A ratio of 1:100 bleach is usable for about 24 hours before it should be discarded. Many EMS agencies prefer to mix a fresh solution before every use. Soiled linens and the like, including soiled uniforms, should be returned to laundry for proper cleaning and any soiled dressing or other bloody materials disposed of in a red biohazard waste container.

CONCLUSION

An enlightened attitude about health and wellness, as well as a "heads-up" attitude about safety, contribute to a Paramedic's wellness and ability to continue practicing paramedicine.

KEY POINTS:

- Wellness is more than an absence of illness and incorporates all aspects—social, spiritual, intellectual, emotional, and physical being—of a person.

- A healthy body is more resistant to both injury and illness.

- A proper diet, one that provides the necessary nutrients in sufficient quantities, is one of the most important components of physical health.

- Exercise is essential to a Paramedic's physical health.

- Stimulation results in stress in the body. The positive form of stress is eustress while the maladaptive reaction to stress results in distress.

- Behavioral and emotional stressors can negatively affect the Paramedic's emotions, way of thinking, and behavior.

- The dominance of the sympathetic nervous system in a chronically elevated state can bring about physical, emotional, and behavioral disorders.

- Maladaptive coping mechanisms include substance abuse, alcoholism, smoking, or the use of other addictive substances.

- Analogous to decompensated shock, people are in crisis when they experience a threatening event but no longer have the capacity to respond.

- Stress management is a process of coping with chronic stress in an effort to recover from its effects.

- Paramedics can learn a number of stress management techniques that will help mitigate the long-term effects of stress.

- The Paramedic may handle acute traumatic stress differently than the layperson; therefore, management may require a different approach.

- Some incidents may require a defusing, or an immediate intervention intended to avert acute stress reactions among responders.

- A typical CIRT (Critical Incident Response Team) has a mental health practitioner as well as emergency responders who are trained in critical incident stress debriefings.

- In many situations, injury can be lessened, or eliminated altogether, with proper preplanning and a safety-conscious attitude on the part of the Paramedic.

- A Paramedic's responsibility is to maintain the safety of both the station and the emergency response vehicle (ERV).

- Paramedics are at greatest risk of personal injury during the initial response to the scene of an emergency.

- Scene safety is an individual responsibility as well as a collective responsibility of the team.

- Whenever possible, two responders should enter the scene together. One responder acts as the contact medic, interacting with the patient and beginning patient care, while the second responder acts in the role of the "cover medic."

- Domestic violence calls are some of the most dangerous calls for law enforcement officers and Paramedics alike.

- Paramedic safety should be kept foremost in mind.

- If attacked, the Paramedic should withdraw immediately.

- Immunizations and proper barrier protection offer Paramedics the best chance in preventing infection for themselves.

- The prevention of exposure to blood and bodily fluid is paramount.

- Contaminated surfaces should be wiped down with a cleaning agent.

- Soiled linens or uniforms should be returned to laundry for proper cleaning.

- Any soiled dressing or other bloody materials should be disposed of in a red biohazard waste container.

- Special operations, such as confined space rescue, vehicle rescue, or water rescue, require special protective apparel as well as training in their proper use.

REVIEW QUESTIONS:

1. What differentiates good stress from bad stress?
2. What are the signs and symptoms of stress?
3. Describe the physiological effects caused by stress.
4. How is the SAFE-R model used as a crisis prevention tool?
5. What are some stress management techniques that are used by prehospital providers?
6. How should a Paramedic lift a heavy load?
7. How can the Paramedic reduce the risk of personal injury when responding to the scene of an emergency?
8. How does scene safety in the roadway of a motor vehicle collision differ from the scene safety of a residential emergency?
9. What is the responsibility of the cover medic? What should the Paramedic do when working alone?
10. What steps should be taken by the Paramedic prior to arrival that can help prevent exposure and/or infection?

CASE STUDY QUESTIONS:

Please refer to the Case Study at the beginning of the chapter and answer the questions below:

1. What stress(es) is/are expressed by the young Paramedic?
2. Describe the body's physiological responses to the stress(es).
3. What stress management techniques could the Paramedic use?
4. In addition to back safety, what other illness and injury prevention techniques should the Paramedic employ?

REFERENCES:

1. Blackwell J. Identification, evaluation, and treatment of overweight and obese adults. *J Am Acad Nurse Pract.* 2002;14(5):196–198.

2. Beebe R. Size matters. Understanding morbid obesity & its associated complications. *Jems.* 2002;27(1):22–28, 30–33.

3. Rashid MN, Fuentes F, et al. Obesity and the risk for cardiovascular disease. *Prev Cardiol.* 2003;6(1):42–47.

4. Scaglione R, Argano C, et al. Obesity and cardiovascular risk: the new public health problem of worldwide proportions. *Expert Rev Cardiovasc Ther.* 2004;2(2):203–212.

5. Mensah GA, Mokdad AH, et al. Obesity, metabolic syndrome, and type 2 diabetes: emerging epidemics and their cardiovascular implications. *Cardiol Clin.* 2004;22(4):485–504.

6. Smith SC, Jr. Multiple risk factors for cardiovascular disease and diabetes mellitus. *Am J Med.* 2007;120(3 Suppl 1):S3–S11.

7. Bray GA, Bellanger T. Epidemiology, trends, and morbidities of obesity and the metabolic syndrome. *Endocrine.* 2006;29(1):109–117.

8. Selye H. Stress and distress. *Compr Ther.* 1975;1(8):9–13.

9. Seematter G, Binnert C, et al. Relationship between stress, inflammation and metabolism. *Curr Opin Clin Nutr Metab Care.* 2004;7(2):169–173.

10. Selye H. The nature of stress. *Basal Facts.* 1985;7(1):3–11.

11. Arun CP. Fight or flight, forbearance and fortitude: the spectrum of actions of the catecholamines and their cousins. *Ann N Y Acad Sci.* 2004;1018:137–140.

12. Wortsman J. Role of epinephrine in acute stress. *Endocrinol Metab Clin North Am.* 2002;31(1):79–106.

13. Crofford LJ. Violence, stress, and somatic syndromes. *Trauma Violence Abuse.* 2007;8(3):299–313.

14. Verschuur M, Spinhoven P, et al. Making a bad thing worse: effects of communication of results of an epidemiological study after an aviation disaster. *Soc Sci Med.* 2007;65(7):1430–1441.

15. Hammer JS, Mathews JJ, et al. Occupational stress within the Paramedic profession: an initial report of stress levels compared to hospital employees. *Ann Emerg Med.* 1986;15(5):536–539.

16. Stanzer M, Guarraci F, et al. Paramedic or EMT-basic partner? Study evaluates preferred partner types & the effect of partners on work-related stress levels. *Jems.* 2007;32(6):72–74.

17. Graham N. Done in, fed up, burned out—part 2: avoiding the short career. *Jems.* 1981;6(2):25–31.

18. Caine RM, Ter-Bagdasarian L. Early identification and management of critical incident stress. *Crit Care Nurse.* 2003;23(1):59–65.

19. Bledsoe BE. Critical incident stress management (CISM): benefit or risk for emergency services? *Prehosp Emerg Care.* 2003;7(2):272–279.

20. Neely KW, Spitzer WJ. A model for a statewide critical incident stress (CIS) debriefing program for emergency services personnel. *Prehosp Disaster Med.* 1997;12(2):114–119.

21. Sterud T, Ekeberg O, et al. Health status in the ambulance services: a systematic review. *BMC Health Serv Res.* 2006;6:82.

22. van der Ploeg E, Kleber RJ. Acute and chronic job stressors among ambulance personnel: predictors of health symptoms. *Occup Environ Med.* 2003;60 (Suppl 1):i40–i46.

23. Alexander DA, Klein S. Ambulance personnel and critical incidents: impact of accident and emergency work on mental health and emotional well-being. *Br J Psychiatry.* 2001;178(1):76–81.

24. Berger W, Figueira I, et al. Partial and full PTSD in Brazilian ambulance workers: prevalence and impact on health and on quality of life. *J Trauma Stress.* 2007;20(4):637–642.

25. http://www.sgsp.edu.pl/sos/mitchel/wyklady/stress.pdf Stress Management, Jeffrey T. Mitchell, PhD, CTS.

26. Foa EB. Psychosocial therapy for posttraumatic stress disorder. *J Clin Psychiatry.* 2006;67 (Suppl 2):40–45.

27. Smith A, Roberts K. Interventions for post-traumatic stress disorder and psychological distress in emergency ambulance personnel: a review of the literature. *Emerg Med J.* 2003;20(1):75–78.

28. *America Burning: Report of the National Commission on Fire Control.* Chapel Hill: U.S. Government; 1973.

29. Mitterer D. Back injuries in EMS. *Emerg Med Serv.* 1999;28(3):41–48.

30. Powers DW, Wagner K. Getting back up from a back injury. *Emerg Med Serv.* 2004;33(2):82–83.

31. Terribilini C, Dernocoeur K. Save your back. Injury prevention for EMS providers. *Jems.* 1989;14(10):34–35, 37–41.

32. Doyle TJ, Vissers RJ. An EMS approach to psychiatric emergencies. *Emerg Med Serv.* 1999;28(6):87, 90–93.

33. Eckstein M, Cowen AR. Scene safety in the face of automatic weapons fire: a new dilemma for EMS? *Prehosp Emerg Care.* 1998;2(2):117–122.

34. Dick T. Bar fight. A mental exercise in scene safety. *Emerg Med Serv.* 2003;32(3):38–39.

35. Carlquist N. Five steps to scene safety. *Emerg Med Serv.* 2007;36(2):82.

36. Carrillo L, Fleming LE, et al. Bloodborne pathogens risk and precautions among urban fire-rescue workers. *J Occup Environ Med.* 1996;38(9):920–924.

37. DiGiacomo JC, Hoff WS, et al. Barrier precautions in trauma resuscitation: real-time analysis utilizing videotape review. *Am J Emerg Med.* 1997;15(1):34–39.

38. Madan AK, Rentz DE, et al. Noncompliance of health care workers with universal precautions during trauma resuscitations. *South Med J.* 2001;94(3):277–280.

39. Sadoh WE, Fawole AO, et al. Practice of universal precautions among healthcare workers. *J Natl Med Assoc.* 2006;98(5):722–726.

40. Eustis TC, Wright SW, et al. Compliance with recommendations for universal precautions among prehospital providers. *Ann Emerg Med.* 1995;25(4):512–515.

41. http://www.cdc.gov

42. Zanni GR, Wick JY. Preventing needlestick injuries. *Consult Pharm.* 2007;22(5):400–402, 404–406, 409.

43. Campos-Outcalt D. HIV postexposure prophylaxis: who should get it? *J Fam Pract.* 2006;55(7):600–604.

CHAPTER 4

RESEARCH AND EMS

KEY CONCEPTS:

Upon completion of this chapter, it is expected that the reader will understand these following concepts:

- Paramedics continually evaluate practices, protocols, and procedures
- Connection between Paramedic practice and evidence-based practice
- Different types of research appropriate for differing research questions
- The research format and ability to identify errors
- Ethical concerns associated with research
- Types of research that can improve "the bottom line"

▶ CASE STUDY:

At a QA/QI meeting a Paramedic presents a case to her coworkers and medical director that introduces the need for medication-facilitated intubation (MFI). This developed after the Paramedic was presented with a patient who—due to the patient's physical condition and medical emergency—could have been greatly aided by MFI. The Paramedic is charged with researching the topic and presenting her findings at the next meeting. The Paramedic has been asked to examine the success or effectiveness of having MFI as an advanced airway skill at other agencies with MFI programs and to consult published research in an effort to support an evidence-based practice change.

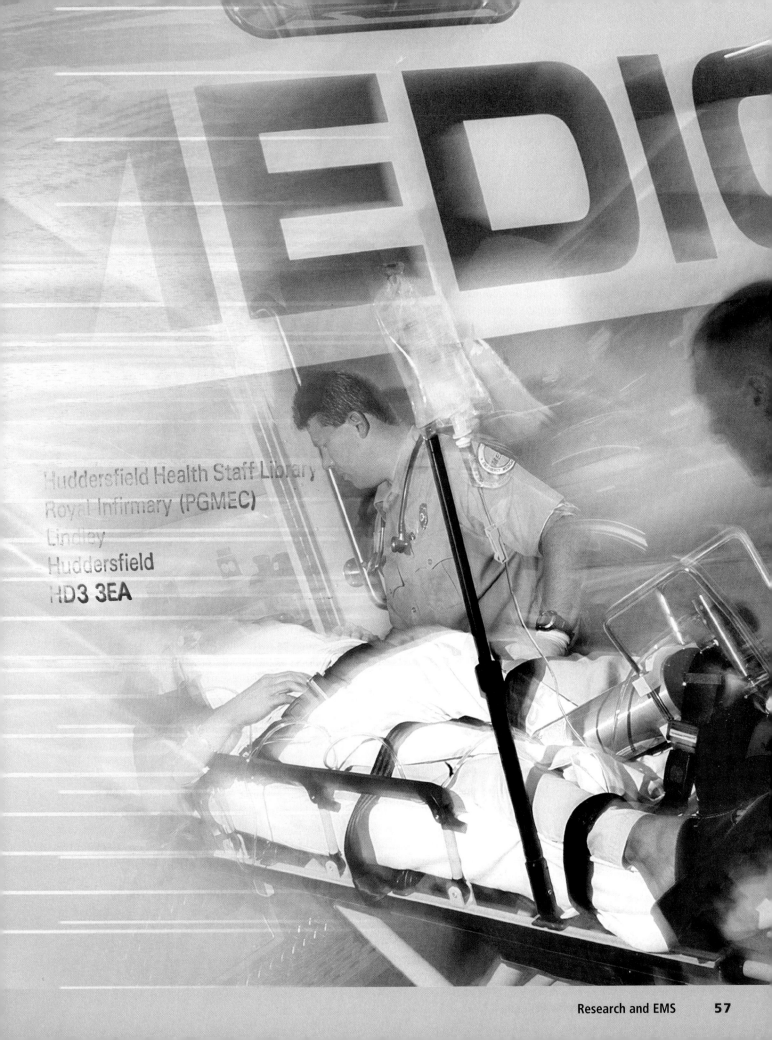

OVERVIEW

Hippocrates stated in his exposition "as to diseases, make a habit of two things—help or at least to do no harm" (Epidemics, Bk I, Section XI). Paramedics driven by the maxim "do no harm" often ask themselves if what they do truly helps, or if, at a minimum, no harm has been caused to the patient.

Practice, Protocols, and Procedures

The question "does it help?" naturally leads to the question of where our practice, protocols, and procedures originated. Most current EMS practice parameters, protocols and procedures, originated from anecdotal experience. These are the result of apparently successful previous practices and of intuitiveness (i.e., this ought to work).

In situations where science did not exist to support a practice, Paramedics and medical directors often used an analogy to think through a situation (i.e., this worked for this other problem in the past and the present situation is similar). Experienced Paramedics call this "common sense" while Paramedic educators refer to it as "pattern recognition" (i.e., comparison of similarities).[1]

Unfortunately, some EMS practices have been driven by correction of earlier misadventures. Practice improvement arrived at by conscious decision (i.e., by committee) is no more reliable because it is simply the group's combined anecdotal experience.

As a result, Paramedic practice is often more likely to be a function of what does not harm the patient. This form of practice can be ineffective and leads to the practice of defensive medicine as well as the misdirected application of resources.

The best way to determine effective Paramedic practices is to look at those practices from a scientific vantage. Use of the scientific method, the acquisition of knowledge through objective observation and considered reasoning, corrects previous misconceptions and integrates new conceptual frameworks for Paramedic practice.[2] The application of the scientific method will lead to the improvement of patient care.

For example, scientific research created the paradigm shift in trauma care that concludes that limited resuscitation (i.e., permissive hypotension) may be more advantageous to the patient than previously thought. Also, in the past it seemed logical that survival chances for trauma patients were increased by replacing blood loss with intravenous solutions in a 3:1 ratio. Well-designed studies have demonstrated the fallacy of that thinking and Paramedics have adjusted their trauma care accordingly—saving lives in the process.[3,4]

While every EMS call can be unique, the purpose of scientific EMS research is to establish a Paramedic practice that is defensible. A Paramedic practice is defendable if it establishes evidence-based medical care is provided in specific circumstances, such care can be independently evaluated by other Paramedics, it can be applied to a number of same or similar circumstances, and it is the most effective means of delivering desired patient outcomes. Such **evidence-based practice** is more likely to weather the scrutiny of cautious public officials and alert community leaders.

Evidence-Based Practice

Emergency medical service in general—and Paramedic practice in particular—are being attacked by some critics who say that EMS is costly to the public and an ineffective means to delivering patient care.

To survive in the current cost-cutting environment Paramedics must prove that their practice is valuable. Paramedicine must prove that Paramedics can decrease morbidity (e.g., through decreased hospital stays or length of stays) and/or decrease mortality and should therefore be seen as valuable.[5–7]

To transform a practice to evidence-based practice, either through updated protocols or continuing education, the first step is to look at the research that already exists.

While EMS research is still limited at this time, Paramedics can look to the research of other allied health professions, such as medicine, nursing, respiratory care, and so on, for support of paramedic practice.

A literature search for research pertaining to shared practice issues (e.g., safety in medication administration) may reveal previous clinical research on the subject that could potentially be applied to the practice of paramedicine.

Similarly, Paramedics can look to the research of other professions, such as business and education, for evidence-based practices. For example, operational issues, such as effective human resource allocation, have already been researched by hospital administrators and major businesses.

Unfortunately, these studies can suggest solutions that are impractical in the out-of-hospital setting or are cost prohibitive for EMS. Furthermore, the practice of out-of-hospital care is unique in many cases and there may be no analogous studies from other allied health professions to draw upon. The best support for Paramedic practice is research done in the prehospital setting, by Paramedics, physicians, and others interested in advancing prehospital patient care. Details on how to start EMS research follows shortly.

Performing a Literature Search

The first step in utilizing research to create evidence-based practice is to ask key questions. These key questions should focus on topics that are important to the Paramedics' practice. An example of a question is: "Does pediatric intubation by Paramedics improve patient outcomes?"

After deciding on the question, the Paramedic should perform a search of the current literature that is available on the topic of interest. By reviewing the published reports of research, called the **literature**, the Paramedic may find studies on the topic or studies that ask a question that is similar to the question at hand.

High-quality EMS research, when completed, is published in various academic journals or works. Unlike the popular press, these journals are peer reviewed.[8–11]

A peer-reviewed journal accepts submissions for publication and circulates them to other experts in the field for inspection and critical analysis. This process is called refereeing. This intradisciplinary review provides readers with a degree of confidence that what they are reading meets the profession's standards and is a scholarly work.

However, even when a work has been properly vetted there may still be some errors. In medicine the saying goes, "One study does not make a practice." It is important that a Paramedic carefully read the entire study to see if the same conditions exist in his or her system such that the study results can reasonably be applied to that practice.

The most effective means of performing a literature search is a computerized search. The most inclusive search engine for medicine is the electronic search engine called MEDLINE, formerly the paper "Index Medicus®." MEDLINE provides a list of most published medical research that is searchable by key words or medical subject headings (MeSH).[12–15]

Other research search engines that can also be used include PubMed, a search engine of the National Library of Medicine (http://www.ncbi.nlm.nih.gov/pubmed/); the Cumulative Index to Nursing and Allied Health (CINAHL – http://www.ebscohost.com/cinahl/); as well as the Educational Resources Information Center (ERIC – http://www.eric.ed.gov/). Even a search of popular search engines like Google® scholar can be helpful.

Hypothetically, a Paramedic could find dozens of citations on a subject, especially if the key words have broad application, like the subject of pediatric intubation.

To separate the "wheat from the chaff," the Paramedic should review the research study's abstract. The **abstract** is an abbreviated "executive" summary that hits a study's highlights.

After reading the abstracts, and eliminating non-related articles, the Paramedic should take the reduced list of studies and review the studies directly. With the reference information (i.e., author's name, journal name, journal volume number, and research title) in hand, the Paramedic may elect to either go directly on-line to read the article or proceed to a medical library.

Most medical libraries, and many university libraries, have a reference librarian. The **reference librarian** is trained in research techniques and can help the Paramedic develop a search strategy to identify which articles will be most helpful.

Reviewing the Literature

After obtaining relevant research articles, the Paramedic needs to identify the kind and type of research that was performed in the study.

Currently, the most common kind of EMS research in the literature is **retrospective research**. A question is raised and Paramedics look at past practice patterns, typically from documentation on the patient care reports, to determine effective versus ineffective practice.

Retrospective data analysis is often used in performance improvement. The danger of retrospective studies are the numerous variables involved in the particular patient scenarios that could account for the patient changes and which are not controlled. For example, if the rate of ventilation in a cardiac arrested patient treated by Paramedics is being measured, how does the researcher know that every Paramedic counts respirations the same way or that every Paramedic even counts respirations, perhaps leaving out the respiratory rate in the documentation by stating that manual ventilation was performed with a bag-valve-mask assembly? As a result, randomness could be an explanation for the results.

Data dredging (data mining) is conducting research without a scientific question in mind (i.e., without a predefined hypothesis). The application of mathematical tests of "statistical significance" to data and trying to observe patterns in that data, and then attempting to form a cause and effect conclusion, is not scientific research.[16]

The most scientifically valid research is **prospective research**. In prospective research, an attempt is made to account for all predictable or known confounding variables, to control those variables, and then add a treatment. If change occurs then it may be reasonable to conclude that the treatment may have caused that change.

The gold standard for research is the **double-blinded randomized clinical trial (RCT)**.[17,18] This technique is a prospective scientific study that controls known and unknown variables (which could result in spurious results), leaving only one variable to be manipulated. Subjects are then chosen at random to be included in either the experimental treatment group or in the control group (the control group receives standard treatment). The key is that the treatment group, those who receive the experimental treatment, are subjects chosen at random.[19]

The results of the treatment of the experimental group subjects is then compared to the results of the control group. Ultimately a conclusion is drawn.

The use of statistically equivalent groups (i.e., patient populations having all the same characteristics [variables] except the one being tested) lends credence to the claim that the procedure/medication/and so on worked as predicted and did not occur as a result of random chance or some other variable.

Clinical Trials

In a **clinical trial** (i.e., experimental medical research), subjects are assigned at random to either the treatment group or to the non-treatment group (i.e., those receiving standard care [control group]).

To limit bias, the participants may not be aware of which treatment group they are in. In a **single-blind study**, the subject does not know which group he is in. In a **double-blind study**, both the researcher and the participants are unaware of which group the subject is in.[17,20,21]

Research often uses inactive drugs, called **placebos**, or ineffective devices, called **shams**, that appear similar to the actual drug or device in order to create blinding for the participants.[22–24]

Statistical Evidence

The key to utilizing experimental research is to understand the statistical methods used to either confirm the hypothesis or reject it.

Classical hypothesis testing compares the results of two treatment groups, statistically, in order to obtain a degree of confidence that the treatment actually caused the effect.

Always skeptical, the researcher's first assumption is that the effect was not caused by the treatment but rather by random chance. With this assumption that the **null hypothesis** is true (i.e., the treatment did not cause the desired effect but rather random chance could account for the change), the probability is calculated. The probability of random chance causing the changes, rather than the treatment, is called the **p value**. An acceptable p value is arbitrarily assigned by the researcher prior to the start of the study and is symbolized as α.

The calculated p value is then compared to the selected α. If the p value is less than the α value, the alternative hypothesis is accepted, and is considered "statistically significant."[25]

Traditionally, in the medical community α values of 0.05 are considered the standard for probabilities.[26] In other words, if the p value in a study is less than 0.05 then this result may be considered to mean that the treatment caused the intended effect and that the researcher is willing to accept the notion that there is a 5% chance that the improvement in outcome occurred by random chance.

Types of Research

Generally, research can be broken down into three types: descriptive studies, observational studies, and experimental studies.

Descriptive Studies

The **descriptive study** simply states the prevalence of a condition and is often illustrative of a problem, without trying to offer an explanation.

A **case report** or case series is an example of a descriptive study. By reporting interesting or unique cases, Paramedics can help other Paramedics gain insight into a problem. The utility in a case study may be the development of theories of causation, leading to further research.

There is precedent for case reports, such as case law. Case law has been used for hundreds of years to support decisions which are based on decisions made by an earlier court. Like case law, case reports may be used in a court of law, or by a Paramedic in front of a medical director, to defend a decision in a highly unusual circumstance.[27]

In dealing with instances of rare diseases, such as Ebola virus, or an exceptional event, such as a plane crash, the case report may be the only means of educating other Paramedics as to the nature and scope of the atypical problem.

Another example of descriptive research is a **cross-sectional survey**. The cross-sectional survey is essentially a snapshot of a certain aspect of a population at a given moment in time that the researcher is interested in. It is obtained by means of observation, usually utilizing a written tool such as a survey. A cross-sectional survey can look at a specific population and a specific disease, for example.

The National Health and Nutrition Examination Survey (NHANES) conducted by the Centers for Disease Control and Prevention has established the prevalence of obesity in the United States and might be used to help support the decision to purchase a bariatric ambulance. By using an analysis of a cross-sectional survey, Paramedics can use the prevalence of certain diseases, conditions, and so on, to determine operational, medical, and educational priorities.

The results of a cross-sectional survey of one population may not be applicable to another patient population. Furthermore, any descriptive study, like the cross-sectional survey, does not prove a cause and effect relationship between various variables.

The final descriptive study is the **ecological study**, also called a correlational study. This type of research design serves to provide information about trends and rates of disease within a population. Often cited as X number of cases of Y disease per 1,000 or per 100,000 of Z population, the ecological study results are often quoted to emphasize the prevalence of a disease and therefore the need for research grants or funding for special projects.

Observational Studies

The **observational study**, in contrast to the descriptive study, asks a question and poses a simple explanation or hypothesis.

To have a scientifically valid result from an observational study, it is necessary to control extraneous confounding variables that could account for the desired change.

One such method of observational study is the **case-control study**. In the case-control study, the Paramedic would compare the cases—those patients with the disease—to the controls—those patients without the disease—and then examine the procedures performed on both to see if there was an association between outcomes.

For example, a case-control study might look at both patients who died and those who survived a cardiac arrest to see if there was a difference in the medications administered to the surviving patients that could have made a statistical difference (i.e., not attributed to chance).

Similar to a case-control study, a **cohort study** examines patients who have been exposed to a treatment and compares them to a group that was not exposed to the same treatment. The patients are followed to determine outcomes.

For example, a group of patients (such as pediatric patients) would be divided into two groups—intubated versus not intubated—and then a review of outcome data (i.e., the patient care report) would be analyzed to determine if one group had a statistically better outcome.

Experimental Studies

Classic research starts with a suggested explanation why something occurs or could occur. For example, a hypothesis might be that administration of oxygen to cardiac patients improves long-term survival for cardiac patients.

With the hypothesis in mind, the researcher uses the experiment to test, under controlled conditions, if a treatment created the predicted change.

When considering the results of the research, the researcher understands that there can be two plausible explanations why the change occurred. The first explanation is that the treatment did not create changes (i.e., any changes are purely random and coincidental). This hypothesis is called the null hypothesis. An **alternative hypothesis**, that the treatment is a plausible explanation for a change, is also considered.

Then a statistical test is applied to the outcome data to determine which hypothesis is most likely correct. The results of the statistical analysis either support the null hypothesis or the alternative hypothesis.

Errors in Research

A common error made in an experiment is to reject the null hypothesis and accept the alternative hypothesis when in fact it is not supported. This is called a **type I error**.

A type I error, also called a false positive, assumes a treatment effect where none exists. An example of a false positive would be the assumption that the administration of oxygen to a patient with carbon monoxide poisoning increased the patient's oxygen saturation.

Alternatively, incorrectly failing to reject the null hypothesis is called a **type II error**, or a false negative. A type II error is a failure to observe the change created by the treatment when one did occur.[28]

An example of a type II error might be ascertaining a patient's blood sugar was low and concluding that treatment is required and subsequently administering glucose, when in fact the glucometer is out of calibration and producing erroneous low readings.

In terms of patient care and test results, a false negative would give patients false reassurance that treatment was effective while a false positive may either lead to a wrong conclusion or may ignore that the patient's condition could have an alternative explanation.

For example, an ST segment elevation on an electro-cardiogram (ECG) tracing suggests myocardial infarction. However, some African Americans have naturally occurring ST segment elevations on their ECG tracing. To state to an African American male that this elevated finding was suggestive of a myocardial infarction would be a false positive.

One cause of a false negative is the limitations that a study group's size places on the experiment. The number of participants in a treatment group, abbreviated N, may not be large enough for the statistical difference to become evident and support the alternative hypothesis. This should not be interpreted to mean that the opposite is true (i.e., that the null hypothesis is true). Instead, the evidence may have been inconclusive.

The results of small studies should be viewed as suspect and lacking **power**. The power of study (i.e., the ability to attribute the changes to the treatment rather than chance) is increased whenever there is an increase in the number of subjects (i.e., sample size) in the study.

Meta-Analysis

In some cases it is difficult to obtain a large population of study subjects, or the event being studied is relatively rare. To overcome the problem of reduced statistical power, a meta-analysis may be performed.

In a **meta-analysis**, the results of several similar small studies are combined and a statistical hypothesis test is applied. Of course, differences in subjects and methods used in the individual studies must be taken into account before a conclusion can be made.[29] For the results of a meta-analysis to be considered valid, it is important that the original research studies are methodologically sound.

Prehospital Research

Contributing to prehospital research can be as easy as being willing to participate in the study. While the person doing the lion's share of the data collection and analysis is usually cited as the lead author, it takes a team to accomplish the goal.

Studies can be as simple as a descriptive study or as complex as a double-blinded randomized clinical trial. In every case participants in a study should carefully consider the study's hypothesis before committing to making a contribution.

At its core, every research project should minimally "do no harm" and should reasonably be expected to improve the patient's condition.[30] If it is lacking either of these two qualities, the study should be considered suspect and perhaps unethical.

Such a critical review of every clinical trial is consistent with the Paramedic's ethical responsibility for beneficence toward patients.[31–33]

Ethical Concerns

The world was witness to the atrocities carried out in Nazi concentration camps, including the inhumane medical studies that were performed, allegedly in the name of science. Following the exposure of these medical studies, during the

Nuremberg trials at the end of World War II, the world scientific community adopted a set of ethical research rules called the Nuremberg code.

The Nuremberg code is a set of guiding principles that limit the scope and nature of experiments using human subjects.[34-36] The United States government, using the 10 principles of the Nuremberg code, created the National Research Act of 1974. This act, found in the Code of Federal Regulations Title 45 Volume 46, speaks to three themes.

The first theme is the respect for the person's freedom and dignity as manifested by informed consent. Implicit in that respect is the patient's right to make an informed choice as to whether to participate.[37-39]

In the past, some convicted criminals would be granted privileges or even amnesty if they were willing to participate in questionable research. By the nature of incarceration, these individuals could not reasonably be expected to make an informed decision that was free of coercion.

The second principle actually speaks to the problem of **diminished autonomy**. Any person who is mentally incapable of making an informed decision (e.g., by virtue of age or infirmity) could not willingly consent to participate in research (21 CFR 50.24). For example, a child could not consent to participate in a study by virtue of age. However, a parent may make the decision whether the child can participate. This is known as substituted judgment. The concept is that a responsible person is substituting her judgment for the child. The parent might determine that if the child had the ability to consent and understood the potential good that could come from such research, the child would agree to participate.

The third principle of ethical research deals with the question of **justice**. In other words, one group of people should not bear all the risks of research when the benefits of said research would benefit all persons in the larger society.

The Tuskegee syphilis project would be an example of injustice in research.[40-42] In the Tuskegee research, poor African American males who contracted syphilis were observed to determine how the disease progresses. This continued even after antibiotics were developed that could have cured the participants and prevented significant complications of syphilis.

Research should not be permitted to begin or continue if researchers reasonably believe that death or permanent disability could occur. In every instance, sensible safeguards should be in place to prevent injury and protect the patient.

Part of this obligation is a willingness to terminate the clinical trial if it can be shown that continuation of the experiment could cause more death or disability than pre-existing standard treatments.

Conversely, if patients receiving the experimental treatment are showing marked improvement over those receiving standard treatment then standard treatment must be stopped and the new experimental treatment offered.

To ensure this last standard, many clinical trials have a **Data and Safety Monitoring Board (DSMB)**. The DSMB

is comprised of individuals who are not directly involved in the research and who can make an objective decision based on the merits of the data.

Institutional Review Board

To protect the rights of patients, and to protect patients from unscrupulous researchers, proposals for research are typically evaluated by an **Institutional Review Board (IRB)**. An IRB is an independent ethics committee that is tasked with ensuring that human rights are not violated and the standards of medical research are upheld.

An IRB review is mandatory for any federally funded research. The activities of these IRBs are monitored by the Office of Human Rights Protection of the Department of Health and Human Services (HHS).[43,44]

Emergency Circumstances

In some cases, such as during an emergency, it would be impractical to obtain informed consent from either the patient or a legally authorized representative (such as a healthcare proxy, if one was available). Recognizing this problem, the United States Code has an emergency exception (21 CFR 50.24).

This exception for patient consent has been applied to numerous clinical trials. If a patient is incapable of consenting due to the medical condition, a form of consent similar to implied consent may be utilized.

Regulations currently require that the public be informed, through various mechanisms of disclosure such as newspaper advertisements or television spots, of clinical trials. This disclosure attempts to establish informed consent before the emergency and advise the population of their right to refuse to participate in the research.

PROFESSIONAL PARAMEDIC

The professional Paramedic should read more about these concepts in the *Belmont Report,* written by the National Commission for the Protection of Human Subjects of Biomedical and Behavioral Research in 1979 (available at http://ohsr.od.nih.gov/guidelines/belmont.html).

Economic Research

Some professional practice questions do not directly involve patient care but rather matters of operational efficiency or cost. Again, research can help to answer the questions.

These research designs are called economic analysis. The classic economic analysis is the **cost-benefit ratio**. A simple cost-benefit analysis asks the question of whether it is advantageous (i.e., cost-effective) to take a particular action or make a change in a procedure.

Business has many statistical methods of determining cost-effectiveness. These same methods can often be applied to EMS.

Absence of Research

Lacking good research to support a practice or procedure, Paramedics often turn to what is referred to as best practice. A **best practice**, a term borrowed from business, suggests that one method of delivering care is the most effective, and therefore a superior, means of providing care.[45]

The use of best practices has two distinct advantages. First, it requires a comparison of one Paramedic's practice against the practice of others. This head-to-head comparison encourages introspection and courage—the courage to accept change.

By questioning current practices, the Paramedic avoids paradigm blindness. **Paradigm blindness** can be summed up by the phrase "because we have always done it this way." Paradigms can sometimes become barriers to innovation and improvement.

Best practices, by definition, speak to improvement—improvement of self and the profession. This concept, continual self-improvement, is best represented by the Japanese concept of kaizen. Kaizen is not only a business principle but a professional attitude for Paramedics.

Kaizen emphasizes process and system thinking. Kaizen is evident when Paramedics participate in performance improvement committees and multi-agency planning.

CONCLUSION

For Paramedics to attain and maintain professional status in the healthcare industry, it is important to continually ask the question, "Does what we do really help?" Paramedics must be prepared to change field practice as evidence, borne of research, demonstrates new and improved means to improve patient care.

KEY POINTS:

- Paramedic practice, protocols, and procedures originated from anecdotal experience. By relying solely on pattern recognition or "common sense," Paramedics ultimately practiced defensive medicine. The use of the scientific method to acquire scientific-based information has helped to correct previous misconceptions and integrate new conceptual frameworks into Paramedic practice.

- Paramedics and medical directors are moving forward from anecdotal-based procedures and protocols toward evidence-based practices. These practices are proven to be logical, independently evaluated, applicable to a number of same or similar circumstances, and are the most effective means of delivering improved patient outcomes. Advantages of evidence-based practice include more cost-effective practices by quantifying how effective certain practices are in delivering patient care. The first step in moving toward evidence-based practice is searching existing research of other allied health professions by performing a literature search.

- In performing a literature search, the first step is to ask a question important to the Paramedic practice. Reviewing abstracts can narrow your search for a specific topic. Because "one study does not make a practice", it is important that several studies relating to a topic be reviewed. A computerized search of peer-reviewed academic journals provides the greatest access to past research as well as the most current information available.

- Retrospective studies are the most common type of research found in EMS literature. This type of research examines past practice patterns to determine effective versus ineffective practices. Though useful, the reliability of retrospective studies is limited due to the numerous variables that may be present but are not accounted for.

- By accounting for predictable or confounding variables, prospective research is the most scientifically valid type of research. The gold standard for research methodology is the double-blinded randomized clinical trial. This method provides a high degree of scientific validity because only one variable is manipulated.

- In clinical trials, the control group is given a placebo or sham, while the experimental group is given the actual treatment. A statistical analysis can then be applied to the data to evaluate whether the treatment caused the desired effect or if the effect occurred by chance. The p value is assigned to provide statistical evidence that a treatment had the desired effect(s).

- Generally, research can be broken down into three types of research: descriptive studies, observational studies, and experimental studies.

- Descriptive studies are studies that involve close or focused examination of a condition or problem that exists. Though not critical of asking "why," or offering an explanation, descriptive studies work to gather valuable and relevant information about the condition or problem at hand. Found in case law, case reports offer insight into a problem through discussion of a particular event or occurrence.

- Further descriptive studies include cross-sectional surveys. Often utilizing a written tool, such as a survey, data is collected to investigate a specific idea. Cross-sectional surveys have the benefits of examining specific populations or diseases that can be applied to a local or national level.

- Often called a correlational study, an ecological study serves to provide information by objectively examining trends and rates. By gathering and analyzing data or reports, both cross-sectional and ecological studies can provide powerful statistics to support a scientific question.

- Observational studies ask a simple question or hypothesis and account for variables in the topic of study. Normally in a case-control study, two or more specific groups are compared and analyzed. A researcher would examine the procedures (for example, to identify any similarities or differences that can be associated between group outcomes regarding a particular situation or condition). A cohort study is similar in methodology; however, instead of examining the treatment or procedures used in specific cases, a specific population is analyzed for statistical significance of treatment.

- All scientific studies essentially begin with a question. In an experimental study the investigation is focused on answering why something occurs or could occur. Null and alternative hypotheses are always formed and variables are limited to the one variable being manipulated.

- If the alternative hypothesis is accepted but is not supported with sufficient scientific evidence, a type I error or false positive result occurs. In contrast, a failure to observe a change may lead to a false negative or type II error. This may be caused by a limited sample size or may occur in a study that has a low statistical power.

- To be confident the data represents changes due to the manipulated variable, (for example, treatment) and not simply because of chance, a larger sample size must be studied. One way researchers overcome this is by performing a meta-analysis. This is done by combining the results of several similar studies and applying a statistical hypothesis test for the variable being studied.

- Outlined in the National Research Act of 1974, the U.S. government established three principles that address ethical concerns of scientific research. The principles exist to protect participants against inhumane and unethical practices.

- The first principle outlines the importance for any study participant to be informed about the study's hypothesis so as to make an informed choice as to whether to participate or not.

- The second principle addresses the problem of diminished autonomy or the ability to consent. A participant may not be able to willingly consent (for example, due to age, infirmity, or mental ability).

- The third principle speaks to maintaining justice for the participants. The idea of fair treatment for both the control and experimental groups is outlined. To ensure justice is upheld, many clinical trials have Data and Safety Monitoring Boards. These boards take an objective approach to evaluating the merit of experimental methodology and data collected. In the case of any federally funded research and for most other research projects, even before research begins a proposal must be submitted to an Institutional Review Board. This independent ethics committee reviews the proposal for any violations of ethics.

- Professional practice questions do not always involve patient care, but can be used to perform economic research. This research provides valuable information through cost-benefit analysis.

- In the absence of research, Paramedics turn to best practice as a way of determining the best method or most effective way of providing patient care.

- Best practice encourages the comparison of practices against others as well as encouraging the examination and constructive criticism of current practices. Questioning one's own practice helps one avoid paradigm blindness.

1. What are the three origins of EMS practice?
2. What are the steps to the scientific method?
3. Describe the process of creating an evidence-based practice.
4. Explain how to perform a literature search.
5. What are the types of research and how do they differ?
6. What are the pitfalls of retrospective data analysis?
7. What type of information is discovered by a researcher from descriptive studies?
8. What are type I and type II errors in experimental research?
9. Explain the ethical concerns and what should be done to safeguard participants of clinical trials.
10. Describe the advantages of a double-blinded randomized clinical trial.
11. How can researchers overcome the problem of reduced stat power?
12. What is best practice and what are its advantages?

► CASE STUDY QUESTIONS:

Please refer to the Case Study at the beginning of the chapter and answer the questions below:

1. Looking back at the task given, investigating the effectiveness of MFI in the prehospital setting, would retrospective or prospective research studies be more helpful?
2. Contacting other agencies and speaking with personnel is much different than gathering information via published reports. What is the difference between the two?
3. What errors in research would you have to be aware of when researching to ensure reliability and validity?
4. You presented your research and both the medical director and QA/QI committee are in favor of an MFI protocol for difficult airway management. However, after several months an important question was brought up about the use of one of the medications in an MFI as it was not statistically used very much. How would you design a research proposal for an experimental study that would evaluate this question?
5. What is the argument behind the statement, "One study does not make a practice"?
6. What are some questions that you should have in mind when evaluating the validity or reliability of a research study?
7. Evaluate the importance of obtaining an objective review of research studies methodology concerning ethics.

► REFERENCES:

1. Theodoridis S, Koutroumbas K. *Pattern Recognition* (3rd ed.). Boston: Academic Press; 2006.
2. Gauch H. *Scientific Method in Practice.* Cambridge: Cambridge University Press; 2003.
3. Mackinnon MA. Permissive hypotension: a change in thinking. *Air Med J.* 2005;24(2):70–72.
4. Dubick MA, Atkins JL. Small-volume fluid resuscitation for the far-forward combat environment: current concepts. *J Trauma.* 2003;54 (5 Suppl):S43–S45.
5. Johnston S, Brightwell R, et al. Paramedics and pre-hospital management of acute myocardial infarction: diagnosis and reperfusion. *Emerg Med J.* 2006;23(5):331–334.

6. Mason S, Knowles E, et al. Effectiveness of Paramedic practitioners in attending 999 calls from elderly people in the community: cluster randomised controlled trial. *BMJ.* 2007;335(7626):919.

7. Davis DP, Peay J, et al. The impact of aeromedical response to patients with moderate to severe traumatic brain injury. *Ann Emerg Med.* 2005;46(2):115–122.

8. Gitanjali B. Peer review—process, perspectives and the path ahead. *J Postgrad Med.* 2001;47(3):210–214.

9. Van Rooyen S, Godlee F, et al. Effect of blinding and unmasking on the quality of peer review: a randomized trial. *JAMA.* 1998;280(3):234–237.

10. Jefferson T, Wager E, et al. Measuring the quality of editorial peer review. *JAMA.* 2002;287(21):2786–2790.

11. Jefferson T, Rudin M, et al. Editorial peer review for improving the quality of reports of biomedical studies. *Cochrane Database Syst Rev.* 2007;2:MR000016.

12. **http://www.nlm.nih.gov/medlineplus/**

13. **http://www.ncbi.nlm.nih.gov/sites/entrez**

14. **http://scholar.google.com/**

15. **http://www.emedicine.com/**

16. Smith GD, Ebrahim S. Data dredging, bias, or confounding. *BMJ.* 2002;325(7378):1437–1438.

17. Lachin JM, Matts JP, et al. Randomization in clinical trials: conclusions and recommendations. *Control Clin Trials.* 1988;9(4):365–374.

18. Eddy DM. Practice policies: where do they come from? *JAMA.* 1990;263(9):1265, 1269, 1272 passim.

19. Rosenberger W, Lachin J. *Randomization in Clinical Trials.* New York: Wiley-Interscience; 2002.

20. Day SJ, Altman DG. Statistics notes: Blinding in clinical trials and other studies. *BMJ.* 2000;321(7259):504.

21. Friedman L, Furberg C, Demets D. *Fundamentals of Clinical Trials.* Berlin: Springer; 1998.

22. Weihrauch TR. Placebo effect in clinical trials. *Med Klin (Munich).* 1999;94(3):173–181.

23. Kienle GS, Kiene H. The powerful placebo effect: fact or fiction? *J Clin Epidemiol.* 1997;50(12):1311–1318.

24. Harrington A. *The Placebo Effect.* Cambridge: Harvard University Press; 1999.

25. Weinberg CR. It's time to rehabilitate the p-value. *Epidemiology.* 2001;12(3):288–290.

26. Whitley E, Ball J. Statistics review 4: Sample size calculations. *Crit Care.* 2002;6(4):335–341.

27. Sinclair M. Precedent, super-precedent. *George Mason Law Review* (14 Geo. Mason L. Rev. 363), 2007.

28. Singh G. A shift from significance test to hypothesis test through power analysis in medical research. *J Postgrad Med.* 2006;52(2):148–150.

29. DerSimonian R, Laird N. Meta-analysis in clinical trials. *Control Clin Trials.* 1986;7(3):177–188.

30. Department of Health and Human Services' Part 46 Protection of Human Subjects [see 46.116, (a),(3)].

31. Pitkin RM, Branagan MA. Can the accuracy of abstracts be improved by providing specific instructions? A randomized controlled trial. *JAMA.* 1998;280(3):267–269.

32. Pitkin RM, Branagan MA, et al. Accuracy of data in abstracts of published research articles. *JAMA.* 1999;281(12):1110–1111.

33. Al-Marzouki S, Evans S, et al. Are these data real? Statistical methods for the detection of data fabrication in clinical trials. *BMJ.* 2005;331(7511):267–270.

34. Weindling P. The origins of informed consent: the International Scientific Commission on Medical War Crimes, and the Nuremburg code. *Bull Hist Med.* 2001; 75(1):37–71.

35. Marrus MR. The Nuremberg doctors' trial in historical context. *Bull Hist Med.* 1999;73(1):106–123.

36. Annas GJ, Grodin MA. The Nazi doctors and the Nuremberg code: relevance for modern medical research. *Med War.* 1990;6(2):120–123.

37. Fisher JA. Procedural misconceptions and informed consent: insights from empirical research on the clinical trials industry. *Kennedy Institute of Ethics Journal.* 2006;16(3):251–268.

38. Palmer BW, Savla GN. The association of specific neuropsychological deficits with capacity to consent to research or treatment. *J Int Neuropsychol Soc.* 2007; 13(6):1047–1059.

39. Evans K, Warner J, et al. How much do emergency healthcare workers know about capacity and consent? *Emerg Med J.* 2007;24(6):391–393.

40. Thomas SB, Quinn SC. The Tuskegee Syphilis Study, 1932 to 1972: implications for HIV education and AIDS risk education programs in the black community. *Am J Public Health.* 1991;81(11):1498–1505.

41. Katz RV, Kegeles SS, et al. The Tuskegee Legacy Project: willingness of minorities to participate in biomedical research. *J Health Care Poor Underserved.* 2006;17(4): 698–715.

42. **http://www.cdc.gov/tuskegee/timeline.htm**

43. Belmont Report: Ethical Principles and Guidelines for the Protection of Human Subjects of Research. Federal Register Document 79-12065.

44. Bankert E. *Institutional Review Board.* Boston: Jones & Bartlett Pub; 2005.

45. Bodmer W. Principles of scientific management. *FASEB J.* 1993;7(9):723–724.

SECTION II

ETHICS AND LAW IN EMS

As a Paramedic, the public as a whole and each individual patient and family entrusts us with their lives to care for them appropriately. Some situations provide dilemmas for the Paramedic, whether it is with a patient, family member, partner, supervisor or medical director. A strong sense of ethics as well as following accepted ethical and legal practices helps allow the Paramedic to maintain the trust and privilege that is placed in us by society.

- **Chapter 5:** Ethics and the Paramedic
- **Chapter 6:** The Law and Paramedics

ETHICS AND THE PARAMEDIC

KEY CONCEPTS:

Upon completion of this chapter, it is expected that the reader will understand these following concepts:

- Conduct and responsibility derived from guiding principles as well as cultural and religious beliefs
- Duty-based ethics founded on principles, not consequences
- Bioethics and their application to day-to-day decision making
- The idea of what is "right"
- Awareness of patient dignity, privacy, and autonomy
- Understanding how ethical principles, and their proper application, can help resolve ethical dilemmas

▶ CASE STUDY:

The Paramedics were called to the home of a 43-year-old man with a history of lung cancer. He was semiconscious with labored breathing. His ex-wife produced an advanced directive stating that he did not want extraordinary means to keep him alive. His mother produced a handwritten will that stated he would accept oxygen and pain medication and any means to deliver them. Many family members were present and they began taking sides and telling the Paramedics what to do.

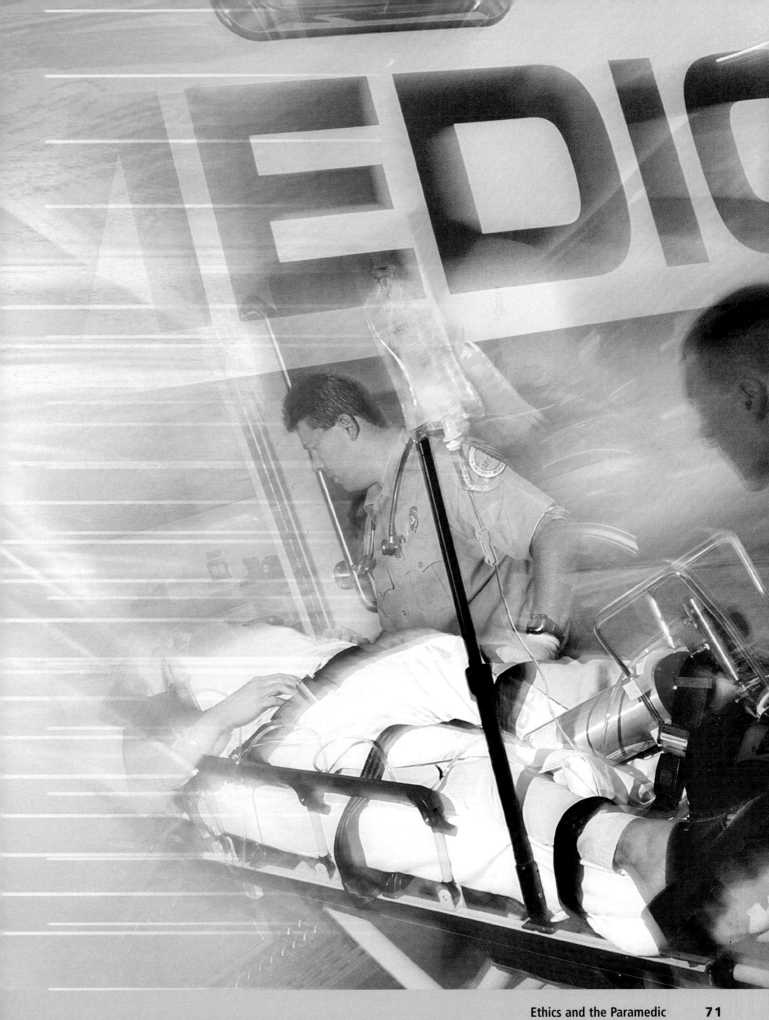

OVERVIEW

Although it is easy to think that the Paramedic operates solely on protocols and guidelines, without thought to real human consequences, a Paramedic's clinical decision making also has a strong ethical component. This chapter evaluates the question of what is "right," versus what is "correct" and draws from two ethical models of decision making. The Paramedic's decisions must also follow established human and legal rights and moral obligations. Paramedics may be asked to apply ethical principles to real life ethical concerns such as end-of-life decisions. To make educated and responsible clinical decisions, the Paramedic should have a well-rounded understanding of the EMS code of ethics.

Ethics Defined

Ethics, from the Greek "ethos" meaning character, is a system of guiding principles that govern a person's conduct. Paramedics use ethical principles to help guide them to make the right decision in a specific situation such as the one depicted earlier.

Factors that can affect a person's ethics are cultural influences and religious beliefs. Religion provides people with a description of what is right and what is wrong. Broadly, these religious beliefs can be applied to a Paramedic's practice. Many Paramedics obtain personal direction from these religious beliefs when confronted with an ethical dilemma.

The culture in which a person lives can also have a great impact on that person's ethics. In this context, culture means those unique activities and symbols that make one group's condition different from another's. Culture can include the way a group of people dress, as well as their unique language and special rituals.

When discussing the concept of culture, images of exotic places and people with strange customs may come to mind. However, a workplace can also have a culture. For example, EMS has a distinctive culture. Paramedics who wear distinctive uniforms separate themselves from the rest of the public. Paramedics also develop phrases and terminology that is often only understood by another Paramedic. Paramedics have certain special rituals and rites of passage, often marked by educational achievement, such as obtaining clinical privileges.

In some EMS organizations, the prevalent culture includes a sense of a higher purpose. For example, the job is viewed as performing a valuable service to the community which is manifested by a positive regard for the patient. These Paramedics obtain positive meaning from their jobs, thus enriching their own lives. The culture of the workplace could be said to be a positive one.

Alternatively, if the prevalent attitude among a group of Paramedics is that EMS is just a "job" and patient care is an onerous task to be endured, then a more negative culture may

exist. The ethics of a Paramedic entering into either one of these two workplaces can be affected by the culture present.

James O. Page, founding editor of the *Journal of Emergency Medical Services,* spoke to the problems of a negative EMS culture in his article entitled "A Call for a Cultural Revolution," written after he witnessed the care provided to his family.[1] Mr. Page emphasized that the problem, as he saw it, was not just with the individuals whose behaviors were unprofessional, but in an EMS system that permitted—even encouraged—this type of behavior, thereby creating an EMS system with a negative culture.

Some Paramedics' personal code of conduct, their **morality**, is a mere reflection of the culture where they work. The influence of others, a so-called worldview, has a significant impact upon most people's decision making and can replace the individual Paramedic's ethics.

Alternatively, other Paramedics have carefully considered and adopted a personal system of beliefs (i.e., professional ethics) which is based upon higher principles, discussed shortly. It takes a strong personal belief system and a strong sense of morality to withstand the ethical challenges from a negative culture.

Medical Ethics

Medical ethics pertains more specifically to how Paramedics behave in regard to patients. The term **bioethics** was originally coined by Van Rensselaer Potter. When speaking of bioethics he was referring to a set of guiding principles for the medical practitioner. Bioethics is a form of applied ethics—that is, ethics applied to the medical situation. Bioethics is used in day-to-day decision making by Paramedics in the field.

Bioethics came to prominence during the 1960s when questions about health care and the implications of medical advances, such as in vitro fertilization and abortion, were forcing theologians, physicians, lawyers, and legislators to consider the morality of certain medical procedures.

Bioethics holds that an unconsidered decision that results in harm to the patient is unethical. However, the answers to questions regarding patient care are often not as clear as they might first appear. Topics of great controversy, such as pediatric intubation, have advocates on both sides, each with valid arguments supporting their position. The role of bioethics is to help guide the Paramedic to make an ethical decision.

One means of coming to the answer is to have Paramedics come to a consensus. When the majority of Paramedics agree to a specific conduct or course of action, determining that it does more good than harm, then the act is considered to be ethical. This **ethical relativism** is in play at all times. Ethical decisions change over time as new conditions, technologies, and knowledge alter the situation's fundamental conditions.

In a number of situations, there is already a consensus as to the ethics concerning a certain conduct. For example, Paramedics agree that diverting drugs for personal use is unethical. In instances when that conduct occurs, the profession has a responsibility to take action. Action must be taken against the offender to prevent a reoccurrence.

If the conduct has risen to the level of criminality then Paramedics have a responsibility to report that crime to the proper authorities. If the conduct is less egregious, but still unethical, then the Paramedic may have a duty to report the conduct to management and/or civil authorities, such as a state EMS office.

Foundations for Value Judgments

When confronted with an ethical conflict the Paramedic must make a decision as to what action to take. He must make a judgment as to which course of action is the correct course of action in terms of right or wrong. That decision making requires that the Paramedic make a **value judgment**. Several models are available to help the Paramedic make that decision.

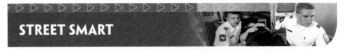

STREET SMART

Some Paramedics, in order to avoid controversy, may elect to not make a decision, deferring to medical direction or to another Paramedic. Even a non-decision is a decision—the same ethical dilemmas still exist.

Teleological Model of Ethics

The **teleological** model of ethics simply states that the end justifies the means. This approach implies that, even though some harm may occur, in the end if the outcome is good then the behavior is ethical. For example, Paramedics do not want to hurt their patients, yet to reverse a drug reaction it may

be necessary to perform a painful needlestick. Teleologically speaking, the benefit of the medication far outweighs the harm of the needlestick.

Generally speaking, the intrinsic good of acts performed by Paramedics should prevent and control disease, relieve pain and suffering, and generally prolong life. These acts should clearly outweigh any suffering, pain, or inconvenience to the patient.

However, when the decision to perform a procedure is complicated then the Paramedic should weigh the outcomes or consequences of performing the act against not performing the act and then make a decision that maximizes the intrinsic good. This approach to ethical decision making is called **act-utilitarianism**.

Underlying this foundation is an implicit understanding that the Paramedic cannot increase her own happiness at the patient's expense. For example, starting an intravenous access on the basis of some future good, such as the Paramedic can keep proficient with obtaining intravenous access by practice, would be an ethical violation.

STREET SMART

The decision to withhold a treatment in favor of transporting the patient to an emergency department where a more experienced physician can perform the skill could be seen as a utilitarian act, provided no harm came to the patient due to the delay.

Deontological Model of Ethics

Other Paramedics maintain that the consequences of an act are relatively unimportant. Their position is that it is more important that decisions be driven by principles.

This approach, the **deontological** approach, acknowledges that harm may occur but that Paramedics must perform their duty. Deontology is duty-based ethics in which the decision as to whether an action is right or wrong is based on principles and not upon the consequences.

A situation that demands action by any person in that situation, as a matter of duty, is called a **universal law**. An example of a universal law would be for one Paramedic to stop another Paramedic from committing an act of violence to a patient in restraints.

There are some universally agreed upon principles to which Paramedics and physicians alike subscribe; for example, the duty to "first, do no harm;" *primum non nocere*. Observance of this rule would be an example of a deontological approach to ethical decision making.

Almost all religions and cultural systems refer to a belief that is commonly called the "golden rule." Also referred to as the ethic of reciprocity, this concept speaks to a basic human right to be treated with decency. Key to the golden rule is that a person attempting to live by this rule treats all people, not just members of one's own group, with consideration.

Virtue Ethics

A somewhat middle ground approach, **virtue ethics**, does not depend on consequence-driven decisions or duty-driven decision making, but upon virtues.

Virtue ethics suggests that a "right-thinking" person will make the best decision for the patient based upon a predetermined set of virtues. The fundamental quality of a virtuous person is to act without regard to the consequences to oneself or to some abstract duty, but rather to act altruistically for the sole benefit of the patient.[2]

The source of one's virtues can be intrinsic, meaning that the virtues come from within the person. Examples of virtues include compassion and kindness. These internalized values are often the result of values instilled in a child by a parent during the child's upbringing. They are considered by some to be innate qualities for a Paramedic.

An extrinsic source of virtues comes from external sources such as religion. Sometimes called **divine command ethics**, extrinsic ethics can be based upon the Bible's Ten Commandments or Buddha's Four Noble Truths and Eight Paths to Righteousness. In both cases, a higher authority has predetermined what qualities a virtuous person would have and calls upon the person to display those virtues through correct action.

Personal Rights and Moral Obligations

The definition of a personal **right** can be somewhat nebulous and hard to define. However, an individual knows when he or she has been deprived of that right. A right could be loosely defined as something to which a person is entitled based on the society's sense of fair play. Rights are not social expediencies that can change as conditions change. Rights are not privileges because privileges depend on the goodwill, or cooperation, of others. Rights are immutable and universal to all people who are designated as possessing them. Some people refer to them as natural rights. Natural rights are a function of existing in the societal group. Because rights are defined by the society, the existence of rights will vary. An example of a natural right in the United States is the freedom of expression. What is a right in one country may be seen as privilege in another. An example is the difference in the freedom of speech in the United States versus the People's Republic of China.

Human rights are easier to understand than natural or personal rights as they are based on a commonly desired human condition (i.e., freedom from want, freedom from pain, and freedom from suffering). Human rights involve universally accepted standards of justice.

A patient's human rights cannot be abridged by a Paramedic without risk of severe social repercussions. These societal remedies are usually in the form of substantial civil penalties or criminal prosecution.

Patients also enjoy some legal rights. These are rights afforded them by the government in the form of laws, statutes, ordinances, and regulations. These legal rights can be affirmative rights in which the person can do something. For example, in the patient's bill of rights the patient has a right to self-determination, such as the right to choose treatment or choose not to have treatment.

These legal rights can also take the form of a prohibition which prohibits others from performing an action affecting the individual. For example, a person has the right to be free from unreasonable searches. The Bill of Patient Rights was recently adopted by the U.S. Congress (Table 5-1).

Mores and Paramedics

What some individuals might argue is a human right is more of a **social norm**. A social norm is a rule of conduct that regulates the interaction between people but is not specific to one individual. Mores are a social custom rather than a universally accepted standard of justice and do not rise to the level of a right. Generally a more is a collective agreement among a group of people on how they will behave in a group and with one another. A more can be thought of as a social contract that states the involved parties will all act in a similar way, or face the condemnation of the collective.

Professional groups, including Paramedics, may adopt certain mores, or **moral obligations**, that go beyond the basic human rights which every patient enjoys. For example, if an off-duty Paramedic fails to stop at the scene of a serious motor vehicle collision to offer aid, the action or omission may not be illegal, but other Paramedics might consider such an act immoral. Some would assert that the Paramedic has a moral obligation to stop. However, the patient does not have a right to care from an off-duty Paramedic.

Foundations of Bioethics

The Hippocratic Oath has stood as the foundation for bioethics for over 2,500 years.[3-5] The Hippocratic Oath defined those ethical principles that a physician was to follow. Inherent in the Hippocratic Oath are the concepts of beneficence and non-malfeasance.

Over time, various philosophers, such as Immanuel Kant, have refined the subject of medical ethics. In the eighteenth century, Thomas Percival developed the first medical code of ethics, which was adopted by the American Medical

Table 5-1 Patient Bill of Rights

- **The Right to Information.** Patients have the right to receive accurate, easily understood information to assist them in making informed decisions about their health plans, facilities, and professionals.

- **The Right to Choose.** Patients have the right to a choice of health care providers that is sufficient to assure access to appropriate high-quality health care including giving women access to qualified specialists such as obstetrician-gynecologists and giving patients with serious medical conditions and chronic illnesses access to specialists.

- **Access to Emergency Services.** Patients have the right to access emergency health services when and where the need arises. Health plans should provide payment when a patient presents himself/herself to any emergency department with acute symptoms of sufficient severity "including severe pain" that a "prudent layperson" could reasonably expect the absence of medical attention to result in placing that consumer's health in serious jeopardy, serious impairment to bodily functions, or serious dysfunction of any bodily organ or part.

- **Being a Full Partner in Health Care Decisions.** Patients have the right to fully participate in all decisions related to their health care. Consumers who are unable to fully participate in treatment decisions have the right to be represented by parents, guardians, family members, or other conservators. Additionally, provider contracts should not contain any so-called "gag clauses" that restrict health professionals' ability to discuss and advise patients on medically necessary treatment options.

- **Care Without Discrimination.** Patients have the right to considerate, respectful care from all members of the health care industry at all times and under all circumstances. Patients must not be discriminated against in the marketing or enrollment or in the provision of health care services, consistent with the benefits covered in their policy and/or as required by law, based on race, ethnicity, national origin, religion, sex, age, current or anticipated mental or physical disability, sexual orientation, genetic information, or source of payment.

- **The Right to Privacy.** Patients have the right to communicate with health care providers in confidence and to have the confidentiality of their individually-identifiable health care information protected. Patients also have the right to review and copy their own medical records and request amendments to their records.

- **The Right to Speedy Complaint Resolution.** Patients have the right to a fair and efficient process for resolving differences with their health plans, health care providers, and the institutions that serve them, including a rigorous system of internal review and an independent system of external review.

- **Taking on New Responsibilities.** In a health care system that affords patients rights and protections, patients must also take greater responsibility for maintaining good health.

Association in 1846.[6] That code of ethics still stands and includes such corollary concepts as respect for human dignity, patient autonomy, privacy, and justice.

Respect for Human Dignity

It almost goes without saying that Paramedics must first have a respect for **human dignity**. Human dignity is not just about patient autonomy and the patient's right to self-determination. Human dignity addresses the right of every person to be treated respectfully, regardless of his or her station in life.

The ideal of human dignity suggests that every Paramedic also has a duty to be **nonjudgmental**. To be nonjudgmental, the Paramedic must resist coming to a decision about someone based on an artificiality such as poverty or race. Prejudice has no place in paramedicine.

In support of this concept, the National Association of EMT code of ethics states, "The Emergency Medical Technician provides services based upon human need, with respect for human dignity, unrestricted by consideration of nationality, race, creed, color or status."[7]

Patient Autonomy

Another tenet central to bioethics is the concept of **patient autonomy**, the patient's ability to control her person and her personal destiny through decision making. Followed to its logical conclusion, patient autonomy implies that patients could decide to do nothing about a fatal illness, a decision that might lead to their own demise. This would be acceptable provided that the patient is capable of understanding and understood the ramifications of such a decision.

Paramedics might otherwise intervene in the previously described case, objectively for the good of the patient, if it were not for the respect that all medical professionals have for patient autonomy. It is understood that the patient's wishes, even without the power to act upon them, would be hollow if it were not for a Paramedic's respect for autonomy. The sanctity of patient autonomy is foundational to medicine.

Privacy

Privacy, a condition of being secluded from the view, opinion, or intrusion by others, is another foundation of the patient–physician relationship. All healthcare providers zealously protect their patients' privacy so that patients may feel at liberty to discuss their medical conditions with health professionals.

If a Paramedic was to violate a patient's privacy, then the patient might not be forthcoming with needed medical information in the future. Such an unauthorized disclosure would not only compromise present patient care but also have a chilling effect on future patient care.

The issue of a patient's right to privacy in an electronic age where personal information can be transmitted to others at the speed of light has become one of national concern, as evidenced by HIPAA federal regulations.[8–10] Paramedics must remain vigilant and attempt to prevent disclosure of private medical information, whether accidental or intentional, in order to maintain the trust of patients.

Veracity

Veracity is not just about truth but an adherence to truthfulness. When a Paramedic practices being truthful with all of her patients, making it a habit to be truthful, then that Paramedic can be said to have veracity. This truthfulness is essential if the Paramedic wants to establish a therapeutic relationship with the patient. For the purpose of treatment, patients reveal facts about themselves that they would not reveal to anyone else.

These revelations are so critical to the physician–patient relationship that the courts, without extraordinary reason, cannot ask the physician to willingly violate that trust. The courts have reasoned that if such a trust was violated then a patient might not confide essential aspects of medical history to the physician. Without that trust patients might not ever seek medical attention. The fallout of a violation of such a fundamental aspect of the physician–patient relationship could lead to widespread illness and untreated injury.

A devotion to the truth, a physician's veracity, burdens the physician with a duty to maintain this relationship until the patient's death—and perhaps beyond. This duty creates a legal bond (a fiduciary relationship) between the physician and the patient.

Fidelity

Inherent within the concept of veracity is the idea of **fidelity**. Fidelity is the obligation of the physician, and therefore the Paramedic, to keep the promises that are made to the patient. Infidelity leads to mistrust and a general deterioration of veracity that is counterproductive to the therapeutic relationship.

Beneficence

The other pillar of a physician–patient relationship is the concept of **beneficence**. Beneficence implies that the physician's actions are acts of mercy and charity, a good act performed for people at a time of need.

The quintessential model of beneficence is the Good Samaritan. The story of the Good Samaritan is that the Good Samaritan cared for another who was injured on the roadside, not out of obligation but out of compassion.

Non-maleficence

Included in every act of beneficence is the idea of **non-maleficence**. While similar, these two concepts are not the same. Beneficence means that an act of good is performed whereas non-maleficence means that no act of harm will be done.

The medical concept of "first, do no harm" is an example of the application of the principle of non-maleficence.[11,12] Harm (for example, in the form of a fever) which results from the physician's inaction is not the physician's responsibility. The patient understands this. Although the patient depends on the physician's mercy and charity to prevent this harm, it is understood that this can only be asked for, not demanded.

However, the Paramedic, like the physician, is responsible for any harmful acts performed and can be held liable (malfeasance). It is therefore important that the Paramedic be prudent, relying on tested or proven methods of treatment when caring for a patient, rather than risk creating harm. There is a greater duty not to injure others than there is to benefit them.

Justice

Justice, the application of the concept of fairness, implies impartiality in the administration of rewards. In the case of medicine, justice might be involved in the distribution of a rare medicine or allocating limited resources on the scene of a multiple casualty incident (MCI).

In some of these instances, a random selection criterion is applied, while in others a standard such as likelihood of medical benefit is applied. In every situation, a recognized standard has to be applied in order to be fair and just.

EMS Code of Ethics

Many healthcare professions, including EMS, have adopted a code of ethics. A code of ethics serves as a standard for the profession and a basis by which practitioners facilitate resolution of ethical dilemmas. Many associations, such as the National Association of EMT (NAEMT), have a code of ethics (Table 5-2).

Moral Rules and Particular Circumstances

Certain trying situations (for example, end-of-life decisions and triage) call upon a Paramedic's morals and ethics. Using the framework of ethical decision making, described earlier, the Paramedic can come to an ethical decision.

Ethical Obligation

The public has come to expect that its emergency medical services system is its "public health safety net." As such, it has placed the ethical burden on EMS systems to respond to all calls for help.

The response to these calls should be immediate and not complicated by concerns of finances. While financial limitations may affect a community's ability to sustain an EMS system, the individual Paramedic should not be burdened with these financial concerns. The Paramedic's duty should be simple: respond to all calls for help.

Allocation of Scarce Medical Resources

Physicians and bioethicists have had many discussions regarding the distribution of limited resources. An example of an allocation of a scarce medical resource is allocation of organs for transplantation. Paramedics are similarly confronted with the same ethical issues when they are on-the-scene of a MCI and must allocate the scarce medical resources.

Most Paramedics rely on the concept of **medical utility** to resolve this ethical dilemma. Simply put, medical utility assumes that those with the best prognosis should be treated with the limited resources. Those with a likelihood of medical benefit are treated first, whereas those who are expected to succumb to their injuries and for whom medical treatment would be futile are left to be treated last.[13–17]

In this situation, medical utility, a form of act-utilitarianism, provides sufficient guidance for Paramedics to act. A problem arises, however, when a fellow emergency responder, such as a firefighter, is injured (Figure 5-1).

Table 5-2 National Association of Emergency Medical Technicians Code of Ethics

EMT Code of Ethics

As adopted by the National Association of EMTs

Professional status as an Emergency Medical Technician and Emergency Medical Technician-Paramedic is maintained and enriched by the willingness of the individual practitioner to accept and fulfill obligations to society, other medical professionals, and the profession of Emergency Medical Technician. As an Emergency Medical Technician-Paramedic, I solemnly pledge myself to the following code of professional ethics:

A fundamental responsibility of the Emergency Medical Technician is to conserve life, to alleviate suffering, to promote health, to do no harm, and to encourage the quality and equal availability of emergency medical care.

The Emergency Medical Technician provides services based on human need, with respect for human dignity, unrestricted by consideration of nationality, race creed, color, or status.

The Emergency Medical Technician does not use professional knowledge and skills in any enterprise detrimental to the public well being.

The Emergency Medical Technician respects and holds in confidence all information of a confidential nature obtained in the course of professional work unless required by law to divulge such information.

The Emergency Medical Technician, as a citizen, understands and upholds the law and performs the duties of citizenship; as a professional, the Emergency Medical Technician has the never-ending responsibility to work with concerned citizens and other health care professionals in promoting a high standard of emergency medical care to all people.

The Emergency Medical Technician shall maintain professional competence and demonstrate concern for the competence of other members of the Emergency Medical Services health care team.

An Emergency Medical Technician assumes responsibility in defining and upholding standards of professional practice and education.

The Emergency Medical Technician assumes responsibility for individual professional actions and judgment, both in dependent and independent emergency functions, and knows and upholds the laws which affect the practice of the Emergency Medical Technician.

An Emergency Medical Technician has the responsibility to be aware of and participate in matters of legislation affecting the Emergency Medical Service System.

The Emergency Medical Technician, or groups of Emergency Medical Technicians, who advertise professional service, do so in conformity with the dignity of the profession.

The Emergency Medical Technician has an obligation to protect the public by not delegating to a person less qualified, any service which requires the professional competence of an Emergency Medical Technician.

The Emergency Medical Technician will work harmoniously with and sustain confidence in Emergency Medical Technician associates, the nurses, the physicians, and other members of the Emergency Medical Services health care team.

The Emergency Medical Technician refuses to participate in unethical procedures, and assumes the responsibility to expose incompetence or unethical conduct of others to the appropriate authority in a proper and professional manner.

Written by Charles Gillespie M. D. Adapted by the National Association of Emergency Medical Technicians, 1978.

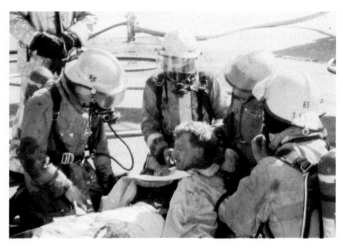

Figure 5-1 Firefighter with injuries on-scene.

transportation would improve operational efficiency and therefore serve a greater good. Others might argue that treating and transporting the firefighter represents a problem of bias and, perhaps more importantly, a breakdown of the concept of medical utility. The key to such ethical problems is to balance benefits with burdens and determine the moral behavior.

Ethics and EMS Research

Following the discovery of the Nazi atrocities of human experiments that were exposed during the Nuremberg tribunals following World War II, there was a strong call for a formal code of ethics for medical researchers. In 1947 the Nuremberg code for the ethical conduct in the use of humans for experiments was advanced and accepted by many countries. Enhancements to this original landmark document were passed in the Helsinki Declaration of 1964 and in subsequent guidelines passed by the World Health Organization.

Currently, all medical research, including EMS research, is governed under the federal regulation 45 CFR 46.111 as well. Medical research is monitored by the U.S. Department of Health and Human Services. The Department of Health and Human Services requires that all medical research be presented to an **Institutional Review Board (IRB)** for acceptance. An IRB consists of experts from the fields of theology, sociology, psychology, and medicine.[18] The IRB is responsible for reviewing all aspects of a proposed research project in terms of the potential psychosocial impact and ensure that all human subject research is ethical.

Before any research is accepted by an IRB, the researcher must demonstrate that the risks to the subjects are minimized and any risks are proportional to the potential gain or benefit, that subject selection is unbiased, and that informed consent is obtained from each subject.

End-of-Life Decisions

End-of-life decisions are complicated by the definition of death. Is death the absence of a heartbeat and breathing (clinical death), as the ancients believed? Or is death the absence of life; that is, those factors that make us uniquely human, such as consciousness, wakefulness, and awareness.

Current technologies permit a patient to be in a **persistent vegetative state (PVS)**, a permanent state of unconsciousness, with an intact brainstem that still produces a heartbeat and breathing. Most medical authorities agree that biological death (death of the human) occurs when the brain is dead. To establish death, most physicians apply the Harvard Medical School criteria: unresponsiveness, lack of movement, no reflexes, and a flatline EEG.

Paramedics encounter patients who are near-death and are sometimes confronted with the question of end-of-life decisions. Without guidance from the patient, in the form of advanced directives, or the presence of a healthcare proxy, the Paramedic may be called on to make the decision to start CPR.

Under the conditions described, and barring the presence of signs of death (i.e., signs that would indicate medical futility, such as rigor mortis or rigor lividity), the Paramedic is generally compelled to perform CPR and leave the end-of-life decision to the family and the physician at a later time.

Ethics Committees

Many healthcare organizations have established an **ethics committee**, a committee which can help individuals, including Paramedics, deal with common ethical concerns. An example of when an ethics committee might help a Paramedic would be with the development of palliative care protocols that provide for appropriate comfort and pain relief at the end-of-life without hastening the patient's death. Also, guidance could be provided as to whether it is appropriate to administer oxygen to a patient with a Do-Not-Resuscitate (DNR) order.

An ethics committee typically has the same make-up as an IRB. Generally its mission is to foster awareness of ethical concerns that might arise during patient care and to guide practitioners, including Paramedics, with decision making.

Other organizations that deal with issues of medical ethics include the Institute of Society, Ethics and the Life Sciences, formed in 1969 and based in Hastings-on-the-Hudson, and the Kennedy Institute of Ethics, established at Georgetown University in Washington, DC.

CONCLUSION

Paramedics are confronted with ethical dilemmas and with health-related questions which raise ethical issues. An understanding of ethical principles, and their proper application, can help the Paramedic to resolve these ethical dilemmas and allow the Paramedic to continue to provide care without hesitation.

▶ KEY POINTS:

- Ethics is defined as a system of guiding principles that govern a person's conduct. Cultural and religious beliefs can strongly affect a person's ethics. There are even workplace cultures in EMS, which can have a positive or negative influence on how Paramedics view their responsibility. It takes a strong personal belief system and a strong sense of morality to withstand the ethical challenges from a negative culture.

- Bioethics is a form of applied ethics (i.e., ethics applied to the medical situation) and is used in day-to-day decision making by Paramedics in the field. When the majority of Paramedics agree to a specific conduct or course of action, saying that it does more good than harm, then the act is considered to be ethical.

- Generally speaking, the intrinsic good of acts performed by Paramedics should prevent and control disease, relieve pain and suffering, and generally prolong life and clearly outweigh any suffering, pain, or inconvenience to the patient.

- Deontology is duty-based ethics where the decision if an action is right or wrong is based on principles and not upon their consequences. A situation that demands action and for which all persons, as a matter of duty, should act unconditionally is called a universal law.

- Virtue ethics suggest that a "right-thinking" person will make the best decision for the patient based upon a predetermined set of virtues. This person will be able to act altruistically for the sole benefit of the patient.

- The definition of what is "right" can vary. Generally, a right is a sense of fairness. Natural rights are inalienable, such as the freedom of expression. Human rights involve universally accepted standards of justice, such as freedom from pain and suffering. Legal rights come in the form of laws, statutes, ordinances, and regulations. Moral obligations may go beyond the basic human rights of the patient, such as the obligation for an off-duty Paramedic to stop at the scene of an accident and offer assistance.

- Human dignity addresses the right of every person to be treated respectfully, regardless of his or her station in life. Paramedics must respect human dignity, and therefore be nonjudgmental.

- The sanctity of patient autonomy is foundational to medicine. Patients have the ability to control their personal destiny through decision making, given that they are capable of understanding the ramifications of their decision.

- The patient's privacy must be maintained in order to sustain patient trust.

- When Paramedics practice being truthful with all of their patients, making it a habit to be truthful, then those Paramedics can be said to have veracity. This truthfulness is essential if there is to be a therapeutic relationship between the Paramedic and the patient. To maintain patient trust, the Paramedic must also practice fidelity, keeping the promises made to the patient.

- Beneficence assumes an act of good is performed, whereas non-maleficence means that no act of harm will be done. It is important that the Paramedic be prudent, relying on tested or proven methods of treatment, when caring for a patient, rather than risk creating harm. There is a greater duty not to injure others than to benefit them.

- In the case of medicine, justice—the application of the concept of fairness—might be involved in the distribution of a rare medicine, or to ration out limited resources on the scene of a multiple casualty incident (MCI). The concept of medical utility assumes that those with the best prognosis should be treated with the limited resources.

- A code of ethics serves as a standard for the profession and a basis by which practitioners facilitate resolution of ethical dilemmas.

- There is a formal code of ethics for medical researchers. An Institutional Review Board reviews proposed research projects, ensuring they meet certain ethical criteria before they can be carried out.

- Paramedics are sometimes confronted with the question of end-of-life decisions. Without guidance from advance directives or a healthcare proxy, and unless there are signs of death (i.e., rigor mortis or rigor lividity), the Paramedic generally performs CPR and leaves the end-of-life decision to the family and physician at a later time.

- An ethics committee's mission is to foster awareness of ethical concerns that might arise during patient care and to guide practitioners, including Paramedics, in their decision making.

- An understanding of ethical principles, and their proper application, can help the Paramedic to resolve ethical dilemmas and allow the Paramedic to continue to provide care without hesitation.

REVIEW QUESTIONS:

1. What influences a person's ethics?
2. What encompasses the term "bioethics," coined by Van Rensselaer Potter?
3. What is necessary for an act to be considered ethical or unethical?
4. How does the teleological foundation of ethics differ from the deontological model?
5. How can the definition of what is "right" vary?
6. What are the foundations of bioethics?
7. What is veracity, and how is it related to fidelity?
8. How is beneficence different than non-maleficence?
9. What concept is demonstrated when limited resources are applied to select people?
10. Explain the role of ethics in EMS research.
11. What professions make up an ethics committee and what is its overarching purpose?
12. When confronted with an end-of-life decision, when is it appropriate for the Paramedic not to perform CPR?

CASE STUDY QUESTIONS:

Please refer to the Case Study at the beginning of the chapter and answer the questions below:
1. How would you decide what care to provide for the patient in the case study?
2. What model of ethics supports your decision?

3. Many educational programs for healthcare providers require a course in ethics. Should Paramedics be required to complete such a course? Why or why not?

REFERENCES:

1. Page JO. *The Paramedics: An Illustrated History of Paramedics in Their First Decade in the U.S.A.* Kfar Sava: Backdraft Publications; 1979.

2. Miller DG, Pellegrino ED, Thomasma DC. *The Christian Virtues in Medical Practice.* Washington DC: Georgetown University Press; 1996.

3. Yeager AL. On Hippocrates. Either help or do not harm the patient. *Bmj.* 2002;325(7362):496.

4. Doherty DJ. Contemporary medical ethics. Would Hippocrates approve—or even understand? *Postgrad Med.* 1985;77(3): 212–216.

5. Cameron NM. Bioethics and the challenge of the post-consensus society. *Ethics Med.* 1995;11(1):1–7.

6. Baker et al. *The American Medical Ethics Revolution: How the AMA's Code of Ethics Has Transformed Physicians' Relationships to Patients, Professionals, and Society.* Baltimore: The Johns Hopkins University Press; 1999.

7. **http://www.naemt.org/about_us/emtoath.aspx**

8. Ouellette A, Reider J. Practical, state, and federal limits on the scope of compelled disclosure of health records. *Am J Bioeth.* 2007;7(3):46–48.

9. Banks DL. The Health Insurance Portability and Accountability Act: does it live up to the promise? *J Med Syst.* 2006; 30(1):45–50.

10. Buppert C. Safeguarding patient privacy. Establish department compliance with new federal regulations on individually identifiable health information. *Nurs Manage.* 2002;33(12):31–35.

11. Meskin LH. Non-maleficence: do no harm! *J Am Dent Assoc.* 1992;123(6):8, 11.

12. Hoyt D. Prehospital care: do no harm? *Ann Surg.* 2003;237(2):161–162.

13. Marco CA, Schears RM. Prehospital resuscitation practices: a survey of prehospital providers. *J Emerg Med.* 2003;24(1): 101–106.

14. Van der Hoeven JG, Waanders H, Compier EA, van der Weyden PK, Meinders AE. Prolonged resuscitation efforts for cardiac arrest patients who cannot be resuscitated at the scene: who is likely to benefit? *Ann Emerg Med.* 1993;22(11):1659–1663.

15. Battistella FD, Nugent W, Owings JT, & Anderson JT. Field triage of the pulseless trauma patient. *Arch Surg.* 1999;134(7):742–745; discussion 745–746.

16. Hawkins ML, Treat RC, Mansberger AR, Jr. Trauma victims: field triage guidelines. *South Med J.* 1987;80(5):562–565.

17. Sharma BR. Triage in trauma-care system: a forensic view. *J Clin Forensic Med.* 2005;12(2):64–73.

18. Garvin C, Landrum RE. (Ed.). *Protecting Human Subjects: Departmental Subject Pools and Institutional Review Boards.* New York: American Psychological Association; 1999.

CHAPTER 6

THE LAW AND PARAMEDICS

KEY CONCEPTS:

Upon completion of this chapter, it is expected that the reader will understand these following concepts:

- The origins of case law
- Civil and tort laws and the elements of a lawsuit
- The complexity of patient consent (both legal and ethical concerns)
- Understanding of patient rights
- Principles of advanced directives
- Acts and laws that impact the Paramedic as an employee

▶ CASE STUDY:

A Paramedic has been subpoenaed to give an affidavit as part of a pretrial investigation into the death of a 45-year-old man. The plaintiff is suing the hospital for malpractice and the untimely death of the patient. The patient was brought to the emergency department by EMS with the complaint of chest pressure and shortness of breath. It is claimed that the patient had to wait 15 minutes to be seen by a physician and had gone into sudden cardiac arrest and died. The lawyers for the plaintiff are looking into the prehospital care given by the Paramedic. The Paramedic's assessment, diagnostic workup, and course of treatment all followed standard protocols. However, despite the Paramedic's best efforts to inform the patient of the necessity for intravenous access, the patient refused, insisting on hospital personnel to perform such treatments. The prehospital care given by the Paramedic was found to have been within the Paramedic's scope of practice despite the patient's unresolved symptoms upon arrival at the emergency room (ER).

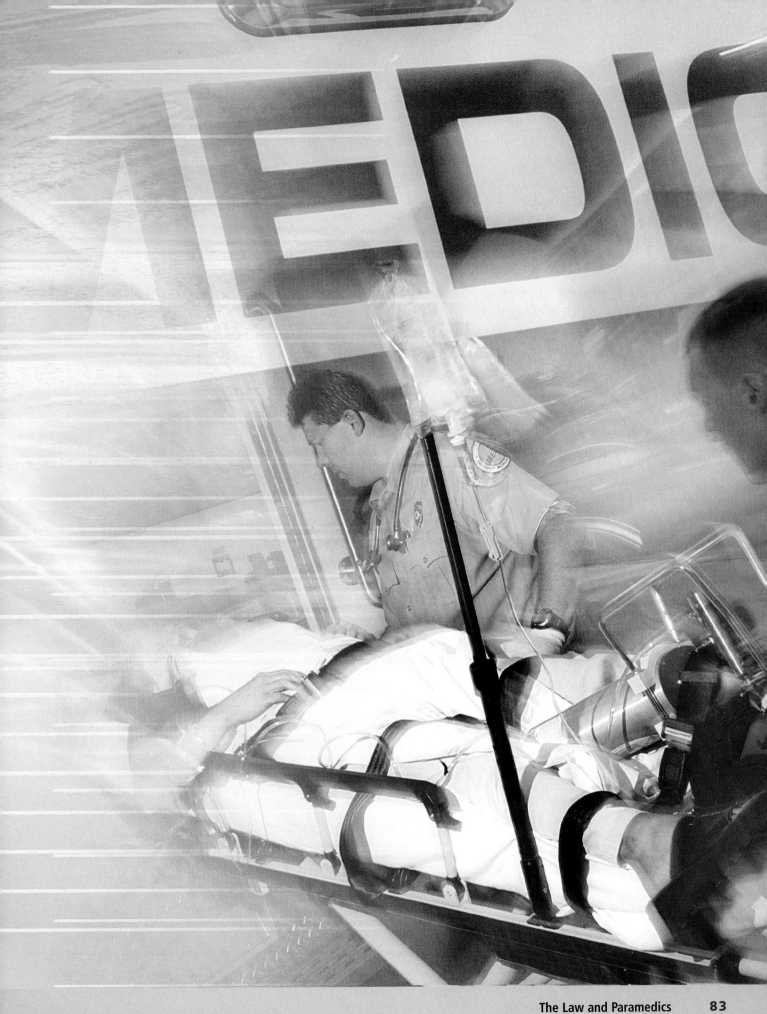

OVERVIEW

The Paramedic is expected to have a commanding knowledge of human physiology, symptomology, and pharmacology, but there is a more sobering side to paramedic practice that even the most knowledgeable Paramedic cannot overlook; the legal side. The legal side of EMS affects almost every Paramedic action from their duty to act to how Paramedics conduct themselves in the field. This chapter examines the origins of case law and the divisions between criminal and civil law. The Paramedic must train for the unknown, and should not wait to be caught in the middle of a legal case before becoming familiar with the legal side of the profession. Paramedics should not have a defensive approach, living in fear of being sued; rather, they should develop a preventative approach through a sound understanding of the law. Often the Paramedic's focus is placed on roles and responsibilities; however, in an almost reverse way of thinking the complexity of patient rights must also be examined and understood. Paramedics must also have an understanding of the legal basis of their actions when managing the day-to-day situations of patients with mental health issues, as well as patients who refuse care.

Origin of Law

In the past, when a transgression occurred against a king, the accused would be brought before the king and be allowed to plead his case. The king would then make a decision, pronounce sentence, and issue an edict (i.e., a public declaration equivalent to law that prohibited others from performing similar acts under certain penalty for such acts).[1] It was in this manner that the rule of law began.

Over time, when the numbers of cases became too numerous for the king, the king would appoint a magistrate (i.e., his majesty's administrator) to handle the minor cases. These magistrates would judge the worthiness of a case and render judgment. They would also make a notation of the resolution to report to the king as well as to preserve the decision for future reference.

Over time a considerable number of these judicial cases were documented and became **case law**. These case laws were arranged in order of date and jurisdiction (i.e., codified) for ease of reference. When another magistrate came across a similar case and needed guidance or wished to render a similar judgment, the magistrate would refer to this case law. By using case law in this manner, the courts helped to assure fairness under the law.[2]

Without a king to issue edicts or a dictator to impose his decrees, democracy required a new means of establishing public policy. Duly elected legislators representing the people of a particular area of the governing state would create new laws, called **statutes**. Using these statutes, the government could govern the population and offenders of the law could be prosecuted under a judicial system. This is the general structure of the government in the United States today.[3]

Government units or departments have also been formed, under statutory authority, and charged with various functions to carry out the business of government. These departments, during the performance of their duties, often find it necessary to regulate the conduct of citizens pursuant to their rule-making authority through the establishment of rules. These rules, or **regulations**, while not being statutory law, carry the same force as law.

Any reported violation of a regulation would need to be investigated and then determined, or adjudicated, in a court having authority (i.e., **jurisdiction**). When a regulation is violated an administrative court generally has jurisdiction.

When a violation of a departmental regulation occurs, the department (the petitioner) brings charges against the alleged wrongdoer (the respondent). The respondent is notified to appear in administrative court and respond to the charges. A hearing would then be conducted before an **administrative law judge (ALJ)** to discuss the merits of the case. A decision would then be rendered by the ALJ. While serious, these cases frequently held less severe penalties for the individual, as opposed to criminal penalties, because it was a violation of a regulation rather than of a statute. However, the penalty may have a significant impact upon the respondent's job or profession.

Criminal Law versus Civil Law

Criminal Law

One of the purposes of criminal law was to replace personal vendettas and blood feuds between groups of people with a general condemnation of an act by a sympathetic public. By removing the aggrieved victim from the process, and replacing her with the state as prosecutor, successive acts of vengeance were prevented and order was maintained.

A crime could therefore be defined as an act done in violation of a person's duties to the community and for which the written law requires the person to provide satisfaction, often in the form of restitution and loss of liberty, to the community. Crimes were defined and codified in the **criminal law**. The outraged community would rise up and, in its capacity as the state, demand prosecution of the individual. Therefore, when a person is charged with a crime the prosecutor is the state (e.g., *the State of Montana v. Joe Citizen*), and the person is tried in a criminal court.

Dependent on the severity of the crime, a citizen could be tried in a local city or town court before a justice, for a violation or infraction of the law, or before a judge in a county or state court, for a misdemeanor or felony charge.

There are two separate criminal court systems; one for the states and one for the federal government. The federal government has courts to adjudicate crimes involving federal laws. In addition, each state has state courts to adjudicate crimes involving violations of state laws.

Each state also has courts which determine appeals from the decisions of trial level state courts. An **appeal** is a request for the appellate court to change the decision issued by the trial level court. The federal court system also has courts which determine appeals from trial level federal courts. In some situations, due to the type of issue presented, decisions of state courts may additionally be challenged in the federal appeals courts. The highest court in the United States is the U.S. Supreme Court. Thus, U.S. Supreme Court is the last court of appeal.

STREET SMART

Many insurance providers/carriers will not protect or pay claims for Paramedics whose conduct rises to the level of criminality.

Civil Law

In order to resolve conflicts between individuals and to help maintain the peace, the states and the federal government have provided a forum in which persons and businesses can adjudicate allegations of civil wrongs which are not of a criminal nature. Every state, as well as the federal government, has civil courts to provide for resolution of disputes involving **civil law**.

Common matters of civil law include contracts (an agreement between parties that is alleged to have been breached), torts (claims involving a duty and allegations of injury, often due to negligence), estates, trusts, wills, real estate matters, commercial matters, and grievances against the government.

A **tort** is a civil or private wrongful act, other than a breach of contract, resulting in some type of injury or harm (not necessarily physical injury).[4] A tort involves some type of duty which arises by law. Duties and responsibilities relating to contracts arise from the relationship as a result of the agreement or contract. Those contract issues are not torts.

Several different types of torts are relevant to a Paramedic. An intentional tort occurs when the Paramedic intentionally and affirmatively performs an act which causes harm to the patient. An **assault** (a threat of violence) or a **battery** (unwanted touching) are examples of intentional torts. (Depending on the severity of the act, an assault and battery can separately constitute a crime and be prosecuted under the criminal law.) Another example of a claim of intentional tort that has been lodged against a Paramedic is the charge of **false imprisonment** (a restriction of movement or a confinement that abridges the patient's right to freedom, such as by the use of restraints).

Paramedics have certain public expectations placed upon them in regard to their conduct and behavior. This **public trust** involves an understanding between the patient and the Paramedic that the patient will be treated with dignity and respect in the same manner a physician would treat the patient. If the Paramedic violates that trust, then the patient may bring a lawsuit against the Paramedic for any damages sustained.

Lawsuits against Paramedics more frequently involve carelessness and an allegation of **negligence**, a failure of the Paramedic to exercise the degree of care that a prudent person would exercise.

Negligence is further divided into simple negligence, the lack of ordinary care that a reasonably prudent person under the same or similar circumstances would exercise, and gross negligence. **Gross negligence** involves intent on the part of the Paramedic to willfully, or with reckless disregard for the patient, cause harm to the patient. Separately, egregious conduct of this type might also give rise to criminal charges which might be leveled against the Paramedic by the district attorney, acting on behalf of the state.

Negligence, either simple or gross, that occurs during patient care can give rise to a charge of **malpractice**, a variation of negligence. Examples of malpractice are discussed later in the chapter.

Elements of a Tort Action

For a tort of malpractice to be **actionable** (i.e., to be the basis for a lawsuit), it must have the four elements of a tort. The elements of a tort are described in the following text.

Duty to Act

The first element of a tort is a **duty to act**. Generally speaking a Paramedic has a duty to act whenever the Paramedic is called to perform patient care (i.e., the Paramedic is "on duty"). The duty arises from her employment or volunteer status as a Paramedic. Generally, a citizen does not have a duty to act toward a patient requesting assistance, regardless of training, unless that person is acting in the capacity as an EMS provider or there is an expectation of the person to act in that role by virtue of job description.

However, once a duty has been undertaken, or an assignment accepted, then the patient can reasonably expect that the Paramedic will continue care until care can be **turned over to** another patient care provider with the same or higher training.[5] If the Paramedic were to prematurely terminate the Paramedic–patient relationship before the other provider assumed responsibility for patient care, thus interrupting patient care and resulting in harm to the patient, the patient could charge the Paramedic with patient **abandonment**.

Abandonment occurs as a result of an overt action—for example, when a Paramedic walks away from the patient without turning over care to another provider who has the same or higher level of training. However, if a Paramedic were to stop and render aid and then left the patient in order to summon further assistance, this would not be abandonment as the Paramedic is attempting to make reasonable arrangements to provide for continued patient care.

Finally, it would not be abandonment if a Paramedic were to render aid, such as CPR, until becoming physically exhausted and incapable of providing further aid.

Good Samaritan Act

Most Paramedics have no duty to respond to medical emergencies when off-duty. However, in an effort to encourage healthcare professionals such as physicians, nurses, and Paramedics to render aid during public emergencies, many state legislatures have created **Good Samaritan statutes**.[6]

The Bible story of the Good Samaritan is found in the Gospel according to Luke (10:25–27). The biblical parable tells of an injured traveler who is cared for by a well-meaning stranger. The Good Samaritan doctrine was established from this story.

In the spirit of the Good Samaritan, legislatures have enacted laws that protect well-meaning healthcare providers who, having no duty to respond, do nonetheless come to the aid of an injured person. These laws protect them from liability for negligent acts which are performed in the course of providing such assistance.

Good Samaritan laws do not provide immunity (exemption from being sued) from lawsuits. Rather, the Good Samaritan acts provide the Paramedic with a legal defense to counter a complainant's claim of negligence. The Paramedic is still required to go to court and demonstrate that he or she was acting in the capacity of a Good Samaritan.

Good Samaritan laws also may not apply when the Paramedic involved created the situation. For example, if an off-duty Paramedic was to be involved in a motor vehicle collision he would likely not be considered a Good Samaritan and might be liable if he does not provide assistance, minimally calling for rescue.[7] He might not enjoy the protections of the Good Samaritan act if he was expected to render first aid.

Every state in the United States has enacted either a Good Samaritan law or volunteer protection act that protects those who, in good faith, attempt to render aid to the sick or injured when off-duty. Of course, there is an assumption that the patient wants the care being provided.

Breach of Duty

Assuming that the Paramedic has a duty to act, the next element to determine in the lawsuit would be if the Paramedic committed a **breach of duty**. A breach of duty occurs when a Paramedic fails to perform patient care in conformance with the standard of care. The **standard of care** is that care and treatment that another Paramedic with the same or similar training would have rendered in the same or a similar situation.

The standard of care is established in court during a lawsuit by the testimony of expert witnesses who would explain the standard of care as relating to the situation in question. The expert would refer to local or regional treatment protocols, authoritative textbooks and perhaps, quality assurance standards.

Once the standard of care is established, the plaintiff's lawyer would then establish that there was a material breach of that standard.

A Paramedic may make an error in one of two ways. An error of commission is the performance of an act which is alleged to be improper or wrong. An error of omission is a failure to do something which she should have done. If the Paramedic performed an inappropriate procedure (e.g., gave a fluid bolus to a head-injured patient), then the charge would be **malfeasance**.

If the Paramedic performed the correct procedure but did so incorrectly, then the charge would be **misfeasance**. For example, if a Paramedic performed an endotracheal intubation on an apneic patient and the endotracheal tube was placed in the esophagus instead of the trachea, then the plaintiff would make an allegation of misfeasance.

Finally, a Paramedic can fail to perform the correct or required procedure, which would be an error of omission. For example, defibrillator batteries are typically checked on a routine basis. If a Paramedic were to arrive on-scene of a cardiac arrest and the defibrillator failed because of a dead battery, the family of the deceased could make an allegation of **nonfeasance**.

In every instance, in order to find negligence the Paramedic must have performed incorrectly.[8] The Paramedic must have either affirmatively committed an error or failed to act appropriately (omission).

Damages

It is not enough that a mistake was made. For the mistake to be actionable, the patient must have experienced some injury or harm from the error. The legal concept *de minimis non curat et lex* is applied to frivolous lawsuits where the patient did not experience any substantial injury. The term translated means: "the law has not a cure for trifles."

Damages are compensation for having suffered some injury or loss. Compensatory damages include both economic and non-economic damages. Economic damages are concrete and can easily be calculated. In other words one can put a fixed price on the loss. Economic damages include such things as the cost of repair, reimbursement for lost wages, and medical expenses. Non-economic damages are compensation for intangibles that one cannot put a fixed price on. These include compensation for pain and suffering, loss of life, injury to a part of the body, and loss of companionship.

Another type of damages are **punitive damages**, which can also be levied by the court against the Paramedic. Punitive damages are akin to a civil fine that is intended as a punishment for egregious conduct or to send a message to others so as to deter such conduct by others in the future.

Proximate Causation

The saying goes that bad things happen to good people and it is unfortunate that patients are forced to endure hardships as a result of misfortune. But the presence of an injury and the commission of an error do not always equal cause and effect.[9]

A tort requires that there be a duty, a breach of that duty, and an injury as a proximate result. Thus, the plaintiff must prove that the Paramedic's actions were the **proximate cause** of the injury.[10]

This is often difficult to prove. In many instances, the injury may already have been present. For example, a patient who experienced a spinal cord injury during a motor vehicle collision may have experienced that injury at the moment of impact (i.e., primary injury). However, the patient may complain that the injury did not occur at the moment of impact but as a result of rough or inappropriate handling of the patient by the Paramedic. The plaintiff would assert that the Paramedic's actions may have caused the injury.

Alternatively, the patient may assert that the injury occurred at the time of the collision but the injury was made worse (i.e., secondary injury) by the Paramedic. In those cases, the patient might argue that the Paramedic should share responsibility for damages with the patient or the individual who caused the accident. This is called **contributory negligence**. In this situation, the Paramedic would only be responsible for a percentage of the damages that were levied by the court.

In other instances, there may be no way to prove that the Paramedic's actions created the harm, despite the fact it can demonstrated that the Paramedic erred and that the patient is injured. Without proximate causation linking the act to the injury, the patient, as plaintiff, cannot prove that the Paramedic is negligent.

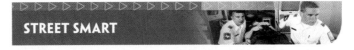
Borrowed Servant Doctrine

EMS practice dictates that the Paramedic with the highest level of education or experience is responsible for patient care. Therefore, the Paramedic is responsible for directing and supervising any patient care performed by any other EMS providers on the team with lower levels of training.

In those circumstances, called the **borrowed servant doctrine**, the Paramedic is not only accepting assistance from those EMS providers but is also accepting responsibility for the actions and the errors of those providers. Therefore, the Paramedic's failure to supervise a subordinate, who in turn makes an error and causes harm to befall the patient, leaves the Paramedic liable for the assistant's actions.

This legal principle, *respondeat superior,* Latin meaning "let the master answer," is well established in case law. Whenever a Paramedic permits another EMS provider to care for a patient, the Paramedic assumes **vicarious liability** for the actions of that provider. Take the case where the Paramedic, while caring for a minor injury, allows the ambulance driver to drive at high rates of speed with lights and siren on. If the ambulance was to have a collision and harm the patient, the public, or the occupants of the other vehicles, the courts might hold the Paramedic vicariously liable for the harm caused because the Paramedic did not instruct the driver to turn off the warning lights and siren or slow to a reasonable speed.

The Process of a Civil Lawsuit

When a patient feels that he has been harmed by the Paramedic's actions (i.e., an actionable cause), the patient generally approaches an attorney. The attorney initiates the legal proceedings in hopes of obtaining a payment for the damages the patient sustained.

The attorney would **serve** (cause to be delivered) papers, called a summons and complaint, on the Paramedic. The summons and complaint identifies some of the specifics of the matter and asks the defendant (the Paramedic being sued) to respond to the allegation contained in the complaint.

Attorneys usually hire a person, called a **process server**, to deliver the summons and complaint to the defendant. In the situation where a reasonable effort has been made to serve the defendant, and the defendant refuses to accept the papers, then the courts can rule that the papers be served in a different manner.

Once the matter is pending in court, the plaintiff or defendant could then ask the court to make a decision based on the facts asserted only in the papers that had been filed in court. The judge, acting as fact finder, might then arrive at a finding in favor of the plaintiff and grant the plaintiff's request for damages. Alternatively, it is also possible the judge might determine that judgment should be awarded to the defendant Paramedic and dismiss the lawsuit. This determination by the judge solely on the papers without conducting a trial is called **summary judgment**.

It is in the Paramedic's best interests to accept the papers and contact his own attorney to avoid being in default. Failing to appear in court or to contest the lawsuit can result in a summary judgment being entered against the Paramedic.

Most malpractice insurance carriers require that any Paramedic served with papers contact the insurance carrier within a specified period of time. This allows the insurance carrier to contact an attorney to represent the insured Paramedic. If the Paramedic's employer is providing the insurance coverage, then the insurance company seeks to protect the interests of both the Paramedic's employer and the insurance company. In some cases, the Paramedic may have his own malpractice insurance coverage. In that case, the Paramedic must contact that insurance carrier.

Pretrial Discovery

In an effort to determine the truth in a matter, the defendant's attorney (the Paramedic's lawyer) and the plaintiff's attorney (the patient's lawyer) will undertake specific prescribed legal proceedings.

One action may be to issue a **subpoena**, which is a legal command or direction issued by the court to appear at a certain place, such as the office of the plaintiff's attorney or the courthouse, at a particular time. The subpoena may direct the Paramedic to appear personally and it can also demand that certain pertinent files and records be brought with the Paramedic. Failure to respond to a subpoena may subject the Paramedic to legal sanctions including a charge of contempt of court.

In some instances, the patient may simply authorize, through a written **release of information**, that the Paramedic's **patient care report (PCR)** be released to the attorney. If this report is released, the Paramedic is not required to appear at that time.

Every report must be authenticated before it can be entered into the court's record as evidence. To authenticate the PCR, for example, the Paramedic may be given a copy in court and asked to testify that the item is a true and accurate copy or that it is the original document. Another means of authenticating the PCR that may be acceptable in some instances is to have a **notary public**, a person who is

recognized by the court, verify the Paramedic's identity. The Paramedic then swears that the copy of the PCR is a true and accurate copy of the original. If using a notary public is permitted, then it may not be necessary for the Paramedic to appear in court to authenticate the document.

As a part of the pretrial investigation, the Paramedic may be requested to give a sworn written statement, called an **affidavit**, which attests to facts involving the case.

In a more formal proceeding prior to the trial stage, the Paramedic may also be called to a **deposition**, which usually occurs in an attorney's office. During a deposition, the Paramedic swears to an oath. Then the plaintiff's attorney asks questions while a stenographer takes minutes of the proceedings. A judge is generally not present during a deposition. The deposition allows the plaintiff's attorney to obtain testimony in an out-of-court setting that will assist in preparing the case. The testimony given at the deposition may or may not be presented later during the trial.

The purpose of the pretrial discovery phase is to provide both parties with sufficient information to decide how to proceed with the case. It is possible that the attorney will learn that the Paramedic is not a party who should be sued. Paramedics have been removed as a named party in a lawsuit during this phase.

If the case has merit, the defendant (i.e., the Paramedic) and the Paramedic's attorney may decide that a trial would be counterproductive, inordinately difficult or expensive and agree to pay the plaintiff a sum of money, called a **settlement**, to the plaintiff in order to conclude the matter.

Quality Assurance and Discoverability

Atypical patient presentations and/or differences in the knowledge base of individual Paramedics can lead to less than desirable practice in the field on occasion. Quality assurance/ improvement (QA/QI) is an effort to improve patient care through uniformity and reliability with the standard of care.

QA/QI is often accomplished through retrospective analysis of the PCR. Disclosure of any deficiencies in the PCR, in a court of law, would have a chilling effect upon the QA/QI process.

In an effort to encourage EMS care, vis-á-vis through the QA/QI process, many states have adopted laws that protect these QA/QI results from disclosure during the discovery process.

Immunity and Defense

Immunity is a special privilege which, as used in the civil law, means that the person or entity with immunity is exempt or cannot be sued or held responsible for torts. The idea is that it is in the public interest that these entities not be sued. The practice of governmental immunity stems from old case law that essentially stipulates that a citizen of the crown cannot sue the king.

Governmental immunity (also called sovereign immunity) means that the government is exempt from liability for torts committed by its employees except to the extent that it has consented by statute to be sued.

As is relevant to the Paramedic, immunity is usually granted when the Paramedic is required by law to report a crime, called **mandatory reporting**, and the Paramedic does so in good faith. Paramedics may be required to report child abuse, sexual assaults, gunshot wounds, certain communicable diseases, and animal bites. In fact, the failure to report these conditions, as required by law, may leave the Paramedic with some personal liability for failing to report.

States have limited or restricted their immunity over the years. It is more infrequent that EMS employees of state, local, or federal government are granted governmental immunity.

Motions in Court

During a trial, both the plaintiff and the defendant can request that the judge accept a **motion**. A motion is a request to the judge for some action (i.e., dismiss the case, order a party to do something, postponement, cease and desist orders, etc.). A motion can be verbal, but is most often a written request that contains pertinent points for the judge to consider.

For example, the attorney for the defendant, the Paramedic, may make a motion for **summary dismissal** based upon the facts in the case, stating that the facts of the case are clear and without dispute. A lawsuit may also be dismissed if the time from the occurrence of the incident to the time of filing the lawsuit has exceeded the **statute of limitations**. The statute of limitations simply states that a plaintiff (usually the patient) cannot commence a lawsuit after a certain amount of time has passed.

The statute of limitations is handled differently in the case of a child. Typically, the state permits the child to reach an age of majority, between 18 and 21 years of age, and then adds the additional time to permit the lawsuit to be commenced. Therefore, in a pediatric case, it may take 10 years or more before a case is commenced and more time for it to be finally resolved.[11]

The defendant's attorney may also request summary dismissal, claiming that the court does not have jurisdiction in the matter. Jurisdiction is usually established early in the case. If there is a jurisdictional problem in that the plaintiff commenced the lawsuit in the wrong place, then the case may be dismissed in that court. However, a new case would likely then subsequently be commenced in a different court or court system which would have jurisdiction.

The plaintiff's attorney may request a summary judgment awarding judgment to the patient based solely on the papers submitted to the court. The concept of **negligence per se** is a case where summary judgment might be granted for the plaintiff. Negligence per se occurs when the Paramedic committed a criminal act, and the patient was injured as a result of that criminal act. The assumption is that the Paramedic's negligence flows from the criminal act. An example of negligence per se might be the case where a Paramedic was diverting narcotics for personal use and substituting sterile water in the drug vial. Later a patient in pain received the substituted sterile water and suffered harm (pain) because there was no drug in the vial.

The incidences of summary dismissal and summary judgment are both low because there are usually issues of fact to be decided at trial. Judges also tend to prefer that each party has its opportunity to present its case in court.

The best defense against a successful lawsuit is to practice within the Paramedic's scope of practice, to practice to the standard of care within the EMS system, to observe the patient's rights, and to document one's actions completely and thoroughly.[12]

Patient Consent

Paramedics have both an ethical and legal responsibility to preserve the patient's right to self-determination. In 1914 Supreme Court Justice Benjamin Cardozo said "every human being of adult years and sound mind has a right to determine what shall be done with his own body."[13] When a Paramedic helps to preserve this right it encourages patient autonomy, which in turn can lead to a more open dialogue and more rational decision making by the patient.

The importance of preserving patient autonomy cannot be overstated. One of the leading causes of lawsuits by patients against physicians, as reported in a National Academy of Sciences study, was the lack of rapport between patient and physician leading to increased mutual mistrust.

Patient-oriented medical care has not always been the policy in medicine. In the past, physicians, in a form of benevolent paternalism, expected patients to comply with their instructions without question and to leave the medical decisions to them.

The landmark 1972 case *Canterbury v. Spence* may have changed the nature of the physician–patient relationship. During that case the judge decided "it is the prerogative of the patient, not the physician, to determine for himself the direction in which his interests seem to lie..."

Implicit in this statement is the concept of patient education and self-disclosure.[14] The trend in medicine is now toward more patient involvement in decisions that directly affect the patient. This is now viewed as a matter of right.

Disclosure

One of the fundamental precepts of patient consent is **disclosure**. Disclosure is an open dialogue between patient and provider in which the provider tells the patient about the procedure, including its attendant risks, and recommends the procedure to the patient. It is therefore implicit that the Paramedic will get the patient's consent, or authorization, before continuing with the procedure.

An issue crucial to disclosure is the extent of the information required to be disclosed. The Paramedic should provide the patient with information that is material to the situation at hand. For example, the patient should be informed how the procedure will help the patient. As an example, before starting an intravenous access, the Paramedic could explain to the patient that having an intravenous access allows the Paramedic to administer drugs more quickly.

The patient should also be told of the risks that can reasonably be expected as a result of the procedure. This is called **foreseeable harm**. It is not necessary to provide the patient with an exhaustive explanation of the risks of the procedure or medication. The patient should be provided a short list of the most common reactions or consequences (e.g., pain at the insertion site of an IV).

Immediately following the explanation, the Paramedic should offer to answer any questions the patient may have. The Paramedic should also advise the patient that he or she can withdraw permission, or withdraw consent, for the procedure at any time.

Understanding

For a valid legal consent to occur, the patient must be of sound mind (possess the intelligence and presence of mind) to understand what is being said to her.[15] An explanation offered to an incoherent patient who then consents is not informed consent. Inherent in the concept of informed consent is that the patient must have the capacity to understand what is being offered.

If the patient is under the influence of drugs or alcohol, that patient may not have the capacity to consent. A question arises when a patient has had a few drinks but is not intoxicated. In those situations, the Paramedic is advised to contact medical control for direction before proceeding.

Other medical conditions can also impair a person's ability to think, and therefore consent. Fever-induced delirium, acute stress reaction, medication-facilitated impairment, and organic brain syndromes are just a few of the medical conditions that can preclude a patient from making an informed decision.

The patient must also have the legal **capacity** to understand what is being offered.[16] Therefore, capacity is not only a matter of the patient's mental state but age as well.

In general, the patient must be of legal age (i.e., the **age of majority**) in order to consent. In most states the age of majority is 18 years of age, though some states have set the age of majority at 21 years old.

There are some notable exceptions to the age of majority and ability to consent.[17] Adolescents below the legal age of majority can consent to limited health care. For example, they can consent to treatment for venereal diseases, drug abuse, and birth control. Otherwise, these youths must have parental permission, discussed further in the chapter, before they can receive health care, including EMS. The reasoning for these special exceptions is that laws provide for them due to societal determinations that they are in the best interest of a greater public good: fewer teenage pregnancies, a decrease in sexually transmitted disease (STD), and decreased drug addiction.

Voluntariness

The patient's consent must be voluntary and the patient cannot be coerced into consenting. However, a limited explanation of the procedure by the Paramedic, without an offer to ask questions or to withdraw permission, might be construed to be coercion. The patient in the back of an ambulance is left with few options. For example, the patient cannot get up and leave when the ambulance is moving and may feel compelled to agree with the Paramedic. The Paramedic should make every effort to ensure that the patient is comfortable with the decision made.

Permission

Following the explanation and an opportunity for the patient to ask questions, the Paramedic should then ask for permission to proceed. In most cases the permission is going to be verbal. Every effort should be made to have the permission confirmed by another person, a **witness**, who can attest to the patient's capacity, the explanation's content, and the patient's consent.

The Paramedic would then follow-up the verbal permission with a notation on the PCR.

BARNACLE

Some Paramedics use the mnemonic BARNACLE to ensure that they have completed all of the necessary steps in obtaining an informed consent (Table 6-1).

The (B) in BARNACLE stands for benefits. Were the benefits of the procedure explained to the patient? Next, were the alternatives (A)—for example, that consent can be withdrawn—explained to the patient? Then, were the reasonably foreseeable risks (R) explained to the patient as well as the nature (N) of the procedure? Then, was the patient given satisfactory answers (A) to the patient's questions? The patient should be advised that he can withdraw his consent (C) at any time. If the patient does withdraw consent, what are the reasonable consequences if he lacks (L) the treatment? Finally, were all explanations (E) offered in terms that the patient could understand?

Emergency Exception

In some cases, the delay created by a lengthy explanation might compromise the patient's health. In those cases it is

Table 6-1 BARNACLE

B	Benefits of procedure
A	Alternatives to procedure
R	Risks of procedure
N	Nature of procedure
A	Answers to patient questions
C	Consent to rights of patient
L	Lack of treatment consequences
E	Explanations understood

understood that, provided the Paramedic is practicing to the standard of care, the patient would want that care. An example would be intravenous access. Intravenous access, seen on television and in the hospital, is so commonplace that patients can reasonably expect to understand that an IV will be started by a Paramedic, and that the patient understood the benefits and risks of such a procedure when 9-1-1 was called.

While an **emergency exception** may clearly be of benefit to the patient during a crisis, not every call for EMS is an emergency. Therefore, a Paramedic should practice obtaining informed consent whenever possible and reasonably practical.

Therapeutic Privilege

In rare instances, it is acceptable to withhold information from a patient for the patient's benefit. For example, it may be inappropriate to disclose unhappy news to a depressed patient who has threatened suicide. The case of *Canterbury v. Spence* established that when the disclosure poses a threat or detriment to the patient, then disclosure is contraindicated from a medical point of view.

At first glance, this may appear to be a form of parentalism, discussed earlier, but the key difference is that the deception has a therapeutic value to the patient in and of itself. Examples of the use of therapeutic privilege include the use of placebos, medically inert drugs and shams, and procedures performed that are not helpful or harmful to the patient.

Waiver of the Right to Consent

Some patients will summarily waive their right to consent, permitting the Paramedic to treat the patient's condition to the standard of care. A statement such as "do what you think is best" is an example of a waiver of the right to consent. This waiver should be noted in the PCR, verbatim if possible, and witnessed by another EMS provider.

Advantages of Consent

Consent protects the patient's right to choose (autonomy) and thereby strengthens the trust between provider and patient. When important patient care decisions are made jointly, it increases the patient's responsibility as well as protects the Paramedic's tolerability for a poor outcome.

Informed consent, as opposed to no consent, also decreases the danger of complaints about fraud, deception, or duress. These charges, once levied, are hard to deny without the presence of an informed consent.

Perhaps more importantly, consent can also have a therapeutic benefit in and of itself. Patients naturally fear the unknown; informed consent provides them with reassurance, decreasing their anxiety of the unknown in the process. The therapeutic impact of knowledge to an anxious patient can reduce some of the negative physiological consequences of sympathetic stimulation generated by fear.

Finally, the American Hospital Association's Patient's Bill of Rights states that the patient has the right to make decisions about health care. Even if the decision is poor, in terms of negative consequences, the patient still has the right to make that decision.

Types of Consent

Expressed Consent

In a typical medical environment, such as a hospital or doctor's office, before performing any medical procedure the physician must provide a complete verbal explanation, or written justification, to the patient and then obtain a written or verbal consent from the patient. Obviously, this takes time as well as requires an alert and aware patient. Thus, it is not always practical during an emergency.

During an emergency, a patient allows a Paramedic to initiate care and indicates consent by either gesture or verbal acknowledgment. Or, if the patient does not object to receiving care, then **expressed consent** is assumed.[18]

When practical, a Paramedic is well-advised to try and obtain a **verbal consent** for specific procedures, such as starting an intravenous access, and particularly for uncommon procedures such as elective cardioversion. A request for permission, accompanied by a simple explanation, can improve patient compliance and decrease the risk of misunderstanding.

The essential aspect of patient consent is the fact that the patient is informed of the benefits and risks of the procedure and then makes a rational decision based on that information. Whenever a patient can make an informed consent it strengthens the physician–patient relationship.

Implied Consent

When a patient is unconscious and unable to speak for himself, then Paramedics can treat the patient under the doctrine of **implied consent**. Under implied consent, it is assumed that the patient would consent if awake and capable of consenting.

Implied consent is assumed even if the patient was refusing care moments before going unconscious because it is thought that the patient, suddenly faced with the reality of his mortality, would have changed his mind.

Implied consent is not applicable if there is a healthcare proxy or an advanced directive available; both are discussed later in the chapter. In those cases, the consent from the healthcare proxy must be obtained. Otherwise, the express wish of the patient, outlined in the advanced directive, is to be honored.

Involuntary Consent

When a law enforcement officer (LEO) places a person in custody, that person no longer has the freedom of movement. This condition makes the person necessarily dependant upon the officer for his or her safety and welfare, including health care, while in custody.

During a life or limb emergency an officer can provide consent for the person in custody (e.g., a prisoner). This type of consent is called **involuntary consent**.[19] Involuntary consent is usually reserved for true emergencies; the police power to provide consent is not generally invoked for minor emergencies or elective procedures.

The patient who is under the control of mental health officials is in a similar circumstance. Some, but not all, mental health patients are admitted involuntarily; that is, they are mandated into treatment. In those cases, permission for treatment is obtained from mental health officials, not the patient, in another form of involuntary consent.[20]

Emancipated Minors

In some special circumstances patients who are below the age of majority are permitted to give informed consent, provided they are capable of understanding the consequences of their decisions and that they are not impaired by alcohol or drugs. This special class of youths is called **emancipated minors.**

In some states youths under the age of 18 may get married with parental permission. Once married, the husband and wife are considered to be adults and are treated, for purposes of health care, as emancipated minors. A similar situation is created when adolescents under 18 years of age enlist in the armed forces.

In the majority of states, once an adolescent female is a mother she is treated as an adult. These teen-aged mothers are capable of consenting for treatment for both themselves and their children and are considered emancipated minors.

An adolescent, living away from home and without support from the family, may also petition the court for status as an emancipated minor. Once the court decree is issued the adolescent can consent to health care.

Pediatric Consent

Children, by virtue of their age, are usually unable to consent, except for the very limited healthcare services that were discussed earlier. A parent or legally appointed guardian must provide consent for them.

Obtaining consent from a parent to treat a child is the same as obtaining consent to treat an adult. The parent must be capable of understanding the consequences of a decision to accept the treatment, the risk/benefit, as well as the consequence if treatment is refused.

However, the Paramedic must be prepared to answer more questions about the procedure and may need to include the child in the discussion, depending on the child's developmental age.

Pediatric Consent without a Parent

Problems occur when a child is hurt and no parent is immediately available to consent to the child's treatment and transportation.

If the child has been left in the custody and care of another adult (e.g., a schoolteacher) then that adult has the authority to provide consent. Parents are frequently asked to complete permission slips, slips that permit the school's agents (e.g., teachers, coaches, and aides) to act in the parent's stead. These adults who have children entrusted to their care can, and are expected to, seek medical attention for the injured or ill child in an emergency. This status is called *loco parentis*.

If there is no parent, relative, guardian, or duly-empowered adult present, then the child can be treated in a modified form of implied consent called the **emergency doctrine**. The emergency doctrine holds that if the parent was present the parent would want the child treated and transported to the hospital. The emergency doctrine is usually invoked only in cases of life or limb-threatening emergencies. Every effort should be made to contact the parent, guardian, or responsible adult to obtain consent.

In rare cases, a parent may refuse treatment and transportation for a child. The difficulty lies when the parent refuses care beyond reason and the child is in obvious need of such care. Paramedics should not become confrontational with the parents but continue to gently, but firmly, insist that a physician see the child. If the parent still refuses, it may be necessary to involve a law enforcement officer and invoke child protective laws.

In these limited cases, the officer may take **protective custody** of the child, citing child protective laws, and the officer will give permission to treat and transport the child pursuant to a form of involuntary consent. In this case, the parents may be charged with child abuse or neglect by appropriate authorities. However, every effort should be made to reason with the parent before such a heavy-handed approach is taken.

Medical Restraint

Paramedics may encounter a patient experiencing a **behavioral emergency**, abnormal or bizarre behavior that may include violence or threats of violence. Paramedics, unsure of the cause of the behavior (e.g., drug intoxication, toxicological emergency, or psychiatric emergency), may need to institute a **medical restraint** and treat and transport the patient against his or her will.

Each state usually has a mental health law which provides for the involuntary restraint and transportation of a mentally disturbed person to a medical facility for treatment. The applicable law may provide for whether or not a law enforcement officer can or must be present. When confronted with such a situation, the Paramedic should use every persuasion to encourage the patient to go voluntarily: a "talk 'em down before taking 'em down" approach.

In a situation in which the patient does not want to go voluntarily, it may be necessary for either the Paramedic or the officer to invoke the mental health law and to restrain a patient in order to protect the patient from himself or herself or to protect others from the patient.

The American College of Emergency Physicians (ACEP), in their position paper on the use of restraints, states that these emotionally disturbed patients, who are usually either homicidal or suicidal, need to be treated with respect while under these trying situations and afforded as much dignity as

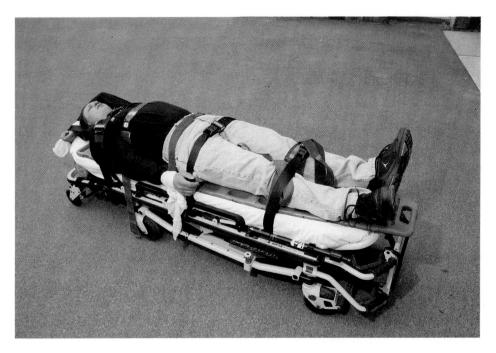

Figure 6-1 Proper use of extremity restraints in opposing directions.

possible. Furthermore, restraints should be applied humanely with only the minimum amount of force needed to effect the medical restraint.

In some instances it is better to leave the actual act of physical restraint to police officers who are trained in restraint procedures. Once restrained, handcuffs and other police restraint devices should be removed as soon as is practical. They should be replaced with other more humane restraint devices, such as padded-leather restraints, wide-band cravats, and the like. Regardless of the restraint device used, the Paramedic should be trained in the use of that device.

Following restraint, it is imperative that the Paramedic periodically reassess the patient and document the continued need and use of restraints. The least restrictive, but effective, restraint should be used (Figure 6-1).

Positional Asphyxia

Sometimes during a restraint a patient will become so agitated and combative that he will enter a state of **excited delirium**. When in excited delirium the patient will be tachycardic, hypertensive, and have hyperpyrexia. In some instances, the condition is worsened by the presence of sympathomimetic drugs such as methamphetamine or cocaine.

Patients in a state of excited delirium who have been restrained and then placed face down rapidly tire from the restricted breathing. They become hypoxic, a process called **positional asphyxia**, and then subsequently go into cardiac arrest. While positional asphyxia is uncommon, there have been "in-custody" deaths of patients who have been physically restrained and placed face down. This is especially so if the patient has been "hog-tied" (ankles and wrists tied together behind the back) (Figure 6-2).

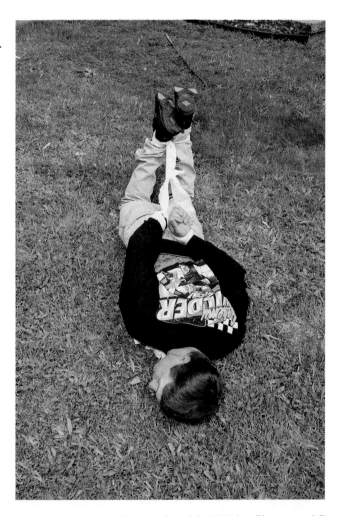

Figure 6-2 Patients should NOT be "hog-tied."

While the exact etiology of this cardiac arrest has been debated, most healthcare providers agree that restraining a patient face down poses a significant risk of positional asphyxia and subsequent cardiac arrest. Whenever possible, the restrained patient should be placed face up or supine and not "hog-tied."

Refusal of Medical Assistance

Every patient has a right to refuse care. Inherent in the right to refuse medical care is the understanding that the patient must first be able to consent to care before he or she can refuse care.[21] In the case where the patient can consent, and yet still refuses care, the Paramedic needs to carefully proceed with a **refusal of medical assistance (RMA)**.

An exploration of the reason for refusal can sometimes reveal issues or problems that can be easily resolved. For example, some patients lack insurance and are concerned about their ability to pay for the services they need. It is important that they understand that their health supersedes any financial considerations and arrangements can always be made to ensure that the patient can get the help that is needed. Most hospitals and many EMS services are obligated, by federal law, to provide free service to impoverished people.

If the patient remains resistant, the Paramedic should proceed with a complete description of the illness or injuries that he or she has sustained and the potential complications that could arise if the illness or injuries are not treated.

STREET SMART

In many cases, an injury or illness, unchecked, can lead to permanent disability and even death. Some agencies require that Paramedics list the foreseeable complications, including death, on the PCR. The Paramedic must then ask the patient to read the PCR out loud and then sign it. The "death warrant," as it is commonly known, serves several functions. For one, the patient must be able to read and understand the English language. Asking for the text to be read aloud establishes that the patient both read and understands the foreseeable consequences of refusal.

If the patient remains adamant in her refusal of treatment and/or transportation, then the Paramedic should advise the patient of alternatives. Alternatives may include seeking private medical care and calling EMS again if desired.

Finally, it is important that Paramedics offer assistance to the limit that the patient will accept. Frequently, patients who initially accept a bandage and then permit vital signs to

be taken will ultimately rescind their refusal when the patient senses the genuine concern on the part of the Paramedic.

Many EMS agencies have a standard refusal of care form, crafted by attorneys, for use in the field (Figure 6-3). To be effective as a form of notification, the patient should receive a copy of the RMA form. Most agencies also require a witness to the patient's signature.

While any adult can serve as a witness, the best witnesses are those who are not interested parties (i.e., someone who does not stand to benefit financially from a lawsuit). A witness is essentially assuring that the refusal was obtained without duress and that the signature is authentic, not that the patient understood the explanation offered.

Against Medical Advice

Some patients refuse care in opposition to all logic when confronted with a clear and immediate danger to their health. These patients are deciding, **against medical advice (AMA)**, to not go to the hospital.[22] In those cases the Paramedic is advised to contact medical control for direction and advice.

In some instances, the patient may still be permitted to refuse care but the input of the physician often provides the patient with the incentive to accept care and transportation.[23, 24] Also, the Paramedic then has the knowledge that he or she did all that could be done to convince the patient to seek medical care immediately.

However, the situation is different in the case of children. A seriously ill or injured child needs to be seen by a physician. If the parents refuse to permit the child to be seen, and it is clearly a life-threatening situation, then a police officer should be summoned to the scene. The officer may have to take the child into protective custody in order to get the child to treatment.

Destination

Generally, patients are transported to the closest appropriate medical facility. If there are several reasonable options within approximately the same distance, then the patient is often given the choice of hospitals.

Increasingly, hospitals are becoming more specialized and the appropriate medical facility may not be the closest or the patient's choice. Under a restricted set of circumstances or conditions, a patient may be diverted from the closest hospital to a hospital equipped to handle the patient's particular emergency.

The first example of a specialty center may have been the trauma center. A trauma center has some very unique capabilities which permit it to provide the highest level of care for certain traumatic injuries. In general, Paramedics are permitted to divert to these trauma centers based upon authority granted within a set of state, regional, or local protocols.

With the likely future development of specialty care centers, at some point Paramedics may divert to such specialty hospitals as cardiac care centers, with interventional

Rensselaer County Emergency Medical Services

REFUSAL OF MEDICAL CARE, TREATMENT, AND/OR TRANSPORTATION

PCR Number: _____ Date: _____ Time: _____

PATIENT: I understand that competent persons maintain the right to refuse medical care, treatment and/or transportation.

I, _____, hereby acknowledge that I have been advised by members of

the _____ [AGENCY], that they recommend that I receive medical care, treatment

and/or transportation to a hospital emergency department for further evaluation by a physician.

I further understand that I may refuse medical care, treatment and/or transportation, but do so at my own risk.

I do not have any known physical or mental condition that would prohibit me from making an informed, competent, and intelligent decision to refuse the medical care, treatment and/or transportation that has been offered and recommended.

THE RISK ASSOCIATED WITH REFUSAL MAY INCLUDE POSSIBLE LOSS OF LIMB OR LIFE

I HAVE ALSO BEEN ADVISED THAT IF I DEVELOP ANY MEDICAL COMPLAINTS OR SYMPTOMS, I SHOULD

IMMEDIATELY CONTACT AN AMBULANCE, HOSPITAL EMERGENCY DEPARTMENT, OR MY PHYSICIAN.

I hereby release _____ [AGENCY], its, officers, agents, personnel, and employees from any and all claims, causes of action or injuries, of whatsoever kind or nature, arising out of or in connection with my refusal of medical care, treatment and/or transportation.

Patient's Signature: _____ Date: _____

Patient's Name (print): _____ Patient's Age: _____ Patient refused signature: _____

FOR MINORS OR PERSONS WHO HAVE GUARDIANS: I am the patient's legal guardian. My relationship to the patient is _____.

I am hereby acting on behalf of the patient, _____ [PATIENT'S NAME]. I have

read the above information and refuse medical care, treatment and/or transportation on behalf of the patient.

Guardian's Signature: _____ Date: _____

Guardian's Name (print): _____ Guardian's Full Address: _____

_____

WITNESS: I, _____, witnessed members of the _____

_____ [AGENCY] recommend to the patient medical care, treatment, and/or transportation to a hospital

emergency department for further evaluation and attention. I further witnessed the above-named patient (or patient's guardian) decline such medical care, treatment, and/or transportation.

Witness Signature: _____ Date: _____

Witness Name (print): _____ Witness' Full Address: _____

Occupation: _____ _____

EMS PROVIDER: I, _____ [EMS PROVIDER], have offered and recommended to

_____ [PATIENT'S NAME OR GUARDIAN'S NAME], emergency medical care and treatment, including transportation to a hospital. The patient (or patient's guardian) has refused my recommendation for medical care, treatment, and/or transportation. I have fully explained the reasons for medical care, treatment, and/or transportation to the patient (or patient's guardian). I have also explained this form to the patient (or patient's guardian) and have requested that he/she personally read it. The patient (or patient's guardian) has expressed to me an understanding of the information contained herein and did not have any questions regarding the content of this form. The patient (or patient's guardian) did not appear to me to be suffering from any illness or injury nor any condition that would affect his/her ability to refuse medical care, treatment, and/or transportation. The patient (or patient's guardian) is alert and oriented to person, place, time, and situation.

EMS Provider Signature: _____ Date: _____

Provider Certification Level / NYS ID Number: _____ Police Agency Present: NO _____ YES _____

Police Officer's Name: _____ Police Agency Name: _____

Figure 6-3 An example of a refusal of medical assistance form. (Reprinted with permission of Rensselaer County Emergency Medical Services)

cardiology capabilities, and stroke centers, with rehabilitation facilities, for example.

Diversion should only occur under express authority of medical control and when the patient has been fully appraised of the risks associated with refusing to go to the specialty hospital.

Advanced Directives

The development of new life-saving technologies is accompanied by questions about the quality of life in terminal illness and prolongation of suffering.[25] These advances have coincidentally occurred at a time when patient autonomy is increasingly being asserted. Together, the two trends have combined to create a conflict between paternalistic physicians who have always had dominion over life and death decisions and the patient's wishes regarding the quality of his or her life.

Several landmark cases have had a tremendous impact upon these decisions, changing the entire fabric of medical decision making in the process.

Case of Karen Ann Quinlan

Karen Ann Quinlan was found unconscious following suspected ingestion of barbiturates and alcohol at a party. Following mouth-to-mouth resuscitation, Ms. Quinlan recovered but remained in a persistent vegetative state (PVS). Her family, witnessing her body waste away and given no hope for a recovery to a meaningful life, requested that the mechanical ventilator supporting her be removed and that Ms. Quinlan be allowed to die peacefully, in other words, "death with dignity."

The state took the position that such an act, removal of the ventilator, would cause her death and therefore constitute criminal homicide. The state sought to prevent the family from removing Ms. Quinlan from the ventilator.

The family felt that Ms. Quinlan, a devout Catholic, would not want to live by these extraordinary means, and that decisions on her behalf were a private family matter. The family also felt the state's position constituted an invasion of privacy (i.e., the patient's right to self-determination).

The New Jersey Supreme Court ruled in favor of the family, stating that the family's right to privacy extends to matters of life and death. Ms. Quinlan was removed from the ventilator, started to breathe spontaneously, and survived for almost a decade.

The importance of the Quinlan case was that it recognized the patient's right to make life and death decisions and preserved the patient's autonomy. That case helped initiate the right to die movement.

Case of Nancy Cruzan

Nancy Cruzan was a young woman left in a persistent vegetative state (PVS) following head injuries sustained in a motor vehicle collision. Faced with the prospect of a bleak future, the family wanted Ms. Cruzan's tube feedings stopped.[26]

The state of Missouri interceded, stating there was no "clear and convincing evidence" that Ms. Cruzan did not want to live this way. The appeals for this decision went all the way to the U.S. Supreme Court, who upheld the lower courts' decision.

Subsequently, several of Ms. Cruzan's friends came forward and testified, under oath, that they had had conversations with Ms. Cruzan in the past and that she indicated she would not want to live in a persistent vegetative state.

Had Ms. Cruzan made her intentions known to others earlier, or in a more definite manner (e.g., in a written letter), the controversy would have been averted.

The Cruzan case helped to establish the concept of **advanced directives**, a central tenant in the right to die movement. Advanced directives, written declarations of patient intent during specific circumstances, are designed to provide guidance when a patient is threatened with an existence in a persistent vegetative state or afflicted with a terminal illness.

Principles of Advanced Directives

Four core principles are included within the concept of advanced directives. These principles provide a foundation which sustains an advanced directive.

The first principle is that competent people can refuse medical treatment, even at their own peril. This statement affirms the patient's right to self-determination.

Next, the interests of the state are subordinate to the will of a competent patient. If the competent patient, meeting all of the conditions of consent described earlier, makes a decision about his or her health care, then that decision is inconvertible.

The third principle supports making healthcare decisions in a healthcare setting as opposed to a court room. The idea is that the best patient care decisions are made by a partnership of physician and patient and that the courts are used only when an impasse is reached.

The fourth principle states that if a patient lacks the ability to make decisions, then the patient may assign a surrogate decision maker in her stead. A surrogate decision maker has the responsibility to know the patient's preferences and must place the patients' wishes before the surrogate's wishes. This level of understanding usually involves a personal dialogue between the two individuals and frequently results in a written statement that helps to support the decision maker.

If the surrogate decision maker knows the patient's wishes, then, in certain situations, the surrogate makes the decision in a process called **substituted judgment**. If the surrogate decision maker does not know the patient's wishes for the specific situation that he or she is being presented with, but does know the patient's wishes for similar situations, then the surrogate must make a decision on the presumption of what is in the patient's best interest.

Patient Self-Determination Act of 1990

In 1990, following the public's growing insistence that the patient should control the personal healthcare decisions, Congress passed the Patient Self-Determination Act (PSDA).[27]

Regulations within the act required hospitals to provide notice to all patients that they have several rights. First, the patient has a right to participate in and direct her own health care. Next, the patient has the right to refuse medical and/or surgical treatments, up to and including the use of life-saving or life-preserving technologies. The patient also has a right to prepare an advanced directive, and the hospital should assist the patient with preparing an advanced directive. Finally, the hospital has a duty to assist the patient with those decision-making activities such as preparation of advanced directives, designation of a healthcare proxy, and assistance with the institution's policies on how to utilize those rights.

Types of Advanced Directives

The intention of an advanced directive is to give the patient control over her own body and to provide guidance to others on how to proceed with healthcare decisions. In addition, these advance directives afford healthcare providers some immunity from criminal or civil prosecution for making decisions or taking actions on the patient's behalf.

There are several advanced directive instruments which meet these objectives. The first, and perhaps original, advanced directive instrument is the living will. The living will, drawn up by a patient, and perhaps an attorney, details the patient's wishes regarding specific healthcare decisions.

A living will might preclude certain treatments using terms such as "extraordinary treatment," "heroic measures," and "artificial life support." The use of these imprecise terms has led to confusion and are ineffective if death is not imminent. The states of New York, Massachusetts, and Michigan have rejected the use of living wills as the language therein was not "precise and convincing." These states and many others preferred the creation of a durable power of attorney for health care (DPAHC). A DPAHC is a surrogate decision maker, one who uses substituted judgment to guide the patient's healthcare decisions.

The **healthcare proxy**, the title for the person who has a DPAHC, has a responsibility to review the medical record, to consult with healthcare providers, and to give consent to either initiate or to refuse care.

Do-Not-Resuscitate Orders

At some stage during the progression of a terminal disease the patient, or healthcare proxy, may decide that any artificial life support would be futile and that death is inevitable. In those cases, the physician, after consultation with the patient or healthcare proxy, will issue a **Do-Not-Resuscitate (DNR)** order (sometimes called a Do-Not-Attempt-Resuscitation (DNAR) order).

Paramedics are expected to honor a DNR order and not commence cardiopulmonary resuscitation (CPR), defibrillation, or other advanced life support measures when presented with a DNR.

The confusion lies in which treatments are life-sustaining versus life-prolonging. The provision of supplemental oxygen (e.g., via a partial rebreather mask) is generally considered to be life-sustaining and therefore acceptable. However, assisting ventilations with a bag-valve-mask assembly is thought to be life-prolonging and therefore unacceptable.

It is important that Paramedics establish with their medical directors, beforehand, which treatments are life-sustaining and which are life-prolonging.

There is general agreement that the provision of pain medication, for the purpose of **palliative care**, is life-sustaining and therefore acceptable. All forms of comfort measures (i.e., palliative care, including suctioning, repositioning, and analgesia) are considered humane and merciful.

Physician's Order of Life-Sustaining Treatment

Physician's Order of Life-Sustaining Treatment (POLST) is a more detailed description of the patient's wishes, placed in the form of a physician's order. This program was started in Oregon in 1991 as an answer to the issues that routinely occur in patients who may have a DNR order, but who have not yet progressed into cardiopulmonary arrest. Most states in the United States only allow Paramedics to honor DNR orders once the patient has become pulseless and apneic. They also do not allow Paramedics to honor living wills or other advanced directives. The advantage of the POLST program is the forms that are generated through a discussion between the patient and their physician that address specific situations including utilizing artificial hydration, nutrition, intubation, antibiotics, and other medical therapies. Many states that have instituted POLST programs allow Paramedics to follow these orders.

Confidentiality

An aspect of patient trust and provider veracity is the patient's assumption of confidentiality. Inappropriate disclosure of sensitive patient information would be a failure on the part of the Paramedic and may well have a chilling effect on future Paramedic–patient relations. For this reason Paramedics share patient information only with those on a need-to-know basis.

The duty of maintaining patient confidentiality stems from a person's right to privacy. In the past, this was more of a professional duty than a legal right. However, current laws protect a patient's confidentiality to a greater extent.

A breach of confidentiality should not be confused with libel or slander. **Libel** occurs when a falsehood which is damaging to a person's reputation is written or printed and then disseminated to the public. **Slander** occurs when defamatory lies about a person are told to others. Libel and slander involve the telling of an un-truth, whereas a breach of confidentiality is an act of unauthorized disclosure of private and personal patient information. Both libel and slander are actionable in a court of law.

Breaches of Patient Confidentiality

A patient's confidentiality can be broken under some very specific circumstances. The American Medical Association (AMA) acknowledged this in a position paper which says that a physician may breach a patient's confidentiality when required to do so by law.

As stated earlier, the courts hold the physician–patient relationship in high regard. Before making a decision to abridge a patient's rights to privacy, the courts weigh the good of the community and the protection of the physician–patient relationship versus the individual's rights. The disclosure is then limited to that which is necessary to the issue so as to protect the patient's privacy rights.

Situations in which a Paramedic might be compelled by law to disclose confidential patient information may include gunshot wounds, contagious diseases, and/or child abuse and those cases where it is necessary to protect the welfare of another individual or the community. Laws in each state or jurisdiction may vary and the Paramedic should be familiar with applicable statutes that may impact him or her.

Limited Disclosure

The number of people who are directly, or indirectly, connected to the care of one patient is incredible. Literally dozens of people, from bedside caregivers to support services, to utilization review, billing, and quality assurance, all have access to a patient's confidential record.

The concept of **legitimate interest** comes into play when deciding if patient information should be shared. A Paramedic should only provide confidential patient information to those who have a need to know, and then only to the extent that that is needed. For example, an admission clerk does not need to know the patient's HIV status, yet does need to know if the patient has been previously admitted. A notable portion of people in the medical chain will need confidential patient information (Table 6-2).

Table 6-2 Information Dissemination

- Paramedic
- ER MD and RN
- Billing clerk
- Utilization reviewer
- Infectious disease RN
- Public health service
- CDC
- Media—reporting outbreak

Health Insurance Portability and Accountability Act

The U.S. Congress passed the Health Insurance Portability and Accountability Act (HIPAA) in 1996.[28, 29] HIPAA provides for criminal penalties for inappropriate disclosure of patient information. It also establishes a number of protections for the patient's right to privacy. HIPAA was enacted, in part, to stem the electronic transmission of patient information to unauthorized parties.

HIPAA restricts the distribution of confidential patient information to only those with a legitimate interest, such as consulted healthcare professionals, those providing patient treatment, coding and billing offices, and specific managerial functions, such as quality assurance and utilization review.[30] Patient information may be used for training and education provided that all identifying information is removed or the patient consents.

HIPAA also requires that every healthcare agency, including EMS, appoint a **privacy officer**. The privacy officer is responsible for patient record security, record security awareness training of all employees, as well as implementing a privacy protection plan within the agency.

In the future, Paramedics may be required to provide patients with a notice of privacy practices for the EMS agency. That may include information about what confidential patient history is considered to be **protected health information (PHI)**.

Disclosure to Law Enforcement

On occasion, law enforcement officers will request specific information about a patient. In most cases, the disclosure of confidential patient information to another could be a violation of the HIPAA regulations. Generally, the officer should be provided with information which is required by law. The patient's name and address can be shared but all other requests for information should be denied until the patient signs a release of information or a subpoena is served.[31]

Employment Law

The Paramedic, whether career or volunteer, is an employee of the EMS agency. As such, the Paramedic is afforded certain protections as a result of Congressional acts. The following is a gross overview of those laws which may pertain to the Paramedic. Other laws, both local ordinances and state statutes, may also apply to the Paramedic. Therefore, every Paramedic is advised to become aware of the relevant legal environment and seek legal counsel when appropriate.

Americans with Disabilities Act

Congress passed the **Americans with Disabilities Act (ADA)** to protect those citizens who had suffered hardship or discrimination from employers. The ADA prohibits discrimination based on disability in hiring, promoting, training, and retiring. To be included in the class of protected persons, the individual must have a permanent disability which limits full participation in the **activities of daily living (ADL)**.

The ADA does not imply that, for example, the hearing-impaired person must be hired as a Paramedic. Clearly, some jobs require specific skills and capabilities. These skills and capabilities are generally described in the position's **functional job description**. The tasks described therein are those that are needed to perform the function and exclude rare or marginal job functions.

Perhaps more importantly, the ADA establishes that **reasonable accommodations** must be made, whenever possible, which would permit the disabled person to function. New technologies are ever increasing the capacity of disabled citizens to perform varied and vital functions, many within EMS.

Title VII

Title VII, the Civil Rights Act, provides the employee with certain rights (e.g., freedom of religious expression, etc.). Recently, a great deal of notoriety has been given to the right of employees to be free of sexual harassment.

Sexual harassment can be as blatant as demands of sex in exchange for career advancement, a *quid pro quo*. In many cases, the charge of sexual harassment stems from a perception of a "hostile working environment." A hostile working environment is one that is intended to humiliate or intimidate the worker because of gender. Examples of a hostile working environment include displays of sexually explicit pictures, uninvited kissing or embracing, or flagrant sexual humor.

Every EMS agency should have a policy forbidding sexual harassment and that policy should include a complaint process. Most complaint processes start with an internal investigation of the inappropriate conduct and end with a resolution that can vary from counseling and reassignment to termination.

Amendments to Title VII

Since its passage through Congress, Title VII has had several amendments added. One of them, the Age Discrimination in Employment Act (ADEA), prohibits the discrimination of those over the age of 40. Another, the Equal Pay Act, requires that pay be based on seniority or merit and not personal preference.

EMS and the Fair Labor Standards Act (FLSA) have come into conflict from time to time. The FLSA is intended to guarantee that all employees are paid the minimum wage as well as receive overtime for working extended hours past the normal workweek.

Over the years, employers have created a large number of work patterns and arrangements in order to meet the public's demand for round-the-clock EMS coverage. These arrangements include on-call pay, per diem pay, stipends, and the like. Some of these arrangements had to be modified to meet the requirements of the FLSA.

Family and Medical Leave Act

The Family and Medical Leave Act (FMLA) requires that employers with more than 50 employees provide their employees 12 weeks of unpaid leave for purpose of childrearing.

Many employers have embraced the FMLA by creating family leave policies, believing that employees who are afforded the opportunity to establish their families and then return to work will be happier and more productive.

CONCLUSION

The acts, laws, and regulations which affect a Paramedic are intended to either protect the Paramedic or to provide for the patient's protection. Careful attention to these laws, both in letter and in spirit, will help the Paramedic provide safe and effective care.

KEY POINTS:

- Case law is developed from compiled case decisions and assures fairness through consistent application of the law.

- Different units or departments carry out various functions of government. Each department may be regulated by rules or regulations that are not statutory laws but carry the same force.

- Criminal law is a violation of a person's duties to the community; therefore, the prosecutor is the state and the case is tried in a criminal court.

- An appeal is a request for the appellate court to change the decision issued by the trial level court.

- Civil law is the system of law concerned with private disputes between members of the community.

- A tort is a civil or private wrongful act, other than a breach of contract, resulting in some type of injury or harm (not necessarily physical injury).

- Simple negligence is the Paramedic's failure to exercise the degree of care that a prudent person, under the same or similar circumstances, would exercise.

- Gross negligence involves intent on the Paramedic's part to willfully or with reckless disregard cause the patient harm.

- For a tort of malpractice to be actionable against a Paramedic, it must have the four elements of tort. First, the Paramedic must have a duty to act. Second, it must be shown that the Paramedic breached his duty (standard of care). Third, there is actual harm or damages as a result. Fourth, proximate cause of harm must be shown.

- Good Samaritan laws protect healthcare providers from liability for negligent acts that are performed in the course of providing assistance when there is no duty to act or respond. Although these laws do not provide immunity from lawsuits, the Good Samaritan acts do provide the Paramedic with legal defense to counter a complainant's claim of negligence.

- Standard of care is the care and treatment that another Paramedic with the same or similar training would have rendered in the same or similar situation.

- Malfeasance is the performance of an inappropriate procedure.

- Misfeasance is the situation when a Paramedic performs the right procedure but performs it incorrectly.

- Nonfeasance is the failure to perform the correct or required procedure, which would be an error of omission.

- Damages are compensation awarded to the patient for some injury or loss.

- The Paramedic is responsible for directing and supervising the patient care performed by any other EMS providers on the team with less training than the Paramedic.

- The process of a civil lawsuit begins with the Paramedic being served papers by a process server.

- The purpose of the pretrial discovery phase is to provide both parties with sufficient information to decide how to proceed with the case.

- Immunity is usually granted when the Paramedic is required by law to report a crime, called mandatory reporting, and the Paramedic does so in good faith.

- A motion is a request to the judge for some action.

- The best defense against a successful lawsuit is to practice within the Paramedic's scope of practice, to practice to the standard of care within the EMS system, to observe the patient's rights, and to completely and thoroughly document one's actions.

- The significance of patient consent is that the patient makes a rational decision based on information that the Paramedic provides.

- To obtain a valid legal consent, the patient must be of sound mind and have the capacity to understand what is being offered.

- The patient's consent must be voluntary and the patient cannot be coerced into consenting.

- In rare instances disclosure is contraindicated from a medical point of view if the disclosure poses a threat or detriment to the patient.

- Consent protects the patient's right to choose, decreases legal charges against providers, and can have a therapeutic benefit in and of itself.

- A law enforcement officer can provide involuntary consent during a life or limb emergency when a patient is in custody. Similar circumstances apply to patients who are under the control of mental health officials.

- Emancipated minors are those youths under the age of 18 who are married, enlisted in the armed forces, or have petitioned and have legal documentation of emancipation. Also, once an adolescent female is a mother she is capable of consenting for treatment for herself and her children.

- Similar to consent for an adult, obtaining consent for a child requires the parent to be capable of understanding the consequences of the decision to accept the treatment, the risk/benefit, as well as the consequence if treatment is refused.

- If the child has been left in the custody and care of another adult, that adult has been given *loco parentis* and has the authority to provide consent.

- In rare cases, a parent may refuse treatment and transportation for a child. If the parent still refuses to give consent after attempts to convince him care is needed, it may be necessary to involve a law enforcement officer and invoke child protective laws.

- Paramedics may encounter a patient experiencing a behavioral emergency. In a situation in which the patient does not want to go voluntarily, it may be necessary for either the Paramedic or the officer to invoke the mental health law and to restrain the patient in order to protect the patient from himself or herself or to protect others from the patient.

- Following restraint, it is imperative that the Paramedic periodically reassess the patient and document the continued need and use of restraints. The least restrictive, but effective, restraint should be used.

- In the case where the patient can consent, and yet still refuses care, the Paramedic needs to carefully proceed with a refusal of medical assistance (RMA). The Paramedic should proceed with a complete description of the illness or injuries that he or she has sustained and the potential complications that could arise if the illness or injuries are not treated.

- Paramedics should offer assistance to the limit that the patient will accept.

- Generally, patients are transported to the closest appropriate medical facility. Circumstances may occur necessitating diversion from the closest hospital to a hospital equipped to handle the patient's particular emergency.

- High-profile cases such as the Quinlan case emphasized a patient's right to self-determination, while the Cruzan case showed that written directives would have provided guidance when in a vegetative state.

- Types of advanced directives include the living will, healthcare proxy, and DNR order.

- In cases of a terminal disease, the patient, or healthcare proxy, may decide that any resuscitation efforts should not be performed. A physician can issue a Do-Not-Resuscitate (DNR) order or a Do-Not-Attempt-Resuscitation order (DNAR).

- Confidentiality is the nondisclosure of sensitive patient information and stems from a patient's right to privacy. Libel occurs when a falsehood, which is damaging to a person's reputation, is written or printed and then disseminated to the public. Slander occurs when defamatory lies about a person are told to others.

- A Paramedic should only provide confidential patient information to those who have a need to know to the extent that that is needed.

- The Health Insurance Portability and Accountability Act (HIPAA) established a number of protections for the patient's right to privacy.

- The Americans with Disabilities Act (ADA) prohibits discrimination based on disability in hiring, promoting, training, and retiring. The ADA also asserts that reasonable accommodations must be made, whenever possible, which would permit the disabled person to function.

- Some jobs require specific skills and capabilities that are generally described in the position's functional job description.

- The Civil Rights Act, Title VII, provides employees the right to be free of sexual harassment in the workplace. Amendments to Title VII include the Age Discrimination in Employment Act that prohibits the discrimination of those over the age of 40 and the Equal Pay Act that requires pay to be based on seniority or merit, not personal preference.

- The Family and Medical Leave Act provides employees 12 weeks of unpaid leave for purposes of childrearing.

REVIEW QUESTIONS:

1. Explain the difference between criminal and civil law.
2. What are tort laws and how do they pertain to the Paramedic?
3. Identify the four elements of a lawsuit.
4. How does the Good Samaritan law protect Paramedics?
5. Describe the three levels of damages.
6. Define four types of consent.
7. What issues are associated with pediatric consent?
8. How do the elements of the mnemonic BARNACLE ensure the Paramedic has completed all of the necessary steps in obtaining an informed consent?
9. Identify the elements of a valid refusal of medical assistance.
10. What is the difference between the refusal of medical assistance and refusal against medical advice?
11. What are the origins of advanced directives?
12. Describe a DNR order and what care a Paramedic can still render.
13. Why is patient confidentiality important and what is limited disclosure?
14. What acts and laws have been established that impact the Paramedic as an employee?

CASE STUDY QUESTIONS:

Please refer to the Case Study at the beginning of the chapter and answer the questions below:

1. Assess whether the patient had the right to refuse intravenous therapy.

2. What indications would require the Paramedic to initiate intravenous access by implied consent?

3. What argument can be made for the Paramedic in regard to being held liable for proximate cause of death?

4. What should the Paramedic have done to prepare for a situation like this?

REFERENCES:

1. Pennington K. *The Prince and the Law, 1200–1600: Sovereignty and Rights in the Western Legal Tradition (A Centennial Book)*. Berkeley: University of California Press; 1993.

2. Irons P. *A People's History of the Supreme Court*. New York: Viking Adult; 1999.

3. **http://www.supremecourtus.gov**

4. Cockburn T, Madden B. Intentional torts claims in medical cases. *J Law Med.* 2006;13(3):311–335.

5. Wiggins CO. Ambulance malpractice and immunity. Can a plaintiff ever prevail? *J Leg Med.* 2003;24(3):359–377.

6. Good Samaritan protection. *Ann Emerg Med.* 2000;35(6): 640–641.

7. Wilson A. On scene, off duty. *Jems.* 1991;16(7):29–30.

8. Augustine J. Can we leave the scene? *Emerg Med Serv.* 2005;34(2):44.

9. Williams K. Medical Samaritans: Is there a duty to treat? *Oxf J Leg Stud.* 2001;21(3):393–413.

10. Kelly GC. Patient privacy lawsuit results in judgment for patient. *Emerg Med Serv.* 2003;32(8):26.

11. Colwell CB, Pons P, Blanchet JH, Mangino C. Claims against a Paramedic ambulance service: a ten-year experience. *J Emerg Med.* 1999;17(6):999–1002.

12. Weaver J. Surviving a lawsuit. *Emerg Med Serv.* 2007;36(9):47–48, 50, 52 passim.

13. Goldberg RJ, Zautcke JL, Koenigsberg MD, Lee RW, Nagorka FW, Kling M, et al. A review of pre-hospital care litigation in a large metropolitan EMS system. *Ann Emerg Me.* 1990;19(5):557–561.

14. Graham DH. Documenting patient refusals. *Emerg Med Serv.* 2001;30(4):56–60.

15. Bedolla M. The Patient's Bill of Rights of the American Hospital Association: a reflection. *Linacre Q.* 1990;57(3):33–37.

16. Schyve PM. Patient rights and organization ethics: the Joint Commission perspective. *Bioethics Forum.* 1996;12(2): 13–20.

17. Selbst SM. Medical/legal issues in pre-hospital pediatric emergency care. *Pediatr Emerg Care.* 1988;4(4):276–278.

18. Ayres RJ, Jr. Legal considerations in pre-hospital care. *Emerg Med Clin North Am.* 1993;11(4):853–867.

19. Grant JR, Southall PE, Fowler DR, Mealey J, Thomas EJ, Kinlock TW. Death in custody: a historical analysis. *J Forensic Sci.* 2007;52(5):1177–1181.

20. Wobeser WL, Datema J, Bechard B, Ford P. Causes of death among people in custody in Ontario, 1990–1999. *Cmaj.* 2002;167(10):1109–1113.

21. Moss ST, Chan TC, Buchanan J, Dunford JV, Vilke GM. Outcome study of pre-hospital patients signed out against medical advice by field Paramedics. *Ann Emerg Med.* 1998;31(2):247–250.

22. Cone DC, Kim DT, Davidson SJ. Patient-initiated refusals of pre-hospital care: ambulance call report documentation, patient outcome, and on-line medical command. *Prehosp Disaster Med.* 1995;10(1):3–9.

23. Stuhlmiller DF, Cudnik MT, Sundheim SM, Threlkeld MS, Collins TE, Jr. Adequacy of online medical command communication and emergency medical services documentation of informed refusals. *Acad Emerg Med.* 2005;12(10):970–977.

24. Knight S, Olson LM, Cook LJ, Mann NC, Corneli HM, Dean JM. Against all advice: an analysis of out-of-hospital refusals of care. *Ann Emerg Med.* 2003;42(5):689–696.

25. La Puma J, Orentlicher D, Moss RJ. Advance directives on admission. Clinical implications and analysis of the Patient Self-Determination Act of 1990. *Jama.* 1991;266(3):402–405.

26. Ashley RC. How can I best protect my family from a Schiavo/Schindler situation? *Crit Care Nurse.* 2005;25(3):60–61.

27. Kring DL. The Patient Self-Determination Act: has it reached the end of its life? *JONAS Healthcare Law Ethics Regul.* 2007;9(4):125–131.

28. Garner JC. Final HIPAA security regulations: a review. *Manag Care Q.* 2003;11(3):15–27.

29. Ludwig GG. HIPAA takes effect. *Emerg Med Serv.* 2003;32(5):46.

30. Wirth S. Privacy matters. *Jems.* 2002;27(11):191–193.

31. Schulman R. HIPAA privacy and security implications for field triage. *Prehosp Emerg Care.* 2006;10(3):340–342.

SECTION III

EMS AND PUBLIC HEALTH

Since September 11, 2001, the Emergency Services community recognizes that there is a strong link between EMS and public health. In some areas of the United States, Paramedics are utilized to augment the public health system, whether as part of a response to a public health emergency or to augment day to day public health activities in areas of need. These chapters provide a foundation in the field of public health and illness and injury prevention to allow the Paramedic to fulfill these important roles in the healthcare system.

- **Chapter 7:** Public Health and the Paramedic
- **Chapter 8:** Illness and Injury Prevention

PUBLIC HEALTH AND THE PARAMEDIC

KEY CONCEPTS:

Upon completion of this chapter, it is expected that the reader will understand these following concepts:

- Improvement of a community's health status—the broad mission of public health
- The international issues relating to public health
- EMS as a "safety net" in public health
- EMS roles in healthcare access and disaster management

▶ CASE STUDY:

The local Paramedic agency had been called upon to assist in a mass flu inoculation program. Several of the inexperienced Paramedics said that while flu inoculation was important, they didn't see the relevance to EMS. Weren't nurses supposed to be doing this?

A senior Paramedic overheard them and suggested that after the program had concluded, they might want to research the relationship of flu immunization programs, public health, disaster management, and EMS. He offered to assist them in their research.

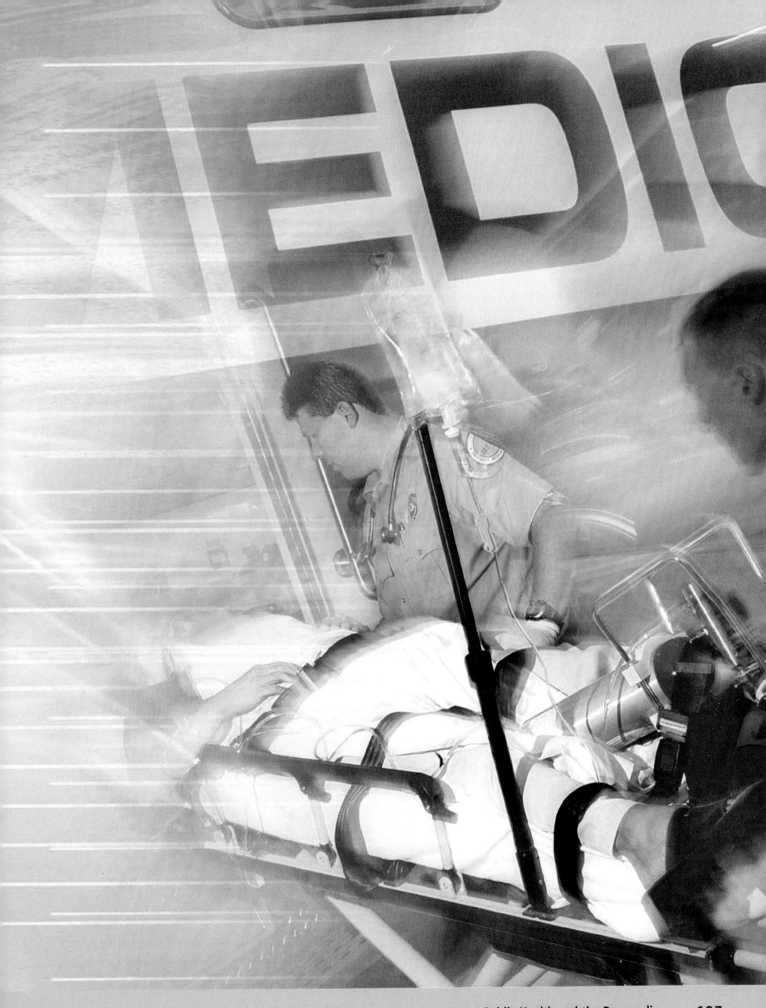

OVERVIEW

Public health extends farther than just the measurement of a community's absence of disease and infirmity. Rather, its broad mission is carried out through prevention and active response to improve the public health of communities. Many organizations exist, both internationally and in the United States, that contribute to the overall goal of public health. These organizations are beginning to recognize the value of EMS and the need to strengthen it as a "safety net" for public health. The growing role of EMS as an integrated part of today's public health system is discussed throughout the chapter.

What Is Public Health?

Health is defined by the **World Health Organization (WHO)**, the most prominent and influential international public health agency, as "a state of complete physical, mental, and social well-being and not merely the absence of disease and infirmity."[1] This state of well-being applies to not only individuals, but extends also to large groups, communities, and nations. Public health, therefore, is defined as the practice and discipline of improving the health of communities, and is focused primarily on **prevention** of illness and injury, discussed in detail in Chapter 8. As a secondary mission, public health agencies respond to disease outbreaks and disasters. In these instances, public health will work closely with Paramedics to prevent such occurrences from reaching catastrophic proportions. Thus, it is important for Paramedics to have an understanding of the organization of public health services in order to fully appreciate their mission and cooperate with their efforts for injury and illness prevention as well as disaster response.

Public Health in History

The concept of community-based disease prevention reaches far back into antiquity. The practice of **quarantine** (isolating diseased individuals from the larger community) can be traced back to biblical times when lepers were forced to live outside city limits and maintain their distance from non-lepers.

The ancient Romans understood the importance of sanitation in preventing the spread of disease throughout the empire and developed separate sewers and water delivery systems. Many of these aqueducts can still be seen throughout Europe, reminding us of the Romans' accomplishments in public health and disease prevention (Figure 7-1).

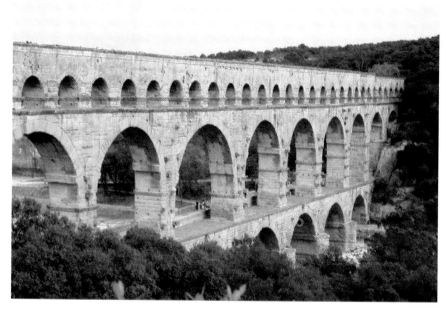

Figure 7-1 Roman aqueduct in Pont du Gard, France. Aqueducts like this one, built circa 19 B.C., would have carried water to supply an entire city. (Image copyright Riekephotos, 2009. Used under license from Shutterstock.com)

Koch's Postulates

1. The organism must be found in all animals suffering from a disease, but not in healthy animals.
2. The organism must be isolated from a diseased animal and grown in pure culture.
3. The cultured organism should cause disease when introduced into a healthy animal.
4. The organism must be reisolated from the experimentally infected animal.

Figure 7-2 Koch's postulates.

Table 7-1 Multidisciplinary Public Health Team

- Biologists
- Sociologists
- Social anthropologists
- Engineers
- Politicians
- Health educators
- Industrial hygienist
- Health reporter
- Sanitarians (Environmental health specialist)
- Physicians
- Nurses
- Paramedics

The practice of quarantine was even more prominent during the period of the bubonic plague (i.e,, Black Death), in fourteenth century Europe. During those times dead bodies were removed from the towns and cities in an attempt to eradicate the spread of the plague, another example of a public health practice.

Despite these early attempts at prevention, communicable diseases continued to spread largely unchecked. This was primarily due to a misunderstanding of the origins of disease. In the late nineteenth century, the germ theory of disease emerged, largely due to the work of the German physician Robert Koch (1843–1910).[2] Koch developed four "postulates" to establish that an organism is the cause of a particular disease (Figure 7-2). This landmark theory permitted public officials the opportunity to incorporate the ancient principles of quarantine while allowing physicians and scientists to identify, isolate, and inoculate the population. This combination of public health medicine and clinical medicine started to have an impact on mortality and morbidity from infectious disease.

Traditional Public Health Missions

The traditional focus of public health has been on women and children's health, substance abuse prevention, and workplace safety, including environmental safety. Accomplishing these public health missions requires the efforts of both healthcare providers such as physicians and nurses, as well as individuals and organizations from many disciplines. Table 7-1 lists some of the individuals involved in public health.

Challenges to the public's health (e.g., the H1N1 outbreak and the looming threat of cross-species infection) have placed a growing emphasis on public health medicine, spotlighting its ability to quickly identify infectious disease and prevent further progression of that disease through immunization.

Public Health Organization

Within public health there are several different subdivisions. These include epidemiology, environmental health, social and behavioral health, occupational health, and disaster planning and response. While there is considerable overlap between these individual subdivisions, their responsibilities

and contributions to the overall well-being of communities and populations are each unique.

Epidemiology/Biostatistics

Public health's mission has been to monitor, identify, and prevent outbreaks of disease. That mission is accomplished through epidemiology. Epidemiology is defined as "the branch of medical science that deals with the incidence, distribution, and control of disease in a population."[3] Epidemiologists are engaged in the surveillance of disease outbreaks and how particular diseases are spread within and between various populations. Based on these observations and the information gained from their research, recommendations can be made regarding public health intervention. The ongoing investigations in HIV are one example in which epidemiologists have been able to track which population groups are at greatest risk of contracting HIV and have assisted in developing prevention programs for these groups. Biostatistics is the application of statistical analysis to biological data, and is the mathematical component of epidemiology.

Environmental Health

Environmental health is considered the physical, chemical, biological, and psychosocial well-being of a person as it is related to the natural environment. It considers whether the environment is healthy for that person. Perhaps the most common subject in the field of environmental health is pollution. While pollution control has been practiced for centuries, it is only in the past 50 years that significant public health agendas have been aimed at reducing environmental pollution. Among these agendas have been programs to reduce noise, air, and light pollution, as evidenced in motor vehicle production standards. Sanitation, specifically human and consumer waste, is a branch of environmental health directed at preventing waste from polluting the soil and water. Finally, industrial and other toxic waste disposal is an important concern of environmental public health. Strict standards, such as the federal clean air act, have been established in an effort to contain such harmful waste and prevent it from contaminating soil, water, and air resources.

Social and Behavioral Health

While social and behavioral health issues may initially seem out of place in the public health sector, addressing these issues is very important to a population's overall well-being. An example of a problem that affects social health is overpopulation. Overcrowding is a significant public health problem in some urban parts of the United States as well as many countries throughout the world, notably China and India. Having a high concentration of people in a small area increases the risk of disease and raises public health concerns over sanitation and safety.

Recently this issue has been addressed in the prison systems, a microcosm of overcrowding, where there are barriers to healthcare access. The European section of the WHO has undertaken a project to improve the conditions in European prisons. Although significant progress has been made, there is still much to be done.[4]

Other social and behavioral health issues to address include adolescent sexual activity, sexually transmitted diseases, substance abuse, and mental health.

Occupational Health

In the past, workplace injury was commonplace. As a result, productivity suffered and the taxpayer's burden to support persons injured and out of work via worker's compensation was staggering. The field of occupational health is responsible for helping to maintain safety within workplaces, to decrease worker injury, and as a result to reduce health-related expenses.

In 1995, the International Labor Organization (ILO) and the WHO established goals for occupational health (Figure 7-3). Common workplace hazards identified included biological or chemical exposure, high noise levels, physical hazards such as falls and dangerous machinery, long hours, and sexual harassment. According to the ILO, the primary purpose of promoting occupational health is to decrease worker injury and to improve worker morale (i.e., a worker should not have to expect to risk life or limb by going to work). The ILO and the WHO, along with many professional organizations, are trying to develop a "culture of safety" where foreseeable risks are eliminated and injuries prevented.

Disaster Planning/Response

Within the past 10 years the world has witnessed numerous disasters, both natural and manmade. Natural disasters such as hurricanes, floods, tornados, and tsunamis have garnered international attention, as have the emergency services responses to these disasters. Since these disasters cannot be prevented, the quick and coordinated response to such events is crucial to prevent death and disability. Through preplanning

1. The promotion and maintenance of the highest degree of physical, mental, and social well-being of workers in all occupations.

2. The prevention amongst workers of departures from health caused by their working conditions.

3. The protection of workers in their employment from risks resulting from factors adverse to health.

4. The placing and maintenance of the worker in an occupational environment adapted to his physiological and psychological capabilities.

5. The adaptation of work to man and of each man to his job.

Figure 7-3 Goals of occupational health as developed by the Joint Committee of WHO/ILO in 1950 (revised 1995).

for predictable public disasters, public health planners can mitigate the resultant harm from these disasters.

Pandemics, outbreaks of diseases that spread throughout a country or a region, are a constant threat to public health.[5-9] These outbreaks of infectious disease may reach disaster proportions if not prevented or controlled in an appropriate fashion. Recent scares have included SARS and H1N1 flu. In addition to these natural disasters, large-scale accidents and mass casualties pose a threat not only for injury, but also for exposure to chemical and other environmental toxins. Witness the increase in asthma among responders to the World Trade Center attack of September 11, 2001.

Public health officials and researchers are involved in planning escape routes, resource mobilization, and response policies for such disasters, and continue to work with EMS providers in order to be prepared for these events if and when they occur.

Public Health Management

Several organizations exist to conduct public health research and implement public health law and policy. From international organizations such as the WHO to local health departments, these organizations work together to meet the goal of public well-being. Since each nation's public health structure is unique, it is not possible to describe the "typical" structure worldwide. Therefore, the remainder of the discussion, aside from an introduction to the international bodies, is based on the configuration in the United States.

International

The World Health Organization (WHO) is the most prominent and influential international public health agency. Founded in April 1948 as a specialized health agency under the United Nations, the WHO lists as its primary constitutional objective the "attainment by all peoples of the highest possible level of health."[1] Based in Geneva, Switzerland, the WHO is governed by 193 member nations and is managed by the

World Health Assembly, its international decision-making body. The WHO focuses efforts on monitoring disease outbreaks such as SARS, influenza, and HIV/AIDS, as well as assisting individual governments with the development and administration of vaccines. Largely through the efforts of the WHO, smallpox was declared eradicated in 1979, and polio is on the horizon to follow suit in the next several years. In addition to infectious disease research, the WHO is actively involved in dozens of other areas of medical and public health interest. These include chronic diseases such as hypertension and diabetes, as well as more indolent disorders such as blindness and birth defects. Further information about WHO can be obtained from their website: **http://www.who.int**

The World Federation of Public Health Associations (WFPHA) is an international nongovernmental organization established in 1967 to bring together multiple international public health workers for professional exchange, collaboration, and action. There are currently 70 member organizations, including the American Public Health Association, who meet annually to discuss partnerships and collaborative efforts in public health research and policy, share information and publications, and assist each other in the implementation of these policies in their respective countries. The WFPHA has an official liaison to the WHO, and they work in close cooperation. Current WFPHA projects include an international hand-washing campaign, global tobacco control and smoking cessation programs, HIV/AIDS research, and persistent organic pollutants eradication.

The American Public Health Movement

In the early 1800s American cities were being ravaged by epidemics of smallpox, yellow fever, and cholera. Quarantines and in-house confinement were the only effective means of preventing the spread of these diseases at the time. As a result, industry suffered from massive sick calls, leading to declines in productivity.[10–12]

In response to these epidemics, and in an effort to get workers back to work, a few wealthy patrons hired graduate nurses to care for the poor in Boston, Cincinnati, and Washington, DC. These nurses were referred to as community nurses. They worked in the ghettos and tenements of major cities to improve the public health and reduce the incidence of disease by teaching simple hygienic practices such as washing food as a part of its preparation.

Like modern day Paramedics, these public health nurses would leave the safety of their homes to go to workplaces, public houses, street corners, and clinics to meet with and teach the public about basic sanitary practices. Ms. Lillian Wald, RN, who was credited with coining the term "public health nurse," opened the Henry Street Settlement, a famous public health clinic, in New York City in 1793.[13]

Another significant problem at the time was infant mortality, particularly in the inner city. Many early public health efforts were meant to improve maternal–child health and decrease infant mortality. One of the earliest pioneers in the American public health movement was Dr. Sara Josephine Baker. Dr. Baker concerned herself with infant mortality. Dr. Baker worked tirelessly in the ghettos of New York City, particularly Hell's Kitchen, and helped to decrease the infant mortality rate through public education of proper maternal health practices.

The Federal Public Health Service

Another early origin of public health was the federal **Public Health Service (PHS)**. The origin of the PHS was preceded by the Marine Hospital Service (MHS). At that time, if a sailor got sick away from home he had nowhere to turn to for help. But if a sailor paid 20 cents a month to the Marine Hospital Service fund, the MHS would provide him with medical care if he should get sick away from home at a distant port of call.

The MHS, and then the PHS, would later became a key portion of the Department of Health and Human Services (DHHS). The current United States Public Health Service (US PHS) has 5,700 commissioned health services officers and 51,000 civilian employees, all led by the Surgeon General. THE US PHS provides logistical support to local, county, and state public health departments. It also provides direct patient health care to medically underserved areas in the United States.

Eight agencies comprise the current United States Public Health Service. These include the National Institutes for Health (NIH), the Food and Drug Administration (FDA), the Agency for Toxic Substances and Disease Registry (ATSDR), and the Centers for Disease Control and Prevention (CDC).

The Centers for Disease Control and Prevention (CDC) is the leading U.S. governmental agency for public health study. According to the CDC website, "since it was founded in 1946 to help control malaria, CDC has remained at the forefront of public health efforts to prevent and control infectious and chronic disease, injuries, workplace hazards, disabilities, and environmental health threats."[14]

Although officially under the auspices of the U.S. Department of Health and Human Services, the CDC is recognized independently worldwide for its significant contribution to public health and safety. Similar to the WHO, the CDC focuses research and policy efforts on emerging infectious diseases as well as chronic medical conditions and environmental health and safety.

Through its various publications, including the *Morbidity and Mortality Weekly Report* (MMWR) and *Emerging Infectious Disease Journal*, the CDC is able to communicate to federal, state, and local governments important relevant topics on an up-to-date basis. Furthermore, the CDC is regarded as an expert panel and its opinions on various public health issues within the United States are frequently cited in public reports and in the news media. Further information about the CDC can be obtained from its website: **http://www.cdc.gov**.

As described earlier, the American Public Health Association (APHA) is one of the member associations in the WFPHA. As a separate, distinct American organization, the APHA works to promote the health of American citizens through preventive efforts, research, and public health practice and policy.[15] While many of the projects are similar in scope and purpose to the CDC, the APHA exists as a nongovernmental agency within the United States and works with individual states and other individual organizations to reach their goals.

The Occupational Safety and Health Administration (OSHA) is the federal government's effort to promote occupational health. Founded in 1971 to reduce and prevent work-related injuries, illness, and death, OSHA is responsible for developing and enforcing various standards of safety in the workplace. Included within these workplace standards are standards for permissible exposure levels to chemicals and dusts, personal protective equipment, confined space conditions, and bloodborne pathogen exposure guidelines, the latter of which is of particular importance to EMS and other healthcare workers. More recently, OSHA has been developing prevention strategies to prevent pandemic influenza outbreak in workplaces.

State and Local

State and local governments are the primary source of public health policy and regulation. In addition, state and local health departments are involved in the enforcement of these regulations. Although national public health and safety guidelines are developed at the federal level (i.e., OSHA and other similar organizations), the state and local governments are responsible for developing and enacting the majority of public health laws in accordance with these accepted international and national standards. Frequently governed by a state's Department of Health, these agencies outline such policies as public smoking policies and laws, vaccination schedules, and restaurant and food service inspection. Many are also responsible for investigating outbreaks of illnesses within the state or local communities. EMS personnel will have the most contact with these local public health agencies and, as described in the following text, the greatest cooperative impact on health care and safety.

Public Health and EMS

In December 2001, a very important paper was published in the *Annals of Emergency Medicine* that outlined the joint efforts of public health and emergency medicine.[16] As an extension of the emergency department, EMS is considered crucial to delivering the highest quality care in both public health surveillance and response.

Because Paramedics are primarily a community-based health organization, they are in a position to assist public health officials with identification of infectious diseases and mass immunization of the public.

This role is just one of many roles that Paramedics could become involved with in public health. This fact was recognized in the report produced by the National Academy's Institutes of Medicine (IOM) entitled, "Emergency Medical Services at the Crossroads." In that report, the IOM spoke of the EMS's evolving role in health care and the need for public health and EMS to cooperate.

The IOM made specific reference to EMS as the "safety net" of the public's health, referring to the juncture where public health and clinical medicine meet. EMS is there, treating and transporting sick and injured patients, when the efforts of public health to prevent illness and injury have been unsuccessful. The IOM report also recognizes the complexity of the public health system and the need for different factions of health care to form strategic alliances in order to accomplish the mission to serve the common good.

With this renewed emphasis, the mission of EMS is now seen as being more in-step with the PHS than previously thought. A relationship between public health's physicians, nurses, scientists, and sanitarians and Paramedics is growing.

The potential intersections between Paramedics and public health care are numerous. For example, Paramedics could share demographic information on symptom patterns which are commonly associated with certain infectious diseases. With this information, public health departments could identify potential outbreaks by identifying groups, or clusters, of patients. Paramedics could also cooperate with public health's prevention education programs, advocate for healthcare changes, and lobby for legislative changes that improve the public's safety.

Healthcare Access

Another focus of public health is healthcare access. Public health is concerned with accessibility of health care to an individual and to a population. Without access to physicians and nurses, the public cannot receive immunizations, health education, and other preventive measures.

For many patients who do not have primary care physicians, the emergency department (ED) serves as a site for preventive (primary) medical care.[17–23] Although this arrangement is not ideal for either the patient or the ED, it nevertheless is a safety net for those patients who would otherwise have no medical care at all.

In addition to serving as a safety net for the underserved populations, the ED also operates in its primary function as a treatment center for acute medical and surgical conditions, providing a necessary service which complements the role of the primary medical provider as the manager of chronic conditions. The role of EMS providers in assisting these persons in transport to ED facilities in times of medical need is obviously an important link in the overall chain of healthcare access. Furthermore, the strategic location of EMS vehicles and personnel in various rural, suburban, and urban communities, an aspect of public health planning, allows Paramedics to be in the appropriate location at the appropriate time for optimal response.

Disaster Response

The partnership between EMS providers and public health officials in preparation for and response to pandemics, natural disasters, and mass casualties is vital to reducing morbidity and mortality in these situations. Joint preparation sessions—whether through drills, didactics, or tabletop exercises—allow individuals from each organization to meet and become familiar with each other and one another's roles. The development of specialized response teams, escape routes, shelter management, and quarantine strategies can be planned and implemented utilizing both public health and EMS resources. Additional cooperation of other governmental and private relief agencies further strengthens the response network and provides greater preparation for an actual event.

CONCLUSION

Health is defined as a state of complete physical, mental, and social well-being. Public health is the practice of maintaining and improving the health of a community, and is focused on primary and secondary prevention of illness and injury. In addition, public health agencies are involved in providing a response to disease and disaster, working closely with EMS personnel to provide the necessary public services when these events occur. It is important for EMS providers to understand the organization and workings of public health on the international, national, state, and especially local levels in order to cooperate and participate in the various prevention and response operations they will collectively encounter.

KEY POINTS:

- Public health is defined as the practice and discipline of improving the health of communities. Although the primary focus is prevention of illness and injury, public health agencies work closely with Paramedics when responding to disease outbreaks and disasters.

- Public health had its roots in community-based practices of quarantine and improved water sanitation, but communicable diseases continued to spread largely unchecked until the development of germ theory of disease.

- The public health team is made up of both healthcare providers and individuals and organizations. Within public health there are several different subdivisions. These include epidemiology, environmental health, social and behavioral health, occupational health, and disaster planning and response.

- Epidemiology is the branch of medical science that deals with the incidence, distribution, and control of disease in a population.

- Environmental health is considered the physical, chemical, biological, and psychosocial well-being of a person as it is related to the natural environment.

- Social and behavioral health addresses issues that are important to the overall well-being of a population, such as adolescent sexual activity, sexually transmitted diseases, substance abuse, and mental health.

- The field of occupational health is responsible for helping to maintain safety within workplaces.

- Disaster planning and response begins with the examination of predictable public disasters such as natural disasters, outbreaks of infectious disease, large-scale accidents and mass casualties, and exposure to chemical and other environmental toxins.

- The partnership between EMS providers and public health officials is vital to reducing morbidity and mortality in disaster situations.

- The World Health Organization (WHO) focuses efforts on monitoring disease outbreaks, developing and administering vaccines, researching infectious diseases, and managing chronic diseases and disorders.

- The public health movement was first started by public health nurses and other individuals who worked to reduce the incidence of disease and infant mortality through public education of proper health practices.

- Led by the Surgeon General, the U.S. PHS provides logistical support to local, county, and state public health departments as well as direct patient health care to medically underserved areas in the United States.

- The Centers for Disease Control (CDC) focuses research and policy efforts on emerging infectious diseases as well as chronic medical conditions and environmental health and safety.

- The Occupational Safety and Health Administration (OSHA) is the federal government agency that is responsible for developing and enforcing various standards of safety in the workplace. OSHA's policies aim at reducing and preventing work-related injuries, illness, and death.

- One of the many roles that Paramedics may become involved with in public health is the identification of infectious diseases and mass immunization of the public.

- Public health is also concerned with the public's access to health care, such as immunizations, health education, and other preventive measures. EMS assists with patient access by responding and transporting patients to the ED to receive appropriate care.

REVIEW QUESTIONS:

1. Other than prevention, what is the focus of public health?
2. How did germ theory affect the treatment of disease?
3. What are the five subdivisions of public health?
4. How can officials better plan for and respond to predictable public disasters?
5. What is the World Health Organization's role in public health?
6. How did the public health movement begin in the United States?
7. What state and federal departments are responsible for public health programs?
8. Describe how the Centers for Disease Control and the Occupational Safety and Health Administration work to improve public health.
9. Explain how the mission of EMS is in-step with the Public Health Service.
10. How does EMS help to improve public access to health care?

CASE STUDY QUESTIONS:

Please refer to the Case Study at the beginning of the chapter and answer the questions below.

1. In addition to increasing the number of people immunized against the flu, what other benefits arise from EMS participation in a mass flu immunization program?
2. How is an immunization program related to the mission of EMS?

REFERENCES:

1. http://www.who.int/en/
2. Brock T. *Robert Koch: A Life in Medicine and Bacteriology.* Berlin, NY: Science Tech Publishers; 1999.
3. http://www.merriam-webster.com/
4. Gatherer A, Moller L, Hayton P. The World Health Organization European Health in Prisons Project after 10 years: persistent barriers and achievements. *Am J Public Health.* 2005;95(10):1696–1700.
5. Smolinski MS, Hamburg MA, Lederberg J. *Microbial Threats to Health: Emergence, Detection & Response.* Washington DC: Natl Academy Pr; 2003.
6. Brundage JF. Cases and deaths during influenza pandemics in the United States. *Am J Prev Med.* 2006;31(3):252–256.
7. Sloan FA, Berman S, Rosenbaum S, Chalk RA, Giffin RB. The fragility of the U.S. vaccine supply. *N Engl J Med.* 2004;351(23):2443–2447.

8. Webby RJ, Webster RG. Are we ready for pandemic influenza? *Science*. 2003;302(5650):1519–1522.

9. Spicuzza L, Spicuzza A, La Rosa M, Polosa R, Di Maria G. New and emerging infectious diseases. *Allergy Asthma Proc*. 2007;28(1):28–34.

10. Bourdelais P. *Epidemics Laid Low: A History of What Happened in Rich Countries*. Baltimore: The Johns Hopkins University Press; 2006.

11. Steel J. Inappropriate—the patient or the service? *Accid Emerg Nurs*. 1995;3(3):146–149.

12. Lee PR. Health policy and the health of the public. A two hundred year perspective. *Mobius*. 1984;4(3):95–113.

13. Wald L. *The House on Henry Street (Philanthropy and Society)*. New Brunswick: Transaction Publishers; 1991.

14. http://www.cdc.gov/

15. http://www.apha.org/

16. Pollock DA, Lowery DW, O'Brien PM. Emergency medicine and public health: new steps in old directions. *Ann Emerg Med*. 2001;38(6):675–683.

17. Bezzina AJ, Smith PB, Cromwell D, Eagar K. Primary care patients in the emergency department: who are they? A review of the definition of the "primary care patient" in the emergency department. *Emerg Med Australas*. 2005; 17(5-6):472–479.

18. Wise M. Inappropriate attendance in accident and emergency. *Accid Emerg Nurs*. 1997;5(2):102–106.

19. Hamlin C, Sheard S. Revolutions in public health: 1848, and 1998? *Bmj*. 1998;317(7158):587–591.

20. Byrne M, Murphy AW, Plunkett PK, McGee HM, Murray A, Bury G. Frequent attenders to an emergency department: a study of primary health care use, medical profile, and psychosocial characteristics. *Ann Emerg Med*. 2003;41(3):309–318.

21. Richardson S. Emergency departments and the inappropriate attender—is it time for a reconceptualisation of the role of primary care in emergency facilities? *Nurs Prax N Z*. 1999;14(2):13–20.

22. Richman IB, Clark S, Sullivan AF, Camargo CA, Jr. National study of the relation of primary care shortages to emergency department utilization. *Acad Emerg Med*. 2007;14(3):279–282.

23. Young GP, Sklar D. Health care reform and emergency medicine. *Ann Emerg Med*. 1995;25(5):666–674.

CHAPTER 8

ILLNESS AND INJURY PREVENTION

KEY CONCEPTS:

Upon completion of this chapter, it is expected that the reader will understand these following concepts:

- Impact of public health prevention programs
- Decision making based on surveillance of injury
- The Haddon matrix and injury countermeasures
- The 4-E's of injury prevention strategy
- Evaluating an injury prevention program
- Recognizing teachable moments for the Paramedic

▶ CASE STUDY:

For the fourth time this month, the Paramedics went to the same address for the same man with the same complaint . . . exacerbation of his chronic obstructive lung disease. The man was a heavy smoker all of his life. Even though he said he had quit, you could still see the yellow on his fingers and smell the smoke on his clothing.

The Paramedics wondered about the numerous stop smoking campaigns that were available. Which ones worked? How could they assist in getting people to quit or, better yet, never start?

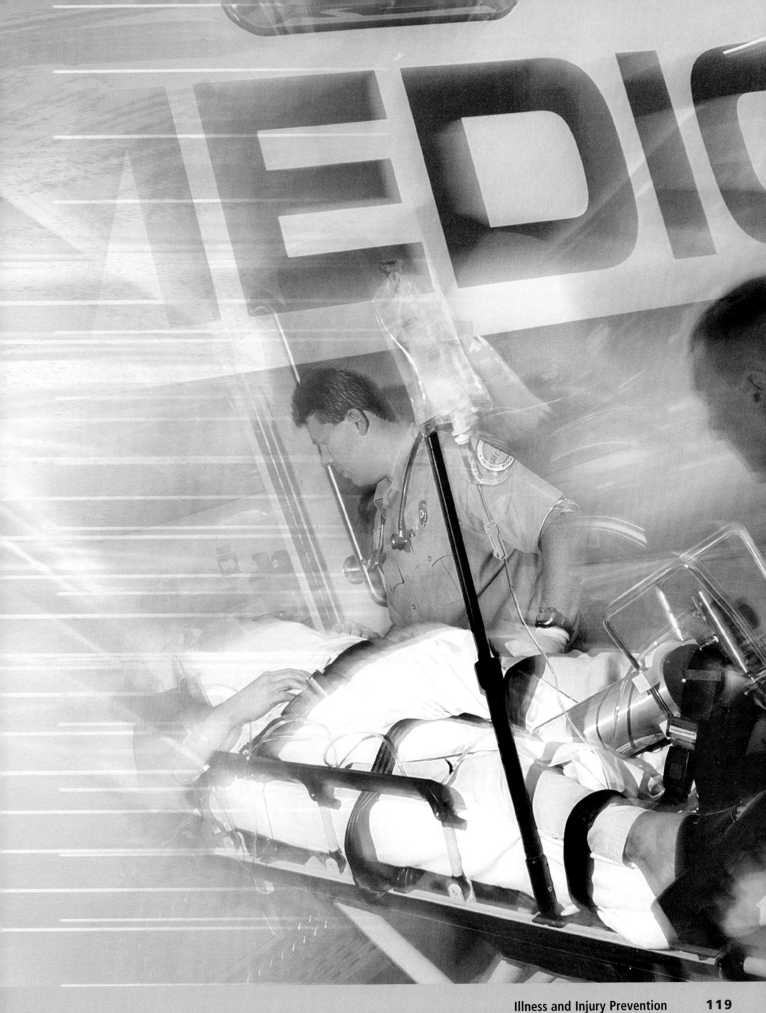

OVERVIEW

Because the Paramedic's goal is to help others, it becomes the Paramedic's mission to help prevent injury as well. Public health promotion programs have proven themselves time and time again. EMS, as a profession, has therefore evolved to include these programs in its mission. Decisions on how to develop public health promotion programs arose from observations, or surveillance of injuries. The Haddon Matrix represents the many opportunities for change and injury countermeasures that can be implemented. Although any of the 4-E's of the injury prevention strategy can be used in a public health program, education is perhaps the best vehicle for making a difference.

Public Health

The focus of public health is to promote the wellness of a community or a people in order to improve the health of the population. The tenants of public health medicine are consistent with the concepts of primary care. Primary care medicine states that it is easier to prevent disease or injury in an individual rather than treat it.[1,2] However, public health differs from primary care because public health treats communities whereas primary care treats individuals. Because of its community focus, public health concentrates on the detection of community-wide disease and the creation of programs for **injury prevention**.

Public health helps to reduce the cost of health care, through prevention and/or reduction of injury and illness, and therefore provides significant economic benefits to the community. Many people believe that public health is rightfully a function of government. Governments, in general, are formed to secure the people's welfare and help ensure a population's prosperity. Therefore, public health can be viewed as a matter of national security in that the country's health provides for that country's social stability.

Impact of Public Health Prevention Programs

In the past, the spread of infectious diseases (such as smallpox and the plague) was rampant and mortality from these diseases was very high.[3] In some instances, public officials would attempt to enforce public health measures, such as quarantine, in an attempt to halt the transmission of these diseases, with varying degrees of success. However, the result of these "after the fact" measures was premature death, evidenced by an average life expectancy of 30 years.

In the last century, the average life expectancy in the western world has steadily increased to the point where it is over 70 years in most industrialized countries. This improvement can be attributed to a combination of improvements in preventive medicine and to broad public health measures such as sanitation systems and water purification plants.

Public Health Prevention Initiatives

Currently public health is involved in many illness and injury prevention initiatives including family planning, smoking cessation programs, workplace safety, and motor vehicle safety (Table 8-1). These initiatives were all chosen because they represented an area of significant mortality for the public.

The success of these initiatives can be seen in the efforts of public health to influence family health and planning. Through education, promotion of well-baby visits, childhood immunization programs, and freestanding clinics, infant mortality has dropped 90% from 1900 to the present and maternal mortality has dropped 99%.[4,5]

Paramedics may recognize the effects of these efforts over the decades in terms of injury from motor vehicle collisions. Improvements in motor vehicle safety through improved motor vehicle engineering (e.g., seat belts and airbags) and improved road design (e.g., civil engineering) have resulted in a marked decrease in mortality and morbidity in motor vehicle collisions.

Injury Surveillance

Injury and illness detection is the first step in injury and illness prevention. Based upon research and statistical data concerning the incidence of a disease or the prevalance of an injury, public health officials can make judgments about the need for new prevention programs or the revision of an existing prevention program. Therefore, for public

Table 8-1 Examples of Paramedic Public Health Initiatives

Pedestrian safety	Bicycle lanes and sidewalks
Bicycle safety	Helmet patrols (ice cream tickets)
SIDS	Back to sleep programs
Drowning prevention	Pool inspections
Child passenger safety	Childseat inspections
Food safety	Health inspections

health officials to make good decisions they need accurate information (surveillance). This process, surveillience and prevention, is consistent with the "plan-do-check-act" cycle of quality improvement.

Early Efforts at Injury Surveillance

One of the early champions for public safety and injury prevention was Ralph Nader. Nader and his associates, referred to as Nader's raiders, would investigate and report to the public items and goods that they deemed unsafe. These early efforts amounted to surveillance of a problem and a recommendation for action to reduce or eliminate the problem. One problem Nader was concerned about was the high incidence of mortality caused by ejection from a motor vehicle.

Largely as a result of Nader's vigorous lobbying of the government and industry, cars were required to have case-hardened steel pins, later called Nader pins, installed in car door locks. These Nader pins prevented passengers from being ejected during a motor vehicle collision, and have therefore saved countless lives. Nader's influence in injury prevention serves as an example of one group's ability to have a positive impact on the community's health through injury surveillance and action.

Trauma Surveillance

While Dr. "Deke" Farrington's article "Death in a Ditch" and the 1966 white paper "Accidental Death and Disability: The Neglected Disease of Modern Society" brought the problem of trauma to the forefront, it took another white paper, "Injury in America: A Continuing Public Health Problem" to emphasize the lack of injury prevention.[6,7]

Written by the National Academy of Sciences in 1983, "Injury in America" emphasized that injury prevention is more cost-effective than injury treatment. As a result, Congress dedicated funding to injury surveillance and prevention. Subsequently, the federal Centers for Disease Control was tasked with injury surveillance and created the Division of Injury Control, which is now called the **National Centers for Injury Prevention and Control** and the name of the federal Centers for Disease Control was changed to the Center for Disease Control and Prevention.

There are 10 national injury prevention and control centers across the country (Table 8-2), each with a focus on regional injury interests, and all are a part of a national network of injury prevention programs.

Injury statistics are also compiled in the National Trauma Registry, which is maintained by regional trauma centers. This registry is an invaluable source of data regarding trauma and trauma trends. Selected data fields, called a data set, are gleaned from the patient care record (PCR) produced by Paramedics.

High-performing EMS agencies typically consult the trauma registry for valuable information regarding topics for continuing medical education and professional development in order to keep current and ensure Paramedics are prepared for

Table 8-2 National Centers for Injury Prevention Programs

1. University of Alabama
2. University of California at Los Angeles (UCLA)
3. University of California at San Francisco
4. Harvard School of Public Health
5. University of Iowa
6. Johns Hopkins University School of Hygiene and Public Health
7. University of North Carolina
8. University of Washington, Harborview Medical Center
9. University of Pittsburgh, Center for Injury Research and Control
10. Colorado State University

the pressing trauma conditions at that time. This information is also used to create injury prevention programs focused on the specific trauma issues encountered in a given region.

EMS and Injury Prevention

As a part of an approach to provide comprehensive prehospital care, Paramedics have been increasingly involved in public health efforts. Injury prevention programs, in particular, have involved Paramedics.

In 1996, the National Highway Safety and Traffic Administration (NHSTA) helped to create a consensus statement regarding EMS and injury prevention. That statement, "Role of EMS in Injury Prevention," affirmed the position of EMS as a legitimate source for injury prevention education.[8] It was hoped that the consensus paper, sent out for peer-review to some 300 leaders in the EMS community, would help to shift some of the focus of EMS toward injury prevention and health promotion.

EMS was specifically identified as a vehicle for this injury prevention campaign because of its unique advantages. EMS agencies are, at their essence, community-based organizations which blend public safety with public health to provide a service, EMS.[9–11] In their role as EMS providers, Paramedics enjoy the public's respect. This high-credibility affords them an effective platform from which to educate and to support changes, especially regarding injury prevention.

Injury Prevention Theory and the Haddon Matrix

Starting in 1963, William Haddon, Jr., the first director of the NHSTA, started work on an injury prevention matrix, an easily understood concept map of injury casuation and prevention. Using a model similar to one used for disease, Haddon plotted the factors that cause injury across a horizontal X-axis and the stages of an injury process along the Y-axis. The result was an injury prevention matrix.

Each square in the **Haddon matrix** represents an opportunity to intervene and either prevent or mitigate the effects of traumatic injury. The matrix helps people recognize that the Paramedic is not limited to affecting traumatic injury only after an injury occurs. It emphasizes that there are other opportunities to affect traumatic injury. The horizontal X-axis contains the elements host, agent, and environment, taken from the **Public Health Model**. In the case of injury, the host is the patient and the host's characteristics are those human factors, such as alcohol intoxication, which come into play during an injury.

The agent is the source of the injury. In broadest terms, it is the source of the mechanical (kinetic), chemical, electrical, thermal, or radiation energy that, when inflicted on someone, causes trauma. For example, a handgun would be the agent of injury in a pediatric gunshot wound.

The final X-axis component is the environment. The environment consists of those circumstances which have an impact on the trauma. The environment can be further subdivided into social environment and physical environment. The physical environment, in the case of pediatric gunshot wounds, would be the presence of a handgun in the home. The social environment would be the combination of the adult's attitude regarding handgun ownership, laws pertaining to handgun registration, and the child's innate curiosity.

Marked along the Y-axis are the stages of injury: pre-event, event, and post-event. These stages correspond with the three levels of medicine: primary care, secondary care, and tertiary care. Table 8-3 illustrates a Haddon matrix, using the problem of accidental shootings in the pediatric population and interventions as an example. These interventions are only theoretical. The appeal of the Haddon matrix is that it allows—and almost encourages—free-thinking (i.e., "thinking outside of the box") about solutions to public health problems.

Injury Countermeasures

In 1970, Haddon produced another paper on injury prevention, entitled "On the Escape of Tigers: An Ecological Note." The paper precisely detailed the 10 levels of **countermeasures** that could be effective in reducing injury. Starting from pre-incident (i.e., preventative medicine) and proceeding through to post-incident or clinical medicine, Haddon lays out the logical points for effective intervention in injury prevention.

The first intervention point for prevention would be elimination of the offending agent. While in some cases, such as handguns, this may appear unreasonable, consider the case that was made for nuclear disarmament. That is, the ability to possess the weapons exists but there is a decision not to possess them.

If the agent (i.e., the hazard) cannot be eliminated, then perhaps it can be reduced to a non-lethal level. For example, a pharmacist is only allowed to fill a limited prescription of tricyclic antidepressants. This limited number of pills dispensed helps to ensure that less than lethal doses are readily available to the potentially suicidal patient with depression.

If the hazard cannot be eliminated or reduced, then perhaps the hazard can be contained in order to prevent its release or use. For example, pools have long been recognized as an attractive nuisance to children. Many accidental drownings have occurred in unsupervised pools. An example of containment of this hazard would be to assemble fences, with padlocked gates, around pools. This containment measure is mandated by law in many communities.

If the hazard cannot be eliminated, nor reduced, nor contained, then perhaps the rate of release can be slowed, and/or distributed over time, in order to decrease the impact of the event. Airbags and padded steering wheels are designed to dissipate the energy in a collision across both a larger area as well as over a longer time.

If the hazard cannot be eliminated, nor reduced, nor contained, nor slowed, then the only alternative is to eliminate the target (i.e., the host). A case in which the host, the patient, is eliminated is highways are closed during snow emergencies. A declared snow emergency, enforced with the force of law, prevents motorists from even being on the highway under potentially dangerous conditions.

In some cases, if the host can be removed, then protecting the host is the best option. Safety engineers have created many barrier devices, ranging from simple gloves to soft body armor, to protect the host (people) from injury.

If contact between the agent and the host is inevitable, then modification of some basic quality of the agent could be considered. For example, enlarging the size of baseballs

Table 8-3 Haddon Matrix for Accidental Pediatric Shootings

Problem Statement:
CDC reports, in the year 2000, that there was a 58% increase in the number of gun accidents in the pediatric population aged 0–4 years of age, or 1,200 accidental pediatric shootings.

	Host	Agent	Physical Environment	Social Environment
	Children age 0–4	Handguns loaded	Home bedside	United States Right to bear arms
Pre-incident	Gun safety education	Trigger locks	Gun lock boxes	Gun regulation
Incident	Pediatric shooting	Restriction Body armor	Gun alarms Fully automatic	Gun ownership Education classes
Post-incident	Pediatric GSW EMS	Automatic confiscation	Trauma systems	Community statistics Pediatric GSW education

to what we now call the softball decreased the incidence of orbital fractures in children playing baseball.

In addition, modifying the host (the patient) to be more resilient to injury can help to decrease the injury's incidence or severity. For example, many healthcare plans offer employee exercise programs to improve the health of their participants and increase the participants' resilence to injury and illness, thereby diminishing the effect of the hazard/agent.

If injury cannot be prevented and yet is foreseeable, then systems for the rapid detection, treatment, and evacuation to definitive treatment need to be in place. This essentially describes the mission of EMS.

However, improvement in these systems can increase the efficiency and the effectiveness of EMS. An example of an improved means of detection is the addition of technology for location identification of cellular telephone users. This can improve the communications specialist's ability to send needed help. OnStar® is one system available in motor vehicles that detects and reports—through impact sensors, cellular technology, and global positioning systems—the location and extent of a motor vehicle collision back to a public safety access point (PSAP).

Finally, efforts to improve tertiary care and rehabilitation will diminish the long-term impacts of injury. Prostethetics, used to treat wounded soldiers of the Irag war, have improved tremendously and offer an improved quality of life to these veterans.

Injury Prevention Strategies

Injury prevention strategies are ways to go about implementing Haddon's countermeasures.[12] These can include engineering safety into products or processes, educating people about the dangers, increasing or improving enforcement of laws and regulations which promote safety, and providing economic incentives for people to use safer products or processes.

Paramedics, when trying to brainstorm injury prevention strategies for inclusion in Haddon's countermeasures, can consider four basic strategies, the "4-E's," of injury prevention.

The first E, engineering, refers to the addition of safety devices during the engineering phase of product design that will prevent injury. The creation of needleless intravenous administration sets is an example of safety engineering. In this case, the injury, accidental needlesticks, is eliminated through a pre-incident intervention which affects the agent.

The next E, education, requires that the educator change the behavior of the host, the population, in a substantial manner. To affect such change, educators usually must energize learners, through motivational speaking, to change behaviors that may have already been engrained into their lives. Understandably, the impact of injury prevention is greatest when the learner has not already learned the behavior and is just initially learning the "correct" behavior, the one that will decrease injury. An example of the impact of education

on injury prevention is seat belt safety seminars. Following public education campaigns about the importance of seat belt use, the use of seat belts remains highest in younger drivers. Older drivers, taught to drive when seat belts were not mandatory, have been more resistant to change.

The third E, law enforcement, is actually a form of learning. Law enforcement provides punishment for nonconformance with safety regulations, a form of operant conditioning. Enforcement of safety regulations, such as speed limits, and the resultant punishment of fees and fines provide the host with a powerful incentive to change behavior.

The fourth and final E is economic incentives. It is also a form of education—positive operant conditioning. Efforts to behave safely or to correct behaviors are encouraged by positive feedback, in the form of economic reward. For example, some EMS systems distribute tickets for ice cream cones to children seen wearing bicycle helmets. Another example might be a rebate after the purchase of a child's car seat or a smoke detector.

Assessment

Whenever Paramedics or an agency become involved in primary injury prevention, using any of the previous strategies, they are improving the quality of health in their jurisdiction. Therefore, like all EMS activities, injury prevention is included in the quality improvement cycle.

The first portion of the PDCA cycle of quality improvement is planning. Several key questions should be answered before implementation of the initiative as the answers may affect the decision-making process. Every suggested improvement, whether it is implementing an educational program or purchasing a product with an engineered safety feature, needs to be weighed in a cost-benefit analysis. The cost, whether financial or otherwise, must be considered in light of the potential benefit to be gained from the proposed change.

For instance, is the cost of the product (for example, a self-protecting intravenous catheter) worth the benefit of reduced needlestick injuries which can cost, by some estimates, as much as $5,000 per incident? Would one potentially preventable needlestick injury pay for the increased costs of the new intravenous catheters?

Intrinsic within the cost-benefit analysis is the question of acceptance by the user. A safer device that is not used offers no benefit. For example, workers must use the safer device in order to prevent injuries. OSHA recognized this fact when it required the participation of nonmanagerial front-line employees in the decision-making process for utilization of personal protective equipment (29 CFR 1910.1030(c)(1)(v).

Also taken into consideration during planning is the concept of equity. Safety changes (e.g., workplace routines) must be equitable. **Equity** is a concept of fairness or evenhandedness. To be accepted, any change must appear to be equitable to all parties concerned.

Changes that are broadly applied to all individuals would be said to have **horizontal equity**. For example, the blood alcohol level of 0.08 is considered the limit in most states for driving while intoxicated. This legal limitation is an example of an effort to prevent alcohol-related collisions by reducing the threshold for law enforcement. The change is then applied to everyone.

However, in some instances it is more appropriate to provide an injury prevention program to one group of people who are unduly affected by a problem. This unequal treatment, preferential or targeted treatment, tends to improve the health of that specific group. However, it also tends to reduce the burden carried by the rest of the population in the form of higher taxes or insurance premiums. This type of injury prevention program would create **vertical equity**. For example, if statistics demonstrate a higher number of accidental shootings among children in low-income households, then public health programs could be justifiably organized to emphasize prevention within that population.

When Paramedics are planning injury prevention programs, they should be sensitive to the problem of **stigma**. Stigma is a negative connotation attached to participation in a program, such as labeling and public embarassment. For example, a prevention program that asks drug abusers to come forward and be identified before participation in a drug treatment program may not meet with much acceptance by the intended beneficiaries. The potential participants may be concerned about persecution and public ridicule as well as labeling. The success of Alcoholics Anonymous is owed, in part, to the anonymity that participants are provided while they recover.

The final question concerns the feasibility of any proposed changes. In some instances, prevention programs require the reallocation of scarce resources, including personnel and funds. The reallocation of essential resources requires the enlightened thinking of EMS leaders who can see the long-term benefit of such programs. Unfortunately, the realities of politics often interfere with these programs. As a result, many prevention programs—both local and federal—have fallen due to budget cuts and other immediacies.

Implementation

To lead successful injury prevention programs, EMS leaders must first get Paramedics to invest, intellectually and spiritually, in these programs. The changing safety paradigm in EMS, placing personal safety above all else, is helping Paramedics see the benefits of injury prevention programs.

Chapter 3 on personal well-being emphasized the importance of safety and injury prevention. Paramedics, cognizant of their roles as models for their community, may minimally demonstrate those safety habits that they would have the public emulate. For example, passing motorists who see a Paramedic wearing a seat belt, driving with headlights on during the daytime, or using headlights along with windshield wipers, may imitate the Paramedic's action. These injury prevention efforts can have a positive impact.

Teaching Injury Prevention

Paramedics appreciate that every call for an injured person has the potential for being a moment to reflect on the activity that caused the injury and consider how to prevent that injury in the future. That moment is called the **teachable moment**. A teachable moment might be defined as the time when the patient has a heightened awareness of a problem and is receptive to information. The positive impact which prevention can have to prevent future injury can be mentioned.

Use of this opportunity to teach, to change the behavior of another person, must be carefully considered. Ill-chosen words can sound accusatory and produce an effect opposite of the intended effect. The patient may perceive the well-intentioned words of a Paramedic as victim blaming. Victim blaming is counterproductive to the goal at hand, preventing a similar occurrence in the future, and tends to cause hostile feelings. For example, lecturing a patient with emphysema about the ill effects of smoking at a time when the patient is short of breath is both ill-advised and counterproductive to the goal of smoking cessation. It would be better if the Paramedic were to offer supportive and nonjudgmental care to the patient at the present time and then leave the card of a smoking cessation program with a family member.

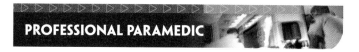

PROFESSIONAL PARAMEDIC

Many behaviors are culturally related. The professional Paramedic should recognize that changing a behavior may be better accomplished through Paramedic cultural or religious networks. The goal is assisting the patient, not the Paramedic's glory.

EMS Injury Prevention Programs

Some Paramedics may still be hesitant about getting involved in public education for injury prevention, citing concerns about this "new" role. But these Paramedics should be aware that other Paramedics have been remarkably successful with public education campaigns in the past. A model for EMS success in injury prevention is the EPIC medic program in San Diego.[13] The San Diego Paramedics created an injury prevention project entitled Eliminate Preventable Injuries of Children (EPIC). Using a combination of home safety assessments, pool safety inspections, child passenger seat safety education, and several other initiatives, these Paramedics have strived to make their community a safer environment for children.

The success of programs like the EPIC medic program has not gone unnoticed by their peers and the community alike. For example, the EPIC Paramedics were awarded the Nicholas Rosecrans Award, a national award recognizing

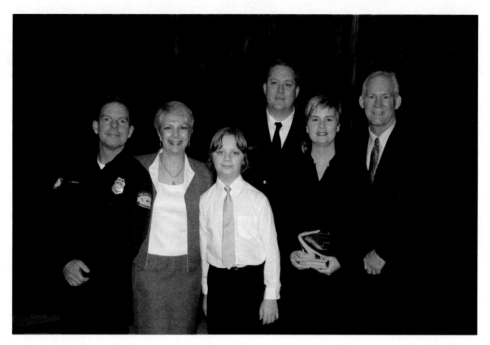

Figure 8-1 The EPIC team receiving the Nicholas Rosecrans Award for excellence in injury prevention. (Courtesy of EPIC medics; photo by Jeff Lucia)

excellence in injury prevention in EMS (Figure 8-1). The Nicolas Rosecrans Award is given to agencies or individuals for community work with injury prevention. Specifically, this prestigious award may be given to those agencies or persons who have either established or expanded a comprehensive injury prevention program, promoted injury prevention within the EMS community, improved the delivery of EMS to injured patients, or successfully created collaborations or partnerships with other public safety organizations to advance injury prevention.

Outcomes

Action without reflection cannot be said to be effective, for there is no measurement of the change. Statements about the effectiveness of an injury prevention program require verification. A process of evaluation, the checking portion in the PDCA cycle, is an integral part of any injury prevention program.

The measurement of any success, including success in injury prevention, is typically data-driven. The measurement should involve both the means and the end. Measuring means,

or **process evaluation**, includes statistics on attendance, among other items, and explains how the program was implemented. This information is vital to a later analysis of cost versus benefit. In some cases, the outcome may be acceptable even though more efficient or effective means of achieving that goal are available or possible.

The measurement of ends, or **outcomes evaluation**, is a matter of comparing the level of injury or illness before and after the program. The initiative is evaluated to determine whether the program made a difference. For example, data about rates of injury in motor vehicle collisions following a seat belt campaign can be obtained from patient care records (PCR) or trauma registry statistics. Statements about the success or failure of injury prevention programs rest on the result of the outcomes evaluation. For example, Pinellas County EMS in Florida established a pool safety campaign after a series of drownings. Kicking off with a media campaign to announce the campaign, the Paramedics of Pinellas County performed public education programs, pool safety inspections, and the like. Following the campaign, Pinellas County EMS was able to show a 43% reduction in drowning.[14] These kinds of hard numbers tend to impress the public and politicians alike.

CONCLUSION

With the specter of Avian flu, the epidemic in obesity, and the proliferation of drug-resistant diseases, there will be many opportunities for Paramedics to work with public health in a strategic alliance that can be synergistic and provide the best outcome for the public.

KEY POINTS:

- Public health is based on the premise that, as a community, it is easier to prevent disease or injury than provide treatment. With public health, the concentration lies on the detection of community-wide disease and the creation of programs for injury prevention.

- Current public health prevention initiatives include family planning, smoking cessation programs, workplace safety, and motor vehicle safety. These initiatives are areas of focus because they have been shown to result in significant mortality for the public.

- In order for public health officials to make good decisions, they need accurate information or surveillance. Ralph Nader pioneered early surveillance efforts by investigating and reporting to the public about items and goods that were deemed unsafe. The Paramedic can appreciate improvements on motor vehicle safety that resulted in the marked decrease in mortality and morbidity in motor vehicle collisions.

- Stemming from several documents that emphasized the lack of injury prevention and the notion that prevention is more cost-effective than injury treatment, the National Centers for Injury Prevention and Control were established. These centers, along with the National Trauma Registry, gather data regarding injury interests.

- The National Highway Safety and Traffic Administration (NHSTA) helped to increase the Paramedic's involvement in public health efforts. This is in part because EMS agencies are community-based organizations, which affords them an effective platform for community education and injury prevention.

- The first director of the NHSTA developed an injury prevention matrix based on the factors that cause injury and the stages of an injury process. The matrix emphasized that there is an opportunity for the Paramedic to affect traumatic injury before injury occurs.

- In another paper on injury prevention, Haddon detailed 10 logical points or countermeasures for effective intervention in injury prevention. An example of Haddon's logic that is pertinent to paramedicine is that, if injury cannot be prevented and yet is foreseeable, then systems for the rapid detection, treatment, and evacuation of definitive treatment need to be in place.

- The "4-E's"—engineering, education, law enforcement, and economic incentives—are basic strategies that the Paramedic can use when brainstorming injury prevention strategies for inclusion in Haddon's countermeasure of injury prevention.

- Injury prevention is included in the quality improvement cycle. For each suggested improvement, a cost-benefit analysis should be made. Equity should also be taken into consideration, as well as any stigma that may be associated with the program. The feasibility of any proposed changes should be assessed.

- Implementation and the success of injury prevention programs depend on how much the Paramedic invests intellectually and spiritually into the program. The changing safety paradigm in EMS, placing personal safety above all else, is helping Paramedics see the benefits of injury prevention programs.

- An appropriate teachable moment might be defined as the time when the patient has a heightened awareness of a problem and is receptive to information given by the Paramedic.

- An evaluation process is an integral part of any injury prevention program. The measurement should include the process evaluation and the outcomes evaluation. These statements about the success or failure can be used to determine how efficient or effective the process was and how effective the program was overall.

REVIEW QUESTIONS:

1. Why is EMS an excellent vehicle for injury prevention programs?
2. What agencies compile injury statistics and why?
3. What does the Haddon matrix emphasize?
4. What is the first point of injury prevention?
5. What injury prevention point is similar to the mission of EMS?
6. How are the 4-E's used in brainstorming injury prevention strategies?
7. Identify the four components of the quality improvement cycle.
8. What do EMS providers need to invest into an injury prevention program for it to be successful?
9. Describe a teachable moment.
10. Why should the evaluation of an injury prevention program measure both the means and the end?

CASE STUDY QUESTIONS:

Please refer to the Case Study at the beginning of the chapter and answer the questions below.

1. Using the Haddon matrix, identify the host, agent, and environment in the case study. Also identify the pre-event, event, and post-event.

2. Identify where the patient in the case study currently is and brainstorm ideas for assisting him in quitting/reducing his smoking.

REFERENCES:

1. Abegunde DO, Mathers CD, Adam T, Ortegon M, Strong K. The burden and costs of chronic diseases in low-income and middle-income countries. *Lancet*. 2007;370(9603):1929–1938.
2. Novick L. *Public Health Administration: Principles for Population-Based Management.* Sudbury, MA: Jones and Bartlett Publishers; 2004.
3. Bollet A. *Plagues and Poxes: The Impact of Human History on Epidemic Disease*. New York: Demos Medical Publishing; 2004.
4. Thompson JB. International policies for achieving safe motherhood: women's lives in the balance. *Health Care Women Int*. 2005;26(6):472–483.
5. Garrett E, ed.,et al. *Infant Mortality: A Continuing Social Problem*. Aldershot: Ashgate Pub Co; 2007.
6. Council N, Sciences D, Sciences N. *Accidental Death and Disability: The Neglected Disease of Modern Society*. Washington, DC: National Academies Press; 2000.
7. Council N, Medicine I. *Injury in America: A Continuing Public Health Problem*. Washington, DC: National Academies Press; 1985.
8. Garrison HG, Foltin G, et al. *Consensus Statement: The Role of Out-of-Hospital EMS in Primary Injury Prevention, Consensus*

Workshop on the Role of EMS in Injury Prevention. Arlington, VA: Final Report; 1995.

9. Garrison HG, Foltin GL, Becker LR, Chew JL, Johnson M, Madsen GM, et al. The role of emergency medical services in primary injury prevention. East Carolina Injury Prevention Program. *Prehosp Emerg Care*. 1997;1(3):156–162.

10. Griffiths K. Best practices in injury prevention: National award highlights programs across the nation. *Jems*. 2002;27(8):60–74.

11. Kinnane JM, Garrison HG, Coben JH, Alonso-Serra HM. Injury prevention: is there a role for out-of-hospital emergency medical services? *Acad Emerg Med*. 1997;4(4):306–312.

12. Christoffel T, Gallagher S. *Injury Prevention and Public Health: Practical Knowledge, Skills, and Strategies*. New York: Jones & Bartlett Pub; 2005.

13. Krimston J, Griffiths K. EMS champions of injury prevention. Highlights from some of the best injury-prevention programs in the United States. *Jems*. 2004;29(11):80–84, 86, 88 passim.

14. Kirkwood HA. Before the call comes in. EMS and injury prevention. *Jems*. 1995;20(6):21, 23.

SECTION IV

SCIENTIFIC PRINCIPLES

The four chapters in this section provide a basic foundation in lifespan development, physiology, pathophysiology, and medical terminology. These areas again help lay a solid foundation for the Paramedic to build upon in the later technical and clinical chapters.

- **Chapter 9:** Lifespan Development
- **Chapter 10:** Basic Human Physiology
- **Chapter 11:** Principles of Pathophysiology
- **Chapter 12:** Medical Terminology

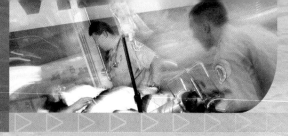

CHAPTER 9

▷ ▷

LIFESPAN DEVELOPMENT

KEY CONCEPTS:

Upon completion of this chapter, it is expected that the reader will understand these following concepts:

- Human development from conception to childbirth
- The psychosocial theories of nature vs. nurture
- The continuous state of physical, cognitive, and psychosocial development from young to old
- The impressionable time of middle childhood and the health concerns that face adolescents
- Moral development and facing adult responsibilities
- A greater understanding of acceptance of the stages of dying

▶ CASE STUDY:

The Paramedics were called to the home of a 13-year-old male with difficulty breathing. When they arrived they were introduced to Erik. His cold had worsened and he was having some difficulty breathing. While one of the Paramedics began interventions, the other planned to obtain a history. As he began with questions about allergies and medication, he realized he didn't know much about what 13-year-olds can do. He made a mental note to review human growth and development. It was like being back in Paramedic school. . . .

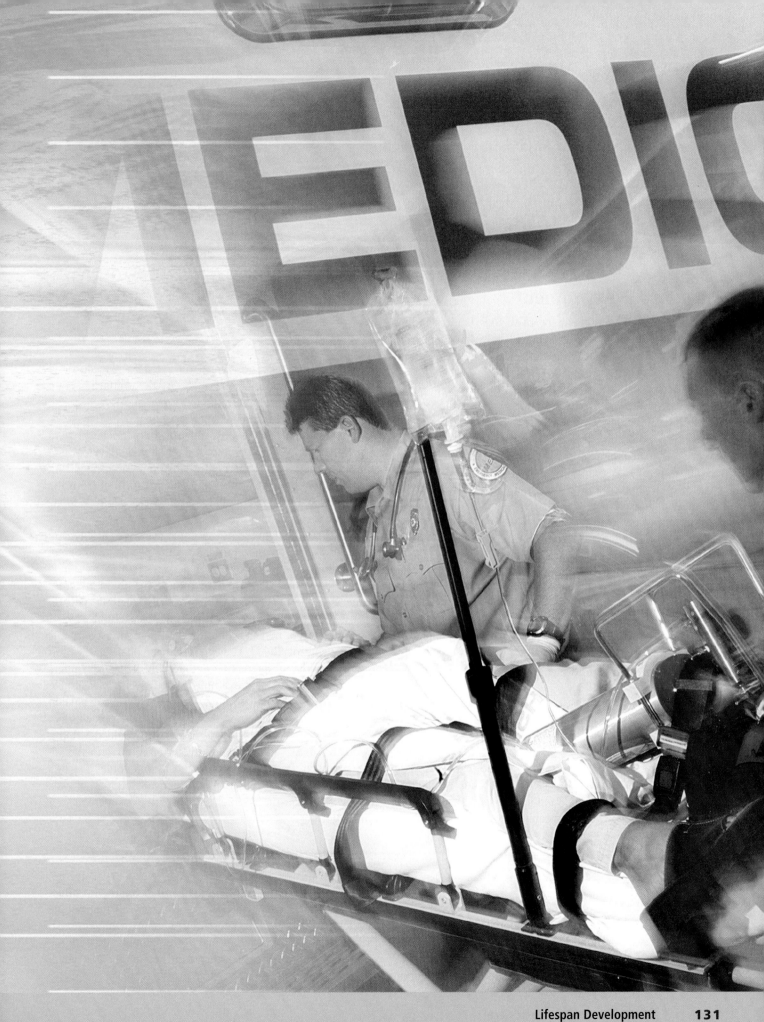

OVERVIEW

The Paramedic may encounter patients ranging in age from newborns to over a hundred years of age. The Paramedic's emphasis is often placed on how to treat the patient medically. This chapter discusses human development. Knowing the patient's age can dictate a Paramedic's approach to assessment and care (for example, the difference between a fussy 3-year-old and an elderly person who is making an end-of-life decision). This chapter discusses the physical, cognitive, and psychosocial development of people from birth to death.

Personal Development

Paramedics will encounter patients of all ages. Understanding the patient's developmental stage will help the Paramedic adjust his approach accordingly and to connect more therapeutically with the patient.

A person's development can be divided into three components. The first and outwardly most evident is the patient's physical development, those bodily changes that occur not just during one's youth but throughout life. The second change is the person's mental or cognitive development and includes the development of reasoning, the ability to think, and memory. Cognitive development also includes language acquisition, that human characteristic which permits communication. The third aspect of personal development is a person's emotions, the affective self. This aspect of development is the result of internal psychological dynamics and external societal influences. The affective portion of the person represents the psychosocial aspect of a person's development.

The changes in a person's patterns of thinking, feeling, and physical growth are all part of the person's development. Each of these elements affect the person, to varying degrees, over the course of a lifetime. These changes, coupled with life experience, combine to create the person that he or she has become.

Theories of Personal Development

Several theories have been advanced over the years to explain human development over a lifespan. These theories take into account the physical, mental, and psychosocial aspects of a person and try to provide a meaningful explanation of the changes that commonly occur.

Theories of Psychosocial Development

The first and most widely known theorist of psychosocial development was Sigmund Freud. Having laid a framework for understanding the human psyche, others—such as Erikson, Skinner, and Piaget—have sought to improve upon it. Each theorist has brought a unique perspective to the study of psychosocial development.

Psychosexual Theory

Sigmund Freud advanced one of the first psychosocial developmental theories in the late 1800s.[1] Freud attached great importance to sexuality and linked a person's psychosocial development to sex. Freud suggested that human psychic development was linked to physical growth, specifically where the sexual energy was centered, and that human development was therefore biologically controlled. Freud suggested that during childhood a person's sexual energy shifted from the oral to the anal to the genital regions as each become a focus in the person's personal life.

Fundamental to Freud's theory are the ideas of id, ego, and superego. A person's id consisted of the person's biological needs, such as water and food. A person's id also contained the will to live and the drive to reproduce, the libido. Inherent in the id is the concept of pleasure; that is, people will do what is pleasurable and avoid what is not pleasurable.

Eventually a person would develop an ego, a conscious state that controls the id. The ego is that personal sense of self as a physical being interacting in the world. The ego tempers the id with reality. For example, while sex is pleasurable (a function of the id), if it were to be pursued to the exclusion of all other social interaction then the ego would prevent that.

Finally, in early childhood the person would develop a superego, those societal values that run counter to the id. The superego works to suppress the id and forces the ego to consider moral behavior. Freud postulated that it was the ego that kept the conflict between id and superego to a minimum.

Psychosocial Theory

Erik Erikson, a student of Freud's psychosexual theory, dismissed the centrality of sexuality in favor of the effect of social influences on the person. Erikson felt that people develop because of social pressures to conform and co-exist. Erikson's view of psychosocial development stressed the role of the ego in direct conflict with Freud's theory, which stressed the role of the id.

In essence, Freud's theory stressed the physical developments and supported the idea that nature controlled one's development. Erikson stressed the social influences and supported the idea that nurturance had a greater impact upon personal development.[2] This is the classic nature vs. nurture argument.

Erikson's theory was also more comprehensive and included eight stages. Erikson's theory takes into account the entire span of a person's lifetime, adding three stages of adulthood to Freud's five stages of psychosexual development.

Conflict is the pivotal event that moves people through the various stages of Erikson's psychosocial development. Each stage is represented by the critical conflicts. For example, Erikson believed that the young person must resolve confusion over one's role in life to form a personal identity.

Behaviorism

While Pavlov's experiments with dogs, where he was able to condition dogs to salivate when a bell was rung, set the stage for a new developmental theory called behaviorism, B. F. Skinner's operant conditioning took center stage. Skinner believed that human behavior is simply a function of an interaction, positive and negative, with the social environment.

Expanding on behaviorism, Albert Bandura, another American psychologist, suggested that people learn in three ways: by direct instruction, direct experience, and observation. Bandura's social learning theory suggested that people developed through learning.

All three of these theorists—Pavlov, Skinner, and Bandura—took the approach that life experiences (nurturance) are the dominant influence in a person's psychosocial development.[3,4]

Cognitive Development Theory

Cognitive development theorists looked at how the mind was developed. Jean Piaget, an early cognitive theorist suggested that people develop in a building block fashion, one learned behavior building upon another. Piaget suggested that people learn schemes (ways to deal with the world) upon which they build new schemes. The earliest schemes are primitive reflexes. A person's intelligence is a function of the ability to create new schemes to successfully adapt to the environmental conditions in which a person finds himself. This process of assimilation (integrating new information into a preexisting matrix) along with accommodation (the changing of preconceptions to allow for new information) was the source of human development over a lifespan.

Topics in Human Development

Central to all discussions of lifespan development is the argument of whether genetics are dominant in a person's development or whether the environment and society play a greater role in human development. Despite the abundance of theories, and an even greater abundance of debate, the argument lives on.

Conception to Childbirth

At the moment of sexual climax, millions of spermatozoa are deposited into the vaginal vault and begin the journey through the cervix and into the fallopian tubes. When the spermatoza reach the egg, called an **ovum** (Figure 9-1), one will penetrate and fertilize the ovum.

The fertilized ovum, now called a **zygote**, starts to divide repeatedly. During this early stage the zygote will form a hollow, fluid-filled ball or **blastocyst**. The cells inside of the blastocyst will form the human, whereas the cells on the outside will form a protective covering that eventually develops into the placenta.

While this development has been occurring, the zygote has been traveling down the fallopian tubes and into the uterus. At the end of the first week, the zygote implants into the uterine lining. The amnion, which makes amniotic fluid, and the chorion, which will make the placenta, start to form along with the zygote. The placenta will provide the infant with nutrition through the **umbilical cord**, which connects the mother and child (Figure 9-2).

In about 30% of pregnancies, the zygote fails to implant and the pregnancy is spontaneously aborted.[5–7] This is referred to as **spontaneous abortion**.

In the weeks following the implantation, the zygote, now called an **embryo**, is rapidly dividing and laying down the foundations for all of the major organ systems. During this period of time, from conception to the end of the ninth week, the infant is at greatest risk for fetal malformation. Potential causes of fetal malformation are toxic substances or agents, called **teratogens**. Examples of teratogens include illegal drugs such as cocaine, alcohol, and infections such as rubella (measles) and toxoplasmosis. Women who drink alcoholic beverages while pregnant can potentially cause a number of birth defects, collectively referred to as **fetal alcohol syndrome**.[8–14.]

Genetics and Human Development

Every person alive is the result of the union of two sex gametes: a spermatozoa and an ovum. Each gamete brings 23 **chromosomes**, a double helix of DNA, into the mix. Together, these chromosomes provide an individual's genetic make-up, the **genotype**. The subsequent division of the cell, called **mitosis**, continues until a person is created. The visible outward expression of the chromosome, the **phenotype**, is therefore the result of the genetic influences of both the parents.

If the gametes each bring an X-chromosome to the union, then the individual will be female. If one of the spermatozoa brings a Y-chromosome to the union, then the person will be a male. Each chromosome provides **genes**. These genes determine the physical characteristics which

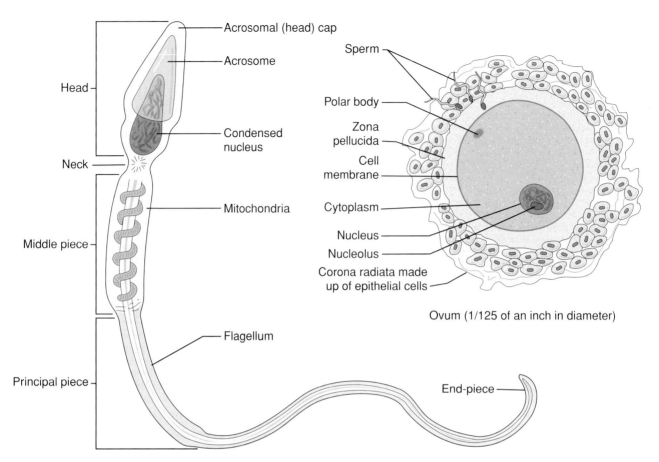

Figure 9-1 The sperm and fertilized ovum.

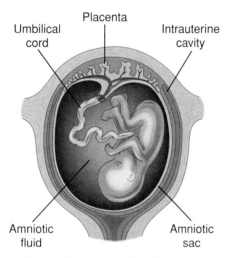

Figure 9-2 Fetus in utero attached to placenta by the umbilical cord.

comprise the individual. If one parent's genes control the child's characteristics, then that gene is said to be dominant. If one parent's chromosome is not dominant, but instead is recessive, then the recessive gene will not control the characteristic. For example, if a blue-eyed mother mates with a brown-eyed father and brown eyes are dominant, then the child will have brown eyes; note eye coloring is not that simple.

Some genetic diseases are linked to the sex chromosomes (i.e., sex-linked transmission). If both parents contribute that abnormal chromosome, then the child will have the disease. Examples of sex-linked diseases include sickle-cell disease, Brugada syndrome, Huntington's disease, and Marfan syndrome. If the child has one sickle-cell disease gene, then the child will be a carrier but will not have the disease. If the child has both genes, then the child will have the disease.

Pregnancy

After the ninth week, the pregnancy is generally viable. The embryo, called a fetus, will come to term in about the ninth month. The stages of a pregnancy are evenly divided into trimesters, each of which has specific characteristics. The first trimester, the germinal period, is a period of high hazard. The second semester sees rapid growth in the fetus and the first signs of life, fetal movements called **quickening**. During the final trimester, at the twenty-sixth week, the pregnancy reaches the point where, if the pregnancy were to terminate prematurely, the infant would be viable.

A number of other factors also combine to increase infant mortality, including advanced maternal age (greater than 35), domestic violence (approximately 8% of pregnant women are battered), and poor health, including a lack of prenatal care

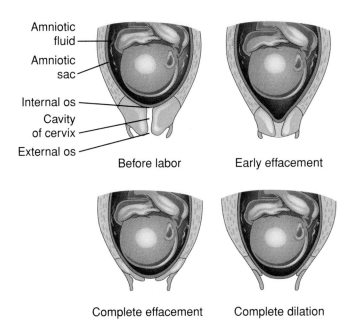

Amniotic fluid
Amniotic sac
Internal os
Cavity of cervix
External os

Before labor   Early effacement

Complete effacement   Complete dilation

Figure 9-3 Childbirth.

and poor nutrition. As a result, the most dangerous time in any human's existence is the time from the moment of conception until birth.

Childbirth

Childbirth, the culmination of nine months of growth and development, begins when the uterus starts to contract in a process called **labor** (Figure 9-3). These strong rhythmic contractions begin to push the fetus into the birth canal and dilate the cervix through a process of widening and thinning. This process takes approximately 12 hours on average. It can range from one hour, called a precipitous delivery, to 24 hours or more.

The infant, with its head engaged in the birth canal, begins a rapid passage down the birth canal in the second stage of delivery. The delivery of the infant may take upwards of an hour, barring any complications.

The third and final stage of the delivery is the delivery of the **placenta**, which marks the end of the pregnancy.

The Newly Born

At the moment of delivery the newly born must undergo dramatic physiological changes in order to adapt to extrauterine life. During this transition period, the newly born's cardiopulmonary system switches from dependence on the mother, via the placenta, to independence.

During the first minute of life the umbilical blood flow diminishes, raising carbon dioxide levels, which in turn stimulate the newly born's first breath. The increase in intrathoracic pressure, from the air-filled lungs, causes the

cardiac shunts (the foramen ovale and the ductus arteriosus) to reverse blood flow and then close.[15–17]

The Infant

The first year of an infant's existence revolves around eating, sleeping, and growing. Initially, the infant spends eight hours in full rest (non-REM sleep), another eight hours in REM sleep (dreaming), and the rest of the time in varying amounts of quiet alertness, drowsiness, and distress.

At about the fourth month, the infant's sleep/wake cycle starts to approximate that of an adult and the child's response to the environment starts to become more determined. Initially, the infant has only primitive survival reflexes, such as the sucking reflex and the swallowing reflex.

Physical Development

The average newborn weighs between 3 to 3.5 kg at birth and will almost triple that weight in the first year of life. Most newborns typically drop between 5% to 10% of their birth weight in the first week due to a combination of fluid loss and consumption of brown fat; brown fat is special baby fat used to generate heat. Normally, if the newborn is feeding properly, the newborn should regain this weight and surpass the birth weight by the end of the second week of life.[18,19]

Table 9-1 Comparison of Vital Signs Between Newborn and 1-Year-Old Infant

Vital Signs	Newborn	1-Year-Old
Heart rate (BPM)	120–160	100–120
Respirations (BPM)	40–60	20–30
Blood pressure (mmHg)	> 60	70–100

At the moment of birth, the newborn is challenged to adapt to the world outside of the womb. At that moment the newborn's heart is racing, between 100 and 160 beats per minute, but soon settles to a sustained tachycardia around 120 beats per minute. In like fashion, the newborn's respirations are between 40 and 60 breaths per minute but become increasingly slower over the first year until they stabilize at about 20 to 30 breaths per minute (Table 9-1).

Maintaining ventilation represents one of the greater challenges for an infant. The combination of a narrower airway, which is more easily obstructed, and the fact that an infant is an obligate nose breather (i.e., primarily breathes through the smaller nasal passages) makes partial airway obstruction more likely and breathing more difficult.

Once air has passed the upper airway into the lungs, there are fewer alveoli to exchange oxygen to meet the high metabolic rate and oxygen demand of the infant's body. To compensate for the mismatch between demand and capacity, the infant increases the respiratory rate. This is not an effective mechanism yet because of the combination of horizontal ribs, which decrease expansion, and weak accessory muscles which force the diaphragm to act as the primary muscle of respiration. The diaphragm is limited in its ability to sustain a rapid respiration. Compounding the problem is the increased heat loss, from rapid respiration, which in turn increases the metabolic demand upon the body to produce heat. The infant can quickly fatigue and then experience respiratory distress and failure.

During the first six months of life, the infant experiences dramatic neuromuscular development. The primitive reflexes (e.g., the Babinski reflex) start to wane at about six months as the motor neurons within the spinal cord mature (Figure 9-4). This neurological development starts in a head-to-toe (i.e., cephalocaudal) fashion and from an inward-to-outward (i.e., proximodistal) fashion.

During the assessment of the infant, the Paramedic should be attentive to the presence of infantile reflexes.[27–29] Upon observation of a healthy infant's general appearance, the Paramedic should note an infant who is interactive with the environment, whose limbs move when stimulated, and who has a strong sucking and gagging reflex. An infant in trouble has limp extremities and a "Raggedy Ann" appearance.

Most infants, when the Paramedic claps his hands, will startle and extend both of their arms. This is called the Moro reflex. An absent Moro reflex on one side may indicate a neurological disorder, such as hemiplegia, or perhaps a fractured clavicle.

Other primitive or infantile reflexes include the rooting reflex, in which the infant turns toward the cheek that is stroked, and the sucking reflex. Both of these reflexes are present at birth and help the infant with breastfeeding.

The next reflex is the palmar grasp reflex. The palmar grasp reflex is seen when the infant's hands grasp an object pressing against the palm. Another reflex is the tonic neck reflex, in which turning the infant's head to the side causes the ipsilateral arm to straighten and the contralateral arm to bend, in the classic fencing posture. Both of these reflex tests are tests of the motor neurons of the upper nervous system. The Babinski reflex, a fanning of the toes and extension of the great toe caused by stroking the lateral soles of the feet, is a test of the lower motor neurons.

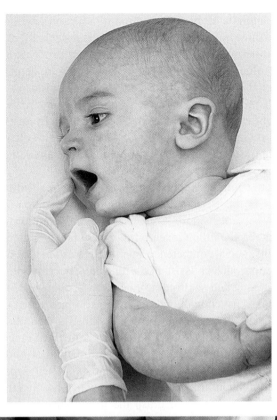
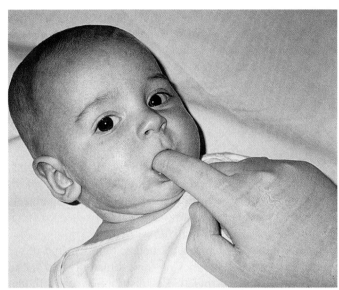
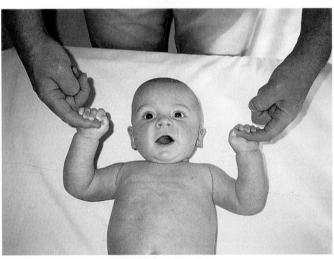
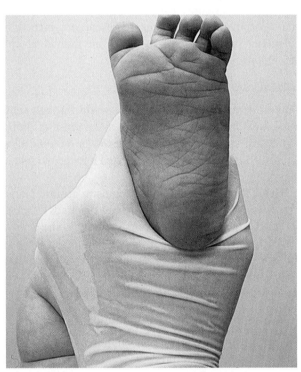
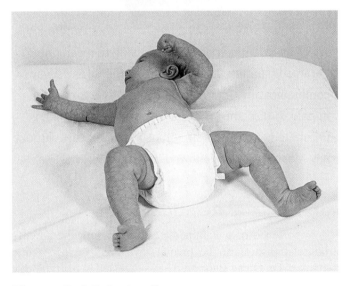
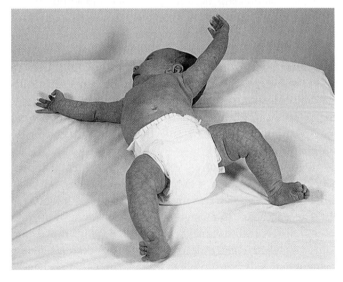

Figure 9-4 Infant reflexes.

At about the time the posterior fontanel closes, at three to four months, these primitive reflexes start to wane. By the time the anterior fontanel closes, in nine months to a year, all of these reflexes should be gone.

The infant experiences the greatest amount of growth during this period of time. Bones grow, influenced by factors such as growth hormone, genetics, and the infant's general health. The infant becomes physically stronger as the muscle mass increases correspondingly.

As the infant gains control over the larger muscle groups, the infant will raise the chest off the floor and then crawl. Later the infant will stand and move about, grasping objects to help with balance while walking. This is called cruising. Eventually, the child will walk unassisted.

Each new skill represents another objective the infant has accomplished while moving toward maturity. Taking an age-related average, Arnold Gesell distributed these different tasks across a timeline, called **developmental milestones**. The developmental milestones represent a typical child's development and are used to gauge an individual child's development against a norm.

Cognitive Development

An infant obtains knowledge of the world through sensory input, which the infant brain tries to make sense of. Initially, the newborn uses his primitive reflexes as building blocks. Then, future experiences are assimilated into the old schemes, thus building all new schemes.

During this phase, the infant begins to acquire language skills. Starting with cooing (simple vowel sounds), the infant proceeds to preverbal gestures (e.g., pointing). The child then utters his or her first words at about 12 months. From that point, and for the remainder of the first two years, speech develops rapidly and the infant's vocabulary expands to over 200 words, mainly consisting of labels of people or things.

Psychosocial Development

The first psychosocial task encountered by an infant is bonding. Bonding is a process that establishes a lasting nurturing relationship between a mother and child. While bonding may begin during pregnancy, it is a reciprocal relationship that involves both mother and child.

Many factors can influence bonding including physical separation from the infant, difficulty in delivery, and absence of breastfeeding. The Paramedic can be witness to this bonding behavior, such as mutual gazing, reflective smiling, and response to touch. Absence of these bonding behaviors (i.e., poor bonding) may be reflective of poor maternal care and even child abuse.

During this formative year, an infant's temperament becomes manifest. For example, the infant may be easy, difficult, or slow-to-warm-up. The majority of infants are cheerful and adapt to change readily. The slow-to-warm-up infant appears inactive, maybe even in a negative mood, and adjusts slowly to changes. The difficult infant does not accept changes and is demonstrative in his disapproval of change.

A smile is often an indication of a person's affect. Until around three months of age, infants smile reflexively, meaning they smile randomly and without apparent provocation. The infant older than three months will start to demonstrate emotional expressivity through a social smile. A social smile is a reflective smile (in response to someone smiling at the infant). It is not a reflexive smile caused by an external stimulus (e.g., the proximity of a person's face). Often social smiling is accompanied by vocalizations such as cooing or by lip movements called mouthing.

The continued social interaction between infant and parents is the start of the process of socialization. As the infant becomes more connected, psychoemotionally, to the mother, the infant is learning behaviors which will affect the child's social competence later in life. Further parent–child interaction, such as assistance with simple psychomotor tasks (a process called scaffolding), helps to further develop both the infant's psychomotor skills and the infant's social skills.

A test of an infant's social skills is the ability to withstand parental separation. During a medical emergency the Paramedic may need to examine the child at a location separate from the mother. This tends to elicit separation anxiety in the infant.[30,31] The infant may be observed to reach out to the mother, or to grasp the mother firmly and resist separation. One theory suggests that the infant has no concept of time. Thus, when a mother leaves the child for even a minute, the child—who depends on the mother for survival—feels abandoned and instinctively cries for the mother. As the infant develops, the infant will be comforted by memories of the mother and self-soothing activities such as thumb sucking during periods of isolation.

During this early period of socialization, autism is often discovered. Autism is a developmental disorder which includes impaired social interactions, an absence of separation anxiety, and problems with both verbal and nonverbal communications. Failure to manifest early signs of socialization, such as reflective smiling, may be indicative of autism.

STREET SMART

While an infant's crying is distressing to most, the Paramedic understands that this is the infant's way of communicating. Infants cry because they are angry, in pain or discomfort, or have a basic need which is unfulfilled. The cry of an infant in pain occurs without any moaning and is followed by breath holding.[32-34]

Parent–Child Relationships

The importance of a Paramedic understanding the parent–child relationship can be pivotal to a positive therapeutic encounter. Dr. Diana Baumrind has suggested in her typology of parenting that there are four styles of parenting, each with a different impact on a child's psychosocial development. The child development literature has suggested that the impact of these parenting styles, both negative and positive, is evident as early as the preschool years.

Each of these parenting styles will have an impact upon the child's social competence and psychosocial development. In some cases, the parenting style is predictive of the problem behaviors. Each of these parenting styles revolves around the emphasis, or de-emphasis, of nurturance. Nurturance is the quality of caring and concern. A nurturing parent provides clarity of communication, makes demands for maturity, and maintains parental control. The last element, parental control, seems to be pivotal in describing a parenting style.

Permissive, or indulgent, parents tend to give control over to the child by not establishing boundaries or routines. While these parents tend to display affection to their children, they fail to consistently enforce or clarify rules, presenting the child with mixed messages. Permissive parents tend to accept all of a child's behaviors, both good and bad, without judgment. Children of permissive parents tend to perform poorly in the structured environment of the school and have problems with authority. However, they have higher self-esteem and better social skills than children of other parenting styles.

In contrast, the authoritarian parent always needs to be in control and tends to demand high levels of maturity. Strict rules are the norm and the display of affection is rare. Authoritarian parents tend to focus on negative behaviors. Children of authoritarian parents tend to be anxious and withdrawn, with poor social skills, but perform moderately well in school. Children of authoritarian parents also tend to have higher levels of depression. As a result of their upbringing, the interaction between Paramedic and child can be difficult as these children are generally mistrustful of adults.

The authoritative parent, sometimes referred to as the democratic parent, has all four qualities in balance. Authoritative parents establish rules, hold children responsible for adhering to those rules, and provide explanations of expectations to the child. Authoritative parents focus on positive behaviors. They try to catch their children being good. Children of authoritative parents tend to be happy, self-confident, and independent, to the point of genuine openness to other adults.

The last parenting style could almost be called a non-parenting style: the uninvolved parent. These indifferent parents have little commitment to parenting. Children of indifferent parents tend to have low tolerance for frustration and exhibit problems with impulse control. This group of children is a particular problem for Paramedics as they also tend to be aggressive, to the point of committing violence.

From a Paramedic's perspective, it may seem reasonable to withdraw from a situation in which a child is aggressive. However, the more constructive approach is to remain steadfast. The Paramedic can acknowledge the behavior as being unacceptable, without becoming aggressive in either words or action, and all the while remain authoritative.

Preschool Children: Early Childhood

The early childhood years, from age 2 to 5, are a period of extraordinary growth. For each year of growth the child, now called a toddler, will add five pounds and three inches of height. The spinal column starts to lengthen and the internal organs start to ascend under the protection of the thoracic cage.

The toddler's pulmonary system continues to grow as terminal airways continue to branch, alveoli develop, and hemoglobin levels climb to near adult levels. Perhaps most remarkably, the toddler's nervous system is almost completed in its development. The peripheral nervous system is myelinated, allowing for the development of fine motor skills, and the brain has attained almost 90% of its adult mass.

While such factors as genetics and wellness can affect a child's height and growth, all children should become larger and taller. Those who fail to grow, exhibiting **failure to thrive**, may be under severe psychosocial pressures or have nutritional deficits. Paramedics need to identify these toddlers and encourage the parent to seek medical attention for the child.

Physical Development

During these early preschool years, a child learns to run, jump, hop, and throw. These complex motor activities are an outward manifestation of the growing neuromuscular system (Figure 9-5).

At or about 3 years of age, children will learn how to toilet themselves. Within another year, children learn how to dress themselves. The 6-year-old child should have developed enough motor dexterity to be able to tie a shoe.

At this age, the impact of sex can be first noted. Males tend to be slightly better at skills emphasizing force or power whereas females tend to be better at fine motor skills, such as balancing and foot movements. Most toddlers, because of improved eye-to-hand coordination, enjoy games such as puzzles or coloring with crayons. These activities can be solitary or enjoyed in groups. When engaged in group activities, toddlers tend to identify with other same sex children and begin to model their behaviors based on the behaviors of others of the same sex.

The play "pals" that toddlers are often placed with are other siblings. It is during this play period that sibling rivalry will be seen. Sibling rivalry is a form of competition, for parental approval or attention, between brothers and/or sisters. Sibling rivalry can, at times, involve unacceptable behaviors such as aggression or "acting out." In general, sibling rivalry should be viewed as the toddler's effort to establish herself as a person and to establish her place within the family hierarchy. While not entirely preventable, toddlers can be taught that violence is not an acceptable means of resolving disagreement and that there are other more positive ways to get attention.

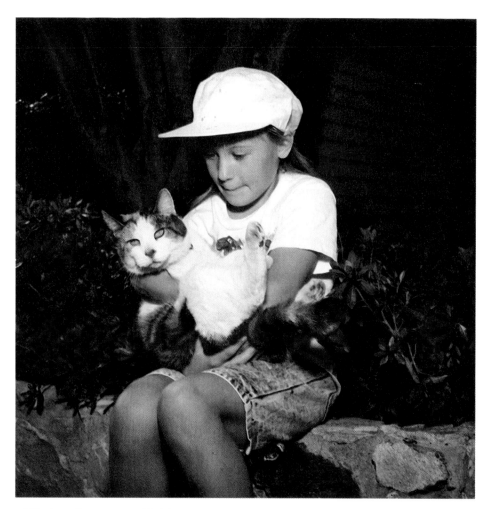

Figure 9-5 Motor skill development: Child.

Cognitive Development

The early childhood individual is in a preoperational stage of cognitive development, as per Piaget's studies. The thinking is concrete and the child cannot think in terms of abstracts. The result is that these children will take what the Paramedic says literally. Therefore, the Paramedic should carefully construct statements in order to avoid misinterpretation and confusion. As time progresses, the children develop more symbolic thought, which helps them remember experiences.

As symbolic thought develops, so does mathematical reasoning. Young children understand that the numbers, names, and objects in a set are related (i.e., 1 = one = a dog). Young children struggle to learn concepts such as ordinality (that numbers occur in an order) and cardinality (that the last number represents the sum of the set of objects).

Also critical at this point in a young child's development is language acquisition. Going beyond the 300 or 400 learned earlier, the young child now learns how to apply **syntax**, the rules of grammar, and **semantics**, the meaning of words. The focus of this language development is upon the practical application of language to social and personal relationships.

Here again, the differences between the sexes become more evident. Females tend to ask questions and make requests more indirectly than males, while maintaining more eye contact. Females also tend to use more nonverbal cues such as body language.

Psychosocial Development

Play has a pivotal role in human development at this age. Psychoanalytic theory suggests that play provides children an opportunity to gain mastery and demonstrate autonomy for the purpose of self-satisfaction.

Cognitive theory suggests that play develops in readily identifiable stages, starting with functional play. Functional play is focused on performance, usually of a simple repeated movement, such as dribbling a ball or shooting a basket.

The next level of play is constructive play. In constructive play, the child takes common objects and attempts to build things. Construction of objects permits the child to move into the next phase of play, pretend play. Pretending to substitute oneself into another character or role permits the child the opportunity to expand horizons without threat; lines like "after all, it wasn't me, it was my dolly," might be heard.

Eventually, children become involved in games with rules at about the fifth year. Games encourage an understanding of interpersonal relationships as well as the relation of abstract concepts to the real world.

School-Aged Children: Middle Childhood

Middle childhood is centered on education, the school years, and personal development. The influence of family starts to wane in the face of growing social involvement and peer pressure.

Physical Development

School age signals a slowing in physical growth for a child. Girls may grow to be taller than their male counterparts for a time until boys enter puberty. Mortality is traditionally lower during this time, with viral illnesses being the largest source of sickness.

Cognitive Development

During middle childhood, children are more interactive with their environment. They experiment, test, and generally assess their life condition and developing concepts about it.

During this time, the child starts to focus on objects and events. The child is able to focus on and comprehend the complexity of multifaceted problems. Piaget refers to this as the concrete operational stage.[35] Children in this stage are able to understand such concrete operational concepts as spatial relations, nature of time, and the sequential nature of certain activities.

Gardner advances the theory by stating that the multiple intelligences of a person become evident during this stage. A person's language skills (many children are—or learn to be—bilingual at this age), musical skills (such as playing an instrument), logical skills (manifest in math or chess), and kinesthetic skills (such as demonstrated in Figure 9-6) may become apparent. Perhaps the most important intelligence a child learns at this age is the ability to form close human bonds as well as a social self (personal and interpersonal skills).

Psychosocial Development

The stage of middle childhood can be one of great upheaval for the individual. There are many challenges to the psychosocial self such as knowing who the child is. The child develops a sense of self and a desire to succeed and achieve.

Peers, school, and family are modifiers of the child's sense of self and often come into conflict with one another. Erikson's psychosocial theory states that middle childhood is a time in which children are concerned about their capacity to do good work (industry versus inferiority) and show initiative.

Children often manifest their differences in achievement motivation during this period. Some are learning oriented, and are focused on attaining competence in an area of study. These children are intrinsically motivated. Other children are more interested in pleasing others (extrinsically motivated) and have a performance orientation.

Peer Relations

According to Piaget, children in middle childhood overcome their egocentrism (i.e., focus on oneself) and start to relate to others more in terms of common interests, goals, and so on. Parents have a lesser influence in this matter, as they are not viewed as peers, and friends start to take on a greater role in shaping the person's personality.

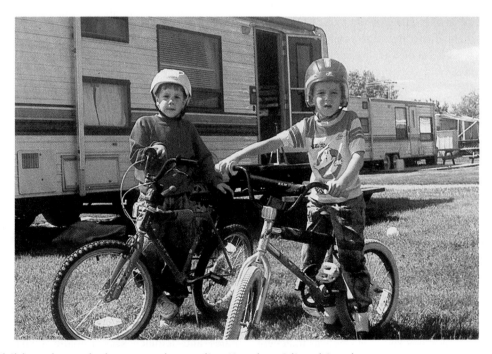

Figure 9-6 Children learn balance and coordination by riding bicycles.

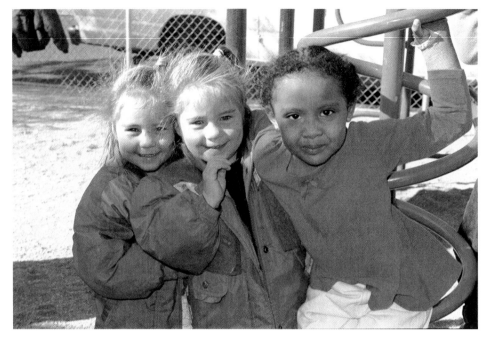

Figure 9-7 Children tend to gravitate to same sex friendships.

Initially, these children are interested in same-sex friends, almost to the exclusion of the opposite sex, and form close friendships (Figure 9-7). Females tend to form close and intimate friendships of one other same-sex friend at this age (dyads) while males tend to include a larger circle of acquaintances.

A child who forms friendships easily is viewed as popular. In addition, popular children are seen as confident, good-natured, and energetic. Physical traits that support athleticism help a child gain popularity and social acceptance.

Conformity to the group is stressed during this time and peer pressure can cause children to make rash decisions which run counter to their personal values or the values taught to them by their parents. This experimentation can be healthy, if not taken to extremes, as it encourages independent thought about values and morals.

Divorce

Dr. Judith Wallerstein, in her landmark work entitled "The Unexpected Legacy of Divorce," described the problems of trust and intimacy that children experience because of divorce.[36] Divided loyalties, inconsistent discipline, and long periods of tension and discord can come together to produce a fear of intimacy, lowered expectations of authority figures, and a sense of powerlessness in a child.

These fears can be problematic if the Paramedic is treating a child with divorced parents. Conflicts may arise during even routine physical assessments and a war of wills may occur. Despite the Paramedic's good intentions, the child may not be willing to accept care and will resent efforts to provide that care, to the point of becoming violent. The Paramedics can only resort to tact and diplomacy and a willingness to accept what the child will permit.

Gender Identity

During the school-age years, children start to attach a gender-role identity to themselves; that sense of being a male or a female. It is difficult to establish which factor has a greater influence on a child's gender-role identity—genetic influences, hormonal factors, or social factors—but it can be a confusing time for a child. In some cases the child's psychological assignment of gender may be in conflict with the child's biological sex assignment. A child may attempt to maintain androgyny for a time (having both masculine and feminine qualities), in an effort to understand the mental and physical changes within themselves, while others experiment with one and then the other gender role.

Regardless of a child's gender-role identity, it is important that the Paramedic remain nonjudgmental in this matter and focus on the patient's medical condition.

Adolescence

Adolescence could best be described as a stormy transition from childhood to adulthood. Societal concerns, such as educational preparation versus industry, have culminated in child labor laws, compulsory education, and a separate judicial system for juveniles. Each is a response to an issue faced by adolescents.

Physical Development

The most remarkable changes in the human physique, the body habitus, occur in adolescence. Entering into puberty, males and females see dramatic sexual changes in their physical bodies.

For males, the development of facial hair, enlargement of the penis, and the first ejaculation represent milestones in their passage to manhood.

For females, the development of breasts, the widening of the hips, and the first menarche (period) represent milestones in their passage to womanhood.

The timing of puberty is widely variable, with some females experiencing menarche at age 12 while some males do not experience ejaculation until age 18.

Females who are early maturing are very concerned about their physical appearance and are often confronted with social situations for which they are not, psychosocially speaking, prepared.

Late maturing males may appear immature and therefore lack social grace and self-confidence, but are actually at more liberty to develop a unique personality, unfretted by social pressures.

Adolescent Health Concerns

The opportunities for freedom, and the accompanying experimentation, coupled with the use of inhibition-reducing drugs, such as alcohol, can potentially create unhealthy situations for adolescents. The Paramedic should keep these health concerns in mind when treating adolescent patients.

Sex and the Adolescent

The advent of sexuality brings the risk of sexually transmitted diseases. It has been estimated that 25% of adolescents leaving high school will have, or have had, a sexually transmitted disease. A combination of early sexual maturing, early sexual activity, drug and/or alcohol use (lowering inhibitions), and inadequate instruction about the use of contraceptives results in a high rate of teenage pregnancy and an epidemic of sexually transmitted diseases (STD) in adolescents.[37-39]

Over the last two decades, the number of cases of chlamydia has risen almost 300% and it is estimated that there will be one million new cases of genital herpes simplex virus type 2 (HSV-2) each year. It is thought that young women are more susceptible to STDs because epithelial cells, which are more susceptible to infection by STDs, extend over the vaginal surface of the cervix and the cervix is unprotected by cervical mucosa. These epithelial cells later retract in an adult woman, exposing the cervical mucosa.

Genital human papillomavirus (HPV), genital warts, is the most common sexually transmitted disease among sexually active adolescents. Genital human papillomavirus has been connected to the incidence of cervical cancer.[40] There is currently a vaccine for HPV and it is hoped that its use will decrease the number of cervical cancer cases.

Obesity

Chaotic schedules, the ease and availability of "junk foods," and peer pressure contribute to poor teenage nutrition. On one extreme is the national epidemic of teenage obesity. Adolescents seeking solace in food eat carbohydrate-high "comfort" foods, instead of healthier choices, leading to weight gain beyond growth. They then become obese.

The United Nation's World Health Organization (WHO) called obesity the "global health epidemic" in 1998 and stated that at that time the health of 6 million children was in jeopardy because of obesity. The health risks associated with obesity are impressive: type 2 diabetes mellitus, secondary hypertension, accelerated coronary artery disease, and stroke.

At the other extreme of teenage weight problems is **anorexia nervosa**. Anorexia nervosa is a psychiatric illness involving problems with self-image and is characterized by self-starvation and **bulimia**, binge-eating and then purging via laxatives or vomiting. Anorexia nervosa affects about 1 in 1,000 young women or 1% of adolescent girls. If untreated, anorexia nervosa can be fatal.[41]

Teenage Suicide

At increased risk for premature death from trauma, secondary to increased risk-taking behaviors and a false sense of invulnerability, teenagers are also at higher risk of death from suicide.

While death from motor vehicle collisions and homicide are still competing for the distinction of most common cause of death for young people age 12 to 22, suicide is still in the top three causes of teenage death. Teenage suicide is frequently the result of a high-stress event (e.g., death of a peer) and/or inadequate coping mechanisms. About 20% to 25% of adolescents report signs of depression at one time or another during adolescence. Among adolescents, 8% report suffering from debilitating or clinical depression. Suicide is the third leading cause of death for teenagers age 15 to 19.[42-44] Therefore, Paramedics should take all teenage depression and suicide attempts seriously.

Cognitive Development

The cognitive development of the adolescent revolves around using logic to solve problems, seeing the possibilities rather than the realities, and engineering new ideas. To turn a phrase, adolescents start to see problems as "less black and white and more as gray."

Piaget referred to this stage of intellectual development as the formal stage. Formal thinking involves the application of logic to abstract ideas to solve problems. This formal thinking allows the individual to find meaning in seemingly confusing data and to apply problem-solving techniques to resolve conflict.

Psychosocial Development

Adolescents return to egocentrism, a stage previously encountered in early childhood. Impressed with their newfound abilities to reason logically and think abstractly, they formulate idealisms without regard for practical reality.

During this time, adolescents turn their attention to morality and their own moral development. Kohlberg divided

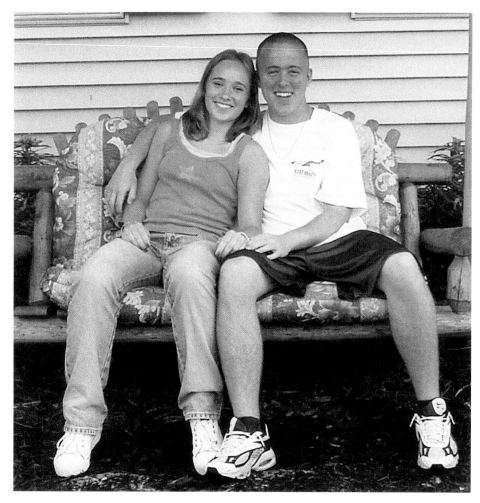

Figure 9-8 Adolescence is a time of growth and experimentation.

the process of moral development into six stages and three levels.

The first level is preconventional morality. This is the first stage of moral development and is simply avoidance of pain. To a person at this level, the morality of an act is defined by the positive or negative outcome (i.e., pain and punishment). Notably, obedience is a function of punishment. Advancing to the next stage, the hedonistic phase, the person conforms less to avoid punishment but more to attain or gain an advantage.

Level two is simply conventional morality. Stage three, conventional morality, involves being seen as a "good person" by friends and family at its lowest stage. Conduct is geared toward that goal. The advanced version of conventional morality, stage four, is also called a "law and order" morality. People at this stage conform to the rules for the sake of the rules.

The third level of moral development is postconventional morality. People at the lowest stage of postconventional morality are concerned with abstract concepts such as justice and democratic principles. Their moral beliefs tend to be more flexible, in concert with the society in which they exist.

The highest level of moral development, and the sixth stage, is principle-based morality. Having developed a strong set of internal principles (e.g., guiding missions), these adolescents conform to their principles rather than face self-condemnation.

Teenagers are challenged to develop their social self, their intellectual self, their moral self, and their sexual self into a socially acceptable personage (Figure 9-8).

Early Adulthood

Early adulthood is a period of striving and accomplishment. It is punctuated with peak life events such as marriage and childbirth.

A fundamental decision made by most young adults is whether to go to college or to start work. Women are more likely to go to college and more likely to complete college within the traditional four-year cycle. Men are more likely to go to work or start college but not complete it.

The young adult immediately entering the workforce will first enter a period of self-exploration, in preparation for work, then try to find an organization or business to enter into. Unions, like the guilds before them, offer these young adults opportunities to train as apprentices. Apprentices have the advantage of gaining competence on the job as well as learning organizational rules and mores.

Physical Development

The majority of people, both male and female, reach their peak height in their early twenties, and their health is generally at its peak as well. Unfortunately, obesity—a growing problem to children and adolescents—is also more common in young adults, with over one-half of all adults being overweight.

As an adolescent reaches maturity, and the age of consent, unhealthy decisions can be made regarding such potentially devastating behaviors as tobacco smoking, alcohol consumption, and unprotected sex. These behaviors may be seen as outlets from the stress of everyday pressures. Some stress can be negative, such as distress or stress caused by creditors trying to collect on unpaid bills. Other stress can be positive (eustress), such as the birth of a child.

Regardless of the type of stress, all stress can be seen as either a chance for harm or as a challenge and the body responds accordingly. The sympathetic nervous system responds by an adrenaline release which leads to hypertension and tachycardia. Persistent or sustained stress eventually takes a toll on the body and the mind, resulting in effects such as hypertension, immune system disorders, and mental disorders.

Cognitive Development

Young adults tend to explore the world and seek out new experiences which engender questions about themselves, the people with whom they associate, and the world in general. Young people explore their world through interaction with others, engaging in dialectical thinking (i.e., discovering the truth through dialogue and appreciating that there may be multiple perspectives).

Psychosocial Development

Entering young adulthood, many people are engaged in finding the "ideal mate," that special someone with whom to share common goals and aspirations. Erikson refers to this stage as the choice between intimacy and isolation. Inherent in this process is a social clock. A social clock can be thought of as a set of expectations, placed on the individual by society, to complete certain tasks (e.g., marriage and childbirth) within a predetermined time (young adulthood). Young adults who fail to accept the social norm are seen as outcasts and tend to become self-absorbed in isolation.

Love and Friendship

The differences between the sexes become more evident when it comes to how they look at friendship and love. Young women are inclined to reveal deep personal feelings to a same-sex friend, and then expect that confidence to be shared exclusively. Young men tend to establish same-sex friendships based on common activities, such as sports.

Regardless of sexual orientation, most young people are seeking a monogamous relationship with a significant other person. According to Dr. Robert Sternberg, love has three aspects or components: intimacy, passion, and commitment. Utilizing these three components, Sternberg has described seven combinations, each a variation of love: friendship, infatuation, empty love, romantic, companionate, fatuous, and consummate love.

For example, intimacy without either passion or commitment is friendship. Infatuation, on the other hand, is passion without intimacy and commitment. Arranged marriages are an example of empty love, where there is commitment but no intimacy or passion. Sternberg goes on to describe romantic love, companionate love, and fatuous love. The greatest and deepest love has all three components—intimacy, passion, and commitment—and is a complete form of love.

Marriage

Hypothetically, marriages are an equal partner relationship in which shared concerns and responsibilities help form the bond. In a conventional relationship, the male is the head of the household and sole provider, whereas the woman is the homemaker and mother. This form of relationship is rapidly waning in the face of growing single-parent households and equal partner relationships, in which both parties work and make the home together. It should be noted that one-third of men and one-fifth of women are single by choice and that singlehood is a viable alternative for some people.

While marriage is a relative constant in a young adult person's life, so is divorce. Divorce occurs in about 50% of first marriages and most divorces occur in early adulthood.[45] And while 82% of divorced people eventually remarry, with about one-half of those marriages ending in divorce, there is a growing lack of commitment in the institution of marriage.

Parenthood

In general, most young adults have less preparation for parenthood than they did for their livelihood. The resulting strain between the expectations of happiness from parenting and the reality of parenting (felt largely by the mother) places an additional burden upon the relationship. As a result, many mothers become single parents and have to depend upon extended families for support and assistance. Paramedics should understand that single mothers may have limited resources and that EMS is one of the few social supports readily available during a time of acute distress.

Middle Adulthood

Middle adulthood could be characterized as a period of maximal productivity as well as a period of readjustment and realignment. Middle adulthood is also a period of physical decline and changes in interpersonal focus.

Physical Development

The impact of aging, which commenced in young adulthood, begins to manifest in more obvious ways. Changes related to age include a decrease in strength, which peaked in the person's thirties, and a loss of muscle mass. The most outward signs of aging—graying of the hair; loss of hair; weight gain, called the "middle-aged spread"; and wrinkled skin—all signal the onset of aging.

Perhaps more disconcerting to the middle-aged adult, and of importance to Paramedics, is the loss of sensory acuity. Most adults by age 50 will need to wear corrective lens, as the lens within the eye thickens and is less able to accommodate for vision. Reading documents, such as permission forms and consents, is more difficult without glasses. Hearing loss is also reported in middle-aged adults.

Climacteric

Climacteric is an age-related decrease in sex hormone production that occurs in both men and women. While men experience a gradual decline in the number and the viability of sperm as a result of decreased testosterone production, men have been known to sire children at age 80.

Women experience a more dramatic decline in their reproductive capabilities. A decline in sex hormone production—estrogen and progesterone—results in **menopause**, the inability to conceive. By definition, menopause is the cessation of a woman's menses for an entire year. However, many women go through a prolonged period of intermittent and irregular menstrual periods until hormone levels stabilize.

The symptoms which often accompany these fluctuating hormone levels—such as hot flashes, night sweats, vaginal dryness, and insomnia—are distressing. Some women elect to have hormone replacement therapy. While hormone replacement therapy can help to reduce menopausal symptoms as well as the incidence or severity of **osteoporosis** (a loss of calcium from the bones secondary to a decrease in hormones), hormone replacement therapy also increases the risk of cancer, particularly breast cancer.[46–48]

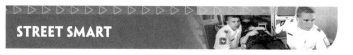
Cognitive Development

Dr. K. Warner Schaie's sequential studies have indicated that while intelligence (the ability to think) peaks at different ages for both men and women, all intellectual abilities show decline at about age 68. The declines are modest in most cases. Significant loss of intellectual capacity does not occur until age 80.

What is different between the intellect of a young adult and a middle-aged adult is information processing. Young adults have the ability to process new information in novel situations (a fluid intelligence) whereas middle-aged adults begin to solidify their understandings (crystallized intelligence). Crystallized intelligence is the person's ability to use long-term memory (experiences and skills) to resolve problems. This dichotomy is represented in the comments of young adults who claim middle-aged adults are "too rigid in their thinking" and middle-aged adults who complain young adults do not take advantage of their "wisdom,"—that is, the middle-aged person's intelligence and experience.

The rapidly changing complexity of the world has forced adults, in record numbers, to return to school. These adult learners are either changing careers, to meet the demands of an overchanging market, or reinforcing their present career choice through life-long learning. Schools that understand the difference between fluid and crystal intelligence are able to respond appropriately to the learning needs of each population of students.

Psychosocial Development

The quintessential milestone of middle age is the "mid-life crisis." The mid-life crisis is in actuality a readjustment from young adulthood, with marriage and children, to middle-aged existence. Central to the concerns of a middle-aged adult is the idea of legacy. Legacy implies that life had meaning—that the dream of young adulthood has come to fruition. Erikson characterized this stage of life as an issue of generativity versus stagnation.

Middle age is therefore a time of reassessment and realignment. If the person is at ease with the progress, then the person may choose to reprioritize, rededicate, and renew. Other persons, overwhelmed by the failure of their dreams, can spiral into depression, anger, and frustration, which can develop into crisis—even suicide.

Aging Parents

At a time when many middle-aged adults are seeing their children become adults, and are looking forward to the "empty nest," they are confronted with aged parents in need of care. Children of aged parents, particularly daughters, are often expected to care for their parents.

For some middle-aged adults, the strain of caring for aged parents, especially if they lack financial means, results in frustration, anger, and, in rare cases, elder abuse.

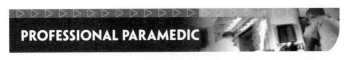

PROFESSIONAL PARAMEDIC

The professional Paramedic recognizes that aging is not a disease but a developmental event beginning before birth.

Late Adulthood

Late adulthood is somewhat synonymous with being elderly. The traditional definition of an elderly person is anyone who is 65 years old or older. This arbitrary cut-off is a poor marker for the onset of **senescence**, the breakdown in the body's ability to monitor for organ system failure and to repair those organs, which is inherent in the concept of being elderly. People less than 65 years of age may have symptoms of senescence whereas others with a chronological age of 80 years may in fact have the health of a 50-year-old.

However, the fact remains, regardless of any cut-offs in age, that the human population is aging. In 1900 only about 1% of Earth's human population was greater than 65 years of age. By 1992 that number had jumped to 6%, or 342 million people. An estimated 2.5 billion, or 20%, of the human population will be older than 65 years by the year 2050.

Paramedics may consider the elderly to be frail or feeble, based upon their interactions with a limited percentage of the entire population of the elderly (i.e., the approximately 1.5 million residents in nursing homes). This stereotypical view of the elderly, called **ageism**, is self-defeating for the Paramedic and fails to recognize the large population of active and vivacious senior citizens. Most Americans ranging from age 65 to 84 years of age have sufficient health to allow them to perform their **activities of daily living** independently, including dressing, feeding, and caring for themselves.

Life Expectancy

The National Center for Health Statistics and the United States Bureau of the Census reports that, on average, a person who has reached the age of 65 in 2000 can expect to live another 18.9 years and that a child born in the year 2000 could expect to be alive at least 86.9 years.

This increased life longevity—29 more years of life in 2000 when compared to a person born in 1900—is the result of a number of factors. These include improved sanitation, better health care, and improved nutrition, as well as reduced death rates in children and young adults.

The most widely circulated theory for senescence is the wear and tear theory. It is assumed that after years of exposure to the elements, toxins, free radicals, and pollution, the human body simply breaks down over time. Others have postulated that the human body has a gene that starts the aging process, ensuring a turnover in the species. For whatever reason, aging has significant effects upon the body.

Physical Development

A quick system-by-system review of organ systems quickly demonstrates the impact of aging (Figure 9-9). The most visible vestige of a person is skin. The skin of an elderly person wrinkles and sags as a result of a decrease in subcutaneous connective tissues. The bones of an elderly person also tend toward demineralization, a process called osteoporosis, leading to spontaneous fractures and falls.

While the cardiovascular system as well as the cardiopulmonary system are in decline, worsened by cardiovascular disease, it is the sensory system that fares worse. Cataracts, glaucoma, and loss of hearing are common to all elderly.

Not a single organ system in the body is spared the ravages of aging. Each organ system, according to the genetic make-up of an individual (sometimes called a person's constitution) fails over time.

Cognitive Development

The changes in mental functioning are generally related to the health of the person, not to age. It is not inevitable that every elderly person will become senile.

When discussing an elderly person's mental state, it is important to differentiate dementia from **delirium**. Delirium is a sudden change in mental function. It is an acute brain syndrome, which is usually associated with reversible metabolic derangements (e.g., hypoxia, or the toxic effects of medications).

Senile dementia is the result of irreversible damage to the brain that typically is manifest over a longer period of time (e.g., a series of brain attacks, such as strokes).[49-51] A common cause of dementia is Alzheimer's disease, a

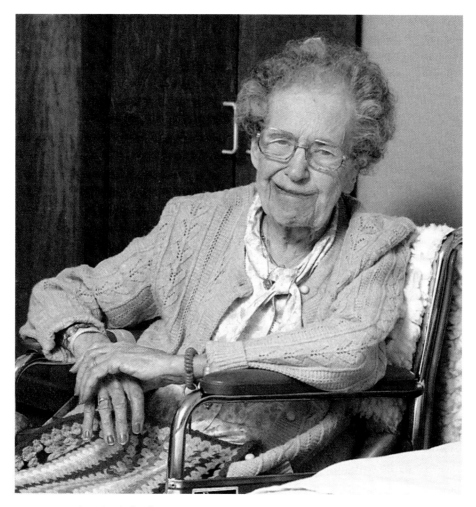

Figure 9-9 With age comes physical decline.

gradual degenerative disease of the brain characterized by confusion, forgetfulness, and ending with coma and death.

While passive senile dementia can occur, due to a loss of brain cells, the majority of elderly patients are in good health and any acute alteration in mental function should be immediately investigated for a potentially reversible cause.

Psychosocial Development

The final stage of human development, per Erikson, is integrity versus despair. Efforts to maintain one's dignity and using one's wisdom for the greater good will lead to feelings of integrity, whereas chronic poor health and substandard living conditions may cause an elderly person to fall into despair.

Most elderly persons want to be self-sufficient and live as independently as possible. In the past, options were generally limited to living at home while being assisted by adult children or living in a nursing home. New assisted-living centers, where meals are prepared for the residents; adult-care programs; and at-home, long-term care programs have provided much-needed steps between independent living and the nursing home. The key to satisfaction with these living arrangements is control of the individual, to the

extent possible, over living conditions and the availability of companionship (Figure 9-10).

Death and Dying

As one ages, one is faced with the inevitability of death. Most aging people begin to plan for it. An acceptance of the inevitability of death should not be confused with a desire to die.

However a desire to die and suicide are closely linked to aging. Unfortunately, a large number of elderly persons, particularly males, are clinically depressed, never seek or obtain the assistance they need, and commit suicide.[52,53] Depression in the elderly, like delirium, is a potentially reversible mental illness which should be confronted and dealt with immediately.

When a terminal disease threatens an elderly person's life, the person will begin the dying process. Kubler-Ross identified five stages of dying in her landmark work on death and dying. While these five stages are presented in a linear order, they can occur in variations. Some people may manifest all of the stages and some may only undergo a few of the stages.[54,55]

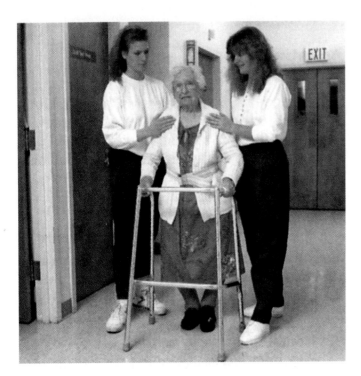

Figure 9-10 Companionship is important to the elderly.

The first stage of dying is denial, a refusal on the part of the patient, or the patient's family, to accept what is happening. Behaviors seen in patients in denial may range from a flat refusal to seek more medical attention to seeking the opinion of multiple physicians.

The next stage of dying is anger: anger at the world, anger at God, anger at family. Self-reproach is sometimes heard from a patient in anger.

The next stage of dying is bargaining. These patients will attempt to bargain with God, promising to stop sinful behaviors or to do some extraordinary good.

The patient eventually falls into a depression. Depression is the natural acceptance of the inevitable and the start of mourning. Patients who are depressed should be given support and observed for signs of suicidal thought.

In time, and in many cases there is not enough time, a patient will reach the final stage, acceptance. Acceptance of death is a reasonable conclusion when faced with the facts of the patient's situation.

Paramedics are, on occasion, called to help care for dying patients. In many instances all that is asked of the Paramedic is to honor a Do-Not-Attempt-Resuscitation (DNAR) order or to follow the wishes of a healthcare proxy who is speaking on the patient's behalf. In some instances, EMS may be called to the scene of a dying person to administer comfort measures, called **palliative care**, such as morphine sulfate. Sometimes this happens at the request of a hospice nurse.

Hospice is a concept of care which differs from mainstream medicine. Traditional medicine's mission is largely curative, whereas hospice medicine is focused on providing for the physical, emotional, and spiritual needs of a terminal patient.

CONCLUSION

From conception to the crypt, a person undergoes dramatic changes over the span of an entire lifetime. Understanding these changes, and their impact upon the person, helps the Paramedic empathize with the patient's situation. It also allows the Paramedic to adjust patient care to the patient's stage of life development in order to help ensure a more therapeutic outcome.

▶ KEY POINTS:

- Understanding the patient's developmental stage will help the Paramedic adjust his approach accordingly and to connect more therapeutically with the patient. The three components of development are (1) physical, (2) mental or cognitive, and (3) emotional or the affective self.

- Sigmund Freud's psychosocial developmental theory attached great importance to sexuality and linked the psychosocial development of a person to sex. Fundamental to Freud's theory are the ideas of a person's id, ego, and superego. Freud's theory stressed the physical developments and supported the idea that nature controlled one's development.

- Erikson stressed the social influences and supported the idea that nurturance had a great impact upon personal development. Conflict is the pivotal event that moves people through the eight stages of Erikson's psychosocial development.

- Pavlov, Skinner, and Bandura took the approach that life experiences (nurturance) are the dominant influence in a person's psychosocial development.

- Jean Piaget suggested that people develop in a building block fashion by developing schemas, one learned behavior building upon another. This process of assimilation, along with accommodation, is considered the source of human development over a lifespan.

- The path of fertilization begins at the moment of sexual climax and ends with the fertilization of the female ovum by a single spermatozoon. The newly fertilized ovum or zygote begins to develop in the fallopian tubes as it travels down to the uterus. The placenta is formed from zygotic cells and provides the fetus with nutrition though the umbilical cord.

- From the moment of conception to the end of the ninth week, the newly developed embryo begins the formation of the major organs. At this point in time the infant is at high risk for fetal malformation. Potential causes of malformation include illegal drug use, alcohol consumption, and severe infections during pregnancy.

- The female gender is a result of both gametes contributing an X chromosome. The male gender is a result of the male gamete contributing a Y chromosome. The child's physical appearance is due to the genetics of both parents. Chromosomes can be considered dominant or recessive, with the dominant contributor controlling the phenotypic or physical appearance.

- Sex chromosomes can also be linked to genetic diseases. If the child carries both genes then he or she will have the disease. If the child has only one gene linked to the disease, the disease will not be expressed, but he or she will be a carrier.

- A developing embryo, now called a fetus, will come to term in about nine months. The stages of pregnancy are divided into trimesters.

- Childbirth occurs in three stages. The first stage begins when the uterus starts to contract in a process called labor. The second stage is the infant's movement down the birth canal, and the third and final stage is the delivery of the placenta.

- During the first minute of life the umbilical blood flow diminishes, raising carbon dioxide levels, which in turn stimulate the newly born's first breath. The increase in intrathoracic pressure, from the air-filled lungs, causes the cardiac shunts—the foramen ovale and the ductus arterious—to reverse blood flow and then close. The newborn's pulse is between 100 and 160 beats per minute, and respirations are between 40 to 60 breaths per minute.

- The Paramedic should recognize that infants can quickly fatigue and experience respiratory failure due to an easily obstructed airway, compensation for increased oxygen demand, weak accessory muscles, and loss of heat.

- The developmental milestones represent a typical child's development and are used to gauge an individual child's development against a norm. During the first six months the infant displays primitive reflexes. During the assessment of an infant the Paramedic should be attentive to the presence of infantile reflexes. Infantile reflexes may include the Moro reflex, palmar grasp reflex, and Babinski reflex.

- Cognitively, primitive reflexes continue to develop as the infant assimilates experiences into old schemas, thus building new schemas. The infant also begins to acquire language skills. The Paramedic may witness bonding or behavior such as mutual gazing, reflective smiling, and response to touch. This behavior is the beginning of psychosocial development between a mother and child.

- The continued social interaction between infant and parents is the start of the socialization process. During this early period of socialization, autism is often discovered.

- Parenting methods may be divided into four styles with an emphasis—or de-emphasis—on nurturance. The styles include the permissive or indulgent parent, the authoritarian parent, the authoritative parent, and the uninvolved parent.

- The child raised by the uninvolved style of parenting may be more aggressive, to the point of violence. When the Paramedic is faced with a situation in which the child is aggressive, the Paramedic should acknowledge the behavior without becoming aggressive in either words or action, all the while remaining authoritative.

- During the period of early childhood, from ages 2 to 5, there is extraordinary growth where all children become larger and taller. Those who fail to grow, exhibiting failure to thrive, may be under severe psychosocial pressures or have nutritional deficits. Paramedics need to identify these toddlers and encourage the parent to seek medical attention for the child.

- The growing neuromuscular system in a toddler is made evident by the toddler's ability to perform more complex motor activities. The toddler is in the preoperational stage of cognitive development and is not able to think abstractly. Young children also develop mathematical reasoning and language acquisition.

- Physical growth slows during the middle childhood stage, although the child is more interactive with his environment. In this concrete operational stage, the child is able to understand such concepts as spatial relation, nature of time, and the sequential nature of certain activities. The multiple intelligences of a person may also become evident.

- Middle childhood is also a time when the child develops a sense of self and a desire to succeed and achieve. At this age children begin to relate to others more in terms of common interests and goals. With less influence by parents, peers take on a greater role in shaping the person's personality.

- During the school-age years, children start to attach a gender-role identity to themselves, that sense of being a male or a female. Regardless of a child's gender-role identity, it is important that the Paramedic remain nonjudgmental in this matter and focus on the patient's medical condition.

- The most remarkable changes in the human physique, or body habitus, occur during adolescent physical development. Entering into puberty, males and females see dramatic sexual changes in their physical bodies as they develop secondary sex characteristics.

- Unhealthy situations can arise as adolescents seek out opportunities for freedom. Because of a desire to experiment, adolescents may engage in drug use and explore their sexuality in unsafe ways. The advent of sexuality brings the risk of acquiring sexually transmitted diseases.

- Chaotic schedules, the ease and availability of "junk foods," and peer pressure contribute to poor teenage nutrition and a national epidemic of teenage obesity. The health risks associated with obesity include type 2 diabetes mellitus, secondary hypertension, accelerated coronary artery disease, and stroke. At the other extreme of teenage weight problems is a psychiatric illness called anorexia nervosa.

- There is an increased risk of premature death among teenagers secondary to engaging in increased risk-taking behaviors and having a false sense of invulnerability. However, teenagers are also at higher risk of death from suicide.

- Cognitive development of the adolescent enters the formal stage and revolves around using logic to solve problems, as well as seeing problems as "less black and white and more gray." The psychosocial development involves a return of egocentrism, a stage previously encountered in early childhood. During this time, adolescents turn their attention to morality and their own moral development.

- Early adulthood is a period of striving and accomplishment that is punctuated by fundamental decisions, like going to college or entering the workforce, and peak life events such as marriage and childbirth.

- The majority of people, both male and female, reach their peak height in their early twenties, and their health is generally at its peak as well. However, obesity is becoming more common and the risk for developing unhealthy behaviors still remains.

- Cognitive development of young adults includes exploration of the world through interaction with others and seeking out new experiences that engender questions about themselves, the people with whom they associate, and the world in general.

- Psychosocial development of young adults involves finding that special someone with whom to share common goals and aspirations. These goals and aspirations may include marriage and parenthood.

- Paramedics should understand that single mothers may have limited resources and that EMS is one of the few social supports readily available during a time of acute distress. Paramedics should also be sensitive to the fact that 5% of married adults cannot, or do not want to, have children.

- Middle adulthood can be characterized as a period of maximal productivity as well as a period of readjustment and realignment. Middle adulthood is also a period of physical decline and changes in interpersonal focus and information processing.

- The quintessential milestone of middle age is the "mid-life crisis," and central to the concerns of a middle-aged adult is the idea of legacy. Legacy implies that life had meaning, and that the dream of young adulthood has come to fruition. Middle-aged adults are also confronted with aged parents in need of care.

- Late adulthood is somewhat synonymous with being elderly, but is marked by the onset of senescence. Most Americans ranging in age from 65 to 84 have sufficient health to allow them to independently perform their activities of daily living. However, due to the stereotypical view of the elderly that exists, called ageism, the Paramedic may fail to recognize the large population of active and vivacious senior citizens.

- Improved sanitation, better health care, and improved nutrition, as well as reduced death rates in children and young adults, have all contributed to increased life longevity. The effects of physical aging include osteoporosis, cardiovascular and cardiopulmonary decline, and a decreased sensory system.

- Changes in mental functioning among the elderly are generally related to the person's health, not to age. Delirium is a sudden change in mental function, which is an acute brain syndrome that is usually associated with reversible metabolic derangements such as hypoxia. Senile dementia is the result of irreversible damage to the brain that typically is manifested over a longer period of time, such as Alzheimer's disease. While passive senile dementia can occur, the majority of elderly patients are in good health. Therefore, any acute alteration in mental function should be immediately investigated for a potentially reversible cause.

- The goal of most elderly persons is to be self-sufficient and live as independently as possible. Independence can be maintained at assisted-living centers, through adult-care programs, and at-home.

- Depression in the elderly, like delirium, is a potentially reversible mental illness that should be confronted and dealt with immediately. When a terminal disease threatens an elderly person's life, the person will begin the dying process marked by what is referred to as the five stages of dying.

- Paramedics are, on occasion, called to help care for dying patients. In many instances, all that

is asked of the Paramedic is to honor a Do-Not-Attempt-Resuscitation (DNAR) order or to follow the wishes of a healthcare proxy who is speaking on the patient's behalf.

- Hospice medicine is focused on providing for the physical, emotional, and spiritual needs of a terminal patient. In some instances, EMS may be called to the scene of a dying person to administer comfort measures, called palliative care (such as morphine sulfate), sometimes at the request of a hospice nurse.

REVIEW QUESTIONS:

1. Describe the main points for each theory of psychosocial development put forth by Freud, Erickson, Skinner, and Piaget.
2. How is the gender of a fetus determined?
3. Explain how two parents, both with recessive genes for a disorder, can potentially have a child that will have the disorder.
4. What are the stages of childbirth?
5. What are some developmental milestones for infants and toddlers?
6. Describe the four different types of parenting.
7. At what stage of development is there extraordinary growth and development?
8. Starting with concrete thinking, what is the progression of cognitive development of a child through young adulthood?

9. What are some health risks that teenagers face and why are they more prone to engage in unhealthy behavior?
10. What confronts an adult when he or she reaches middle age?
11. Why is the stereotypical view of elderly people inaccurate?
12. What factors have helped to increase our life expectancy?
13. Differentiate between delirium and dementia.
14. What are the five stages of dying per Kubler-Ross?
15. Discuss the importance of palliative care and the effects of hospice.

CASE STUDY QUESTIONS:

Please refer to the Case Study at the beginning of the chapter and answer the questions below.

1. Based on lifespan development, what expectations should Paramedics have for the following considerations in a 13-year-old male?

- Physical development
- Cognitive development
- Affective development

REFERENCES:

1. Erikson E. *Identity and the Life Cycle*. New York: W. W. Norton & Company; 1980.

2. Greenberg-Edelstein R. *Nurturance Phenomenon: Roots of Group Psychotherapy*. Norwalk, Conn.: Appleton & Lange; 1986.

3. Hall C. *A Primer of Freudian Psychology*. New York: Plume; 1999.

4. Slater L. *Opening Skinner's Box: Great Psychological Experiments of the Twentieth Century*. New York: W. W. Norton & Company; 2005.

5. Sanders B. Uterine factors and infertility. *J Reprod Med*. 2006;51(3):169–176.

6. Vercammen EE, D'Hooghe TM. Endometriosis and recurrent pregnancy loss. *Semin Reprod Med*. 2000;18(4):363–368.

7. Szamatowicz M, Grochowski D. Fertility and infertility in aging women. *Gynecol Endocrinol*. 1998;12(6):407–413.

8. ACOG. ACOG Committee Opinion No. 383: Evaluation of stillbirths and neonatal deaths. *Obstet Gynecol*. 2007;110(4):963–966.

9. Mathews TJ, MacDorman MF. Infant mortality statistics from the 2004 period linked birth/infant death data set. *Natl Vital Stat Rep*. 2007;55(14):1–32.

10. Sharps PW, Laughon K, Giangrande SK. Intimate partner violence and the childbearing year: Maternal and infant health consequences. *Trauma Violence Abuse*. 2007;8(2):105–116.

11. Ashdown-Lambert JR. A review of low birth weight: predictors, precursors and morbidity outcomes. *J R Soc Health*. 2005;125(2):76–83.

12. Boy A, Salihu HM. Intimate partner violence and birth outcomes: a systematic review. *Int J Fertil Womens Med*. 2004;49(4):159–164.

13. Berenson AB, Wiemann CM, Wilkinson GS, Jones WA, Anderson GD. Perinatal morbidity associated with violence experienced by pregnant women. *Am J Obstet Gynecol*. 1994;170(6):1760–1766; discussion 1766–1769.

14. Lipsky S, Holt VL, Easterling TR, Critchlow CW. Impact of police-reported intimate partner violence during pregnancy on birth outcomes. *Obstet Gynecol*. 2003;102(3):557–564.

15. Polgar G. The first breath: A turbulent period of physiologic adjustment. *Clin Pediatr (Phila)*. 1963;2:562–571.

16. Scarpelli EM. Perinatal lung mechanics and the first breath. *Lung*. 1984;162(2):61–71.

17. 2005 American Heart Association. AHA guidelines for cardiopulmonary resuscitation (CPR) and emergency cardiovascular care (ECC) of pediatric and neonatal patients: Pediatric basic life support. *Pediatrics*. 2006;117(5):e989–1004.

18. Ehrenkranz RA. Early, aggressive nutritional management for very low birth weight infants: what is the evidence? *Semin Perinatol*. 2007;31(2):48–55.

19. Brown JE, Murtaugh MA, Jacobs DR, Jr., Margellos HC. Variation in newborn size according to pregnancy weight change by trimester. *Am J Clin Nutr*. 2002;76(1):205–209.

20. Aylott M. The neonatal energy triangle. Part 2: Thermoregulatory and respiratory adaption. *Paediatr Nurs*. 2006;18(7):38–42.

21. Sherman TI, Greenspan JS, St. Clair N, Touch SM, Shaffer TH. Optimizing the neonatal thermal environment. *Neonatal Netw*. 2006;25(4):251–260.

22. Stern L. The newborn infant and his thermal environment. *Curr Probl Pediatr*. 1970;1(1):1–29.

23. Sedin G, Agren J. Water and heat—the priority for the newborn infant. *Ups J Med Sci*. 2006;111(1):45–59.

24. Shott SR, Myer CM, III, Willis R, Cotton RT. Nasal obstruction in the neonate. *Rhinology*. 1989;27(2):91–96.

25. Coates H. Nasal obstruction in the neonate and infant. *Clin Pediatr (Phila)*. 1992;31(1):25–29.

26. Hanson LA, Adlerberth I, Carlsson B, Zaman S, Hahn-Zoric M, Jalil F. Antibody-mediated immunity in the neonate. *Padiatr Padol*. 1990;25(5):371–376.

27. Zafeiriou DI. Primitive reflexes and postural reactions in the neurodevelopmental examination. *Pediatr Neurol*. 2004;31(1):1–8.

28. Futagi Y, Tagawa T, Otani K. Primitive reflex profiles in infants: differences based on categories of neurological abnormality. *Brain Dev*. 1992;14(5):294–298.

29. Zafeiriou DI. Plantar grasp reflex in high-risk infants during the first year of life. *Pediatr Neurol*. 2000;22(1):75–76.

30. Suveg C, Aschenbrand SG, Kendall PC. Separation anxiety disorder, panic disorder, and school refusal. *Child Adolesc Psychiatr Clin N Am*. 2005;14(4):773–795, ix.

31. Jurbergs N, Ledley DR. Separation anxiety disorder. *Pediatr Ann*. 2005;34(2):108–115.

32. Manworren RC, Hynan LS. Clinical validation of FLACC: preverbal patient pain scale. *Pediatr Nurs*. 2003;29(2):140–146.

33. Hummel P, van Dijk M. Pain assessment: current status and challenges. *Semin Fetal Neonatal Med*. 2006;11(4):237–245.

34. Johnston CC. Pain assessment and management in infants. *Pediatrician*. 1989;16(1–2):16–23.

35. Bjorklund DF. In search of a metatheory for cognitive development (or, Piaget is dead and I don't feel so good myself). *Child Dev*. 1997;68(1):144–148.

36. Blakeslee J, Lewis S, Lewis J, Wallerstein J. *The Unexpected Legacy of Divorce: A 25 Year Landmark Study*. Westport, Conn.: Hyperion Books; 2000.

37. Johnson HL, Erbelding EJ, Zenilman JM, Ghanem KG. Sexually transmitted diseases and risk behaviors among pregnant women attending inner city public sexually transmitted diseases clinics in Baltimore, MD, 1996–2002. *Sex Transm Dis*. 2007;34(12):991–994.

38. Gray-Swain MR, Peipert JF. Pelvic inflammatory disease in adolescents. *Curr Opin Obstet Gynecol.* 2006;18(5):503–510.

39. McKinzie J. Sexually transmitted diseases. *Emerg Med Clin North Am.* 2001;19(3):723–743.

40. Rambout L, Hopkins L, Hutton B, Fergusson D. Prophylactic vaccination against human papillomavirus infection and disease in women: a systematic review of randomized controlled trials. *Cmaj.* 2007;177(5):469–479.

41. Sodersten P, Bergh C, Bjornstrom M. Prevalence and recovery from anorexia nervosa. *Am J Psychiatry.* 2008;165(2):264–265.

42. Steele MM, Doey T. Suicidal behaviour in children and adolescents. Part 1: etiology and risk factors. *Can J Psychiatry.* 2007;52(6 Suppl 1):21S–33S.

43. Steele MM, Doey T. Suicidal behaviour in children and adolescents. Part 2: treatment and prevention. *Can J Psychiatry.* 2007;52(6 Suppl 1):35S–45S.

44. Wintersteen MB, Diamond GS, Fein JA. Screening for suicide risk in the pediatric emergency and acute care setting. *Curr Opin Pediatr.* 2007;19(4):398–404.

45. Furstenberg FF, Jr. History and current status of divorce in the United States. *Future Child.* 1994;4(1):29–43.

46. Espie M, Daures JP, Chevallier T, Mares P, Micheletti MC, De Reilhac P. Breast cancer incidence and hormone replacement therapy: results from the MISSION study, prospective phase. *Gynecol Endocrinol.* 2007;23(7):391–397.

47. Rossouw JE, Anderson GL, Prentice RL, LaCroix AZ, Kooperberg C, Stefanick ML, et al. Risks and benefits of estrogen plus progestin in healthy postmenopausal women: principal results from the Women's Health Initiative randomized controlled trial. *Jama.* 2002;288(3):pp. 321–333.

48. Rossouw JE, Prentice RL, Manson JE, Wu L, Barad D, Barnabei VM, et al. Postmenopausal hormone therapy and risk of cardiovascular disease by age and years since menopause. *Jama.* 2007;297(13):1465–1477.

49. Kirshner HS. Delirium: a focused review. *Curr Neurol Neurosci Rep.* 2007;7(6):479–482.

50. Rummans TA, Evans JM, Krahn LE, Fleming KC. Delirium in elderly patients: evaluation and management. *Mayo Clin Proc.* 1995;70(10):989–998.

51. Borja B, Borja CS, Gade S. Psychiatric emergencies in the geriatric population. *Clin Geriatr Med.* 2007;23(2):391–400, vii.

52. Heisel MJ. Suicide and its prevention among older adults. *Can J Psychiatry.* 2006;51(3):143–154.

53. Manthorpe J, Iliffe S. Suicide among older people. *Nurs Older People.* 2006;17(10):25–29.

54. Kubler-Ross E, Wessler S, Avioli LV. On death and dying. *Jama.* 1972;221(2):174–179.

55. Curry LC, Stone JG. The grief process: a preparation for death. *Clin Nurse Spec.* 1991; 5(1):17–22.

CHAPTER 10

BASIC HUMAN PHYSIOLOGY

KEY CONCEPTS:

Upon completion of this chapter, it is expected that the reader will understand these following concepts:

- Cellular physiology and the need for homeostasis
- Fluid movement as dynamic driven by concentrations and hydrostatic pressure
- The body's general adaptation syndrome
- Cell-mediated sympathetic and parasympathetic responses
- The body's thermoregulatory mechanism
- The cell's ability to adapt to variable conditions

▶ CASE STUDY:

"Hey, take a look in today's paper. Remember that man from the auto crash two weeks ago? He died!" The Paramedics remembered the man. He was in a serious auto crash and had suffered some serious injuries. On-scene, it took a while before they could get him out of the car so he could be properly ventilated with a bag-mask assembly. He kept asking for a glass of water during the extrication and thought he could get up and walk away. They got a couple of large IVs into him. By the time he was transferred to the hospital, he had a blood pressure of 100/80 and a heart rate of 100. "Wonder what happened to him?"

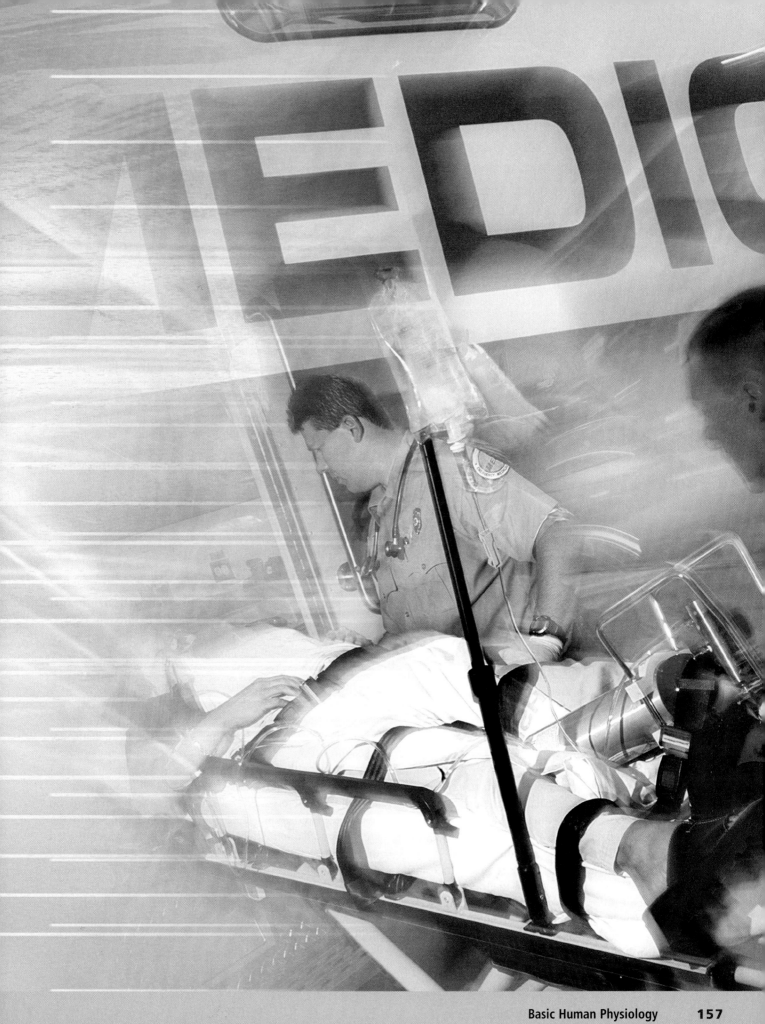

OVERVIEW

The systems of the body work together to carry out the body's functions. These systems can be broken down into individual organs, then to specific tissues, and further into specialized cells. This chapter begins with a look at cellular physiology and the process of maintaining an internal equilibrium. This balance or homeostasis is seen throughout systems of the body in response to internal and external stimuli. For the Paramedic, this includes the sympathetic and parasympathetic responses of the nervous system, the body's thermoregulatory mechanism, and the cell's ability to adapt to variable conditions.

Physiology

The study of the body's functions, in its normal human condition, is called **physiology**. Different from anatomy, which studies human form, physiology studies the physical, mechanical, and biochemical processes that go on inside the body every day (i.e., how the body works). This chapter is a brief overview of human physiology, with an emphasis on physiology that may have particular importance to the Paramedic.

Cellular Milieu

The human body is actually a complex association of independent cells which, together, form tissues. The tissues in turn become organs, and ultimately all the cells comprise a person. Therefore, a person's overall well-being is dependent on the health of all of the person's constituent cells.

To survive and thrive (i.e., to be healthy), cells need an environment, a **milieu**, that has (1) water, the most abundant substance in the body; (2) food stuffs, in the form of glucose, amino acids, and fatty acids; and (3) oxygen. All of these essential elements must be maintained in an internal environment where there is sufficient heat and acidity for biochemical reactions, or **metabolism**, to occur and life processes to go on.

Homeostasis

One of the primary functions of the human body is to maintain a relatively even state of temperature, acid load, oxygenation, blood glucose, and so on, for internal life processes. When the goal is achieved it is called **wellness**, a state of physiologic equilibrium free of disease. The body's process to attain this state of internal equilibrium is called **homeostasis**.

Coined by Cannon in 1939, the term "homeostasis" attempts to describe the processes that the body undertakes to try to maintain a constant state of equilibrium.[1] Key to understanding the complex concept of homeostasis is an understanding of the regulatory mechanisms that the body utilizes to help to maintain homeostasis, namely the endocrine system and autonomic nervous system.

Resisting homeostasis are a myriad of external factors, such as cold and heat, lack of food, and infectious diseases. Abnormal internal conditions, broadly called diseases, also challenge homeostasis. The body must overcome them in order to maintain homeostasis. Because these factors are always changing, the human body is in a constant state of flux, resisting and adapting to external and internal conditions, while trying to maintain normalcy within a certain set of acceptable parameters called a **range**. Because of this ever-changing internal milieu, some scientists and physicians have suggested that the more correct term for this process would be "homeodynamics," in recognition of the ever-changing conditions.

The sum of the biological processes within the body—circulation, ventilation, and so on, through symbiosis—support the cells of the body.

Cellular Physiology

The outside of a cell is made up of a **cell wall membrane**, a porous semipermeable dual layer lipid–protein matrix. Inside the cell is an internal fluid called **cytoplasm**, which is primarily water and organelles, subunits with a specific cellular function(s).

In the center of the cell is the first organelle, the nucleus, which contains chromosomes and DNA. These are the blueprints for cellular protein production and reproduction.

Outside of the nucleus, but inside the cytoplasm, are **lysosomes**, tiny sacs that contain enzymes which can break down proteins. Lysosomes can break down foreign proteins in bacteria, called **antigens**, or the cell's own chromosomes.

The largest organelle in the cell is the **mitochondria**. Inside the mitochondria, glucose is transformed into the energy source **adenosine triphosphate** (ATP), which is used to power the rest of the cell's functions. This function, the production of ATP, earned the mitochondria the nickname of the cell's "powerhouse" (Figure 10-1).

For the all important mitochondria to work properly, the body must maintain a complex set of conditions—including fluid balance, acidity, oxygenation, and temperature. The body depends on the nervous system, the endocrine system, and the immune system to maintain that crucial balance.

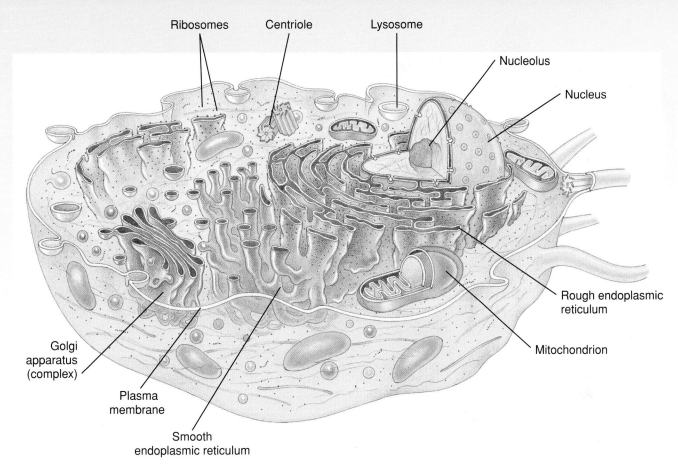

Figure 10-1 Cross-section of a typical cell.

Labels on figure:
Ribosomes
Centriole
Lysosome
Nucleolus
Nucleus
Rough endoplasmic reticulum
Mitochondrion
Smooth endoplasmic reticulum
Plasma membrane
Golgi apparatus (complex)

Sodium Potassium Pump

To make adaptations to the constantly changing conditions that exist within the body, the cells need energy. For the cell, that energy is in the form of adenosine triphosphate (ATP).

The phase of glucose metabolism does not utilize oxygen and is called **anaerobic metabolism**. During anaerobic metabolism, the cell changes glucose into pyruvate acid, which is in turn converted into lactic acid by an enzyme called lactate dehydrogenase (de- – "without"; hydrogen; -ase – indicating an enzyme).

Although anaerobic metabolism is relatively inefficient in that it only yields two ATP, or about 2% of the energy that is available from glucose if oxygen were to be used, it is 100 times faster than aerobic metabolism. For this reason, cells that need quick energy in a short amount of time (i.e., skeletal muscles) use anaerobic metabolism.

Interestingly, red blood cells (erythrocytes) that carry oxygen cannot use the oxygen they carry. They depend on anaerobic metabolism and save the oxygen for the cells of the body instead.

Anaerobic metabolism only yields two ATP but can still release 619 kCal of heat. This amount of heat is comparable to the amount of heat released by aerobic metabolism (696 kCal). Thus, anaerobic metabolism can help keep the body warm (a very important factor discussed later) while not

requiring the complex interactions of other organs required in aerobic metabolism.

Under ideal conditions, and in the presence of sufficient glucose and oxygen, the cell uses oxygen in the next step of its metabolism, a process called **aerobic metabolism**, to create ATP from glucose (Figure 10-2).

During this process, the body uses eight different enzymes to divide glucose, a process called **glycolysis** (glycol- – "sugar"; -lysis – "to divide"), to create a chemical called pyruvate. Pyruvate and oxygen enter into the citric acid or Krebs cycle, another complex series of changes facilitated by enzymes, and there they undergo a process that creates ATP.

The end result of this chemical reaction creates carbon dioxide (CO_2), water (H_2O), energy (in the form of ATP), and heat from the carbohydrate glucose. Aerobic metabolism produces about 36 ATP for the cell to use as energy compared to the 2 ATP produced from glucose during anaerobic metabolism.

Glucose Storage

When glucose is abundant, such as after a meal of carbohydrates, any glucose which is not needed immediately by the body is stored in the liver and muscles as a dual molecule called **glycogen** (glycol- – "sugar"; -gen – "create"). When glucose levels fall, then the body liberates some glucose from

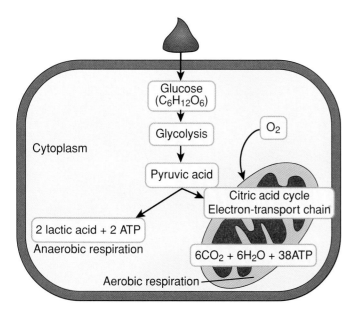

Figure 10-2 First aerobic then anaerobic metabolism.

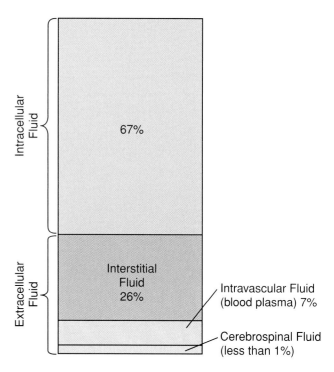

Figure 10-3 Distribution of water in the body.

these glucose stores. These two bonded glucose molecules (glycogen) are broken down by an enzyme called **glucagon** into individual glucose molecules.

In the absence of other readily available glucose stores, the body can use other food sources to create glucose, a process called gluconeogenesis (glycol- – "sugar"; neo – "new"; genesis – "creation"). For example, the body can release glucose from fats, and in the process leave fatty acids behind. In extreme cases when glucose is not readily available, the body can even break down muscles, liberating proteins in the process. These proteins are then further broken down into amino acids and glucose, leaving urea behind.

The process of aerobic metabolism is dependent upon many organ systems working together in synchrony in order to be effective. To make ATP, the mitochondria needs ideal conditions of temperature and acidity. The body temperature must be maintained at a fairly constant range of 99.6°F +/− 1°F by a complex system of cooling and heat preservation which uses bodily fluids in the same way as an automobile engine uses radiator fluid. Acidity is also maintained by a complex system of dilution and diuresis (Greek "to pass urine"). Central to maintaining both of these conditions is fluid balance.

Fluid Balance

The body is primarily made up of water—some 50% to 55% of total body weight (TBW) in women and 55% to 60% of TBW in men.[2] The water within the body can be divided into two portions or compartments. The water that is within the cells is **intracellular water** and the water that is outside of the cells is **extracellular water**.

The majority of body water is intracellular. This amounts to about 35% to 40% of the TBW, or 25 liters (L) in the average 70 kilogram (kg)/154 pound male (Figure 10-3). The remaining fluid is extracellular water which is in one of two types. **Interstitial fluid** is the fluid between cells. It is about 16% of the TBW, or 11 L. The second type of extracellular water is fluid found in the blood, which is called **intravascular fluid**. It is primarily made of plasma and constitutes about 4% of the TBW or 3 or 4 L. (For clarification, the blood volume in the 70 kg male is about 6 L but only a portion of the blood is plasma, the rest being formed elements.)

Anatomists in the past referred to the volume of fluid inside the cells (intracellular) as the first space, the volume of fluid in the bloodstream (intravascular) as the second space, and the volume of blood in between the cells (the interstitial space) as the third space.

While these volumes of fluid in each compartment are illustrative of the general distribution of fluids within the body, it should not be thought that fluid levels between body compartments are static. In fact, there is a constant movement of fluids between compartments, an ebb and flow of living sustaining water laden with glucose, oxygen, and other chemicals necessary for life. This is also known as nutritional flow.

Fluids can move from outside to inside the cells and from compartment to compartment by diffusion or osmosis. What controls the amount of fluid transferred from one compartment to another is either the pressure behind the fluid or the salts or the proteins in the fluid of the other compartment. In both cases, nature is trying to reach a balance between the amounts of solutes in the two compartments.

For example, when the interstitial fluid volume is low, such as during dehydration, then fluids are drawn out of the intravascular compartment into the interstitial space. This pressure created by the force behind the volume of water is called the **hydrostatic pressure**. An analogy can be made to the garden hose. A garden hose can flow so many liters of water per minute (lpm) and this flow can be measured as a pressure (mmHg). Interestingly, as the circumference of the opening narrows, such as when one places a thumb over the end of the hose, the pressure increases but the volume of fluid (lpm) remains the same. However, when the hose is narrowed to a critical point, about 70% to 90%, then the volume starts to decline. Therefore, when the capillary hydrostatic pressure is greater than the tissue hydrostatic pressure, which is near zero, then fluid freely moves, or diffuses, across the capillary wall and into the tissues.

Resisting this infusion of fluids into the interstitial space is the tissue's hydrostatic pressure. This pressure is a combination of factors including maximal interstitial fluid volume and compliance of the tissue (i.e., its elasticity). In short, the tissues have mechanisms that stop the free infusion of fluids once the tissues are adequately hydrated; adequate hydration being a function of the cells' needs at the time.

Constantly draining the tissues (the interstitial space) is the venous system and the lymphatic system. The venous system does the bulk of the elimination of the fluids from the interstitial space. The lymphatic system acts as a storm sewer of sorts, ridding the tissue of excess fluid beyond what the venous system can drain. Therefore, any backup of the venous system, or blockage of the lymphatic system, can result in dramatic fluid buildup in the tissues called **edema**.

As a result of this constant filling of the interstitial space with nutrient-laden fluids and the subsequent drainage of those tissues, a flow is created. Another factor in this flow is osmotic pressure. Osmosis occurs whenever a semipermeable membrane exists and there is a concentration of a substance, typically salt, on one side. Since the salt cannot cross a semipermeable membrane, water diffuses across the semipermeable membrane to try to balance the solution.

If the solution being infused into the bloodstream has the same amount of salt (solute) and water (solvent) as the solution on the other side of the capillary membrane, then osmosis will not occur. Such a fluid is said to be a balanced solution. Another name for a balanced solution is an **isotonic** solution (iso- – "equal"; tonic – "tension"). An example of a balanced solution that is used for intravenous infusions is "normal saline"; termed "normal saline" because it has approximately the same amount of saline (sodium chloride 0.9%) as exists in blood and is therefore isotonic.[1,3,4]

Therefore, when a fluid has more water and less salt (electrolytes) than the solution on the other side of a semipermeable membrane, then the fluid is labeled **hypotonic**. In an effort to obtain a balance of concentrations, the water from the hypotonic solution will cross the membrane until the two solutions are balanced (i.e., equal parts water and salt). An example of a hypotonic solution is 5% dextrose in sterile water (D_5W). Since there is more water in intravenous D_5W than in the interstitial space, the water passes into the tissues. This is useful when treating dehydration.

Alternatively, when a fluid has less water and more salt (electrolytes), then the solution is called **hypertonic**. A hypertonic fluid on the other side of a semipermeable membrane will pull fluids into itself (Figure 10-4). The military has made limited use of hypertonic solutions during resuscitation of wounded soldiers who have hemorrhaged and are in need of intravascular volume replacement.

The capillary membrane, however, is relatively permeable to electrolytes, such as sodium chloride. For this reason, electrolytes in the blood, for example, do not create a great deal of osmotic pressure. However, capillary membranes are semipermeable to proteins. These proteins can be found in both the intercellular and extracellular space, including the intravascular space. These proteins create a force similar to osmotic pressure called **oncotic** pressure.

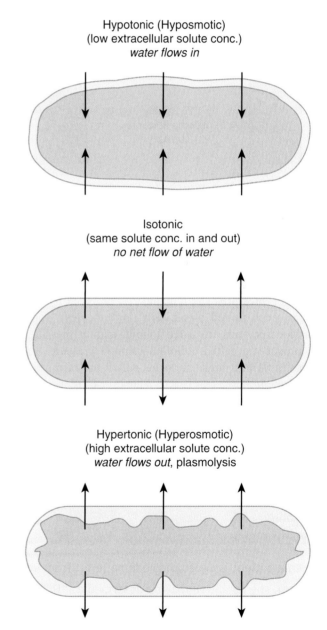

Figure 10-4 Effects of isotonic, hypotonic, and hypertonic fluids across a semipermeable membrane.

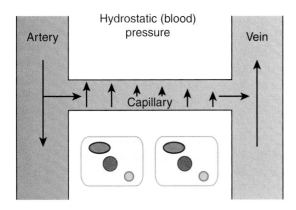

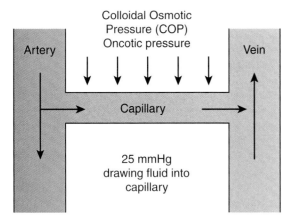

Figure 10-5 The effects of oncotic and hydrostatic pressure upon intravascular volume.

The most common intravascular protein is albumin, principally made in the liver. Albumin creates about 70% of the oncotic pressure. The remainder is provided by formed elements such as red blood cells (erythrocytes). Together these blood proteins are called colloids and the pressure that they produce is called colloidal osmotic pressure (COP). Whenever COP is high fluids are pulled out of the tissues and into the intravascular space. Whenever COP is low (e.g., when albumin levels are low during liver failure) fluid leaks from the intravascular space and into the interstitial space, a process called **third spacing** (Figure 10-5).

Temperature Regulation

The enzymes within the cells operate best in a narrow temperature range of 98.6°F +/− 1°F. All endothermic (i.e., warm-blooded) animals create heat during cellular metabolism and use that heat to maintain a relatively constant core temperature. However, at least 90% of all cellular metabolism is used to maintain that heat production, leaving little for other life processes.[8] While this may seem like an enormous cost, the benefit is that it permits people to move about freely regardless of the environmental conditions. However, this ability to adapt to conditions is not unlimited.

If too much heat builds up in the body's core, a condition called **hyperthermia**, then the cell walls become more fluid-like and cannot maintain their integrity. If there is too little heat, a condition called **hypothermia**, then the cell walls become gel-like, almost crystalline, and all cell wall activities stop. Thus, the body takes measures to both accumulate heat as well as dissipate heat.

The anterior hypothalamus regulates the body's temperature, acting as a thermostat and controlling heat loss mechanisms. With a set point of approximately 99°F, if the body gets warmer than 99°F the hypothalamus engages certain heat loss mechanisms including rapid breathing, sweating, and vasodilatation.

Vasodilatation is perhaps one of the most effective heat-dissipating mechanisms that the body has. Controlled by the parasympathetic nervous system, surface capillaries under the skin react to dissipate the heat. Surface capillaries normally hold about 300 mL of blood but can be dilated to accommodate as much as 3,000 mL of blood. This causes the skin to act as a massive radiator to allow heat to dissipate by conduction, convection, and radiation.[9,10]

If the body should start to cool, then the hypothalamus can either increase heat production by causing shivering, an involuntary contraction of muscles, and/or by vasoconstriction. Alpha receptors of the sympathetic nervous system cause peripheral vasoconstriction by contracting the capillary sphincters (round muscles) that control the blood flow in the capillary bed. Vasoconstriction can reduce blood flow in the skin from 300 mL to as little as 30 mL for short periods of time.

Temperature and the Oxyhemoglobin Curve

Increased body temperature (i.e., a fever) has been maligned by laypersons as being harmful to the body. Nothing could be further from the truth. Fever is actually beneficial to the healing process at many levels.

The hypothalamus, located in the brain, controls the mean temperature of the body and maintains it at a steady state of approximately 99.6°F. During an infection, poisons from the bacteria, called **endotoxins**, stimulate chemical mediators (such as interleukin and interferon) to affect the hypothalamus. In essence, these chemical mediators reset the hypothalamus thermostat, thereby causing it to raise the body's temperature.

These **pyrogens** (fever producers) therefore create a **pyrexia** (Greek—fever) which makes the environment hostile to bacteria, increases motility of macrophages, and enhances phagocytosis (cell eating) of bacteria by white blood cells.[11–13]

The increased temperature also moves the oxyhemoglobin dissociation curve to the right, improving oxygen off loading to the cells. Also, metabolism is increased at the site of a localized infection vis-á-vis Hoff's law where a 1°C temperature rise results in a 13% increase in metabolism.

While fever can be helpful in mild infections, in the case of a severe systemic infection high fever can lead to delirium and/or convulsions. One possible cause of these convulsions is cerebral hypoxia. While hemoglobin readily releases oxygen to the cells whenever the tissues are acidotic or hyperthermic, hemoglobin picks up less oxygen in the lungs. Tissues that are sensitive to even small drops in oxygen saturation of hemoglobin, such as nervous tissue, will suffer from the resultant systemic hypoxia.

Stress

Stress and Cellular Response

Environmental conditions, both internal and external, are constantly changing and therefore can cause an imbalance within the body (i.e., a disruption in the homeostasis of the body). These constantly changing conditions, called **stress**, cause the body to respond in an effort to regain homeostasis.

In 1946 Hans Selye noted this physiologic response in lab rats while injecting them with an ovarian extract. He quickly noted the physiologic response was not limited to injections only but to cold and injury as well. Selye labeled these noxious stimuli as **stressors**.

Selye noted that when a person was stimulated with a sufficient stressor there was a predictable progression of responses by the body. These responses occurred in stages, and involved the central nervous system, the endocrine system, and the immune system. Selye labeled the body's predictable pattern of response to these stressors as the **general adaptation syndrome**.[14,15]

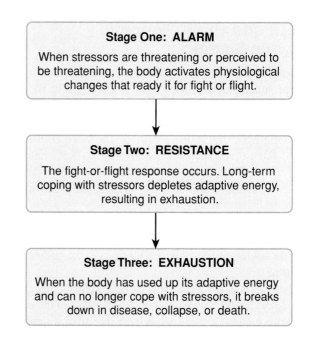

Stage One: ALARM

When stressors are threatening or perceived to be threatening, the body activates physiological changes that ready it for fight or flight.

Stage Two: RESISTANCE

The fight-or-flight response occurs. Long-term coping with stressors depletes adaptive energy, resulting in exhaustion.

Stage Three: EXHAUSTION

When the body has used up its adaptive energy and can no longer cope with stressors, it breaks down in disease, collapse, or death.

Figure 10-6 The stages observed in the general adaptation syndrome.

The first stage of the general adaptation syndrome is the **alarm stage**. During this stage, the body responds to the stressor via the central nervous system. The next stage is the stage of **resistance** in which the body attempts to reestablish homeostasis, utilizing the endocrine and/or the immune system. The final stage is **exhaustion** or recovery. Exhaustion occurs when the body's response is insufficient to meet the challenge of the stressor (Figure 10-6).

Stress that overcomes the body's innate defenses, and leads to exhaustion, is termed **distress** and heralds the onset of disease. However, not all stress is harmful. Stress is a condition of daily living. Daily stress essentially keeps body defenses on guard for larger stress threats. This daily stress is called **eustress**. An example of stress being purposefully introduced is the vigorous physical training in military boot camps. This activity prepares the body for the physical challenges or stressors that await the soldier on the battlefield.

From a physiologic perspective, stress creates a physical or chemical disturbance at the cellular level. However, to the layperson stress implies a psychological origin. There is a connection between the body's response to psychological stress and the resulting physiological response. Any emotional stress (e.g., fear or joy) can trigger the same response as a physical stress.

As might be assumed, the body goes through the three stages of the general adaptation syndrome whether the stressor is physical or psychological. This includes the final stage, exhaustion, and the beginning of certain disease states. There is ample evidence that persistent psychological stress upon the body can lead to hypertension, coronary artery disease, strokes, asthma, stomach ulcers, obesity, and impotence, to name just a handful of stress-related diseases.

Stress and the Autonomic Nervous System

The autonomic nervous system controls the moment-to-moment functions of most of the organs within the body and is composed of two divisions: the sympathetic and the parasympathetic nervous systems. Some have compared the sympathetic nervous system to the accelerator on a car and the parasympathetic to the brake. This analogy is not accurate. The better analogy for the parasympathetic nervous system would be the idle adjustment on the carburetor.[16]

Many organs have dual innervations from these two divisions of the autonomic nervous system and the dominance of one division over the other is a function of the body's needs at the time.

The effects of the parasympathetic system can be grossly characterized as the "feed and breed" regulation of the organs. The parasympathetic nervous system increases digestion in the gut, slows the heart rate down, and causes erections in males. The control of the parasympathetic nervous system is maintained primarily by the vagus (Latin – wander) nerve, the 10th cranial nerve, through its many branches.

The sympathetic nervous system is reactive, stimulated by stressors, and promotes protection of the body. For this reason, the responses of the body's organs to stimulation from the sympathetic nervous system has been described as "fight or flight."

The sympathetic nervous system (Figure 10-7), originating from the thoracic–lumbar region (thoracolumbar division) of the spinal cord, causes a litany of bodily responses.

Neurotransmitters

Both the sympathetic and parasympathetic systems affect organ function by their virtual connection at the motor endplate. It is a virtual connection because neurons do not physically contact the organs that they innervate, the neurons being separated by a gap called the **synapse**. The nervous signal is transmitted across this synapse by a chemical messenger called a **neurotransmitter** to awaiting chemical receptors across the synapse called **neuroreceptors** (Figure 10-8).

The sympathetic nervous system, at the motor endplates, uses the neurotransmitter **norepinephrine**, or adrenaline (ad- – "above"; renal – "kidneys"; -ine – for hormone). The transmission of a nervous signal using adrenaline as the neurotransmitter is called an **adrenergic transmission**.

In a typical sympathetic nervous system transmission, an electrical stimulus releases norepinephrine from storage in pockets, or vesicles, within the neuron that travel to the synapse. The chemical neurotransmitter norepinephrine then travels across the synapse to occupy neuroreceptors on the next neuron. These neurotransmitters cause increased permeability of the affected neuron, specifically to potassium,

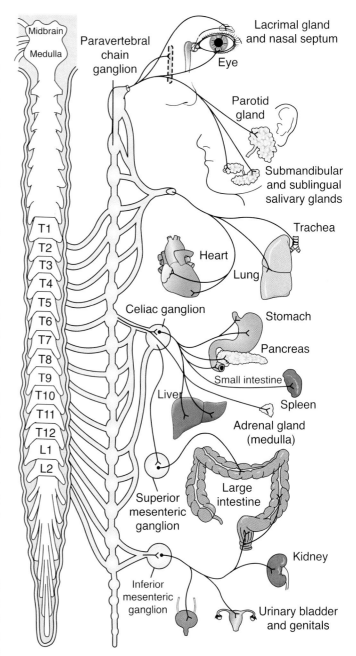

Figure 10-7 Sympathetic nervous system.

creating an electrical transference across the cell wall membrane that propagates the nervous signal or stimulates the affected organ.

The parasympathetic nerve uses the neurotransmitter **acetylcholine**. Originally acetylcholine was called vagusschtuff by German physiologists because it was released by the vagus nerve and affected the heart rate. The transmission of a nervous signal using acetylcholine as the neurotransmitter at the motor endplate is called a **cholinergic transmission** (Figure 10-9).

Note that acetylcholine is the prime neurotransmitter for all preganglionic fibers of the autonomic nervous system.

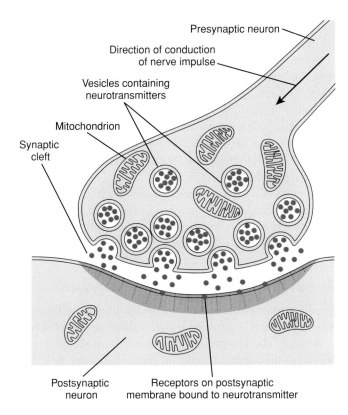

Figure 10-8 Neurotransmission across a synapse.

Paramedics are interested in the postganglionic neurons, those that connect with the target organs, of the autonomic nervous system.

There are different neurotransmitters in the different portions of the nervous system throughout the body: monoamine class neurotransmitters like norepinephrine, dopamine, histamine, and serotonin; amino acid class neurotransmitters like glycine and gamma aminobutyric acid (GABA); and neuropeptide class neurotransmitters like endorphins. These are just some examples of the over 30 major neurotransmitters in the body. Many current drug therapies affect these neurotransmitters by simply supplanting or blocking them. Atropine, for example, blocks the neurotransmitter acetylcholine and thus impairs the parasympathetic nervous system conduction.

Neuroreceptors

Each division of the autonomic nervous system joins with the target organs at the motor endplate via neuroreceptors. Each division has two neuroreceptors.

The parasympathetic nervous system has nicotinic and muscarinic receptors, named after the first chemicals that initially were used to stimulate them.

Nicotinic receptors are found in the central and peripheral nervous system as well as the neuromuscular junction with skeletal muscles. Certain paralytic drugs, like curare and succinylcholine, are nicotinic antagonists. They act by blocking the nicotinic receptors and are called neuromuscular blocking agents. Cholinergic stimulation of nicotinic receptors is quick

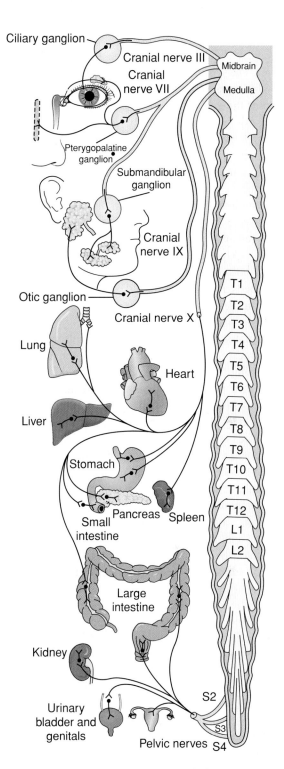

Figure 10-9 The innervations of the parasympathetic nervous system.

in onset and short in duration, causing a sodium influx and local depolarization.

The other parasympathetic neuroreceptors, **muscarinic receptors**, are slower and indirectly open ion channels that cause depolarization. Muscarinic receptors, by definition, are more sensitive to muscarine, a naturally occurring chemical found in mushrooms, than to nicotine.

The effects of muscarine poisoning, from poisonous mushrooms, provides a clue to the location of muscarinic receptors. The symptoms of muscarine ingestion are contained within the mnemonic SLUDGEM: Salivation, Lacrimation (tearing of the eyes), Urination, Defecation, Gastrointestinal pain, Emesis (vomiting), and Miosis (pinpoint pupils). While these symptoms can be severe, the stimulation of muscarinic receptors in the heart, affecting cardiac contraction, and the lungs, causing bronchial constriction, can be more life threatening.

The sympathetic neuroreceptors are also divided into two types of receptors. These receptors, called alpha receptors and beta receptors, are further divided into type 1 and type 2 receptors. **Alpha$_1$ adrenergic receptors** are primarily involved with excitation. They are located in the peripheral vascular beds, on the arteriole side, and control the sphincters (round muscles) of the bladder, intestine, and the iris of the pupil.

Stimulation of alpha$_1$ receptors results in constriction of the precapillary sphincters of the peripheral vascular bed, resulting in a displacement of blood volume to the core circulation, a phenomenon known as **shunting**. The result is that the skin, drained of blood, appears pale. Vasomotor regulation may be one of the most important functions of the sympathetic nervous system, ensuring perfusion to the body's core organs. The shunting of blood, during crisis, provides for increased blood flow to the vital organs of the heart, lung, and brain, while decreasing the chance of excessive hemorrhage from external trauma.[17–19]

Alpha$_2$ adrenergic receptors are found in the gastrointestinal tract where they decrease bowel motility, via relaxation of the smooth muscles within the intestinal walls.

Paramedics are generally more interested in the effects of the beta adrenergic receptors because they affect the heart and lungs. Beta adrenergic receptors are also subdivided into beta$_1$ adrenergic receptors and beta$_2$ adrenergic receptors.

Beta$_1$ adrenergic receptors are found in abundance in the heart, though not exclusively, as there are beta$_2$ adrenergic receptors in the heart as well. Beta$_1$ adrenergic receptors cause the muscle of the heart, the myocardium, to beat harder (i.e., **inotropy**) and stimulate the heart to beat faster (i.e., **chronotropy**) as well. Beta$_1$ adrenergic receptors are also found in the kidneys where they cause the secretion of renin, which is converted into angiotensin, a powerful vasoconstrictor. The addition of angiotensin increases the shunting of blood to the core organs (i.e., the heart, lungs, and brain), which was started by alpha$_1$ adrenergic receptors.

Beta$_2$ adrenergic receptors act upon the smooth muscles found in the bronchial walls, the level of the terminal bronchioles, and cause bronchodilation. The original bronchodilator was racemic epinephrine (EP), which was a potent bronchodilator that also caused unintended tachycardia. Newer bronchodilators are more beta-specific, implying that they are more active on the beta$_2$ adrenergic receptors than beta$_1$ adrenergic receptors.

A certain class of drugs that imitate epinephrine, called sympathomimetic, will affect adrenergic neuroreceptors. However, each has a predilection for one of the specific adrenergic receptors. For example, norepinephrine is more active with alpha adrenergic receptors. Because alpha adrenergic receptors affect peripheral vascular beds, norepinephrine is effective in states of massive vasodilation such as septic shock.[20–22]

Isoprenaline hydrochloride (isoproterenol) is almost exclusively a beta adrenergic receptor stimulant and increases heart rate (chronotropy) and strength of contraction (inotropy), making it useful in treating cardiogenic shock.[23–25]

Stress and the Endocrine System

The endocrine system can also be stimulated by stress. When the endocrine system is activated by stress there are two effects.

Initially, the sympathetic nervous system stimulates the medulla of the adrenal glands, an endocrine organ, to secrete the hormone, adrenaline. Adrenaline is physiologically and chemically the same as the neurotransmitter epinephrine (EP). Circulating adrenaline then goes to the liver and muscles where it stimulates glycolysis of glucogen stores and liberates glucose into the bloodstream.

Simultaneously, the sympathetic nervous system stimulates the release of corticotrophin-releasing factor (CRF) from the hypothalamus. In turn, CRF stimulates the pituitary gland to release several important stress hormones including antidiuretic hormone (vasopressin), from the posterior pituitary gland, and adrenocorticotropic hormone (ACTH), from the anterior pituitary gland.

Vasopressin is a powerful **vasopressor**, a chemical that causes vasoconstriction particularly on the arterioles. Vasopressin's first action is to prevent diuresis by vasoconstricting the distal arterioles in the kidneys and preventing diuresis.[26–28] This helps to maintain blood volume, which is especially important if one is hemorrhaging.

At the same time adrenocorticotropic hormone (adreno-–"adrenals"; cortico–"cortex"; -tropic–"affecting") stimulates the cortex of the adrenal glands to secrete **cortisol**. Cortisol is a glucocorticoid hormone that stimulates the production of glucogen from amino acids and fatty acids contained in lipids, a process called **glyconeogenesis** (gluco-–"glucose"; neo-–"new"; genesis–"creation"). Cortisol helps to ensure that there are adequate levels of glucose circulating in the bloodstream once the immediately available glucose from the liver is exhausted.

Other hormones also excreted during times of stress include endorphins, naturally occurring opiates within the body that reduce the perception of pain, and growth hormone. Growth hormone or somatotropin (soma-–"body"; tropin–"affecting") affects the metabolism of carbohydrates, proteins, and lipids.

Stress and the Immune System

The last leg of the neuro–endo–immune axis of the stress response is the immune system. The major organs of the immune system—the thymus, spleen, and lymph nodes—are directly innervated by the nerve fibers of the autonomic nervous system.

The hypothalamus, located in the brainstem, acts through the pituitary gland and then the adrenal gland to modulate the immune response. The now-activated adrenal glands increase levels of glucocorticosteroids, which in turn suppress white blood cells, the macrophages and the monocytes.

An important function of the immune system may be to alert other organs, through the release of inflammatory mediators such as interferon, of an impending systemic threat, be it from infection, cancer, or trauma. This mechanism is discussed more fully in the section on systemic inflammatory response syndrome.

Cellular Adaptation

Cells live in a highly volatile environment where changes in conditions, such as acidity or temperature, are constant even as the body strives to maintain homeostasis. Even the availability of basic materials—such as glucose, oxygen, proteins, carbohydrates, and fats—for metabolism and reproduction are highly variable. In order to survive in such a hostile environment, cells must adapt to the conditions. Cells must overcome those hostile conditions or be overcome themselves. Cells have developed some unique methods of adaptation.

Atrophy

Atrophy is the reduction of cells. A physical loss of cells as a result of the normal changes of aging or simple disuse is considered **physiologic**, a natural development of cells. An example of physiologic atrophy is the reduction in uterus mass following childbirth. Cell atrophy can also be the result of disease, or **pathologic**. For example, the atrophy can be due to diminished blood flow.

Muscle atrophy secondary to disease can be broken down in two general categories: (1) atrophy due to a neuromuscular disease and (2) atrophy due to diseases that affect the muscles directly. Examples of diseases that cause problems at the neuromuscular junction include poliomyelitis, amyotrophic lateral sclerosis (Lou Gehrig's disease), and Guillain-Barré. Primary muscle wasting diseases include muscular dystrophy and other congenital diseases.

The most common sources of muscle atrophy, secondary to disuse, are stroke (cerebrovascular accident), spinal cord injury with resulting paralysis, and peripheral neuropathy secondary to diabetes mellitus.[29–32]

Hypertrophy

Hypertrophy is an increase in either the weight or functional capacity of a tissue or organ beyond what is normal. It should not be confused with hyperplasia, which is an actual increase in the number of cells. Cells that hypertrophy cannot normally divide to increase their numbers and therefore must increase in size to accommodate demands upon them. The classic example is the bodybuilder who undergoes resistance training to create enlarged, or hypertrophied, biceps muscles. A more pertinent example would be myocardial hypertrophy (i.e., an enlarged heart), where the heart has to overcome hypertension.

Cell Replacement

Metaplasia is replacement of one adult cell type with another type of adult cell. For example, tobacco smoke causes a decrease in the number of cilia in the bronchial airways and an increase in the number of mucus-producing goblet cells. Metaplastic cell changes are typically due to chronic irritation and may develop into precancerous cells.

Hyperplasia (hyper- – "increase"; genesis – "creation") is an abnormal increase in the number of cells due to frequent cell division/reproduction which causes the tissue or organ to increase in size. Examples of common hyperplasia are callouses on the hands and benign prostatic hyperplasia, more commonly known as prostate enlargement, which commonly affects men over 50 years of age.

Some cellular hyperplasia is physiologic. Breast enlargement during pregnancy is an example of a hormone-driven hyperplasia.

Some cellular hyperplasia is compensatory. For example, after the surgical removal of a portion of the liver, a procedure called a **hepatectomy**, the various human growth factors encourage the liver to regenerate itself.[33,34]

Some cellular hyperplasia can be pathologic. A form of hyperplasia that is of concern to women is lobular carcinoma in situ (carcinoma – "tumor"; in situ – "in place"). While the word "tumor" is thus included within the term "lobular carcinoma in situ," it seldom progresses to invasive cancer. However, the woman is at great risk for other types of breast cancers.

A tumor, a form of hyperplasia, is an abnormal mass of cells which result from excessive cell division but serve no useful purpose in the body. Tumors may be **benign** (kind, no danger) or they may be **malignant** (disposed to do evil). Malignant tumors are always cancerous; in fact, the term "malignancy" means cancer. Cancer is not a single disease but a collection of over 100 varieties of malignancies.

Dysplasia

Cells in the body are in a constant state of turnover, with new cells replacing old cells. When there are too many new, or immature, cells that are not functional then **dysplasia** has occurred. In some instances (e.g., cervical cancer), the presence of dysplasia is an early warning of future malignancy.

Apoptosis

To prevent intrinsic biochemical errors from accumulating within a cell, or to simply replace old worn out or **senescent** cells, all of the cells in the body are programmed to commit suicide. This process of planned cell death, called **apoptosis** (Greek – apo- –"from"; ptosis – "falling"), is controlled by genes in the nucleus and involves a systematic disassembly of the cell. Approximately 10 billion cells die every day, without endangering other cells, so that new, more perfect cells can replace them.[35–37]

Apoptosis serves several vital functions, such as maintaining relatively even numbers of cells among rapidly dividing cells (e.g., the epithelial cells of the skin or bowels). Removal of cells that have been damaged by virus or damaged by exposure to radiation or toxins is also beneficial.

Apoptosis can also be a pathological condition when it is stimulated by DNA damage caused by oxygen-free radicals. Oxygen-free radicals have been implicated in neurodegenerative diseases, such as amyotrophic lateral sclerosis, Parkinson's disease, and Alzheimer's disease. Apoptosis can also be stimulated by stress conditions, an important comorbid factor.

CONCLUSION

A review of the conditions necessary to maintain cellular viability or wellness, and thus human life, shows that physiology is a complex process. The body's failure to maintain that internal milieu, through a dynamic, ongoing process called homeostasis, leads to illness and disease.

▶ KEY POINTS:

- Physiology is the study of the body's functions in its normal human condition. Functions include the physical, mechanical, and biochemical processes that are carried out inside the body. Together cells form tissues that in turn become organs and the organ systems that ultimately comprise a person.

- The essential elements water, glucose, amino acids, fatty acids, and oxygen are used in biochemical reactions. Together these biochemical reactions become the body's metabolism that is carried out in order for life processes to occur.

- To achieve a state of wellness, the body must maintain a physiologic equilibrium. The body's process to attain this state of internal equilibrium is called homeostasis. Though in a constant state of flux, the body uses regulatory mechanisms to maintain temperature, acidity, oxygenation, and fluid balance within a certain range.

- The cell is made up of an outer semipermeable membrane that encompasses cytoplasm and organelles. The nucleus is a membrane organelle containing DNA that provides the blueprints for cellular reproduction and protein synthesis.

- Found outside the nucleus but inside the cytoplasm are several organelles that serve different functions. Lysosomes can break down the cell's own proteins and foreign proteins called antigens. Mitochondria transform glucose into the usable energy source adenosine triphosphate (ATP).

- Anaerobic metabolism occurs without the use of oxygen and yields only two ATP. Though it generates a small amount of ATP, the process is much faster than aerobic metabolism and releases a greater amount of heat energy.

- Aerobic metabolism utilizes oxygen and glucose under ideal conditions to first carry out glycolysis that produces pyruvate. Pyruvate and oxygen then enter the Krebs cycle that generates 36 ATP. The products for both forms of metabolism are carbon dioxide, water, and energy in the form of ATP.

- Glucose that is not needed for immediate use is stored in the liver and muscles as glycogen. When there is a demand for glucose, glycogen can be broken down into individual glucose molecules by the enzyme glycagon. For a cell to carry out aerobic metabolism, the body must maintain ideal temperature and acidity. The body can use other food sources to carry out gluconeogenesis if there is an absence of readily available glucose.

- Water comprises the greatest percentage of our total body weight and can be found in two basic compartments: intracellular and extracellular. The majority of body water is intracellular. Extracellular water is found in either interstitial fluid or intravascular fluid.

- Fluid volumes are not static. They can move from outside to inside the cells and from compartment to compartment by diffusion or osmosis. In the past the volume of fluid inside the cells (intracellular) was considered as the first space, the volume of fluid in the bloodstream (intravascular) as the second space, and the volume of blood in between the cells (the interstitial space) as the third space.

- Fluid distribution from one compartment to another is controlled by hydrostatic pressure and the concentrations of dissolved salts or proteins. Fluid flow is restricted by hydrostatic pressure, which is the combination of factors including maximal interstitial fluid volume and compliance of the tissue, or elasticity.

- The venous system serves to eliminate fluids from the interstitial space while the lymphatic system drains excess fluid not carried away by the venous system. A dramatic fluid buildup in the tissues called edema can develop from a backup of the venous system.

- Osmosis is the diffusion of water through a selectively permeable membrane. The amount of solute (salt) dissolved in water (solvent) determines the osmotic pressure. Osmotic pressure is dependent on the concentration of salt on one side of a membrane. This pressure determines the net movement of water across the membrane by osmosis.

- Saline with 0.9% sodium chloride is an isotonic solution because it has approximately the same concentration of salt that exists in blood. A hypotonic solution is a fluid with more water and less salt than a solution on the other side of a semipermeable membrane. Conversely, a hypertonic solution on one side of a semipermeable membrane has less water and more salt than the other solution.

- Warm-blooded animals have a constant core temperature of $98.6°F +/- 1°F$. To some extent, this temperature remains constant through a large range of environmental conditions. This heat is created by cellular metabolism and is controlled by the anterior hypothalamus. The most effective heat loss mechanism controlled by the hypothalamus is vasodilation. This dilates the skin surface capillaries, allowing heat to dissipate. Under hypothermic conditions, vasoconstriction is used to increase heat production.

- Pyrexia, or fever, is an essential part of the healing process. Endotoxins, or bacterial poisons, affect the hypothalamus by raising the body's temperature, producing a fever. An increase in body temperature creates an unfavorable environment for bacteria. It increases macrophage motility and signals the defense of white blood cells.

- A rise in body temperature also increases one's metabolism vis-á-vis Hoff's law. Though very beneficial for mild infections, high fevers during severe infections can lead to delirium or convulsions.

- Stress is the constant change in the environmental conditions within the body. General adaptation syndrome is the body's response to environmental, chemical, and physical changes that disrupt homeostasis.

- General adaptation syndrome comes in three stages: the alarm stage, the resistance stage, and the exhaustion stage. Stress that exhausts the body's defenses is termed distress. Everyday stresses that help the body's defenses stay on guard are called eustresses. Any psychological stress can in turn trigger a physical stress such as cardiac, respiratory, or gastrointestinal disease.

- The autonomic nervous system is divided into the sympathetic and parasympathetic nervous system. The sympathetic nervous system, originating from the thoracic and lumbar region, is described as the body's "fight or flight" regulator. The sympathetic nervous system is highly reactive and promotes protection of the body.

- The parasympathetic nervous system, originating from the vagus nerve, opposes the effects of the sympathetic nervous system. It is characterized as the body's "feed and breed" regulator and controls bodily processes such as digestion in the gut, slowing of the heart rate, and erection in males.

- Both the sympathetic nervous system and the parasympathetic nervous system are virtually connected to their affected organs by way of a synapse. Nervous signals travel across the synapse by a chemical messenger called a neurotransmitter. Neuroreceptors await across the synapse to receive the signals.

- Norepinephrine or adrenaline is used by the sympathetic nervous system as a neurotransmitter that creates a transmission called an adrenergic transmission. Norepinephrine is released by electrical stimuli and travels across the synapse to occupy the neuroreceptors and the receiving neutron. This neurotransmitter then causes an increase in permeability of the neuron to potassium, stimulating the affected organ.

- Acetylcholine is used by the parasympathetic nervous system as a neurotransmitter which creates a transmission called cholingeric transmission. There are over 30 major neurotransmitters in the body, some being categorized within the monamine class, the amino acid class, and the neuropeptide class. These neurotransmitters can be blocked by the use of simple drug therapies such as atropine.

- The neuroreceptors of the parasympathetic nervous system are nicotinic and muscarinic receptors. Nicotinic receptors are found in the central nervous system, peripheral nervous system, and neuromuscular junction within skeletal muscles. The stimulation of this neuroreceptor has a quick onset and is short lived. Muscarinic receptors, in comparison, are much slower.

- The neuroreceptors of the sympathetic nervous system are divided into $alpha_1$ and $alpha_2$ and $beta_1$ and $beta_2$. Shunting occurs when the $alpha_1$ receptors are stimulated. The sphincters of the peripheral vascular beds are constricted and the blood volume rushes to the core circulation. Shunting ensures good perfusion to the body's core organs while decreasing chances of excessive bleeding from external trauma. $Alpha_2$ receptors relax the smooth muscles of the intestinal walls, causing a decrease in bowel motility.

- $Beta_1$ receptors are found in the heart and cause its muscles to beat harder and faster. $Beta_1$ receptors are also found in the kidneys where they aid in the shunting of blood due to the secretion of angiotensin, a vasoconstrictor. $Beta_2$ receptors cause bronchiodilation by acting upon the smooth muscles of the bronchial walls.

- Sympathomimetic drugs are a class of drugs that imitate epinephrine. These drugs affect adrenergic receptors, with each drug affecting a specific type of receptor.

- The endocrine system can also be activated by stress. During times of stress, the adrenal gland, an endocrine organ, first secretes adrenaline. After being stimulated, this hormone travels to the liver where it stimulates glycolysis. At the same time, corticotropin-releasing factor (CRF) is released after being stimulated by the sympathetic nervous system. In turn, CRF stimulates the pituitary gland to release an antidiuretic hormone (vasopressin). This vasopressor vasoconstricts to prevent diuresis.

- Simultaneously, ACTH stimulates the adrenal glands to secrete cortisol. Cortisol is a hormone that stimulates the glyconeogenesis process to ensure adequate circulation of glucose in the bloodstream.

- The major organs of the immune system are the thymus, spleen, and lymph nodes. The hypothalamus regulates the immune system through the adrenal gland by increasing the production of glucocorticosteroids. The glucocorticosteroids suppress white blood cells, macrophages, and monocytes.

- Cells constantly live in highly variable conditions which they must adapt themselves to by developing very unique methods.

- Atrophy is the reduction of cells due to aging, disuse, or disease. Muscle atrophy is broken down into neuromuscular disease and diseases that affect the muscles directly. Secondary to disease causing muscle atrophy are stroke, spinal injury, and peripheral neuropathy.

- Hypertrophy is an increase in tissue or organ weight beyond normal limits. Myocardial hypertrophy is an enlarged heart, making hypertension an issue to overcome.

- Metaplasia is the replacement of one adult cell type with another. Hyperplasia is an abnormal increase in cell number due to cell division that causes an increase in tissue size. Some cellular hyperplasia is physiologic, or hormonally driven. Some cellular hyperplasia is compensatory due to a removal of cells. Tumors can be either benign or malignant.

- Dysplasia occurs when cells are nonfunctional due to an overabundance of new cells. This can be an early warning of cancer.

- Apoptosis is the process of planned cell death. Its functions include maintaining even cell numbers and removing damaged cells. Apoptosis can also be a harmful condition due to oxygen-free radicals. This may cause neurodegenerative disease.

REVIEW QUESTIONS:

1. How does understanding the body's regulatory mechanisms help to define homeostasis?
2. Describe the parts of the cell.
3. Compare and contrast aerobic and anaerobic metabolism.
4. If more glucose is taken into the body than is needed, where and how is it stored in the body?
5. How does increasing the salt concentration of a solution on one side of a semipermeable membrane affect the net movement of water?
6. Why is edema called third spacing of fluid?
7. Describe the body's mechanism of thermoregulation.
8. How is fever beneficial to the healing process?
9. Name the stages of the general adaptation syndrome.
10. What is the difference between distress and eustress?
11. Would it be possible for acetylcholine to carry out an adrenergic transmission? Why or why not?
12. What are three types of neuroreceptors?
13. Describe the functions that alpha and beta receptors are involved in.
14. What is the effect of stress on the endocrine system?
15. Compare atrophy to hypertrophy.

CASE STUDY QUESTIONS:

Please refer to the Case Study at the beginning of the chapter and answer the questions below.

1. Explain the importance of preventing heat loss in a patient who has suffered a severe injury.
2. What effect does stimulation of the sympathetic nervous system have on blood vessels?
3. Explain why a seriously injured patient may request a drink of water.

REFERENCES:

1. Cannon WB. *The Wisdom of the Body*. New York: Norton; 1932.
2. Martinoli R, Mohamed EI, Maiolo C, Cianci R, Denoth F, Salvadori S, et al. Total body water estimation using bioelectrical impedance: a meta-analysis of the data available in the literature. *Acta Diabetol*. 2003;40 (Suppl 1):S203–S206.
3. Gala GJ, Lilly MP, Thomas SE, Gann DS. Interaction of sodium and volume in fluid resuscitation after hemorrhage. *J Trauma*. 1991;31(4):545–555; discussion 555–546.
4. Orlowski JP, Abulleil MM, Phillips JM. The hemodynamic and cardiovascular effects of near-drowning in hypotonic, isotonic, or hypertonic solutions. *Ann Emerg Med*. 1989;18(10): 1044–1049.
5. Gunnar WP, Merlotti GJ, Barrett J, Jonasson O. Resuscitation from hemorrhagic shock. Alterations of the intracranial pressure after normal saline, 3% saline and dextran-40. *Ann Surg*. 1986;204(6):686–692.
6. Young ME, Flynn KT. Third-spacing: when the body conceals fluid loss. *Rn*. 1988;51(8):46–48.
7. Perel P, Roberts I. Colloids versus crystalloids for fluid resuscitation in critically ill patients. *Cochrane Database Syst Rev*. 2007;4:CD000567.
8. Rolfe DF, Brown GC. Cellular energy utilization and molecular origin of standard metabolic rate in mammals. *Physiol Rev*. 1997;77(3):731–758.
9. Sessler DI, Moayeri A, Stoen R, Glosten B, Hynson J, McGuire J. Thermoregulatory vasoconstriction decreases cutaneous heat loss. *Anesthesiology*. 1990;73(4):656–660.
10. Song CW, Chelstrom LM, Haumschild DJ. Changes in human skin blood flow by hyperthermia. *Int J Radiat Oncol Biol Phys*. 1990;18(4):903–907.
11. Haahr S, Mogensen S. Function of fever in infectious disease. *Biomedicine*. 1978;28(6):305–307.

12. Blatteis CM. Fever: is it beneficial? *Yale J Biol Med.* 1986;59(2):107–116.

13. Ryan GB. Inflammation and localization of infection. *Surg Clin North Am.* 1976;56(4):831–846.

14. Selye H. The general adaptation syndrome and the diseases of adaptation. *Practitioner.* 1949;163(977):393–405.

15. Goldstein DS, Kopin IJ. Evolution of concepts of stress. *Stress.* 2007;10(2):109–120.

16. Appenzeller O, Oribe E. *The Autonomic Nervous System.* Amsterdam: Elsevier Publishing Company; 1997.

17. Little RA, Stoner HB. Body temperature after accidental injury. *Br J Surg.* 1981;68(4):221–224.

18. Fahim M. Cardiovascular sensory receptors and their regulatory mechanisms. *Indian J Physiol Pharmacol.* 2003;47(2):124–146.

19. Van Corven EJ, van Rijswijk A, Jalink K, van der Bend RL, van Blitterswijk WJ, Moolenaar WH. Mitogenic action of lysophosphatidic acid and phosphatidic acid on fibroblasts. Dependence on acyl-chain length and inhibition by suramin. *Biochem J.* 1992;281 (Pt 1):163–169.

20. Groeneveld AB, Girbes AR, Thijs LG. Treating septic shock with norepinephrine. *Crit Care Med.* 1999;27(9):2022–2023.

21. Singer M. Catecholamine treatment for shock—equally good or bad? *Lancet.* 2007;370(9588):636–637.

22. Vincent JL, De Backer D. Inotrope/vasopressor support in sepsis-induced organ hypoperfusion. *Semin Respir Crit Care Med.* 2001;22(1):61–74.

23. Mueller HS. Inotropic agents in the treatment of cardiogenic shock. *World J Surg.* 1985;9(1):3–10.

24. Eichna LW. The treatment of cardiogenic shock. 3. The use of isoproterenol in cardiogenic shock. *Am Heart J.* 1967;74(6):48–52.

25. Worthley LI, Tyler P, Moran JL. A comparison of dopamine, dobutamine and isoproterenol in the treatment of shock. *Intensive Care Med.* 1985;11(1):13–19.

26. Farrow S, Banata G, Schallhorn S, May R, Mers A, Cadaret L, et al. Vasopressin inhibits diuresis induced by water immersion in humans. *J Appl Physiol.* 1992;73(3):932–936.

27. Meybohm P, Cavus E, Bein B, Steinfath M, Weber B, Hamann C, et al. Small volume resuscitation: a randomized controlled trial with either norepinephrine or vasopressin during severe hemorrhage. *J Trauma.* 2007;62(3):640–646.

28. Tsuneyoshi I, Onomoto M, Yonetani A, Kanmura Y. Low-dose vasopressin infusion in patients with severe vasodilatory hypotension after prolonged hemorrhage during general anesthesia. *J Anesth.* 2005;19(2):170–173.

29. Trudel G, Uhthoff HK. Muscle atrophy in stroke patients. *Arch Phys Med Rehabil.* 2003;84(4):623; author reply 623.

30. Giangregorio L, McCartney N. Bone loss and muscle atrophy in spinal cord injury: epidemiology, fracture prediction, and rehabilitation strategies. *J Spinal Cord Med.* 2006;29(5):489–500.

31. Baldi JC, Jackson RD, Moraille R, Mysiw WJ. Muscle atrophy is prevented in patients with acute spinal cord injury using functional electrical stimulation. *Spinal Cord.* 1998; 36(7):463–469.

32. Andersen H, Gjerstad MD, Jakobsen J. Atrophy of foot muscles: a measure of diabetic neuropathy. *Diabetes Care.* 2004;27(10):2382–2385.

33. Kobayashi M, Ogata T, Araki K, Hayashi T. Human liver regeneration after major hepatectomy. *Ann Surg.* 1992;216(5):616.

34. Yamanaka N, Okamoto E, Kawamura E, Kato T, Oriyama T, Fujimoto J, et al. Dynamics of normal and injured human liver regeneration after hepatectomy as assessed on the basis of computed tomography and liver function. *Hepatology.* 1993;18(1):79–85.

35. Beutler E. The relationship of red cell enzymes to red cell life-span. *Blood Cells.* 1988;14(1):69–91.

36. Kay M. Immunoregulation of cellular life span. *Ann N Y Acad Sci.* 2005;1057:85–111.

37. Taylor RC, Cullen SP, Martin SJ. Apoptosis: controlled demolition at the cellular level. *Nat Rev Mol Cell Biol.* 2007;9:231–241.

CHAPTER 11

PRINCIPLES OF PATHOPHYSIOLOGY

KEY CONCEPTS:

Upon completion of this chapter, it is expected that the reader will understand these following concepts:

- The interplay between modifiable and nonmodifiable risk factors and disease and its impact on mortality
- Impact of physical and chemical injury on cell physiology
- Infectious disease and the body's response to pathogens
- The concept and etiologies of shock using the Hinshaw–Cox classification
- The pathophysiology of shock and the body's response
- Biochemical changes and cellular death

▶ ## CASE STUDY:

The Paramedics responded to a man who had collapsed. Upon their arrival, they found him unconscious with a slow pulse and agonal breathing. Despite their best resuscitative efforts, he had no vital signs when they transferred him to the hospital, yet they continued CPR during the transport. Both Paramedics were perplexed when the ED physician requested the transplant team. What organs would be available now? Wasn't the man dead?

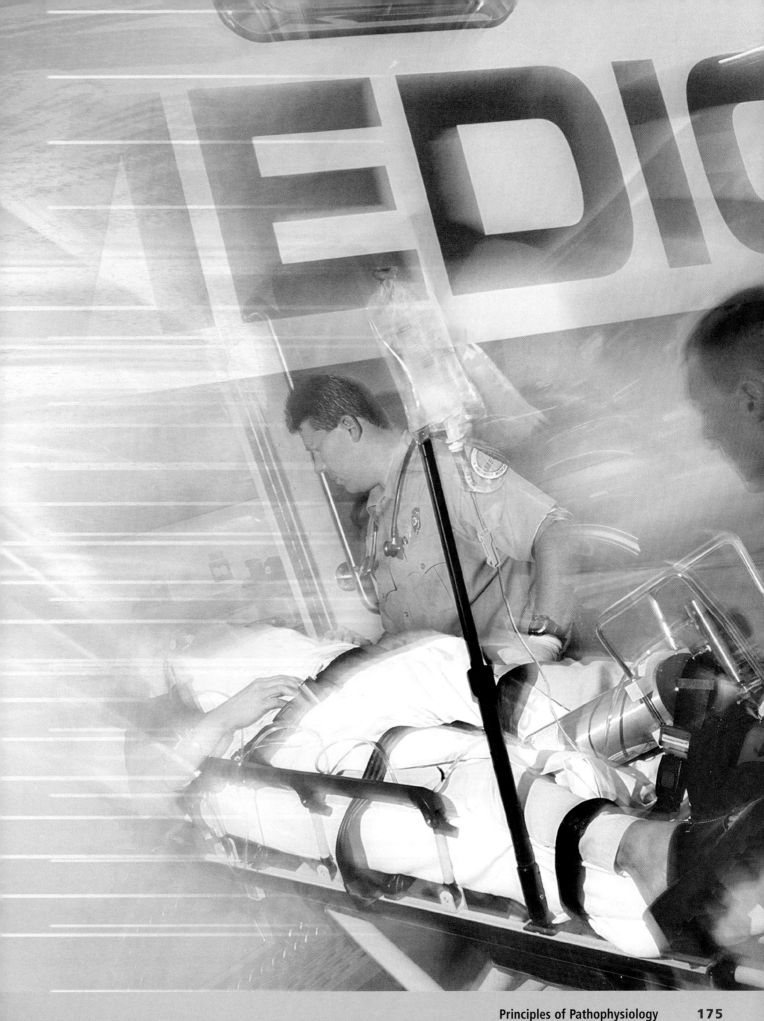

OVERVIEW

There is a physiological cause for every illness or disorder that the Paramedic encounters. Although it's not the Paramedic's job to determine the exact cause of the disease, it is the Paramedic's job to recognize the signs and symptoms and treat the patient appropriately based on an assessment. This chapter provides the background knowledge the Paramedic needs to better understand the disease process and treatment. After examining disease risk factors, the focus is on how the body is impacted by injury and its response to pathogens. Although the Paramedic should be familiar with the signs of shock, he or she should also know the pathophysiology causing the body's response to determine its etiology. Often the Paramedic's treatment reverses the pathogenesis of an illness or disorder.

Pathophysiology Defined

Pathos (Greek - "to suffer") is the prefix added to physiology, the study of the normal human condition, to make the term **pathophysiology**. The origins of the term define pathophysiology: to study the causes of suffering in the normal human condition. While the causes of disease are numerous, they share a few common mechanisms, making the study of pathophysiology somewhat easier.

This chapter is a discussion of those mechanisms and the body's reactions to illness or injury. Discussions of the many illnesses and ailments of humans, related to specific organs, or **systemic pathology**, is contained in all of the chapters that follow. This chapter will serve as the foundation for understanding those chapters while the previous physiology chapter serves as the foundation for understanding this chapter.

Disease: Defined

Disease can be defined as an abnormal change in the function of cells, tissues, or organs. An example of each is cancer in cells, emphysema in tissues, and acute myocardial infarction in organs. These changes interfere with homeostasis of the body, making the body ill at ease—or literally diseased (dis- – "not"; ease – "rest").

Paramedics are often more interested in the **pathogenesis** (patho- – Greek "suffering"; genesis – "beginning") of a disease, the sequence of events—at the molecular and cellular level—that lead to organ dysfunction. By understanding these underlying conditions, treatment can be directed toward removing the cause and not just treating the symptoms.

Etiologies of Disease

All diseases have an assumed origin, an **etiology**. In the case of an infection the etiology is a microbe.

The occurrence of disease has many other compounding factors, such as malnutrition, overcrowded living conditions, poverty, lack of immunizations, and so on, which influence the incidence of disease. For example, poor sanitation, poverty, and overcrowding make cholera infection one of the leading causes of death, or **mortality**, in the world.[1,2]

The many causes of cellular death due to disease can be categorized as either known causes or unknown causes. Unknown causes of cellular death are primarily due to an incomplete understanding of the disease and/or because of a lack of evidence of the disease. The "Black Death" is one example of an unknown cause of cellular death. Typically, the cause of an emergent disease is unknown until scientists have a sufficient number of cases to study so as to identify the source. A more recent example is the Severe Acute Respiratory Syndrome (SARS) epidemic. Initially the cause of SARS was unknown; however, it has now been identified as a coronavirus, the same type of virus that causes the common cold.[3–5]

Known Causes of Disease

The known causes, or etiologies, of cellular injury can be broken down into two categories: the extrinsic (external) causes and the intrinsic (internal) causes. Extrinsic causes include chemical causes, physical causes, infection/inflammation, and metabolic imbalances. The intrinsic (internal) causes are causes such as genetic derangements.

Of the three general chemical causes of cellular injury, hypoxia is ranked number one and receives the largest portion of a Paramedic's attention. Other chemical causes of cellular injury include the creation of free radicals and toxins.

The physical cause of cellular injury is trauma. Trauma encompasses any mechanical injury, heat or cold injury, radiation, electrical injury, or barotrauma.

At the molecular level, there can be metabolic derangements (an extrinsic cause) and genetic derangements (intrinsic cause) that lead to disease. Inappropriate immunological response, the so-called autoimmune response, and an exaggerated inflammatory response can also cause disease.

Risk Factors

Frequently, medical professionals will speak of the **incidence** of a disease, the incidence being the number of new cases per standardized group per time. An example would be 1 case per 100,000 per year of x disease.

The incidence of disease (prevalence) is not the same as the risk of a disease. **Risk**, the likelihood that a situation could lead to harm—that is, that the person would contract a disease—is a function of an individual's life circumstances. And everyone's life circumstances are different.

Every person has some **risk factors** that tend to make that person more or less vulnerable to a disease as compared to another person. Some risk factors are functions of the human condition and are therefore modifiable. Others are nonmodifiable risk factors which are, essentially, a fact of life for the individual.

An example of nonmodifiable risk factors is heredity. Heredity is a significant risk factor. If a woman has breast cancer then her offspring are at risk for breast cancer. It is thought that more diseases can be partially or completely explained by genetics. With the unraveling of the DNA mystery by the Human Genome Project, some 35 diseases have been directly linked, or at least partially attributed to, genetic origins. Cystic fibrosis, a disease of the lungs, is due to a malfunctioning gene. Sickle-cell anemia, a disease of red blood cells, also has a genetic origin.

Another nonmodifiable risk factor is a person's gender. For example, the overwhelming majority of patients with breast cancer are women, though breast cancer is a reality for a small subset of men. There are a number of other gender-related diseases (e.g., prostate cancer) that are exclusive to one gender. There are other diseases that tend to be more prevalent in one gender. In some cases, gender helps protect a person from disease, as is the case with acute coronary syndrome.

A person's race may be a risk factor, especially in cases of infectious disease. For example, Europeans were generally more resistant, and therefore had a lower risk of contracting smallpox due to centuries of exposure to smallpox. This risk is considered lower when compared to the first Americans who had no exposure experience with smallpox until the arrival of Europeans. They suffered staggering losses of life due to smallpox.

Some risk factors are conditions that predispose a person to another disease. For example, African Americans have a higher incidence of hypertension. Hypertension has been directly linked to an increased risk of coronary syndrome secondary to the disease of atherosclerosis.

Age as a Risk Factor

Outward signs of aging include wrinkles, secondary to loss of the underlying layer of fat, and gray hair. These signs indicate the presence of the changes of aging that are occurring within the body. The multitude of hormonal, biochemical, and physiologic changes that accompany aging combine to make the elderly person more at risk for all diseases in general. In addition, specific diseases, such as dementia, are age-related.

Modifiable Risk Factors

The term "modifiable" would seem to indicate that the person has some control of the existence of factors. In some cases, such as tobacco smoking, obesity, and alcohol consumption, the person does have control over these risk factors. However, eliminating these risk factors is seldom as simple as it might appear.

Some risk factors are a function of one's lifestyle or occupational choices. These modifiable risk factors are called **environmental risk** factors. Farmers, for example, inhale dust from moldy hay that leads to a pulmonary disease called farmer's lung. Wearing a simple dust mask can help to modify or eliminate the risk of acquiring farmer's lung.

 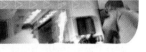

Prognosis

The expected outcome from a disease is called the **prognosis**. A good prognosis, or the likelihood of recovery and survival, or a poor prognosis, which suggests death or disability, is a culmination of modifiable risk factors (such as nutrition), nonmodifiable risk factors (such as age), and the availability of treatments. For example, a middle-aged male who experiences sudden cardiac death in an airport has a better prognosis than the same male stricken while in a rural community, owing to the rapid availability of automated external defibrillators in airports.

Iatrogenic Disease

Iatrogenic (iatro- – "physician"; genic – "cause") disease is a previously known cause of disease that was introduced to the patient as a result of medical intervention.[11]

The classic example of an iatrogenic disease was described by Dr. Ignaz Semmelweis, the father of microbiology. While attending to patients at Vienna General Hospital, Dr. Semmelweis noted a connection between childbed fever (then referred to as puerperal fever) and the dirty hands of birth attendants. He immediately ordered that hands be washed with "chlorine liquida," a chlorinated lime solution (calcium hypochlorite). As a result, the death rate from puerperal fever immediately dropped after the institution of this simple intervention. Unfortunately, fellow physicians failed to heed his advice until the emergence of the germ theory some 40 years later.

Death from a hospital-acquired infection, called a **nosocomial** infection (in this case, childbed fever), was the direct result of medical intervention. Hippocrates, in his treatise "Epidemic," advised aspiring physicians that their first responsibility was to "do no harm," an edict that has been maintained to this day.

Drug-resistant strains of diseases, grown in the hospitals and the intensive care units, can be easily transmitted by unwitting healthcare professionals, including Paramedics, to

PROFESSIONAL PARAMEDIC

Whenever a medical intervention is being considered, the Paramedic must consider the risk/benefit of the procedure before making a decision. Even with the best of intentions and using the best techniques, iatrogenic disease—which can be caused by an infiltration of an intravenous line—will occur in every Paramedic's practice. The key is to identify and consider the risk, monitor for its occurrence, and mitigate its harm as soon as possible.

unsuspecting and physically weakened patients. This can occur simply because a healthcare professional failed to wash his or her hands or take proper infection control precautions.[12–14]

Iatrogenic disease does not end with infections. Every medical intervention carries with it some risk of harm to the patient and the potential to cause disease. Patients, as was discussed in Chapter 6 on medicolegal responsibilities, have a right to know about these risks and to make an informed decision (i.e., informed consent).

Disease as a Process

The origin and development of a disease follows an ordered sequence of events at the cellular, biochemical, and molecular level, which is called its pathogenesis. Thus, the disease has predictable effects upon the patient. When a patient becomes diseased, one of three outcomes is inevitable: recovery, death, or survival with remission.

For cells, **recovery** means a return to a former functional capacity. For a person, recovery means a return to health. To be cured, the patient must have no remnant of the disease.

Recovery does not necessarily mean that the patient is unchanged. Some patients recover with physical or chemical changes remaining after the encounter with the disease; these changes are called **residuals**. Scars, called poxmarks, are a visible residual left after recovery from the disease smallpox. Hemiplegia (hemi- – "half"; plegia – "paralyzed") is a residual that can remain after a stroke.

Some people learn to co-exist with their disease having learned to compensate for their disease. Often with the help of medications, a patient may become asymptomatic.

Periodically patients will decompensate and become symptomatic. These episodes in which a chronic disease returns, or flares up, is called an **exacerbation**. Asthma, a chronic disease of the airways, is largely managed by the use of bronchodilators and anti-inflammatory drugs. Occasionally, the patient will experience an exacerbation of his or her asthma, usually triggered by some stimulus. This patient will present to EMS emergently with an acute exacerbation of the chronic disease asthma.

In some cases, after a person has become diseased, the body's defense, or medical treatment, may force the disease into a non-active state called **remission**. Remission does not mean the patient has been cured, but rather that the disease has been stopped.

Some diseases, particularly certain infections, become **dormant** (Latin – "to sleep") and remain in a state of biological rest. These diseases remain dormant until favorable conditions exist for them to reanimate. Tuberculosis is an excellent example of a disease that can infect a person and then remain dormant. It remains in spore form for years—and even decades—only to re-infect the person when the person is aged or debilitated.[15]

Ultimately disease will kill everyone. When a body's defense mechanisms become overwhelmed, and the body cannot compensate, the patient will succumb to disease and death will ensue. The process of death is described at the end of this chapter.

Morbidity and Mortality

Physicians, nurses, and allied health professionals monitor the incidence of disease (called the **morbidity**) and death rate (or mortality) for trends. Awareness of these leading indicators of disease (i.e., death and disability) provide healthcare professionals an opportunity to prepare for outbreaks of these diseases and to properly treat the population when an outbreak occurs.

Epidemiology deals with the study of the causes, distribution, and control of disease in populations. Advances in epidemiology permit public health authorities to stockpile needed antibiotics, medicines, and the like in anticipation of epidemics and other public health emergencies.

In the United States, the federal Centers for Disease Control and Prevention (CDC), located in Atlanta, Georgia, has taken the lead in this area and regularly disseminates epidemiological information through its publication of Morbidity and Mortality Reports (MMR). These reports appear both on-line and in print.[16]

Chemical Causes of Cell Injury

Chemical causes of cellular injury can be divided into hypoxia (the leading cause of cell injury and death), free oxygen radicals, and toxins, which include poisons. Each of these sources of cellular injury is unique because it works primarily at a biochemical level, the foundation level of cellular physiology.

Hypoxic Injury

The classic cause of cell injury is low oxygen concentrations, a condition called **hypoxia**. Hypoxia causes cells to redirect their metabolic processes to anaerobic respiration in an effort to sustain the cell. While this response can be effective for a time, eventually anaerobic metabolism proves insufficient to sustain the cell.

Hypoxia and Dr. Fick

Key to effective cellular metabolism is the ready availability of oxygen for the cells. The process of getting oxygen to the cells is outlined by the **Fick principle** (Figure 11-1). Fick, in his monograph *Medical Physics,* described the function of the lungs; the hemodynamics of the body, including the work of the heart; and the properties of the gasses oxygen and carbon dioxide. The Fick principle can be summed up in five key concepts: oxygenation, ventilation, respiration, circulation, and cellular respiration.

The Fick principle places hypoxia at the center of disease and makes the resolution of hypoxia the first priority in the treatment of disease. Too little oxygen in the blood perfusing the cells causes hypoxemia (hypo- – Greek "under"; ox – "oxygen"; -emia – "blood") and leads to disease.

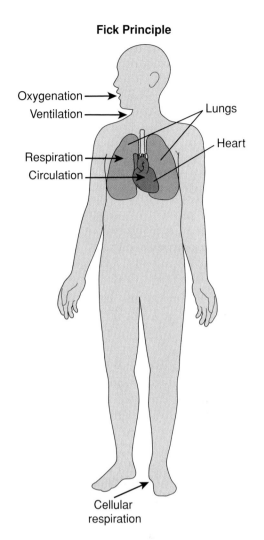

Fick Principle

Figure 11-1 The Fick principle.

The first element of the Fick principle addresses the availability of oxygen in the ambient air going into the lungs. Lack of oxygen, due to an oxygen poor environment, can lead to hypoxia and is categorized as **hypoxic hypoxia**.

The next element in the Fick principle is ventilation. Even high flow oxygen via nonrebreather mask is useless if the airway is compromised.

With oxygen-laden air in the lungs, the process of respiration can occur. Respiration depends on an intact capillary–alveolar interface. An interruption of blood flow (e.g., by a pulmonary embolism) or alveolar filling (e.g., pneumonia) will interfere with respiration and create hypoxic hypoxia.

An adequate volume of circulating red blood cells is needed to carry the oxygen to the various organs of the body. The volume of red blood cells is expressed as the percentage of red blood cells in the blood and is called the **hematocrit**. A low hematocrit, or other red blood cell abnormality, can lead to oxygen deprivation at the cellular level. This is called **anemic hypoxia**.

With the hemoglobin loaded with oxygen, the body now must move the blood about the body via the circulatory system.

Problems of circulation can lead to oxygen deprivation at the cellular level and is called **ischemic hypoxia**. Examples of circulation problems include occlusion of blood vessels, such as a deep vein thrombus, or heart failure.

Finally, the cells must be able to accept the oxygen; that is, oxygen must be able to be diffused across the cell membrane and utilized in the Krebs cycle. The inability of the cells to accept or use oxygen, such as in cyanide poisoning, is called **histoxic hypoxia**.

Paramedic practice involves preventing hypoxia by supporting the different elements of the Fick principle. For example, the administration of oxygen via nonrebreather face mask supplements the available oxygen in the air. Intravenous fluids help to support circulation.

ACLS View of Hypoxia

Some Paramedics simplify the causes of cellular hypoxia by referring to problems with the pipes, the pump, or the fluid—a familiar mantra in Advanced Cardiac Life Support (ACLS).

Problems of the pipes include vasodilatation, such as that which occurs with neurogenic shock and anaphylactic shock (discussed later). Problems with the pipes can also include leaky pipes which may occur during severe infections.

Problems with the pump include acute myocardial infarction leading to pump failure (**cardiogenic shock**). Also, an impaired heart cannot meet the body's demands for perfusion, which is called **heart failure**.

Problems with fluids imply problems with the oxygen-carrying capacity of the blood itself. This can be caused by a condition called **anemia**.

Ischemic Cascade

When cells are deprived of oxygen, and subsequently convert to anaerobic respiration, a cascade of biochemical changes start to take place which can eventually lead to cell death.

The first step in the pathogenesis of hypoxia is called **ischemia**. The cells, fully dedicated to anaerobic respiration, rapidly deplete available glucose. Lactic acid, the by-product of glycolysis, is all that then remains.

With an abundance of acid present, the cytoplasm pH drops rapidly and cellular proteins start to denature. At this point the cell is **injured** and recovery is questionable.

As the cell's proteins continue to denature, the lysosomes within the cell swell and burst, releasing proteases, which hasten the cell's destruction. The now dead cell is said to have **necrosis** (Greek for dead). If a large number of cells are involved, then the term **infarction** is applied.

Reperfusion Injury and Free Radicals

Acute interventions during a medical emergency can reverse hypoxia and prevent permanent injury and even infarction. Emergency interventions that have an impact on the Fick principles of oxygenation, ventilation, respiration, circulation, and cellular respiration can reestablish perfusion to the cells and tissues. The key is to provide oxygenation via perfusion to the affected cells before the lysosomes swell.

These near-miss events are not completely harmless. During the course of reperfusion, products of incomplete metabolism (hydrogen peroxide and other reactive oxygen chemicals) are created.[17] The analogy of a smoldering fire is useful. A smoldering fire results in products of incomplete combustion such as cyanide, which are dangerous. In the same manner, the reactive oxygen chemicals which are products of incomplete metabolism, such as hydrogen peroxide, wreak havoc in the cell.

Reactive oxygen chemicals consist of an electrically uncharged atom with an unpaired electron. This unpaired electron is unstable, by nature, and looks for another electron with which to pair up and thus stabilize. Unfortunately the reactive oyxgen chemicals tend to either pair up with amino acids within the DNA, causing their destruction, or pair up with lipids in the cell wall, a process called lipid peroxidation, which also results in destruction.

As a result, these reactive oxygen chemicals fragment DNA, thus impairing the cell's ability to make proteins and to reproduce itself. They may also cause cell wall damage, making the cell walls more permeable to sodium. Increased intracellular sodium leads to cell swelling and autolysis (auto--"self"; lysis – "divide").

STREET SMART

One therapy that has been given consideration is the co-administration of drugs called antioxidants during a resuscitation. Antioxidants, like vitamin C and vitamin E, absorb reactive oxygen chemicals and effectively neutralize them before they can do damage.[18]

Toxins

Some substances are so lethal that they are called poisons. As little as a few micrograms of these substances can kill a person. However, any substance taken in excess—even water—can be toxic to the body. The definition of a **toxin** is any substance capable of causing cell injury and death, and that includes poisons. Toxins injure cells by one of two basic mechanisms: by direct reaction with the cell or through metabolites.

Metabolites are the by-products of drugs and chemicals after the cell has reacted with them. The biochemical changes that occur in the cell can convert a previously harmless drug or chemical into a toxin. For example, acetaminophen is harmless to the liver until after the liver metabolizes it. Thereafter, excessive amounts of metabolites of acetaminophen can build up to toxic levels, causing liver necrosis.[19–21]

Toxins that affect the cells directly usually react with a molecular component of the cell. By mutating or neutralizing that molecule the toxin impairs the cell's function, thereby injuring the cell. By way of example, the poison cyanide works by inactivating an enzyme, cytochrome oxidase, which is needed in cellular metabolism for the cell to use oxygen in the mitochondria.[22] Without this enzyme the mitochondria cannot make ATP. In essence, cyanide suffocates the cell by making the abundantly available oxygen useless.

Physical Causes of Cellular Injury

Those forces that exist outside of the body, in the physical world, can cause injury to the body and the cells within. Such forces include mechanical forces, referring to those injuries sustained by physical force or violence; extremes of temperature; radiation, including electromagnetic radiation; and changes in atmospheric pressures.

Mechanical Injury

Mechanical injury is due to abrupt and sudden physical forces acting upon the body, such as friction, blunt force, or penetrating force. This mechanical injury is referred to as **trauma** (Figure 11-2). These traumatic injury-producing forces tend to either stretch, tear, or crush tissues. Examples of traumatic injury, ranging from superficial to deep, are abrasions, lacerations, punctures, and fractures.

Heat or Cold Injury

The body has excellent mechanisms for keeping itself within the range of normal temperatures needed for cellular metabolism. When these mechanisms fail, cellular metabolism is affected and cells die. Examples of some heat-related diseases include heat cramps, exhaustion, or heat stroke.

Initially, in the case of heat exhaustion, the body is unable to compensate for the heat load that it is being exposed to and most of the emergency medical care is supportive of the body's efforts to correct it. When the heat becomes excessive, the lipid–protein cell membrane starts to liquefy. This allows sodium and water into the cell, as well as intracellular proteins such as enzymes, and DNA starts to break down. These conditions lead to cell death.

Concurrent conditions that result from heat stroke include **rhabdomyolysis** (rhabdo- "rod like"– ""; myo – "muscle"; -lysis – "split"), a breakdown of muscle, and **myoglobulinuria** (myo- – "muscle"; globin – "protein"; -uria – "urine"), a condition in which the protein products of muscle breakdown clog the kidneys. This leads to renal failure.

The opposite situation, hypothermia and cold-related injury, can lead to some localized injury (Figure 11-3) as a result of freezing and coagulation of the microcirculation, as well as the potential for more systemic injury. When the body's core temperature drops, cells suffer hypothermic injury from two mechanisms.

The first mechanism of injury is a disturbance in the ion concentrations of the cell, particularly sodium. As the cell wall starts to gel, eventually becoming crystalline, the sodium–potassium pump fails and sodium and water rush in. If the hypothermia is reversed in a timely fashion, the result will be edema. Cellular death can also occur.

Even as the cells start to cool, the cells continue with metabolism. This slowed metabolism is akin to the smoldering fire and smoke analogy used earlier. Partial products of metabolism—the reactive oxygen chemicals and particularly the oxygen-free radicals—start to accumulate. These chemicals have their greatest potential for cellular injury during the reperfusion stage or recovery phase.

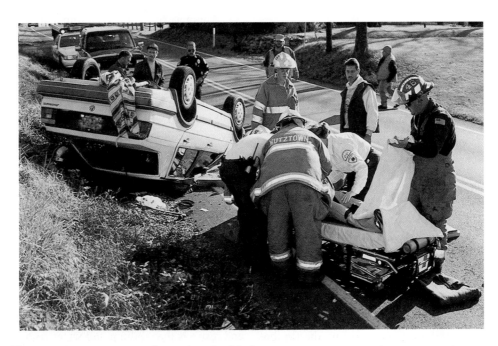

Figure 11-2 Trauma as a source of mechanical injury. (Courtesy of David J. Reimer Sr.)

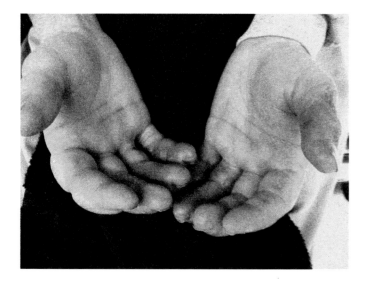

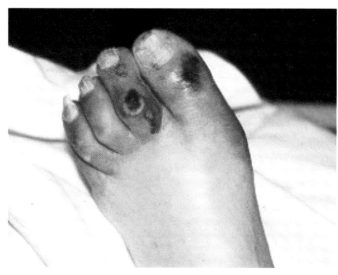

Figure 11-3 Frostbite as a result of cold injury.

Burn Injury

Burn injury (Figure 11-4) involves exposure to large amounts of energy from sources along the electromagnetic spectrum. Burns can be caused by five sources of electromagnetic energy: thermal (infrared), radiation (gamma), light (ultraviolet), radio, and electricity.

The most widely known source of thermal burns is direct contact with fire. However, other sources of thermal energy—such as superheated steam, boiling liquids, and heated objects—can also cause thermal injury.

Sources of nuclear radiation (e.g., uranium or plutonium) can also cause burns. Radiation exposure can be divided into particulate exposure (i.e., alpha and beta particles), and electromagnetic energy in the form of X-rays and gamma rays. The electromagnetic energy exposure (Figure 11-5) is considered to be more dangerous.

Intense light, which includes the light of the sun, contains photons (Greek – light) and are represented by the symbol of gamma. High-intensity photons are called gamma rays.

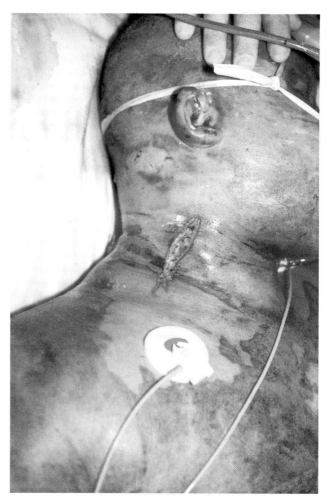

Figure 11-4 Burn injury.

Therefore, the exposure to sunlight (visible light) is actually exposure to celestial radiation. There are many sources of photons and all can cause photo burns.

Another form of electromagnetic radiation is radio frequency radiation (RFR), or radio waves. Contact with a noninsulated source of radio waves, such as a microwave antenna, can cause burns. However, RFR (including microwaves) are generally non-ionizing. The danger of radio frequency radiation is with the production of thermal energy.

Electrical energy, the movement of electrons, is what powers the cell's metabolic processes (i.e., electron transport). However, when massive amounts of electron energy enter the tissues then injury will occur. The cells suffer from thermal burns as well as electrolysis (electro- – "electron"; lysis – "divide"). The buildup of thermal energy occurs as a result of the flow of electricity overcoming resistance from the tissues and creating heat, called **joule heat** as a by-product of that reaction.

More problematic can be **electroporation**, the effect of electrical current passing through the tissue. The effect of electricity upon the lipid–protein layer of the cell membrane is to denature the proteins that are in the cell's pores. The end result is that sodium and water rush into the cell and the cell lysis.

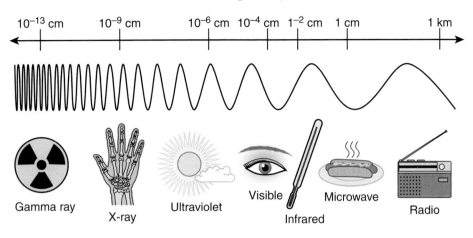

The Electromagnetic Spectrum

| 10^{-13} cm | 10^{-9} cm | 10^{-6} cm | 10^{-4} cm | 1^{-2} cm | 1 cm | 1 km |

Gamma ray   X-ray   Ultraviolet   Visible   Infrared   Microwave   Radio

Figure 11-5 Electromagnetic spectrum.

Mechanism of Injury

The major mechanism of injury for a burn is either direct heat transfer or ionization. Heat placed in direct contact with the cells **denatures** their proteins. That is, it breaks down the protein's complex folded structure. This can be seen when the clear liquid protein of an egg white is cooked on a griddle. The egg white coagulates, becoming solid and turning white.

Ionization, on the other hand, strips away electrons, leaving highly reactive chemicals to break down chemical bonds and alter cellular chemistry. High levels of ionization lead to conditions such as radiation poisoning or sun poisoning. Low levels of ionization, particularly the penetrating radiation of gamma rays, can alter amino acids in the DNA and cause long-term complications.

The likelihood of long-term complications from ionizing radiation exposure, the **stochastic effects**, is a function of the length (duration of time) of exposure and/or the strength of the radiation. Ionizing radiation is thought to cause cancers in individuals. Frequent exposure to radiation, such as sunburns while sun tanning, can lead to an increased susceptibility to cancer. Exposure to ionizing radiation can also cause birth defects and cancer in subsequent generations, called the **teratogenic effect**, as a result of changes in the structure of that all important protein, the DNA.

Barotrauma

Barotrauma is physical damage to tissues, an injury caused by an imbalance between pressures in the environment and those within the body. The pathophysiology of barotraumas revolves around the fact that gasses, in the air or within the blood, are more compressible, or distensible, than the surrounding tissues.

The classic example of direct barotrauma is injury due to the shock wave of an explosion.[23–25] During an explosion there is a rapid rise in atmospheric pressure that can cause mechanical damage to any air-filled organs such as the lungs and eardrums. It occurs in the same manner that slapping an air-filled paper bag destroys the paper bag.

There is also indirect barotrauma secondary to dissolved gasses. Gasses such as oxygen, carbon dioxide, and nitrogen are dissolved in blood. When there is increased pressure, such as occurs during deep sea diving, then the gasses compress. As the diver ascends, the gasses "come out of solution" and take up volume in the bloodstream, causing occlusions. At the same time, the volume of air within the lungs expands (Boyle's law) thereby overpressurizing the lungs and creating a risk of a ruptured lung or pneumothorax (Figure 11-6).

Barotrauma is not restricted to diving incidents only. The same pathophysiological processes in decompression illness occur in mountain sickness.

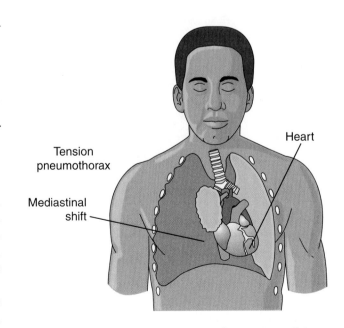

Tension pneumothorax

Heart

Mediastinal shift

Figure 11-6 Tension pneumothorax possibly secondary to barotrauma.

Metabolic Disorders

Nutritional deficiencies can lead to metabolic derangement and disease. Scurvy, for example, is an ancient disease, having been recorded by the Egyptians in 1559 B.C., which became more problematic when early sailing voyages became prolonged. In 1520 Magellan lost more than 80% of his crew to scurvy while trying to circumnavigate the globe. British Navel Surgeon Sir James Lind linked scurvy with a deficiency of vitamin C, ascorbic acid, in 1746. He immediately ordered citrus fruit, known to be high in vitamin C, aboard every British Navy ship; hence the origin of the British sailors' nickname "limeys."

Nutritional excess can also lead to disease. The current epidemic of obesity in America (Figure 11-7) has led to an increase in obesity-related disease, such as diabetes mellitus, as well as an increase in obesity-linked diseases such as sleep apnea and Pickwickian syndrome.

Genetic Disorders

The existence of genetic diseases has been recognized for centuries. These disorders were described as running in a family. What was missing was an understanding of why these disorders ran in families. Abnormalities in a person's genes can cause a genetic disorder. Within the DNA, genes carry the blueprint for protein production which is the life work of most cells. These proteins are essential to cell health.

If the DNA sequence of one gene is altered, called a **mutation**, then protein production can be altered. Examples of monogenic disorders include Marfan syndrome, sickle-cell anemia, and cystic fibrosis.

In some instances the entire chromosome is structurally defective. Gross breaks in some chromosomes with subsequent

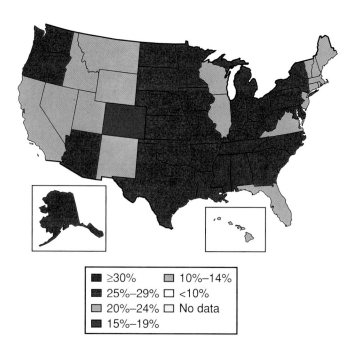

Figure 11-7 Obesity in the United States. (Courtesy of Centers for Disease Control and Prevention)

Legend:
- ≥30%
- 25%–29%
- 20%–24%
- 15%–19%
- 10%–14%
- <10%
- No data

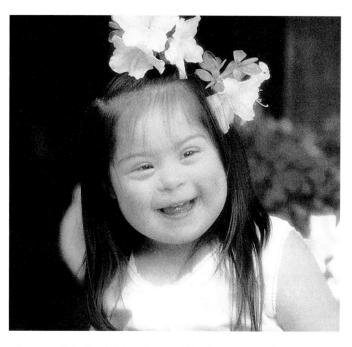

Figure 11-8 This child with Down syndrome is encouraged to develop psychomotor skills. (From Down Right Beautiful 1996 Calendar, Marijone's Designer Portraits)

rejoinings at new locations, called **translocations**; extra copies of chromosomes; or missing copies of chromosomes leads to genetic disorders. Down syndrome is a common genetic disorder linked to having three copies of the 21st chromosome.[26,27] A child with Down syndrome (Figure 11-8) may have a flattened nose and widely spaced eyes.

However, most genetic disorders are complex and involve a combination of environmental and multiple genetic mutations. Many chronic diseases—such as Alzheimer's disease, heart disease, arthritis, and obesity—are thought to have genetic underpinnings.

Not all genetic differences necessarily lead to disease. In fact, some genetic changes may be evolutionary in nature. In an incredible case of genetic detective work, it has been discovered that some people cannot contract human immunodeficiency virus (HIV), the cause of AIDS. The reason is because of a genetic mutation which prevents the white blood cells from creating the receptor, CCR5, that permits the HIV virus to gain entrance into the white blood cell.

Infection

The majority of deaths during recorded history have been due to infectious diseases. Infectious diseases, referred to in medical circles as **pathogens**, stem from a number of sources. Listed from smallest to largest, they are prions, viruses, bacteria (Figure 11-9), fungi, protozoa, and helminthes (worms). All of these microorganisms are parasites, dependent on the host for survival.

Infectious diseases have three pathogenic mechanisms. Some infectious agents (e.g., herpes simplex) replicate themselves inside the host cells. Eventually these

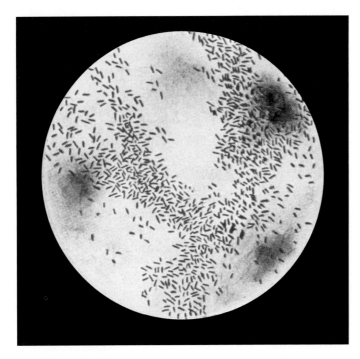

Figure 11-9 Common microorganisms that can cause disease. (Courtesy of Centers for Disease Control and Prevention Public Health Image Library)

microorganisms destroy the cell's structural integrity, thereby killing the cell, which is a direct **cytopathic** effect. The microorganisms are then released to infect other cells or other potential hosts.

Other microorganisms are dangerous to the host because they produce a toxin that is harmful (poisonous) to the cell. Toxins can be categorized as either being exotoxins or endotoxins. **Exotoxins** are proteins that are produced by bacteria and released into the interstitial fluid where they are absorbed, because they are highly soluble, into surrounding cells. Exotoxins can be cell specific. For example, the toxins that produce tetanus and botulism affect nervous tissue whereas the toxins of the streptococcus bacteria affect vascular tissue.

Some bacteria produce toxins by their death. These toxins, called **endotoxins**, are the result of the breakdown of the bacteria's cell wall membrane.[28,29] Endotoxins are complex substances made up of polysaccharides or phospholipids and are attracted to other cell wall membranes. The bacteria Clostridium tetanus produces a phospholipase (phospholipids make up cell wall membranes and the suffix -ase means enzyme) which breaks down cell walls.

Finally, some infections are dangerous because they trigger an immune response that causes damage to the host, an **autoimmune response**. For example, the causative agent of rheumatic fever, streptococcus, triggers an undifferentiated immune response that destroys healthy tissue (frequently the heart valves) in the process.

Immune Reactions

Immune reactions can be classified as either exaggerated immune responses or autoimmune responses. In the first case,

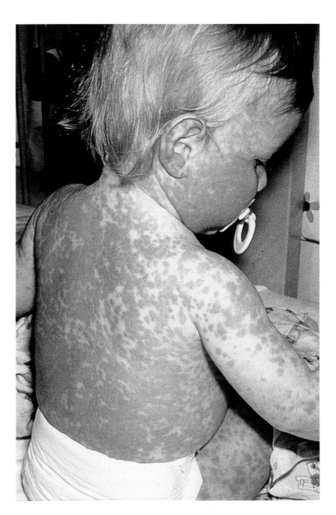

Figure 11-10 Patient experiencing an allergic reaction. (Courtesy of Robert A. Silverman, M. D., Clinical Professor, Department of Pediatrics, Georgetown University, Georgetown, MD)

the body has a disproportionate response to a foreign protein or polysaccharide, an **antigen** (anti- – "not"; gen – "self") and the results are life-threatening to the patient. This exaggerated immune response, called an **anaphylactic response**, can lead to severe airway compromise and/or cardiovascular collapse secondary to relative hypovolemia. This may be exemplified by a patient with an allergic reaction (Figure 11-10).

In the case of the autoimmune response, described earlier, the body sets upon itself and starts to destroy normal cells along with infected cells. Autoimmune response has been implicated in the diseases multiple sclerosis, diabetes mellitus, scleroderma, Crohn's disease, lupus erythematosus, rheumatoid arthritis, and gluten sensitivity.

Effect: Systemic Defense

The body's defenses to disease start with general nonspecific barriers and end with targeted cellular attacks against the offending disease. If these defenses are overwhelmed, then the patient is diseased.

Patients with disease go into shock, a condition of deranged metabolic functions that have systemic effects described later in this chapter. The shock **syndrome**, a predictable pattern of signs and symptoms, can either culminate with recovery or death. The Paramedic's mission is to support the body in its struggle against shock.

Nonspecific Defenses

While the analogy is not glamorous, the truth is that the body is essentially two hollow tubes, with one tube being a cul de sac. The outside of the tube is covered by skin, the largest organ of the body. Skin is a barrier to physical attack by trauma, chemicals, and so on and from biological attack from microorganisms such as fungus, bacteria, and virus.

The key to the skin's effectiveness as a barrier lies in the fact that the outermost layer of skin is dead. Most microorganisms depend on the host cells being alive. The layers of dead epithelial cells, contained in the epidermis, prevent infection from reaching the live cells deeper in the tissue. Barrier devices, such as gloves (Figure 11-11), are simply adjuncts to the first defense, the skin.

But the defense does not stop there. Sebaceous glands excrete acidic (pH 3–5) secretions—lactic acid and fatty acids—which act as a biochemical barrier and create a hostile environment for fungi and bacteria.

Finally, if any infection obtains a foothold in the skin it is only temporary. Skin is sloughed off, or mechanically abraded, continuously, and replaced as quickly. The combination of these three mechanisms culminates in a very effective barrier defense against outside sources of disease.

Internally, the body is lined with mucous membranes that cover the pulmonary tree, the cul de sac mentioned earlier, and the gastrointestinal tract that extends the length of the human torso. Mucous membranes secrete mucus, a sticky liquid that entraps foreign invaders, such as bacteria. Bacteria-laden mucus in the lungs is either expectorated, and thus sputum may be infectious, or ingested, where the bacteria meet their fate in the stomach's acid.

Infectious trespassers in the oropharynx are first greeted by lysozyme-carrying saliva, which breaks down cell walls. If any remain alive, they are carried to the acidic environment of the stomach to be destroyed. Note that external bodily fluids such as perspiration, tears, and ear wax are either mucus-like, trapping potentially infectious materials, or contain the enzyme lysozyme.

Like the skin, the internal organs can be protected from foreign invaders by mechanical means such as regurgitation, defecation, menstruation, and urination.

Inflammatory Response

If the nonspecific defenses of the skin or the mucosa are breached and internal cells and tissues are injured, the second-string defenders, the inflammatory system, responds. The inflammatory system is made up of white blood cells and chemical intermediaries that act as messengers.

A variety of causes can stimulate the inflammatory response. Causes include infections that lead to systemic infections; trauma, such as burn trauma; anaphylactic reactions; complications of childbirth; and eclampsia, to name just a few.

Inflammation: Acute Phase

Forward scouts, the mast cells contained in the bloodstream, are triggered by trauma, hypoxia, toxins, or any source of cellular injury. They respond from the bloodstream almost immediately. Outwardly, the response of the inflammatory system is visible as redness (rubor), swelling (tumor), pain (dolor), and warmth (calor) at the injury site.

Looking beneath these outward manifestations, a complex process of inflammation is revealed. Mast cells, containing granules of chemical mediators like histamine and serotonin, break down or **degranulate**, releasing their contents into the surrounding interstitial fluids (Figure 11-12).

The chemical mediators histamine and serotonin cause vasoconstriction of the smooth muscle in the surrounding arterioles, thereby limiting the spread of injury. They also dilate the postcapillary venules, resulting in swelling and pain. Dilation of the capillary beds is important because it increases the permeability of the capillary walls and allows more white blood cells to migrate out of the blood and into the interstitial space surrounding the cells. The collection of white blood cells and fluids is called an **exudate**.

Mast cells also release two chemical messengers: **chemotactic factors**, which attract specific leukocytes (white blood cells) to the injury site. These chemotactic factors—neutrophil chemotactic factor and eosinophil chemotactic factor of anaphylaxis (ECF-A)—bring out the workhorses of inflammation—neutrophils and eosinophils—during the early stages of the inflammatory response.

Neutrophils destroy bacteria by engulfing them in a process called **phagocytosis** (Figure 11-13). Then the neutrophils break down the bacteria with their lysosomes. Eosinophils destroy parasitic infestations, such as helminthes (worms), and release enzymes that slow the inflammatory response.[30] Chief amongst these enzymes is histaminase, an enzyme that breaks down histamine.

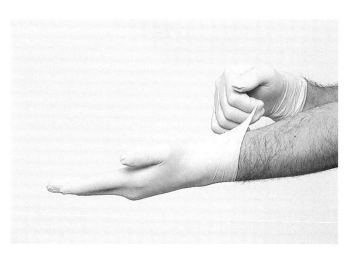

Figure 11-11 Barrier devices, such as gloves, support the body's own nonspecific defense, the skin.

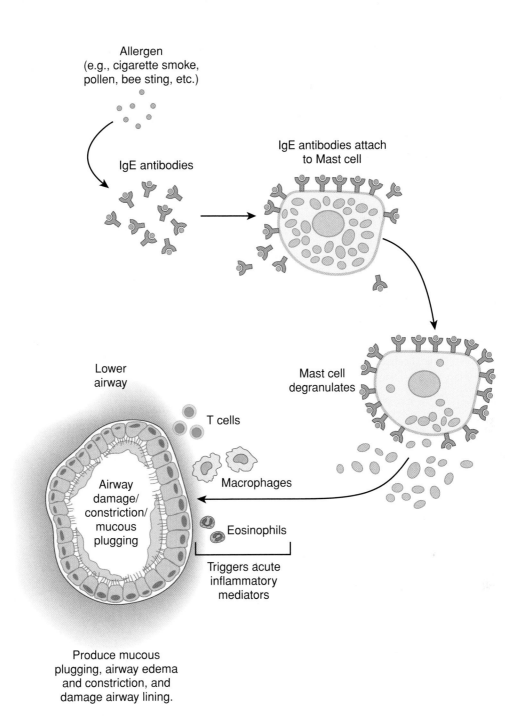

Allergen
(e.g., cigarette smoke,
pollen, bee sting, etc.)

IgE antibodies

IgE antibodies attach
to Mast cell

Mast cell
degranulates

Lower
airway

T cells

Macrophages

Airway
damage/
constriction/
mucous
plugging

Eosinophils

Triggers acute
inflammatory
mediators

Produce mucous
plugging, airway edema
and constriction, and
damage airway lining.

Figure 11-12 Mast cell degranulation.

Inflammation: Prolonged or Chronic

Mast cells also create chemical mediators such as **leukotrienes** (slow acting substances of anaphylaxis—SRS-A). Leukotrienes produce chemical effects which are similar to histamine and help to prolong the inflammation, if necessary. Leukotrienes could be considered as long-acting histamine.

Perhaps most notable to the patient is the presence of **prostaglandins**, a chemical mediator released from the mast cell that creates the sensation of pain. However, the primary function of prostaglandins is not to create pain but to increase

vascular permeability and smooth muscle contraction later in the inflammatory response.

If the infection is persistent (i.e., greater than 24 hours), then monocytes, which later become macrophages, come to the aid of the neutrophils and a similar process continues.[31] At this stage the body typically mounts a fever response. The fever is induced by chemicals from the neutrophils and the macrophages, which are released after exposure to the bacterial remains (endotoxins).

The cellular remnants of this battle, containing dead and dying leukocytes and bacterial remains, either migrate to the

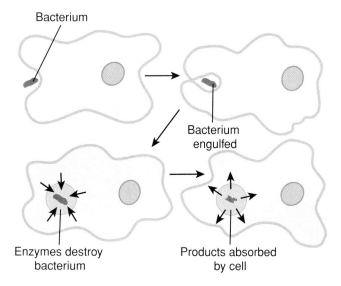

Figure 11-13 Neutrophils engaged in phagocytosis of an invading bacteria. (Diagram by Ruth Lawson, Otago Polytechnic, licensed under the Creative Commons Attribution-Sharealike versions 3.0, 2.5, 2.0 and 1.0)

skin's surface as pus or are carried away in the lymphatic system as purulent exudate. If the purulent exudate is walled off in a specific area, then it is called an **abscess**. Abscesses can be difficult to resolve without a surgical procedure such as **incision and drainage** (I&D).[32]

Support for Inflammation: The Complement System

The complement system, as the name suggests, supports and controls the inflammatory response. Plasma proteins circulate in the blood and make up almost one half of the blood proteins. The other half of the blood proteins are albumin. The blood proteins comprise the complement system and can be activated by either one of two mechanisms.

The first mechanism includes the classic pathway, an **immune complex**, in which an antibody (e.g., IgG or IgM) has attached to an antigen and stimulates the complement system. The activated plasma proteins of the complement system act as **anaphylatoxins**, increasing the degranulation of mast cells and attracting other white blood cells (leukocytes) to the site. The plasma proteins mark resistant bacterium by attaching fragments of themselves to the bacterial cell wall, a process called **opsonization**, thus enhancing the impact of the leukocytes.

With the second mechanism, the alternative pathway, toxins secreted by the bacterium or fungi stimulate the complement system and cause all of the same effects as the classic pathway.

In some cases the body does not recognize the bacteria and cannot mount an effective antigen–antibody defense. In those cases, the complement system creates a **membrane attack complex (MAC)**, which attaches itself to the cell's walls and forms a tube from the outside to the inside. The tube allows water to enter the cell, the cell to swell, and the cell to lysis (Figure 11-14).

Support for Inflammation: The Coagulation System

The term "coagulation" evokes thoughts of blood clots and hemorrhage. However, during the inflammatory response the coagulation system acts to entrap fluids (exudates) and foreign bodies (Figure 11-15).

Both endotoxins (via the extrinsic pathway) and kinins (via the intrinsic pathway) can stimulate the coagulation cascade to begin. Circulating prothrombin, a plasma protein, is converted into thrombin, which in turn is converted into fibrinogen and then fibrin. The resulting fibrin net prevents the spread of the infection to adjunct tissues by essentially walling off the site.

Perhaps as important as preventing the spread of infection, the fibrin net keeps the offending microorganisms confined to a smaller area for phagocytic action by neutrophils and macrophages. Finally, the fibrin net serves as scaffolding for scar formation and healing.

Support for Inflammation: The Kinin System

Another class of circulating plasma proteins is the kinin group, made up of chains of amino acids. Like the coagulation cascade, kallikrein is activated and converted to bradykinin in a cascade. However, kallikrein is present in sweat, tears, saliva, urine, and feces and can be converted into bradykinin.

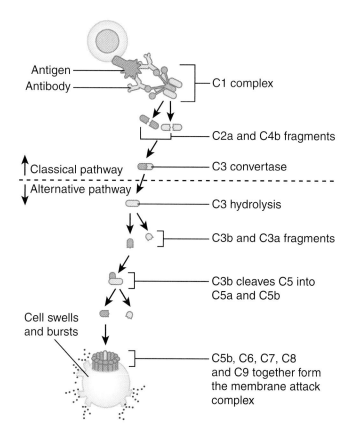

Figure 11-14 The complement system creating a membrane attack complex.

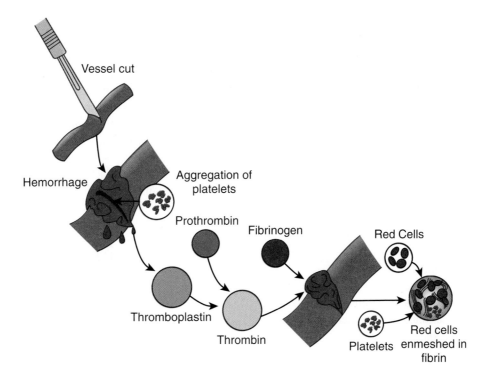

Figure 11-15 Coagulation.

Bradykinin is similar to histamine in its actions. It causes vasodilation, increased permeability of the vascular bed, and works with prostaglandins to produce pain. Bradykinin was first discovered in Brazil by three pharmacologists working with snake venom which caused circulatory collapse. Using this early work, scientists developed a new class of antihypertensive drugs called ACE inhibitors.

Immune Response

The immune response is the body's specific defense against substances that are not part of the body (by definition, antigens). Antigens can be **exogenous**, from outside of the body, and enter the body by injection, ingestion, or inhalation. Antigens can also be **endogenous**, from within the body (e.g., a virus that has replicated within a cell). Whatever the source of the antigen, the body's immune system reacts.

Lymphocytes within the body respond to the site of injury and, depending on the type of lymphocyte, incapacitate the antigen. B lymphocytes, from bone marrow, produce antibodies that then attack the cell. T lymphocytes, from the thymus gland, recognize the antigen and attack it directly.

B Lymphocytes

After an infection, some remaining B lymphocytes remain in contact with the antigen. This contact stimulates the B lymphocyte to divide. The resulting clones can either have a memory of the antigen, called **memory cells**, or they become **plasma cells**. Plasma cells generate antibodies, a type of protein globulin called **immunoglobulins**.

Five types of immunoglobulins have been identified: IgA, IgD, IgE, IgG (gamma globulin), and IgM, and each immunoglobulin fits into the surface of an antigen in a key and lock fashion, linking them together. The result of this union is to either neutralize bacterial toxins or activate the complement system. Complement proteins then cause the swelling and rupture of the cells via membrane attack complexes.

If the same antigen is introduced again, circulating memory cells will recognize the antigen and plasma cells will start to release antibodies. This phenomenon is called **humoral immunity**.

T Lymphocytes

Originating in the bone marrow with B lymphocytes, T lymphocytes travel to the thymus where they mature and exit the thymus **immunocompetent** (i.e., capable of providing immunity) and travel to the lymphatic system. Once in the lymphatic system, specific cytotoxic T lymphocytes, or killer T cells, attack antigens which antibodies could not bind to. They form an antigen–antibody complex (i.e., antigens for which the patient does not yet have immunity).

Cytotoxic T cells can release lymphokine, a chemical that attracts macrophages, or they can release cell-killing toxins. Some even release interferon, a glucoprotein that inhibits cell growth.

Helper T cells bind to macrophages or B lymphocytes and together produce a protein (interleukin) which stimulates more production of both B and T lymphocytes. The resulting activity of T lymphocytes produces **cell–mediated immunity**.

Outcomes: Shock Syndrome

Whenever a Paramedic approaches a patient, the quintessential question in the Paramedic's mind should be, "Is the patient in shock?" Shock is of great significance in emergency medicine. While seemingly a simple question to answer, the definitions of shock are as different as the causes of shock.

The common layperson definition of shock might be any condition that could potentially lead to death. In 1862, Samuel Gross, a surgeon, described shock as the "rude unhinging of the machinery of life." John Collins Warren made the statement that shock is but "a momentary pause in the act of death." If asked to define shock, a Paramedic might describe a state of hypoperfusion and inadequate tissue circulation, and this would be technically correct. Yet all of these definitions are insufficient for the Paramedic's purposes.

A better definition of shock is the "body's inability to provide the necessary substrates, oxygen and glucose, for example, to the cells for cellular life and the inability of the body to maintain homeostasis."[33–36]

This definition emphasizes the body's complexity and interaction and the singular importance of maintaining the viability of cells. The importance of identifying shock to a Paramedic's practice cannot be overemphasized. Failure to identify declining trends in the vital signs and subtle signs of hypoperfusion can lead to missed rescues and increased morbidity and mortality. Shock deserves aggressive treatment from the moment subtle signs are identified.

Classifications of Shock

Henri Francois Le Dran, a French surgeon, first originated the term "choc," meaning jolt or impact, when describing the fatal syndrome that was associated with gunshot wounds. The term was later expanded to include any lethal deterioration in a patient's condition.

As time progressed, additional etiologies besides trauma for the shock syndrome were identified. These included severe infections and shock of a cardiac origin. In 1972 Hinshaw and Cox advanced a universal system for inclusion of all causes of the shock syndrome.

The Hinshaw–Cox shock classification included four major categories. The first, **hypovolemic shock**, included shock that arose from trauma (hemorrhagic shock) but also included other etiologies where there was a loss of circulating blood volume.[37]

The next category of shock was **cardiogenic shock**, or shock of a cardiac origin. Cardiogenic shock could include diseases of the muscle (e.g., cardiomyopathy), diseases of the coronary arteries, and diseases of cardiac conduction. Whatever the cause, there has to be a failure of the heart as an effective pump.

Originally called vasogenic shock, the classification was renamed **distributive shock**, a term that is more descriptive of the problem of poor blood distribution. Distributive shock included shock caused by the widespread vasodilatation seen with severe infections and during anaphylactic reactions, to name a few causes.

The final classification of shock, **obstructive shock**, dealt with the physical impairment of forward blood flow despite an effective pump, an adequate blood volume, and a normal vasculature. Examples of obstructive shock include massive pulmonary clots, embolism, and a collapsed lung (pneumothorax), which proceeds to crush the heart as well.

Recently a fifth classification has been added, **endocrine shock**. Endocrine shock recognizes the importance of hormones in maintaining homeostasis. The classic endocrine shock is hypoglycemic shock.

Regardless of the etiology of shock or its classification, all shock leads to cell injury. Cellular injury is generally owed to ischemia, whether it is from a lack of oxygen (hypoxia) or glucose (hypoglycemia), the creation of inflammation as well as free radical injury.

Pathophysiology of Shock

The body's homeostatic mechanisms engage at the first sign of hemodynamic instability in an effort to maintain adequate tissue perfusion. Chemoreceptors in the carotid arteries and the medulla oblongata, as well as baroreceptors in the aortic arch and the carotid arteries, sense variations in blood pressure, oxygenation, and acidosis. This early hemodynamic instability activates the sympathetic nervous system and starts the body's compensatory mechanisms, which compensate for shock.[38–40]

Organs in Shock

The earliest organs to suffer in shock are the organs of the gastrointestinal system. Hypoperfusion of the gut leads to erosions of the stomach (erosive gastritis), irritations of the pancreas (pancreatitis), cessation of peristalsis (paralytic ileus), and fine hemorrhage of the bowel (colonic hemorrhage).

The next set of organs—the liver, spleen, and kidneys—enjoy the protection of the thoracic cage and are important to short-term survival. These are often referred to as core organs.

The first organs to be affected by hypoperfusion are the paired kidneys which attempt to conserve volume and produce small amounts of urine (i.e., **oliguria**), sometimes less than 0.5 mL/kg per hour. This conservation of volume is mainly created by sympathetic stimulation and angiotensin that combine to create vasoconstriction. The net effect of prolonged hypoperfusion is **acute renal failure (ARF)** secondary to tubular ischemia.

The liver also fails, a condition called **shock–liver**, and is associated with massive ischemic changes that peak in one to three days and resolve in three to ten days, provided the cause of the shock has been resolved.[41,42] Systemically, the loss of liver function leads to decreased blood proteins, especially albumin.

Without albumin in the bloodstream to help maintain colloidal osmotic pressure (COP), intravascular fluids leak into the third space, creating total body edema or **anasarca** (ana- – "throughout"; sacra – "flesh").

Blood proteins created from the liver are also critical to the coagulation cascade. Blood clotting factors are stimulated by the inflammatory response. After initial blood clotting factors are partially consumed by massive coagulation throughout the body, the remaining clotting factors are insufficient to protect the body, a condition called **disseminated intravascular coagulation (DIC)**.

The paradox of DIC is that the patient's body forms clots where they are not needed, leading to localized tissue ischemia. The patient does not form clots where they are needed, which leads to hemorrhage.

Splenic injury can be either direct parenchymal injury, such as blunt trauma, or cellular injury induced by ischemia that leads to impaired cellular or humoral immunity. Subsequent dysfunction of the immune system leaves the patient prone to massive infections and life-threatening **sepsis** (Greek – putrefaction).

Sepsis involves the widespread activation of both the inflammatory response as well as the coagulation cascade and generally indicates the body's failure to control the infection.[28, 43–46] The subsequent massive shift of fluids into third space, with resulting anasarca, leads to hypotension, hypoperfusion, and widespread cellular ischemia.

Systemic infections involving the whole body which lead to sepsis can cause **multiple organ dysfunction syndrome (MODS)**, a failure of two or more organ systems.

MODS can also be caused by an uncontrolled inflammatory response from any disease. Diseases could include pulmonary embolism, electrocution, and complications of childbirth, such as amniotic embolism.

During infection, MODS is the final step in a process known as **systemic inflammatory response syndrome (SIRS)**. The evolution of SIRS is localized infection leading to systemic infection leading to sepsis, then on to septic shock and MODS.

Shock: Vital Organs

The differentiation of decompensated and irreversible shock may be academic for Paramedics because the timetable for recovery from ARF, DIC, MODS, and SIRS is often days or weeks. What may have more utility to the Paramedic is distinguishing shock that affects the vital organs: the lungs, heart, and brain.

Lungs

The first system to respond to hypoperfusion, to shock, is the pulmonary system. Increased acid production from anaerobic respiration stimulates chemoreceptors in the carotid artery and in the medulla oblongata. The resulting **tachypnea** (rapid breathing) and **hyperpnea** (deep breathing) increases the work of breathing for the muscles, particularly the diaphragm.

Eventually, a mismatch occurs between the increasing work of breathing and the muscle impairment from ischemia, resulting in respiratory failure.

Impaired gas exchange at the alveolar level causes an inflammatory response. The resultant leaky pipes of the alveolar capillaries spill into the alveolar space, filling it with exudate that is appreciated as rales (crackles) by the Paramedic. The combination of alveolar edema, from inflammation and pulmonary hemorrhage, from disturbed coagulation causes **adult respiratory distress syndrome (ARDS)**.[47,48]

As time progresses, the resulting difference between the amount of lungs filled (alveolar ventilation) and the capillary circulation (pulmonary perfusion) results in a mismatch, termed a **V/Q mismatch**. Blood, now unoxygenated, bypasses whole sections of the lung, a process called **shunting**, producing systemic hypoxia from **acute respiratory failure**.

Heart

Hypovolemia (from hemorrhage), vasodilatation (from sepsis), and hypoxia all drive the heart to try to compensate and maintain cardiac output, which equals stroke volume times heart rate.

The primary mechanism is sympathetic stimulation, an adrenergic surge which races the heart and increases the blood pressure. Catecholamines, such as adrenaline/epinephrine, work to support the sympathetic nervous system.

The sympathetic nervous system, in turn, starts to constrict capillary sphincters, effectively closing off capillary beds, thereby shunting blood to the core organs. The order of the shunting, sometimes called the pecking order of shock, starts with the fetus. The mother's body will sacrifice the fetus in order to save the mother; hence, the EMS axiom "to save the baby, you have to save the mother first."

The alpha receptors of the sympathetic nervous system then close down the skin, leading to pale, cool, and clammy skin. Then the gastrointestinal tract is closed down, producing nausea. Thereafter, the remaining core organs are affected.

The sympathetic nervous system also stimulates the vital organs through the beta receptors. Adrenaline/epinephrine stimulates the beta$_2$ receptors in the two lungs to breathe faster (tachypnea) and to breathe deeper (hypernea), increasing available oxygen to balance the oxygen demand of the tissues.

The heart's beta$_1$ receptors are stimulated by the sympathetic nervous system to increase the heart's strength of contraction (inotropy) as well as the rate of contraction (chronotropy).

A factor working against the heart is the health of the coronary arteries. Coronary arteries can be narrowed by chronic inflammation or occluded by a blood clot (**thrombus**) in a condition called **acute coronary syndrome (ACS)**, leading to coronary ischemia. For this reason, and as a matter of practice, ACS should be suspected as a comorbid factor in high-risk patients with shock syndrome.[49–51]

In a corollary to ACS, increased demands upon the heart can induce tachydysrhythymias. Both tachycardias of a ventricular origin and those of a supraventricular (supra- – "above"; ventricles – Latin "belly" of the heart) do not permit adequate ventricular filling time, affecting cardiac output (CO = SV X HR) adversely. The target heart rate should be less than 150 beats per minute.

Conversely, heart rates that are too slow can also reduce cardiac output, adversely affecting the patient's hemodynamic status. Vagally mediated bradycardias occur with head injuries, with neurogenic shock, in end-stage hemorrhage shock, and under certain conditions with acute coronary syndrome. The resultant cardiac output is insufficient to meet demands and global ischemia occurs. The target heart rate should be greater than 50 beats per minute (BPM).

Finally, during sepsis or hemorrhagic shock, toxic circulating myocardial depressant factors cause myocardial depression. Also, there is a decrease in the strength of myocardial contraction (inotropy), which results in profound hypotension as well.

Brain

The brain requires an almost steady state of perfusion to ensure adequate oxygen and glucose because neurons are extremely sensitive to any ischemia or hypoxia. The brain needs a mean arterial blood pressure (MAP) of approximately 50 to 60 mmHg to maintain adequate perfusion, and the brain is highly adaptive in its efforts to maintain perfusion. Without adequate perfusion, sufficient oxygen and/or glucose becomes unavailable and brain damage starts to occur.

Starting with irreversible damage in the cerebral cortex, ischemic changes will start to progressively affect all areas of the brain. Outwardly, the manifestations of these changes will include symptoms of anxiety and urgency before descending into feelings of doom and confusion, with concomitant combativeness followed by unconsciousness.

Maintenance of cerebral perfusion is the target goal of all Paramedics. Every effort is made to either support the brain directly, via oxygen and/or glucose administration, or to support auxiliary organs, such as the heart and lungs, in order to support the brain.

Decompensated Shock

Decompensated shock is the end-stage of a series of cumulative physiologic derangements typically involving one organ system which goes on to affect the entire body. Affected are the inflammatory system and the complement system, leading to coagulation, and culminating in a pathological process called the shock syndrome.

Key to survival from shock is the maintenance of perfusion to the vital organs, particularly the brain. The body, through the sympathetic nervous system, attempts to maintain perfusion, but reaches a break point where it fails.[52] This failure has been attributed to several mechanisms.

The leading theory of decompensated shock involves the body's production of acid, both carbonic acid (respiratory acid) and lactic acid (metabolic acid). This acid accumulates, called an **acid load**, to the point that tissues are acidotic. The round muscles of the capillary sphincters, that have until that moment been shutting down capillary beds and shunting blood to core organs, can no longer remain closed in an acidotic environment and the muscles relax. The result of this relaxation is massive vasodilatation and a relative hypovolemia as blood leaves the central circulation for the periphery.

Another theory, either working alone or in concert with the acid load theory, states that catecholamine depletion (loss of the neurotransmitters of the sympathetic nervous system) leads to relaxation of capillary sphincters and a rapid decline in peripheral vascular resistance.

The last theory suggests that there is a decrease in sympathetic tone due to loss of perfusion to the central nervous system. The significant finding in all three conditions is the sudden loss of peripheral vascular resistance (closed capillary beds that shunt blood to the core) and subsequent loss of blood pressure and perfusion to the core organs.

Axioms of Shock Treatment

Paramedic care largely revolves around making a **tentative field diagnosis** of shock syndrome based upon the symptom complex and then directing treatments toward supporting the patient's body in its efforts to maintain homeostasis.

The traditional approach to treatment follows the same line as assessment: airway, breathing, and circulation. The therapeutic goals, following this ABC system, are universally applicable to all forms of shock and are as follows.

First, it is important to provide and optimize the unloading of oxygen at the cellular level. The provision of supplemental oxygen, as needed, is essential in order to prevent hypoxia. Perhaps more importantly, ventilation must be assured. Ventilation is critical in the **acid**–base balance mechanisms. Profound acidosis, respiratory or metabolic, not only shifts the oxyhemoglobin curve, but also causes capillary sphincter relaxation and massive vasodilatation.

The next goal is the maintenance of an adequate circulatory pressure for perfusion. The end goal is to maintain adequate cerebral perfusion pressure (CPP). Cerebral perfusion pressure is the difference between the mean arterial pressure (MAP) and the intracranial pressure (ICP). Its range should be greater than 10 to 15 mmHg in adults. The normal CPP range is 70 to 100 mmHg, and when the CPP falls to less than 50 mmHg acutely, or 70 mmHg for a prolonged period of time, the brain suffers ischemia secondary to hypoperfusion.[53–55]

In the out-of-hospital environment, it is difficult to monitor some of these values. Therefore, Paramedics focus on monitoring the mean arterial pressure, when automated noninvasive oscillometric technique is available, or the pulse pressure (systolic pressure minus diastolic pressure) when auscultatory manual sphygmomanometry is used. Then, making a reasonable estimate of the ICP, the Paramedic measures the MAP, typically in a range of 50 to 150 mmHg, and estimates the CPP.

The average ICP in a conscious and alert adult is approximately 10 to 15 mmHg. When the patient starts to become confused or drowsy (a Glasgow Coma Scale (GCS) of 13 to 15) then the ICP is approximately 20 mmHg. If the patient's GCS drops to 8 or less, then the ICP is approximately 30 mmHg. These values assume that the patient has not been medicated with sedatives such as diazepam.

The importance of oxygenation and ventilation cannot be overemphasized enough. Hypoxia and **hypercapnia** (increased carbon dioxide) levels raise cerebral blood flow (CBF), which in turn raises intracranial pressure. Hypoxia is poorly tolerated and hypercapnia, in the form of carbonic acid (respiratory acid) with values greater than 45 mmHg should be avoided.[56–60]

Next, cardiac function should be maximized, in large part to maintain the MAP in a range that supports adequate cerebral perfusion pressures. Typically, the first objective is to normalize the heart rate within the range of 50 to 150 BPM, with 60 to 80 BPM being optimal.[61]

If the MAP remains suboptimal, then the use of vasopressors, such as dopamine, may be needed to support the sympathetic nervous system. Vasopressors should be titrated, keeping the CPP and the MAP in mind.

The final goal should be to redistribute blood flow to ensure perfusion of vital organs. The kidneys help to maintain intravascular volume by reducing urine output and by utilizing the renin–angiotensin–aldosterone mechanism. This mechanism helps ensure not only that there is reabsorption of sodium at the kidneys but also that adrenal epinephrine release increases.

From a prehospital point of view, the need is to provide optimal intravascular volume, particularly **preload** (the volume of venous blood entering the heart during diastole), to optimize stroke volume and cardiac output. This is achieved through intravenous infusions of crystalloid- or colloid-containing solutions.

These goals are not in treatment priority order. Rather, they should be individualized to each patient. It should be clear that the overarching mission is to support the body while it tries to provide oxygen delivery to the vital organs.

Pathological Cell Injury

Cellular injury, due to any of the previously discussed causes, can be reversible in the early stages. Reversible cellular injury is characterized with cellular swelling, from an accumulation of sodium and water, and changes in the cell wall membrane called **blebs**, which have the appearance of bubble wrap commonly used for packing.

There comes a point when the lysosomes rupture, emptying their contents of enzymes, which begin to autolysis proteins (i.e., denature the proteins). Eventually the nucleus starts to shrink and fragment and the cell undergoes the final processes of necrosis, a cascade of cellular changes that lead to death.

After the lysosomal rupture, there is a free efflux of calcium. The efflux of calcium joins unused phosphate, from the remains of the ATP, and precipitates (i.e., falls out of solution) as a solid mass. At this point, the cell has experienced irreversible hypoxic injury. Free oxygen radicals, such as hydrogen peroxide, perforate the cell wall membrane, making it defective. Finally, the combination of mitochondrial damage, leading to the release of oxygen-free radicals, and cytoskeletal damage, as seen on the cell wall membrane, cause the cell to fragment.

Patterns of Necrosis

When a mass of cells within a tissue or organ die there are characteristic changes that affect the remaining tissues. When muscle cells die, such as in myocardial infarction, the skeleton of the cell remains and the tissue remains firm.[62,63] This state is called **coagulative necrosis**.

Coagulative necrosis permits the dead cells to act as a scaffolding for other tissue, but the tissue no longer functions. In the case of an acute myocardial infarction, the affected portion of the muscle mass is considered to be **akinetic** (without motion) and does not contribute to the heart's work.

Cells that are largely lipid in content, such as the neurons of the brain, simply liquify upon death and leave a pool in their place. This process is called **liquifactive necrosis**. When a patient experiences a series of small ischemic strokes, the dead tissue undergoes liquifactive necrosis and leaves a small cavity, called a lacuane (Latin – lacuna).

When tissues die from ischemia (e.g., the toes of a patient with diminished distal circulation secondary to complications of diabetes mellitus), tissues undergo gangrenous necrosis. In this type of gangrene, called dry gangrene, the affected portion generally blackens and then simply falls off the body.

If a secondary infection sets in, resulting in toxin-producing bacteria such as clostridium, then the condition is called wet gangrene. Wet gangrene can lead to systemic infections and systemic inflammatory response syndrome.

If the tissues involved are invaded by anaerobic bacteria, typically secondary to wounds, then gasses form and the gangrene is called gas gangrene. Gas gangrene must be aggressively treated with antibiotics, for without treatment gas gangrene is invariably fatal.

Death

When the body's compensatory mechanism fails to maintain homeostasis, and the cells of the body are irreversibly injured, first the tissues, then the organs, and then the organism will die. Somatic death (soma—"body") is the death of the organism. There are specific changes within the body that are associated with death, referred to as **postmortem** changes.

Initially, the patient experiences what is called **clinical death**, the absence of vital signs. Clinical death is characterized by unresponsiveness to loud verbal and painful stimuli, absence of breathing, and an absence of a central pulse. Barring any restrictions to the contrary, cardiopulmonary resuscitation is usually indicated.

Although a patient may be dead, it is possible for some tissues or organs to still be alive. These tissues and/or organs can be harvested for transplantation if the remaining living tissue is removed quickly.

In certain circumstances the patient is beyond resuscitation. These patients have undergone **biological death**. Biological death is associated with irreversibility, meaning that any resuscitative efforts would be futile. Biological death is usually associated with an absence of brain activity, as evidenced by an electroencephalogram. The patient is termed **brain dead**. This definition has limited utility to Paramedics.

Paramedics rely on other signs to determine biological death. Initially, Paramedics confirm clinical death and then proceed to confirm biological death. Paramedics use the findings of the three "mortis" to help confirm biological death.

The first mortis (Latin – death) is **rigor mortis**, a stiffening of the muscles. Muscles stiffen following **anoxia** (a- – "without"; ox – "oxygen"; -ia – "state") from acid buildup in the tissues that interferes with the release of the contractile protein actin from myosin. Initially, the short muscles of the body (e.g., the muscles of the jaw) are affected. In about 12 hours the entire body is rigid and afterwards (about 36 hours after clinical death) the breakdown of the proteins returns the body to a flaccid condition.[64-66]

The second mortis is **livor mortis**. Livor mortis, or lividity, is a condition caused by relaxation of the vascular bed and a pooling of blood in dependant portions of the body.[67,68] All bleeding stops and fluids start to drain from the body. Often the most notable changes occur when the fluids drain from the face, leaving gaunt cheekbones and a peaked nose with a beak-like appearance.

The third mortis is **algor mortis**. Algor mortis is the body's natural cooling. As the body's metabolic processes cease, so does the production of heat. On average, the body cools about 1°F to 1.5°F an hour until the body reaches room temperature, usually about 24 hours.[69-71]

The presences of the three mortis, as well as the signs of clinical death, are often felt to be sufficient to withhold resuscitative efforts. Some EMS systems include other conditions, such as decapitation, incineration, and **hemicorporectomy** (amputation at the waist) for inclusion in their criteria for obvious death.

When the body has undergone **putrefaction**, it is assumed that the patient is dead. Putrefaction is a process of decomposition within the body characterized by greenish discoloration, secondary to hemolysis of blood, and slippage of the skin from the skeleton, due to breakdown of subcutaneous fat. Putrefaction starts between 24 and 48 hours after clinical death.

CONCLUSION

From birth to death, disease is a constant in the human condition. The study of pathophysiology, the study of the suffering of the human condition wrought by disease, provides Paramedics with an understanding on how to intercede and reduce suffering through medical therapeutics.

KEY POINTS:

- Pathophysiology is the study of the causes of suffering in the normal human condition.

- Disease is an abnormal change in the function of cells, tissues, or organs which in turn interferes with homeostasis.

- All diseases have an origin or etiology.

- Each person has certain risk factors—some modifiable and some not—that make that person more or less vulnerable to a disease.

- Modifiable risk factors are factors over which a person has some control.

- Nonmodifiable risk factors include family (genetics), aging, and gender.

- Prognosis is the expected outcome from a disease.

- Iatrogenic disease is produced as a consequence of medical intervention.

- Nosocomial infection is death from a hospital-acquired infection.

- Pathogenesis is the origin and development of a disease followed in a sequential order at the cellular, biochemical, and molecular level.

- Exacerbation of a disease may occur where the disease returns or flares up. In remission, the disease may be forced into a nonactive state.

- Morbidity (the incidence of disease) and mortality (death rate) are constantly monitored for trends.

- Hypoxia is a low oxygen concentration in the body.

- The Fick principle can be summed up in five concepts: oxygenation, ventilation, respiration, circulation, and cellular respiration.

- Paramedics work to prevent hypoxia by supporting the elements of the Fick principle.

- Ischemia is the first step in the pathogenesis of hypoxia, followed by injury and then death.

- A toxin is defined as any substance capable of causing cell injury and death.

- Metabolites are the by-products of drugs and chemicals after they interact with a cell.

- Outside forces such as trauma, extreme temperature, radiation, and atmospheric pressures can all cause injury to the body and its cells.

- During heat emergencies, the body has difficulty compensating for excessive heat.

- Burns can be caused by five sources of electromagnetic energy: thermal, radiation, light, radio, and electricity.

- A burn uses the method of either direct heat transfer or ionization as its mechanism of injury.

- Stochastic effects are the long-term complications from exposure to ionizing radiation. Teratogenic effects are the harmful effects of ionizing radiation on future generations.

- Low temperatures, or hypothermia, lead to impaired cell walls.

- Barotrauma is physical damage to tissues due to pressure imbalances between those in the environment and those in the body. A common condition found in the prehospital setting is a pneumothorax.

- Either a deficiency of nutrition or excess of nutrition can lead to metabolic disease.

- A genetic disorder is an abnormality in a person's genes which may be passed on through future family generations.

- Infectious diseases stem from prions, viruses, bacteria, fungi, protozoa, and helminthes, all of which are parasites.

- Skin is the body's first defense against physical, chemical, and biological attacks.

- Mucous membranes line the internal "tubes" of the body with mucus, engulfing any foreign predators.

- Various acids and saliva create another line of defense.

- Mechanical defenses include regurgitation, defecation, menstruation, and urination.

- The inflammatory system defends the body when nonspecific, external defenders are weakened.

- Complement, coagulation, and kinen proteins support inflammation.

- The immune response is an internal, specific method of defense.

- The immune response consists of B lymphocytes (humoral immunity) and T cells (cell-mediated immunity).

- Shock is the body's inability to provide the necessary substrates to the cells, which makes the body unable to maintain homeostasis.

- The Hinshaw-Cox shock classification system includes four categories:
  1. Hypovolemic
  2. Distributive
  3. Cardiogenic
  4. Obstructive

- The body begins compensating for the shock state by activating the sympathetic nervous system.

- Multiple organ dysfunction is a failure of two or more organs due to total body systemic infection leading to sepsis.

- The Paramedic must identify shock affecting the core organs.

- The pecking order of shock is the order of shunting which begins with the fetus. The skin is then closed down, followed by the gastrointestinal tract. The core organs are the last to be affected.

- In order to adequately perfuse the brain, a mean arterial blood pressure (MAP) of 50 to 60 mmHg is needed. Cerebral perfusion pressure can be estimated from mean arterial pressure.

- Decompensated shock is the body's inability to maintain perfusion.

- Attention to airway, breathing, and circulation is necessary in all forms of shock.

- Hypoxia and hypercapnia can result in increased intracranial pressure.

- Vasopressors such as dopamine are used to maximize cardiac function and to support the sympathetic nervous system during times when the mean arterial pressure is suboptimal.

- Cellular injury can be reversible.

- Cellular injury occurs in steps: swelling, cell wall changes, lysosome changes, cellular death.

- Coagulative necrosis occurs when muscle cells die but remain firm.

- Liquifactive necrosis occurs when lipid cells liquify when they die.

- Dry gangrene occurs when tissues die from ischemia.

- Wet gangrene forms when secondary infections invade the ischemic tissues.

- Gas gangrene forms when the tissues are invaded by anaerobic bacteria.

- Somatic death is the death of an organism.

- Death occurs in stages.

- Clinical death is when a person no longer has vital signs.

- Biological death is the absence of any brain activity.

REVIEW QUESTIONS:

1. Define pathophysiology.
2. How is a tentative field diagnosis helpful to the Paramedic in the treatment of a patient?
3. What is the difference between a disorder and a syndrome?
4. List several modifiable and nonmodifiable risk factors.
5. Choose one modifiable risk factor and discuss its impact on an associated disease.
6. What is meant by the term "iatrogenic disease"?
7. What term is used to describe the crossover from recovery toward death?
8. Describe how hypoxia impacts cellular function and the resultant consequences.
9. Describe how trauma impacts cellular function and provide an example of resultant harm.
10. Initially, how does the body respond to an infection on the skin? (*Hint:* Think of the three cardinal signs.)
11. What are the four classifications of shock using the Hinshaw–Cox descriptions?
12. How does the sympathetic nervous system support the body in shock?

CASE STUDY QUESTIONS:

Please refer to the Case Study at the beginning of the chapter and answer the questions below.

1. Describe the changes that occur in cells as perfusion ceases.
2. What type of death has been described with the absence of vital signs?
3. Why might some organs in a deceased individual still be viable for transplant?

REFERENCES:

1. Atkins D. *Reports of Hospital Physicians and Other Documents in Relation to the Epidemic of Cholera of 1832.* New York G. & C. & H. Carvill; 1832.
2. Guerrant RL, Carneiro-Filho BA, Dillingham RA. Cholera, diarrhea, and oral rehydration therapy: triumph and indictment. *Clin Infect Dis.* 2003;37(3):398–405.
3. van der Hoek L. Human coronaviruses: what do they cause? *Antivir Ther.* 2007;12(4 Pt B):651–658.
4. Cheng VC, Lau SK, Woo PC, Yuen KY. Severe acute respiratory syndrome coronavirus as an agent of emerging and reemerging infection. *Clin Microbiol Rev.* 2007;20(4):660–694.
5. Gu J, Korteweg C. Pathology and pathogenesis of severe acute respiratory syndrome. *Am J Pathol.* 2007;170(4):1136–1147.
6. Kohl BA, Deutschman CS. The inflammatory response to surgery and trauma. *Curr Opin Crit Care.* 2006;12(4):325–332.
7. Pallister I. Current concepts of the inflammatory response after major trauma: an update. *Injury.* 2005;36(1):227–229; author reply 229–230.
8. Plank LD, Hill GL. Sequential metabolic changes following induction of systemic inflammatory response in patients with severe sepsis or major blunt trauma. *World J Surg.* 2000;24(6):630–638.
9. Nafziger SD. Smallpox. *Crit Care Clin.* 2005;21(4):739–746, vii.
10. Parrino J, Graham BS. Smallpox vaccines: past, present, and future. *J Allergy Clin Immunol.* 2006;118(6):1320–1326.
11. Fleming ST. Complications, adverse events, and iatrogenesis: classifications and quality of care measurement issues. *Clin Perform Qual Health Care.* 1996;4(3):137–147.
12. Jefferson T, Foxlee R, Del Mar C, Dooley L, Ferroni E, Hewak B, et al. Physical interventions to interrupt or reduce the spread of respiratory viruses: systematic review. *Bmj.* 2008;336(7635):77–80.
13. Hart S. Using an aseptic technique to reduce the risk of infection. *Nurs Stand.* 2007;21(47):43–48.

14. Larson EL, Quiros D, Lin SX. Dissemination of the CDC's Hand Hygiene Guideline and impact on infection rates. *Am J Infect Control.* 2007;35(10):666–675.

15. Cardona PJ. New insights on the nature of latent tuberculosis infection and its treatment. *Inflamm Allergy Drug Targets.* 2007;6(1):27–39.

16. **http://www.cdc.gov/mmwr**

17. Yellon DM, Hausenloy DJ. Myocardial reperfusion injury. *N Engl J Med.* 2007;357(11):1121–1135.

18. Hamilton KL. Antioxidants and cardioprotection. *Med Sci Sports Exerc.* 2007;39(9):1544–1553.

19. Tang W. Drug metabolite profiling and elucidation of drug-induced hepatotoxicity. *Expert Opin Drug Metab Toxicol.* 2007;3(3):407–420.

20. Park BK, Kitteringham NR, Maggs JL, Pirmohamed M, Williams DP. The role of metabolic activation in drug-induced hepatotoxicity. *Annu Rev Pharmacol Toxicol.* 2005;45:177–202.

21. Prescott LF. Reactive metabolites as a cause of hepatotoxicity. *Int J Clin Pharmacol Res.* 1983;3(6):437–441.

22. Way JL, Leung P, Cannon E, Morgan R, Tamulinas C, Leong-Way J, et al. The mechanism of cyanide intoxication and its antagonism. *Ciba Found Symp.* 1988;140:232–243.

23. Eastridge BJ. Things that go boom: injuries from explosives. *J Trauma.* 2007;62(6 Suppl):S38.

24. Garner MJ, Brett SJ. Mechanisms of injury by explosive devices. *Anesthesiol Clin.* 2007;25(1):147–160, x.

25. Bridges EJ. Blast injuries: from triage to critical care. *Crit Care Nurs Clin North Am.* 2006;18(3):333–348.

26. Roubertoux PL, Kerdelhue B. Trisomy 21: from chromosomes to mental retardation. *Behav Genet.* 2006;36(3):346–354.

27. Gardiner K, Davisson M. The sequence of human chromosome 21 and implications for research into Down syndrome. *Genome Biol.* 2000;1(2):REVIEWS0002.

28. Munford RS. Severe sepsis and septic shock: the role of gram-negative bacteremia. *Annu Rev Pathol.* 2006;1:467–496.

29. Bahador M, Cross AS. From therapy to experimental model: a hundred years of endotoxin administration to human subjects. *J Endotoxin Res.* 2007;13(5):251–279.

30. Dombrowicz D, Capron M. Eosinophils, allergy and parasites. *Curr Opin Immunol.* 2001;13(6):716–720.

31. *Surgical Wound Healing and Management.* Stockholm: Informa Healthcare; 2007.

32. Bryant R, Nix D. *Acute and Chronic Wounds: Current Management Concepts.* St. Louis, MO: Mosby; 2006.

33. Greenhalgh DG, Saffle JR, Holmes JHT, Gamelli RL, Palmieri TL, Horton JW, et al. American Burn Association consensus conference to define sepsis and infection in burns. *J Burn Care Res.* 2007;28(6):776–790.

34. Levy MM, Fink MP, Marshall JC, Abraham E, Angus D, Cook D, et al. 2001 SCCM/ESICM/ACCP/ATS/SIS International Sepsis Definitions Conference. *Crit Care Med.* 2003;31(4):1250–1256.

35. Robertson CM, Coopersmith CM. The systemic inflammatory response syndrome. *Microbes Infect.* 2006;8(5):1382–1389.

36. Haljamae H. The pathophysiology of shock. *Acta Anaesthesiol Scand Suppl.* 1993;98:3–6.

37. Bongard F, Sue D. *CURRENT Critical Care Diagnosis & Treatment.* New York: McGraw-Hill Medical; 2002.

38. Little RA, Jones RO, Eltraifi AE. Cardiovascular reflex function after injury. *Prog Clin Biol Res.* 1988;264:191–200.

39. Shepherd JT, Vanhoutte PM. Role of the venous system in circulatory control. *Mayo Clin Proc.* 1978;53(4):247–255.

40. Sanz G, Nadal-Ginard B, Malpartida F, Froufe J. Hemodynamics of myocardial infarct (critical analysis of experimental studies). *Rev Esp Cardiol.* 1971;24(6):575–584.

41. Seeto RK, Fenn B, Rockey DC. Ischemic hepatitis: clinical presentation and pathogenesis. *Am J Med.* 2000;109(2):109–113.

42. Henrion J. Hypoxic hepatitis: the point of view of the clinician. *Acta Gastroenterol Belg.* 2007;70(2):214–216.

43. O'Brien JM, Jr., Ali NA, Aberegg SK, Abraham E. Sepsis. *Am J Med.* 2007;120(12):1012–1022.

44. Hollenberg SM. Vasopressor support in septic shock. *Chest.* 2007;132(5):1678–1687.

45. Lever A, Mackenzie I. Sepsis: definition, epidemiology, and diagnosis. *Bmj.* 2007;335(7625):879–883.

46. Gentili A, Iannella E, Giuntoli,L, Baroncini S. System for predicting outcome and for clinical evaluation in sepsis and septic shock: could scores and biochemical markers be of greater help in the future? *Med Sci Monit.* 2006;12(6):LE11–12.

47. Hardaway RM. A brief overview of acute respiratory distress syndrome. *World J Surg.* 2006;30(10):1829–1834; discussion 1835.

48. Lasky M, Puyo C. Acute respiratory distress syndrome update. *Mo Med.* 2005;102(5):469–474.

49. Gowda RM, Fox JT, Khan IA. Cardiogenic shock: basics and clinical considerations. *Int J Cardiol.* 2008;123(3):221–228.

50. Aymong ED, Ramanathan K, Buller CE. Pathophysiology of cardiogenic shock complicating acute myocardial infarction. *Med Clin North Am.* 2007;91(4):701–712; xii.

51. Iakobishvili Z, Hasdai D. Cardiogenic shock: treatment. *Med Clin North Am.* 2007;91(4):713–727; xii.

52. Peitzman AB, Billiar TR, Harbrecht BG, Kelly E, Udekwu AO, Simmons RL. Hemorrhagic shock. *Curr Probl Surg.* 1995;32(11):925–1002.

53. Meybohm P, Cavus E, Bein B, Steinfath M, Weber B, Hamann C, et al. Small volume resuscitation: a randomized controlled trial with either norepinephrine or vasopressin during severe hemorrhage. *J Trauma.* 2007;62(3):640–646.

54. Earle SA, de Moya MA, Zuccarelli JE, Norenberg MD, Proctor KG. Cerebrovascular resuscitation after polytrauma and fluid restriction. *J Am Coll Surg.* 2007;204(2):261–275.

55. Alspaugh DM, Sartorelli K, Shackford SR, Okum EJ, Buckingham S, Osler T. Prehospital resuscitation with phenylephrine in uncontrolled hemorrhagic shock and brain injury. *J Trauma.* 2000;48(5):851–863; discussion 863–864.

56. Stiefel MF, Udoetuk JD, Spiotta AM, Gracias VH, Goldberg A, Maloney-Wilensky E, et al. Conventional neurocritical care and

cerebral oxygenation after traumatic brain injury. *J Neurosurg.* 2006;105(4):568–575.

57. Young JS, Blow O,Turrentine F, Claridge JA, Schulman A. Is there an upper limit of intracranial pressure in patients with severe head injury if cerebral perfusion pressure is maintained? *Neurosurg Focus.* 2003;15(6):E2.

58. Jeremitsky E, Omert L, Dunham CM, Protetch J, Rodriguez A. Harbingers of poor outcome the day after severe brain injury: hypothermia, hypoxia, and hypoperfusion. *J Trauma.* 2003;54(2):312–319.

59. Plurad D, Brown C, Chan L, Demetriades D, Rhee P. Emergency department hypotension is not an independent risk factor for post-traumatic acute renal dysfunction. *J Trauma.* 2006;61(5):1120–1127; discussion 1127–1128.

60. Manley G, Knudson MM, Morabito D, Damron S, Erickson V, Pitts L. Hypotension, hypoxia, and head injury: frequency, duration, and consequences. *Arch Surg.* 2001;136(10): 1118–1123.

61. Cotton BA, Snodgrass KB, Fleming SB, Carpenter RO, Kemp CD, Arbogast PG, et al. Beta-blocker exposure is associated with improved survival after severe traumatic brain injury. *J Trauma.* 2007;62(1):26–33; discussion 33–35.

62. Baroldi G. Different morphological types of myocardial cell death in man. *Recent Adv Stud Cardiac Struct Metab.* 1975;6:383–397.

63. Baroldi G. Anatomy and quantification of myocardial cell death. *Methods Achiev Exp Pathol.* 1988;13:87–113.

64. Henssge C, Madea B, Gallenkemper E. Death time estimation in case work. II. Integration of different methods. *Forensic Sci Int.* 1988;39(1):77–87.

65. Krompecher T. Experimental evaluation of rigor mortis. VIII. Estimation of time since death by repeated measurements of the intensity of rigor mortis on rats. *Forensic Sci Int.* 1994;68(3):149–159.

66. Krompecher T. Experimental evaluation of rigor mortis. V. Effect of various temperatures on the evolution of rigor mortis. *Forensic Sci Int.* 1981;17(1):19–26.

67. Sannohe S. Change in the postmortem formation of hypostasis in skin preparations 100 micrometers thick. *Am J Forensic Med Pathol.* 2002;23(4):349–354.

68. Bockholdt B, Maxeiner H, Hegenbarth W. Factors and circumstances influencing the development of hemorrhages in livor mortis. *Forensic Sci Int.* 2005;149(2–3):133–137.

69. Bisegna P, Henssge C, Althaus L, Giusti G. Estimation of the time since death: sudden increase of ambient temperature. *Forensic Sci Int.* 2007;176(2):196–199.

70. Green MA, Wright JC. The theoretical aspects of the time dependent Z equation as a means of postmortem interval estimation using body temperature data only. *Forensic Sci Int.* 1985;28(1):53–62.

71. Henssge C. Death time estimation in case work. I. The rectal temperature time of death nomogram. *Forensic Sci Int.* 1988;38(3–4):209–236.

CHAPTER 12

MEDICAL TERMINOLOGY

KEY CONCEPTS:

Upon completion of this chapter, it is expected that the reader will understand these following concepts:

- Understanding the origins of medical terminology
- How prefixes and suffixes complement a root word's meaning
- The importance of standard abbreviations
- Using topographic anatomy to accurately describe the body's position and direction

▶ CASE STUDY:

As a new member to the agency's quality improvement committee, the young Paramedic was assigned to review patient run records. He complained that many providers abbreviated terms haphazardly or misspelled medical or anatomical terms. Relying on his previous educational degree, he devised a game to teach medical terms, acceptable abbreviations, and terms to describe a body's position or location.

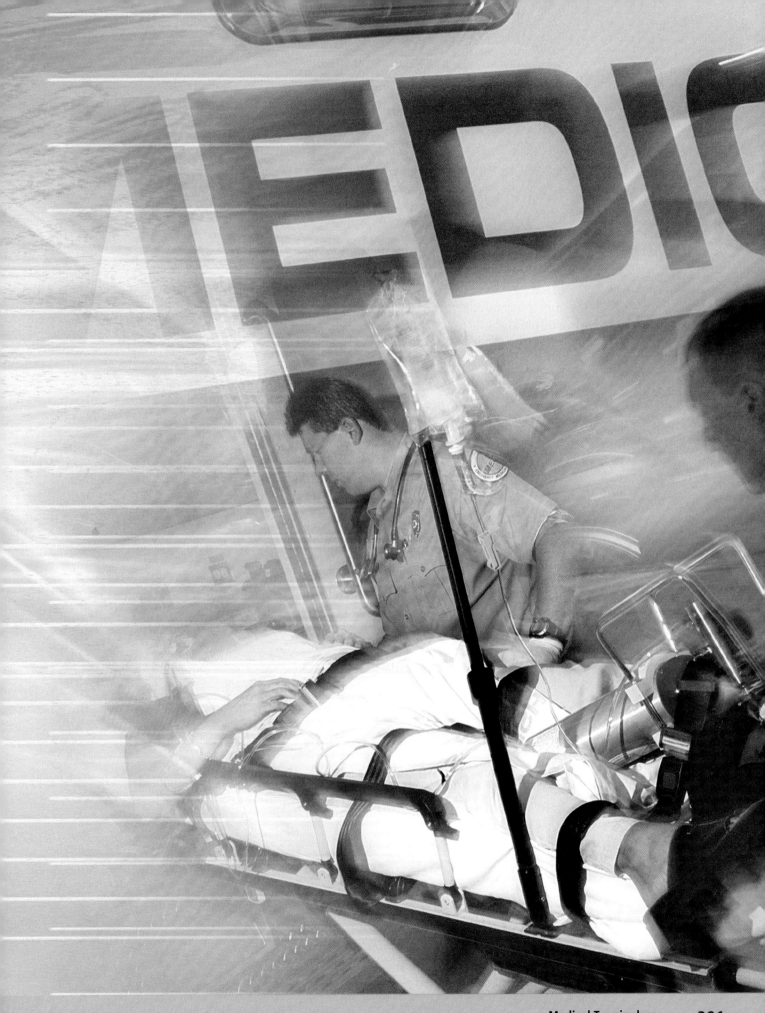

OVERVIEW

To communicate accurately and clearly to other healthcare providers, the Paramedic needs to use proper medical terminology. By examining common grammatical rules and the breakdown of words, terms can be used more efficiently and accurately. A clear and accurate report includes a body's location via topographic anatomy and the standard anatomical position.

Medical Terminology

While reading the medical literature, the fledgling Paramedic may come across many unfamiliar terms and wonder about their meaning. These medical terms may appear difficult to learn and even more difficult to pronounce. One might even think one is learning a second language. That would actually be correct.

The language of medicine is called medicalese.[1] By understanding a few rules of medical terminology, the Paramedic can quickly learn a term's meaning. The Paramedic's vocabulary will expand and the Paramedic will become fluent in medicalese.

This chapter is an overview of terms and abbreviations commonly used by Paramedics.

Medicalese

Medicalese has its roots in Greek and Latin words. In the ancient past these two dialects were common to all men of science, regardless of their national origins, and it was through this common medium that scientists were able to share ideas. As medicine began to embrace science it also adopted the Latin and Greek vocabulary for the same purpose, as a medium for communication.

As time went on, medicine started to develop an extensive vocabulary (a lexicon) of medical expressions and terminology. The use of the medical lexicon continues to the present day as a means for communication between medical professionals of differing practice.

▷ ▷ ▷ ▷ ▷ ▷ ▷ ▷ ▷ ▷ ▷ ▷ ▷ ▷ ▷ ▷
PROFESSIONAL PARAMEDIC

The professional Paramedic, when mentoring healthcare students, should use the correct medical term and then follow that up with the common term. This helps teach medicalese as well as reinforces medical terminology for the Paramedic.

Anatomy of Medical Terminology

By following several basic rules, the Paramedic can understand and learn medical terminology. First, most medical terms consist of four parts: the root word, a prefix and/or a suffix, and a combining form. These parts can be thought of as the building blocks of medical terminology.

A **root** word relates to the main idea and often describes the organ involved or the key symptom. For example, "cardi" is Latin, meaning the heart. Learning root words means memorizing these words.[2] Fortunately, using prefixes and/or suffixes, many terms are built from a relative handful of root words (Table 12-1). Prefixes and/or suffixes build on a root word, giving it a new meaning.

When a **prefix** complements a root, it is placed at the beginning of the root (Tables 12-2 to 12-5). Take, for

Table 12-1 Common Word Roots Used in EMS

Root	Meaning
Aden/o-	Gland
Arthr/o-	Joint
Card/o-	Heart
Cephal/o-	Head
Cerebr/o-	Cerebrum
Cyst/o-	Bladder
Encephal/o-	Brain
Enter/o-	Intestines
Erythr/o-	Red
Gastro/o-	Stomach
Gloss/o-	Mouth
Hem/o-	Blood
Hepat/o-	Liver
Ile/o-	Small intestine
Lingu/o-	Tongue
Nephr/o-	Kidneys
Neur/o-	Nerves
Onc/o-	Cancer
Oste/o	Bone
Ot/o-	Ear
Path/o-	Disease
Ped/o-	Children
Ren/o-	Kidneys
Splem/o-	Spleen
Thromb/o-	Clot
Trach/o-	Trachea

Table 12-2   Partial List of Medical Prefixes

Prefix	Meaning	Origin
a/-	"without"	Greek
ab/-	"from"/"away from"	Latin
ad/-	"toward"	Latin
ambi/-	"both"	Greek
dextro/-	"right side"	Latin
levo/-	"left"	Latin
dia/-	"throughout"	Greek
entero/-	"within"	Greek
hetero/-	"different"	Greek
homo/-	"same"	Greek
hyper/-	"beyond"/"high"	Greek
hydro/-	"water"	Greek
hypo/-	"beneath"/"low"	Greek
iatr/-	"healer"	Greek
leuko/-	"white'	Greek
macro/-	"large"/"long"	Greek
mega/-	"great"	Greek
micro/-	"small"	Greek
neo/-	"new"	Greek
oligo/-	"scant"	Greek
orth/-	"straight"	Greek
osteo/-	"bone"	Greek
oto/-	"ear"	Greek
patho/-	"suffering"	Greek
phlebo/-	"vein"	Greek
pneumo/-	"air"	Greek
poly/-	"many"	Greek
pro/-	"before"	Latin
tachy/-	"rapid"	Greek
toc/-	"childbirth"	Greek
trans/-	"across"	Latin

Table 12-3   Prefixes of Color

Prefix	Color
<Alb/-	"White"
Chlor/-	"Green"
Cirr/-	"Yellow"
Cyan/-	"Blue"
Erthr/-	"Red"
Glauco/-	"Grey"
Leuk/-	"White"
Melan/-	"Black"

Table 12-4   Prefixes of Position

Prefix	Position
Ad/-	"toward"
Ante/-	"in front"
Anti/-	"against"
Apo/-	"separate"
Circum/-	"around"
Contra/-	"against"
Dia/-	"through"
Dis/-	"apart"
Dorso/-	"back"
Epi/-	"upon"
Later/	"side"
Eco/-	"out"
Endo/-	"in"
Exo/-	"out"
In/-	"in"
Opistho/	"backwards"
Peri/-	"around"
Posto/-	"after"
Pre/-	"in front"
Pro/-	"in front"
Re/-	"again"
Retro/-	"backwards"
Trans/-	"through"
Ventro/-	"in front"

Table 12-5   Prefixes of Numbers

Prefix	Amounts
Aniso/-	"unequal"
Diplo/-	"double"
Hyper/-	"above"
Hypo/-	"below"
In/-	"none"
Iso/-	"equal"
Macro/-	"large"
Mega/-	"large"
Micro/-	"small"
Multi/-	"many"
Oligo/-	"few"
Pan/-	"all"
Poly/-	"many"
Prim/-	"first"
Prot/-	"first"

example, the word "pericardium." The root, on the right, is "cardi," meaning heart. The prefix, "peri," means around. Therefore, the term "pericardium" would mean "around the heart."

When a **suffix** complements a root, it is placed after the root and changes the meaning of the term (Tables 12-6 to 12-9). Using the term "myocarditis," for example, and reading from right to left, the term "-itis" means infection, the term "cardi-" means heart, and the prefix "myo-" means muscle. The term "myocarditis" means an infection of the cardiac muscle.

When two or more roots are placed together, they must be separated by a vowel. Physicians often use these **combining forms** to explain a complex process. For example, the term "cardiomyopathy" has as its roots "cardia-," meaning heart, "my," meaning muscle, and "patho," meaning disease. The letter "O" separates the roots "cardia," "my," and "path." "Cardiomyopathy," reading from right to left, means disease of the muscle of the heart.

Combining Forms

Sometimes two root terms are used and a combining vowel must be used to make the two root terms distinguishable but connected (Table 12-10). Typically the letter "o" is used. For example, "cardi-: "o" "-logy" is the study of the heart.

However, if the root word ends with a vowel, then it is unnecessary to use a combining vowel. For example, combining "cyst-" with "-itis" would be "cystitis," not "cystoitis."

Plural Forms

To establish a plural meaning from a singular word, the Paramedic only needs to apply a few rules (Table 12-11). For example, if the singular word ends with "ax" then remove the "ax" and replace it with "aces" to make the meaning of the word plural.

Table 12-6 Partial List of Common Suffixes for Diagnosis

Suffix	Meaning	Used	Meaning
-algia	Pain	Neuralgia	Nerve pain
-cele	Swelling	Hydrocele	Water cyst
-emia	Blood	Anemia	Without blood
-ectasis	Expansion	Bronchiectasis	Enlarged bronchi
-dynia	Pain	Angiodynia	Pain with IV
-edema	Swelling	Laryngoedema	Swollen throat
-gen	Begin	Carcinogen	Cancer causing
-iasis	Formation	Cholelithiasis	Gall stone
-itis	Inflammation	Pharyngitis	Sore throat
-megaly	Enlargement	Cardiomegaly	Enlarged heart
-oma	Tumor	Carcinoma	Cancer
-pathy	Disease	Myopathy	Disease of muscle
-phasia	Speech	Aphasia	Speechless
-plegia	Paralysis	Hemiplegia	Help paralysis
-phobia	Fear	Agoraphobia	Fear of places
-rrhagia	Flow	Dysmenorrhagia	Excessive menstrual flow
-rrhage	Burst	Hemorrhage	Bleeding
-rrhea	Discharge	Otorrhea	Discharge from ear
-scopy	Examine	Bronchoscopy	Examine the bronchi
-spasm	Contraction	Bronchospasm	Contraction of bronchi

Table 12-8 Diagnostic Suffixes for Medical Instruments

Suffix	Meaning	Used
-gram	Record	Electrocardiogram
-graph	Recording tool	Electrocardiograph
-meter	Measurement tool	Capnometer
-scope	Instrument	Laryngoscope

Table 12-9 Medical Suffixes

Suffix	Meaning	Used
-iac	Afflicted	Hemophiliac
-ia	Unhealthy	Anesthesia
-ism	Condition	Alcoholism
-ist	Expert	Cardiologist

Table 12-7 Surgical Suffixes

Suffix	Meaning	Used
-clasis	Breakdown	Osteoclasis
-ectomy	Removal	Appendectomy
-centesis	Tap or drain	Pericardial centesis
-lysis	Loosen/divide	Fibrinolysis
-plasty	Formation	Rhinoplasty
-stomy	Opening	Tracheostomy
-tripsy	Crush	Lithotripsy
-tomy	Cut	Tracheotomy

Table 12-10 Examples of Combining Terms

Root	Suffix	Use
Cardiology	-ist	Cardiologist
Enter	-lysis	Enterolysis
Bronchi	-scopy	Bronchoscopy
Lith	-tripsy	Lithotripsy
Ortho	-pnea	Orthopnea
Trachea	-tomy	Tracheotomy
Trachea	-stomy	Tracheostomy

Table 12-11 Making Plural Forms of Terms

Singular Form	Plural Form
-a	add -e
-ax	drop –ax, add -aces
-en	drop –en, add -ina
-is	drop –is, add -es
-ix	drop –ix, add -ices
-sis	drop –sis, add -ses
-um	drop –um, add -a
-us	drop –us, add -i
-x	drop –x, add -es
-y	drop –y, add -ies

Reading Medical Terminology

When both a suffix and a prefix are used in a word, then the suffix is read first, then the prefix, and then the root (read last, first, and middle). For example, the term "hypoglycemia" has "gly" as its root and "gly" refers to glucose. To read this term correctly, first read the suffix, "-emia," referring to blood, then "hypo-," meaning low, and then "gly." Together the term means blood with low sugar.

All medical terms are interpreted with the suffix read first, prefix next, and root last (last, first, and middle). This concept is difficult for those Paramedics who have been educated to read from left to right. It takes practice to become proficient at deciphering medical terminology. With a little practice, the Paramedic rapidly becomes proficient at learning the meaning of these terms and can incorporate them into the documentation.

Pronunciation

Proper pronunciation of medical terms is key to understanding. While verbalizing these terms may seem difficult, dissection of the term to its constituent parts (prefix, root, and suffix) and careful articulation will likely produce satisfactory results.

Often other medical professionals will help to correct errors in inflection or in pronunciation. By repeating the corrected pronunciation, the Paramedic helps to commit the term to memory.

Spelling

Many medical terms have a similar sounding constituent but are spelled differently. Spelling them correctly can be difficult, especially if the Paramedic hears the word spoken and then must spell it. For example, the "si" sound can be spelled with "psy," as in "psychiatry," "sy" as in "symptom," or "cy" as in "cystitis."

To avoid errors and confusion the term should be spelled correctly. When in doubt, the Paramedic should consult a medical dictionary for the correct spelling.

Abbreviations

The basis for abbreviations is brevity, meaning short and concise. Paramedics strive to be short and concise in their medical writing. Correct use of abbreviations can help with that process, provided that the meaning of the communication is not lost in the process. For example, the abbreviation "Ca" can mean both "calcium" and "cancer."

Emergency physicians, allied healthcare professionals, EMS managers, educators, and attorneys are just a few of the people who may read a PCR. Without a common translation, abbreviations can become meaningless to the reader, and the PCR loses its potency as a vehicle for communication.

As a result of common medical errors, some abbreviations are no longer accepted.[5] For example, the abbreviation for morphine sulfate is MSO_4. Unfortunately, during transcription, the MSO_4 may be confused with $MgSO_4$, which is magnesium sulfate. For this reason clinicians, including Paramedics, should spell out MSO_4 as morphine in order to decrease confusion and prevent errors.[6-9]

To help resolve the problem, many EMS agencies have a list of accepted abbreviations (Table 12-12). This list is usually gleaned from a similar list of abbreviations used by the healthcare professionals at the local hospital(s). Paramedics should obtain and utilize their agency's abbreviation list.

Table 12-12 List of Common Abbreviations

/a	Before	DOE	Dyspnea on exertion
AAA	Abdominal aortic aneurysm	DPT	Diphtheria, pertussis, tetanus
AAL	Anterior axillary line	DTs	Delirium tremens
AB	Abortion	Dr.	Doctor
ABCs	Airway, breathing, circulation	Dx	Diagnosis
Abd	Abdominal	ECG/EKG	Electrocardiogram
AC	Antecubital fossa	EEG	Electroencephalogram
ACLS	Advanced cardiac life support	EENT	Ears, eyes, nose, throat
ADL	Activities of daily living	EID	Esophageal intubation detector
AED	Automatic external defibrillator	EJV	External jugular vein
A fib	Atrial fibrillation	EMD	Emergency medical dispatch
AIDS	Acquired immune deficiency syndrome	EMS	Emergency medical service
ALS	Advanced life support	EMT	Emergency medical technician
AMA	Against medical advice	EPI	Epinephrine
AMI	Acute myocardial infarction	Eq	Equivalents
AMS	Altered mental status	ET	Endotracheal tube
A/O	Alert and oriented	ETA	Estimated time of arrival
A/P	Anterior–posterior	EtOH	Ethyl alcohol
ASA	Aspirin	°F	Fahrenheit
ASHD	Arteriosclerotic heart disease	FU	Follow up
ARDS	Adult respiratory distress syndrome	FUO	Fever of unknown origin
ATV	Automatic transport ventilator	Fx	Fracture
AV	Atrioventricular	GCS	Glasgow coma scale
BAC	Blood alcohol content	GI	Gastrointestinal
BBB	Bundle branch block	GSW	Gun shot wound
BG	Blood glucose	gtt	Drops
Bid	Twice per day	GU	Genitourinary
BLS	Basic life support	GYN	Gynecologic
BM	Bowel movement	H	Hour
BP	Blood pressure	HBO	Hyperbaric oxygen
Bpm	Beats per minute	HBV	Hepatitis B virus
BSA	Body surface area	HIV	Human immunodeficiency virus
BVM	Bag valve mask	h/o	History of
Bx	Biopsy	HPI	History of the present illness
/c	With	HTN	Hypertension
C	Celcius/Centigrade	Hx	History
Ca	Cancer	I&D	Incision and drainage
CABG	Coronary artery bypass graft	ICP	Intracranial pressure
CAD	Coronary artery disease	ICU	Intensive care unit
C/C	Chief complaint or concern	IDDM	Insulin dependent diabetes mellitus
cc	Cubic centimeters	IM	Intramuscular
CCU	Critical care unit	IO	Intraosseous
CHF	Congestive heart failure	IPPB	Intermittent positive pressure breathing
CNS	Central nervous system	IUD	Intrauterine device
c/o	Complained of	IV	Intravenous
CO	Carbon monoxide	IVP	IV push (medication)
CO_2	Carbon dioxide	JVD	Jugular venous distention
COBS	Chronic organic brain syndrome	KED	Kendrick extrication device
COPD	Chronic obstructive pulmonary disease	kg	Kilogram
CP	Chest pain	KVO	Keep vein open
CPR	Cardiopulmonary resuscitation	L	Liter
CSF	Cerebrospinal fluid	Lac	Laceration
CSM	Circulatory/sensory/motor function	LLQ	Left lower quadrant
CT	Computerized tomography	LMP	Last menstrual period
CVA	Cerebral vascular accident	LPN	Licensed practical nurse
D_5W	5% Dextrose	LOC	Loss of consciousness or level of consciousness
d/c	Discontinue	LR	Lactated ringers solution
DKA	Diabetic ketoacidosis	LUQ	Left upper quadrant
DM	Diabetes mellitus	mcg	Microgram
DOA	Dead on arrival	MCI	Multiple casualty incident
DOB	Date of birth	MCL	Modified chest lead

Table 12-12 (*continued*)

MD	Physician		RMA	Refused medical assistance
mEq	Milliequivalents		RN	Registered nurse
mg	Milligram		ROM	Range of motion
MI	Myocardial infarction		RUQ	Right upper quadrant
mL	Milliliter		r/o	Rule out
mm	Millimeter		ROM	Range of motion
mmHg	Millimeter Mercury		RR	Respiratory rate
MRI	Magnetic resonance imaging		Rx	Prescription or treatment
MVA	Motor vehicle accident		/s	Without
MVC	Motor vehicle collision		SSS	Sick sinus syndrome
MVP	Mitral valve prolapsed		S1	First heart sound
N/A	Not applicable		S2	Second heart sound
NAD	No apparent distress		S3	Third heart sound
NC	Nasogastric		S4	Fourth heart sound
NKA	No known allergies		SA	Sinoatrial
NPA	Nasal pharyngeal airway		SIDS	Sudden infant death syndrome
NPO	Nothing by mouth		SE	Sublingual
NRB	Nonrebreather face mask		SOB	Shortness of breath
NS	Normal saline		SQ/SC	Subcutaneous
NSR	Normal sinus rhythm		SSCP	Substernal chest pain
NTG	Nitroglycerine		STD	Sexually transmitted disease
N/V	Nausea and vomiting		STAT	Immediately
O_2	Oxygen		SVT	Supraventricular tachycardia
OB/GYN	Obstetrics/gynecology		TB	Tuberculosis
OD	Overdose		TIA	Transient ischemic attack
OPA	Oral pharyngeal airway		Tid	Three times a day
OR	Operating room		TKO	To keep open
OTC	Over-the-counter		TOT	Turned over to
oz.	Ounce		Tx	Treatment or traction
P	Pulse		URI	Upper respiratory infection
/p	After		UTI	Urinary tract infection
PA	Physician assistant		VD	Venereal disease
PAC	Premature atrial contraction		VS	Vital signs
PAT	Paroxysmal atrial tachycardia		VF/VFib	Ventricular fibrillation
PCN	Penicillin		VT/VTach	Ventricular tachycardia
PE	Physical exam		w/	With
PEA	Pulseless electical activity		WNL	Within normal limits
PEARL	Pupils equal and reactive to light		w/o	Without
PIAA	Personal injury auto accident		WPW	Wolff-Parkinson White Syndrome
PID	Pelvic inflammatory disease		y/o	Year old
PJC	Premature junctional contraction		xport	Transport
PMH	Past medical history			
PND	Paroxysmal nocturnal dyspnea		**Approved Symbols**	
PO	By mouth		♂	Male
Pm	As needed		♀	Female
PSVT	Paroxysmal supraventricular tachycardia		=	Equal
Pt	Patient		+	Positive
PVC	Premature ventricular contraction		−	Negative
Q	Every		>	Increase
Qd	Every day		<	Decrease
Qh	Every hour			Change
Qid	Four times a day		R	Right
Qod	Every other day		L	Left
RLQ	Right lower quadrant		×	Times or multiply

Topographic Anatomy

Medical terminology includes a number of positional and directional terms (Tables 12-13 to 12-16). These terms direct a Paramedic to an area of the body or the organs involved. To serve as a reference, the body is divided into three planes. The frontal plane divides the body in half front from back. The sagittal plane divides the body from left to right, whereas the transverse plane divides the body into upper and lower. With these reference points in place, the Paramedic can more accurately describe a specific location on the body using topographic anatomy.

In every case, the assumption is that the patient is standing in the standard anatomical position; that is to say, the patient is standing upright, eyes forward, hands to the side with the palms of the hand forward and feet together.

Table 12-13 Directional Terms

Term	Plane	Relation	Description
Caudal	Transverse	Inferior	Toward the feet
Cephalic	Transverse	Superior	Toward the head
Dorsal	Frontal	Inferior	Toward the back
Ventral	Frontal	Anterior	Toward the front

Table 12-14 Relational Terms

Term	Description
Apex	Top of the pyramid
Base	Bottom of the pyramid
Distal	Away from the structure
Lateral	To the side of the structure
Medial	Toward the structure
Deep	Away from the surface
Superficial	Toward the surface

Table 12-15 Terms Describing Patient Positions

Term	Description
Prone	Lying on belly
Supine	Lying on back
Left lateral	Lying on left side
Fowlers	Sitting up right
Trendelenburg	Supine with legs elevated
Sims	Side lying knee to chest

Table 12-16 Terms Describing Movement

Term	Description
Abduction	Away from midline
Adduction	Toward the midline
Circumduction	Circular motion
Dorsiflexion	Backwards
Eversion	Turn outward
Extension	Straightening
Flexion	Bending
Inversion	Turn inward
Pronation	Turn downward
Supination	Turn upward

CONCLUSION

Abbreviations and medical terminology, when used inappropriately, only serve to confuse the message. With practice and attention to detail, the Paramedic can learn medicalese and become conversant with fellow healthcare professionals.

KEY POINTS:

- Medicalese has its roots in Greek and Latin words.

- Medical terms may consist of four parts: the root word, a prefix and/or a suffix, and a combining form.

- A prefix complements a root; it is placed at the beginning of the root.

- A suffix complements a root; it is placed behind the root.

- Sometimes when two root terms are used a combining vowel must be used to make the two root terms distinguishable but connected.

- All medical terms are interpreted with the suffix being read first, then the prefix, and then the root (last, first, and middle).

- Terms should be spelled correctly. Use a medical dictionary for the correct spelling.

- Paramedics should use appropriate and accepted abbreviations.

- The body can be divided up into three planes: frontal, sagittal, and transverse planes.

- The standard anatomical position is when a patient is standing upright, eyes forward, hands to the side with the palms of the hand forward, and feet together.

- Using the three planes and standard anatomical position, the Paramedic can use topographic anatomy to describe a specific location.

REVIEW QUESTIONS:

1. What are the origins of medical terminology?
2. Explain how a prefix complements a root word's meaning.
3. Explain how a suffix complements a root word's meaning.
4. List several examples of commonly accepted medical abbreviations.
5. What is standard anatomical position?

CASE STUDY QUESTIONS:

Please refer to the Case Study at the beginning of the chapter and answer the questions below.

1. Why would the correct use and spelling of medical terms be of concern to the quality improvement committee?

2. How would you perceive the care given by a Paramedic if the only documentation available contained misspelled words, as well as inappropriately used words or abbreviations?

3. Using topographical anatomy, describe a bruise located on the left arm between the elbow and wrist on the same side of the arm as the palm of the hand.

REFERENCES:

1. Waife SO. Medicalese. *Miss Valley Med J.* 1958;80(1):10–11.

2. Dzuganova B. Word analysis—a useful tool in learning the language of medicine in English. *Bratisl Lek Listy.* 1998;99(10):551–553.

3. Williams N, Ogden J. The impact of matching the patient's vocabulary: a randomized control trial. *Fam Pract.* 2004;21(6):630–635.

4. Zeng Q, Kogan S, Ash N, Greenes RA. Patient and clinician vocabulary: how different are they? *Medinfo.* 2001;10(Pt 1): 399–403.

5. Nagel KR. Prohibited abbreviations. *Am J Health Syst Pharm.* 2005;62(15):1559.

6. JCAHO says: watch your p's and q's. *Nursing.* 2004; 34(3): 55.

7. Brunetti, L., J. P. Santell, et al. The impact of abbreviations on patient safety. *Jt Comm J Qual Patient Saf.* 2007; 33(9): 576-83.

8. Scalise, D. Clinical communication and patient safety. *Hosp Health Netw.* 2006; 80(8): 49-54, 2. JCAHO says communication problems were the leading root cause of sentinel events in 2005. The reasons are manifold: a harried environment, a hierarchical staffing system and illegible handwriting, to name a few. This gatefold examines the scope of the problem, including data and risk factors, and offers some strategies for improvement.

9. National Patient Safety Goal on abbreviations clarified, implementation revised. *Jt Comm Perspect.* 2003; 23(12): 14-5.

SECTION V

PRINCIPLES OF CLINICAL PRACTICE

Communication with and assessment of the patient is essential to every encounter. Through this process, the Paramedic gains the information needed to form a differential diagnosis and develop an appropriate treatment plan for the patient. These seven chapters provide the Paramedic with the base skills to obtain an effective history and perform a thorough physical examination.

CHAPTER 13

SCENE SIZE-UP AND PRIMARY ASSESSMENT

KEY CONCEPTS:

Upon completion of this chapter, it is expected that the reader will understand these following concepts:

- Thorough scene size-up
- An algorithmic approach to carry out the primary assessment
- Determining level of consciousness, airway, breathing, and circulation status plus treatment of life-threatening conditions
- The value of vital signs

► CASE STUDY:

Two Paramedic crews were called to the scene of a motor vehicle versus bicycle collision. When the first crew arrived, they notified dispatch that there was a teenager, down on the ground, apparently unresponsive; the driver of the pickup truck was complaining of shortness of breath; and an elderly gentleman was leaning against a tree complaining of chest pain.

A witness stated that the bicycle darted out from between two parked cars. She did not see an airbag deploy in the truck and didn't believe that the truck was moving very fast as it had been stopped for a traffic signal just before the incident. As soon as the bike was struck, she said the elderly gentleman yelled that he was his grandson and immediately slumped down against a tree.

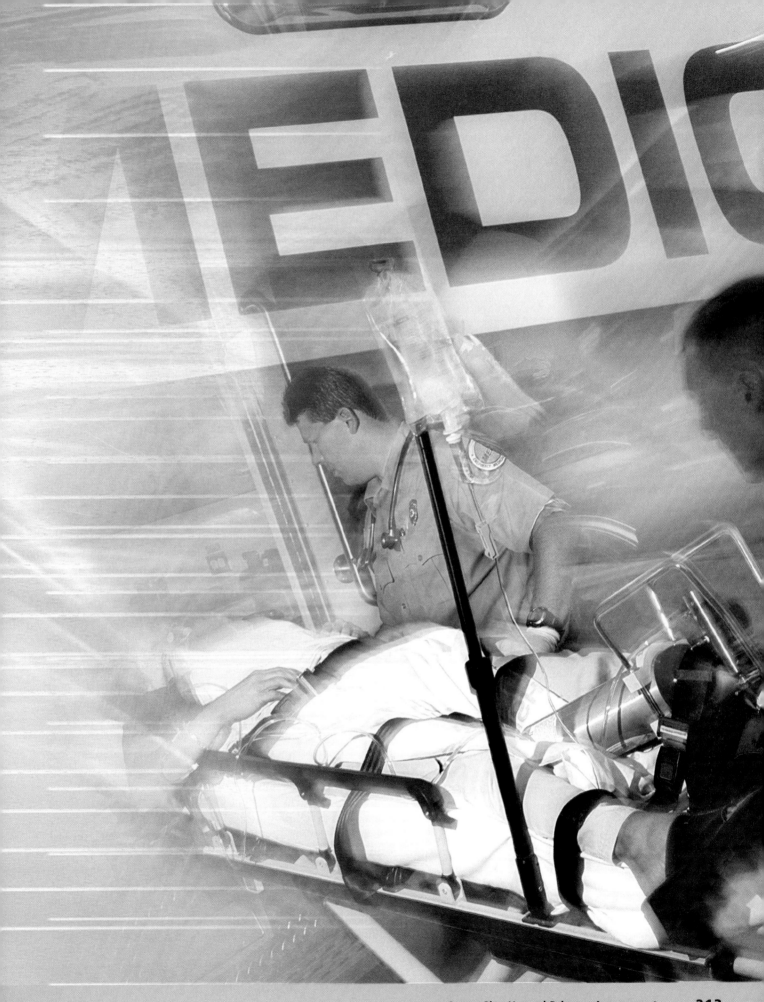

OVERVIEW

An experienced care provider at any level may take only minutes to complete a primary assessment. However, in those moments he or she may acquire pertinent information that will dictate further care. This chapter outlines the methods used to carry out this valuable assessment. Paramedic safety and patient safety are paramount when arriving on-scene and treating the patient. Knowing how to size-up a scene reduces the risk for injury or exposure and offers an organized way to assess environmental conditions, type and number of patients, and need for additional resources. Each component is vital in determining any life-threatening conditions that require immediate interventions.

Patient Assessment

Patient assessment is required as part of every patient contact. During a medical emergency, time is of the essence—environmental conditions may be less than ideal, sometimes even dangerous, and the sights and sounds stressful. In these situations the Paramedic must quickly and thoroughly form an impression of the patient's medical condition and assess the need for any additional resources, all while continuously assessing the safety of the scene. This requires both the science of medicine and the art of crisis and resource management. Regardless of skill level, an algorithmic approach to these situations will assist the Paramedic to provide assessment in the safest, most efficient, most effective, and most consistent manner.

Initially, the Paramedic must assess the scene to evaluate its safety and determine the need for other resources. Next, she must determine the general problem, and then perform a primary assessment of the patient (Figure 13-1).

The goal of the **primary assessment** is to find and manage any life-threatening injuries or conditions the patient might have by assessing for, and correcting, if possible, any threats to airway, breathing, and circulation. Once life threats have been assessed for and managed within the skills of the Paramedic, he/she identifies patients in need of immediate transport.[1-3]

High priority patients are generally transported immediately, with further assessment being performed en route. The assessment of **low priority patients** is typically conducted in a more focused manner while remaining on the scene. If time and personnel allows for it, a full set of vital signs can be obtained at any point during the primary assessment. This process should, however, never interfere with the performance of the primary assessment.

Scene Size-Up

Every scene that the Paramedic responds to requires an assessment of safety, environmental conditions, type and number of patients, and need for specialized resources to assist in scene management. Some of this information may be obtained, and some at least anticipated, before the Paramedic arrives at the scene. What was the dispatch information? Did the dispatch give any hints of possible scene hazards, such as fire or hazardous materials? What is the area like that the Paramedic is responding to? Is it possible that there may be multiple patients or the need for specialized rescue services? All of these issues should be considered while on the way to the scene.

Scene Safety

The first step in any patient assessment is to assure that the scene is safe to enter. **Scene safety** assures the Paramedic's well-being. An injured Paramedic is not helpful to anyone. Likewise, unsafe scenes must never be entered. The Paramedic must continually ask if the conditions remain safe enough for continued work on the scene. It must be remembered that even dangerous scenes may initially appear safe and that conditions may deteriorate quickly.

When assessing scene safety, the first priority should always be that of personal protection.[4-7] Many of the scenes where EMS is called have the potential for danger. Vehicular crashes, industrial accidents, and rescue scenes all expose the Paramedic to potential injury from moving vehicles, sharp surfaces, pinching or crushing hazards, and electric shock or exposure to fire.

Certain situations involve hazardous materials, toxic gasses, or an environment without adequate oxygen. These can lead to injury or death. Crime scenes and calls for assistance to emotionally disturbed persons always carry the risk for violence.

Often Paramedics are injured at scenes by far less obvious hazards. Falls from slips on unstable surfaces, ice, puddles, and unseen trip hazards are quite common. Domestic animals, often agitated by the unusual and chaotic activities at emergency scenes, have also been known to injure emergency personnel.

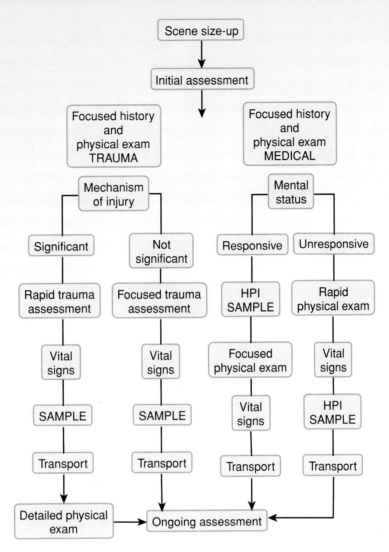

Figure 13-1 Algorithm of scene size-up and primary assessment.

Body Substance Isolation

Along with the visible safety hazards at an emergency scene, one should always remember the unseen potential for exposure to blood- and airborne pathogens. The Paramedic should apply body substance isolation (BSI) precautions to all patient encounters regardless of the suspected diagnosis. BSI creates a barrier between the Paramedic and possibly infectious materials through the use of gloves, masks, gowns, and eye protection (Figure 13-2).[8-11] Gloves should always be worn when the Paramedic is interacting with body fluids, non-intact skin, and moist body surfaces.[12-14]

The use of a mask and eye protection or a face shield to protect the eyes, nose, and mouth is imperative whenever performing procedures or patient care activities that might generate splashes or sprays of blood or body secretions. A gown should also be worn to protect skin and prevent soiling of clothing whenever the possibility of splashes of blood or body secretions exists.

Proper hand washing is one of the most important things that the Paramedic can do to prevent the spread of infection.[15,16] For an in-depth review of infection control techniques and exposure management, please refer to Chapter 3.

STREET SMART

For hands that are not visibly soiled, waterless hand cleaner is a good option. The Paramedic should wash with soap and water as soon as time and location permit.

Mechanism of Injury or Nature of Illness

After assuring the safety of the scene, the next step is to assess the patient's **mechanism of injury (MOI)** or the patient's **nature of illness**. For patients who have experienced

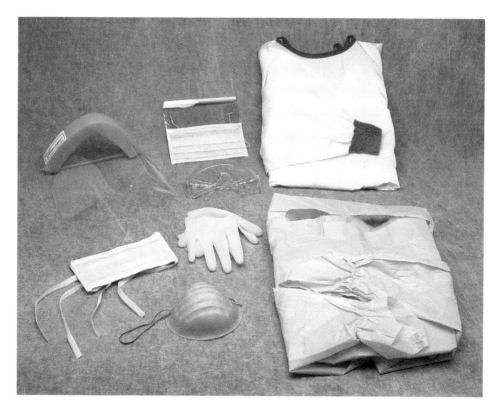

Figure 13-2 Personal protective equipment for body substance isolation includes gloves, gown, goggles, and a mask.

traumatic events, the Paramedic must determine the MOI by obtaining information from the patient, family, or bystanders, as well as from an inspection of the scene. The MOI is the instrument or event which resulted in harm to the patient. Often, the MOI is obvious, such as a motor vehicle collision (MVC) or a fall. Sometimes, however, it is not so clear.

When in doubt, it is safest to assume that the condition is related to trauma and take appropriate precautions to avoid worsening possible injuries which might not be immediately obvious (Figure 13-3).

When assessing the MOI, remember to note the environmental surroundings so as to make a report of these findings to hospital staff who are unable to determine these conditions for themselves. The nature of illness is essentially the history of present illness.

Number of Patients

Every scene must be investigated to determine the actual number of patients.[17] Although this probably seems intuitive, it is not unusual to have "tunnel vision" and focus efforts immediately on caring for the first patient found rather than determining if there are more patients. It is essential to make a determination of how many patients will need care on the scene.

If there are more patients than the responding units can effectively care for, then a mass casualty plan should be initiated. Any additional resources required should be called for. In these situations, it is important for the first responding unit to establish command and begin triage. A Paramedic is less likely to organize an adequate response of additional resources if directly involved in patient care activities.

The Primary Assessment

After assuring the scene is safe to enter and making a scene size-up, the Paramedic can begin the primary assessment. The primary assessment—the first evaluation performed on every patient—is the beginning of "hands on" patient assessment and is performed to address life-threatening problems.

The primary assessment involves forming a **general impression** of the patient, assessing the patient's mental status, airway, breathing, and circulation and determining which patients require immediate transport. Any immediate life threats found in the primary assessment must be addressed as they are discovered and then reassessed on a regular basis.

General Impression

The first step of the primary assessment is to integrate the observations obtained in the scene survey into a general impression of the patient's condition. The Paramedic should concentrate on the patient and ask himself if this patient appears very ill or severely injured. Experienced providers often can identify critically ill patients within a few seconds of entering the room (Figure 13-4). This initial impression has been called "the look test" or "gut impression" by some experienced clinicians attesting to the speed at which these providers can determine through observation if a patient is critically ill or not. Some demographic information can also be obtained by observation, and the Paramedic should note the patient's approximate age, sex, and race.

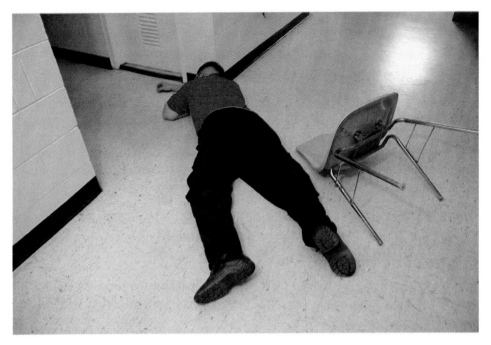

Figure 13-3 Questionable mechanism of injury: The Paramedic must assume a traumatic cause until proven otherwise.

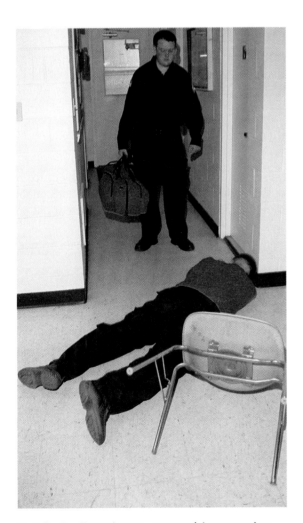

Figure 13-4 Forming a general impression.

Mental Status

Completely normal mental status is considered to be a good indication of adequate perfusion, and therefore an important parameter to evaluate in the primary assessment.[18] Upon approaching a patient, it is often fairly easy to determine a patient's general state of consciousness.

Most of the time patients will be awake and aware of the Paramedic's approach. Of course, some patients will not be awake upon the Paramedic's arrival, and it is important to try to determine how impaired their mentation may be.

Even when a patient appears alert, it is also important to try and quantify how oriented he is to his surroundings. The abbreviation **AVPU** is often used to report the patient's general level of consciousness. A stands for alert, V stands for responsive to voice, P stands for responsive to pain, and U stands for unresponsive.[19]

Alert

If the patient's eyes are open and he appears aware of the Paramedic, then he is referred to as alert. Any patient determined to be alert should have the level of consciousness further qualified by eliciting how well the patient is oriented. To determine orientation, the Paramedic commonly asks three questions relating to person, place, and time.

After introductions to the patient, ask him what his name is, where he is, and what the date is. If he can correctly answer all three questions, then he is determined to be alert and oriented to person, place, and time or "alert and oriented times three."

The statement "alert and oriented times three" is often abbreviated as A&O. If the patient cannot correctly answer all three questions, then he is determined to be disoriented. It is useful for the purpose of reassessment to report which questions the patient cannot answer upon primary evaluation.

For example, the patient who is oriented to person, but unsure of place or time, would be reported as "alert and oriented to person only."

Voice

If the patient does not seem to be awake upon approach, the Paramedic should attempt to awaken the patient before making physical contact with him. Before closing in on the patient's personal space, the Paramedic should say in a loud clear voice, "Sir, can you hear me?" If the patient opens his eyes to the Paramedic's voice, but shuts them again, he is determined to be responsive to voice.

Pain

If the patient does not awaken or respond to the Paramedic's voice, the Paramedic should attempt to awaken him with physical stimuli. The Paramedic should first firmly tap him on the shoulder while asking in a loud clear voice, "Can you hear me?" If this does not arouse the patient, a more noxious physical stimuli must be used.

Several techniques can be used to elicit a painful stimulus. One common technique is the sternal rub. The sternal rub is performed by applying the knuckles of one hand on the patient's sternum and moving it in a firm, circular motion (Figure 13-5a). Other methods include squeezing the trapezius muscle on either side of the base of the neck (Figure 13-5b), applying pressure above the eyes (supraorbital pressure—Figure 13-5c), or pressure with one finger to the soft area just behind the angle of the mandible (Figure 13-5d). The Paramedic assesses for purposeful movement by the patient to stop the painful stimulus.[20]

Unresponsive

If the patient does not respond in any way to verbal or painful stimuli, then he is considered unresponsive. The unresponsive patient is considered to be very ill until proven otherwise.

Airway

After determining the patient's level of consciousness, the Paramedic must next assess the status of the patient's airway. If the patient is conscious and alert, then the airway is most likely being maintained without difficulty. The Paramedic should confirm this assumption by observing the patient's effort to breathe and listening to the patient's speech.

If the patient has normal speech and noiseless, effortless breathing, then the airway is patent and unlikely to need any immediate interventions. If the patient is not awake or has noisy or difficult breathing, then the airway must be further evaluated for possible obstruction. The number one cause of airway obstruction is simply the patient's tongue.

The protective reflex and muscle control of the upper airway decreases as the level of consciousness decreases. This loss of control leads to relaxation of the soft tissues of the pharynx and occlusion of the upper airway. The ability to swallow is affected and this condition leads to a buildup of airway secretions. Simple positioning maneuvers such as a head-tilt chin-lift used for medical patients or a jaw thrust for trauma patients may relieve the obstruction and open the airway (Figure 13-6). Once open, the airway must be reassessed to make sure it is clear. Listen for noises such as gurgling, which may indicate fluid in the airway, or snoring or high pitch whistling, which may indicate continued obstruction of the airway. If there is fluid in the airway, suction should be used to evacuate it.

If the airway remains obstructed after positioning and suctioning, then an attempt at repositioning the airway is warranted. If repositioning does not resolve the obstruction, then the Paramedic should consider the possibility that there may be a foreign body in the airway. This obstruction must be relieved before continuing with the assessment.

If repositioning the airway only temporarily relieves the obstruction, or there continues to be a partial obstruction, consider the use of an airway adjunct. As a general rule, it makes sense to start with less invasive devices such as oropharyngeal or nasopharyngeal airways. However, if a less invasive device does not maintain the patency of the airway, the Paramedic must consider a more definitive method to control the airway.

The Paramedic may need to consider immediate endotracheal intubation, a blindly placed supraglottic airway device, or a surgical airway. Remember that the patient's survival depends on achieving and maintaining a patent airway.[21]

Breathing

Once the airway has been determined to be patent, assessment should continue to evaluate the adequacy of the patient's breathing. The Paramedic should also check for any possible threats to adequate breathing. To remember what to assess, think "Look, listen, and feel."

Look

The chest should be exposed enough to inspect for wounds and for the work of breathing. Any open wounds on the chest wall should be immediately covered to prevent the potential

CULTURAL/REGIONAL DIFFERENCES

The chest must be exposed to allow a visual exam for wounds and effort of breathing. Additionally, the stethoscope should be placed directly on the skin. Efforts should be made, whenever possible, to protect the patient's modesty. A sheet or towel can be loosely placed over the patient's chest or a bystander can be employed to hold a sheet up as a visual barrier. Depending upon local custom, it may be prudent to have a Paramedic of the same gender, if available, examine the patient.

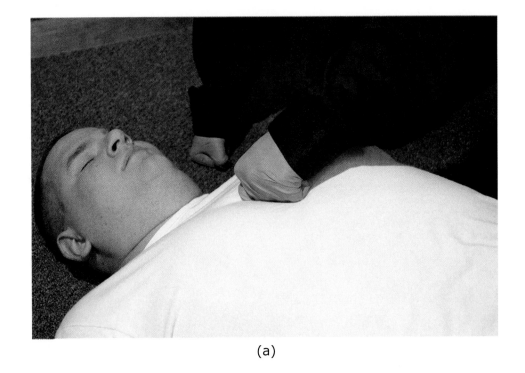

(a)

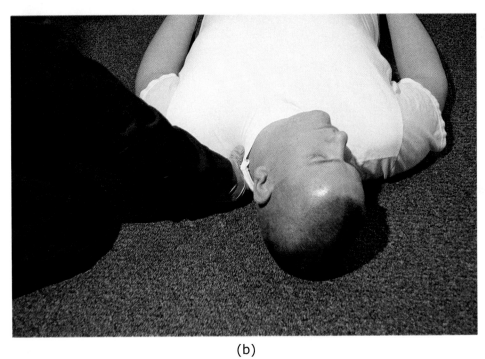

(b)

Figure 13-5 Methods used to assess response to painful stimulus: (a) Sternal rub (b) Trapezius squeeze.

for sucking chest wounds. Bruising should be noted as it may be a sign of significant underlying injury.

If two or more ribs are broken in two or more places, the segment may move out when the chest wall moves in with exhalation and in when the chest wall moves out with inspiration. The paradoxical movement of this flail segment is quite

painful, can cause decreased ventilation, and should be stabilized as soon as possible. The Paramedic should also observe the chest to determine the respiratory rate.[22,23]

Ventilatory rates which are either too fast or too slow will not allow for adequate gas exchange in the lungs. If the patient's ventilatory rate is less than 10 or greater than

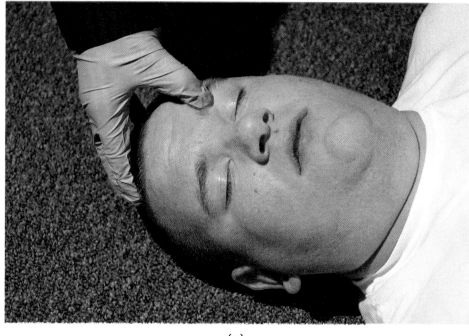

(c)

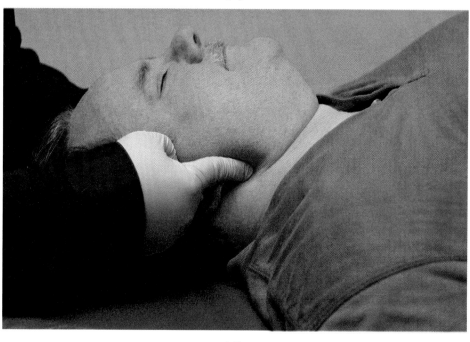

(d)

Figure 13-5 Methods used to assess response to painful stimulus: (c) Supraorbital pressure (d) Mandibular pressure.

30 breaths per minute, then the Paramedic should consider the possible need for ventilatory support.

A quick way to ascertain that the patient's respiratory rate is between 10 and 30 is to observe the chest and start counting the seconds between the first breath and the second. If the time between the first and second breath is 6 seconds or greater, then the respiratory rate is 10 breaths per minute or less. If the time between the first and second breath is 2 seconds or less, then the respiratory rate is 30 breaths per minute or more.

Listen

After inspecting the chest, the Paramedic should listen to the chest with a stethoscope to determine the effectiveness of air movement. At this point in the assessment it is important to determine that air is entering each lung and that the air entry is equal on both sides. The best place to listen during the primary assessment is just below the axilla on each side (Figure 13-7). One inhalation/exhalation cycle is generally enough to assess the depth and equality of breath sounds.

The Paramedic should make note of any unusual or abnormal breath sounds heard, but a full assessment of breath sounds can be made later after life threats are ruled out. If air exchange is inadequate, all measures should be taken to correct the deficit. The patient may require positive pressure ventilation, thoracic decompression, or medication administration to correct problems.

Feel

After listening to the chest to assure adequate and equal air entry, the Paramedic should palpate the chest to assess for potential life threats. Place a hand on each side of the chest and feel full inspiration and expiration. If the patient is conscious, ask her to take a deep breath and ask about pain. While palpating the chest, evaluate for tenderness, crepitus, or subcutaneous air. Any of these conditions may indicate a significant underlying chest injury. Also feel for equal expansion of the chest wall.

Circulation

After securing the patient's airway and breathing, the next step in the primary assessment is to evaluate the effectiveness of circulation. As with the airway and breathing steps, any life threats discovered must be corrected whenever possible during the primary assessment.

Pulse

The Paramedic should evaluate the presence of a radial pulse. If a radial pulse is present, it is reasonable to assume that the patient's blood pressure is adequate to supply perfusion to that peripheral site.[24,25] If there is no radial pulse, immediately

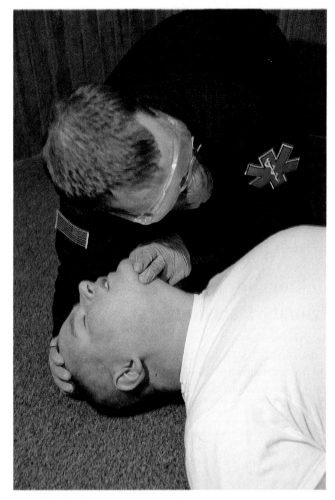

Figure 13-6 Assessing the airway can be simplified to the mantra "Look, listen, and feel."

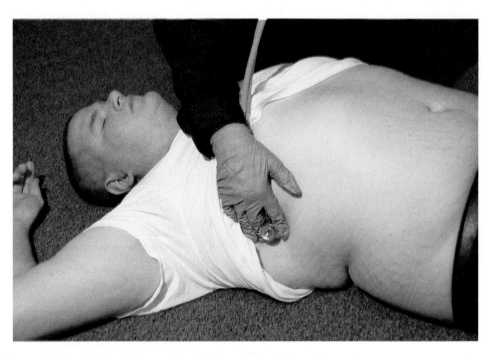

Figure 13-7 Auscultation of lung sounds at the axilla during the primary assessment.

assess the carotid pulse. If the carotid pulse is present, but the radial pulse is not, the patient's blood pressure should be assumed to be quite low.

Bleeding

After assessing for the presence and quality of pulses, the next step is to check for external bleeding. Any active bleeding should be further evaluated and any life-threatening hemorrhage must be corrected immediately whenever possible.

With gloved hands, the Paramedic should sweep under all non-visible parts of the patient's body and expose the patient enough to assure that any external bleeding site can be adequately assessed (Figures 13-8).

After assessing for the presence of external bleeding, the patient's skin should be evaluated for signs of internal bleeding. Pale, cool, and clammy skin may be signs of significant hypoperfusion.

Vital Signs

As time, available personnel, and patient condition allows, a full set of vital signs should be taken during the primary assessment. In no way should obtaining vitals take precedence over—or interfere with—the completion of the primary assessment. However, a complete and accurate set of vital signs can be a useful triage tool to estimate the severity of the patient's condition.

Some life-threatening conditions can be identified by the vital sign abnormalities they cause. Taking vital signs at this time establishes a set of **baseline vital signs** to which all subsequent vital signs are compared.

All other sets of vital signs taken are considered to be **serial vital signs** and are useful to illustrate trends in vital sign changes. For example, a low normal blood pressure discovered when the first set of vital signs is taken is not as significant as a blood pressure which gets slightly lower with each measurement.

A set of vital signs should include, at a minimum, an assessment of pulse, respirations, and blood pressure.[26]

Sick or Not Sick: Priority Decision Making

Once the primary assessment has been completed, the Paramedic must make a determination of the patient's priority. This determination is made by integrating all of the findings gathered in the primary assessment to make a decision

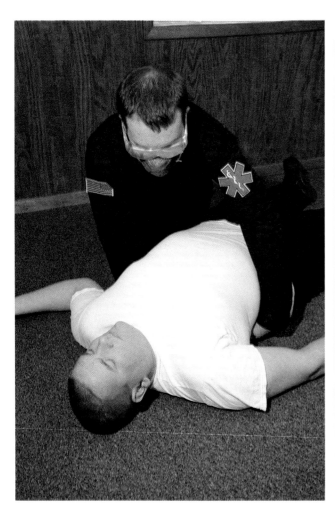
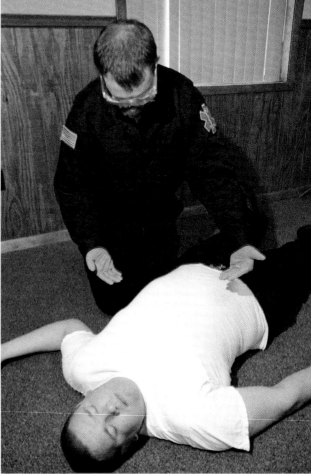

Figure 13-8   A Paramedic performing a sweep for blood during the primary assessment.

whether or not the patient has any life-threatening complaints which would require immediate, rapid transport to the hospital (Table 13-1). These patients are considered high priority patients and require that only life-saving interventions and appropriate packaging take place before they are expeditiously moved to the hospital.

All other assessments and interventions performed on high priority patients should take place en route to the hospital. This type of patient generally receives a minimal amount of interventions while on scene.

Table 13-1 Clues to Life-Threatening Conditions

- Poor general impression
- Unresponsiveness
- Decreased level of consciousness
- Difficulty breathing
- Shock (Hypoperfusion)
- Complicated childbirth
- Chest pain
- Uncontrolled bleeding
- Severe pain anywhere
- Multiple injuries

Those patients who are not determined to have potential life threats may be considered low priority and should have full assessment and any necessary treatments performed on the scene prior to being packaged for transport. Although scene time should never unnecessarily be delayed to complete these tasks, it is appropriate to spend time on-scene with these patients managing their condition as local medical authority allows.

Focused History and Physical Exam

Once the primary assessment has been performed and a priority determined, the appropriate focused history and physical exam may be performed. For medical patients who are responsive, the Paramedic should conduct a focused history and physical exam. For unresponsive patients, the Paramedic should use a rapid physical exam.

For trauma patients with significant mechanism of injury, the Paramedic should carry out a rapid trauma assessment with a detailed physical exam being performed en route to the hospital. For trauma patients without significant mechanism of injury, the Paramedic should conduct a focused trauma assessment.

CONCLUSION

As described in this chapter, the Paramedic's assessment starts the moment she pulls onto the scene. Observation skills are key to rapidly identifying hazards, determining if additional resources are needed, and determining when to move quickly into a rapid transport mode with a critically ill patient.

▶ KEY POINTS:

- Patient assessment is necessary for each patient contact and offers an algorithmic approach to quickly and thoroughly form an impression of the patient's condition; determine the need for any additional resources, and continuously assess the safety of the scene.

- The primary assessment is the first "hands on" assessment of the patient and is performed to address life-threatening problems.

- Responding to an emergency requires an assessment of safety, environmental conditions, type and number of patients, and need for specialized resources.

- Scene safety is the first priority before initial patient contact.

- The Paramedic should use body substance isolation (BSI) precautions in all patient encounters regardless of the suspected diagnosis.

- Proper hand washing is one of the most important things that the Paramedic can do to prevent the spread of infection.

- The Paramedic must determine the mechanism of injury (MOI) for patients who have experienced traumatic events.

- The Paramedic must determine the number of patients in order to determine if adequate resources are available.

- Regardless of whether the patient appears alert, the Paramedic should quantify orientation to surroundings.

- Alert refers to responding appropriately to questioning relative to person, place, and time.

- A patient alert to voice will respond to verbal stimuli.

- A patient who is not responsive to voice but responds to a painful stimulus is said to be alert to pain.

- A patient that does not respond in any way to verbal or painful stimuli is considered unresponsive.

- A patient with normal speech and noiseless, effortless breathing has a patent airway.

- The patients' airway may be obstructed by the tongue, foreign body object, or buildup of airway secretions.

- In opening the airway, consider simple positioning first. Use suction as needed.

- Evaluate the need for airway adjuncts such as oro- or nasopharyngeal devices or more invasive devices such as an endotracheal tube or alternative airway device.

- After an airway is established, assess depth, rate, and effort of breathing.

- After auscultation of the chest, the Paramedic should inspect the chest for wounds such as bruising or flail segments as well as tenderness, crepitus, or subcutaneous air.

- If the patients' respiratory rate is less than 10 or greater than 30 breaths per minute, ventilatory support may be needed to treat inadequate gas exchange in the lungs.

- The presence of a radial pulse represents a blood pressure that is adequate to supply perfusion to that peripheral site.

- Circulation also includes evaluating for any active bleeding or life-threatening hemorrhage that must be corrected immediately whenever possible.

In addition, skin color, temperature, and condition should be noted.

- Vital signs are assessed to establish a baseline to which all subsequent vitals are compared.

- After integrating all of the findings from the primary assessment, the Paramedic

must make a determination of the patient's priority.

- After an primary assessment is performed and a priority is determined, the Paramedic may perform appropriate further exams.

REVIEW QUESTIONS:

1. What is the primary goal of the primary assessment?

2. When the Paramedic arrives on-scene, what should be assessed?

3. Who is the Paramedic responsible for while on-scene?

4. Name the pieces of personal protective equipment the Paramedic can use for body substance isolation.

5. Describe what the Paramedic is looking for when conducting the "look test."

6. Name four different painful stimuli that can be used to determine a patient's level of consciousness.

7. After performing a head-tilt chin-lift on the nontraumatic patient, ventilations on the unconscious patient do not go in. What should be done?

8. What does a weak and thready radial pulse say about a patient's perfusion?

9. What is included in a complete set of vital signs?

10. What information is used to assign a priority to the patient's transport?

CASE STUDY QUESTIONS:

Please refer to the Case Study at the beginning of the chapter and answer the questions below.

1. Describe the scene size-up needed for this incident.

2. Describe the primary assessment of the three different patients.

3. Name the further exams that will be conducted for each of the three patients.

REFERENCES:

1. Koenig KL. Quo vadis: "scoop and run," "stay and treat," or "treat and street"? *Acad Emerg Med*. 1995;2(6):477–479.

2. Seamon MJ, Fisher CA, Gaughan J, Lloyd M, Bradley KM, Santora TA, et al. Prehospital procedures before emergency department thoracotomy: "scoop and run" saves lives. *J Trauma*. 2007;63(1):113–120.

3. Cone DC, Wydro GC. Can basic life support personnel safely determine that advanced life support is not needed? *Prehosp Emerg Care*. 2001;5(4):360–365.

4. Eckstein M, Cowen AR. Scene safety in the face of automatic weapons fire: a new dilemma for EMS? *Prehosp Emerg Care*. 1998;2(2):117–122.

5. Corbett SW, Grange JT, Thomas TL. Exposure of prehospital care providers to violence. *Prehosp Emerg Care*. 1998;2(2):127–131.

6. Grange JT, Corbett SW. Violence against emergency medical services personnel. *Prehosp Emerg Care*. 2002;6(2):186–190.

7. Neely KA. Scene control in prehospital care. *Top Emerg Med*. 1987;9(1):79–86.

8. Carrillo L, Fleming LE, Lee DJ. Bloodborne pathogens risk and precautions among urban fire-rescue workers. *J Occup Environ Med*. 1996;38(9):920–924.

9. Marcus R, Srivastava PU, Bell DM, McKibben PS, Culver DH, Mendelson MH, et al. Occupational blood contact among prehospital providers. *Ann Emerg Med.* 1995;25(6):776–779.

10. Eustis TC, Wright SW, Wrenn KD, Fowlie EJ, Slovis CM. Compliance with recommendations for universal precautions among prehospital providers. *Ann Emerg Med.* 1995;25(4): 512–515.

11. Hellinger WJ, Gonsoulin SM. Risking everything. EMTs, universal precautions, and AIDS. *Jems.* 1998;23(7):56–59.

12. Lund S, Jackson J, Leggett J, Hales L, Dworkin R, Gilbert D. Reality of glove use and handwashing in a community hospital. *Am J Infect Control.* 1994;22(6):352–357.

13. Kaczmarek RG, Moore RM, Jr., McCrohan J, Arrowsmith-Lowe JT, Caquelin C, Reynolds C, et al. Glove use by health care workers: results of a tristate investigation. *Am J Infect Control.* 1991;19(5):228–232.

14. Wolfe FD. Wearing gloves: is it protection or punishment? *Rdh.* 1998;18(9):22–24, 26, 30 passim.

15. Larson EL, Quiros D, Lin SX. Dissemination of the CDC's Hand Hygiene Guideline and impact on infection rates. *Am J Infect Control.* 2007;35(10):666–675.

16. Bubacz MR. Community-acquired methicillin-resistant Staphylococcus aureus: an ever-emerging epidemic. *Aaohn J.* 2007;55(5):193–194.

17. Zoraster RM, Chidester C, Koenig W. Field triage and patient maldistribution in a mass-casualty incident. *Prehosp Disaster Med.* 2007;22(3):224–229.

18. Limmer D, Monosky K. Assessment of the altered mental status patient. *Emerg Med Serv.* 2002;31(3):54–58, 81.

19. Gill M, Martens K, Lynch EL, Salih A, Green SM. Interrater reliability of 3 simplified neurologic scales applied to adults presenting to the emergency department with altered levels of consciousness. *Ann Emerg Med.* 2007;49(4):403–407, 407, e401.

20. Mistovich JJ, Krost W, Limmer DD. Beyond the basics: patient assessment. *Emerg Med Serv.* 2006;35(7):72–77; quiz 78–79.

21. Krost WS, Mistovich JJ, Limmer D. Beyond the basics: airway assessment. *Emerg Med Serv.* 2006;35(1):85–89; quiz 90–91.

22. Pettiford BL, Luketich JD, Landreneau RJ. The management of flail chest. *Thorac Surg Clin.* 2007;17(1):25–33.

23. Davignon K, Kwo J, Bigatello LM. Pathophysiology and management of the flail chest. *Minerva Anestesiol.* 2004;70(4):193–199.

24. McManus J, Yershov AL, Ludwig D, Holcomb JB, Salinas J, Dubick MA, et al. Radial pulse character relationships to systolic blood pressure and trauma outcomes. *Prehosp Emerg Care.* 2005;9(4):423–428.

25. Benson M, Koenig KL, Schultz CH. Disaster triage: START, then SAVE—a new method of dynamic triage for victims of a catastrophic earthquake. *Prehosp Disaster Med.* 1996;11(2):117–124.

26. Mistovich JJ, Krost WS, Limmer DD. Beyond the basics: interpreting vital signs. *Emerg Med Serv.* 2006;35(12):194–199; quiz 200–201.

CHAPTER 14

THERAPEUTIC COMMUNICATIONS

KEY CONCEPTS:

Upon completion of this chapter, it is expected that the reader will understand these following concepts:

- The process of effective communication
- Cultural competence when serving others
- Definitions of space
- Common strategies for establishing patient rapport
- Interview techniques for the Paramedic

▶ CASE STUDY:

Paramedics were called to the home of Susan Garratt for her 22-month-old daughter, who had fallen from the swings and injured her leg. When they arrived, the toddler was crying and wouldn't let her mother touch her right leg. The new Paramedic spoke to Mrs. Garratt but she didn't turn toward him. He yelled her name, which caused the toddler to cry even harder. His partner quickly wrote a short note which asked, "Are you deaf? If so, do you sign or read lips?"

Mrs. Garratt appeared relieved and her answer to the questions was, "Yes I am deaf and I do both." The Paramedic then introduced himself by name and function using both sign language and voice, which was normal toned and well articulated. The interview proceeded smoothly and the child was transported for evaluation of an injured ankle.

Later, the new Paramedic inquired as to where his partner had learned sign language. His reply was, "The community college."

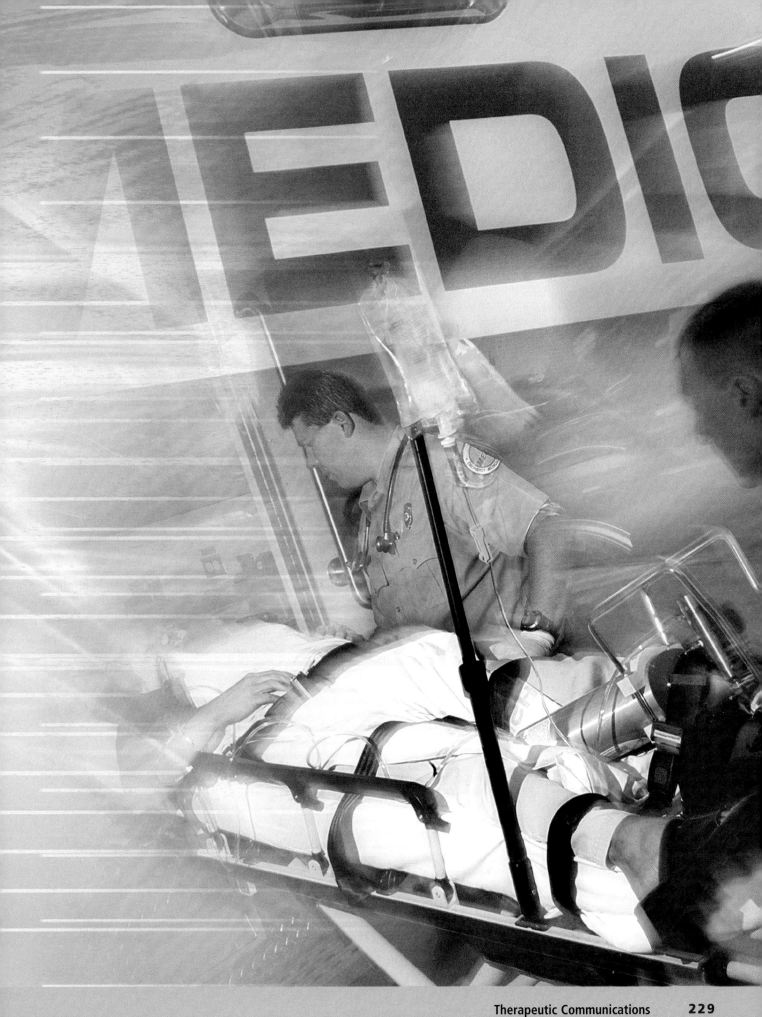

OVERVIEW

Communication goes beyond articulate speech and good handwriting. The Paramedic's actions, as well as those of the patient, can speak louder than words. This chapter examines how the Paramedic can be compassionate and understanding while still effectively performing his duties. The Paramedic must also be able to recognize nonverbal behaviors and establish patient rapport. To make the most of patient communication, several interview techniques are discussed.

Therapeutic Communications

Carefully chosen words and a gentle hand on a patient's shoulder—actions which bring comfort to a patient—help define Paramedics as compassionate caregivers. Caregivers are aware of the limitations of medicine to cure disease and reduce suffering as well as the power of interpersonal communication as a therapeutic tool. As healthcare providers, Paramedics bring both high touch as well as high technology to the patient's bedside.

Human Communications

People communicate with one another directly through speech (verbal) or indirectly, through a medium such as the written word, in order to convey a message. For the communication to be successful, the message must first be encoded, transmitted by the sender, then received and decoded by the receiver (Figure 14-1). This process, which occurs similarly in radio communications, can experience transmitter failure, interference, and poor reception. Identifying those problems and resolving them before they occur improves the quality of

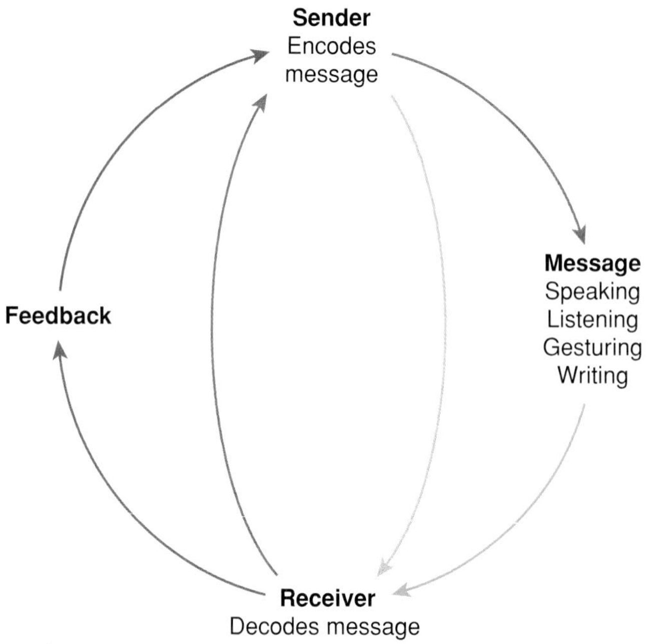

Figure 14-1 The process of communications.

the communication and improves the chance that the message conveyed and the message received are the same.

Encoding

Before conveying the message, the Paramedic needs to assemble the message carefully. Ill chosen words can send an incorrect message to the patient and can also elicit an unwanted response.

Take the word "pain," for example. All patients have some pain history. When the word "pain" is used it can subconsciously bring back memories of prior painful events. As a result, the patient's sympathetic nervous system responds to the stimulus (i.e., fear engendered by the word "pain,") and causes the patient's heart rate and blood pressure to rise. The word "discomfort," on the other hand, does not necessarily conjure the same memories. Therefore, the word may be less inflammatory than pain and allows the patient to avoid the physiological response that the word "pain" elicits.

Dr. Gnatt, of Johns Hopkins Medical School, has studied the human physiological response to words and has advanced the theory of **schizokinesis**.[1,2] A student of Ivan Pavlov, Dr. Gnatt's theory suggests that past painful experiences, unconsciously recalled by trigger words, can elicit an autonomic nervous system response. In some cases, this response could be harmful to the patient.

STREET SMART

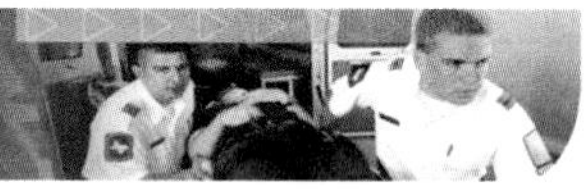

Examples of words that trigger a negative response include the statement "he's walking with a time bomb in his chest," or "those are tombstone ST changes on the ECG." Whether intended for the patient's ears or not, the effect is the same. The patient is left to feel fearful.

Transmission

The process of conveying a message, its **transmission**, can be either a true and accurate representation of the sender's thoughts (i.e., the message expressed is the message meant to be conveyed) or may be conveyed in such a way that the meaning is misconstrued by the receiver. Factors that affect whether a message's transmission is true include the choice of words as well as the sender's **body language**. Body language is the transmission of a message by nonverbal visual cues. Experts suggest that 70% of any spoken message is conveyed by body language. Body language is important and discussed in more detail shortly.

Reception

Factors that influence the receiver's **reception** of the message, what the patient understands the message to be, include both physical and cultural influences. An example of a physical influence that would have an impact on the message's reception is the presence of pain. The patient in pain tends to be self-absorbed and shuts out the outside world. Therefore, pain can be a powerful distracter that interferes with the patient's reception of the message. To get the patient's attention it may be necessary to speak loudly or to first provide some form of analgesia to remove the pain.

Cultural influences, in the form of customs, and language barriers can also affect the reception of the message. For example, a person of Japanese descent may nod in agreement. However, the nod may be a consequence of respecting authority rather than of understanding. In such a case, the nod may not mean that the patient understands the message sent by the Paramedic.

Decoding

An intangible in the process of communication is the receiver's ability to understand, or **decode**, the message. That ability to decode a message is based upon intelligence, the person's basic knowledge of language, life experience (which varies from person to person), and maturity, among many other variables.

The statement "I know what you heard, but that's not what I said," illustrates how two people can take two different meanings from the same statement. Many humorous stories have been told of children who hear an allegorical message and take it literally.

An obstacle to decoding the message is the use of medicalese. Paramedics who choose to use medical terminology when speaking to patients are at risk of being misunderstood or not understood at all. During a Paramedic–patient conversation, the Paramedic should attempt "double–speak," offering lay terms to explain medical terminology to the patient. Then it will be easier for the patient to understand what is being said.

Key to decoding the message is the patient's mental capacity. Medical conditions, such as stroke, can impair the patient's ability to decode the message, a condition called receptive aphasia.

Other conditions that can impair the patient's ability to understand include hypoxia, hypoglycemia, hypoperfusion, and poisoning.[3-5] In fact, any condition which causes the patient to have an altered mental status can interfere with the patient's ability to decode the message.

Feedback

Feedback is the mechanism by which the Paramedic can ensure that the message sent was the message received and decoded; that is, the message heard was the message sent. Feedback is obtained by asking the patient some simple questions.

To use feedback effectively, the Paramedic must practice active listening. It has been estimated that the average person can hear 500 words per minute yet can only speak about 125 to 150 words per minute. Therefore, in an average conversation the listener is only listening, receiving, and decoding the spoken word about one-third of the time. The remainder of the time the listener is left to think. The active listener uses that time to note nonverbal cues such as body language, as well as cognitive gestures, such as facial expressions and fidgeting, to add depth of comprehension to the feedback.

To practice active listening skills, the Paramedic should stop talking. Interruptions are disruptive to the communication process. The Paramedic should also take a non-defensive posture, with arms open, and a genuine look of interest on the Paramedic's face. The Paramedic should proceed to ask clarifying questions which add detail to the patient's responses. The use of encouraging words, such as "I understand," and hand gestures will encourage the patient to be forthright with answers.

STREET SMART

Patients expect Paramedics to take notes.[6] It would be unreasonable for a Paramedic to remember everything that was said. However, when the Paramedic appears to be "treating the clipboard" (taking more interest in completing a form than what the patient has to say), the patient tends to ignore the Paramedic.

Hermeneutics

The overarching goal of communications is to obtain clinically relevant information about the patient so that a diagnosis can be made and treatment offered.

Key to a successful interview is for the Paramedic to put himself in the patient's situation, with all of the accompanying physical and cultural influences, in order to understand the patient better. This approach is called **hermeneutics**.

By taking a "first person" perspective, the Paramedic gains understanding, as well as empathy, for the patient's plight.

Improving Communications

Improving communications starts with an awareness of personal factors which have an impact on communications. Everyone is shaped and changed by personal life experience; these influences and experiences, in turn, color our perception of ourselves and other people. By being **self-aware**, having a conscious understanding of one's life influences and prejudices, the Paramedic can factor those influences into the process, suppress negative influences, and augment positive influences.

A key feature of self-awareness is the person's physical being, which is a manifestation of one's genetics. A person's **genetic make-up**—those physical characteristics that make up a person, including appearance, disposition, and so on—can have a tremendous impact on one's outward appearance. For example, a man who has a large stature and stands over six feet tall may appear to be very intimidating to a short elderly woman. The self-aware Paramedic compensates for this by kneeling on one knee, bringing himself to the patient's eye level.

Culture, that culmination of life experiences in a locality or region that affects the way a person thinks and behaves, also has an impact on how the Paramedic acts toward, and is perceived by, the patient. The self-aware Paramedic is not only aware of how culture affects behavior but also is aware of how the patient's culture influences the patient's interaction with the Paramedic.

Culture relates in part to countries and areas within countries. There are tremendous variations among people from a particular region. For example, among the first Americans, the native American population, there are over 700 different cultures. People of Asian descent originally came from over a dozen countries. One cannot identify a person as being of a particular culture based simply on one characteristic.

It is estimated that over 14% of the United States population, or 31.8 million Americans, do not speak English as their primary language.[7] In New York and California, it is estimated that 30% of the population speak Spanish. This cultural diversity makes communications a formidable challenge to the Paramedic.

Paramedics who view their own cultural practices and customs as superior, a form of **ethnocentrism**, may have difficulty communicating with people from other cultures.

A person's education also can have a great deal of influence over one's ability to communicate. It is estimated that 50% of the U.S. population communicate at or below the eighth-grade literacy level.[8]

To be culturally aware, the Paramedic must first be aware of all of his or her own biases and attempt to eliminate their impact upon the Paramedic–patient interaction. Bias can not only prevent effective communication but it can cause the patient to mistrust the Paramedic and thus harm the Paramedic–patient relationship.

Interview Techniques

The goal of every patient communication is to be complete, clear, concise, courteous, and cohesive. A number of techniques can help improve the probability of success.

When approaching a patient, the Paramedic should make an estimate of the degree of distress that the patient is presently experiencing in order to modify his or her approach to the patient. For example, the patient "in extremis" is not likely to want long-winded conversations about past medical history. On occasion, it is better to reassure the patient that relief is coming and that conversation, for the moment, is not needed.

However, in most cases the patient is not in extreme distress and the Paramedic needs to engage the patient in a meaningful conversation to ascertain a symptom pattern for diagnostic determination.

> ### CULTURAL/REGIONAL DIFFERENCES
>
> The Paramedic must take care in judging a degree of distress. Many persons express their culture's stoicism in the face of discomfort while others are more vocal or effusive.

> ### CULTURAL/REGIONAL DIFFERENCES
>
> While language is an important component of culture, simply speaking the same language does not mean persons are of the same culture. People from South and Central America may speak Spanish as the primary language but their cultures are very different from that of Spain. In many cases their cultures are quite different from each other.

Proxemics

The physical distance between a Paramedic and a patient during the history gathering can have either a positive impact or a chilling effect on the dialogue. The idea that interpersonal distance affects communication was advanced in a theory by Edward T. Hall in 1959. Dr. Hall studied the effect of interpersonal space upon communications and advanced the theory of **proxemics**.[9]

The theory of proxemics is based on the concept of four spaces that surround a person. The first space, the **intimate** space, about the size of a beach blanket or one-half to one and one-half feet, is that space where patients feel most vulnerable. Entry into that space is only permitted to those people whom the patient trusts. All Paramedics must work toward being permitted into that intimate space in order to perform invasive treatments and routine patient care.

The second space is the **personal space**, that area where a patient would engage in a one-on-one conversation. The personal space, about one and one-half feet to four feet, is the distance within which most Paramedics initially interview patients for a history.

The third space is the **social space**, an area of relative safety where strangers can enter, with certain expectations of conduct. A dining room in a restaurant is an example of the use of social space, where everyone is expected to eat politely and maintain a conversational tone.

The fourth space, greater than 12 feet, is called the **public space**. It is that area one would occupy with a stranger without fear but with an ability to flee if danger should arise (Figure 14-2).

When walking in a public space (e.g., in a shopping mall), people become immediately aware of an unknown person who is closing the public space and entering the social space. The expectation is that the person will step aside and allow the other person to pass unhindered.

Dr. Hall's theory of proxemics is based upon American cultural practices and traditions. A Paramedic must also be aware of other cultures which may have larger spaces. An area that a Paramedic might consider a social space may be perceived by the patient as within the personal space.

Similarly, when a person (e.g., a mental health patient) feels threatened, the distances tend to grow larger. Intimate space, normally defined as one to one and one-half feet, might be four feet for a patient with schizophrenia. Invading that intimate space may result in violence.

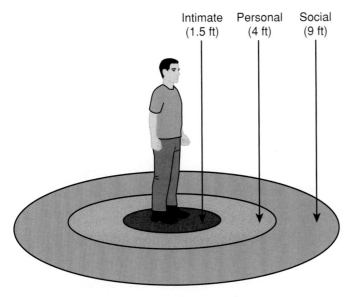

Intimate (1.5 ft)   Personal (4 ft)   Social (9 ft)

Figure 14-2 Proxemics illustrated.

Kinesics

Dr. Ray Birdwhistell suggested that body language may constitute 70% of a person's interpersonal communication.[10,11] This statement makes it clear that effective communication is more than just the spoken word (Figure 14-3). A Paramedic should be aware of the messages, intended and unintended, which the body language is sending to the patient. A knowledge of **kinesics**, the study of nonverbal behavior for communications, can help the Paramedic improve communication skills

The simplest example of kinesics might be nodding one's head yes or shaking one's head no. However, kinesics includes all the movements of the body including facial expression, posture, stance, and gestures. Understanding the concepts of kinesics, a Paramedic knows that standing above a seated patient and speaking down to the patient is conveying a message of superiority or strength. This position may be counterproductive to the task at hand (e.g., gathering a patient history).

Similarly, when a Paramedic, unwittingly or purposefully, blades a patient (stands in front of but at a tangent to the patient) to limit exposure and in preparation for a fight or flight, the Paramedic is telegraphing the patient a message of distrust.

Gestures and mannerisms can also have unintended meanings. For example, most patients will perceive finger-pointing as an aggressive act and that finger-tapping is a sign of impatience. The O.K. sign made with the thumb and forefinger means alright in New England. However, the O.K. sign in Japan means money and in France means zero. Perhaps more alarming, the O.K. sign is an insult in Brazil and Turkey. Lacking knowledge of the patient's background and heritage, it is best not to use hand gestures and other mannerisms during patient care.

Compassionate Touch

Nurses have known about the power of the human touch to bring comfort and solace to patients for years. Whether in the form of handholding, stroking a forearm, or rubbing a back, the compassionate touch is very human and therapeutic. Studies performed in critical care units have shown that intracranial pressure, heart rate, and blood pressure can lower toward normal with compassionate touch.

Dr. Dolores Krieger, RN, has researched and spoken about the power of touch to heal, or **therapeutic touch**.[12,13] Dr. Krieger states that therapeutic touch is first established in the human experience when a mother strokes the soft cheek of a distressed infant. It is developed throughout life during interactions with others. Therapeutic touch is intentional touching that mimics these earlier experiences and telegraphs reassurance, understanding, and caring to the patient.

Paramedics should consider using therapeutic touch, such as hand-holding, to help calm patients and as a means to transmit a message of compassion to the patient. The key to success with therapeutic touch is to recognize the opportunity and to intervene at that time. However, some caution is advised. Misapplied, therapeutic touch can be perceived as an unwanted intrusion into the patient's privacy.

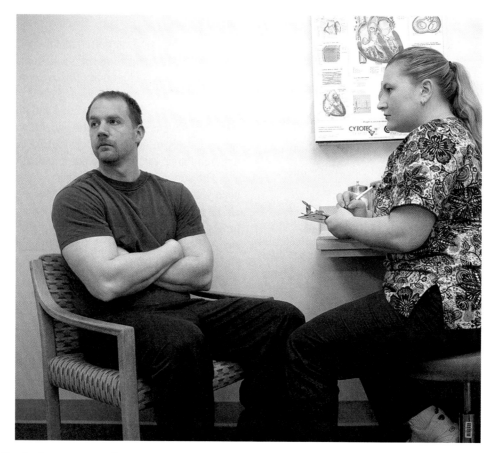

Figure 14-3 Body language often speaks louder than words.

Hearing Impaired

Conveying a message to the patient who is either hearing impaired or hard of hearing (HOH) requires the Paramedic to take deliberate action. While communicating with the hearing impaired can be difficult, demanding patience and persistence from the Paramedic, the end result (improved communication) ultimately results in better patient care.

The first step in communicating with this patient population is recognizing that the patient is hearing impaired. In some cases the patient may be forthright and tell the Paramedic that he is hearing impaired. In other cases subtle clues, such as inattention to the Paramedic during a conversation or inappropriate answers to questions, may lead the Paramedic to suspect that the patient is hearing impaired.

If the patient is hearing impaired, the Paramedic should inquire if the patient can read lips, uses sign language, or would prefer to write down his or her responses.

If the patient is a lip reader then the Paramedic should position himself in front of the patient, so that his lips can be clearly seen, and enunciate words carefully. Some EMS services have special language boards available to improve communication with the hearing impaired patient.

Whenever possible, the Paramedic should consider moving the patient to a quiet area or attempt to eliminate background noises, such as squawking radios or idle conversation. While hearing people automatically and subconsciously filter out ambient background noise, the hearing aids of the hearing impaired amplify all noise. The resulting mass of noise is difficult for the patient to decipher into an intelligent message.

Having identified that there may be a potential impediment to communication (i.e., that the patient is hearing impaired), the Paramedic should be especially conscious of the messages being sent to the patient by body language. Patients with a hearing impairment often utilize facial expressions, hand gestures, and the person's general posture to assist in ascertaining the meaning of a message.

Next, the Paramedic should attempt to gain the patient's attention before speaking. Sitting directly in front of the patient is often all that is needed to get the patient's attention. The Paramedic should be cautious about tapping the patient

STREET SMART

Some patients with a hearing impairment have working dogs. These working dogs listen for and protect their masters; they are the ears of their masters. It is inappropriate to touch or pet a working dog without the master's permission.

on the shoulder or waving his hands in front of the patient's face. These actions could be misconstrued as aggressive. If needed, a simple touch of the hand or forearm will get the patient's attention.

When speaking to the patient, the Paramedic should speak slower than normal, carefully enunciating words, and avoid putting her hands in front of her face. The Paramedic should avoid the use of "yeah" or "nah" as these two words are difficult to distinguish. Instead, the Paramedic should clearly say "no" or "yes," taking time to enunciate (hiss) the letter s.

The Paramedic should avoid the temptation to shout. Shouting not only makes the Paramedic appear impatient but also strains the vocals cords, thereby distorting sounds and making comprehension more difficult.

The Paramedic may want to inquire if the patient can read lips. If the patient is a lip reader then the Paramedic should position herself in front of the patient, so that the lips can be clearly seen. It is important that the Paramedic's face be well-lighted so that the patient can clearly see the Paramedic's lips. A common error made which can reduce the visual cues available is standing in front of a window or a light source. The result is that the Paramedic is silhouetted and the Paramedic's face cannot be seen clearly.

After the message has been conveyed to the patient, the Paramedic should ask the patient to repeat the message back. This "echo" technique helps to ensure that the intended message was transmitted and the patient understands.

In some cases a hearing interpreter may accompany the patient. If the patient has an interpreter, the Paramedic should introduce herself to the interpreter and briefly discuss the intent of the conversation. Even though the interpreter is present, the Paramedic should still speak directly to the patient. The interpreter will then use American sign language or signed English to convey the message to the patient after the Paramedic is done speaking. The Paramedic should speak in short sentences and then allow time for translation. After receiving the message, the patient will use sign language to speak to the interpreter and then turn to face the Paramedic as the interpreter translates the message to the Paramedic.

If the patient has difficulty understanding the message, the Paramedic should repeat the question or restate the message in other words.

A large number of hearing aids are available for the hearing impaired patient including those that are worn behind the ear (BTE) and in the ear (ITE). If the patient has a hearing aid, then the Paramedic should talk to the side of the patient in which the hearing is best; the patient often indicates this by turning that side of the head toward the Paramedic. It is appropriate to ask the patient if he or she has a good side and then to direct conversation to that side.

In some cases, the easiest method of communication is to write down the message. While time-consuming, this method can help reduce errors. The Paramedic should write plainly and avoid the use of cursive handwriting. To facilitate visual communications, some EMS services have special language boards available for use by the Paramedic. These language boards provide visual cues that permit the Paramedic and the patient to communicate quickly.

STREET SMART

When possible, the Paramedic should move the patient with a hearing aid indoors or to the back of the ambulance. The blowing wind generates a whistling sound in the ear of the patient, making it almost impossible for the patient to hear what is said.

Introductions

It is not only a common courtesy to introduce oneself to a patient, but it is a professional responsibility for the Paramedic to advise the patient who he is and what qualifications he possesses to care for the patient. Some states even mandate that all healthcare providers identify themselves to the patient by name and title. Frequently this can be accomplished by use of identification tags or name badges.

But for the professional Paramedic, it is more than compliance with the law. The tradition of introducing oneself helps to set the groundwork for future dialogue between the patient and the Paramedic. Some Paramedics prefer to shake the patient's hand, a generally accepted activity that is seen as nonthreatening. Besides conveying a message of goodwill, the Paramedic has the first opportunity to assess the patient's physiologic state. Cold and sweaty palms may indicate shock while a weak grasp may indicate exhaustion. When the courtesy is returned and the patient gives the Paramedic his name, the Paramedic can further assess the patient's speech and mental status.

STREET SMART

The Paramedic should inquire as to the patient's preferred manner of address. If the patient states that his name is Joe Smith, the Paramedic can immediately ask if he prefers Joe or Mr. Smith.

The saying goes that a "picture is worth a thousand words." The image of the patient seated in a chair, obtained during the introduction, helps the Paramedic immediately gauge the severity of the illness or injury (Figure 14-4).

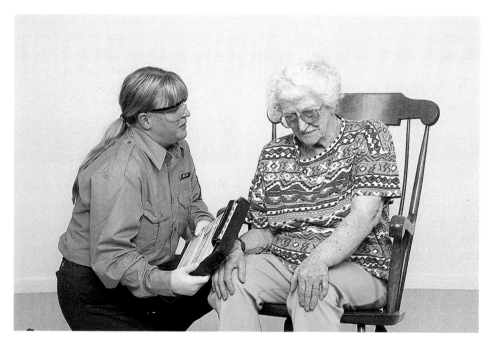

Figure 14-4 A Paramedic's first opportunity for assessment.

Selecting the Correct Questions

The Paramedic should carefully select questions that maximize patient information and provide for a free flow of dialogue. The Paramedic may elect to use either open-ended questions or closed-ended questions to obtain the patient's history during the interview. Each type of question has its merits.

Open-ended questions allow the patient to express himself without restriction and the answers can be used as a springboard to other questions. Open-ended questions usually begin with words like "how," "what," or "could" and ask for an explanation. Patients with limited patience may find these questions frustrating, but generally speaking open-ended questions provide the greatest yield of information.

Closed-ended questions require the person to answer a question with a limited number of options. Closed-ended questions are used when specific information is needed quickly. A closed-ended question generally starts with words like "do," "is," or "are" and result in **automatic answers**— single word responses such as "yes" or "no"—that add small amounts of information.

During an emergency Paramedics often prefer to use closed-ended questions in order to obtain succinct answers. However, the use of closed-ended questions can lead to a limited history from the patient.

Some Paramedics prefer to use an **indirect statement** to obtain needed patient information. An indirect statement is a question that asks for an explanation that is not constrained by the question. An example of an indirect statement would be, "Please tell me about your pain."

Using Proper Tone

The tone of voice is thought to transmit some 23% of the spoken message (the remaining 77% is left to the actual words spoken). When talking to a patient, the Paramedic should be aware that the inflection of the voice can transmit a meaning altogether different than the one intended.

Encouraging Behaviors

By practicing certain behaviors, a Paramedic can help facilitate the dialogue. For example, **acknowledging** the patient's response, either verbally or nonverbally, can encourage the patient to volunteer more information.

In certain instances, when the patient is making what appears to be a painful disclosure, it may be appropriate for the Paramedic to remain silent. Silence, in this instance, is comforting to the patient and shows that the Paramedic respects the patient's privacy.

Sharing one's observations with the patient can also help focus the patient's thoughts as well as direct the dialogue. For example, the statement "You seem upset" may bring the patient's behavior to the patient's attention and allow the patient to correct the impression or explain the behavior.

Conveying empathy, the message that "I am with you" can be as simple as acknowledging the patient's feelings or asking for clarification. Both approaches show the patient that the Paramedic is interested and cares.

Clarification is an excellent tool when the Paramedic is sensing a mixed or confusing message. Clarification asks the patient to restate the message in other words. By asking the question (e.g., "What do you mean when you say . . . ?") the Paramedic is bringing the previous statement to the patient's attention and asking for further explanation.

At the end of a patient interview, the technique of **summarization** can be helpful to ensure the Paramedic's understanding of the information in the interview. Summarization involves taking the patient's own words, then paraphrasing the patient's words to ensure that the message sent was received correctly. Summarization allows the Paramedic to focus on specifics of a patient history. Summarization also reassures the patient that the Paramedic was attentive during the patient interview.

Behaviors Detrimental to Dialogue

A Paramedic should keep in mind that certain behaviors can be detrimental to the Paramedic–patient dialogue. For example, inappropriate slang words, curse words, and laughter can have a devastating effect upon the conversation between patient and Paramedic. While patients do sometimes get themselves into genuinely humorous situations, the laughter is best left for after the call. During the call, all providers should be professional and polite.

Patient Conduct

Patients may exhibit self-protective behaviors, called **blocking behaviors**, which inhibit free dialogue with the Paramedic. Many of these blocking behaviors are manifestations of psychological defense mechanisms. For example, when a patient slams a door he may be displacing his anger from a threatening object (e.g., the Paramedic) to a nonthreatening object (e.g., the door).

Similarly, the patient may deny the feelings. Denial, a strong defense mechanism, is commonly used and is an unconscious refusal to acknowledge feelings or situations. An example of denial is the patient who appears to be having an acute coronary event but keeps telling the Paramedic that it is just indigestion. The patient fears the truth and all of the consequences that would accompany an acute coronary event, including a loss of independence.

Fear is a powerful feeling. Patients overwhelmed with fear may experience debilitating panic attacks or exhibit outright hostility toward the Paramedic. When confronted with a hostile patient, the Paramedic is under no obligation to remain in danger. However, if the Paramedic can recognize the source of the fear or anger and help the patient recognize that fear or anger, the Paramedic could potentially defuse the situation and continue providing patient care.

To deescalate an angry or frightened patient, the Paramedic should permit the patient some control of the situation and then, using a problem-solving approach, analyze and neutralize the cause of the fear.[14]

On rare occasions, a Paramedic may be confronted with inappropriate sexual behavior, often in the form of sexual innuendo. It is important that the Paramedic separate the patient from the behavior, and accept the patient but reject the behavior. The Paramedic should understand that the patient is expressing genuine feelings (care) in an inappropriate manner. The Paramedic needs to express his feelings (e.g., "I am uncomfortable with what you just said.") and then proceed to establish boundaries. In most cases, the patient needs the help that EMS can provide and will demonstrate correct behavior.

Provider Errors in Interviewing

Sometimes the Paramedic is his or her own worst enemy when it comes to facilitating a dialogue. The following are a few behaviors that are counterproductive to the task of gathering a patient history and maintaining a therapeutic communication.

Some Paramedics take pride in their ability to use medical terms and professional jargon. However, when speaking to a patient such medicalese is confusing and erodes the patient's confidence that the Paramedic can relate to the situation or problem.

Another common pitfall is frequent interruptions. When a patient is frequently interrupted by the Paramedic, the patient gets the sense that the Paramedic does not really care about the patient.

Paramedics should also avoid giving false assurances. While reassuring clichés, such as "everything will be alright," can come glibly off the tongue, these words are altogether meaningless to the patient and undermine the trust that the patient has in the Paramedic.

Similarly, Paramedics should avoid giving advice. Such statements usually begin with "If I were you," or "You should do this." Such advice is generally not based upon a sufficient knowledge base and assumes authority. Even physicians generally couch their words of advice with statements like, "It is my recommendation that," or "You might want to consider this," leaving the decision to the patient.

As a rule, Paramedics should also avoid "why" questions. Questions prefaced with the word "why" imply judgment. When a patient senses judgment, a sense of futility prevails and the patient tends to become uncooperative. Moralizing also falls along the same lines as giving advice and asking "why" questions.

STREET SMART

The Paramedic should listen carefully to the words of the patient's spouse. Generally speaking, the spouse of a patient is genuinely concerned and can often add important information about the situation which the patient may not know or may be withholding.

Statements by Friends and Family

Friends and family can offer a rich source of information about a patient, but such information should always be looked at with a skeptical eye. The Paramedic cannot be sure of the motives of friends and families and such hearsay information can be inaccurate.

Special Communication Situations

There are many situations which require the Paramedic to use specific techniques or actions to handle communications with the patient.

Drugs and Alcohol

Paramedics commonly encounter drug- or alcohol-intoxicated patients. These patients, despite distasteful mannerisms or behaviors, are deserving of care and may not be aware of the danger to their health.[15-17]

When confronted with an intoxicated patient, the Paramedic should not moralize about the patient's conduct, but rather recognize that the patient may have unresolved problems. This recognition paves the way for the Paramedic to separate patient from behaviors and provides the start of a therapeutic relationship with the patient.

Alternative Medicine

Paramedics may also encounter patients who lack faith in western medicine. These patients may have already used **alternative medicine** or **complementary medicine** before calling EMS. Unsure of the Paramedic's reaction, the patient may withhold such vital information from the Paramedic.

Paramedics should recognize that alternative medicine is becoming increasingly popular and is more commonplace in some cultures. A study in the *New England Journal of Medicine* indicated that some 34% of Americans have tried alternative medicine.[18] The domain of alternative medicine includes mega-vitamins, therapeutic massages, chiropractic medicine, and acupuncture, to name just a few.

In some cultures, the practice of folk medicine is the prevalent medical care. Special practitioners may use concoctions of herbs and special rituals to cure illness. The Mexican folk healer, for example, is called a "Curandero." In one study of 405 Hispanics in Denver, Colorado, 29% indicated that they had visited a Curandero in the past.[19]

All Paramedics should strive for **cultural competence**, an ability to function effectively within the populations that they serve. Cultural competence requires an awareness and knowledge of common medical practices in the communities.

Death and Dying

No situation puts the Paramedic's therapeutic communication skills to the test more than a patient's death. A caring Paramedic can support the patient's family during this stressful moment in a person's life through therapeutic communications.

The Paramedic should first listen. Listening, nonjudgmentally, to the patient's spouse or loved one allows the process of grieving to begin. If the patient's family is in denial, the Paramedic should gently reestablish reality by refocusing the person to the reality of the situation (i.e., that the patient has died).

Any displays of anger or criticism from the family should not be taken personally. The professional Paramedic can separate the behavior from the person and understands that the behaviors are part of the mourning over the patient's death.

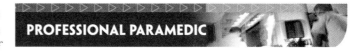

PROFESSIONAL PARAMEDIC

Some allied health programs including paramedicine offer courses in thanatology, the social and psychological study of death and dying.

CONCLUSION

While Paramedics are in many respects taught to "romance the technology," EMS is—above all else—a caring profession. Therapeutic communication helps to establish Paramedics as professionals in the minds of their patients, other healthcare team members, and the general public.

KEY POINTS:

- The overarching goal of communications is to obtain clinically relevant information about the patient so that a diagnosis can be made and treatment offered. Communication should be complete, clear, concise, courteous, and cohesive.

- Successful communication depends on correctly sending and receiving the message. The reception of the message can be affected by physical, cultural, and educational differences between the message's sender and receiver.

- A common obstacle to successful communication is the use of difficult to understand medical terminology. It is good practice to offer lay terms to explain medical terminology to ensure that the patient understands.

- Any medical condition causing the patient to have an altered mental status can interfere with the patient's ability to understand the message.

- The Paramedic should check for patient understanding by looking for feedback in the form of body language, facial expressions, and questions and answers.

- Active listening skills include taking a nondefensive posture, keeping arms open, having a genuine look of interest, asking clarifying questions, and not interrupting the patient responses.

- Paramedics should put themselves in the patient's situation in order to understand the patient better (hermeneutics).

- The theory of proxemics illustrates the importance of keeping the appropriate physical distance between Paramedic and patient. Different people require differing amounts of space to feel comfortable.

- Knowledge of kinesics, the study of nonverbal behavior for communications, can help the Paramedic improve communication skills.

- Applied correctly, therapeutic touch, such as hand-holding, can help calm patients and transmit a message of compassion to the patient.

- Conveying a message to the patient who is either hearing impaired or hard of hearing (HOH) requires the Paramedic to take deliberate action.

- The Paramedic should carefully select questions that maximize patient information and provide for a free flow of dialogue.

- Open-ended questions allow a patient to give more thorough answers, while closed-ended questions result in fast responses and limited information.

- Clarification and summarizing are both excellent ways to ensure that the message sent was received correctly.

- Patients may exhibit self-protective behaviors, called blocking behaviors, which inhibit free dialogue with the Paramedic.

- The Paramedic should not give false assurances or advice.

- In interviewing, avoid "why" questions, as they imply judgment.

- Paramedics should strive for cultural competence, an ability to function effectively within the populations that they serve.

- Therapeutic communication is crucial when dealing with a patient's death.

REVIEW QUESTIONS:

1. What theory explains how words can trigger unpleasant memories and subsequent physical reaction?

2. Describe how the process of radio communications is similar to communication between two people.

3. Define the study of kinesics and explain why it makes up a majority of person-to-person communication.

4. Describe the four types of space that the theory of proxemics outlines.

5. What are some blocking behaviors the patients or family members might display?

6. In an interview with an elderly woman who has mild dementia and is slow to respond, what techniques can the Paramedic use to promote effective communication?

7. Explain how cultural competence allows Paramedics to function effectively within the populations that they serve.

8. How should the Paramedic conduct him- or herself when dealing with the spouse of a patient who just died?

CASE STUDY QUESTIONS:

Please refer to the Case Study at the beginning of the chapter and answer the questions below.

1. Explain why speaking louder may increase the anxiety of persons present on a scene.

2. How does "yelling" affect lip reading?

3. How should the speaker position himself for the lip reader?

4. In addition to Mrs. Garratt's hearing impairment, what other factors are likely to interfere with communication?

REFERENCES:

1. Gantt WH. Principles of nervous breakdown-schizokinesis and autokinesis. *Ann N Y Acad Sci*. 1953;56(2):143–163.
2. Gantt WH. Pain, conditioning and schizokinesis. *Cond Reflex*. 1973;8(2):63–66.
3. Barratt K, von Briesen JD. The continued vitality of a patient's informed consent, or, when the patient says "no." *Wmj*. 1999;98(2):60–61.
4. Sturman ED. The capacity to consent to treatment and research: a review of standardized assessment tools. *Clin Psychol Rev*. 2005;25(7):954–974.
5. Tunzi M. Can the patient decide? Evaluating patient capacity in practice. *Am Fam Physician*. 2001;64(2):299–306.
6. Johnson A. Note to self: tips on internal & external communication. *Jems*. 2007;32(6):26–27.
7. National Institute For Literacy. Available at: http://www.nifl.gov/nifl/facts/facts.html Accessed May 16, 2009.
8. Kaestle C, Damon-Moore H. *Literacy in the United States*. New Haven: Yale University Press; 1991.
9. Meade DM. Mixed messages: interpreting body language. *Emerg Med Serv*. 1999;28(9):59–62, 73.
10. Birdwhistell RL. *Introduction to Kinesics: An Annotation System for Analysis of Body Motion and Gesture*. Louisville: University of Louisville; 1952.
11. Birdwhistell RL. *Kinesics and Context: Essays on Body-Motion Communications*. London: Lane Press; 1970.
12. Krieger D. Alternative medicine: Therapeutic touch. *Nurs Times*. 1976;72(15):572–574.

13. Krieger D. Therapeutic touch: two decades of research, teaching and clinical practice. *Imprint.* 1990;37(3):83, 86–88.

14. Hills LS. Working with anxious or fearful patients: a training tool for the medical practice staff. *J Med Pract Manage.* 2007;23(1):50–53.

15. Dick T. Stinky people. Respecting your limitations & other people's predicaments. *Emerg Med Serv.* 2005;34(11):26.

16. Nordberg M. Mixed emotions. EMTs and Paramedics are often ambivalent about treating the homeless. *Emerg Med Serv.* 1992;21(5):39–45, 48–39, 75.

17. Remy JD. Prehospital care of the intoxicated individual. *Emerg Med Serv.* 2004;33(12):88–89, 91.

18. Eisenberg DM, Kessler RC, Foster C, et al. Unconventional medicine in the United States. Prevalence, costs, and pattern of use. *N Engl J of Med.* 1993;328(4):246–252.

19. Padilla R, Gomez V, Biggerstaff SL, Mehler PS. Use of curanderismo in a public health care system. *Archives of Internal Medicine.* 2001;161(10):1336–13340.

CHAPTER 15

HISTORY TAKING

KEY CONCEPTS:

Upon completion of this chapter, it is expected that the reader will understand these following concepts:

- The need for an accurate medical history to provide competent patient care
- Using a comprehensive medical history to discover as much information about a patient's complaints, interpersonal relationships, and medical history as possible
- Using a focused health history to generate the historical findings necessary to manage an emergent medical condition
- The benefits of asking open-ended questions so patients are allowed to answer in their own words and generate a less-biased history

CASE STUDY:

The Paramedics approached Mrs. Jones, an elderly woman who called EMS frequently. One Paramedic said quietly, "Let's just get her into the bus and get going. She always has the same complaint and her history doesn't change."

His partner said, "No, we'll use a history gathering mnemonic to work this through. There's something different here but I'm not sure what it is." Mrs. Jones always complained of shortness of breath. However, this time the onset was slower and it was accompanied by extreme fatigue. Her physical exam was essentially the same as always but the pair worked her up for a possible myocardial infarction, which was later confirmed at the hospital.

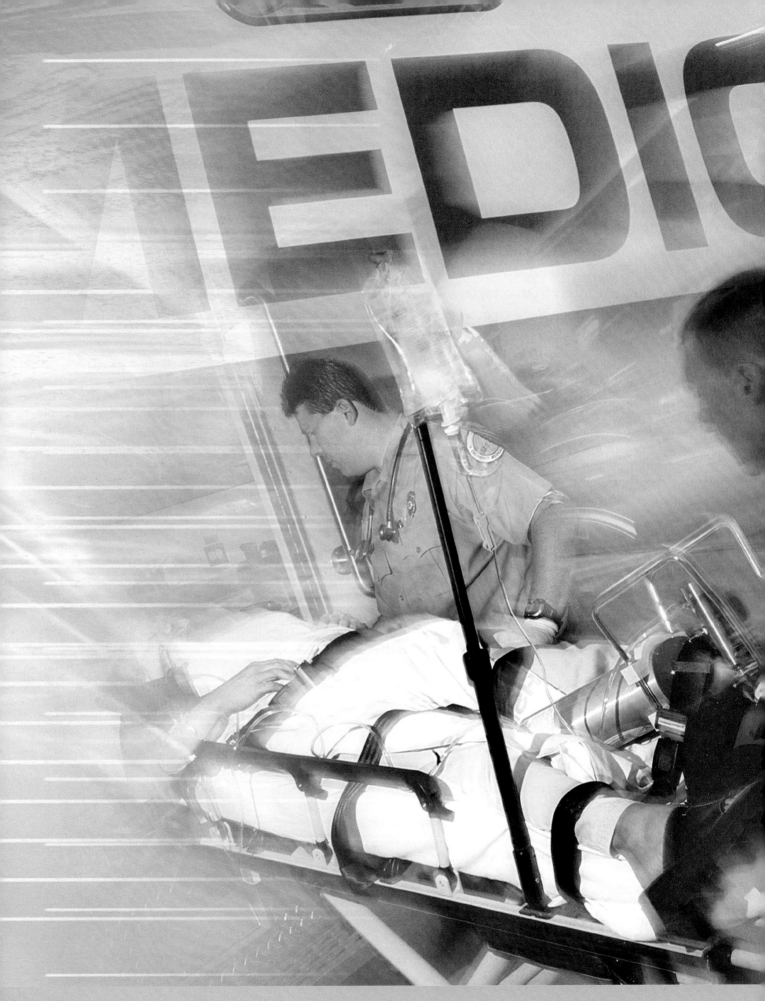

OVERVIEW

Obtaining an accurate medical history is an essential provision of quality patient care. This chapter discusses the art and science behind history taking. A patient's medical history is best obtained by asking the right questions and developing a rapport that allows for a free exchange of information. Asking questions in an open-ended manner allows patients to answer in their own words and generates a history that is less biased by the Paramedic's own interpretation. Once the dialogue has been opened, the Paramedic should guide the patient through the interview using the techniques of facilitation, reflection, clarification, interpretation, and direct questioning to gather the history without diverting the patients from their own account. Using the information generated from a focused health history, the Paramedic is able to expose historical findings necessary to manage a patient's emergent medical condition.

History Taking

History taking is the most important skill for a Paramedic to master. History taking is defined as the medical questioning of a patient to determine the disorder, syndrome, or condition affecting the patient that resulted in the call for assistance. With most patients, the medical condition related to their chief concern can be correctly identified by history taking alone.[1] Often physical exam findings and other tests assist in confirming the paramedical **diagnosis**. If a Paramedic listens to the patient, she will tell the Paramedic what is wrong, and if the Paramedic really listens, the patient will tell the Paramedic how to fix it![2] If history taking is improperly performed, however, the Paramedic can be led to a completely different conclusion about the patient's illness. Therefore, the history must be conscientiously gathered on a patient-by-patient, case-by-case basis. The history and chief concern must also be confirmed with the patient and not be taken for granted from dispatch information or other EMS providers.

The Art and Science of History Taking

The science in history taking is asking the right questions of the patient and interpreting the answers to those questions. The art in history taking is developing a relationship with the patient that allows the Paramedic to ask the right questions and also allows the Paramedic to trust that the patient will provide open and honest answers to those questions.

Emergency medicine is a field of medical practice which often requires a great deal of data to be gathered in a very limited amount of time.[3-5] To achieve this goal, the Paramedic must combine art and science to a great degree. Patient care experience is the best teacher in the art of history taking. However, some basic tenets apply.

Setting the Stage

Any medical records available should be briefly reviewed; for example, a Vial of Life® (Figure 15-1). Important data such as previous illnesses and treatments can often be easily obtained from such records. If the patient is in the care of another provider upon arrival, then a brief report should also be obtained from that person. The Paramedic should also consider the environment in which the interview takes place, as a proper atmosphere can greatly enhance effective communication.

The Paramedic should try to make the patient as comfortable as possible and be respectful of personal space. Generally, there should not be any obstacles, but a distance of a few feet should lie between the Paramedic and the patient. During the interview, the Paramedic should be alert to the patient's comfort level.[6,7] The Paramedic should watch for any signs of

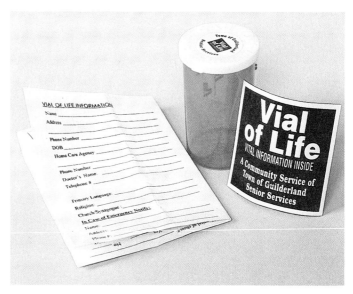

Figure 15-1 The Vial of Life® can provide important patient information.

uneasiness and, if necessary, ask the patient directly about his feelings. Standing over a supine or sitting patient implies a position of power and can be detrimental to good communication. Remember that just as the Paramedic watches the patient for nonverbal clues, so is the patient watching the Paramedic. Paramedics must always be aware of the messages transmitted by both words and actions. Paramedics must be sensitive to those messages and control them as well as possible.

The Paramedic only has one chance to make a good first impression. A clean, neat, and professional appearance implies to a patient that the Paramedic will be a proficient medical provider. A slovenly appearance, in contrast, leaves the patient wondering if the Paramedic will take better care of him than the patient can give himself. Due to the volume of information contained in the patient's history, it may be necessary for the Paramedic to take notes during the interview. Most patients are just fine with note taking, but it should never divert the Paramedic's attention from the patient. If note taking is necessary, the Paramedic should try to make "shorthand" notes which she can then later transcribe onto the final report.

When the Paramedic meets the patient for the first time, he should formally introduce himself and explain his job function. For example, a Paramedic might say, "Good morning sir, I'm Marvin, a Paramedic with the ambulance." If the patient does not identify himself, then the Paramedic should ask for her name. The Paramedic might ask, "What would you like us to call you?"

The Paramedic should pay close attention to the way the patient responds. People who introduce themselves with titles or their full name usually expect the Paramedic to address them that way. Avoid using demeaning terms like "Honey" "Sweetheart" or "Bud."

Starting the Interview

After introductions are made, the Paramedic should ask the patient open-ended questions in an effort to help determine the problem.[6] An open-ended question is one which cannot be answered simply with yes or no. This type of question allows the patient to answer in his or her own words and generates a history which is less biased by the Paramedic's own interpretation. A good example of an open-ended question would be: "What's seems to be the trouble today?" or "Why did you call for EMS today?" Once a dialogue has been opened, the Paramedic should follow the patient's lead and guide him through the interview without diverting the patient from his own account. Some follow-up questions might be: "Can you tell me any more about that?", and "Anything else you can think of?" Some techniques which might assist the Paramedic in this process include **facilitation**, **reflection**, **clarification**, **interpretation**, and **direct questioning** about feelings (Table 15-1).

Table 15-1 Interviewing Techniques

Facilitation

Actions such as the Paramedic nodding his head in acknowledgement and saying "Go on," as well as trying to make eye contact, may encourage the patient to continue talking about a subject.

Reflection

Repeating the patient's words may encourage additional responses. An example would be: Paramedic: "You said it was a crushing pain?" Patient: "It felt like a vise around my chest." Reflection is helpful because it typically doesn't interrupt the patient's train of thought.

Clarification

Make sure to clarify statements which are unclear or vague.

Empathetic Response

Try to show the patient acceptance and understanding of how he or she feels.

Confrontation

When the patient's story has been inconsistent, directly presenting the patient with the inconsistencies about the words or actions can sometimes be helpful. An example might be when a patient tells the Paramedic that the topic they are discussing is not disturbing to him, but then begins to cry. The Paramedic could then directly question the patient about this inconsistency.

Interpretation

A step beyond confrontation in which the Paramedic, as the history taker, actually makes an interpretation of the patient's words or actions and presents it to the patient. For example, as in the previous case in interpretation the Paramedic might state why the Paramedic thinks the story is inconsistent.

This results in direct questioning about feelings.

Unless asked, patients may not offer how their chief concern makes them feel.

The Structure and Content of the Patient History

The patient history consists of several individual elements, each of which serves a specific purpose. Together these parts provide the structure of the history. A comprehensive medical history (Table 15-2) is taken to discover as much information about a patient's concerns, interpersonal relationships, and medical history as possible.

The Focused History

The comprehensive history, due to the extensive amount of data it collects, is often not used in emergent situations. When time is of the essence, a focused history concentrating on the **chief concern (CC)**, **history of present illness (HPI)**, significant **past medical history (PMH)**, and pertinent current health status information is obtained.

The mnemonic SAMPLED can be used to help remember the different historical components that are important to obtain (Table 15-3).

Chief Concern

The chief concern is the main reason for which the patient is seeking medical care. It is best discovered by asking an open-ended question. Whenever feasible, it should be expressed

Table 15-3 SAMPLED History

S	Signs and symptoms (chief concern plus OPQRST AS/PN)
A	Allergies
M	Medications
P	Past medical history
L	List whatever is important based on chief concern: meal, MD visit, menses, and so on
E	Events leading up to chief concern
D	Does the patient have any advance directives (e.g., healthcare proxy, POLST)?

Table 15-2 Elements of a Comprehensive History

Date and time	• Psychiatric illnesses
Identifying data	• Accidents and injuries
• Age	• Operations
• Sex	• Hospitalizations
• Race	Current health status focuses on present state of health
• Birthplace	• Current medications
• Occupation	• Allergies
Source of referral	• Tobacco use
• Who called the ambulance?	• Alcohol, drugs, and related substances
Source of history	• Diet
• Patient	• Screening test
• Family	• Immunizations
• Friends	• Sleep patterns
• Police	• Exercise and leisure activities
• Others	• Environmental hazards
• Reliability	• Use of safety measures
• Variable reliability	Family history
• Memory, trust, and motivation	Psychosocial history
• Assessed at the end of the interview	• Home situation and significant other
Chief concern	• Daily life
History of present illness	• Important experiences
Past history	• Religious beliefs
• General state of health	• Patient's outlook
• Childhood illnesses	Review of body systems
• Adult illnesses	

and documented in the patient's own words. Occasionally a patient's own words will be too vulgar or ambiguous to use directly. In these cases, it is often best to paraphrase the comments in more precise medical language.

History of Present Illness

Once the Paramedic has determined the main symptom that is causing the patient's distress, it is important to gather as many attributes of that symptom as possible. The responses given by the patient allow the Paramedic to think about associated body systems and develop an idea of the nature of the illness. Several mnemonics can be used to help the Paramedic recall the essential elements of the history based on the chief concern.

The mnemonic OPQRST AS/PN (Table 15-4) can be used for any concern of pain. The severity of pain can be measured using a simple "mild, moderate, severe" scale or using a 0 to 10 or Faces scale (Figure 15-2). Other mnemonics can also be useful for specific chief concerns (Table 15-5).

To gather further information, the Paramedic often needs to directly ask the patient questions about the symptoms. When asking a direct question of the patient, the Paramedic should be careful not to ask a **leading question**.

A leading question is one which may direct the patient toward an answer that might not necessarily have been given if asked in another manner. For example, instead of asking "Was the pain crushing?" the Paramedic should ask, "Tell me what the pain in your chest was like." The Paramedic should also be careful to ask only one question at a time to avoid confusing the patient. The Paramedic should remember to use language that is appropriate to the patient's education and knowledge level. When in doubt, it is always best to use plain language instead of medical jargon. An example might be, "Do you ever feel like your heart is racing?" as opposed to "Do you have palpitations?"

Table 15-4 OPQRST AS/PN Mnemonic to Help Obtain a History about Painful Concerns

Onset	When did the pain start?
Provoke	What caused the pain? What makes it worse?
Quality	Describe the pain.
Region	Where is the pain? Where did it start?
Radiation	Does the pain radiate or migrate?
Relief	Is there anything that improves or relieves the pain?
Recurrence	Is there anything that makes the pain return?
Severity	How severe is the pain?
Timing	When did it start?
Associated Symptoms	What other symptoms does the patient have along with the chief concern?
Pertinent Negatives	Associated symptoms important to the chief concern that *are not* present; for example, chest pain without shortness of breath.

Past Medical History and Current Health Status

Certain information about the patient's past medical history and current heath status should be obtained with every patient contact. However, there are many aspects of one's medical history, most of which are not necessary to obtain during a medical emergency. The key is to focus on significant historical information or those aspects necessary to determine the nature and potential severity of the patient's illness or injury. All patients should be questioned about chronic illnesses, medications taken, allergies, and tobacco, alcohol, or other drug use.

Some medical conditions are specific to related body systems (Table 15-6). Most patients should be specifically asked about heart problems, hypertension, breathing problems, and diabetes.

Universal Pain Assessment Tool

This pain assessment tool is intended to help patient care providers assess pain according to individual patient needs. Explain and use 0–10 Scale for patient self-assessment. Use the faces or behavioral observations to interpret expressed pain when patient cannot communicate his/her pain intensity.

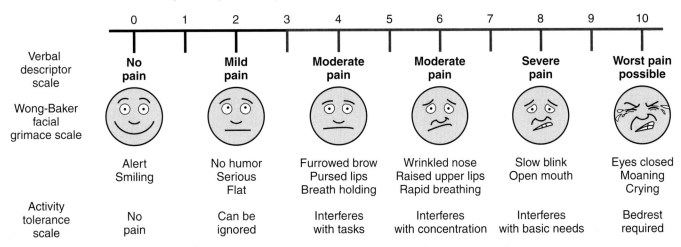

Figure 15-2 Example of several different pain assessment scales in one reference. (Photo courtesy of UCLA Department of Anesthesiology, David Geffen School of Medicine at UCLA)

Table 15-5 Other Useful Mnemonics for Obtaining the History of Present Illness

System	Elements
Any concern of pain	OPQRST AS/PN as described previously
Altered mental status	AEIOU-TIPS A – alcohol E – epilepsy/seizure I – insulin (hyper- and hypoglycemia) O – overdose U – uremia/metabolic T – trauma I – infection P – psychiatric S – stroke
Shortness of breath	HAPI-SOCS H – history of pulmonary disease A – activity at onset P – pain on inspiration I – infection symptoms (chills, night sweats, fever) S – smoker (# packs per day x number of years = # pack years O – orthopnea C – cough? productive? S – sputum (and color)?
Psychiatric/Depression	IN SAD CAGES IN – interest (apathy, withdrawn, disinterested) S – sleep disorder (insomnia, night walking) A – appetite D – depression/mood swings C – concentration A – activity G – guilt E – energy S – suicidal ideation

Table 15-6 Past Medical Conditions Related to Specific Body Systems

System	Past Medical History
Neurological	Stroke, seizure, head injury
Cardiovascular	Acute myocardial infarction, angina, coronary artery bypass graft (CABG), angioplasty/cardiac catheterization
Respiratory	Asthma, emphysema, smoking, hospitalization, intubation
Gastrointestinal	Surgery, abdominal aortic aneurysm, appendicitis, small bowel obstruction
Genitourinary	STD, pregnancy, abortions, kidney stones
Musculoskeletal	Fractures, surgery, multiple sclerosis, sports injuries
Psychiatric	Depression, suicide attempts, admission, medications, drug and alcohol use
Endocrine	Diabetes, thyroid disorder, surgery
Hematologic	Leukemia, infection, travel, transfusion
Allergic	Known allergies, allergy testing, anaphylaxis history

Allergies

The Paramedic should determine if the patient has any allergies to medications. If an allergy is reported by the patient, the Paramedic should inquire what type of reaction the patient had to the medication. In some cases, a reported allergy is actually a common side effect or a familial "allergy" in which the patient's relative is allergic, so the patient avoids a certain medicine. If related to the chief concern, such as a bee sting, the Paramedic should inquire about environmental allergies.

Medications

The Paramedic should ask the patient about any medication use and inquire about prescription, over the counter, and homeopathic or nutritional substances. The Paramedic should also determine if the patient is compliant with medication use and how long the patient has been taking each medicine. It is important to ask about recent changes in medications, such as dosage.

Tobacco, Alcohol, and Drug Use

The use of tobacco, alcohol, or other recreational drugs is a significant risk factor for many diseases.[8-22] Knowledge of their use may raise the Paramedic's index of suspicion for certain illnesses such as heart or vascular disease, COPD, and cirrhosis.

Clinical Reasoning

Based on the patient's chief concern, history of present illness, and answers to direct questioning, the Paramedic can develop a general sense of the body systems that may be involved in the patient's problem. Forming this impression

STREET SMART

Occasionally when Paramedics ask a patient if he has any medical problems, some patients will tell the Paramedic that there are not any, even though there is a history of a chronic disease. People sometimes feel that, since they are under care for an illness, it is no longer "a problem." The best approach is to ask if the patient has any medical problems and then ask if the patient has ever been under a health provider's care for any reason.

will allow the Paramedic to decide which other questions she should ask and which physical exams she should perform to confirm the Paramedic's conclusion. Clinical decision making is discussed further in Chapter 17.

Special Challenges to History Taking

The Paramedic can face difficulty in obtaining an accurate medical history in some situations. Application of several simple techniques can assist the Paramedic in obtaining a history in these situations.

Sensitive Topics

It is often imperative to question the patient about topics that may be embarrassing or socially sensitive in order to learn more about factors which may have contributed to the illness. These topics might include such issues as drug and alcohol use, physical abuse, and sexual history. Much of the difficulty in asking sensitive questions lies with our own biases, embarrassment, or perceptions with these topics. Some patients will readily answer these questions when asked in a professional manner. Questioning a patient about these topics becomes easier with experience. It is often helpful for each individual Paramedic to observe more seasoned providers obtaining this information and then develop an effective method which works.

Silence

For many of us, silence is uncomfortable. Nonetheless, it must be remembered that silence has many uses and possible meanings. Patients may use silence to collect their thoughts or remember details about their concerns. Silence may be the result of insensitivity by the Paramedic in asking questions, or the patient may be taking some time to decide whether or not to trust the Paramedic.

Whenever confronted with unexpected silence, the Paramedic should be alert for nonverbal clues of distress and try to determine if anything in his interview technique might be responsible for them.

Overly Talkative Patients

It is easy to become impatient with an overly talkative patient when time is of the essence. A few techniques may be helpful in this difficult situation.

Although not ideal, the Paramedic may have to lower expectations and accept a less comprehensive history. It may be helpful for the Paramedic to allow the patient free reign for the first few minutes and then directly question the patient about the most important details. If necessary, he should interrupt the patient as gently as possible and summarize the history as succinctly as possible. Phrases such as "I'd like to hear more about the chest pain you had before you called us" may help to refocus the patient on the chief concern.

Regardless of the situation, the Paramedic should not let impatience show. If necessary, he should explain to the patient that time is short and that the current discussion will be continued later.

Patients with Multiple Symptoms

Some patients seem to have every possible symptom. Although it's possible that this patient might have multiple organic illnesses, it's more likely that other confounding factors are present. The Paramedic should refocus the patient on one concern by asking the patient about the most important concern, for example, "You told me many concerns. Which is the most important concern, or the reason you called us to help you today?"

Anxious Patients

It is natural for a patient to be anxious during a medical emergency. For some patients, anxiety has significant implications in their reaction to their illness or even may have contributed to their illness. The Paramedic should be conscious of nonverbal clues to the patient's anxiety and, when he senses anxiety, encourage the patient to talk about his or her feelings.

Reassurance

Providing reassurance to patients can be both beneficial and harmful depending on the way it is provided. In an emergency situation, many patients worry not only about their condition, but also how it affects others they care for or love. By providing reassurance, the Paramedic can help calm the patient down, allowing him to make appropriate medical decisions or be more cooperative with the assessment and treatment. Conversely, reassurance can provide false hope if provided improperly. Statements like, "Everything will be OK" and "You have nothing to worry about" are detrimental when patient receive the news that they have developed a severe condition. It is more appropriate to acknowledge that there are factors that are of concern, but state that it is better to focus on getting well first and take it a step at a time. Reassurance that the patient is in good hands or going to see a good physician can also help the Paramedic provide positive reassurance to the patient without creating a false expectation.

Anger and Hostility

It is not unusual for patients to exhibit anger toward healthcare personnel for a variety of reasons, including feeling unwell, suffering anxiety, or developing a feeling they have lost control over their lives. Paramedics should not take this behavior as anger against them personally. They can attempt to defuse the patient's anger by identifying that, although they understand he is angry, you are there to help him. Paramedics should always remember that their safety and that of their crew are paramount, and thus they should retreat from any situation which becomes dangerous.[23,24]

The Intoxicated Patient

Acutely intoxicated patients who are belligerent, angry, or uncooperative can be some of the most difficult patients to interview. Paramedics should use a calm, direct voice and simple directions to encourage the patient to allow himself to be assessed and treated. The Paramedic should try to avoid talking to the patient in a confined area, as the patient may feel trapped and react with hostility. Intoxicated patients can be unpredictable; as a result, sudden violence is always a possibility.[25] Paramedics should always have an escape route planned and retreat from any situation which cannot be easily de-escalated.[26] Patients who appear clinically intoxicated do not have the capacity to refuse care. Signs of clinical intoxication include slurred speech, disorganized thinking, inappropriate responses to your questions, combativeness, and staggering gait. A Paramedic may need to enlist the aid of local law enforcement to assist in bringing the patient to the emergency department for evaluation if the patient refuses to go.

Crying

Crying is an important clue to emotions.[27–29] The Paramedic should be supportive and wait for the patient to recover. Quiet acceptance or a supportive comment may assist the patient in composing herself and continuing the interview. Handing the patient tissues is a gesture that is always appreciated.

Depression

Depression is a common medical problem and can have multiple manifestations. The Paramedic should always maintain a high index of suspicion for depression in patients complaining of multiple, vague symptoms. If the patient is depressed, one should be concerned for the possibility of self-harm and question the patient directly about suicidal thoughts.[30] Any patient with the potential for self-harm must be transported to an emergency department for further evaluation.

Seductive Patients

Occasionally a provider may feel attracted to a patient. If the Paramedic becomes aware of such feelings, one should realize that these thoughts are normal responses. However, one must prevent these feelings from affecting her professional interaction with the patient. Some patients may make sexual advances toward the Paramedic. Paramedics need to make clear to these patients that the relationship with them is purely professional. It is unethical, and in some states illegal, for a Paramedic to have a personal and/or sexual relationship with a patient who is under his or her care.

Confusing Behaviors or Histories

Occasionally, despite best efforts, the patient's history does not appear to make sense and the Paramedic may feel baffled or confused. While many of these situations involve an emotional component, the Paramedic should avoid dismissing the patient's concerns and instead attempt to focus in on a single chief concern.

Limited Intelligence

Most patients with even moderately limited intelligence can usually give adequate histories. When patients suffer from severe mental impairment, however, most of the history will have to be derived from other sources, such as family, friends, or medical charts. The Paramedic should use simple language when interviewing the patient and listen closely as the patient describes tests or other elements of his medical history.

However, the Paramedic should be careful about making assumptions about the patient's level of functioning. The best technique, just as with any other patient, is to establish a relationship first with the patient and then, if necessary, seek other sources for history.

Language Barriers

When confronted with a patient–provider language barrier, the Paramedic should make every effort to obtain a translator. The best translator is a neutral, objective observer who is fluent in both languages. Using a family member often leads to distorted meanings and may present a confidentiality problem.[31,32] The Paramedic should look at the patient when talking, and not the translator. Also, he should ensure that the translator asks the patient the question and is not just answering the question for the patient.

CULTURAL/REGIONAL DIFFERENCES

In many regions and cultures, it is disrespectful for children to question their elders, especially in personal matters. Usually, however, the children are fluent in the two languages. If it is necessary to use children as translators, one should ask as few questions as possible and alert the staff at the hospital so that a more thorough and accurate history can be obtained.

Hearing Impaired Patients

Patients with hearing impairments may present as many issues as those with language barriers. The Paramedic should look at the patient directly while talking and speak slowly. Often the patient is able to read lips well enough to answer the Paramedic's questions. He should avoid shouting or raising his voice unless the patient indicates it helps her hear the questions. If the patient has a "good ear," the Paramedic should make a point of speaking toward that ear. Communication through written notes, although time-consuming, may be the only solution to obtaining an adequate history.

Vision Impaired Patients

When talking to a patient with limited vision, the Paramedic should make sure to identify herself, alert the patient to her location, and explain what is being done. She should remember to always respond vocally to the patient and avoid raising her voice while speaking. The Paramedic may need to explain procedures and actions in more detail than is needed for patients with normal vision. If walking with a patient with vision impairment, the patient should grasp the Paramedic's arm rather than the Paramedic grasping his or hers. The Paramedic should avoid making any sudden movements that may increase the patient's anxiety in what is likely already a stressful situation.

Family and Friends

Sometimes the Paramedic may need to elicit the history from family, friends, or other bystanders.[33] Whenever possible, the Paramedic should get the patient's permission to discuss the condition with the other person. If the Paramedic cannot get permission, then he should remember that all medical information derived from the patient interview or exam must be held confidential and not shared with the third party.[34–37]

CONCLUSION

The novice Paramedic must master the skill of history taking in order to be effective at providing care to the vast array of patients encountered during one's career. With practice and by observing other experienced healthcare providers obtain a history from a patient, the novice Paramedic will soon develop and refine her skill.

KEY POINTS:

- History taking is the medical questioning of a patient for purposes of ascertaining the disorder, syndrome, or condition affecting the patient that resulted in the activation of EMS.

- The Paramedic must be aware of the messages transmitted by words and actions and have a professional appearance and calm demeanor.

- The Paramedic should formally and respectfully introduce himself and explain his job function.

- The Paramedic should inquire as to the patient's preferred manner of address.

- An open-ended question allows the patient to answer in his or her own words rather than give a simple answer of yes or no.

- Interviewing techniques which assist the Paramedic in developing questions and promote dialogue include facilitation, reflection, clarification, interpretation, and direct questioning.

- A comprehensive medical history is taken to discover as much information as possible about a patient's concerns, interpersonal relationships, and medical history. However, it is often not used in emergent situations due to the extensive amount of data it collects and time required.

- A focused history can be conducted by the Paramedic to concentrate on the chief concern, history of present illness, significant past medical history, and pertinent current health status. The mnemonic SAMPLE is used to remember the different historical components of a focused history.

- The chief concern is the main reason EMS was activated and should be expressed and documented in the patient's own words using quotation marks.

- Several methods can be used to assess a patient's pain, from a simple "mild, moderate, severe" scale to a 0 to 10 or faces scale.

- The mnemonic device OPQRST AS/PN can be used for any concern of pain. The mnemonic AEIOU-TIPS is used for altered mental status.

- The mnemonic HAPI-SOCS is used for shortness of breath.

- The mnemonic IN SAD CAGES is used for psychiatric issues/depression.

- The mnemonic SAMPLE is used for gathering past history. Ask additional questions for clarification.

- The Paramedic should be conscious of nonverbal clues to anxiety or anger.

- When communicating with an acutely intoxicated patient, the Paramedic should use a calm direct voice, and give simple directions to encourage patient access to evaluation and treatment.

- Strong emotions exhibited by the patient during an interview may require the Paramedic to assist the patient through quiet acceptance or a supportive comment.

- The Paramedic should always keep the patient relationship professional.

- The Paramedic should use simple language, listen closely, and not make assumptions about a patient's level of function when interviewing patients with mental impairments.

- When confronted with a patient–provider language barrier, the Paramedic should make every effort to obtain a translator.

- The Paramedic should explain who he is, where he is, and what he will be doing in a clear, normal tone of voice for the vision impaired patient.

- All medical information derived from the patient interview or exam must be held confidential and not shared with a third party.

REVIEW QUESTIONS:

1. How can the Paramedic set the stage for an effective patient interview?
2. List the interviewing techniques that can assist the Paramedic in developing questions and promote dialogue with a patient.
3. A male patient makes sexually suggestive statements to a female Paramedic. How should the Paramedic handle this patient?
4. List the components of the focused history and the information acquired by asking those questions.
5. Why is it critical for the Paramedic to ask about tobacco, alcohol, and other recreational drugs? How might the Paramedic do so?
6. You are called to a nursing home to transport an elderly male patient who is febrile, barely responsive, and hypoxemic on room air. You attempt to obtain a history from the patient without success due to his mental status. What other sources of information can be helpful to you and the emergency department? What questions are important to ask?
7. If confronted with an overly talkative patient, what can the Paramedic do to effectively gather a medical history?
8. Using a translator, a Paramedic is speaking with a patient with a language barrier. What should he be conscious of when asking and receiving responses to questions?

CASE STUDY QUESTIONS:

Please refer to the Case Study at the beginning of the chapter and answer the questions below.

1. What mnemonic is best for
   - Shortness of breath
   - Pain
   - Altered mental status
   - Psychiatric disorders or depression
2. What is the value of a mnemonic in history gathering?

REFERENCES:

1. Bickley LS, Szilagyi PG. *Bates' Guide to Physical Examination and History Taking* (9th ed.) with E-Book *(Guide to Physical Exam & History Taking (Bates))*. Philadelphia: Lippincott Williams & Wilkins; 2007.

2. Trautlein JJ, Lambert RL, Miller J. Malpractice in the emergency department—review of 200 cases. *Ann Emerg Med*. 1984; 13(9 Pt 1):709–711.

3. Considine J, Botti M, Thomas S. Do knowledge and experience have specific roles in triage decision-making? *Acad Emerg Med*. 2007;14(8):722–726.

4. Croskerry P, Sinclair D. Emergency medicine: a practice prone to error? *Cjem*. 2001;3(4):271–276.

5. Juckett G. Cross-cultural medicine. *Am Fam Physician*. 2005;72(11):2267–2274.

6. Novack DH, Dube C, Goldstein MG. Teaching medical interviewing. A basic course on interviewing and the physician–patient relationship. *Arch Intern Med*. 1992;152(9):1814–1820.

7. McGuire BN, Ahmed AH, Regan T. Methods of obtaining a medical history in the emergency department. *Academic Emergency Medicine*. 2001;8(5):469–470.

8. O'Keefe JH, Bybee KA, Lavie CJ. Alcohol and cardiovascular health: the razor-sharp double-edged sword. *J Am Coll Cardiol*. 2007;50(11):1009–1014.

9. **http://www.cdc.gov/alcohol/**

10. Boffetta P, Garfinkel L. Alcohol drinking and mortality among men enrolled in an American Cancer Society prospective study. *Epidemiology*. 1990;1(5):342–348.

11. Beulens JW, Hendriks HF. Alcohol and ischaemic heart disease. *Lancet*. 2006;367(9514):902; author reply 902.

12. Chao A, Thun MJ, Jacobs EJ, Henley SJ, Rodriguez C, Calle EE. Cigarette smoking and colorectal cancer mortality in the cancer prevention study II. *J Natl Cancer Inst*. 2000;92(23):1888–1896.

13. Villeneuve PJ, Mao Y. Lifetime probability of developing lung cancer, by smoking status, Canada. *Can J Public Health*. 1994;85(6):385–388.

14. Calle EE, Miracle-McMahill HL, Thun MJ, Heath CW, Jr. Cigarette smoking and risk of fatal breast cancer. *Am J Epidemiol*. 1994;139(10):1001–1007.

15. Pinto BM, Rabin C, Farrell N. Lifestyle and coronary heart disease prevention. *Prim Care*. 2005;32(4):947–961.

16. Hughes JR. Clinical significance of tobacco withdrawal. *Nicotine Tob Res*. 2006;8(2):153–156.

17. **http://www.cancer.gov/cancertopics/factsheet/Tobacco/cessation**

18. Daniel JC, Huynh TT, Zhou W, Kougias P, El Sayed HF, Huh J, et al. Acute aortic dissection associated with use of cocaine. *J Vasc Surg*. 2007;46(3):427–433.

19. Jager G, de Win MM, van der Tweel I, Schilt T, Kahn RS, van den Brink W, et al. Assessment of cognitive brain function in ecstasy users and contributions of other drugs of abuse: results from an FMRI study. *Neuropsychopharmacology*. 2008;33(2):247–258.

20. Swahn MH, Bossarte RM. Gender, early alcohol use, and suicide ideation and attempts: findings from the 2005 youth risk behavior survey. *J Adolesc Health*. 2007;41(2):175–181.

21. Cunningham R, Walton MA, et al. Past-year violence typologies among patients with cocaine-related chest pain. *Am J Drug Alcohol Abuse*. 2007;33(4):571–582.

22. Levis JT, Garmel GM. Cocaine-associated chest pain. *Emerg Med Clin North Am*. 2005;23(4):1083–1103.

23. Hodge AN, Marshall AP. Violence and aggression in the emergency department: a critical care perspective. *Aust Crit Care*. 2007;20(2):61–67.

24. Ray MM. The dark side of the job: violence in the emergency department. *J Emerg Nurs*. 2007;33(3):257–261.

25. Allely P, Graham W, McDonnell M, Spedding R. Alcohol levels in the emergency department: a worrying trend. *Emerg Med J*. 2006;23(9):707–708.

26. Ferns T, Cork A, Rew M. Personal safety in the accident and emergency department. *Br J Nurs*. 2005;14(13):725–730.

27. Casement PJ. *Learning from the Patient*. New York: The Guilford Press; 1992.

28. Tateno A, Jorge RE, Robinson RG. Pathological laughing and crying following traumatic brain injury. *J Neuropsychiatry Clin Neurosci*. 2004;16(4):426–434.

29. Murube J, Murube L, Murube A. Origin and types of emotional tearing. *Eur J Ophthalmol*. 1999;9(2):77–84.

30. Dominguez OJ, Jr. What's so unusual? *Emerg Med Serv*. 2001;30(3):102.

31. Dunckley M, Hughes R, Addington-Hall J, Higginson IJ. Language translation of outcome measurement tools: views of health professionals. *Int J Palliat Nurs*. 2003;9(2):49–55.

32. Rollins G. Translation, por favor. *Hosp Health Netw*. 2002;76(12):41, 46–50.

33. Herman M, Le A. The crying infant. *Emerg Med Clin North Am*. 2007;25(4):1137–1159, vii.

34. Campbell SG, Sinclair DE. Strategies for managing a busy emergency department. *Cjem*. 2004;6(4):271–276.

35. Moskop JC, Marco CA, Larkin GL, Geiderman JM, Derse AR. From Hippocrates to HIPAA: privacy and confidentiality in emergency medicine—part II: challenges in the emergency department. *Ann Emerg Med*. 2005;45(1):60–67.

36. Moskop JC, Marco CA, Larkin GL, Geiderman JM, Derse AR. From Hippocrates to HIPAA: Privacy and confidentiality in emergency medicine—part I: conceptual, moral, and legal foundations. *Ann Emerg Med*. 2005;45(1):53–59.

37. Olsen JC, Sabin BR. Emergency department patient perceptions of privacy and confidentiality. *J Emerg Med*. 2003;25(3):329–333.

PHYSICAL EXAMINATION AND SECONDARY ASSESSMENT

KEY CONCEPTS:

Upon completion of this chapter, it is expected that the reader will understand these following concepts:

- The four components of each physical exam
- When a focused history and physical exam should be conducted on the scene or a rapid physical exam is appropriate
- Detailed physical examination and its appropriate use
- Matching the proper physical assessment with the patient's presentation or chief complaint
- The ongoing assessment as a repeat of the initial assessment and used to detect trends

▶ CASE STUDY:

Two new students were in the back of the room, bored. They asked each other, "Why do we bother doing a physical exam? The nurses don't pay attention to us and the docs just repeat everything." The instructor for the class, a senior Paramedic, said," Come over here. I'll bet that after a few minutes, you can figure out whether this 'patient' has pneumonia or congestive failure. You can also select the correct treatment as the wrong one can worsen your patient's condition."

After practicing for a while, the students were convinced!

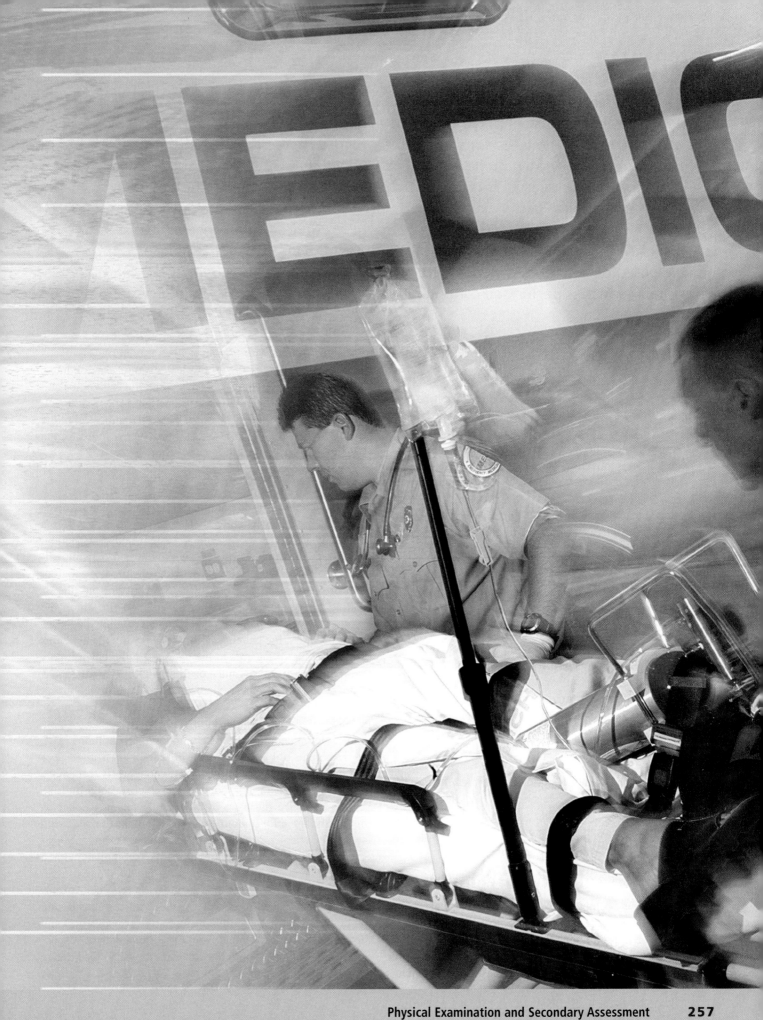

OVERVIEW

After performing the initial assessment and determining patient priority, the next step in patient assessment is to conduct the appropriate history and physical exam. This chapter reviews the basic components of a focused assessment. It also provides techniques for gathering a patient's vital signs. In this chapter physical assessments are identified by mechanism of injury or the patient's chief concern. The detailed physical examination is performed on a patient to determine additional information. However, it may not be appropriate for all patient encounters. The ongoing assessment is also a critical component that allows the Paramedic to alter the treatment plan if needed based on established trends. The ongoing assessment is a repeat of the initial assessment, which is performed continuously throughout the patient encounter.

Physical Examination

During a **physical examination** (also called exam), the Paramedic performs an assessment of the patient from head to toe in an effort to detect **signs** associated with a disease or condition. This may include signs that confirm that a disease or condition is present, thus helping the Paramedic decide which condition is most likely causing the patient's chief concern during this encounter. One example is auscultation of the breath sounds to decide whether the patient's shortness of breath is due to heart failure or asthma. The physical exam may also detect signs of a disease or condition that is present and not related to the patient's chief concern, but which may need to be addressed by the Paramedic. For example, when evaluating a patient who complains of chest pain, the Paramedic may determine, by the patient's history, that the condition is cardiac in nature. This could lead the Paramedic to decide that the patient has developed heart failure during this cardiac event after auscultating the breath sounds.

By developing excellent physical examination skills, the Paramedic can determine a treatment plan when the history does not clearly provide a guide. These skills are also important in situations where the history is not obtainable, as in the case of an unconscious patient. Excellent physical examination skills develop through practice, understanding the pathophysiology of disease, and understanding how diseases commonly present themselves.[1] Whether performing clinical rotations or being a practicing Paramedic, it is helpful to ask the ED practitioners to point out interesting examination findings. This helps Paramedics recognize them on future patients.

Physical Examination Techniques

There are four components to every physical exam: (1) inspection, (2) auscultation, (3) palpation, and (4) percussion. These four components are the essential "hands on" techniques used to assess the patient. In addition to these four techniques, the Paramedic routinely measures the patient's vital signs to complete the physical examination. The Paramedic then combines these physical examination findings, the vital signs, and the history (discussed in Chapter 15) and formulates a treatment plan for the patient. These skills are critical. Although these skills were probably addressed in the Paramedic's basic EMS classes, they will be expanded for the Paramedic as a higher skill level is required.

Inspection

Inspection is a physical examination technique that involves looking at the patient (Figure 16-1). This can take many forms depending upon the specific body system under inspection. The Paramedic should observe the patient and her immediate environment. Observing the patient's posture and apparent level of distress can give clues to the severity of the illness. Making observations about the environment in which the Paramedic finds the patient can help in determining the mechanism of injury, the patient's ability to carry out the activities of daily living, or hazards in the patient's living environment that may lead to future injury or illness. Observing the environment may allow the Paramedic to discover information that leads to additional history taking. Make note of such things as mechanism of injury, medication bottles, any evidence of any illicit drug or alcohol use, and general living conditions.[2,3]

Examples of body system-specific findings from inspection include discovering **lacerations**, **ecchymosis** (bruising), or **abrasions** in an injured extremity; observing **jugular venous pressure** during a cardiovascular exam; or observing the abdomen for **distention**. These findings are discussed later in the chapter during the system specific examinations.

As inspection is difficult to fully accomplish with a clothed patient, it typically requires the patient to be exposed. Judgment is required to balance the need for a complete examination and the need to keep the patient warm (considering the environment in which the examination is occurring) and the patient's modesty intact. Certain components of inspection may need to wait until the patient is moved to the relative privacy of the ambulance.

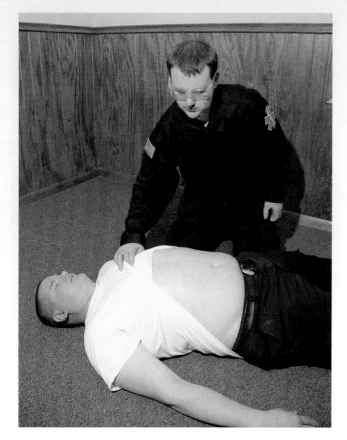

Figure 16-1 Inspection of a trauma patient's abdomen for ecchymosis.

Auscultation

Auscultation is assessing the patient through listening. The assessment tool used during auscultation, the **stethoscope**, is made up of a hollow flexible tube connected to ear pieces that are placed in the Paramedic's ears. The other end of the stethoscope comes in several different sizes (depending on whether the patient is a neonate, adolescent, or adult) and typically consists of two heads: one that is flat (called the diaphragm) and one that is cup-shaped (called the bell) (Figure 16-2). The diaphragm is covered with a thin plastic membrane and acts like the tympanic membrane (eardrum) to amplify and transmit sounds up the stethoscope to the Paramedic's ears. The diaphragm is placed firmly against the bare skin (Figure 16-3a) and is used to pick up higher pitched sounds (e.g., breath sounds). In contrast, the bell is placed lightly on the bare skin (Figure 16-3b) and is used to pick up lower pitched sounds (e.g., the whoosh of a carotid bruit). If the bell is held too tightly against the skin, the skin will stretch tight and act like the diaphragm. In this case, it will lose the ability to detect the lower pitched sounds.[4,5]

When auscultating the patient, note both normal or abnormal sounds, the location of the sounds, and the intensity of the sounds. Specific auscultation techniques and findings will be detailed later in this chapter when discussing specific body system exams.

Palpation

Palpation is the most frequently used physical exam technique. It involves the provider placing his hands or fingers on the patient's body in an effort to detect any abnormalities. Palpation can take many forms depending upon the abnormality the Paramedic is assessing. Different forms of palpation can be used to assess for stability and assess for tenderness. Deep palpation can be used to assess deeper structures (e.g., deep palpation of the abdomen to detect

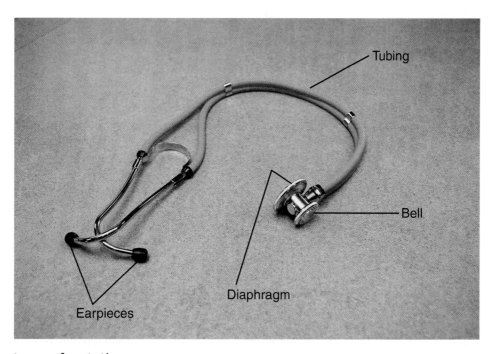

Figure 16-2 Anatomy of a stethoscope.

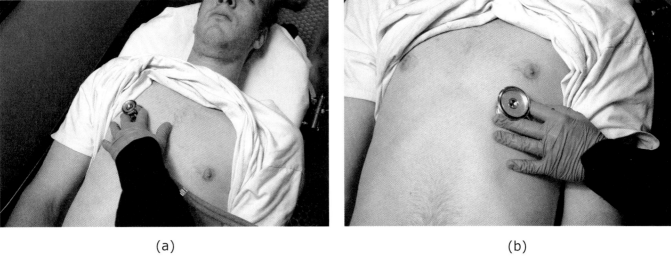

(a)   (b)

Figure 16-3 (a) Auscultation using the diaphragm. (b) Auscultation using the bell.

tenderness or **masses**) (Figure 16-4a), while light palpation can be used to assess for superficial findings (e.g., light palpation of the anterior chest wall to detect subcutaneous emphysema) (Figure 16-4b). Firm palpation along a bony structure can assess for tenderness or **crepitus** (Figure 16-4c). The stability of a joint may be assessed by firmly grasping the bones distal and proximal to the joint and applying stress to the joint's connective tissues (Figure 16-4d). Specific findings and palpation techniques are discussed later in this chapter.

Percussion

Percussion is the act of lightly but sharply tapping the body surface to determine the characteristics of the underlying tissue. It is performed by sharply striking the hyperextended distal joint of one middle finger with the tip of the partially flexed middle finger of the other hand (Figure 16-5). Percussion assesses whether the underlying tissues are air-filled, fluid filled, or solid by the quality of the **percussion note**. Air-filled structures will produce a hollow, tympanic percussion note similar to that of a drum. Fluid-filled structures will produce a dull percussion note. This can be simulated by taking a full plastic bottle of water, laying it on its side, and percussing the bottle. Solid structures will provide a loud, well-defined percussion note. This can be simulated by performing percussion on a table or desk.

Due to the high level of background noise in the field, it is often difficult to hear the percussion note generated during percussion. In that event, the Paramedic may be able to modify the percussion technique and use her stethoscope to amplify the percussion note (Figure 16-6). Percussion can add valuable information to the patient examination. Specific percussion findings and techniques will be discussed later in the chapter.

Vital Signs Measurement

Vital signs are objectively measured characteristics of basic body functions. Vitals signs provide the Paramedic with an indication as to how well the patient's body is functioning or compensating for an injury or illness. Historically, the vital signs included pulse, respirations, blood pressure, and temperature. In the late 1990s, with the emphasis on appropriate assessment of pain and discomfort by all medical professions, the Joint Commission on Hospital Accreditation suggested adding the assessment of the patient's pain as the fifth vital sign, even though pain is technically classified as a **symptom**.[6,7] Finally, some consider measurement of the patient's peripheral oxygen saturation (SpO2), also known as pulse oximetry, as the sixth vital sign. Assessment of the patient's vital signs is reviewed in the following text and the concept of assessing for **orthostatic hypotension** is discussed.

Pulse

The pulse can be assessed at one of several locations where a major artery lies close to the surface of the skin (Figure 16-7). The most easily accessed area for conscious patients is the **radial pulse** at the wrist over the radial artery. For unconscious patients, the **carotid pulse** in the anterior neck is often used during the initial assessment. Other pulses the Paramedic may utilize are the **femoral pulse** at the patient's groin and the **dorsalis pedis (DP) pulse** over the dorsum of the foot. Assess the pulse for *rate*, *rhythm*, and *quality*. The pads of the fingers are used to assess for the pulse by placing light pressure over the location of the pulse. The pads of the fingers are used as they have more nerve endings than the tips and can better detect the presence and quality of the pulse.[8] Firm pressure can alter the perception of the pulse quality and rhythm, or in some cases occlude the pulse completely.

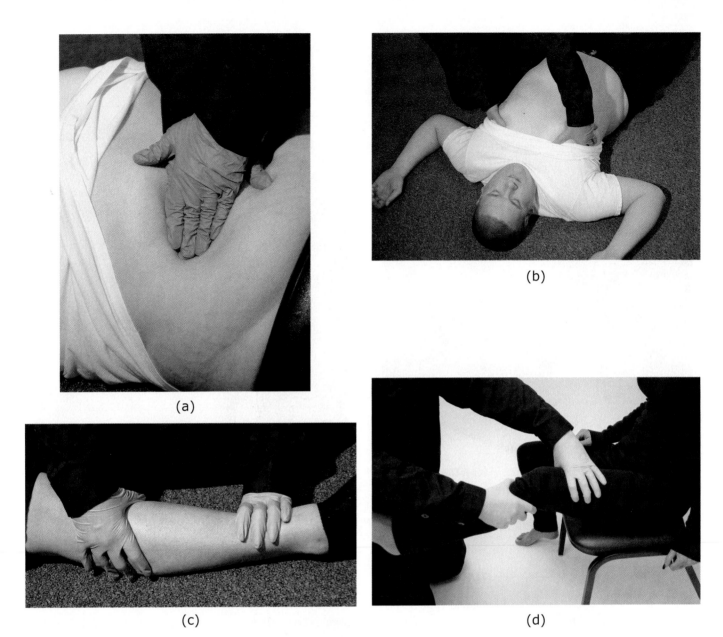

(a)

(b)

(c)

(d)

Figure 16-4 Examples of palpation. (a) Deep palpation of the abdomen. (b) Light palpation of the anterior chest wall. (c) Palpation along a bony structure. (d) Assessing joint stability.

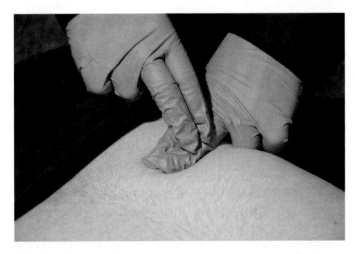

Figure 16-5 The technique of percussion. Note the finger position used by the Paramedic.

STREET SMART

While it is relatively easy to detect a pulse in a normal patient, it can be very difficult to detect a carotid pulse when the patient is in cardiac arrest.[9,10] This fact is emphasized by research that indicates laypeople could not reliably find a pulse in patients in cardiac arrest. Subsequently, the American Heart Association removed pulse checks from its citizen CPR program and replaced it with "signs of life."

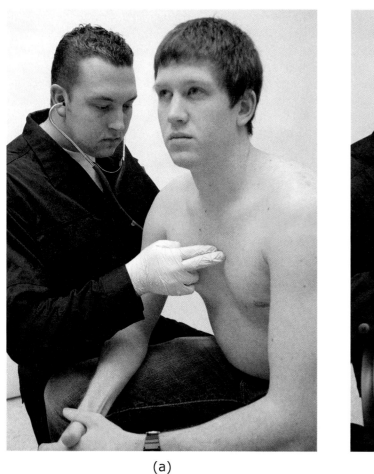

(a)

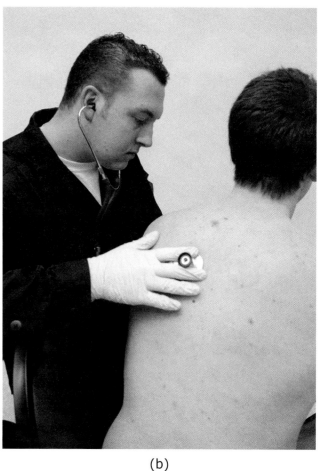

(b)

Figure 16-6 Modification of the percussion to allow improved detection of the percussion note.

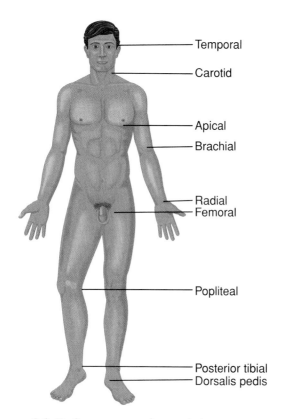

— Temporal

— Carotid

— Apical

— Brachial

— Radial
— Femoral

— Popliteal

— Posterior tibial
— Dorsalis pedis

Figure 16-7 Common pulse points.

Table 16-1 Normal Pediatric Heart Rates by Age

Patient Age	Beats/Minute
Newborn	120–160
Infant (0–5 months)	90–140
Infant (6–12 months)	80–140
Toddler (1–3 years)	80–130
Preschooler (3–5 years)	80–120
School-ager (6–10 years)	70–110
Adolescent (11–14 years)	60–105
Young or middle-aged adult (15–64 years)	60–100

A normal pulse rate for an adult is considered anywhere from 60 to 100 beats per minute. The normal pulse rates are different for children (Table 16-1). **Bradycardia** is defined as a heart rate that is under 60 beats per minute for an adult or below the lower limit of normal for a child. **Tachycardia** is defined as a heart rate that is over 100 beats per minute for an adult or above the upper limit of normal for a child. While the most accurate way to determine the patient's pulse rate is to count the number of beats that occur in one minute, two other methods also provide a reasonable determination of pulse rate. One method is to count the number of heartbeats in a 15-second time period and multiply that by four. A second is to count the number of beats in a 30-second time period and multiply that by two. If the patient's pulse is regular, the shorter time can be used to determine an accurate pulse rate. The more irregular the patient's pulse, the longer time is required to determine an accurate estimate of the pulse rate. In some cases, the pulse is so irregular or the rate changes so rapidly that a range of pulse rates is reported (e.g., the patient's pulse rate varies between 120 and 140 beats per minute).

Generally, the Paramedic can assess the pulse rate by palpating the pulse at one of the locations previously described. However, when the patient is significantly tachycardic, in the 180 to 220 beats per minute range, it can be difficult to count the pulse rate using palpation. In this situation, the Paramedic may need to use a stethoscope to listen to the heart and count an **apical pulse**, or the pulse rate at the chest. In infants and toddlers, where the normal heart rate is well over 100 beats per minute, the Paramedic may also need to assess the apical pulse rate (Figure 16-8).

Assess the rhythm of the pulse to determine its regularity. Is the rhythm regular or does the timing between individual beats vary significantly? Are there premature beats that occasionally and briefly interrupt the underlying regular rhythm, or is the rhythm chaotically irregular, one that does not follow any pattern? This chaotically irregular pulse is sometimes termed an irregularly irregular pulse to indicate the complete absence of a pattern to the pulse rhythm.

Pulse quality is a description of the amplitude or strength of the pulse at that particular location. Pulse quality is often described as normal, absent, strong, bounding, weak, or thready. The term "thready" is usually given to pulses which are both weak and very rapid, as seen with heart rates that are significantly tachycardic. Pulse quality may be different depending on the location of the pulse and the patient's condition. In a healthy individual free of disease or complaint, the pulse quality should be the same regardless of the location of the pulse. However, some conditions will affect the pulse

quality. An injury to an upper extremity may cause the radial pulse to be absent in that extremity. Peripheral vascular disease in a lower extremity, which decreases blood flow to that extremity, can cause a decrease in pulse quality compared to the upper extremities.

Finally, it is important to note that the pulse rate palpated by the Paramedic, which determines the patient's mechanical pulse rate, may be different than the heart's electrical rate as shown on an electrocardiogram (ECG) rhythm monitor.

STREET SMART

During shock, the patient will lose distal pulses first (i.e., radial before femoral and femoral before carotid). A quick survey of pulses can be helpful in establishing the presence of shock. However, no statement can be made about the patient's blood pressure based upon the presence or absence of distal pulses.

Respirations

Respirations are assessed by observing the respiratory rate, depth, pattern, and work of breathing. The respiratory rate is assessed by watching chest rise or auscultating breaths with a stethoscope and counting the number of breaths (Figure 16-9). The normal adult respiratory rate at rest is between 12 and 24 breaths per minute. The respiratory rate can be determined by counting the number of respirations in either a full minute or the number of respirations in 30 seconds and multiplying that count by two. In general, the respiratory rate is best counted when the patient is not aware that the Paramedic is counting the rate. In contrast to the pulse rate, a patient can control his respiratory rate much easier than his pulse rate (Table 16-2).

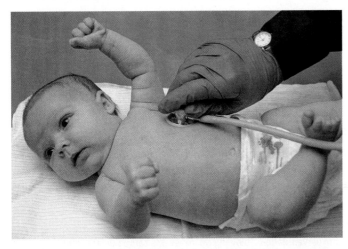

Figure 16-8 Paramedic assessing an apical pulse in a child. The stethoscope is held over the lower sternum to the left and the pulse rate is counted as described in the text.

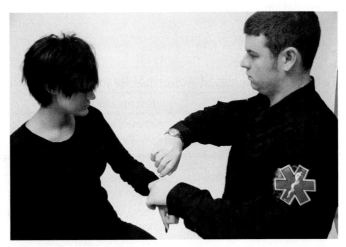

Figure 16-9 Paramedic assessing a patient's respirations.

Table 16-2 Normal Respiratory Rate by Age

Patient Age (yr)	Breaths/Minute
Infant (birth–1)	Initially 40–60; rate drops to 30–40 after a few minutes; slows to 20–30 by 1 year
Toddler (1–3)	20–30
Preschooler (3–5)	20–30
School-ager (6–10)	15–30
Adolescent (11–14)	12–20
Young or middle-aged adult (15–64)	12–20
Older adult (65+)	Depends on patient's health

Along with the rate, the Paramedic should note the depth of respiration. The depth can be described as shallow, normal, or deep. A shallow respiration is less than the normal chest excursion and typically produces an inadequate respiration. Another term used to describe shallow respirations is **hypoventilation**. Hypoventilation can be caused by drug overdose, head injury, or other conditions that can cause coma. A deep respiration is deeper than normal and is termed **hyperventilation**. Examples of conditions that can cause hyperventilation include respiratory distress, a metabolic condition, or drug overdose.

The respiratory pattern is considered the rhythm of the respirations. The respiratory pattern is the combination of the timing of the respirations and the depth of respirations (Figure 16-10). Different causes exist for many of these abnormal patterns (Table 16-3).

The Paramedic should be prepared to assist ventilations whenever a patient is either hypoventilating or hyperventilating, as both of these respiratory situations can represent ineffective ventilation.[11,12]

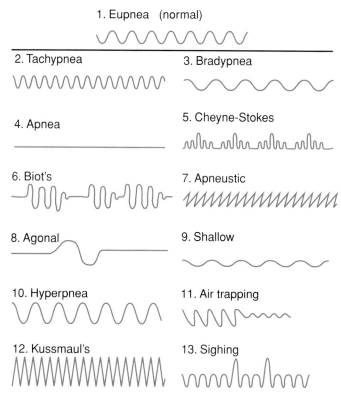

1. Eupnea (normal)
2. Tachypnea
3. Bradypnea
4. Apnea
5. Cheyne-Stokes
6. Biot's
7. Apneustic
8. Agonal
9. Shallow
10. Hyperpnea
11. Air trapping
12. Kussmaul's
13. Sighing

Figure 16-10 Abnormal respiratory patterns.

Table 16-3 Selected Abnormal Respiratory Patterns, Their Description, and Cause

Pattern	Description and Cause
Cheyne-Stokes	Gradually increasing rate and tidal volume, which increases to a maximum, then gradually decreases; occurs in brain stem injuries
Biot's	Irregular pattern and volume, with intermittent periods of apnea; found in patients with increased intracranial pressure
Agonal	Slow, shallow, irregular respiration; results from brain anoxia
Kussmaul's	Deep gasping respirations, representing hyperventilation, "blowing off" of excess carbon dioxide and compensation for an abnormal accumulation of metabolic acids in the blood; though possible in any patient with metabolic acidosis, best known with diabetic ketoacidosis
Central neurogenic hyperventilation	Deep, rapid, regular respiration; found in patients with increased intracranial pressure

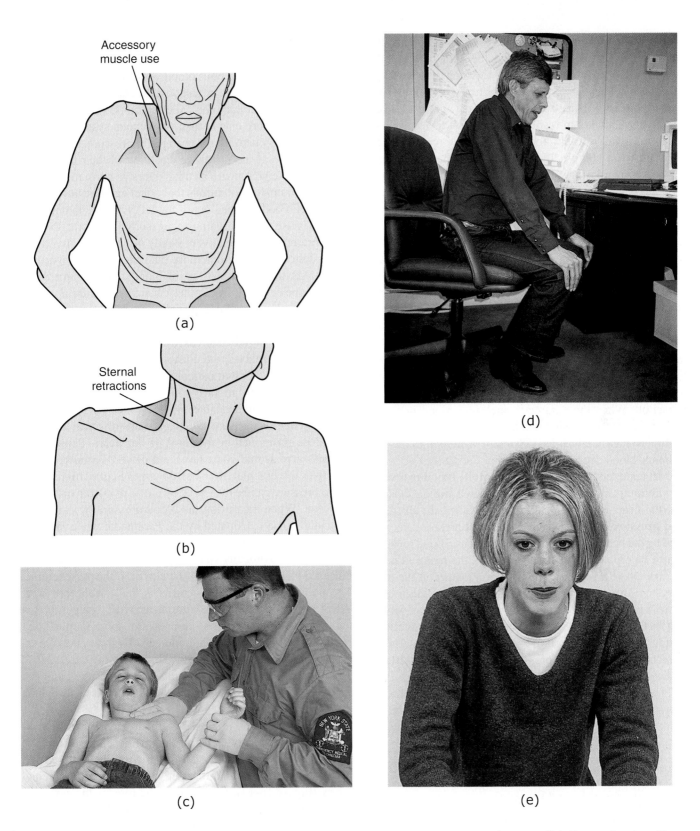

Figure 16-11 Signs of increased work of breathing. (a) Accessory muscle use. (b) Sternal retractions. (c) Rib retractions. (d) Tripod position. (e) Pursed lip breathing.

The patient's work of breathing is also assessed to measure the level of respiratory distress. There are several signs that indicate an increased work of breathing. During normal respiration, the chest expands effortlessly. When a patient is in respiratory distress, more effort is required to breathe and **accessory muscles** are recruited to help expand the rib cage, allowing the patient to inhale. When these muscles are used, they tend to become more defined (Figure 16-11a). When the work of breathing increases, more effort is needed to generate the negative pressure in the thorax required for inspiration. When this happens, the skin at the top of the sternum and the skin between the ribs are pulled inwards because of this negative pressure in the chest. These findings are termed **sternal retractions** (Figure 16-11b) and **rib retractions** (Figure 16-11c), respectively. Patients in respiratory distress also will position themselves in a way to help improve breathing. The **tripod position** (Figure 16-11d) is a sign that the patient is in severe respiratory distress. This position allows the overworked accessory muscles to work better, although most patients begin to tire when they are in such severe respiratory distress. **Pursed lip breathing** (Figure 16-11e) is another sign of increased work of breathing. When the exhalation pressure is high, the alveoli tend to collapse during exhalation. The patient puckers his or her lips while exhaling, providing some resistance to exhalation that provides pressure to keep the alveoli open.[13–16]

Blood Pressure

Blood pressure is a measure of the pressure within the blood vessels that make up the circulatory system. The pressure will vary depending upon the type of vessel and the phase of heart contraction. When the Paramedic measures blood pressure, he is measuring the pressure within the arterial system. Blood pressure is measured at its maximum and minimum. The maximum blood pressure is measured during systole when the heart contracts, and is called the **systolic blood pressure**. The minimum blood pressure is measured during diastole when the heart relaxes and fills, and is called the **diastolic blood pressure**. These two levels of blood pressure are generated by the heart's intermittent contractions. Blood pressure can also be reported as a single pressure, the **mean arterial pressure** (MAP), which is the average pressure in the arterial system over time (Figure 16-12). A typical mean arterial pressure that will maintain adequate cerebral perfusion is about 60 to 80 mmHg.[17] An adequate blood pressure is necessary for adequate perfusion of the body's organs; however, a chronically elevated blood pressure can lead to increased risk of catastrophic cardiovascular events.

The **pulse pressure** is defined as the difference between the systolic and diastolic pressures. The pulse pressure can provide the Paramedic with an indication about the blood volume status or compensation for illness in a given patient. Both the arterial and venous blood vessels have elasticity and change vessel diameter in response to changes in fluid volume, pressure, and pathological conditions, with the arterial system much more elastic than the venous system. Younger patients can compensate for changes in pressure and volume status because of the increased elasticity of their blood vessels. The pulse pressure in an adult at rest is normally approximately 40 mmHg. Conditions that affect **cardiac output**, the volume of blood pumped out of the left ventricle in one minute, can cause a decreased pulse pressure. In general, the diastolic pressure holds relatively steady or drops slightly, while the systolic pressure drops more than the diastolic pressure. Conditions that cause a drop in blood fluid volume (e.g., hemorrhage or shock from other causes) can cause a widening of the pulse pressure, especially in younger or otherwise fit patients.[18] Those patients may be able to initially sustain a near normal or slightly decreased systolic pressure. However, when the heart relaxes, the diastolic pressure is significantly less than normal for that patient. Pulse pressure may provide the Paramedic with an early clue to shock in patients who otherwise appear to be stable.

To properly measure blood pressure, the patient's arm should be positioned at the level of her heart. Support the patient's arm at mid-chest level and center a properly sized cuff over the brachial artery of the arm (Figure 16-13). The blood pressure can be measured by either palpation or by auscultation. When measuring the blood pressure by palpation, the radial pulse is palpated by the Paramedic while inflating the blood pressure cuff. The Paramedic inflates the blood pressure cuff approximately 10 to 20 mmHg above the loss of the pulse, and then slowly deflates the cuff until the pulse returns. The point where the pulse returns is the systolic pressure. When reporting a blood pressure measured by palpation, the Paramedic verbally reports the pressure "by palpation" (for example, "124 by palpation") and records the systolic pressure as a fraction with a P as the denominator (e.g., 124/P). The palpation method is useful in situations where there is a lot of ambient noise that would make it difficult to auscultate the blood pressure.

The auscultation method is a more accurate method of measuring blood pressure. The Paramedic places the blood pressure cuff on the patient's arm as previously described and places the diaphragm of the stethoscope over the brachial artery (Figure 16-14).[19] The Paramedic inflates the cuff until the sound of the heartbeat disappears and inflates the cuff an additional 10 to 20 mmHg. Next, the Paramedic slowly deflates the cuff at a rate of approximately 2 to 3 mmHg per second and notes the pressure at which she hears the sounds of at least two consecutive beats. This is the systolic blood pressure. The **Korotkoff sounds** heard during the inflation and deflation of the cuff are caused by the change in the nature of blood flow though the artery.[20,21] To obtain the diastolic blood pressure, the Paramedic continues deflating the cuff slowly, until she notes a muffling and then a disappearance of the

$$MAP = \frac{SBP + (2 \times DBP)}{3}$$

MAP = mean arterial pressure

SBP = systolic blood pressure

DBP = diastolic blood pressure

Figure 16-12 Computing mean arterial pressure (MAP). Many automated noninvasive blood pressure monitors automatically calculate and display MAP.

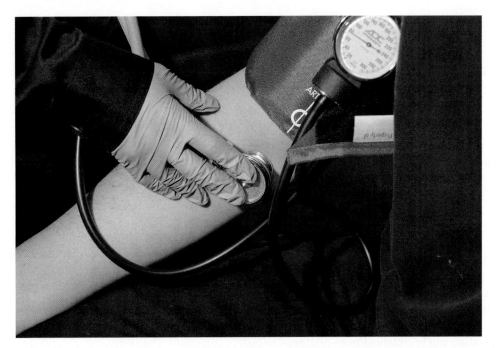

Figure 16-13 Proper placement of a blood pressure cuff helps ensure accurate measurement.

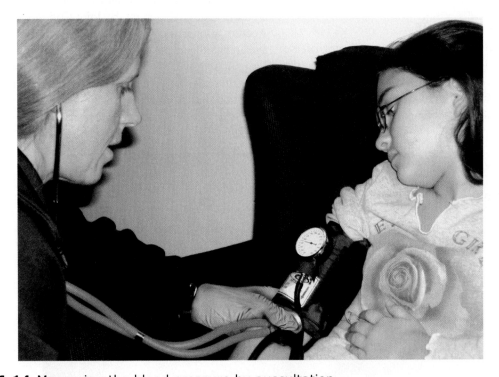

Figure 16-14 Measuring the blood pressure by auscultation.

Korotkoff sounds. This is the diastolic blood pressure. The Paramedic records both systolic and diastolic blood pressure readings to the nearest 2 mmHg.

Blood pressure readings vary significantly with patient age, underlying physical and medical conditions, and current medications. A systolic blood pressure that is above the upper limit of normal indicates **hypertension**. A systolic blood pressure below the lower limit of normal indicates **hypotension**. In an adult, a blood pressure greater than 139 mmHg systolic or 89 mmHg diastolic are always considered abnormally elevated and a systolic pressure below 90 mmHg is considered abnormally low (Table 16-4).

Table 16-4 Normal Blood Pressures

Patient Age (Years)	Blood Pressure (mmHg)	
	Systolic	Diastolic
Infant and toddler (0–3)	80 + (2 times age in years)	Two-thirds systolic
Preschooler (3–5)	78–116	average 55
School-ager (6–10)	80–122	average 57
Adolescent (11–14)	88–140	average 59
Young and middle-aged adult (15–64)	90–150	60–90
Older adult (65+)	Depends on patient's health	Depends on patient's health

Temperature

The body's normal core temperature ranges from 36.1°C to 37.7°C (97°F to 99.8°F). A temperature above 38°C (100.4°F) is considered a fever. An elevated body temperature is called **hyperthermia**. In contrast, **hypothermia** is defined as a body temperature less than 35°C (95°F). Relatively accurate estimates of core temperature can be obtained from oral, rectal, or tympanic thermometers (Figure 16-15), with the rectal temperature as the most accurate estimate of the core body temperature.

Skin Condition and Color

Skin condition and color is an important indicator of the patient's ability to provide sufficient oxygen-rich blood to the tissues. While there is a wide range of normal skin tones, normally many fair skinned individuals will have a pink color or tone to the skin. The Paramedic may need to assess the color of the mucous membranes in the mouth, the palms of the hands and soles of the feet, or the **conjunctiva** (Figure 16-16) in darker skinned patients to determine skin color. Skin condition is generally categorized as normal, dry, moist, or **diaphoretic**. A patient with diaphoretic skin is sweating profusely. This state is associated with many different conditions.

Pain

As previously discussed, assessment of pain was considered the fifth vital sign by the Joint Commission on Hospital Accreditation in the late 1990s in an effort to strongly encourage all healthcare providers to adequately assess every patient for pain and reassess the patient after interventions.[22,23] Various pain scales have been developed in an attempt to quantify the amount of pain. However, pain assessment is still a subjective report that varies between patients. A more detailed

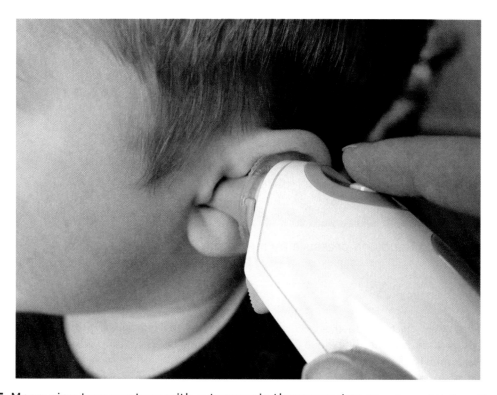

Figure 16-15 Measuring temperature with a tympanic thermometer. (Courtesy of Melissa King/iStockphoto)

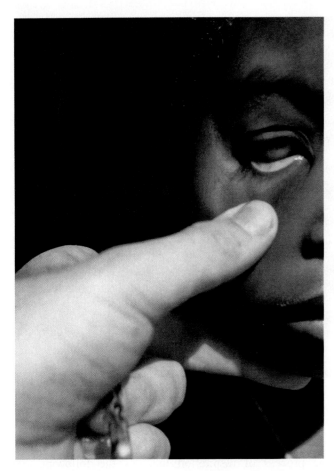

Figure 16-16 Assessing the conjunctiva for pallor that may indicate anemia or blood loss.
(Courtesy of CDC/Dr. Lyle Conrad)

discussion of the pain scales useful for the prehospital environment can be found in Chapter 15.

Pulse Oximetry

Hemoglobin is the molecule in red blood cells that accepts oxygen in the lungs and carries it to the body's tissues to allow cellular respiration. **Pulse oximetry** is a noninvasive measurement of the percentage of hemoglobin in arterial blood that is bound to oxygen molecules.[24] An accurate reading provides the Paramedic a good measure of the patient's **oxygenation**, or his ability to move oxygen from the air in the lungs into the blood. It does not provide an indication of how well the patient is using that oxygenation. It also does not provide an indication of the patient's **ventilation**, or note how well the patient is moving air in and out of the lungs during inhalation and exhalation. A normal pulse oximetry value in a healthy individual without lung disease is between 96% and 100% saturation. For individuals with chronic lung diseases, the patient's personal normal pulse oximetry may actually be as low as 85% without supplemental oxygen.[25]

Pulse oximetry is determined by measuring the change that occurs when a beam of red light and infrared light is directed across a capillary bed. When hemoglobin binds to oxygen, it will cause an imperceptible change in the red and infrared light as it passes through the pulsating capillary bed. This change is translated into a percentage of oxygen saturation that is displayed for the Paramedic. Some pulse oximeters provide a waveform display in addition to the numerical value (Figure 16-17). This waveform fluctuates with changes in the patient's blood flow during normal contraction of the patient's heart. Because it is simple to measure the rate of these fluctuations, most oximeters will provide the patient's pulse rate in addition to the oxygen saturation.

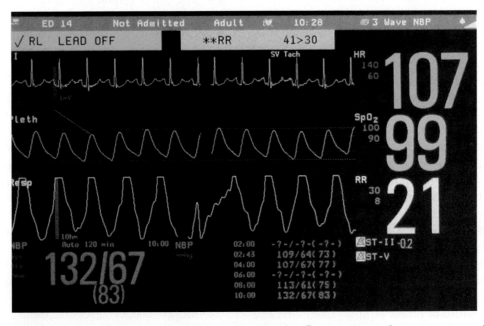

Figure 16-17 Normal pulse oximetry waveform. Notice the fluctuations that correspond with the patient's pulse rate (red arrow).

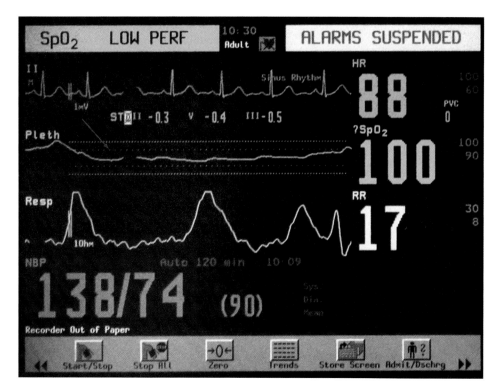

Figure 16-18 Poor oximetry waveform (red arrow).

Several factors may affect the accuracy of the pulse oximetry reading. In order for the reading to be accurate, the patient must have sufficient blood flow in the capillary bed of the body part where the probe is attached. If the waveform is poor (Figure 16-18), then the oximeter will either not read or will provide an inaccurate reading. Blood flow to the capillary bed is decreased if the limb is cool, if the patient is **hypovolemic** (decreased circulating blood volume), or the patient is hypotensive. Traditional pulse oximeters only detect whether or not the hemoglobin is bound to another molecule. Other compounds (e.g., carbon monoxide) can also bind to hemoglobin in the red blood cells. If carbon dioxide is present, the pulse oximeter will still read a normal saturation level, even though the patient's tissues do not receive sufficient oxygen and are **hypoxic**.[26] Newer co-oximeters utilize additional wavelengths of light and can detect the presence of carbon monoxide and other compounds that can bind to hemoglobin.

It is important to note that even patients who present with a pulse oximetry reading within a normal range can benefit from supplemental oxygen. In many conditions, the surface capillary beds utilized to measure oxygen saturation may have fully saturated blood; however, due to blood loss or hypotension, deeper vessels—including those supplying the heart, brain, kidneys, and the intestines—may not have an adequate supply of oxygen. Blood itself not only carries oxygen by hemoglobin in red blood cells, but can also carry dissolved oxygen molecules within the plasma, or liquid portion of the blood. Patients who are in respiratory distress or suffering from a significant illness or injury should receive supplemental oxygen to ensure the organs continue to receive a sufficient amount of oxygen.

Capnography

The process of respiration includes the following steps (Figure 16-19):

- Inhalation of oxygen-containing air into the lungs
- Movement of oxygen from the air across the alveolar membrane into the blood
- Movement of oxygen through the blood to the tissues
- Absorption of oxygen into the cells
- Production of carbon dioxide by the cells as they use the oxygen and glucose for fuel
- Delivery of carbon dioxide back to the lungs
- Movement of the carbon dioxide back across the alveolar membrane into the lungs
- Exhalation of the carbon dioxide into the atmosphere.

From a respiratory system standpoint, the amount of exhaled carbon dioxide is related to the patient's ability to move air in and out of the lungs. If the patient cannot ventilate adequately, the concentration of exhaled carbon dioxide will increase because the patient exhales a smaller amount with each breath, allowing the carbon dioxide level to build up in the lungs. If the patient hyperventilates, the exhaled carbon dioxide level will decrease because a larger amount of carbon dioxide is exhaled with each breath, decreasing the overall concentration of carbon dioxide in the lungs. In situations where the patient is able to circulate the blood adequately, capnography provides an indication of how well the patient is able to ventilate.

From a circulatory standpoint, the amount of exhaled carbon dioxide is directly related to the body's ability to perfuse the tissues, or carry oxygen, glucose, and other nutrients to

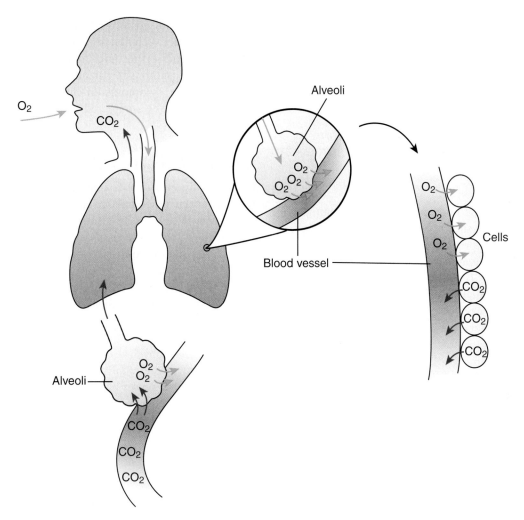

Figure 16-19 The process of respiration.

the cells in order to carry on the metabolic processes required to sustain life.[27] If the patient is perfusing well, the carbon dioxide produced by the metabolic processes inside the cells will be transported back to the lungs for exhalation. Conditions that decrease the patient's ability to circulate the blood (e.g., shock and cardiac arrest) will decrease the level of carbon dioxide in the lungs.

Waveform capnography provides a graphical representation of the exhaled carbon dioxide level over time.[28,29] The level of carbon dioxide will vary with inhalation and exhalation (see the curve shown in Figure 16-20). The normal level of exhaled carbon dioxide is approximately 40 mmHg. End-tidal carbon dioxide levels ($EtCO_2$) below 10 mmHg in the setting of cardiac arrest is associated with a 0% chance of survival. Elevated levels are seen in patients who are not ventilating adequately. A decrease in $EtCO_2$ level during mechanical ventilation may indicate the patient has become hypotensive. It could also mean the ventilation rate is too high and should be slowed to a lower rate. The waveform's shape and pattern can provide clues to the disease process in patients complaining of shortness of breath. Finally, using $EtCO_2$ with patients who are intubated is an excellent patient safety tool, as the Paramedic can immediately detect a dislodged endotracheal

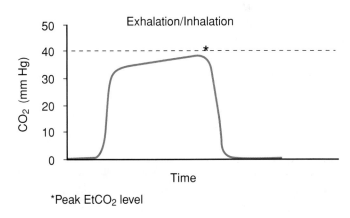

*Peak $EtCO_2$ level

Figure 16-20 Typical capnography waveform.

tube by the change in waveform before the patient's oxygen saturation is affected (Figure 16-21).[30–32] The use of waveform capnography is discussed further in Chapter 25.

Orthostatic Vital Signs

Orthostatic vital signs are vital signs that change with position. When an individual changes position from lying down to standing, the blood pressure normally has a tendency to

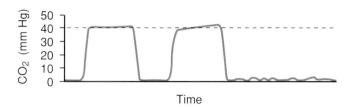

Figure 16-21 Sudden loss of the waveform in an intubated patient likely indicates endotracheal tube dislodgement.

drop due to gravity. The body will compensate initially for this drop in blood pressure by constricting the arterial system.[33] If that does not provide sufficient compensation, then the heart rate will increase in an effort to maintain an adequate blood pressure. If the patient has a decreased blood volume, whether through hemorrhage or through dehydration, the body will not be able to completely compensate for this change by decreasing the size of the blood vessels alone. Therefore, measuring orthostatic vital signs can assess the patient for subtle volume loss that may not be evident during a supine or a seated set of vital signs. To measure orthostatic vital signs, the Paramedic measures the blood pressure and heart rate in the supine, sitting, and standing positions with at least one minute rest between position changes to allow the body to compensate for the change. Although this may be difficult to achieve in the prehospital environment, it is inadvisable with patients who have sustained sufficient trauma to require spinal motion restriction.

Positive orthostatic vital signs are defined as a heart rate increase of 20 beats per minute or greater, a systolic blood pressure drop of greater than 20 mmHg, a diastolic blood pressure increase of 10 mmHg, and/or dizziness or lightheadedness with position change.[34,35] While orthostatic vital signs have been traditionally used as a means of determining blood loss or hypovolemia in patients who had otherwise normal vital signs, other factors—including medication, age, ingested substances (e.g., alcohol), and other medical conditions—can also produce orthostatic changes. In several studies specifically looking at blood loss, changes

in pulse rate with position change could reasonably detect blood loss of between 500 mL and 1 L.[36] Care must be taken when measuring orthostatic vital signs on a patient, especially when assuming the standing position. If the patient develops severe symptoms on changing position, measurement should not be completed, as it puts the patient at risk for fall and injury.

Concern-Based Physical Exam

Conceptually, every call for assistance begins with a patient's **chief concern** or complaint. This is true whether the call was received emergently through the 9-1-1 system or non-emergently through a secondary system. From a dispatch perspective, the algorithms used to determine response resources are keyed from the patient's or caller's chief concern. From a Paramedic perspective, the chief concern is used to help focus the history and physical examination to find the most likely cause of the patient's chief concern and detect life- or limb-threatening conditions that are associated with that condition. Detailed physical examinations are time-consuming and often provide more information than what is useful to the Paramedic. During most patient contacts, the Paramedic will perform a focused physical exam based upon the patient's chief concern.

Focused Exam Matrix

In the prehospital environment, detailed head to toe exams are not practical for many patients. Instead, a focused physical exam is performed on the systems associated with the patient's chief concern. The Paramedic performs a detailed examination of one or two related body systems and a brief examination of other relevant body systems. In this way, the Paramedic can efficiently use her time during the patient contact and assess for findings that can help confirm the paramedical diagnosis suspected by the history or suggest alternate conditions that require assessment.

The physical examination is also guided by the complexity of the patient's chief concern. A patient who is complaining of ankle pain after twisting his right ankle on the sidewalk and did not strike any other part of his body may be appropriate for a single system-focused exam on that ankle. A patient with a strong cardiac and respiratory history complaining of general weakness may require a more extensive physical examination. The discussion throughout the rest of the chapter will provide a guide to the elements of the physical examination that should be covered based upon the patient's chief concern. It is not meant to be all inclusive, and should be modified by the Paramedic based upon clinical judgment, the specific patient's presentation, and examination findings that suggest other conditions that may contribute to the chief concern.

Both the focused and detailed physical examinations take place after correcting life-threatening conditions that were discovered during the primary assessment. Some of the items assessed during the focused or detailed examinations are items that were assessed during the primary assessment.

Table 16-5 Physical Examination by Chief Concern (CC)

Chief Concern	Primary System	Secondary System	Tertiary System
Chest pain	Cardiovascular	Respiratory	Neurological
			Gastrointestinal
Shortness of breath	Respiratory	Cardiac	Neurological
Abdominal pain	Gastrointestinal	Cardiac	
Loss of consciousness	Neurological	Cardiac	Musculoskeletal
Altered mental status	Neuorological	Psychiatric	
Musculoskeletal	Musculoskeletal	Skin	
Psychiatric	Psychiatric	Neurological	

They should be reassessed during the focused exam as necessary to provide the Paramedic with the information needed to efficiently and adequately treat the patient.

Examination Matrix

An examination matrix (Table 16-5) provides a guide to the systems the Paramedic should assess based upon the patient's chief concern. The table is divided into columns that indicate the primary system to focus upon during the exam, as well as a secondary and a tertiary system to include in the examination. The primary system is most closely associated with the conditions that produce the chief concern listed in the first column. The secondary system is also associated with conditions that can produce that chief concern, but not as closely. The tertiary system generally can be affected by disease conditions from the other systems that cause the chief concern. For example, the chief concern of shortness of breath has the respiratory system as its primary system. However, cardiovascular conditions (e.g., angina) can cause shortness of breath. The cardiovascular system is listed as the secondary system. The neurological system may have findings associated with shortness of breath, so it is listed as the tertiary system in the matrix under the shortness of breath chief concern.

As previously discussed, this matrix should be used to guide the Paramedic's focused physical examination based upon the patient's chief complaint. The systems and features examined in a specific patient may be different based upon the history obtained from the patient as well as the Paramedic's findings.

General Exam

In Chapter 13, an algorithmic approach was discussed for performing the primary assessment in every patient. During the overall scene assessment, the Paramedic assesses the scene to determine and call for appropriate resources to handle the situation. On each individual patient, the goal of the primary assessment is to rapidly detect and treat any life-threatening conditions (e.g., inadequate respirations, shock, or massive bleeding). Triage algorithms based on the primary assessment exist to help the Paramedic treat and transport patients in order of severity.

Once the primary assessment is completed, the focused assessment follows. As part of the focused physical exam, some general features should be assessed for every patient. These features include vital signs, appearance, and the scene. All three of these features are part of the Paramedic's initial impression; an assessment of these features should be performed during every single patient encounter.

The constitutional examination consists of the assessment of the patient's vital signs. At a minimum, this includes the blood pressure, pulse, and respirations. The Paramedic should obtain a baseline set of vital signs on every patient after completing the primary assessment. A room air pulse oximetry reading should also be obtained on patients with chief concerns that involve the respiratory system. If a thermometer is available, the patient's body temperature can be assessed. The patient's approximate weight is also important in determining medication dosages for certain medications. At least two sets of vital signs should be taken during every patient encounter as an assessment of stability and to identify changes during treatment.

The patient's appearance can also provide an indication of her ability to compensate for the disease process. Document the position in which the patient was found (e.g., "seated on the couch" or "supine on the ground 50 feet from the vehicle"). The level of distress experienced by the patient on initial contact should also be noted as part of the constitutional examination. This may include distress from painful conditions or respiratory distress. Skin condition and color can also provide clues toward level of distress and compensation for the disease process causing the chief concern. The patient's position may provide clues to the level of distress. For example, a patient in severe respiratory distress may be leaning forward in a tripod position to help ease her breathing. A patient experiencing the pain from a kidney stone may not be able to sit still and will pace or roll on the stretcher in an attempt to find a comfortable position.

Observations made about the scene also provide important clues to the Paramedic and the ED staff. During the primary assessment, the Paramedic views the scene for hazards to his health and safety. As part of the focused exam, the scene should be viewed for evidence of the patient's ability to care for herself. A patient with a disheveled appearance with torn and dirty clothing in an unkempt apartment may not be able to care for herself. Empty pill bottles present at the scene of a patient who has altered mental status may suggest an intentional overdose. For trauma patients, the scene can provide important clues as to the mechanism of injury that can help focus the Paramedic's examination to areas most likely injured. Position in the vehicle, restraint use, or proximity to hazards all provide the Paramedic with important information.

Chest Pain

Approximately 15 million Americans suffered from cardiovascular diseases in 2004, with half of those people suffering a myocardial infarction.[37] Heart disease remains the top cause of death in the United States. Chest pain is one of the more common chief concerns which patients provide to dispatchers during the 9-1-1 call and tell Paramedics during the patient interview. As part of the focused examination, the Paramedic should assess the cardiovascular system as the primary system, and the respiratory, gastrointestinal, and neurological systems as the secondary and tertiary systems. The physical examination elements for a patient with a chief concern of "chest pain" are inspection, auscultation, and palpation.

Cardiovascular System

Inspection of features related to the cardiovascular system starts with an assessment of jugular venous pressure (JVP). The jugular veins run on either side of the neck at an angle from the corner of the mandible to the mid-clavicle on the same side. The jugular veins feed into the large veins that feed into the superior vena cava and into the right atrium. When the heart is not pumping effectively or when the patient has a significant amount of extra fluid in the circulation, the external jugular veins will distend, or stretch and become larger. This can be measured by positioning the patient in a semi-Fowler's position at approximately a 45-degree angle, asking her to turn her head away from you, and inspecting the external jugular vein for distention (Figure 16-22a).[38] It can be helpful for the Paramedic to shine a penlight perpendicular across the vein to improve visualization. In a patient with a normal jugular venous pressure, the external jugular vein will be distended about three centimeters above the **sternal notch**. Distention greater than three centimeters above the sternal notch is considered an elevated JVP (Figure 16-22b).

Inspect the patient's extremities for peripheral edema, a condition that also can indicate heart failure. The most common areas where peripheral edema occurs are in the ankles and feet. However, edema can occur up into the thighs and scrotum in males and external labia in females, as well as in the upper extremities. **Pitting edema** is a term that refers to the amount of indention produced when the edematous limb is pressed over the tibia by the examiner's finger (Figure 16-23). The level of pitting edema is often described as trace, mild, moderate, or severe based upon the size and duration of the indention.

Auscultation of the heart involves listening to the heart with the diaphragm of the stethoscope in four locations (Figure 16-24). Lightly hold the diaphragm of the stethoscope against the chest for approximately 20 seconds in each area. The normal sounds heard at these locations correspond to the heart valves closing during the contraction and relaxation phases of the heart. The two normal heart sounds are called the S1 and S2 sounds (Figure 16-25a). The S1 sound corresponds to the closing of the mitral and tricuspid valve at the beginning of **systole**, or ventricular contraction. The S2 sound corresponds to the closing of the aortic and pulmonic valves at the end of systole, marking the beginning of diastole, or ventricular relaxation and filling. Two extra heart sounds, S3

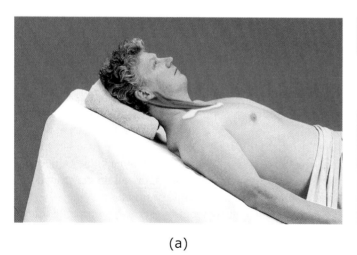
(a)

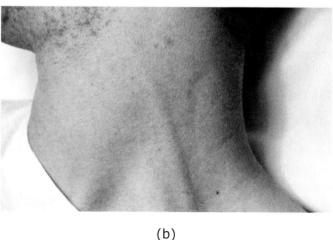
(b)

Figure 16-22 (a) Patient positioning for evaluation of jugular venous pressure. (b) Elevated jugular venous pressure.

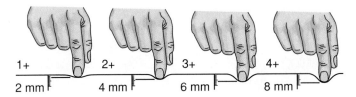

Figure 16-23 Assessment of the severity of peripheral edema.

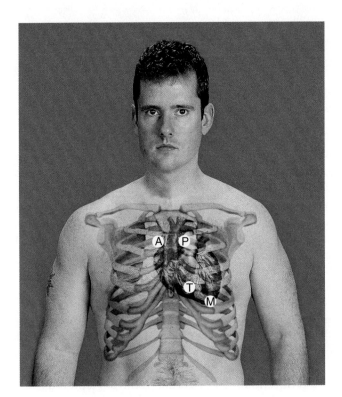

Figure 16-24 Locations for auscultation of heart sounds. A = aortic area. P = pulmonic area. T = tricuspid area. M = mitral area.

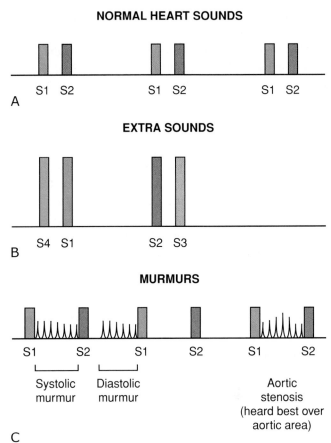

Figure 16-25 Heart sounds. (a) Normal. (b) Extra sounds. (c) Murmurs.

and S4, are diastolic sounds that occur with changes in ventricular filling (Figure 16-25b). When either sound is present it is often called a **gallop**, as the combination of the normal and extra sounds produces a galloping rhythm, similar to hearing a horse gallop. The S3 sound is sometimes normal in children and young adults as the heart fills quickly. In patients with a chief concern of chest pain or shortness of breath, it can indicate fluid overload associated with heart failure. The S4 sound occurs close to the S1 sound and can indicate the ventricles are stiff and are not filling properly.

Murmurs are abnormal heart sounds produced by turbulent blood flow across the four valves. Different types of murmurs are associated with different conditions and can occur during both systole and diastole. Many murmurs are described as a low pitched "whoosh" sound. This sound is sometimes separate from, and sometimes integrated with, the normal heart sounds (Figure 16-25c). A discussion of all the different murmurs is beyond the scope of this text; however, one that may be clinically important to the Paramedic is the

murmur associated with **aortic stenosis**. Aortic stenosis is a condition in which the leaflets of the aortic valve become scarred over time and the pathway through the valve narrows. The murmur associated with aortic stenosis is best heard over the aortic area and is a high-pitched, sometimes loud sound that begins just after the S1 sound and runs until just before the S2 sound. This is clinically important because, in patients with severe stenosis, a higher pressure is required to propel blood out of the left ventricle and into circulation. The patient tends to have significant hypertension; however, this hypertension is necessary for the patient to circulate blood. Medications that can lower the blood pressure should be used with caution in patients with a loud murmur from aortic stenosis (one that can almost be heard before the stethoscope is placed on the chest) as that higher blood pressure is essential to maintain circulation.

Another abnormal heart sound that is sometimes heard is called a **rub**. A rub is a low-pitched, soft scratching sound that occurs at any time during the cardiac cycle and indicates **pericarditis**, or an inflammation of the pericardial sac that surrounds the heart. The sound of the rub is produced when the inflamed pericardium rubs against the heart muscle during heart contraction or relaxation. This sound can be difficult to hear in the loud prehospital environment.

Several features of the cardiovascular system are assessed by palpation. While auscultating the chest for heart sounds, the Paramedic can spread her fingers out over the diaphragm and simultaneously palpate the chest for a **thrill**, or vibration of the chest associated with heart contraction. Forceful contractions can produce a significant pounding inside the chest wall, causing a **heave**. Peripheral pulses are also assessed by palpation for strength and equality in the left and right extremities.

Capillary refill is a measure of the patient's ability to perfuse the extremities with oxygenated blood. Capillary refill is assessed by squeezing the tip of a digit hard enough to blanch it, releasing it, and then counting the number of seconds for it to return to a normal color. A normal capillary refill is two seconds or less. A delayed capillary refill indicates poor perfusion.[39]

Blood pressure is normally equal in both arms. If pulses are unequal in both arms, assess the arms for a difference in systolic pressures. A significant difference in blood pressure in both arms can indicate a problem with the aorta.

Respiratory System

Assessment of the respiratory systems begins with inspecting the patient for respiratory effort. Assessment findings that indicate the patient has increased respiratory effort include use of accessory muscles, sternal or intercostal retractions, increased respiratory rate, or tripod positioning. Accessory muscles of respiration include the muscles in the front of the neck. When the patient is in severe respiratory distress, these muscles contract to help lift the upper portion of the rib cage during inspiration (Figure 16-11a). Sternal and intercostal retractions occur when the patient struggles to move air into the lungs (Figures 16-11b and 16-11c). Patients in severe respiratory distress will frequently assume a tripod position where they sit leaning slightly forward resting their hands on their knees (Figure 16-11d) in an effort to improve their ability to inhale.

The patient's skin and mucous membranes should also be inspected for color. In a well-oxygenated patient, the mucous membranes will be pink. **Cyanosis** is a bluish hue that develops when the patient develops **hypoxemia**, or a decreased oxygen level in the blood (Figure 16-26). In patients with a darker complexion, the Paramedic may have to inspect the oral mucous membranes or the nail beds to assess for cyanosis. In severe hypoxemia, the patient's entire skin becomes cyanotic. The Paramedic needs to intervene rapidly with supplemental oxygen, airway management, and ventilatory support to correct the hypoxemia.

The Paramedic should then auscultate the lungs for lung sounds. Lung sounds should be assessed posteriorly and on both sides of the chest, assessing both the left and right lung at the same level, so that sounds can be compared between the left and right lung. Normal sounds differ depending on the location in the chest. Lung sounds auscultated over the peripheral, smaller airways are called **vesicular sounds**, and sound like leaves rustling in the wind. Lung sounds auscultated

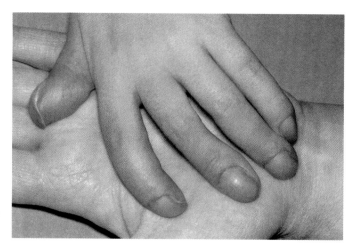

Figure 16-26 A cyanotic patient. (Courtesy of Wellcome Trust/Custom Medical Stock Photo)

over the larger airways are called **bronchial sounds**. These sounds are louder and sound like air rushing through a hollow tube. Normal respiration involves an inspiratory phase that is longer than the expiratory phase. In addition, there is good movement of air in and out of the lungs. Certain conditions cause a prolongation of the expiratory phase. For example, several abnormal lung sounds can indicate specific conditions that help guide the Paramedic toward determining a cause for the patient's chief concern (Table 16-6).

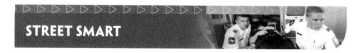

STREET SMART

To differentiate a pericardial rub from a pleural rub, have the patient hold his breath. Pleural rubs are heard when the patient is breathing while pericardial rubs occur with each heartbeat.

Percussion of the chest can also offer additional information about lung findings (Figure 16-5). One figure is placed against the chest wall in-between two ribs while the other taps the first finger. This should be performed at several levels on both the left and right side of the chest, comparing sides for equality. A normal chest percussion note is a somewhat hollow sound. A **hyperresonant** percussion note sounds similar to striking a drum and indicates an increased amount of air in the chest. This is often seen with a **pneumothorax** on the side of the hyperresonant percussion note. A **hyporesonant** percussion note is dull in character, and often indicates fluid in the lung from either a **pleural effusion** or **hemothorax**. Due to noise at the scene of the call, it may be difficult to assess a percussion note until the patient is in the back of the ambulance.

Palpation of the chest is used to assess for stability of the rib cage, tenderness, equal expansion of the chest, and

Table 16-6 Abnormal Lung Sounds

Sound	Description	Conditions Associated
Wheezing	High-pitched sounds, often heard in inspiration, but can be present on expiration	Asthma Chronic obstructive pulmonary disease (COPD) Heart failure
Rales	Crackles similar to Rice Krispies™ crackling in milk	Fluid in smaller airways Heart failure
Rhonchi	Coarse crackling in larger airways	Mucus in larger airways Acute bronchitis Pneumonia
Consolidation	Bronchial sounds heard over periphery, unequal compared to same field on opposite lung	Pneumonia
Stridor	High-pitched inspiratory upper airway sound	Upper airway obstruction from upper airway edema or foreign body
Absent	• Specific field	• Pleural effusion, pneumonia, lower airway obstruction
	• Entire lung	• Pneumothorax, hemothorax, massive pleural effusion
Friction rub	Intermittent coarse rubbing sound similar to sandpaper rubbing with inspiration or expiration	Indication of inflammation of pleura

the presence of subcutaneous emphysema. Point tenderness along the rib or sternum may indicate a fracture in the setting of an injury to the chest. Place the hands on either side of the lower rib cage. During inspiration and expiration, the chest should expand equally with inspiration. **Subcutaneous emphysema** is the presence of air between the layers of the skin and indicates a leak in the respiratory system. Most often this is due to a pneumothorax with air escaping into the skin. At other times, it can occur after a tracheal or larger airway rupture. Subcutaneous emphysema is often described as feeling like bubble wrap underneath the skin. Subcutaneous emphysema can become extensive, traveling up the neck into the face or down the abdomen into the genitals.[40]

Gastrointestinal

The abdominal exam in a patient with a chief concern of chest pain is limited to assessing for pain and signs of fluid overload related to right heart failure. The abdomen is palpated to assess for tenderness, especially over the epigastrium, which may indicate a gastrointestinal origin for the patient's chief concern. **Hepatojugular reflux** is assessed by placing the patient in a semi-reclined position at approximately a 45-degree angle. The jugular vein is first assessed for level of distention (Figure 16-22). The Paramedic then applies firm pressure to the patient's right upper quadrant over the liver. The hepatojugular reflux is positive if the jugular vein distention increases. This is seen in conditions that cause the patient to become fluid overloaded, including heart failure and kidney failure.[41,42]

Neurological

The patient's mental status is the best indicator of the brain's perfusion with oxygenated blood. All of the body systems are designed to support adequate blood flow and oxygen delivery to the brain. A normal mental status indicates that the brain is receiving a sufficient amount of oxygenated blood. An altered mental status, which may vary from confusion to unconsciousness, can indicate that the brain is not receiving enough oxygenated blood.

Put It All Together

The assessment of a patient presenting with the chief concern of chest pain includes many possibilities (Figure 16-27).

Shortness of Breath

Shortness of breath is another common chief concern of patients calling EMS. Shortness of breath occurs primarily from respiratory causes (e.g., asthma or pneumonia), but can also occur from cardiac causes (e.g., heart failure or angina). The physical exam for a patient with a chief concern of "shortness of breath" is similar to that of patients who have a chief concern of chest pain. However, the emphasis is on the respiratory system.

Respiratory

The Paramedic starts by inspecting the patient for respiratory effort and cyanosis. As previously discussed, findings of severe respiratory distress are significant and require rapid

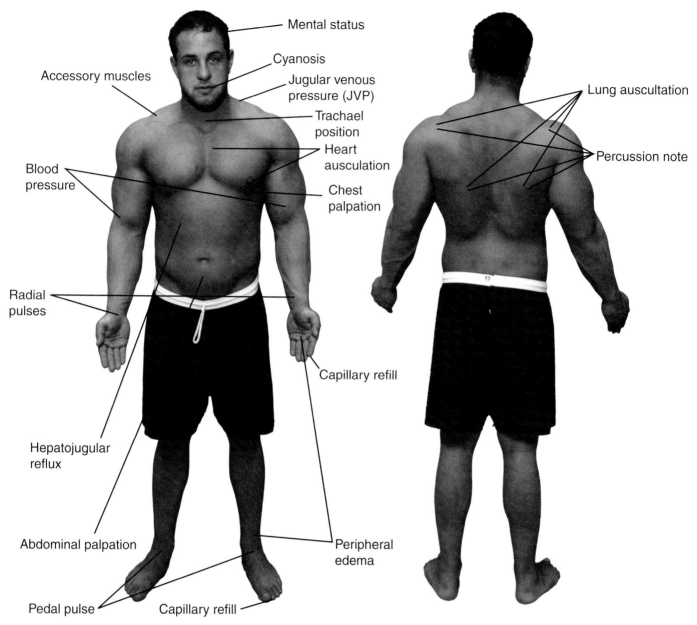

Figure 16-27 Assessment of a patient with the chief concern of chest pain.

intervention. Also note if the patient appears to be tiring. As the respiratory distress progresses, the patient will begin to grow weary of breathing. Immediate intervention at this point with airway management is key to preventing respiratory arrest. One additional feature to assess is the tracheal position. Tracheal position is assessed just above the sternal notch (Figure 16-28). Normally, the trachea is found in the center of the neck, centered in the sternal notch. Deviation of the trachea toward one side can indicate conditions that cause a shift of the heart and lungs to one side, and is usually a late sign of the condition.

The Paramedic assesses the patient using auscultation to identify normal and abnormal lung sounds as previously described. Rales can indicate a cardiac cause for the shortness of breath while many of the other sounds indicate a respiratory cause. As previously described, a hyperresonant percussion note can indicate a pneumothorax while a dull percussion note can indicate fluid or pneumonia if present in one lung field. When palpating the chest, ask the patient to speak. Vibrations palpated on the chest wall that occur with speech are called **tactile fremitus**, and can also indicate an infective process in that portion of the lung. These abnormal vibrations are produced as the vocal sounds are transmitted into the lung and are altered in the area of the infection, causing a vibration that can be palpated over that portion of the lung.

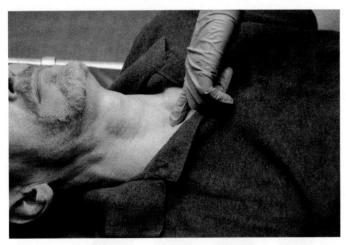

Figure 16-28 Assessing for tracheal position.

Cardiovascular

The Paramedic should inspect the patient for an elevated jugular venous pressure and the presence of peripheral edema. These may indicate a cardiac cause for shortness of breath. The Paramedic then auscultates the heart sounds for the presence of additional heart sounds and murmurs. These may also indicate a cardiac cause for the shortness of breath. Finally, the Paramedic assesses the peripheral pulses and capillary refill to determine the patient's perfusion. Poor perfusion with a lack of oxygen to the body's organs can produce the sensation of shortness of breath without respiratory disease.

Neurovascular

The Paramedic assesses the patient's mental status to determine the level of alertness. As respiratory distress worsens and the patient becomes tired, the patient's mental status will begin to decline.[43] This can result from lack of energy, but also may be due to the buildup of the blood's carbon dioxide (CO_2) level. Patients in respiratory distress use more energy to breathe, thus producing more CO_2. As the level of distress increases, the ventilation becomes poorer and the patient is not able to exhale the CO_2 that is produced. The CO_2 levels increase in the blood. When the CO_2 levels become high enough, the patient's respiratory drive and mental status is further depressed, again impairing the patient's ability to remove the CO_2 from the blood. This cycle continues until the patient becomes unconscious and develops respiratory arrest. Patients with a chief concern of shortness of breath who have an altered mental status require aggressive airway management and ventilatory support in order to halt this dangerous cycle.

Put It All Together

The assessment of a patient presenting with the chief concern of shortness of breath includes many possibilities (Figure 16-29).

Abdominal Pain

Sorting out the cause of abdominal pain is challenging as the abdominal cavity contains many organs with a multitude of causes for pain. There are many conditions that cause abdominal pain; some are life-threatening while others are not. Following is the physical assessment for a patient who has a chief concern of "abdominal pain."

Gastrointestinal

The focused examination of a patient with the chief concern of abdominal pain begins with an examination of the gastrointestinal system. The abdomen is inspected for distention, or protruding of the abdomen past its normal size (Figure 16-30). Localized protrusions at the umbilicus or in the midline of the abdomen may be a **hernia**, or openings in the muscle and tissue layers that allows the intestines to protrude through the opening. The abdomen is also inspected for prominent surface veins, especially around the umbilicus, that may indicate a history of liver failure. The skin is also inspected for **jaundice**, a yellowish hue of the skin, which can indicate liver failure or obstruction of the bile duct (Figure 16-31). Ecchymosis, or bruising, may also be present in several locations on the abdomen, including the umbilicus, the flanks, or across the lower abdomen, and can indicate internal bleeding from either a medical condition or traumatic injury.

The bowels produce sounds from the rhythmic movement of material through the gastrointestinal tract. These sounds can be auscultated by the Paramedic and may provide some clue as to the cause of the patient's abdominal pain. Bowel sounds are generally softer pitched gurgling sounds as compared to lung sounds and may be difficult to hear in the prehospital environment.[44] In order to declare bowel sounds completely absent, the Paramedic would be required to listen for sounds for approximately three minutes, which is not realistic in the prehospital environment. High-pitched, loud sounds that sound like water dripping may indicate a bowel obstruction.

The Paramedic can also assess the abdomen using percussion. The percussion note over the liver and spleen, which are solid organs, should be dull. The percussion note over other parts of the abdomen should be a normal sound similar to that of the lung. If the abdomen is distended, a percussion note can help differentiate between a fluid-filled abdomen and an air-filled abdomen. If the distended abdomen is distended with **ascites**, or fluid, the percussion note will be dull. If the distended abdomen is filled with air, as in the case of a bowel obstruction, then a tympanic percussion note will be heard. Tenderness with percussion over a portion of the abdomen may indicate irritation of the **peritoneum**, the inner lining of the abdomen. Irritation of the peritoneum can occur with infection, inflammation, or blood in the peritoneal cavity. Finally, **costovertebral angle** tenderness, also known as CVA tenderness, can indicate kidney irritation from a kidney stone or infection. The costovertebral angle is located over the lower ribs just medial to the posterior axillary line (Figure 16-32).

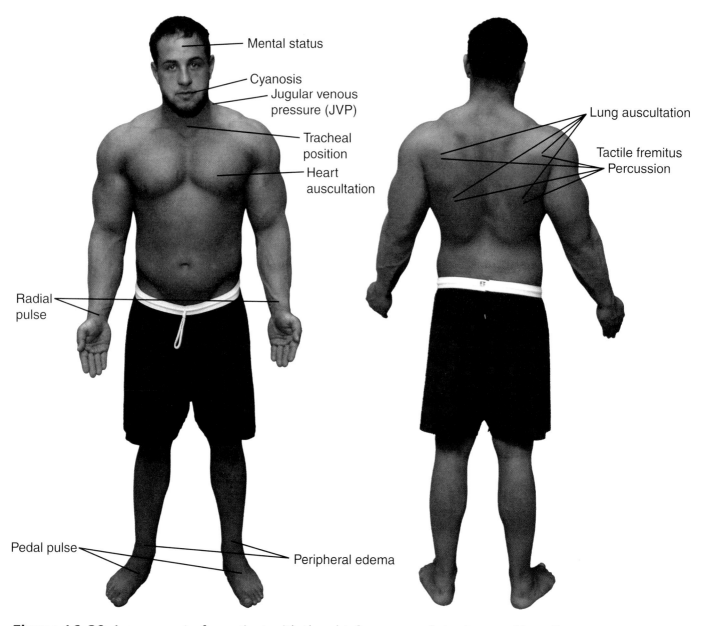

Figure 16-29 Assessment of a patient with the chief concern of shortness of breath.

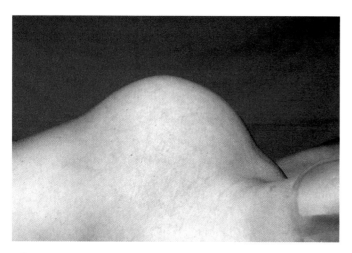

Figure 16-30 Abdominal distention. (Courtesy of Michael English, M.D./Custom Medical Stock Photo)

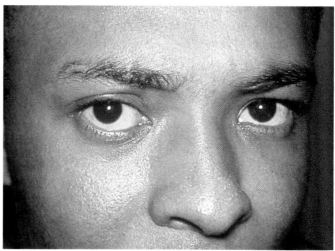

Figure 16-31 Jaundice of the skin and scleral icterus.

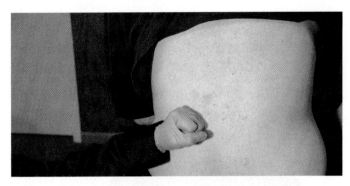

Figure 16-32 Percussion of the costovertebral angle.

Two different methods are used to divide the abdomen. One method utilizes quadrants and the other method uses "nines." Quadrants are made by running both an imaginary vertical line and an imaginary horizontal line through the umbilicus (Figure 16-33a) such that there are four quadrants. Nines are made by dividing the abdomen into three horizontal sections and three vertical sections, similar to a tic-tac-toe board (Figure 16-33b) such that there are nine sections. Either method is acceptable. When the abdomen is divided up into quadrants, findings correspond to the quadrant where the finding was discovered. The Paramedic should decide which method to use and stick with it. Each section should be palpated at least one time by applying gentle, but firm pressure with one hand while the other hand lies on top and helps guide the first. **Rebound tenderness** is tenderness that becomes worse when the pressure is suddenly released

during palpation and may indicate irritation of the peritoneum. **Rovsing's sign** is pain in the right lower quadrant that occurs when the left lower quadrant is palpated, and is often associated with appendicitis. **Murphy's sign** is right upper quadrant tenderness that worsens when the patient takes a deep breath while the quadrant is palpated and may indicate gallbladder inflammation.

In addition to looking for tenderness, the abdomen is palpated to detect masses. An abdominal mass is a general term used to describe an abnormally firm area of the abdomen. Masses can be tender or nontender, firm or soft, or pulsatile. Pulsatile masses in the setting of hypotension raise concern for vascular rupture of the abdominal aorta. Protrusions through the patient's midline are likely related to a ventral hernia.

Cardiovascular

A limited cardiovascular examination is performed in patients with a chief concern of abdominal pain. For patients who have epigastric pain, the Paramedic should be diligent and perform a more extensive cardiovascular examination.[45]

Inspect the patient's skin for color and perfusion. Auscultate the heart for heart tones and murmurs. Palpate the extremities for equality of the pulses, especially in the lower extremities that may indicate a vascular problem with the abdominal aorta. When the abdomen is palpated, also assess the patient for hepatojugular reflux.

Put It All Together

The assessment of a patient presenting with the chief concern of abdominal pain includes many possibilities (Figure 16-34).

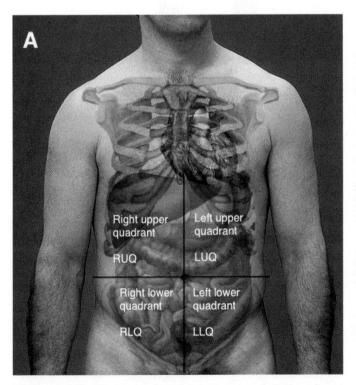

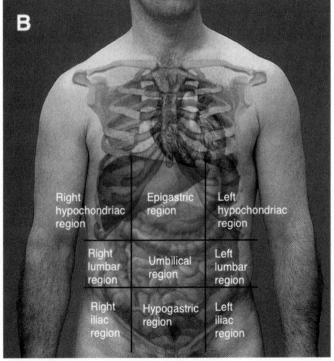

Figure 16-33 Abdominal territories. (a) Quadrants. (b) Nines.

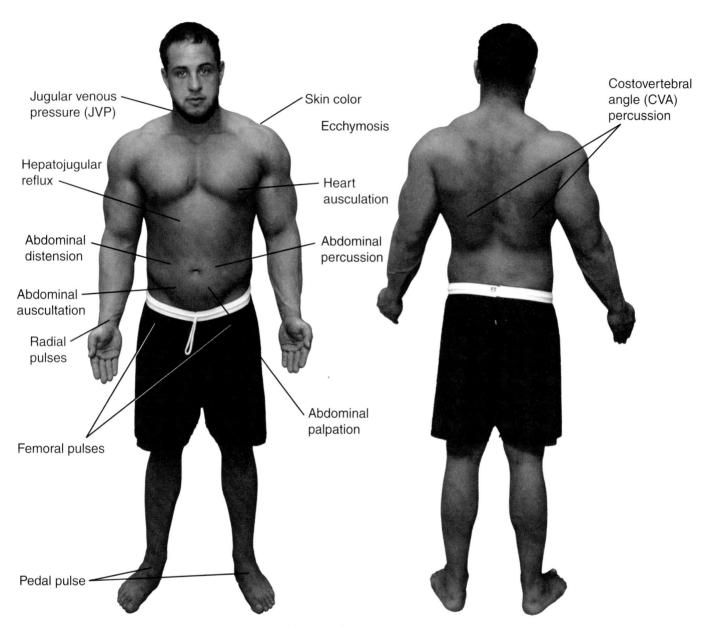

Figure 16-34 Assessment of a patient with the chief concern of abdominal pain.

Labels (clockwise from upper left):
- Jugular venous pressure (JVP)
- Hepatojugular reflux
- Abdominal distension
- Abdominal auscultation
- Radial pulses
- Femoral pulses
- Pedal pulse
- Skin color
- Ecchymosis
- Heart ausculation
- Abdominal percussion
- Abdominal palpation
- Costovertebral angle (CVA) percussion

Syncope

Syncope is a transient loss of consciousness that resolves spontaneously. Near syncope is the feeling that one is going to pass out, although one does not actually lose consciousness. Though these are two separate conditions, both are treated the same in regard to assessment and treatment. While there are many causes of syncope—ranging from benign to life-threatening—the Paramedic should focus her examination on the more life-threatening ones. Following is the physical examination of a patient with a chief concern of syncope or near syncope.

Neurological

The neurological exam begins with assessing the patient's mental status. The Paramedic assesses the patient for responsiveness, alertness, and orientation to self (person), location (place), and time. She also assesses the patient's memory for the events leading up to the call for assistance. Amnesia to the events can indicate a trauma patient sustained a head injury. The Paramedic then assesses the patient's attention by observing whether the patient follows the conversation or is easily distracted. Next, the Paramedic assesses the patient for appropriate language. Do the sentences make sense? Is the speech garbled or clear? Are the responses to questions in the proper context?

The remainder of the neurological exam is divided up into the cranial nerve exam, the peripheral nerve exam, assessment of deep tendon reflexes, and assessment of coordination. The cranial nerves are a set of 12 paired nerves that begin within the brainstem and are responsible for movement and sensation in the head and neck. The first cranial nerve provides the sense

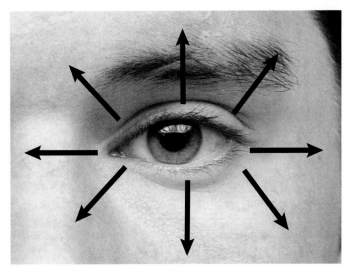

Figure 16-35 Examination of the eyes for extraocular movements.

of smell, which is difficult to assess in the prehospital environment. The second cranial nerve is examined by assessing the patient's visual acuity. This can be as simple as asking him to read something printed and held at a normal reading distance or assessing the visual acuity through a Snellen eye chart. Light perception is the ability to see light only. If the patient has enough vision only to count the number of fingers held up in front of the eye, the visual acuity is measured as counting fingers. The third, fourth, and sixth cranial nerves are assessed by examining the patient's extraocular movements (EOM). Ask the patient to look at a finger, pencil, or the unlit penlight and follow that object with just his eyes. Make an H in the air and watch the patient's eyes (Figure 16-35). If there is normal EOM (sometimes documented as EOM intact or EOMI), the eyes will follow the object smoothly and with full range of motion. Abnormalities may include unequal movement or oscillating movements at the end of the excursion. These oscillating movements are termed **nystagmus**. A few beats of nystagmus are normal. Sustained or prolonged nystagmus may be a sign of intoxication or central nervous system problems. The third cranial nerve also controls the pupillary response, which is assessed by shining a penlight into the patient's pupils one at a time, looking for constriction of both pupils.

Sensation and motor function to the face are carried by the fifth and seventh cranial nerves, respectively. Sensory function is assessed by touching the forehead, cheeks, and lower jaw on the left and right side of the face and looking for equality of sensation. Motor function is assessed by looking for symmetry of certain actions. The Paramedic should ask the patient to smile and then look for a symmetrical smile. The patient should be asked to open his eyes as wide as he can while the Paramedic looks for symmetry in the wrinkles in the forehead. The patient should also be asked to close his eyes as hard as he can, as the Paramedic looks for symmetry.

The eighth cranial nerve is examined by assessing the patient's hearing. The ninth and twelfth cranial nerves are assessed by asking the patient to stick out his tongue and say "ah." The tongue should protrude in the midline, and the soft palate near the pharynx should elevate symmetrically. The last part of the cranial nerve examination is to ask the patient to shrug his shoulders while observing for symmetry, which tests the eleventh cranial nerve.

Peripheral sensation of the skin is organized into dermatomes that correspond to the spinal nerve roots (Figure 16-36). The trunk can be rapidly assessed by running one finger down each side of the thorax, looking for equality of sensation. Lack of sensation below the same level on both sides of the trunk may indicate a spinal cord injury. A similar method can be used to assess sensation in the extremities. A difference in sensation between the extremities may indicate nerve root compression, a stroke, or damage to the peripheral nerve itself.

The **deep tendon reflexes (DTRs)** are tested by tapping a large tendon and looking for involuntary muscle contraction in the muscle associated with that tendon. The biceps tendon DTR is tested by supporting the patient's flexed forearm and tapping over the biceps tendon in the antecubital fossa (Figure 16-37a). The arm should quickly flex in response to tapping the tendon. The patellar tendon DTR is tested by flexing the patient's knee and allowing it to hang unsupported with the patient is seated. The patellar tendon is tapped just below the patella (Figure 16-37b). The knee should quickly extend in response to the tap. The plantar reflex is assessed by running a blunt object along the sole of the foot and observing

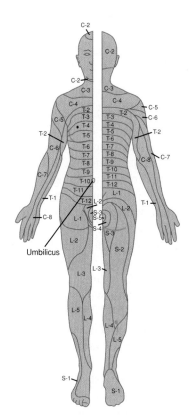

Figure 16-36 Dermatomes.

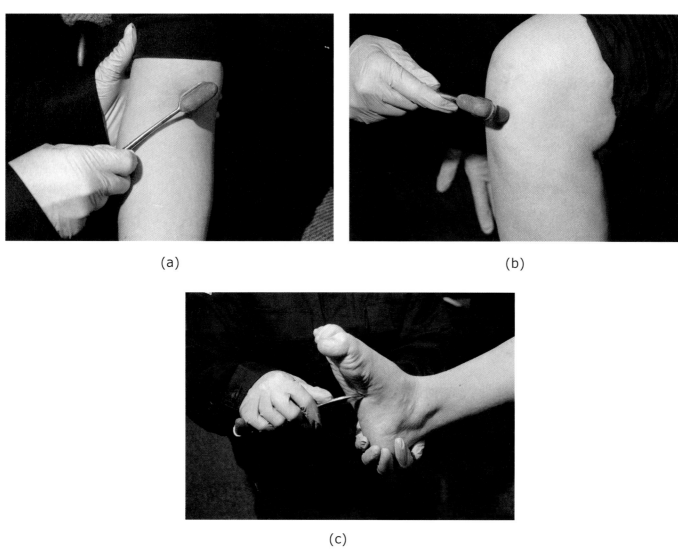

(a)

(b)

(c)

Figure 16-37 Testing deep tendon reflexes. (a) Biceps. (b) Patella. (c) Plantar.

toe movement (Figure 16-37c). In a normal response, the toes flex and move downward. An abnormal response is when the great toe pulls upward and the other toes fan out, indicating spinal cord injury or a problem with the brain.

The final portion of the neurological examination tests the patient's coordination. **Pronator drift** is tested by asking the seated patient to hold her arms out with the palms facing the ceiling and then close her eyes (Figure 16-38a). The test is positive if one arm drifts away from the starting position. The arm that drifts also tends to begin to rotate toward a palm-down position. Coordination is also tested by asking the patient to touch her nose with one pointer finger and then to touch the Paramedic's finger and move back and forth several times (Figure 16-38b). This is repeated with the opposite hand. The lower extremities can be tested by asking the semi-reclined patient to touch the heel of one leg to the opposite leg just below the knee and slide it down the tibia (Figure 16-38c). Abnormalities in coordination often indicate a problem in the **cerebellum**, the portion of the brain responsible for balance.

Cardiovascular

Auscultate the heart sounds for tone, murmurs, and extra heart sounds that may provide a clue as to the reason for syncope. Loud or harsh murmurs that are new may indicate valve scarring or **papillary muscle** rupture that may contribute to the patient's chief concern.[46,47] The papillary muscles stabilize, open, and close the valve leaflets with each myocardial contraction. The carotid arteries are auscultated to assess for **carotid bruits**. A bruit is a whooshing sound heard in a blood vessel that has plaque buildup on the vessel walls. This buildup causes turbulent blood flow. The Paramedic places the bell of the stethoscope over the carotid artery on one side of the neck and asks the patient to take in and hold a deep breath. The Paramedic then listens for the bruit. If a bruit is present, it may indicate atherosclerosis in the carotid artery that puts the patient at risk for a stroke.

Pulses are palpated for strength and equality. Weak or absent peripheral pulses may indicate hypotension as a cause of syncope. Unequal pulses may indicate a vascular

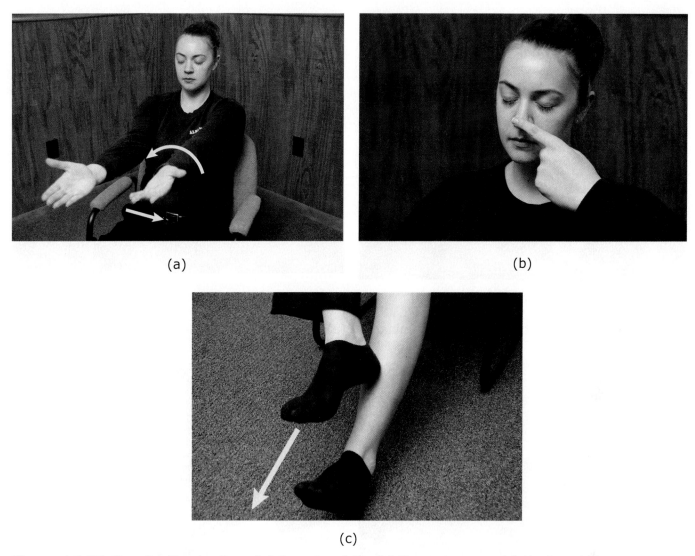

Figure 16-38 Coordination testing: (a) Pronator drift. (b) Finger to nose. (c) Heel to shin.

problem as a cause of the patient's syncope. Perfusion is also assessed using capillary refill and strength of the pulses in the extremities.

Finally, orthostatic vital signs may be helpful in assessing for hypovolemia that is not present with the resting vital signs. Care should be taken when positioning the patient in a standing position so the patient does not fall and injure herself a second time.

Musculoskeletal

The goal of the musculoskeletal examination is to assess for weakness and detect injury sustained during the syncopal episode. The Paramedic examines any painful areas closely for injury using palpation and inspection. Muscle strength of the upper extremities is tested by asking the patient to grip the Paramedic's finger (Figure 16-39a). The proximal portion of the upper extremities is tested by asking the patient to flex her elbows against resistance (Figure 16-39b). Lower extremity muscle strength is also tested distally and proximally. Distally, the Paramedic asks the patient to both **plantarflex**

and **dorsiflex** the feet (Figures 16-40a and 16-40b) against resistance. If the patient is lying or reclined, the Paramedic tests proximal muscle strength by asking her to lift her leg against resistance. If the patient is seated, the Paramedic tests proximal muscle strength by asking the patient to lift or raise her flexed knee against resistance (Figure 16-40c). Unequal muscle strength may indicate stroke, injury to the extremity muscles, or a spinal cord problem.

The bony surfaces of the upper and lower extremities are palpated for tenderness with special attention to the joints and areas that the patient complained were painful during the interview. Assess the stability of straight extremities by placing opposing forces over the bony surfaces and the joints (Figure 16-41). **Angulated** extremities where the long bone is obviously fractured and displaced at an abnormal angle should not be stressed (Figure 16-42). In patients who have sustained an injury, palpate the patient's spine along the bony prominences in the midline while maintaining spinal motion restriction to assess for tenderness that may suggest a spinal fracture.

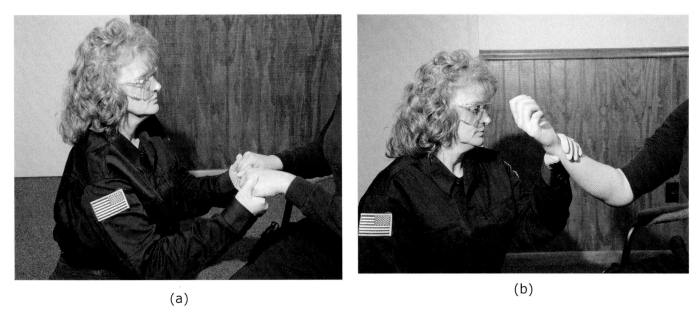

Figure 16-39 Upper extremity motor examination. (a) Grip strength. (b) Elbow strength.

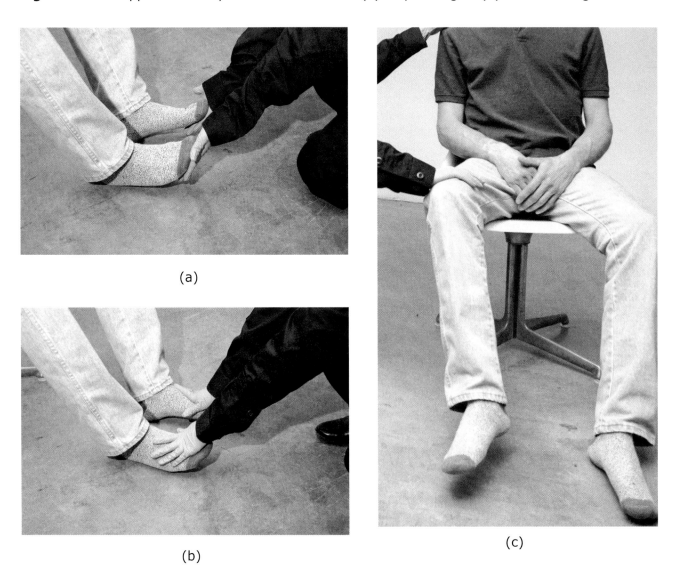

(a)

(b)

(c)

Figure 16-40 Lower extremity motor examination. (a) Plantarflexion against resistance.
(b) Dorsiflexion against resistance. (c) Proximal lower extremity muscle strength examination.

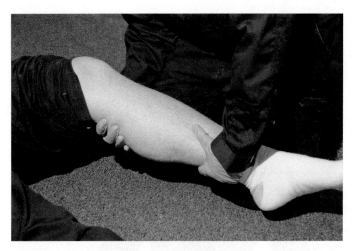

Figure 16-41 Applying oppositional forces over an extremity to test stability.

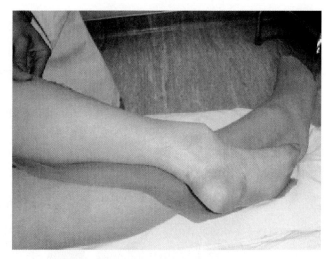

Figure 16-42 Example of an angulated extremity fracture. (Courtesy of Deborah Funk, MD, Albany Medical Center, Albany, NY)

If the patient is **ambulatory** at the scene, the Paramedic should observe the patient's **gait**, or the way the patient walks, for abnormalities. Normally, a steady gait appears balanced with the feet approximately shoulder width apart and flows smoothly as the patient ambulates. A multitude of gait disturbances are possible. It is best to describe and document what you see. The patient may stagger or appear off balance. The patient's feet may be spread far apart. The gait may not be smooth or may include additional movements. If the patient is ambulatory, then the Paramedic should comment on the patient's gait. If he decides to ambulate a patient who is not already ambulating, he should do so with care that the patient does not fall, causing further injury, or worsening the medical condition related to the chief concern. The Paramedic should follow the service policies as some services do not ambulate patients who are not already ambulating at the scene.

Put It All Together

The assessment of a patient presenting with the chief concern of syncope includes many possibilities (Figure 16-43).

Altered Mental Status

"Altered mental status" is a phrase used to describe any change from a normal mental status. This may range from "feeling fuzzy" or mild "confusion" up to complete loss of consciousness. The number of causes of altered mental status varies widely, with some causes being the result of aging, infection, intoxication, toxic substances, or hypoxia. The chief concern of altered mental status is often provided by family members, bystanders, or other individuals as the patient may not even be able to express this as a chief concern. Often at the extremes of age—the elderly and the very young—fever is a cause of altered mental status. **Hypoglycemia** is one of the most

common causes of altered mental status and is immediately treatable by the Paramedic. The Paramedic's goal in assessing the patient with altered mental status is to identify reversible causes while providing supportive care to the patient.

Neurological

The objective of the neurological exam in a patient with a chief concern of altered mental status is to identify signs of a focal neurological issue.[48–50] For example, unequal motor strength or unequal sensation may indicate a localized disruption in brain function, which may be caused by a stroke or a cerebral hemorrhage. A focal neurological issue differs from a condition that causes a global disruption such as low or high blood sugar or fever. The exam is carried out as previously described. Some components of the exam may be difficult to perform if the patient is not able to follow the Paramedic's commands.

Cardiovascular

The objective of the cardiovascular examination in a patient with a chief concern of altered mental status is to identify issues with perfusion that can lead to altered mental status. A rapid method of assessing perfusion is to palpate the peripheral pulses for strength and check the capillary refill in a hand or foot. The Paramedic should auscultate the heart for new murmurs. An irregular heartbeat may indicate atrial fibrillation, a rhythm that is associated with stroke, another potential cause of altered mental status.

Respiratory

The objective of the respiratory system examination is to detect respiratory conditions that can cause altered mental status, most commonly hypoxia and pneumonia. As

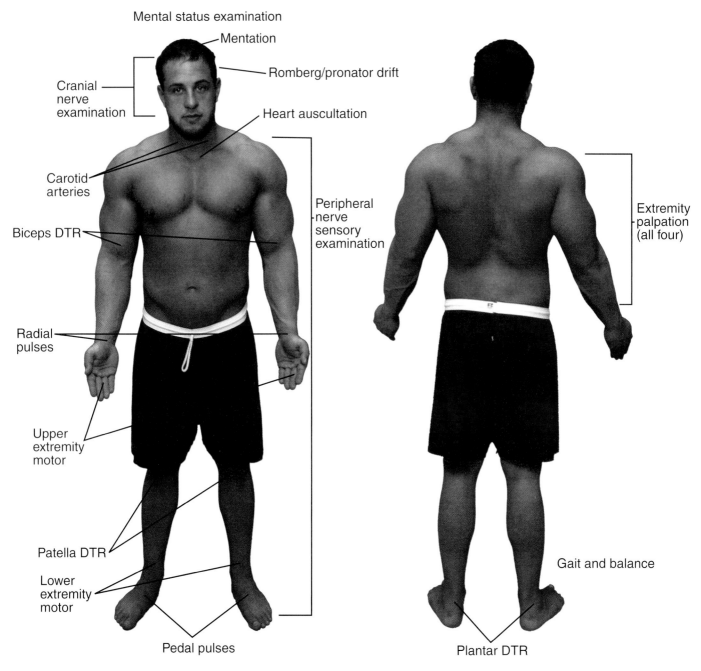

Mental status examination
— Mentation
— Romberg/pronator drift
Cranial nerve examination
Heart auscultation
Carotid arteries
Biceps DTR
Peripheral nerve sensory examination
Radial pulses
Upper extremity motor
Patella DTR
Lower extremity motor
Pedal pulses

Extremity palpation (all four)
Gait and balance
Plantar DTR

Figure 16-43 Assessment of a patient with the chief concern of syncope.

discussed before, a buildup in the level of carbon dioxide in the blood will cause sleepiness and altered consciousness. The Paramedic should assess the patient's respiratory rate and effort, observing for signs of increased work of breathing, poor ventilation, and respiratory failure. She should also assess the lung sounds for abnormal sounds that may indicate a cause of respiratory distress. Measurement of the patient's pulse oximetry will provide an indication of hypoxemia. Percussion of the chest may help detect signs of pneumothorax or pneumonia.

Skin

The skin is assessed for color, condition, and temperature, all features that may indicate infection, fever, or dehydration as a cause of altered mental status. In bedbound patients, including patients with paraplegia or past strokes with an inability to ambulate, **decubitus ulcers** (also known as pressure ulcers) can form and become another source of infection. Skin that is cyanotic indicates severe hypoxemia requiring immediate ventilatory support by the Paramedic. Ecchymosis, lacerations, or abrasions indicate trauma and suggest a traumatic cause for the altered mental status.

Psychiatric

Psychiatric conditions or worsening dementia can also cause an altered mental status. The first episode of a psychiatric disorder may present with altered mental status. Patients with a history of a psychiatric disorder may present with altered mental status if they decompensate, either through a worsening of their chronic disease or through noncompliance with taking their medications. Components of the psychiatric exam include assessment of speech, thought processes, suicidal or homicidal ideation, judgment, insight into medical condition, and mental status. Much of this examination is required to ensure a patient who wishes to refuse medical attention has sufficient **capacity** (i.e., mental ability) to understand the potential medical condition and the consequences of refusing treatment or transport.

The Paramedic should listen to the patient's speech. Abnormal speech may be either fast or very slow compared to a normal rate. **Pressured speech** occurs when the patient is speaking so fast it appears she has an urgency or pressure to speak quickly. The volume of speech may be decreased in a patient who is depressed, while it may be significantly increased in a patient exhibiting pressured speech. The speech may not be understandable in a patient with an altered mental status. For example, a patient may mumble or only grunt in response to questions or stimulus.

For the verbal patient, the Paramedic should assess the patient's thought process. A normal thought process will be clear, understandable, and logical. Abnormalities in the patient's thought process include psychotic or paranoid thoughts and auditory or visual hallucinations. Patients with hallucinations should be asked what they are seeing or what the voices are telling the patient to do. All patients who exhibit signs of depression should be asked about intent to harm themselves or others, as well as if they have a plan to carry out this suicidal or homicidal ideation.[51]

Another component of the psychiatric examination assesses the patient's **insight** into the medical condition and judgment, or ability to make reasonable decisions. Insight is an understanding of the patient's current or chronic medical condition, as well as the consequences of inappropriate treatment. An example of poor insight into one's medical condition is a patient who has insulin-dependent diabetes, packs up her insulin when moving, then cannot find her medications and waits several days until she is sick with an elevated glucose to call for an ambulance. A patient with good insight into her condition would have kept medications separate in a known location so they could be accessed and taken as directed.

The mental status exam is often thought of only as an assessment of the patient's **orientation** to person, place, and time; however, it involves several other components. The patient's memory is tested when the Paramedic asks the patient to remember three distinct objects (e.g., an apple, a table, and a penny). Then, continuing the examination a few minutes later, the Paramedic asks the patient to repeat back those three objects. The patient's language and knowledge is examined as previously described. Abnormalities in the patient's mood and affect may also indicate a psychiatric origin for his altered mental status. A flat affect occurs when the patient's face is absent of an expression. Mood can be described as depressed, elated, or normal.

Put It All Together

The assessment of a patient presenting with the chief concern of altered mental status includes many possibilities (Figure 16-44).

Extremity Pain

Extremity pain as a chief concern can have a traumatic origin or a medical origin. The most common cause of extremity pain is an injury. In order to assist in determining the cause, the pain should be localized to a particular joint, muscle, or bony landmark.

Musculoskeletal

The painful extremity should be inspected for signs of an obvious injury, including a laceration, abrasion, ecchymosis, or edema that can indicate an underlying bone injury. Inspection may indicate signs of an obvious fracture or dislocation, including angulation of that extremity. The Paramedic should assess both the left and right extremities for edema. **Bilateral**, or both left and right, extremity edema tends to indicate a systemic cause while **unilateral**, or one, extremity edema indicates a cause within that extremity. The extent of the edema should be noted, as edema localized to a joint or to a small area may indicate an underlying localized injury. Extensive unilateral edema may indicate an acute problem with the blood supply to that extremity. The extremity should also be palpated for stability as well as to help localize the pain. Edema is assessed for pitting, as discussed in the section on focused cardiovascular examination for patients with a chief concern of chest pain (Figure 16-23).

Skin

Skin color and temperature may also indicate the origin of the patient's extremity pain. Erythema, or redness in the skin, along with warmth may be an indication of **cellulitis**, or a skin infection. Erythema and warmth over a joint may indicate an infection in the joint or an arthritis caused by inflammation within the joint. Finally, abrasions, lacerations, and ecchymosis can indicate trauma to the extremity.

Cardiovascular

The Paramedic should palpate the peripheral pulse to ensure it is present and the extremity is well perfused, especially in the situation of trauma to the extremity. He should check the pulse before and after splinting to detect overtightening of the splint or loss of pulse from vessel damage during the

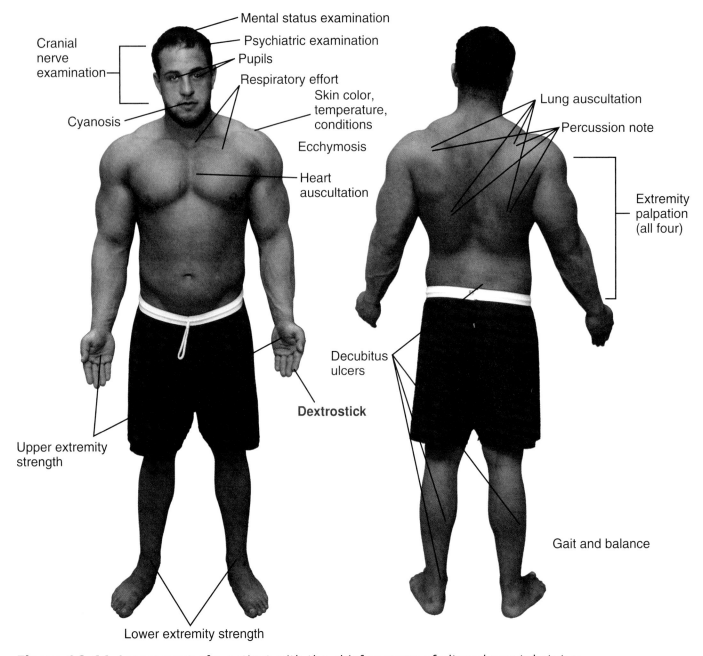

Figure 16-44 Assessment of a patient with the chief concern of altered mental status.

splinting process. In patients with nontraumatic extremity pain and edema, the Paramedic should perform a cardiovascular examination to assess for signs of heart failure as the cause of the patient's chief concern.

Neurological

The Paramedic should assess the painful extremity for sensation and motor function distal to the injury both before and after splinting. Sensation and motor function should also be assessed in the situation of nontraumatic extremity pain.

Put It All Together

The assessment of a patient presenting with the chief concern of extremity pain includes many possibilities (Figure 16-45).

High Blood Pressure

According to the American Heart Association, approximately 72 million people in the United States are diagnosed with high blood pressure, with an even greater number of people unaware their blood pressure is high.[52] Blood pressure can be elevated due to pain or the condition the patient is experiencing. It is estimated that in the year 2004, hypertension caused approximately 54,000 deaths in the United States. High blood pressure is a significant risk factor for kidney failure and heart disease, and a primary cause of stroke. Many patients do not exhibit symptoms for a long time prior to diagnosis.

The Paramedic's goal in assessing patients with the chief concern of high blood pressure is to look for signs that

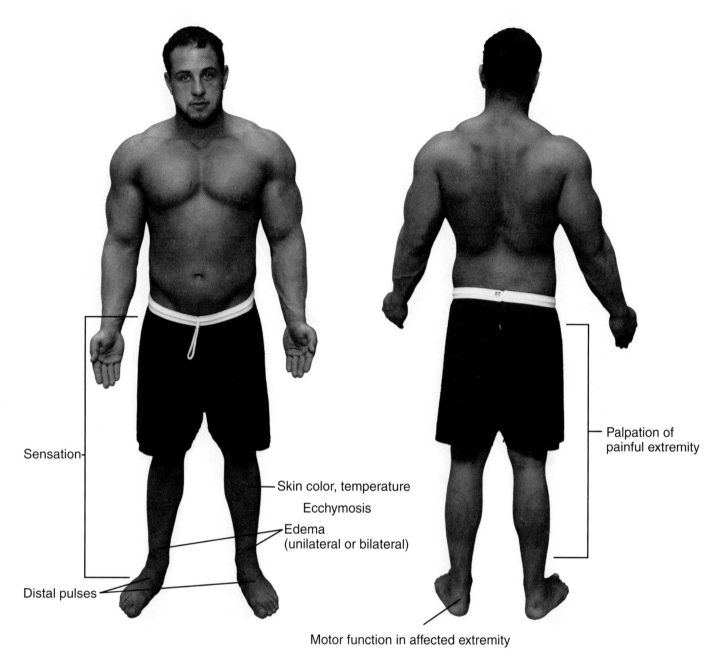

Sensation

Skin color, temperature
Ecchymosis
Edema
(unilateral or bilateral)

Distal pulses

Palpation of
painful extremity

Motor function in affected extremity

Figure 16-45 Assessment of a patient with the chief concern of extremity pain.

the high blood pressure is causing organ damage, including damage to the brain, heart, lungs, and kidneys. The majority of patients encountered by the Paramedic do not require acute lowering of their blood pressure in the prehospital environment. For patients who have a chief concern other than high blood pressure, refer to the section of this chapter that covers a focused examination related to that chief concern.

Cardiovascular

The cardiovascular examination focuses on detecting signs of heart failure. The Paramedic should inspect the patient for an elevated jugular venous pressure as well as peripheral edema. If peripheral edema is present, the Paramedic should

palpate to determine the amount of fluid present. Auscultate the heart for murmurs or extra heart sounds that may indicate fluid overload. He should palpate the peripheral pulses for equality and limb perfusion, and assess the blood pressure in both arms to detect a significant difference that may indicate a problem with the aorta.

Respiratory

The Paramedic should inspect the patient for signs of increased respiratory effort and work of breathing that indicate difficulty breathing, as this may be related to heart failure or cardiac disease. The Paramedic should auscultate the lungs for rales or wheezes that may indicate fluid in the lungs from heart failure.

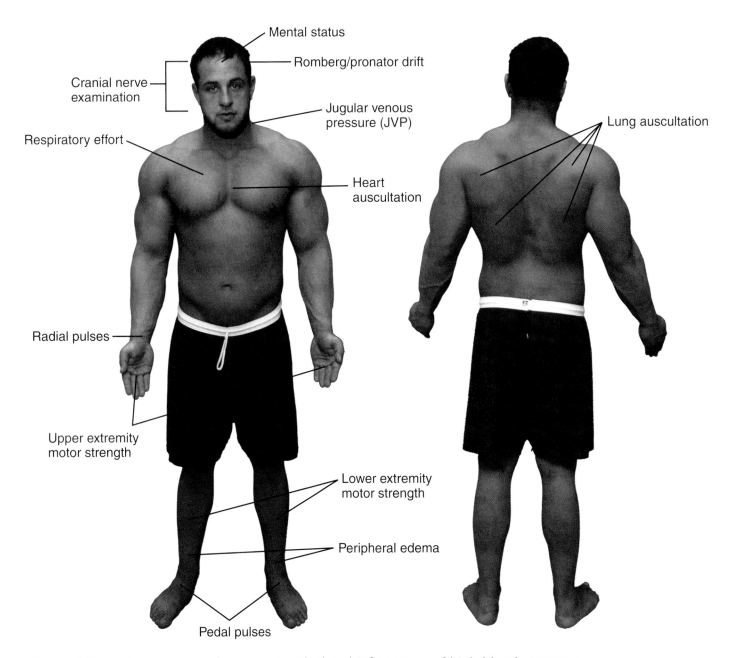

Figure 16-46 Assessment of a patient with the chief concern of high blood pressure.

Neurological

The objective of the neurological examination is to assess for deficits that may be caused by a stroke or other brain event that may be related to the high blood pressure. The Paramedic should assess the patient's cranial nerves and peripheral nerves for function. She should assess muscle strength and coordination for issues that are unilateral, as these may indicate a brain lesion. Altered mental status can result from severe hypertension that disrupts the perfusion of blood to the brain.

Put It All Together

The assessment of a patient presenting with the chief concern of high blood pressure includes many possibilities (Figure 16-46).

HEENT

Patients may complain of a variety of chief concerns related to the head, eyes, ears, nose, and throat, with the most common concern being pain. This may be associated with fever, vision changes, sore throat, foreign body sensation, or other symptoms. In the setting of trauma, there is also a concern of an underlying head injury.

Head

Assess the head for evidence of trauma, including abrasions, lacerations, ecchymosis, and obvious deformities. For patients with a chief concern of headaches or facial pain, the Paramedic should percuss the sinuses (Figure 16-47) to elicit tenderness that may indicate a sinus infection.

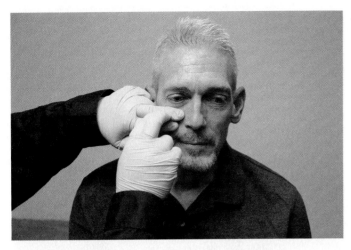

Figure 16-47 Percussion of the sinuses.

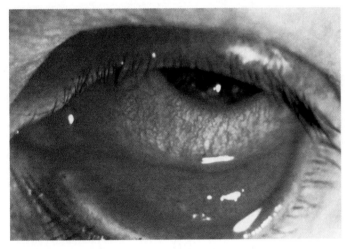

Figure 16-48 Conjunctival erythema. (Courtesy of Custom Medical Stock Photo)

Eyes

The eyes are inspected for **erythema** on the conjunctiva that indicates irritation of the eye (Figure 16-48). Pupillary reaction is tested for responsiveness and equality using a penlight. If a foreign body sensation is present, or signs of irritation exist, the eye is stained using fluroescein to inspect for a foreign body or corneal abrasion (Figure 16-49).

Ears

The Paramedic should inspect the external ear for erythema, signs of trauma, discharge, or edema. She should palpate the external ear for tenderness. Using an otoscope (Figure 16-50), the Paramedic should inspect the ear canal and middle ear for erythema, discharge, fluid behind the **tympanic membrane**, or signs of **otitis media**, a middle ear infection (Figure 16-51).

Nose

The **nares**, or nostrils, are inspected for erythema and edema of the mucous membranes or turbinates If an **epistaxis**, or nosebleed, is present, the Paramedic should inspect the mucous membrane for a source of the bleeding in the anterior portion of the nare. In the setting of nasal trauma, a **septal hematoma** (Figure 16-52) is a finding that requires attention) at the emergency department to ensure permanent damage to the nasal cartilage does not occur. Discharge from the nose may indicate a viral or bacterial infection of the sinuses.[53–55]

Throat

The examination of the throat is important with any patient who has a concern related to the upper airway, including those patients with neck trauma or a suspected allergic reaction. The throat is examined for erythema and **exudates**, whitish discharge on the mucous surface, of the posterior pharynx (Figure 16-53). Swelling in the pharynx may also indicate an impending airway issue. The **uvula** typically hangs in the midline of the pharynx. Deviation of the uvula from the midline may indicate an **abscess** or **hematoma** that can potentially threaten the airway. The external aspects of the anterior neck and mandible are also assessed for edema that may indicate a potential airway issue.

The oral mucous membranes are also examined for signs of dehydration. Normally, the mucous membranes should be pink and glisten with the usual amount of moisture in the mouth. Patients who are dehydrated will lose that glisten in the mucous membranes as less saliva is produced. In extreme dehydration, the lips will become chapped.

Neurological

The Paramedic should perform a cranial nerve examination to ensure proper function of the cranial nerves. Abnormalities in cranial nerve function can indicate an underlying brain concern or compression of an individual cranial nerve.

Put It All Together

The assessment of a patient presenting with the chief concern related to the head, eyes, ears, nose, or throat includes many possibilities (Figure 16-54).

Fever

Fever is a common chief concern for both young and old, with the extremes of age more likely to develop **sepsis**, the inflammatory response to a systemic infection, or **septic shock**, where the patient develops hypotension from the systemic infection. Fever is also a common cause of altered mental status, especially in the elderly. Altered consciousness or personality in the very young can also indicate a severe illness that requires further evaluation at the emergency department. While fever is most often caused by an infection, fever can also be caused by other conditions including toxic ingestion, environmental related illness, and disorders of a patient's thermoregulatory system.

Respiratory

The respiratory exam focuses on searching for a cause of the fever, especially when combined with hypoxemia determined

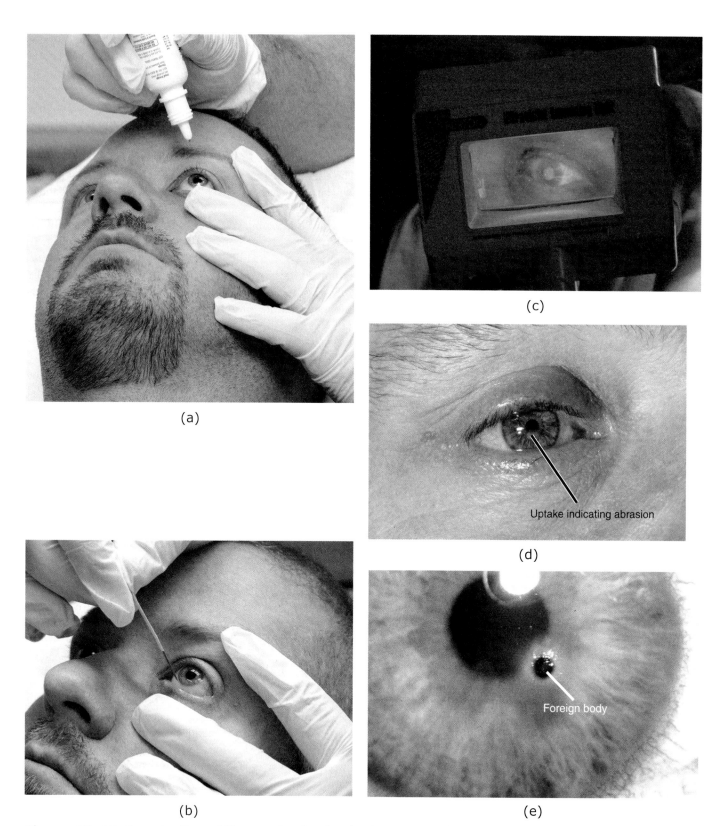

(a)

(b)

(c)

Uptake indicating abrasion

(d)

Foreign body

(e)

Figure 16-49 Examination of the eye for foreign body or corneal abrasion. (a) Instill two drops of tetracaine into the eye to be examined. (b) After 30 to 60 seconds, apply the fluorescein strip, asking the patient to blink several times. (c) Examine the eye under a Wood's lamp or using the cobalt blue filter on an ophthalmoscope. Direct the patient to move through the full range of motion of the eye. (d) Uptake of the dye indicates a corneal abrasion. (e) Foreign body present on the cornea. (Photo (d) is Courtesy of SPL/Custom Medical Stock Photo, (e) Courtesy of Michael Friedburg, O.D.)

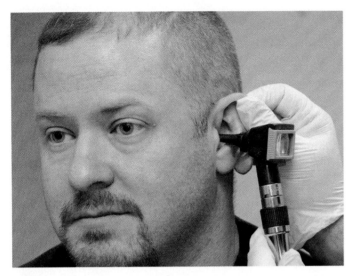

Figure 16-50 Paramedic assessing the ear with an otoscope.

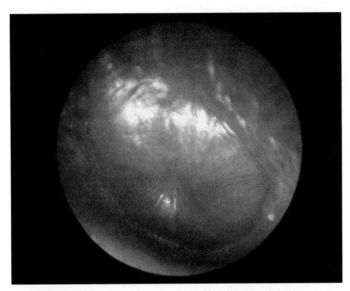

Figure 16-51 Appearance of the tympanic membrane in a patient with a middle ear infection (otitis media). (Courtesy of B. Welleschik; licensed under the Creative Commons Attribution ShareAlike 2.5)

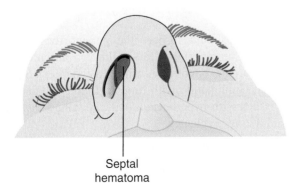

Septal hematoma

Figure 16-52 Septal hematoma.

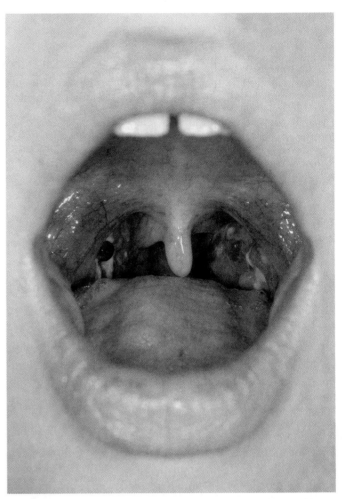

Figure 16-53 Erythema and exudates on the posterior pharynx. (Courtesy of Scott Camazine/ Phototake USA)

from the vital signs. The Paramedic should inspect the patient for signs of increased respiratory effort. He should auscultate the lungs for signs of focal consolidation that may indicate pneumonia. Auscultation may also reveal wheezing from associated **bronchospasm**, or constriction of the smaller air passages that sometimes accompanies a respiratory infection. A dull percussion note over one area of the chest may also indicate a pneumonia in that portion of the lung.

Gastrointestinal

A gastrointestinal source of the fever is often suggested in a patient who is vomiting or has diarrhea. The Paramedic should inspect the patient's abdomen for distention and discoloration. She should auscultate the abdomen to assess the patient's bowel sounds, and palpate the abdomen, assessing for tenderness starting with the quadrant or section furthest away from the area of pain. The Paramedic should also palpate for the signs of peritoneal irritation as previously described. Tenderness to percussion over the abdomen may also indicate peritoneal irritation. A dull percussion note indicates ascites that can be the source of infection. A tympanic percussion note can indicate bowel obstruction or

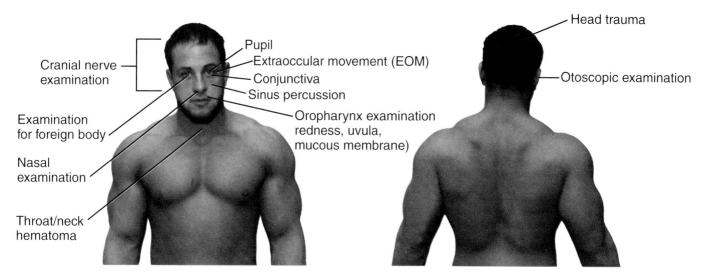

Figure 16-54 Assessment of a patient with the chief concern of related to the head, eyes, ears, nose, or throat.

rupture that may be the source of infection. Tenderness with percussion of the costovertebral angle can indicate **pyelonephritis**, or an infection of the kidney as a possible source of the fever.

Skin

The skin is inspected for signs of infection. Cellulitis can present with erythema over an area of the skin. Patients with a history of diabetes are more likely to develop cellulitis over the lower extremities.[56,57] Streaking, also known as **lymphangitis**, is inflammation of the lymphatic channels in the skin and occurs when there is spread of an infection located distal to the streaking. As discussed earlier, decubitus ulcers can develop and become infected in patients who are bed or chair ridden. Finally, assessing the skin **turgor**, or elasticity, can indicate dehydration.[58]

HEENT

Examine the oropharynx for signs of infection and dehydration in patients who have a chief concern of fever.

Put It All Together

The assessment of a patient presenting with the chief concern of fever includes many possibilities (Figure 16-55).

Pregnancy

While most pregnancies are uneventful, at times the Paramedic will care for patients who have, or potentially have, a chief concern related to their pregnancy. Some of the common concerns include vaginal bleeding, abdominal cramping or pain, trauma in pregnancy, or impending childbirth. Many chronic medical conditions (e.g., asthma or diabetes) can worsen during pregnancy and may require more frequent medical care.[59] Seizures can occur secondary to issues with hypertension in pregnancy.

Gynecological

A brief gynecological examination is indicated when imminent delivery is considered. While maintaining privacy with a sheet or other covering, the Paramedic should briefly inspect the vaginal opening for the presence of bleeding or discharge. **Crowning** occurs as the infant's head begins the passage into the birth canal (Figure 16-56), indicating delivery will occur within several minutes.

The abdomen is palpated to assess for tenderness and signs of peritoneal irritation in the pregnant female patient complaining of abdominal pain. The uterus can often be palpated as a firm mass in the midline of the lower abdomen. It is first detected at approximately 12 to 15 weeks of gestation and grows until almost reaching the **costal margin** of the lower portion of the rib cage by full term. Contractions can also be detected by the Paramedic during palpation as the uterus tightens and constricts. Contractions are measured for duration and timing. The duration contraction is the length of time the uterus is contracted. The timing is measured as the number of minutes between the beginning of one contraction and the beginning of the next, to include both one cycle of uterine contraction and relaxation. This information is often reported as "contractions of one minute in duration, three minutes apart."

Respiratory

The Paramedic should inspect the patient for signs of increased respiratory effort. He should also auscultate the lungs for abnormal sounds (e.g., wheezes and rales). Significant rales in combination with lower extremity edema may indicate issues with hypertension or heart failure that have developed during pregnancy.

Cardiovascular

The Paramedic should inspect the patient for increased jugular venous pressure and significant peripheral edema that may indicate problems with hypertension or heart failure related to

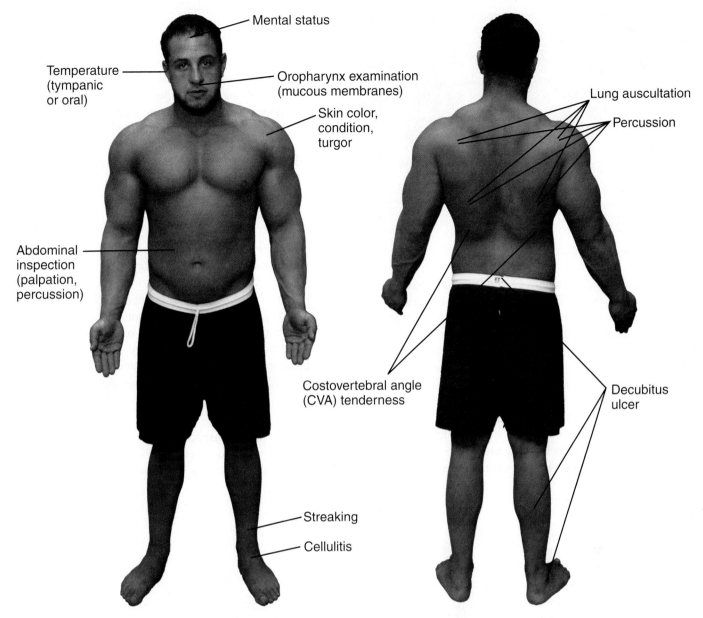

Figure 16-55 Assessment of a patient with the chief concern of fever.

pregnancy. Gallops and certain murmurs are normal in pregnancy as the blood volume increases and the growing fetus compresses pelvic and abdominal blood vessels. However, these conditions may be of concern in patients with a chief concern of chest pain or shortness of breath. The Paramedic should palpate the peripheral pulses or assess capillary refill to assess perfusion, then palpate the edematous extremities to assess the level of edema.

Neurological

Neurological issues during pregnancy are often related to the patient's underlying seizure disorder or can be related to hypertension in pregnancy. In a pregnant patient with hypertension, the Paramedic should assess the deep tendon reflexes. Deep tendon reflexes that are **hyperreflexive**, or produce a

response significantly more brisk than normal, can indicate impending neurological issues. For pregnant patients treated with magnesium, one indication of too much magnesium is deep tendon reflexes that are **hyporeflexive**, or significantly less brisk than normal.

Put It All Together

The assessment of a patient presenting with the chief concern related to pregnancy includes many possibilities (Figure 16-57).

Trauma

Trauma-related concerns are a significant portion of the requests for assistance encountered by Paramedics. The examination of patients who have sustained a suspected traumatic

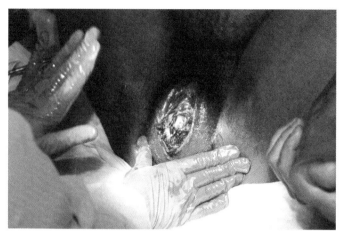

Figure 16-56 Crowning.

injury follows a systematic head to toe approach after the primary survey is completed to ensure detection of injuries based on the mechanism of injury. Even with a minor mechanism, the Paramedic needs to be thorough to ensure the presence of life-threatening injuries is detected as early as possible. Prehospital trauma triage guidelines have been developed to provide guidance to Paramedics in determining which patients should be transported directly to a trauma center and which patients can be cared for at a community hospital (Figure 16-58). Once the primary survey is completed and any life-threatening airway, breathing, or circulatory concerns are addressed, the Paramedic begins a more detailed head to toe examination.

Head

Starting with the patient's head, the Paramedic should inspect the scalp and face for lacerations, abrasions, ecchymosis, or obvious deformities that indicate the presence of a head injury. She should also inspect the mouth to assess for foreign material and unstable or missing teeth that may occlude the airway if untreated. The Paramedic should palpate the skull and face to assess for stability of the bony structure. She should also assess pupil reaction and gross cranial nerve function to look for abnormalities that may indicate cerebral hemorrhage.

Neck

While maintaining spinal motion restriction, the Paramedic should inspect the anterior neck for signs of trauma or edema that may affect airway management or compromise the airway. She should also palpate the trachea and larynx, assessing for stability, tenderness, and position of the trachea. The Paramedic should palpate the neck for subcutaneous emphysema caused by a leak in the respiratory system, and palpate the cervical spine in the midline posteriorly, assessing for tenderness and deformity from a cervical spine injury.

Chest

The Paramedic should inspect the chest for respiratory effort, abnormal chest wall movement, and signs of trauma, including wounds and ecchymosis. He should also auscultate the

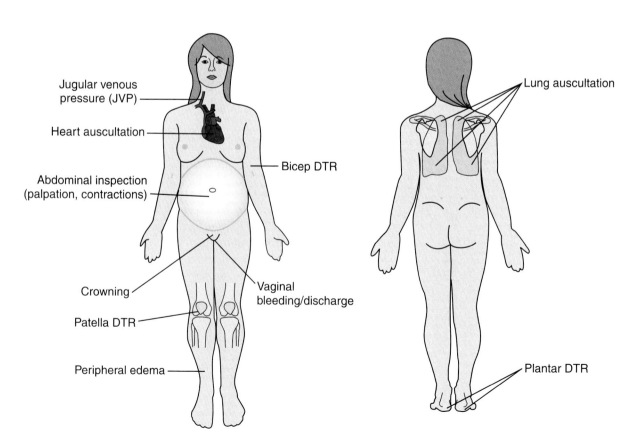

Figure 16-57 Assessment of a patient with the chief concern related to pregnancy.

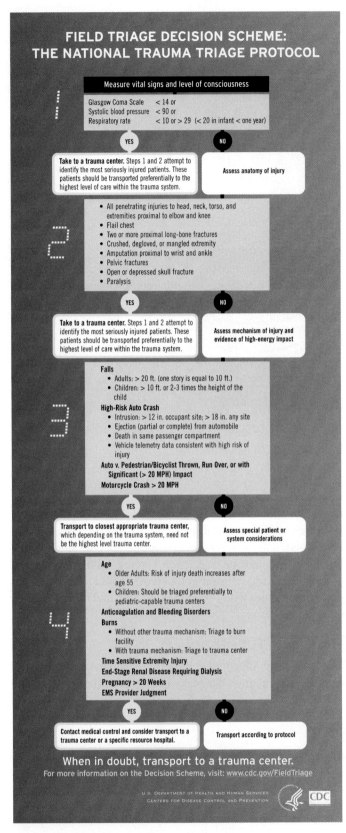

FIELD TRIAGE DECISION SCHEME: THE NATIONAL TRAUMA TRIAGE PROTOCOL

Measure vital signs and level of consciousness

Glasgow Coma Scale < 14 or
Systolic blood pressure < 90 or
Respiratory rate < 10 or > 29 (< 20 in infant < one year)

YES → **Take to a trauma center.** Steps 1 and 2 attempt to identify the most seriously injured patients. These patients should be transported preferentially to the highest level of care within the trauma system.

NO → Assess anatomy of injury

- All penetrating injuries to head, neck, torso, and extremities proximal to elbow and knee
- Flail chest
- Two or more proximal long-bone fractures
- Crushed, degloved, or mangled extremity
- Amputation proximal to wrist and ankle
- Pelvic fractures
- Open or depressed skull fracture
- Paralysis

YES → **Take to a trauma center.** Steps 1 and 2 attempt to identify the most seriously injured patients. These patients should be transported preferentially to the highest level of care within the trauma system.

NO → Assess mechanism of injury and evidence of high-energy impact

Falls
- Adults: > 20 ft. (one story is equal to 10 ft.)
- Children: > 10 ft. or 2-3 times the height of the child

High-Risk Auto Crash
- Intrusion: > 12 in. occupant site; > 18 in. any site
- Ejection (partial or complete) from automobile
- Death in same passenger compartment
- Vehicle telemetry data consistent with high risk of injury

Auto v. Pedestrian/Bicyclist Thrown, Run Over, or with Significant (> 20 MPH) Impact

Motorcycle Crash > 20 MPH

YES → Transport to closest appropriate trauma center, which depending on the trauma system, need not be the highest level trauma center.

NO → Assess special patient or system considerations

Age
- Older Adults: Risk of injury death increases after age 55
- Children: Should be triaged preferentially to pediatric-capable trauma centers

Anticoagulation and Bleeding Disorders

Burns
- Without other trauma mechanism: Triage to burn facility
- With trauma mechanism: Triage to trauma center

Time Sensitive Extremity Injury

End-Stage Renal Disease Requiring Dialysis

Pregnancy > 20 Weeks

EMS Provider Judgment

YES → Contact medical control and consider transport to a trauma center or a specific resource hospital.

NO → Transport according to protocol

When in doubt, transport to a trauma center.

For more information on the Decision Scheme, visit: www.cdc.gov/FieldTriage

U.S. DEPARTMENT OF HEALTH AND HUMAN SERVICES
CENTERS FOR DISEASE CONTROL AND PREVENTION

CDC

Figure 16-58 National EMS trauma triage protocol. (Courtesy of Centers for Disease Control and Prevention, CDC)

chest for the presence and equality of lung sounds in addition to abnormal sounds. The Paramedic should palpate the chest for the presence of subcutaneous emphysema, for tenderness, and instability. A **flail segment** develops when two or more adjacent ribs are fractured in two or more places (Figure 16-59). This produces an unstable area of the chest that impedes normal respiration. During inhalation, the flail segment is drawn inward by the negative pressure in the chest rather than expanding outward with the rest of the chest wall. During exhalation, the opposite occurs due to the increased pressure in the thorax during exhalation. This movement opposite of the normal chest wall movement is called **paradoxical respiration**. A hyperresonant percussion note can indicate a pneumothorax, where air is trapped between the pleural layers surrounding the lung, while a hyporesonant percussion note may indicate a hemothorax, or blood filling the space between the pleural layers.

Abdomen

The abdomen is inspected for wounds and other signs of direct trauma. Ecchymosis along either flank can indicate internal bleeding. A seat belt sign, or ecchymosis along the lower abdomen corresponding to the position of the lap belt, indicates enough force to produce internal damage.[60–62] The Paramedic should note any distention present and palpate the abdomen for tenderness and firmness. Tenderness over the upper quadrants may indicate injury to the solid organs. A firm and distended abdomen is worrisome for internal bleeding that is not controllable in the prehospital environment.

Pelvis

The bony pelvis is assessed for stability and tenderness using palpation. After taking firm hold of the iliac wings (Figure 16-60), the Paramedic gently applies pressure to compress the pelvis. Tenderness may indicate a pelvic fracture, whereas instability is indicative of life-threatening internal pelvic bleeding and requires stabilization by the Paramedic.

Extremities

Finally, each extremity is inspected for obvious deformity, angulation, or wounds. The Paramedic should palpate each extremity for tenderness and stability (Figure 16-41). She should also palpate each extremity for the presence of a distal pulse or capillary refill to assess perfusion. The Paramedic should perform a rapid motor and sensory assessment on each extremity to ensure full function, then assess and document circulation, sensation, and motor function both before and after splinting injured extremities.

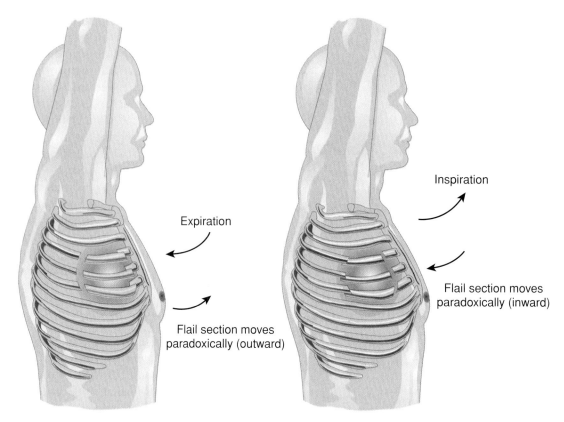

Figure 16-59 A flail segment paradoxically moves opposite the rest of the chest during inspiration and expiration.

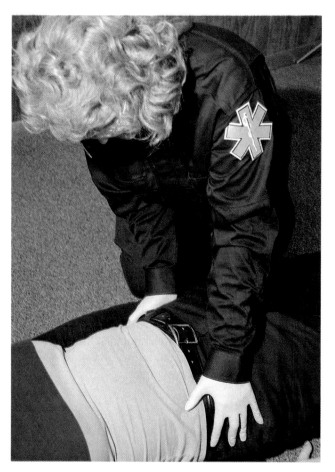

Figure 16-60 Assessing the pelvis for stability.

Spine

The Paramedic should inspect the back for signs of lacerations, abrasions, and ecchymosis. He should palpate the spine for tenderness, stability, and alignment. This is often performed with the patient log-rolled to one side, maintaining spinal motion restriction (Figure 16-61) during the assessment. Any deformity or step off should be treated as a potential fracture with full immobilization and transport to an appropriate facility.

Put It All Together

The assessment of a patient presenting with the chief concern of major trauma includes many possibilities (Figure 16-62).

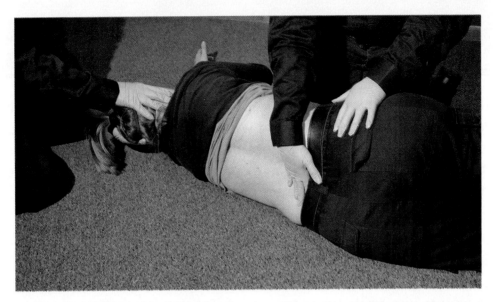

Figure 16-61 Assessment of the back and spine in a patient who was involved in a traumatic event.

Primary survey: Focus on airway, breathing, circulation

Secondary survey: Systematic head to toe approach after the primary survey is completed

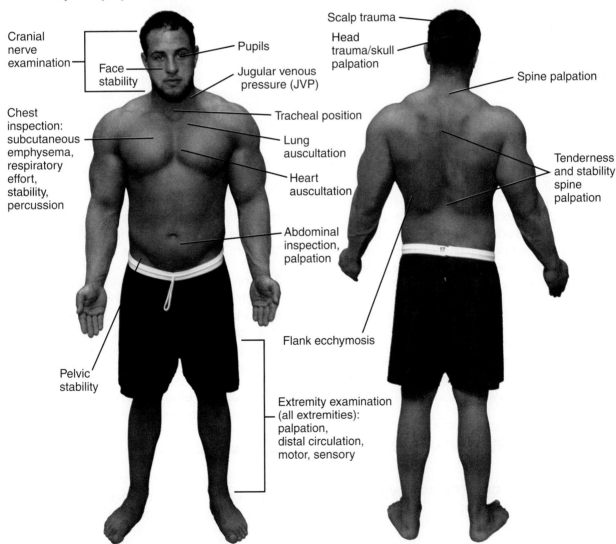

Cranial nerve examination

Face stability

Pupils

Jugular venous pressure (JVP)

Tracheal position

Chest inspection: subcutaneous emphysema, respiratory effort, stability, percussion

Lung auscultation

Heart auscultation

Abdominal inspection, palpation

Pelvic stability

Flank ecchymosis

Extremity examination (all extremities): palpation, distal circulation, motor, sensory

Scalp trauma

Head trauma/skull palpation

Spine palpation

Tenderness and stability spine palpation

Figure 16-62 Assessment of a patient with the chief concern of major trauma.

CONCLUSION

While these common chief concerns will cover the majority of patients that the Paramedic will encounter, there will be some patients that do not have one of these chief concerns. By using these principles to perform a physical assessment, a Paramedic can perform an examination on patients in an efficient manner which allows a full patient assessment.

KEY POINTS:

- The four components to every physical exam are inspection, auscultation, palpation, and percussion.

- Inspection is a technique that involves looking at patients and their surroundings.

- Auscultation of the patient is performed using a stethoscope.

- Palpation is touch used to assess the stability of bony structures and tenderness of muscle and tissue.

- Percussion is lightly but sharply tapping the body surface to determine the characteristics (air-filled, fluid-filled, or solid) of the underlying tissue.

- Vital signs are objectively measured characteristics of basic body functions and include pulse, respirations, blood pressure, and temperature. Assessment of a patient's pain level and peripheral oxygen saturation (SpO_2) may also be included in the Paramedic's assessment of vital signs.

- The pulse is assessed for rate, rhythm, and quality.

- For patients with significant tachycardia, 180 to 220 beats per minute, or infant and toddlers, the Paramedic may use a stethoscope to listen to the heart and count an apical pulse.

- Respirations are assessed by observing the respiratory rate, depth, pattern, and work of breathing.

- Depth of respirations can be described as shallow (hypoventilation), normal, or deep (hyperventilation).

- The respiratory pattern or rhythm of the respirations is the combination of the timing of the respirations and the depth of respirations.

- Blood pressure is the pressure within the arterial vessels of the circulatory system.

- The mean arterial pressure (MAP) is the average pressure in the arterial system over time while the pulse pressure is the difference between the systolic and diastolic pressures.

- The patient's core temperature can be measured from oral, rectal, or tympanic thermometers.

- Skin condition and color is an important indicator of perfusion.

- Pulse oximetry is a noninvasive measurement of the percentage of hemoglobin in arterial blood that is bound to oxygen molecules.

- Factors that may affect the accuracy of the pulse oximetry reading include poor blood flow due to hypovolemia or hypotension, and other compounds (e.g., carbon monoxide) that can also bind to hemoglobin and interfere with pulse oximeter readings.

- The amount of exhaled carbon dioxide is related to the patient's ability to move air in and out of the lungs and is directly related to the patient's level of perfusion.

- Orthostatic vital signs are signs that change when an individual changes position from lying down to a standing position due to the heart's inability to compensate and maintain an adequate blood pressure and pulse.

- Positive orthostatic vital signs are defined as a heart rate increase of 20 beats per minute or greater, a systolic blood pressure drop of greater than 20 mmHg, a diastolic blood pressure increase of 10 mmHg, and/or dizziness or lightheadedness with position change.

- A patient's chief concern or chief complaint is used to focus the history and physical examination on specific body systems.

Chest Pain

- The inspection of a patient with the chief concern of chest pain begins with the assessment of jugular venous pressure (JVP) and signs of peripheral edema.

- Auscultation of heart sounds proceeds systematically and should note the normal heart sounds (S1 and S2), potential extra sounds (S3 and S4), and abnormal heart sounds such as murmurs and rubs.

- Palpate the chest for a thrill or cardiac heave. Assess a patient's peripheral pulse for strength and equality in the left and right extremities.

- Indications of a patient's respiratory effort include use of accessory muscles, evidence of sternal or intercostal retractions, increased respiratory rate, or tripod positioning. The patient's skin, mucous membranes, and nail beds can be assessed for cyanosis developed from hypoxemia.

- When auscultating lung sounds, the Paramedic should auscultate posteriorly and the left and right sides of the chest, comparing the same levels from apex to base. The Paramedic may be able to determine conditions associated with certain abnormal lung sounds (e.g., wheezing, which is associated with asthma or COPD).

- Percussion of the chest may reveal normal hollow sounds, a hyperresonant note often seen with a pneumothorax, or hyporesonant notes that may indicate fluid in the lung from either a pleural effusion or hemothorax. The Paramedic should palpate the chest to assess the stability of the rib cage, tenderness, equal expansion, and the presence of subcutaneous emphysema.

- The abdominal exam in a patient with a chief concern of chest pain is limited to palpation for pain and signs of fluid overload. Positive hepatojugular reflux is a sign of fluid overload related to right-sided heart failure. A normal mental status indicates that the brain is receiving a sufficient amount of oxygenated blood. An altered mental status, which may vary from confusion to unconsciousness, can indicate that the brain is not receiving enough oxygenated blood.

Shortness of Breath

- The physical exam for a patient with a chief concern of shortness of breath is similar to the exam performed for chest pain and begins with the assessment of respiratory effort and cyanosis. Deviation of the trachea is also assessed and is usually a late sign of conditions that can cause a shift of the heart and lungs to one side.

- The Paramedic assesses the patient using auscultation to identify normal and several abnormal lung sounds that can indicate a respiratory cause of shortness of breath. Other lung sounds, elevated venous blood pressures, and peripheral edema may also indicate a cardiac cause of shortness of breath. Peripheral pulses and capillary refill can be used to assess a patient's level of perfusion.

- Patients in respiratory distress use more energy to breathe; thus, they produce more CO_2. As the level of distress increases, the ventilation becomes poorer and the patient is not able to exhale the CO_2 that is produced. The CO_2 levels increase in the blood. When the CO_2 levels become high enough, the patient's respiratory drive and mental status are further depressed, again impairing the patient's ability to remove the CO_2 from the blood. Patients with a chief concern of shortness of breath who have an altered mental status require aggressive airway management and ventilatory support in order to halt this dangerous cycle.

Abdominal Pain

- The abdomen is inspected for distention and prominent surface veins and the skin is inspected for jaundice or ecchymosis. Bowel sounds can be auscultated by the Paramedic and may provide some clue as to the cause of the patient's abdominal pain. Percussion can also be used by the Paramedic to assess the abdomen for ascites or fluid, as well as tenderness indicative of irritation of the kidney or peritoneum.

- The abdomen can be divided into either four quadrants or by a method of nines. Each section found in either method is palpated by applying gentle, but firm pressure with one hand while the other hand lies on top and helps guide the first. Patients may demonstrate rebound tenderness or exhibit different signs associated with specific conditions. The abdomen is also palpated for any masses that can be tender or nontender, firm or soft, or pulsatile.

- For patients who have epigastric pain, the Paramedic should be diligent and perform a more extensive cardiovascular examination. Skin color and perfusion should be inspected, accompanied by auscultation of heart tones and murmurs. The Paramedic should palpate for hepatojugular reflux and assess the extremities for equality of the pulses, especially in the lower extremities. An inequality may indicate a vascular problem with the abdominal aorta.

Syncope

- Syncope is a transient loss of consciousness that resolves spontaneously. Near syncope is the feeling that one is going to pass out, although one does not actually lose consciousness. Assessment of syncope or near syncope begins with the determination of the patient's level of responsiveness, alertness, and orientation to person, place, and time. It also assesses the patient's memory for the events leading up to the call for assistance and whether the patient is able to pay attention or is easily distracted in conversation. The patient should exhibit appropriate language with clear speech and respond to questions in an appropriate context.

- The remainder of the neurological exam is divided up into the cranial nerve exam, the peripheral nerve exam, assessment of deep tendon reflexes, and assessment of coordination. The cranial nerves are a set of 12 paired nerves that begin within the brainstem and are responsible for movement and sensation in the head and neck.

- The second cranial nerve is evaluated through assessment of the patient's visual acuity. The third,

fourth, and sixth cranial nerves are assessed by examining the patient's extraocular movements (EOM). Sustained or prolonged nystagmus may be a sign of intoxication or a central nervous system problem. The third cranial nerve also controls the papillary response, which is assessed by shining a penlight into the patient's pupils one at a time, looking for constriction of both pupils.

- Sensation and motor function impulses to the face are carried by the fifth and seventh cranial nerves, respectively, and are assessed by looking for any asymmetry in sensation or movement of the face. The eighth cranial nerve is examined by assessing the patient's hearing. Asking the patient to stick out his tongue and say "ah" assesses the ninth and twelfth cranial nerves. The last part of the cranial nerve examination is to ask the patient to shrug his shoulders while observing for symmetry, which tests the eleventh cranial nerve.

- Peripheral sensation of the skin is organized into dermatomes that correspond to the spinal nerve roots. Differences in sensation between extremities may indicate nerve root compression, a stroke, or damage to the peripheral nerve itself. Deep tendon reflexes (DTRs) are tested by tapping a large tendon and looking for involuntary muscle contraction in the muscle associated with that tendon. The bicep tendon DTR and patellar tendon DTR, along with the plantar reflex, are reflexes that can be evaluated during an assessment.

- The Paramedic can assess a patient's coordination by testing the patient for pronator drift. Further assessment of coordination can be carried out by asking the patient to touch her nose with one finger and then touch the Paramedic's finger, or asking the patient to touch the heel of one leg to the opposite leg just below the knee and slide it down the tibia.

- The cardiovascular assessment for syncope or near syncope involves auscultation of heart sounds for tone, murmurs, and extra heart sounds. Pulses should be palpated for strength and equality. Orthostatic vital signs may help assess for hypovolemia that is not present with the resting vital signs.

- The musculoskeletal examination is used to assess for weakness and detect injury sustained during the syncopal episode. The Paramedic should palpate and inspect any areas that are painful while testing the muscle strength of both the upper and lower extremities. Bony surfaces and joints should also be assessed for stability. The Paramedic should also observe and document any abnormalities in the patient's gait.

Altered Mental Status

- Altered mental status can be described as any change from a normal mental status. Some causes of altered mental status can be aging, infection, intoxication, toxic substances, hypoxia, hypoglycemia, or trauma. The Paramedic's goal in assessing the patient with altered mental status is to identify reversible causes while providing supportive care to the patient.

- The objective of the neurological exam in a patient with a chief concern of altered mental status is to identify signs of either a focal neurological issue, such as a stroke or a cerebral hemorrhage, or a global disruption, such as low blood sugar or fever. For the respiratory system examination, one of the most common causes of altered mental status is hypoxia. The Paramedic should again focus on the patient's ability to oxygenate and ventilate.

- The assessment of skin color, condition, and temperature may indicate infection, fever, or dehydration as causes of altered mental status. Ecchymosis, lacerations, or abrasions indicate trauma and suggest a traumatic cause for the altered mental status.

- Psychiatric conditions or worsening dementia can also cause an altered mental status. Components of the psychiatric exam include assessment of speech, thought processes, suicidal or homicidal ideation, judgment, insight into medical condition, and mental status. Much of this examination is required to ensure a patient who wishes to refuse medical attention has sufficient capacity (i.e., mental ability) to understand the potential medical condition and the consequences of refusing treatment or transport.

Extremity Pain

- Extremity pain as a chief concern can have a traumatic origin or a medical origin. To determine the cause, the Paramedic should inspect the painful extremity for signs of an obvious injury,

including a fracture or dislocation, laceration, abrasion, ecchymosis, or edema that can indicate an underlying bony injury. Erythema, or redness in the skin, along with warmth may be an indication of cellulitis, or a skin infection.

- The Paramedic should palpate the peripheral pulse of the extremity for adequate perfusion in a trauma situation. Assessment of sensation and motor function should be performed in situations of nontraumatic as well as traumatic extremity pain. Sensation and motor function distal to the injury should also be performed with a pulse check before and after splinting.

High Blood Pressure

- The majority of patients encountered by the Paramedic do not require acute lowering of the blood pressure in the prehospital environment. However, it is the Paramedic's goal in assessing the patient to look for signs that the high blood pressure is causing organ damage, including damage to the brain, heart, lungs, and kidneys.

- The cardiovascular examination focuses on detecting signs of heart failure. The Paramedic should palpate for peripheral edema and pulses, auscultate for heart murmurs or extra heart sounds, and assess the patient's blood pressure.

- The Paramedic should auscultate lung sounds and inspect the patient for signs of difficulty breathing that may be related to heart failure or cardiac disease. Assessment of the cranial nerves and muscle strength and coordination may identify deficits that may be caused by a stroke or other brain event that may be related to high blood pressure. Severe hypertension that disrupts the perfusion of blood to the brain can result in the patient presenting with altered mental status.

HEENT

- A variety of chief concerns are related to the head, eyes, ears, nose, and throat, with the most common concern being pain. The Paramedic should inspect the head for evidence of trauma and the eyes for responsiveness to light, erythema on the conjunctiva, and signs of irritation or a foreign body present.

- Ears should be inspected for erythema, signs of trauma, and discharge or edema. The nares, or nostrils, are also inspected for erythema and edema. If an epistaxis is present, the Paramedic should inspect the mucous membrane to find a source of the bleeding in the anterior portion of the nare.

- The throat is examined by the Paramedic for erythema, exudates, swelling, and deviation of the uvula from the midline of the pharynx. Oral mucous membranes are also examined for signs of dehydration.

Fever

- Fever is a common chief concern for both young and old, with the extremes of age more likely to develop sepsis, or septic shock. Fever is also a common cause of altered mental status, especially in the elderly, but fever may also be caused by toxic ingestion, environmental related illness, and disorders of the patient's thermoregulatory system.

- The respiratory exam focuses on searching for a cause of fever. The Paramedic should inspect the patient for signs of difficulty breathing, and auscultate lungs for signs of focal consolidation and constriction of the smaller airway passages.

- The Paramedic should have a high index of suspicion of a gastrointestinal source of fever with patients who present with vomiting or diarrhea. Palpation of the abdomen should be performed to assess pain, inflammation, ascites, and the possibility of pyelonephritis.

- Besides assessing the patient's skin color and temperature, the skin should be inspected for signs of infection as well as skin turgor that can indicate dehydration. The oropharynx should also be examined for signs of infection and dehydration.

Pregnancy

- Some of the common concerns for a patient who is pregnant include vaginal bleeding, abdominal cramping or pain, trauma in pregnancy, or impending childbirth. The patient may also have a history of medical conditions such as diabetes or hypertension, although she may also have developed these conditions as a result of her pregnancy.

- A brief gynecological examination is indicated when imminent delivery is considered. It involves the Paramedic briefly inspecting the vaginal opening for

the presence of bleeding or discharge and evidence of crowning. The abdomen is palpated to assess for tenderness and signs of peritoneal irritation. Contractions may also be detected and should be measured for duration and timing.

- Significant rales in combination with lower extremity edema may indicate issues with hypertension or heart failure that have developed during pregnancy. Significant peripheral edema, increased jugular venous pressure, and chest pain or shortness of breath may also indicate problems with hypertension or heart failure.

- Neurological issues during pregnancy are often related to the patient's underlying seizure disorder or can be related to hypertension in pregnancy. For pregnant patients treated with magnesium, one indication of too much magnesium is deep tendon reflexes that are hyporeflexive, or significantly less brisk than normal.

Trauma

- The examination of patients who have sustained a suspected traumatic injury follows a systematic head to toe approach after the primary survey is completed to ensure detection of injuries based on the mechanism of injury. Starting with the patient's head, the Paramedic inspects the scalp and face for lacerations, abrasions, ecchymosis, or obvious deformities that indicate the presence of a head injury. Inspection of the skull, face, and mouth is performed along with evaluating pupil reaction and gross cranial nerve function.

- With proper spinal motion restriction in place, the Paramedic should inspect the anterior neck for signs of trauma or edema that may affect airway management or compromise. The cervical spine should be assessed for midline position and palpated for tenderness and deformity.

- Assessment of the chest for patients with a chief concern of trauma involves inspection of the chest for respiratory effort, abnormal chest wall movement, and signs of trauma. A flail segment develops when two or more adjacent ribs are fractured in two or more places. This results in paradoxical respirations whereby the flail segment moves opposite of the normal chest wall movement. Further inspection and auscultation may indicate a pneumothorax or hemothorax.

- The abdomen is inspected by the Paramedic for wounds and other signs of direct trauma such as ecchymosis and distention. Tenderness or firmness upon palpation of the abdomen may indicate injury to solid organs or internal bleeding. Pressure applied to the iliac wings of the pelvis is performed to assess the stability of the pelvis.

- Assessment and documentation of circulation, sensation, and motor function is performed before and after splinting injured extremities. Each extremity should be assessed for the presence of a distal pulse, sensation, and motor function. Inspection and palpation of the spine is often performed with the patient log-rolled to one side with proper spinal motion restriction carried out. Any deformity or step off should be treated as a potential fracture with full immobilization and transport to an appropriate facility.

REVIEW QUESTIONS:

1. You are called to the scene of a 55-year-old female with the chief concern of chest pain. Describe the elements of the physical examination that you will perform during your patient assessment.
2. During your patient examination, you find that she has tenderness to palpation of her abdomen. Describe what you should do.
3. You are called to a construction site to care for a 25-year-old male patient with eye pain. He states he may have gotten a piece of metal in his eye and his eye is in pain. How do you assess the eye for a foreign body?
4. You are called by the husband of a 32-year-old female patient who is obviously pregnant. The patient has a chief concern of shortness of breath with a history of asthma. During your assessment, you find she is also having severe, crampy lower abdominal pain. What should you do?

CASE STUDY QUESTIONS:

Please refer to the Case Study at the beginning of the chapter and answer the questions below.

1. What are the four components of each physical exam?
2. When examining a patient, what elements of a patient's condition can you see? Hear? Feel? Detect by the return of sound?
3. Describe a situation in which the incorrect treatment could actually worsen your patient's condition.

REFERENCES:

1. Rock, M. Underexposed. The neglected art of the physical exam. *Jems.* 2006;31(5):40, 42–43.

2. Dickinson ET, O'Connor RE, Krett RD. The impact of prehospital instant photography of motor vehicle crashes on receiving physician perception. *Prehosp Emerg Care.* 1997;1(2):76–79.

3. Scott LA, Brice JH, Baker CC, Shen P. An analysis of Paramedic verbal reports to physicians in the emergency department trauma room. *Prehosp Emerg Care.* 2003;7(2):247–251.

4. Kantola I, Vesalainen R, Kangassalo K, Kariluoto A. Bell or diaphragm in the measurement of blood pressure? *J Hypertens.* 2005;23(3):499–503.

5. Welsby PD, Parry G, Smith D. The stethoscope: some preliminary investigations. *Postgrad Med J.* 2003;79(938):695–698.

6. Lanser P, Gesell S. Pain management: the fifth vital sign. *Healthc Benchmarks.* 2001;8(6):62, 68–70.

7. Mularski RA, White-Chu F, Overbay D, Miller L, Asch SM, Ganzini L. Measuring pain as the 5th vital sign does not improve quality of pain management. *J Gen Intern Med.* 2006;21(6):607–612.

8. Ochoa FJ, Ramalle-Gomara E, Carpintero JM, Garcia A, Saralegui I. Competence of health professionals to check the carotid pulse. *Resuscitation.* 1998;37(3):173–175.

9. Eberle B, Dick WF, Schneider T, Wisser G, Doetsch S, Tzanova I. Checking the carotid pulse check: diagnostic accuracy of first responders in patients with and without a pulse. *Resuscitation.* 1996;33(2):107–116.

10. Bahr J, Klingler H, Panzer W, Rode H, Kettler D. Skills of lay people in checking the carotid pulse. *Resuscitation.* 1997;35(1):23–26.

11. American Academy of Orthopedic Surgeons. *Emergency Care and Transportation of the Sick and Injured* (Book with Mini CD-ROM for Windows & Macintosh, Palm/Handspring, Windows CE/Pocket PC eBook Reader, Smart Phone). Boston: Jones & Bartlett Publishers; 2002.

12. Hermansen CL, Lorah KN. Respiratory distress in the newborn. *Am Fam Physician.* 2007;76(7):987–994.

13. Bianchi R, Gigliotti F, Romagnoli I, Lanini B, Castellani C, Grazzini M, et al. Chest wall kinematics and breathlessness during pursed-lip breathing in patients with COPD. *Chest.* 2004;125(2):459–465.

14. Ritz T, Roth WT. Behavioral interventions in asthma. Breathing training. *Behav Modif.* 2003;27(5):710–730.

15. Holloway E, Ram FS. Breathing exercises for asthma. *Cochrane Database Syst Rev.* 2004;1:CD001277.

16. Truesdell S. Helping patients with COPD manage episodes of acute shortness of breath. *Medsurg Nurs.* 2000;9(4):178–182.

17. Lang EW, Chesnut RM. Intracranial pressure. Monitoring and management. *Neurosurg Clin N Am.* 1994;5(4):573–605.

18. White WB. Systolic versus diastolic blood pressure versus pulse pressure. *Curr Cardiol Rep.* 2002;4(6):463–467.

19. Singer AJ, Kahn SR, Thode HC, Jr., Hollander JE. Comparison of forearm and upper arm blood pressures. *Prehosp Emerg Care.* 1999;3(2):123–126.

20. Naqvi NH. A universal celebration: 100 years of Korotkoff sounds, 1905–2005. *Vesalius.* 2005;11(2):59–60.

21. Shlyakhto E, Conrady A. Korotkoff sounds: what do we know about its discovery? *J Hypertens.* 2005;23(1):3–4.

22. Phillips DM. JCAHO pain management standards are unveiled. Joint Commission on Accreditation of Healthcare Organizations. *Jama.* 2000;284(4):428–429.

23. Noe C, et al. New JCAHO standards for pain management. *Tex Nurs.* 2001;75(4):7.

24. Kelleher JF. Pulse oximetry. *J Clin Monit.* 1989;5(1):37–62.

25. Weg JG, Haas CF. Long-term oxygen therapy for COPD. Improving longevity and quality of life in hypoxemic patients. *Postgrad Med.* 1998;103(4):143–144, 147–148, 153–155.

26. Thrush D, Hodges MR. Accuracy of pulse oximetry during hypoxemia. *South Med J.* 1994;87(4):518–521.

27. Soubani AO. Noninvasive monitoring of oxygen and carbon dioxide. *Am J Emerg Med.* 2001;19(2):141–146.

28. Benumof JL. Interpretation of capnography. *Aana J.* 1998;66(2):169–176.

29. Grmec S, Klemen P. Does the end-tidal carbon dioxide ($EtCO_2$) concentration have prognostic value during out-of-hospital cardiac arrest? *Eur J Emerg Med.* 2001;8(4):263–269.

30. Hatlestad D. Capnography as a predictor of the return of spontaneous circulation. *Emerg Med Serv.* 2004;33(8):75–80; quiz 115.

31. Werner SL, Smith CE, Goldstein JR, Jones RA, Cydulka RK. Pilot study to evaluate the accuracy of ultrasonography in confirming endotracheal tube placement. *Ann Emerg Med.* 2007;49(1):75–80.

32. Ahrens T, Wijeweera H, Ray S. Capnography. A key underutilized technology. *Crit Care Nurs Clin North Am.* 1999;11(1):49–62.

33. Medow MS, Stewart JM, Sanyal S, Mumtaz A, Sica D., Frishman WH. Pathophysiology, diagnosis, and treatment of orthostatic hypotension and vasovagal syncope. *Cardiol Rev.* 2008;16(1):4–20.

34. Burri C, Henkemeyer H, Passler HH, Allgower M. Evaluation of acute blood loss by means of simple hemodynamic parameters. *Prog Surg.* 1973;11:108–131.

35. Gauer OH, Henry JP, Sieker HO. Changes in central venous pressure after moderate hemorrhage and transfusion in man. *Circ Res.* 1956;4(1):79–84.

36. Shenkin HA, Cheney RH, Govans SR, et al. On the diagnosis of hemorrhage in man: a study of volunteers bled large amounts. *Am J Med Sci.* 1994;25(5):421.

37. Roger VL. Epidemiology of myocardial infarction. *Med Clin North Am.* 2007;91(4):ix, 537–552.

38. Sinisalo J, Rapola J, Rossinen J, Kupari M. Simplifying the estimation of jugular venous pressure. *Am J Cardiol.* 2007;100(12):1779–1781.

39. Lima A, Bakker J. Noninvasive monitoring of peripheral perfusion. *Intensive Care Med.* 2005;31(10):1316–1326.

40. Sanchez LD, Ban KM, Bramwell K, Sakles JC, Davis D, Wolfe R, et al. A 29-year-old man with subcutaneous emphysema of the neck following blunt trauma. *Intern Emerg Med.* 2007;2(1):50–52.

41. Pullen RL, Jr. Assessing for hepatojugular reflux. *Nursing.* 2006;36(2):28.

42. Mueller C, Frana B, Rodriguez D, Laule-Kilian K, Perruchoud AP. Emergency diagnosis of congestive heart failure: impact of signs and symptoms. *Can J Cardiol.* 2005;21(11):921–924.

43. Sydow M. Ventilating the patient with severe asthma: nonconventional therapy. *Minerva Anestesiol.* 2003;69(5): 333–337.

44. Eskelinen M, Ikonen J, Lipponen P. Contributions of history-taking, physical examination, and computer assistance to diagnosis of acute small-bowel obstruction. A prospective study of 1333 patients with acute abdominal pain. *Scand J Gastroenterol.* 1994;29(8):715–721.

45. Culic V, Miric D, Eterovic D. Correlation between symptomatology and site of acute myocardial infarction. *Int J Cardiol.* 2001;77(2-3):163–168.

46. Goldberg R, Goff D, Cooper L, Luepker R, Zapka J, Bittner V, et al. Age and sex differences in presentation of symptoms among patients with acute coronary disease: the REACT Trial. Rapid early action for coronary treatment. *Coron Artery Dis.* 2000;11(5):399–407.

47. Davis N, Sistino JJ. Review of ventricular rupture: key concepts and diagnostic tools for success. *Perfusion.* 2002;17(1):63–67.

48. Guhathakurta S, Chen Q, Nalladaru Z, Squire BH, Sharma AK. Delayed traumatic mitral regurgitation after blunt chest trauma. *J Trauma.* 1999;47(5):982–984.

49. Kothari R, Barsan W, Brott T, Broderick J, Ashbrock S. Frequency and accuracy of prehospital diagnosis of acute stroke. *Stroke.* 1995;26(6):937–941.

50. Kothari RU, Pancioli A, Liu T, Brott T, Broderick J. Cincinnati Prehospital Stroke Scale: Reproducibility and validity. *Ann Emerg Med.* 1999;33(4):373–378.

51. Bray JE, Martin J, Cooper G, Barger B, Bernard S, Bladin, C. Paramedic identification of stroke: community validation of the Melbourne ambulance stroke screen. *Cerebrovasc Dis.* 2005;20(1):28–33.

52. Ekker T. When hope is lost . . . dealing with the suicidal patient. *Jems.* 1991;16(11):64–67.

53. Whelton PK, Beevers DG, Sonkodi S. Strategies for improvement of awareness, treatment and control of hypertension: results of a panel discussion. *J Hum Hypertens.* 2004;18(8): 563–565.

54. Scheid DC, Hamm RM. Acute bacterial rhinosinusitis in adults: part I. Evaluation. *Am Fam Physician.* 2004;70(9): 1685–1692.

55. Wald ER. Purulent nasal discharge. *Pediatr Infect Dis J.* 1991;10(4):329–333.

56. Louie JP, Bell LM. Appropriate use of antibiotics for common infections in an era of increasing resistance. *Emerg Med Clin North Am.* 2002;20(1):69–91.

57. Frykberg RG. Diabetic foot ulcers: pathogenesis and management. *Am Fam Physician.* 2002;66(9):1655–1662.

58. Popov T. Review: capillary refill time, abnormal skin turgor, and abnormal respiratory pattern are useful signs for detecting dehydration in children. *Evid Based Nurs.* 2005;8(2):57.

59. Torgersen KL, Curran CA. A systematic approach to the physiologic adaptations of pregnancy. *Crit Care Nurs Q.* 2006;29(1):2–19.

60. Chandler CF, Lane JS, Waxman KS. Seatbelt sign following blunt trauma is associated with increased incidence of abdominal injury. *Am Surg.* 1997;63(10):885–888.

61. Samoilenko MV, Magomedov MK, Shabalkin BV. Arteriosclerosis of the right gastro-omental artery. *Kardiologiia.* 1992;32(1):16–18.

62. Randhawa MP, Jr., Menzoian JO. Seat belt aorta. *Ann Vasc Surg.* 1990;4(4):370–377.

CHAPTER 17

CLINICAL DECISION MAKING AND TEAMWORK

KEY CONCEPTS:

Upon completion of this chapter, it is expected that the reader will understand these following concepts:

- Paramedic approach to clinical decision making
- Developing a Paramedic field diagnosis
- The importance of enveloping a mechanism of injury or nature of illness
- Differentiating between emergent and urgent
- Methods of improved clinical decision making

▶ CASE STUDY:

The Paramedics saw both patients approach the ambulances parked at the first aid station at the county fair. Each patient had the same complaint—chest pain which was worse when they took a deep breath. In obtaining a brief history, they found that Joseph Gonterman, a tall lanky 19-year-old, had just developed the pain after some coughing. He had a history of simple pneumothoraxes and currently had normal vital signs and oxygen saturation. Guiseppe Ferrari, a 68-year-old with a history of chronic lung disease, had been ill for several days before the fair. Since his granddaughter was showing her prized calf, he had decided to come to the fair anyway. Now it was difficult for him to breathe and he felt a little faint.

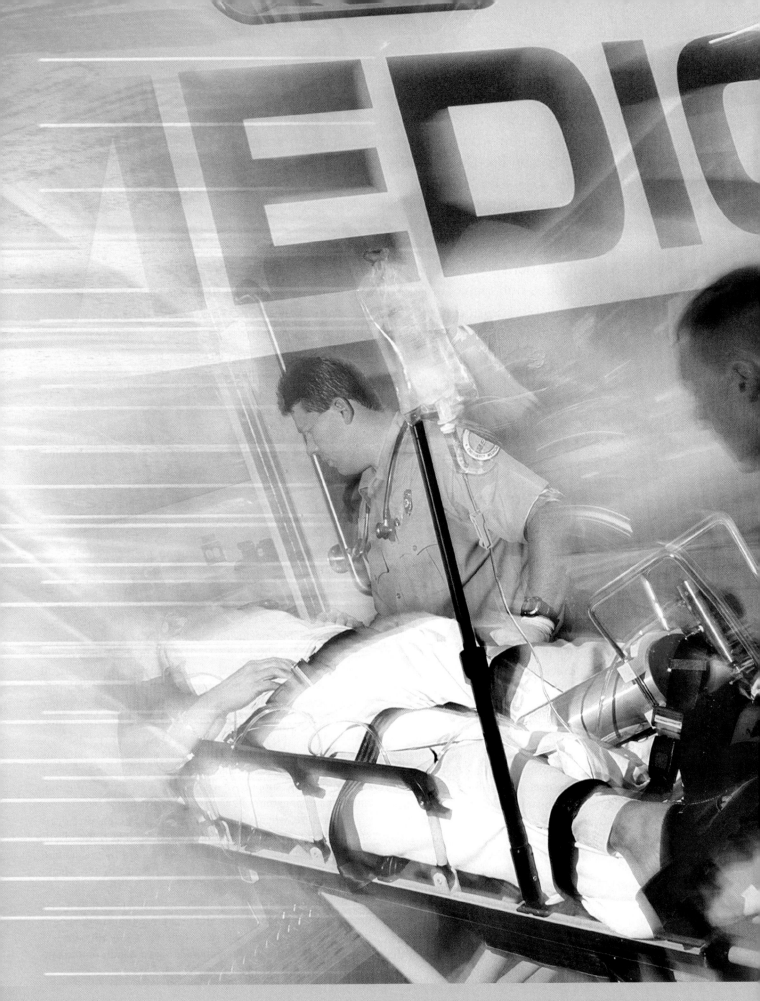

OVERVIEW

The out-of-hospital environment is heavily influenced by factors that create an environment like no other where medicine is practiced. The spectrum of patient care in the out-of-hospital environment ranges from obvious critical life threats and potential life threats to non life-threatening presentations. Effective practice in this environment requires the gathering, evaluating, and synthesizing of a great deal of information. The Paramedic must apply independent decision-making skills to make judgments and work effectively under immense pressure. Protocols, standing orders, and patient care algorithms can greatly assist the Paramedic in decision making. This approach has limitations, however: (1) It only addresses "classic" patient presentations, (2) it does not speak to those patients with multiple disease etiologies or those requiring multiple treatment modalities, and (3) it promotes linear thinking or "cookbook medicine." The components of critical thinking include concept formation, data formation, application of principle, evaluation, and reflection on action.

Clinical Decision Making

Using a process of systematic analysis and critical thinking, the Paramedic makes clinical decisions that will be incorporated into a patient's treatment plan. This process of assessment and treatment planning is called **clinical decision making**.

Medical Intelligence

Using his intelligence (i.e., past experience and medical knowledge), the Paramedic takes a systematic approach to investigating a problem and coming to a decision. This systematic approach to clinical decision making is called **medical intelligence**. In essence, it is how Paramedics think. It has been suggested that medical intelligence—the process of learning from experience and past practice and then coming to a decision—is what separates healthcare providers from the lay public.

Medical intelligence starts with information gathering. For the Paramedic, this means taking a patient history and performing the physical exam. With the facts in hand, the Paramedic compares the data against his own previous experiences, anecdotal information, and formal medical education.[1-3] This is called the **knowledge base**. The Paramedic then starts to form ideas about what is causing the patient's condition.

This process of forming ideas, called **concept formation**, is based on inductive logic. Inductive logic begins with observations, such as the history and physical exam. The facts are then incorporated with the knowledge base. Then the Paramedic reduces it all to a single theory, a hypothesis. In the case of patient care, the hypothesis is the cause of the patient's illness or the Paramedic's diagnosis.

A Paramedic's diagnosis is based upon a collection of the patient's signs and symptoms, called the **symptom complex,** obtained by the Paramedic during the history and physical exam.

The Paramedic then compares the patient's symptom complex against her knowledge base of diseases, disorders, and syndromes to find a similar grouping of signs and symptoms and matches the **symptom patterns** to derive a diagnosis.

Ordinarily, a Paramedic is hard pressed to make a diagnosis of a disease in the field. Generally, a medical diagnosis of a disease is made after exhaustive medical tests lead a physician to one irreducible conclusion which excludes all other possible conclusions. The physician arrives at this medical diagnosis as a result of a deductive process that eliminates, or **rules out**, all other possible known explanations for the patient's condition.

Paramedics do not have the resources or the time to use deductive logic in the field. Paramedics instead rely on their faster, but less precise, inductive logic to make a diagnosis. This diagnosis tends to be broad in its scope, and treatments derived from the diagnosis tend to be **palliative** in nature (i.e., providing supportive care and relief from suffering, rather than being curative).

Therefore, whenever a Paramedic makes a tentative decision, called a **Paramedic field diagnosis**, it is a broad all-encompassing conclusion. A Paramedic field diagnosis is a complaint-based conclusion about the nature of the illness or injury.

A Paramedic's field diagnosis generally identifies a disorder or a syndrome. A **disorder** is a physiological deviation from a normal homeostasis (e.g., hypoxia). A **syndrome** is a collection of symptoms that characterize a condition or state (e.g., acute coronary syndrome).

When conditions prohibit a more intensive history and physical, the Paramedic should elect to treat the patient with supportive care based upon the chief concern.[4-6] This is referred to as symptom-based care.[7] The Paramedic should then strive to obtain more clinical information when conditions improve. For example, a Paramedic confronted with a patient with air hunger should elect to treat the hypoxia first and then proceed to provide rapid transport and perform further assessment en route.

The Method of Paramedic Practice

Starting with the patient's chief complaint, or concern, the Paramedic forms a cognitive map of the potential etiologies of the chief concern. For example, if the patient's chief concern is chest pain, that elicits thoughts of numerous conditions which could account for the chest pain, including acute coronary syndrome, costracondritis, and pulmonary embolism, to name a few.

The thought of each of these conditions, and their accompanying symptom complex, is contained in the Paramedic's mind as a **script**. A script can be thought of as an idea which has an associated symptom complex and an associated field diagnosis and treatment plan.

For example, when thinking of acute coronary syndrome, the Paramedic thinks of not only those signs and symptoms in the symptom complex which are coupled with the diagnosis of acute coronary syndrome (such as substernal chest pain, ST segment elevation, and so on), but the associated treatments as well.

Initial Impression

Upon arrival at the patient's side, the Paramedic must first make a decision whether the call is medical or trauma in nature. To make that decision, the Paramedic considers if there is a **mechanism of injury**, suggesting trauma, or a **nature of illness**, suggesting the call is medical.

In the case of trauma, the mechanism of injury can provide some valuable clues to underlying injuries. The mechanism of injury includes those forces (e.g., shearing or tearing) that create physical harm to the patient.

Certain mechanisms of injury have characteristic injuries that are associated with that mechanism. These characteristic injuries are referred to as the **predictable injury pattern**.

When arriving on a potential trauma call, the Paramedic uses his knowledge of **kinematics**, the study of motion, and the mechanism of injury to derive a predictable injury pattern.[8-14] For example, a front-end motor vehicle collision would propel a patient forward against the windshield and cause head and neck injuries.

The patient's chief complaint, or concern, and the lack of a mechanism of injury helps establish the medical nature of a call. The Paramedic then goes about ascertaining the nature of the illness. The nature of the illness is the sum of the patient's chief complaint, or concern, and the history of the present illness.

Urgent or Emergent

Early in the assessment process, the Paramedic makes a general decision whether the patient is **emergent** (i.e., arising unexpectedly and in need of immediate medical attention) or **urgent** (i.e., not emergent and in need of further assessment and evaluation before treatment is initiated).

This general assessment of the patient's condition is termed the **initial impression**. An initial field impression is based on a myriad of factors such as patient presentation, environmental factors, gross observation, and resources on-scene. These factors assemble in the Paramedic's mind to create a sense of emergency or urgency.

If the patient is emergent, then initial life-saving maneuvers during the primary assessment must be performed on-scene. The patient is then rapidly moved to the ambulance for transportation to definitive care.

If the patient is urgent then, after a primary assessment is completed, a more detailed history and physical is performed.

Some experienced Paramedics come to this decision very quickly. These master Paramedics use what is termed **Gestalt**, a way of seeing a pattern in the patient observation as a whole. It is not obtained by a summation of symptoms but rather from patterns having been observed in similar situations in past practice and experience.

Following the general impression, the Paramedic proceeds with obtaining the history and performing a physical examination in order to ascertain the symptom complex. Using a standardized approach, such as the mnemonic OPQRST, reveals the symptom complex.

Some findings, such as nausea or headache, are non-specific (i.e., not indicative of any one disease), and are often common to all sick patients. These general findings of illness are often referred to as **constitutional signs**. While constitutional signs help to establish that the patient is not well and in need of supportive care, they do not assist the Paramedic toward reaching a clinical decision.

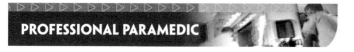

PROFESSIONAL PARAMEDIC

Savvy patients may inquire about the necessity of field tests. Questions will arise regarding the accuracy of the test and whether the test delays transportation. The professional Paramedic knows how often the test gives a correct positive result (its sensitivity) but also how often it fails to give a correct positive result (its specificity). Paramedics must be able to describe the time the procedure takes and how it will enhance overall care.

Tests

Owing to the urgent nature of a medical emergency, the Paramedic must choose those tests that have the greatest yield of information. A random test, such as obtaining a 12 lead ECG, without conscious consideration of what the results might reveal is wasteful. Before implementing any test, the Paramedic should ask, "Will this test affect my decision making?" If the answer is no, or unknown, then the test may be a waste of time.

Whenever a test is performed, the Paramedic should be aware of its specificity and the sensitivity, the test's predictive value.

For example, when the 12 lead ECG machine analysis states "acute myocardial infarction suspected" the Paramedic can have confidence that the patient is having an acute myocardial infarction. In other words, the Paramedic can assume the machine is correct, based on research that has shown good sensitivity (97% accurate in one study).[15,16]

However, the Paramedic must also be skeptical of the results as well. The 12 lead ECG machine may lack specificity (i.e., the machine may not read "acute myocardial infarction suspected" when in fact one does exist).

Understanding the limitation of every machine or test, the Paramedic should never rely on one test result to make a clinical decision. Instead, the Paramedic should consider the entire patient presentation, coupled with the test results, to arrive at a field diagnosis.

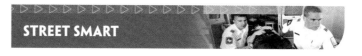

STREET SMART

Paramedics who routinely perform tests, such as blood glucose analysis, without consideration of the meaning of the results may be practicing defensive medicine. The practice of performing random tests in order to limit liability, or criticism from the medical director, rather than performing just those tests that benefit the patient should not be encouraged.

Differential Diagnosis

After gathering the facts in the case (the symptom complex), comparing that to similar symptom patterns, and recognizing the similarity, the Paramedic advances a field diagnosis.

On occasion, the Paramedic may be conflicted whether to state one field diagnosis or another. In those cases, the Paramedic should consider applying **Ockham's razor**. Ockham's razor, simply stated, says that if all things are equal, the simplest solution tends to be the best one. In other words, common things occur commonly. While exotic diseases do exist, the probability is low that these diseases are involved.

STREET SMART

The saying goes "When one hears hoof beats think horses not zebras." While the physician is tasked with "ruling out" these diagnoses, the Paramedic should focus on the more common and predictable causes of illness.

When the Paramedic is faced with a situation in which several plausible explanations for a disorder exist and the Paramedic cannot narrow the causes down to one disease or another, then the Paramedic should treat the patient aggressively. The Paramedic should assume that the disorder which can harm the patient the most exists. For example, while epigastric discomfort could be gastric esophageal reflux disease, it might also be connected to an inferior wall acute ischemic event.[17,18] Keeping the patient's best interests in mind, the Paramedic should treat the patient as if he were having an acute coronary event and consider the possible cardiac origin for this discomfort.

If the Paramedic errs in the field and treats the patient with GERD as a cardiac patient, then the patient will most likely be no worse for the care. However, if the Paramedic treats the cardiac patient for heartburn only, missing the potential for an acute coronary event, then the patient could have a catastrophic event and the opportunity for timely intervention may be lost.

The Paramedic's treatment philosophy could be summed up with the saying "Hope for the best but treat for the worst."

The Paramedic must become a good clinical decision maker. The Paramedic's ability to take all of the clinical information and separate out irrelevant information from critical data is important for clinical decision making. Prepared with a well-conceived field diagnosis, the Paramedic can then proceed with a treatment plan.

Barriers to Effective Clinical Decision Making

Skill in good clinical decision making is a function of formal education and practical experience. It is essential that graduate Paramedics have a formal education which provides both depth and breadth in achieving a comprehensive understanding of paramedicine.

However, the knowledge base of the Paramedic who graduated, even with highest honors, is soon outdated. Every Paramedic must understand and accept the need for continuing education for competency assurance and professional development. This attitude can be best summed up by the Japanese idea of **Kaizen**, meaning continuous performance improvement.

Improved clinical decision making can also be obtained from practical experience with a master Paramedic. **Mentors**, experienced master Paramedics, accept graduate Paramedics as their protégés to teach good clinical decision making. These mentors often depend on intuition when making decisions in ambiguous or complex situations. This clinical intuition, borne of experience, can be described as understanding without rationale, as opposed to irrational guessing. Sharing intuition with novice Paramedics permits the novice Paramedic to develop expert judgment.

With limited education, and even more limited experience, the novice Paramedic may resort to applying protocol-driven care in every circumstance. **Protocols** are a set of mandatory behaviors meant to be applied in specific clinical conditions. Protocols, almost by definition, assume that the one patient's situation is the same or similar to another patient's condition in the same situation.

In many cases this approach is acceptable, and has advantages in a time-sensitive emergency. However, some patients do not fit the prescribed clinical condition. That is, the patient does not fit into the mold.

In those cases, the Paramedic should view the protocols as a set of **guidelines**. Guidelines provide direction while permitting use of knowledge and experience to shape clinical decisions. Implicit with the use of guidelines is accountability. Whenever guidelines are in use, the Paramedic must be willing to discuss and defend the clinical decisions.

Every Paramedic should look forward to the opportunity to defend a clinical decision. These conversations with fellow Paramedics or the medical director permit the Paramedic the opportunity to improve clinical decision making. Emergency medicine is a dynamic field that requires flexibility in thought and a willingness to see a different point of view.

Paramedics who are unwilling to consider alternatives to patient care, other than the routine care, because it has always been done this way, are experiencing **paradigm blindness**.[19] Good clinical decision making depends on a willingness to accept new ideas and to practice creative thinking in the field (i.e., thinking outside of the box).

The greatest danger to any Paramedic's clinical decision making is fear. Whenever a Paramedic feels unsure, or even threatened, by a clinical situation, the response will be an adrenaline surge. Adrenaline can help to sharpen the Paramedic's senses, improving the patient assessment, but it can also narrow the Paramedic's focus. This narrow focus of attention (e.g., to a task) causes the Paramedic to miss seeing the larger picture and therefore miss important clinical information.

Paramedics should strive to see situations as challenging, not threatening, and maintain a sense of control from within. This **internal locus of control** (i.e., the idea that one has the ability to control the situation) gives the Paramedic a sense of control over the situation. This sense of control can translate to a feeling of confidence and improved clinical decision making. Others, seeing the confidence evident in the Paramedic, tend to follow the Paramedic's lead.

Improved Clinical Decision Making

The Paramedic's best ally for clinical decision making is the patient. While the patient always has a right to make informed decisions about patient care, **shared decision making** goes beyond consent and engages the patient in a conversation about clinical decision making whenever possible. The patient is seen as not being dependent (a paternalistic view), but rather interdependent with the Paramedic. In a shared decision-making model, the patient is consulted about clinical decisions. Providing the patient with current information about his or her state of health and offering medically reasonable alternatives empowers both the patient and the Paramedic.

Obtaining **patient concordance**, the process of shared decision making, includes a communication of risk, the advantages of compliance, and a shared responsibility to report changes. Shared clinical decision making fosters openness and trust between the patient and the Paramedic. In addition, shared clinical decision making decreases patient dissatisfaction, even allowing the patient to decide to withhold treatment until arrival at the hospital.

It should be noted that while younger and better educated patients prefer to share clinical decision making, cultural and ethnic differences may decrease patient cooperation. This lack of cooperation should not be viewed as resistance to care but rather as a trust in the Paramedic's decision.

Treatment

Paramedics typically start patient care with **empiric therapy**, treatment based on initial observations obtained during the primary assessment. For example, a person with obvious difficulty breathing may receive oxygen immediately. Such treatments are considered basic life support. Though they may be complex, such as intravenous therapy, they are not intended to treat a specific disorder. Rather, they are intended to support the body (palliative care).

Evaluate

Some novice Paramedics are compelled to act either by training or cultural influences within an organization. This action imperative (i.e., don't just stand there, do something) is sometimes ill advised and can lead to catastrophic events.

Illnesses are progressive. Watchful waiting while providing supportive care can sometimes make a cloudy clinical picture clearer or may demonstrate the ineffectiveness of a particular treatment. This may lead the Paramedic to consider other treatment pathways.

This process of assessment, treatment, and then reassessment is consistent with the quality improvement cycle (plan–do–check–act). Attention to evaluation of treatments and then consideration of further interventions leads to higher quality of care.

Disposition

Paramedic care is the beginning of the continuum of care which is continued in the emergency department, critical care units, rehabilitation floors, and homecare services. In many cases, the Paramedic's decision in the field puts the patient onto a **treatment pathway**. For example, the Paramedic's field diagnosis might activate a "cardiac team" at a center for interventional cardiology, alert a critical care unit of an impending arrival, and set about a cascade of events, all designed to return the patient to the best state of health possible.[20–25] Key to this process is good clinical decision making.

Clinical decision making is a process of systematic analysis, using medical intelligence and critical thinking, aided by input from the team, which in the end is the basis for a plan of care. It always has the patient's best interests in mind.

CONCLUSION

The Paramedic of the future is a thinking practitioner who essentially operates almost independently in the prehospital environment. By using the methods discussed in this chapter, the Paramedic can move away from blindly following protocols and toward a thinking, professional practitioner.

KEY POINTS:

- "Medical intelligence" is a term used to describe the Paramedic's systematic approach to clinical decision making.

- The symptom complex is compared to the Paramedic's own knowledge base to determine if any familiar symptom patterns exist.

- Gathering information and reducing it to a single theory is called inductive logic. The Paramedic uses this line of thinking to investigate a problem and develop an appropriate treatment plan.

- When presented with a chief complaint or concern, the Paramedic should begin to develop a list of possible etiologies of the chief concern. This cognitive list is then associated with a field diagnosis and treatment plan.

- To determine whether an emergency call is medical or trauma in nature, the Paramedic must consider either the mechanism of injury or the nature of illness.

- The initial impression of a patient is based on factors such as patient presentation, environmental factors, and resources available.

- The initial impression is used in conjunction with the primary assessment to determine if the patient is emergent or urgent.

- Some findings, such as nausea or headache, are referred to as constitutional signs because they are nonspecific and are often common to all sick patients.

- Before implementing any test, the Paramedic should determine whether the test will affect the decision-making or treatment plan.

- Before the test is performed, the Paramedic should be aware of its specificity and sensitivity.

- The idea of preparing or treating for the worst and hoping for the best is one way the Paramedic can keep the patient's best interests in mind while developing an appropriate field diagnosis and treatment plan.

- Skill in good clinical decision making is a function of formal education and practical experience.

- Protocols should be viewed as a set of guidelines that provide direction while permitting the Paramedic to use knowledge and experience to shape clinical decisions.

- Good clinical decision making depends on a willingness to accept new ideas and to practice creative thinking in the field (i.e., thinking outside of the box).

- An internal locus of control, or one's sense of control over a situation, can translate to a feeling of confidence and improved clinical decision making. Shared decision making goes beyond consent and engages the patient in a conversation about clinical decision making whenever possible.

- Treatment may begin with empiric therapy, based on the initial assessment. Further interventions should be based on a reassessment of treatments given.

REVIEW QUESTIONS:

1. Explain the process of medical intelligence.
2. Defend the concept of Paramedic field diagnosis.
3. Explain mechanism of injury and its relationship to a predictable injury pattern.
4. Explain the difference between emergent and urgent.
5. List the barriers to effective clinical decision making.
6. Explain the difference between protocols and guidelines.
7. List methods of improved clinical decision making.
8. Explain how identifying inaccurate field diagnoses can lead to improved patient care.

CASE STUDY QUESTIONS:

Please refer to the Case Study at the beginning of the chapter and answer the questions below.

1. Name the symptom complex for Joseph Gonterman. Name the symptom complex for Guiseppe Ferrari.
2. Are each of these patients suffering from a trauma event or a medical one? Explain your answers.
3. Do Mr. Gonterman and Mr. Ferrari have the same priority? Why or why not?

REFERENCES:

1. Glick TH. Evidence-guided education: patients' outcome data should influence our teaching priorities. *Acad Med.* 2005;80(2):147–151.
2. Kilminster SM, Jolly BC. Effective supervision in clinical practice settings: a literature review. *Med Educ.* 2000;34(10):827–840.
3. Dornan T, Littlewood S, Margolis SA, Scherpbier A, Spencer J, Ypinazar V. How can experience in clinical and community settings contribute to early medical education? A BEME systematic review. *Med Teach.* 2006;28(1):3–18.
4. Fleischer AB, Jr., Gardner EF, Feldman SR. Are patients' chief complaints generally specific to one organ system? *Am J Manag Care.* 2001;7(3):299–305.
5. Rottman SJ, Schriger DL, Charlop G, Salas JH, Lee S. On-line medical control versus protocol-based prehospital care. *Ann Emerg Med.* 1997;30(1):62–68.
6. Kothari R, Barsan W, Brott T, Broderick J, Ashbrock S. Frequency and accuracy of prehospital diagnosis of acute stroke. *Stroke.* 1995;26(6):937–941.
7. MacDonald GS, Steiner SR. Emergency medical service providers' role in the early heart attack care program: prevention

and stratification strategies. *Md Med J, Suppl.* 1997;7(1)(Suppl):79–84.
8. Eid HO, Abu-Zidan FM. Biomechanics of road traffic collision injuries: a clinician's perspective. *Singapore Med J.* 2007;48(7):693–700; quiz 700.
9. Mackay M. Mechanisms of injury and biomechanics: vehicle design and crash performance. *World J Surg.* 1992;16(3):420–427.
10. Green RN, German A, Nowak ES, Dalmotas D, Stewart DE. Fatal injuries to restrained passenger car occupants in Canada: crash modes and kinematics of injury. *Accid Anal Prev.* 1994;26(2):207–214.
11. Kumar S, Ferrari R, Narayan Y. Kinematic and electromyographic response to whiplash loading in low-velocity whiplash impacts—a review. *Clin Biomech (Bristol, Avon).* 2005;20(4):343–356.
12. Kumar S, Ferrari R, Narayan Y. The effect of trunk flexion in healthy volunteers in rear whiplash-type impacts. *Spine.* 2005;30(15):1742–1749.
13. Mikhail JN. Side impact motor vehicular crashes: patterns of injury. *Int J Trauma Nurs.* 1995;1(3):64–69.

14. Loo GT, Siegel JH, Dischinger PC, Rixen D, Burgess AR, Addis MD, et al. Airbag protection versus compartment intrusion effect determines the pattern of injuries in multiple trauma motor vehicle crashes. *J Trauma*. 1996;41(6):935–951.

15. Sekiguchi K, Kanda T, Osada M, Tsunoda Y, Kodajima N, Fukumura Y, et al. Comparative accuracy of automated computer analysis versus physicans in training in the interpretation of electrocardiograms. *J Med*. 1999;30(1-2):75–81.

16. Willems JL, Abreu-Lima C, Arnaud P, van Bemmel JH, Brohet C, Degani R, et al. The diagnostic performance of computer programs for the interpretation of electrocardiograms. *N Engl J Med*. 1991;325(25):1767–1773.

17. Sheps DS, Creed F, Clouse RE. Chest pain in patients with cardiac and noncardiac disease. *Psychosom Med*. 2004;66(6):861–867.

18. Miller CD, Lindsell CJ, Khandelwal S, Chandra A, Pollack CV, Tiffany BR, et al. Is the initial diagnostic impression of "noncardiac chest pain" adequate to exclude cardiac disease? *Ann Emerg Med*. 2004;44(6):565–574.

19. Camp R. *Benchmarking: The Search for Industry Best Practices That Lead to Superior Performance*. Portland: Productivity Press; 2006.

20. Le May MR, Dionne R, Maloney J, Trickett J, Watpool I, Ruest M, et al. Diagnostic performance and potential clinical impact of advanced care Paramedic interpretation of ST-segment elevation myocardial infarction in the field. *Cjem*. 2006;8(6): 401–407.

21. Feldman JA, Brinsfield K, Bernard S, White D, Maciejko T. Real-time Paramedic compared with blinded physician identification of ST-segment elevation myocardial infarction: results of an observational study. *Am J Emerg Med*. 2005;23(4):443–448.

22. Strauss DG, Sprague PQ, Underhill K, Maynard C, Adams GL, Kessenich A, et al. Paramedic transtelephonic communication to cardiologist of clinical and electrocardiographic assessment for rapid reperfusion of ST-elevation myocardial infarction. *J Electrocardiol*. 2007;40(3):265–270.

23. Adams GL, Campbell PT, Adams JM, Strauss DG, Wall K, Patterson J, et al. Effectiveness of prehospital wireless transmission of electrocardiograms to a cardiologist via hand-held device for patients with acute myocardial infarction (from the Timely Intervention in Myocardial Emergency, NorthEast Experience [TIME-NE]). *Am J Cardiol*. 2006;98(9):1160–1164.

24. Wojner-Alexandrov AW, Alexandrov AV, Rodriguez D, Persse D, Grotta JC. Houston Paramedic and emergency stroke treatment and outcomes study (HoPSTO). *Stroke*. 2005;36(7):1512–1518.

25. Qazi K, Kempf JA, Christopher NC, Gerson LW. Paramedic judgment of the need for trauma team activation for pediatric patients. *Acad Emerg Med*. 1998;5(10):1002–1007.

COMMUNICATIONS

KEY CONCEPTS:

Upon completion of this chapter, it is expected that the reader will understand these following concepts:

- Duality of EMS communications
- A history of radio communications from ground to satellite
- Breakdown of radio architectures, bandwidths, and technology
- Phases of EMS communications, from the initial call for help to turning the care over to hospital staff
- The standardized radio report for communicating with physicians

► CASE STUDY:

The Paramedic was the first on-scene of a two-car motor vehicle collision with possible patient entrapment. A first due report was relayed to the dispatcher and different members of the public safety team began to arrive. A fellow Paramedic took up EMS command and the Paramedic was directed to care for a critically ill trauma patient. After a primary assessment and treatment of life-threatening injuries, the patient was extricated and moved to an ambulance. While en route to the hospital, the Paramedic contacted medical control for advanced procedures and to initiate a trauma alert.

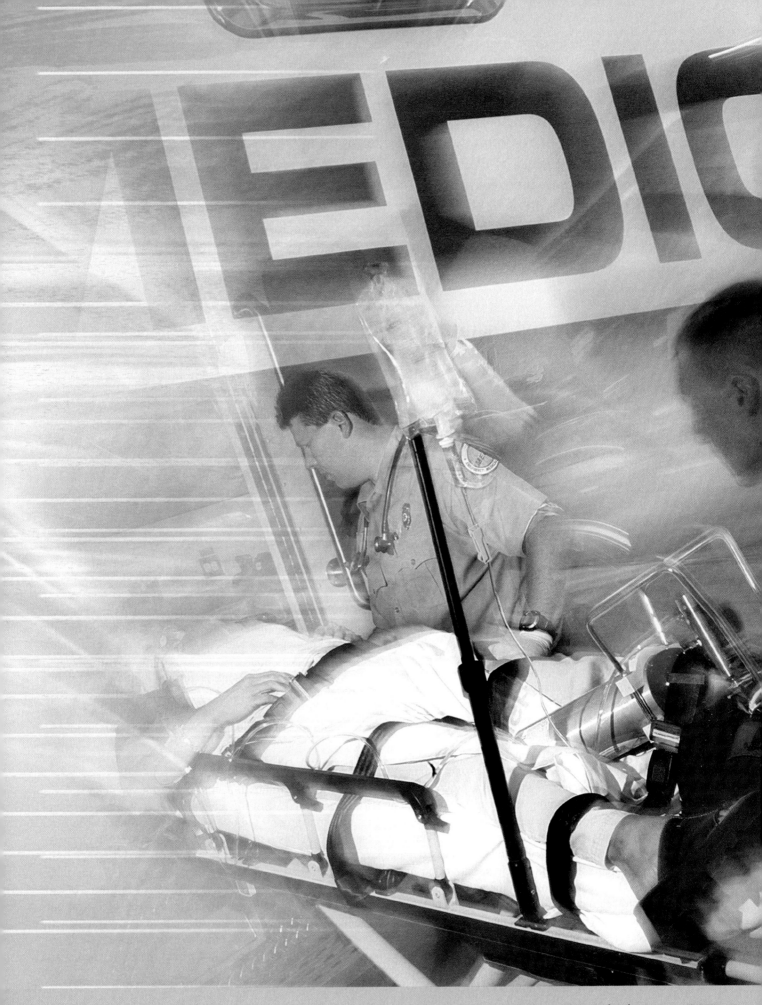

OVERVIEW

Communication can involve the exchange of ideas or interactions between two parties, as well as the technology that is behind sending and receiving information. Both of these aspects of communication are examined in this chapter. First, the chapter looks at the duality of EMS communications. A fundamental part of the Paramedic's day-to-day operations involve interacting with fellow members of a public safety team as well as healthcare providers at hospital care facilities. Because the Paramedic relies on technology to perform these functions, the Paramedic should have an understanding of radio communications and the technology used in the prehospital setting.

Communications and Teamwork

Teamwork is an outward demonstration of the power of communication. Health care is a team activity; its goal is the patient's health. Paramedics, in the prehospital phase, actually play for two teams. The first team is the public safety team, a triad made up of law enforcement officers (LEO), firefighters (FF), and Paramedics. This team's goal is to provide for the public's safety through control and command of public emergencies. As with any team, communication is essential. Communications are essential to maintain the threefold concerns of the rescuer's safety, the public's safety, and the patient's safety as the Paramedics go about accomplishing their mission.

While Paramedics are part of the public safety team, a Paramedic is also part of a healthcare team. Healthcare teams, ranging from primary care providers to rehabilitation services, are dedicated to helping the patient through a medical emergency. A Paramedic's communication with the healthcare team serves the patient's interests by providing the patient's past medical history, information about the history of the patient's present illness, and the patient's response to prehospital treatment. The Paramedic's communication with the healthcare team also represents a hand-off of the patient, or the transfer of care, from the prehospital team to the emergency department team.

Communication occurs between team members within the team as well as with other teams. Instances of communication, called interfaces, occur in both oral and written forms, and take place at many times during the duration of the patient contact. The first interface may be between lay first responders or emergency medical responders and the Paramedic. The next interface may be between prehospital and emergency department personnel (Figure 18-1). In fact, there are often many interfaces with other members of both the public safety team and the healthcare team during the course of a patient's care.

For the sake of expediency, most of these communications are either face-to-face or via a mobile communications device such as a radio or cellular telephone. In every case, these contacts are then recorded in a written document which

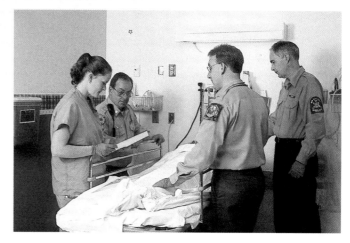

Figure 18-1 A Paramedic giving a verbal report to a nurse.

has both medical and legal importance.[1–7] This chapter deals with the first communication, verbal communication, while the next chapter deals with the second, written communication or documentation.

Verbal communications is further divided into mobile communications and face-to-face exchanges. Before discussing the first, mobile communications, it is important to have a foundation in radio theory.

History of Radio

Since the first radio transmission, from St. John's, Newfoundland, to Cornwall, England, the potential for communication through radio has been ever growing. The early theorists, such as James Clark Maxwell, a Scottish physicist, hypothesized that an electrical or magnetic disturbance could spread across the "ether" (ether was invisible substance thought to fill space) like waves on the ocean from a distant storm. This theory was substantially correct. Electrical current passing through a wire creates a field of electromagnetic energy around it as it passes. Alternating current, electricity that flows to and fro through a wire, repeatedly creates and increases these fields.

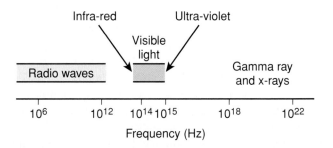
At smaller frequencies, these fields tend to collapse, or dissipate, over time. However, scientists learned that when electricity approaches 10,000 CPS the electromagnetic field tends to radiate outwards and the electromagnetic field is sustained. These radiating waves of electromagnetic energy, or radio waves, can be detected at great distances In other words, radio waves are a part of the spectrum of electromagnetic energy (Figure 18-2).

The discovery of radio was a great breakthrough, especially for remote settings, such as at sea. Previously, sailors, soldiers, and merchants depended on semaphore, a system of flag signals that can be seen over great distances. Later, they depended on the hardwired telegraph before the advent of the wireless radio.

Telegraph has a close relationship with the development of radio. Telegraph, a system of communication transmitted over wires, was the predominant communication method during the 1800s. The first telegraph message, sent by Samuel F.B. Morse in 1844, carried the message, "What hath God wrought?"[8] From that point, telegraph messages using Morse code were the predominant means of rapid communication. Original telegraphs often used multiple wires, one for each letter in some cases. There was a continuous effort to reduce the number of wires. Eventually, the telegraph required only two wires—one to signal and the other a return. Some scientists, thinking that electricity could travel through the ground for thousands of kilometers, buried the return wire into the ground, and found that the telegraph still worked.

These developments gave strength to the theory of a ground wave and to the idea that a signal could be transmitted across the ground. The first "wireless" communication system used a ground wave for signal transmission. Efforts to create a ground-based wireless system were met with frustration, primarily because the use of alternating current was still in its infancy, until Marconi intervened.

Guglielmo Marconi, of Bologna, Italy, utilized the works of Heinrich Hertz. In 1887, Hertz caused a spark to leap across a gap and create an electromagnetic wave.[9] At that time, this phenomenon was known by various terms including "ether waves" and "Hertzian waves." Using this idea of an electric spark, Marconi invented a spark transmitter, a primitive black box with an antenna that could transmit the "spark," or signal, over a distance to a receiver that would produce an audible snap. That snap, in turn, could be used similarly to the telegraph's Morse code. This black box, developed in December 1894, was eventually brought to England. After obtaining a patent, the Wireless Telegraph and Signal Company was formed. Marconi, 23 years old at the time, would later receive the Nobel Prize for physics in 1908 for his invention.

After the first transatlantic wireless transmission in 1915, wireless communications, a branch of telecommunications, grew rapidly. The U.S. Navy, interested in the potential of wireless communications for ship-to-ship communication as well as ship-to-shore interactions, investigated Marconi and his device. Before long, many U.S. warships had a radio. Often the radio was placed in hastily constructed wooden sheds, later called the "radio shack," on deck.

Earlier radios, restricted by the technology of the time, operated in either low-frequency (LF) or medium-frequency (MF) ranges. They were subject to a great deal of atmospheric interference and were therefore reduced to using Morse code. Later developments in radio technology, by such notables as Reginald Fessenden of Canada and Harold D. Arnold, permitted both voice transmission and transatlantic transmission.

Radio Technology

Radio technology has eclipsed even the wildest dreams of those early radio pioneers. The first mechanical radio wave generators were restricted to a maximum of 100 KHz,

Infra-red   Ultra-violet

Visible light

Radio waves

Gamma ray and x-rays

10^6 10^{12} 10^{14} 10^{15} 10^{18} 10^{22}

Frequency (Hz)

Figure 18-2 Radio waves in the electromagnetic spectrum.

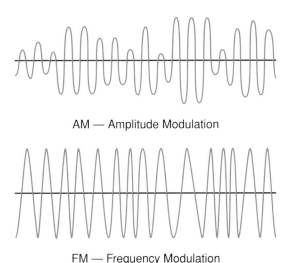

AM — Amplitude Modulation

FM — Frequency Modulation

Figure 18-3 AM radio transmission versus FM radio transmission.

severely restricting their usefulness. Later, electronic generators, or oscillators, markedly expanded the properties of the radio wave. To achieve voice transmission, an audio signal produced from a microphone was "impressed upon" a radio signal, called a radio frequency (RF) carrier. This heralded the era of radio telecommunications.

To understand how an audio signal might be impressed upon a radio frequency, consider the analogy of flotsam and waves. While the waves continue to crash on the beach, the flotsam, or audio signal, slowly washes to shore. Through modulation techniques which modify the wave by either changing the wave's height (**amplitude modulation** [AM]) or by changing the wave's speed (**frequency modulation** [FM]), the message can be carried through antennas to be transmitted (Figure 18-3).

Often the key to adequate radio transmission was the size of the receiving or transmitting antenna. The length of an antenna is a function of the length of the wave. The lower the frequency, the longer the radio wave and, therefore, the longer the antenna. In some cases the radio wave was over 20 feet, often making mobile radios impractical. To shorten radio antennas from being 9- or 10-foot-long "whips," a radio antenna would be cut down to one-half the wavelength, a half-wave antenna, or even one-quarter of the wave length. An antenna which was correctly matched to a radio greatly improved radio transmission.

However, despite an adequate antenna, the quality of many radio transmissions suffered from **interference**. Interference can be thought of as extraneous electromagnetic energy heard on the radio as crackles and dead spots, sometimes called **static**. Sources of static include other unshielded electrical devices emitting 60 cycle interference, lightning in the atmosphere, bursts of radio waves from sunspot activity, and even the spark plugs in an automobile.

To reduce static interference heard between radio transmissions, called white noise, electrical engineers developed **squelch control**. Squelch control reduces the amount of signal received between transmissions, narrowing the reception of radio waves, and eliminating background interference. There are two types of squelch control. **Carrier squelch** eliminates background static during pauses in a transmission, essentially muting the radio between transmissions and thereby improving the message's overall quality. **Coded (or tone) squelch** permits the radio to receive only the intended signal. Sometimes also called **private line (PL)**, coded squelch eliminates reception of near-broadcast messages by only accepting signals with the correct code. The quality and the privacy of radio transmissions are thus improved.

STREET SMART

In the past, public health nurses would take a portable AM transistor radio and dial it between radio stations and then place it over a pacemaker. The electric spark of the pacemaker could be heard distinctly on the radio.

Radio Frequency

Radio waves are transmitted literally at the speed of light. The difference in radio waves is not in the speed but rather in the frequency of the waves in the radio transmission. These radio waves, measured in cycles per second, are called **Hertz**, after the scientist who discovered them. A Hertz is an international unit of measurement. One thousand Hertz, or cycles per second, equals a kiloHertz, labeled kHz. Similarly, one million Hertz is called a megaHertz (mHz), and one billion is called a gigaHertz (gHz). New electronic technology, using lasers, is able to generate a trillion Hertz, or a teraHertz (tHz) radio wave.

The various radio waves are all part of the overall radio spectrum (Figure 18-4). The human ear is able to detect sound in the form of waves in the 15 Hz to 20,000 Hz range. The human voice is able to produce sound in the 200 Hz to 2,500 Hz range.[11] However, the radio spectrum goes from 3 Hz to over a trillion Hertz. The lowest radio frequency, termed extremely low (ELF), is between 3 and 30 Hz and is able to be transmitted over 5,000 miles or more. Perhaps more importantly, extremely low radio frequencies can penetrate water for a distance of several hundred feet. The ELF is therefore useful for submarine communications.

The next band of radio frequency, by international designation, is the super-low (SLF) frequencies between 30 to 300 Hz. The earliest radios were only capable of creating about 100 Hz, thus limiting them to the SLF frequency band.

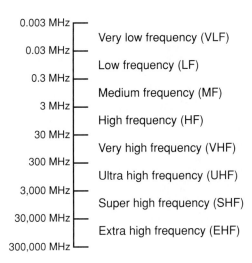

0.003 MHz		
0.03 MHz	—	Very low frequency (VLF)
0.3 MHz	—	Low frequency (LF)
3 MHz	—	Medium frequency (MF)
30 MHz	—	High frequency (HF)
300 MHz	—	Very high frequency (VHF)
3,000 MHz	—	Ultra high frequency (UHF)
30,000 MHz	—	Super high frequency (SHF)
300,000 MHz	—	Extra high frequency (EHF)

Figure 18-4 The radio frequency spectrum.

The next three radio bands—ultra-low frequency (ULF), very-low frequency (VLF), and low frequency (LF)—also have limited utility because of extreme radio interference. The medium frequency (MF), 300 to 3,000 kHz, was the first to see extensive use because the problem of interference was being overcome. Early commercial radio stations, using AM technology that would transmit on RF carriers in the 550 to 1,600 kHz range, started to broadcast entertainment programs to the public using these new technologies.

After the advent of crystal-oscillator radios, high-frequency (HF) radio transmissions, in the 3 to 300 mHz range, that were capable of "crystal-clear" transmission blossomed. These tighter radio waves were capable of being transmitted over the land, as a **ground wave**, from point A to point B. These waves provided remarkable quality as long as there were no obstacles in the **line of sight** (LOS) to block the transmission.

To overcome the problem of obstacles to LOS, the HF radio antenna could be directed toward the sky. The HF radio signal would rise until it struck the ionosphere, a layer of atmosphere where the sun's ultraviolet rays ionize the gasses, and the signal would be reflected back to Earth.[12] This phenomenon, known as **skip**, could permit HF transmissions to travel over 300 miles on a **sky wave**.

Amateur civilian short-wave radio operators, using this phenomenon to their advantage, can now communicate with other short-wave radio operators all the way around the world under the right atmospheric conditions by skipping signals from one receiver to another.[13] These "ham operators," as short-wave radio operators have come to be known, have assisted during disasters and can be instrumental in other public safety emergencies.

The principal radio frequency band used by emergency services is very-high frequency (VHF). VHF, from 30 to 300 mHz, can be cleanly transmitted over 25 to 50 miles. VHF is useful to EMS because it takes less power to transmit using the higher frequencies. This is an advantage for emergency services telecommunications devices that depend on batteries. VHF is also the bandwidth used by commercial television broadcasts.

CULTURAL/REGIONAL DIFFERENCES

In rural and frontier environments, a transmission distance of 100 miles is too short. To overcome the problem of distance, some radio systems have resorted to the use of radio repeaters. Repeaters—radios that pick up, amplify, and then retransmit a radio transmission—can extend the range of a VHF almost indefinitely. The transmission's distance is a function of the number of repeaters available.

Ultra-high frequency (UHF) radios, in the 300 to 3,000 mHz range, can transmit in a LOS for 15 to 100 miles, dependent on terrain. If the UHF radio antenna is on-board an airplane, the distance can be boosted to over 300 nautical miles, and if the radio transmitter is in a satellite the signal can travel literally thousands of miles. Super-high frequencies (SHF), otherwise known as microwave transmissions, within the 3 to 30 gHz bandwidth and extremely-high frequencies (EHF), within the 30 to 300 gHz bandwidth, are used for satellite transmissions. While a SHF or EHF radio may be limited to a LOS of about 40 miles, a SHF or EHF radio can literally bounce a signal off a satellite and back to Earth, bypassing obstructions such as mountains. This feature makes these **satellite phones**, also called Earth stations, extremely useful in frontier communities with little or no development, as well as in wilderness situations.

At present, there are two satellite phone systems in place. One uses satellites in a geosynchronous orbit. With as few as four satellites, these satellite phone systems can provide worldwide coverage. Unfortunately, obstacles such as high terrain can block the view of satellites on the horizon. To resolve this problem, newer low Earth orbit (LEO) satellite technology was developed. A LEO satellite is not geosynchronous and orbits the Earth at a high rate of speed, with an average orbital time of 80 minutes. A LEO satellite phone system, such as Globalstar or Iridium, has a larger number of satellites in orbit, which are constantly crossing the sky and creating a grid with interlocking cells of coverage.

Besides the obvious advantage of satellite phones in rural and frontier EMS, satellite phones are also useful during disasters. During a disaster, traditional telephone wires may be down and cellular towers "locked up" from overwhelming use. During these times, dedicated satellite phones could be used.

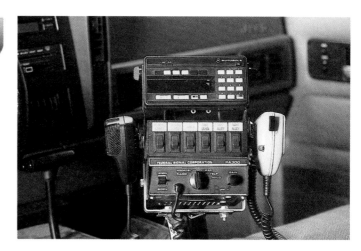

Figure 18-5 Mobile radio.

Wave Propagation

As mentioned earlier, there are two types of wave propagation: ground and sky. The distance that a ground wave travels is a function of its length. A longer wave will roughly follow a surface path. However, it is diminished by each obstacle it meets (called **fading**) until either it is too weak to be received or it reaches its target (the receiver's antenna). A ground wave is also affected by the surface over which it travels. Soils that are poor conductors will shorten the length of the transmission whereas a HF radio transmission may travel 700 miles over the open water of the ocean.

Shorter waves (e.g., UVF), when using a ground wave, are easily blocked by any obstacle in the LOS such as foliage and buildings. Using a UVF radio in rough terrain, such as a city, requires that the operator either build a tall antenna to overcome the obstacles, or depend on a phenomenon called **bounce**. Bounce occurs whenever a short wave strikes a reflective surface and is redirected in another direction. With enough reflective surfaces, the **reflected path** will roughly result in the intended direction of travel.

Radios that use the sky wave, tropospheric (TROPO) radios bounce the radio signal off the ionosphere in the direction of the receiver antenna. As radio signals are wave-like, a sky wave will scatter, permitting worldwide reception.[14] The United States military has used troposcatter radio systems since the 1950s for long distance radio.

Radio Systems

Radio systems consist of components that permit a radio message to be transmitted and received. The arrangement of radio components is referred to as the **system architecture**. Currently, two radio architectures exist in EMS: traditional land mobile radio (LMR) architecture and cellular system architecture.

Land Mobile Radio Architecture

A traditional land mobile radio (LMR) architecture has many components, in varying numbers, depending on the size, location, and complexity of the EMS system. Factors include the existence of base station(s), mobile radio(s), portable radio(s), and repeater(s).

A base station is a fixed facility which generally serves as a focal point in an EMS system. Base stations generally have more powerful transmitters because they do not rely upon batteries. **Hard-wired** in the electric power supply, a base station is vulnerable to power outages. For this reason, many EMS agencies have a backup power supply, such as a generator, to ensure reliable operation.

Mobile radios (Figure 18-5) are affixed to vehicles and use the vehicle's battery for power. Often the radio itself is secured inside a trunk, or behind a seat, protected from impact in case of collision. A small remote radio control panel, called a **radio head**, is placed in the driver's and/or patient compartment.

The simplest radio system is **simplex**. A simplex radio only allows communication in one direction at a time. The oldest example of a portable simplex radio may be the Motorola walkie-talkie used in World War II. These handy **portable radios** permitted communication between platoons and regimental command in the same manner that modern radios permit communication "car-to-car" between emergency vehicles (Figure 18-6).

The difficulty with simplex radio is that it requires one party to complete the message before the other party can respond. In some instances, it is desirable to have a dialogue. Thus, **duplex** radios were invented. A duplex radio operates in the same manner as a hard-wired telephone, referred to as a **landline**. Using two frequencies—one to transmit and one to receive—an operator could talk and listen at the same time, permitting more rapid communications. Communication was enhanced since clarification questions could be asked at the time they were germane to the discussion.

Multiplex radios permit the transmission of both audio signals as well as data. The transmission of an electrocardiogram (ECG), called **telemetry**, during patient report is an example of the use of a multiplex radio.[15,16]

Transmission via a handheld radio is affected by the size of the battery. A larger battery, while providing more power, may be too bulky to be portable, thus limiting its use in the field.

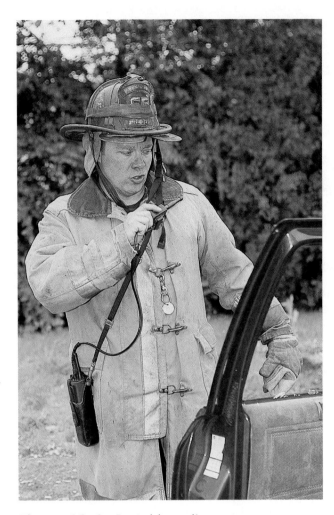

Figure 18-6 Portable radio.

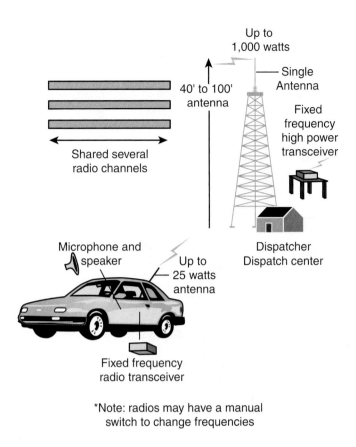

Up to 1,000 watts
Single Antenna
40' to 100' antenna
Fixed frequency high power transceiver
Shared several radio channels
Dispatcher Dispatch center
Microphone and speaker
Up to 25 watts antenna
Fixed frequency radio transceiver
*Note: radios may have a manual switch to change frequencies

Figure 18-7 Standard land mobile radio architecture.

To improve the transmission distance of a portable radio, some EMS systems depend upon repeaters to boost the signal (Figure 18-7).

Computer-Assisted Radios

The overwhelming public demand for general radio frequencies within the available radio band set aside by the federal government has forced some EMS agencies to have to share radio frequencies with school buses, livery services, and public works departments. The resultant **channel crowding** may cause a high priority EMS radio transmission from a portable radio to be suppressed (**walked on**) by a more powerful mobile transmitter from another department. In examining the problem, engineers realized that the majority of time there are no radio transmissions on any one channel and that this so-called **dead airtime** could be used to greater efficiency if it was controlled. Using computers, engineers devised a technique whereby multiple users could communicate over fewer frequencies, with the computer selecting the frequency to be used based on availability.

This technique of computer-assisted radio communications, called **trunking**, has several other advantages. For example, a computer-assisted mobile or portable radio allows an administrator (e.g., a city manager) to talk to all departments within a city at once, via a **simulcast**, or to all public services leaders, or to an individual department such as EMS. Trunking also prevents one message from blocking another message. The computer, in the example used earlier, would detect that an EMS message from a portable radio, a high-priority communication, was more important than the water department's transmission. The computer could elect to either switch the water department radio to another radio frequency or to store the message in the computer's short-term memory, so it could be rebroadcast when airtime became available. This in effect gives emergency radio transmissions a higher priority.

Cellular System Architecture

The advent of cellular telephones may have revolutionized emergency communications during day-to-day operations (Figure 18-8). **Cellular telephones** are actually low-powered wireless transmitters (radios) that work within close proximity to a radio tower. Each tower provides service to an area referred to as a **cell**. Each mobile radio (cellular telephone) has a forward link to the tower as well as a reverse link and operates as a duplex radio within that cell. As the cellular phone reaches the boundaries of the cell, the next tower (linked by computer) automatically transfers the call

Components of a Cellular System

Radio telephony systems

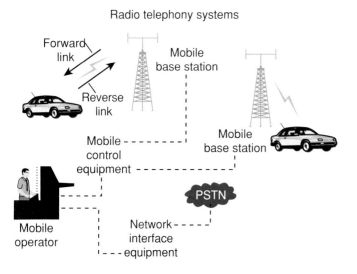

Figure 18-8 Cellular radio system architecture.

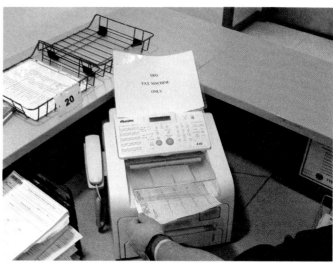

Figure 18-9 Facsimile (FAX) machines can receive high-quality electrocardiograms (ECG) from the field.

to another radio channel, without interruption of service. As each tower switches, or **hands-off**, the transmission to the next tower, there is no interruption in transmission.

The first cellular systems, created in the late 1970s, were analog systems operating at 800 mHz and quickly became mainstream in the public. Unfortunately, transmissions between cellular telephones could be picked up by multiband receivers called **scanners** that monitor several radio frequencies, including those used by cellular telephones. This practice of scanning for conversations breached patient confidentiality and made cellular telephone use problematic for Paramedics.

The subsequent generations of cellular service, such as the personal cellular service (PCS), used digital service instead of analog. Digital cellular systems have encrypted voice and data features that increase security and help maintain the confidentiality of patient information.[17,18]

Cellular Telephone

There are three varieties of cellular phones or **mobile subscriber units (MSU)** for use within a cellular radio system. The most common MSU is the portable cellular telephone which boasts about 0.6 watts of power. These small, personal cellular telephones are convenient but often lack the range necessary to reach towers outside of a service area.

The transportable cellular telephone boasts more power, 1.6 watts. However, its larger battery makes it less convenient to carry. The mobile telephone, with its 4.0 watts of power, is powerful and dependable. The mobile telephone is usually mounted to the interior of the vehicle and has an external antenna to improve reception.

New satellite mobile telephones, formerly the sole domain of the military, are seeing increased use, especially in remote and rural areas where cellular service is often undependable or nonexistent. Satellite telephones offer the promise of dependable and secure (encrypted digital) connectivity

with distant medical centers where Paramedics may be able to benefit from the available expertise.

Alternative Communication Devices

Both the **facsimile machine** (Figure 18-9) and the computer have seen use as an alternative means of communication. The facsimile machine, using digital technology, can transmit a high-quality copy from one location to another (e.g., an electrocardiogram (ECG) can be sent to an emergency department or a cardiologist's office).

The advent of the computer has added a number of possibilities. By using laptop or handheld computers inside a vehicle, called a **mobile data terminal**, a Paramedic can create a document and then download it for transmission over a telephone line, via modem, over the Internet, or by using wireless technologies including Bluetooth®. Paramedics can also use palm-sized **personal digital assistants (PDA)** or personal palm computers (Figure 18-10) and move about the patient compartment at will, all the while transmitting and receiving critical patient information.

Public Safety Communications

The first use of a telephone to call for emergency medical assistance may have occurred when Alexander Graham Bell spilled acid on himself and called out over the telephone, "Mr. Watson, come here, I want your help." From those early beginnings, telecommunications, and especially radio, have grown enormously.

The easy availability of either radio transmitters or radio components created a surge of amateur radio enthusiasts, many of whom competed with commercial radio providers for the limited radio bands. To stem this growing problem, Congress passed a resolution, the **Communications Act of 1934**, which states that the President of the United States has control over all government radios and that the **Federal**

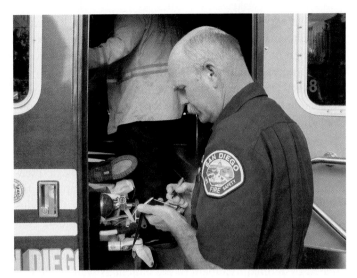

Figure 18-10 Paramedic using a PDA on-scene. (Courtesy of Computerworld Honors Program)

Communications Commission (FCC) has control over the civilian use of radios.[19,20]

The FCC, the agency with rule-making and enforcement responsibility, quickly began allocating frequencies to specific interest groups and then required them to license with the FCC for permission to use those frequencies. The earliest frequencies assigned to public safety included those in the VHF and UHF bandwidth.[21]

Early EMS Radio Communications

Despite the availability of a number of designated radio frequencies for public use, a 1970 study showed that less than 5% of ambulances had a mobile radio. In the seminal white paper, "Accidental Death and Disability," one recommendation spoke of the need for dedicated frequencies for EMS: frequencies to be used between the ambulance and the hospital as well as between the dispatch center and the ambulance. Another recommendation advocated for a centralized radio and telephone communications center. During that era, it was not uncommon for a citizen to either call the operator for help or call a seven-digit emergency **hotline**. These hotlines, dedicated telephone numbers, usually rang into someone's house. That person would then use a call-down tree to summon an emergency crew. Some hospitals still maintain an emergency hotline (Figure 18-11) as a backup to radio communications. While other emergency notification systems also evolved, they all had one thing in common: inefficiency.

The final recommendation of the white paper called for the creation of a single nationwide telephone number for all emergency services. The practice at the time was that every jurisdiction had its own seven-digit emergency telephone number. Unfortunately, the telephone company's service area did not always line-up with the boundaries of a particular EMS service. This resulted in frequent errors.

Despite the recognition of communications as an integral component of EMS and a growing public awareness of

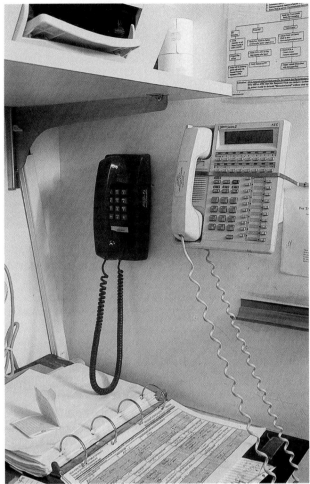

Figure 18-11 Dedicated emergency hotline.

the importance of communications to the "chain of survival," EMS communications continue to be problematic.

Phases of EMS Communications

There are three phases of communication in every EMS incident: (1) the occurrence and the detection of the occurrence, (2) the notification and response of responders, and (3) the treatment and transportation of the patient. Delays due to communications problems during any one of these three phases can result in increased harm, and even death, for the patient.

Detection

In 1967, the President's Commission on Law Enforcement and Administration of Justice recommended that there be a single universal emergency number in the United States. Britain had used a national three-digit emergency number, 9-9-9, since 1937 and had a great deal of success with a universal number. In November of 1967, the FCC and the American Telegraph and Telephone Company (AT&T) announced that AT&T would use 9-1-1 as its universal emergency number in all of the areas served by AT&T. The number 9-1-1 was chosen, in part, because no exchange or area code in the AT&T system used the number 9-1-1.

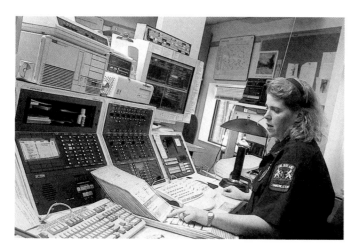

Figure 18-12 Communciations center or public safety access point.

Shortly thereafter, on February 16, 1968, Representative Rankin Fite, Speaker of the House of Representatives, placed the first 9-1-1 call in Haleyville, Alabama. Since that fateful first call, 9-1-1 service has been extended to over 96% of the United States. Canada has also adopted the 9-1-1 emergency number, making it an international emergency number.

When a 9-1-1 call is placed, a specially trained "call-taker" takes down information regarding the nature of the emergency to pass along to fellow workers or responders. The entire 9-1-1 operation is generally located in a centralized communications center called a **public safety access point (PSAP)** which runs 24 hours a day, seven days a week (Figure 18-12).

Subsequent generations of 9-1-1 service have been enhanced (E9-1-1) to include a call-back feature as well as location identifier. These features allow emergency **communications specialists (COMSPEC)** to dispatch emergency responders to people who are unable to speak or who have lapsed into unconsciousness.

At its inception, 9-1-1 service was very effective in getting help to those in need of assistance. However, the widespread use of mobile cellular telephones has reduced some of the advantages of the E9-1-1 system. Communications specialists receiving a 9-1-1 call from a cellular telephone do not have a call-back number nor do they have a location identifier to assist them with rushing aid to the patient's side. Recognizing this problem, the telecommunications industry has agreed to rectify the problem in two phases. During phase I, cellular telephones will not only provide a call-back number to the PSAP but also provide the location of the transmitting tower. During phase II, the cellular telephone will be able to emit a location finder, a homing beacon of sorts, which multiple towers can use to triangulate the position and give the cellular telephone's exact location in terms of latitude and longitude.

Prearrival Instructions

In 1975, Phoenix firefighter Paramedic Bill Tune successfully coached a woman while she performed CPR on her infant. After reviewing the incident, Chief Allen Brunacini of the Phoenix Fire Department ordered that callers receive instruction on how to self-rescue before responders arrived. Most current EMS dispatch procedures include some form of prearrival instruction. This instruction, called **medical self-help**, added another dimension to the role of communications specialists—being the "first" first responder.

Notification and Response

The next phase of emergency communications is the notification phase. During the notification and response phase, the greatest danger is posed for a Paramedic. Using the lights and siren in response to an emergency, the Paramedic is at risk of bodily harm secondary to motor vehicle collision. This danger is accepted in light of the potential good which can be created by prompt treatment of the patient as well as the fact that the danger can be mitigated by the cautious operation of the emergency response vehicle. Nevertheless, in many cases, Paramedics and the public are put in harm's way during a call for assistance in which a delayed response would not harm the patient. Concerned about the widespread practice of sending all EMS units out with lights and sirens on to the scene regardless of the nature of the emergency, in 1977 Dr. Jeff Clawson went about systematically placing EMS calls in a priority classification.

Dr. Clawson's objective was to send the right response to the right person at the right time. Original trials of the new **Medical Priority Dispatching™** were successful in Salt Lake City, Utah, and the system proliferated across the United States and Canada.[22,23] According to **emergency medical dispatch (EMD)** protocols, the communication specialist was to interrogate the caller, give prearrival instructions, and use preset criteria to make a response determination before dispatching the appropriate EMS responder units.

The use of EMD has become so widespread in the United States that the American Society of Testing and Materials (ASTM) issued a practice standard in 1990. In addition, the National Association of Emergency Medical Services Physicians (NAEMSP) advanced a position paper that essentially states that EMD is the standard of care for dispatching EMS calls.

First-Due Report

Almost all Paramedics notify the PSAP of their departure from their assigned post or station and their arrival on-scene. In some cases, particularly where there are multiple casualties, a **first-due report** is important for scene command and control. A first-due report is a brief synopsis of the scene size-up obtained by the first arriving EMS responder. Typically it includes the exact location of the call, the nature of the incident, known or suspected hazards, and the anticipated number of patients. If special resources (e.g., heavy rescue) are needed, they would be requested at that time.

In the 1920s, police officers used **10-codes**. These police departments often had one radio frequency and used

10-codes as abbreviated messages designed to minimize airtime. In 1940, the Associated Police Communications Officers, now the Association of Public Safety Communications Officials (APCO), published its first 10-code list. Since that publication, and despite efforts at standardization, dozens of versions of the 10-code have been created. These 10-codes are useful when only used intradepartmentally; however, the use of 10-codes can be confusing in cross-jurisdictional communications, and especially to responding mutual aid companies that do not use the same codes. Therefore, many EMS systems and disaster planners prefer the use of **plain English transmissions** and discourage the use of 10–codes.

Radio Conduct

While plain English transmissions can be clear, the ability to use plain English has caused some emergency personnel to take free license and use vulgarity over the air. The FCC has the authority to fine, suspend, or terminate any radio license for failure to comply with the standards for radio operation, including the misuse of radio or use of profanity while on-the-air. As a result, and as part of the culture of EMS, a characteristic form of spoken communication has arisen. Frequently, Paramedics will use a standard nomenclature, such as the terms "affirmative," "negative," and "stand-by," as well as the use of concise radio reporting style, to ensure that a clear message gets through. It is also common for Paramedics to suspend pleasantries, such as saying "please" or "thank you" during a transmission. There is an implicit understanding among Paramedics that the Paramedic is both courteous and professional when foregoing the use of pleasantries in favor of conserving airtime.

Treatment and Transportation Communications

The Paramedic shares a special relationship with an emergency physician that requires a more complete disclosure of the patient's condition than would be expected from an EMT. This duty is owed, in part, because of the invasive procedures that a Paramedic is allowed to perform. Typically, when a Paramedic is contacting medical control for guidance and instruction, the report begins with the Paramedic's identifier. Many systems assign numbers to Paramedics which indicate that the person on the radio is a recognized Paramedic with clinical privileges. The following format is an example of a standardized radio report. Each EMS system varies with regard to the information required and the order of presentation.

Starting with patient demographics (age, sex, and weight in kilograms) and the patient's chief concern (in the patient's own words, if possible), the Paramedic would provide a history of the present illness (HPI). Mnemonics such as AEIOU TIPS or PQRST can be helpful in organizing the mass of patient health information into a meaningful whole.

What follows is the patient's **past medical history (PMH)**. The mnemonic **AMPLE** can be useful for organizing the patient's information. While advising the physician about every allergy, every medication, and the patient's

complete past medical history may appear helpful, this amount of information may serve to only confuse the physician who is trying to understand the underlying problem. A Paramedic uses judgment to select the information that is pertinent to share with the physician in order to optimize time and increase efficiency.

The Paramedic would then proceed to the physical examination. Paramedics will have already completed an initial survey. If the patient is high priority, then all life-saving interventions should be conveyed to the physician in a standard ABC order. Provided that all life-threatening conditions have been treated and temporarily stabilized, the Paramedic would then proceed to report the patient's **vital signs**: temperature, pulse, respirations, and blood pressure. Following the initial assessment and vital signs, the Paramedic should report the findings of a **focused/vectored physical examination (PE)**. The Paramedic understands that he is the emergency physician's eyes and ears in the field. The Paramedic should anticipate what observations the physician will likely request. Clinical practice, working side-by-side with the emergency physician, can help educate the Paramedic as to the expectations that a physician will have for a physical examination report.

In the case of a medical patient, the **history of present illness** plays a pivotal role in the decision-making process. In the case of a trauma patient, the mechanism of injury coupled with the physical examination findings is of paramount importance. Paramedics learn through experience to emphasize the appropriate findings according to the patient's presentation. Once the patient presentation is complete, it is appropriate for the Paramedic to make a **field diagnosis** of the patient's condition. Providing a field diagnosis over the radio helps the emergency physician understand the Paramedic's direction and intent. At this time, the EMS physician can ask for more assessment findings, both history and physical, as well as redirect the Paramedic's attention to alternative conclusions.

What follows is usually a discussion of the treatments provided up to that point in time, including their effect, and a dialogue about how to proceed. Whenever a Paramedic accepts a medical order, he or she should practice the **echo technique**. With echo technique, when the physician gives an order the Paramedic should repeat the order back to the physician exactly as received. The physician should then confirm the accuracy of the read-back.

To prevent confusion, some EMS systems only allow a Paramedic to accept one order at a time. Stacking orders, each received one at a time, is acceptable provided that adequate time is permitted between interventions to assure that the therapeutic goal has been met, or not met as the case may be, before proceeding.

Many systems also require an **alert report** be sent to the triage station or a charge nurse. In some EMS systems, the Paramedic is tasked with alerting the receiving facility. The information in the alert report is brief and concise: age, sex, **chief complaint**, mental status, vital signs, treatments in progress, and an estimated time of arrival (ETA).

Radio Difficulties

Paramedics frequently encounter problems while trying to operate their radio systems. The Public Safety Wireless Network study indicated that some 15% of public safety providers had problems with static, batteries, or both, while another 23% complained of signal fading. Despite the fact that 24 more mHz of bandwidth has been dedicated for public safety use, some 32% of public safety providers complained about channel crowding.

The question of interagency interoperability is important in the post September 11, 2001 era. It is imperative that all public safety agencies be able to communicate with one another in order to more efficiently carry out their mission with the maximum degree of safety. The Fire and EMS Communications Interoperability study indicated that less than 35% of the agencies surveyed—some 1,045 agencies nationwide—indicated confidence in the interoperability of their radios during a large scale task force operation typically seen at a multiple casualty incident.

CONCLUSION

Whether communicating with other members of the healthcare team or the public safety team, the quality of communications is important to overall teamwork. Working as a team, and optimizing communications at both levels, will help facilitate patient care and the patient's recovery from a medical emergency.

▶ KEY POINTS:

- Paramedics are a part of both the public safety team and the healthcare team. Communication within the public safety team, made up of law enforcement officers, firefighters, and Paramedics, serves to provide safety to the rescuer, the public, and the patient.

- The Paramedic's communication with the healthcare team serves the patient's interests by providing the patient's past medical history, information about the history of the patient's present illness, and the patient's response to prehospital treatment.

- Communication occurs between team members as well as with other teams.

- Interfaces can occur in both oral and written forms.

- AM and FM radio signals are generated through modulation techniques which modify a wave by either changing the wave's height (amplitude modulation [AM]) or by changing the wave's speed (frequency modulation [FM]). The message can then be carried through antennas to be transmitted.

- The antenna's length is a function of the wave's length; therefore, an antenna correctly matched to a radio greatly improves radio transmission. The difference in radio waves is not in the speed but rather in the frequency of the waves in the radio transmission, measured in cycles per second or Hertz.

- To overcome obstacles in the line of sight that can block transmissions, high-frequency radio waves are directed toward the atmosphere and the signal is reflected back to Earth, covering great distances with great quality.

- The principal radio frequency band used by emergency services is very-high frequency (VHF). VHF, from 30 to 300 mHz, can be cleanly transmitted over 25 to 50 miles.

- To overcome the problem of distance, repeaters—which pick-up, amplify, and then retransmit a radio transmission—can extend the range of a VHF almost indefinitely.

- Two radio architectures exist in EMS today: traditional land mobile radio (LMR) architecture and cellular system architecture.

- The simplest radio system, simplex (or a walkie-talkie), only allows communication in one direction at a time.

- A duplex radio is similar to a landline and uses two frequencies. One frequency is used to transmit and one is used to receive, allowing an operator to talk and listen at the same time.

- Multiplex radios permit the transmission of both audio signal as well as data such as telemetry.

- To reduce channel crowding, computers allow multiple users to communicate over fewer frequencies by selecting the frequency to be used based on availability, a process called trunking.

- Cellular telephones are actually low-powered wireless transmitters (radios) that work within close proximity of a radio tower.

- Technology today allows Paramedics to use laptop or handheld computers along with personal digital assistants (PDA) before, during, and after calls to gather, transmit, and receive critical patient information using cable or wireless technologies.

- The Communications Act of 1934 granted the Federal Communications Commission (FCC) control over all civilian use of radios.

- The 9-1-1 system that we use today, which covers over 96% of the United States, was adapted from the British 9-9-9 national emergency number and initially put in place by AT&T.

- The first phase of communication in an EMS incident is a call received at a centralized communications center or public safety access point.

- The next phase of emergency communications is the notification and response phase.

- The third phase of emergency communications is the treatment and transport of the patient.

- Paramedics need a formalized radio report method.

REVIEW QUESTIONS:

1. What is meant by the duality of EMS communications?
2. Where did radio communications get its start?
3. What is the principal radio frequency band used by emergency services?
4. What is the difference between amplitude modulation and frequency modulation?
5. Describe ways the transmission and reception of a radio signal can be improved.

6. Compare the two radio architectures that exist in EMS.
7. Who has control over the civilian use of radios?
8. Describe early EMS radio communications and the development of public safety access points.
9. List and describe the elements of a radio report.

CASE STUDY QUESTIONS:

Please refer to the Case Study at the beginning of the chapter and answer the questions below.

1. What should be included in the radio report to the medical control physician?
2. How important was the first-due report given by the first member of the public safety team on-scene?

3. How does communication improve a Paramedic's clinical decision making?
4. If you were asked to manage and provide EMS for a large event in your area, how would you assess the importance of communication between the public safety team and healthcare team?

REFERENCES:

1. Kelly CG. The ways and whys of documentation. Good documentation is more than what's on a PCS form. *Emerg Med Serv.* 2007;36(7):30.
2. Perkins TJ. Tell me a story. The importance of good documentation. *Emerg Med Serv.* 2007;36(9):30, 32–33.
3. Krentz MJ, Wainscott MP. Medical accountability. *Emerg Med Clin North Am.* 1990;8(1):17–32.
4. Lazar RA, Schappert RJ, 3rd. Presumed insufficient. The importance of the prehospital care report. *Jems.* 1991;16(1):101–104.
5. Harkins S. Documentation: why is it so important? *Emerg Med Serv.* 2002;31(10):89–90, 93–94.
6. Maltz HM. EMS documentation. A legal necessity to avoid liability claims. *Emerg Med Serv.* 2002;31(10):96, 98, 146.

7. Erich J. Documenting your life away: common EMS report errors. *Emerg Med Serv.* 2003;32(11):47–49, 52.

8. Mabee C. *The American Leonardo: A Life of Samuel F. B. Morse.* Fleischmanns: Purple Mountain Press; 2000.

9. Hertz H. *Electric Waves: Being Researches on the Propagation of Electric Action with Finite Velocity Through Space.* New York: Cornell University Library; 1893.

10. http://www.nal.usda.gov/speccoll/collectionsguide/mssindex1.shtml

11. Fausti SA, Erickson DA, et al. The effects of impulsive noise upon human hearing sensitivity (8 to 20 kHz). *Scand Audiol.* 1981;10(1):21–29.

12. Sizun H. *Radio Wave Propagation for Telecommunication Applications (Signals and Communication Technology).* New York: Springer; 2004.

13. http://www.arrl.org

14. Tse D, Viswanath P. *Fundamentals of Wireless Ccommunication.* New York: Cambridge University Press; 2005.

15. Sillesen M, Sejersten M, et al. Referral of patients with ST-segment elevation acute myocardial infarction directly to the catheterization suite based on prehospital teletransmission of 12-lead electrocardiogram. *J Electrocardiol.* 2008; 41(1):49–53.

16. Adams GL, Campbell PT, et al. Effectiveness of prehospital wireless transmission of electrocardiograms to a cardiologist via hand-held device for patients with acute myocardial infarction (from the Timely Intervention in Myocardial Emergency, NorthEast Experience [TIME-NE]). *Am J Cardiol.* 2006;98(9):1160–1164.

17. Nazeran H, Setty S, et al. A PDA-based flexible telecommunication system for telemedicine applications. *Conf Proc IEEE Eng Med Biol Soc.* 2004;3:2200–2203.

18. Kline JA, Johnson CL, et al. Prospective study of clinician-entered research data in the emergency department using an Internet-based system after the HIPAA Privacy Rule. *BMC Med Inform Decis Mak.* 2004;4,(17):1–16.

19. Granados MR, Sr. New FCC rules affect EMS radio frequencies. *Emerg Med Serv.* 1996;25(2):24–25.

20. Johnson MS, Van Cott CC. The FCC may be listening. An update on EMS communications. *Jems.* 1992;17(5):19–24, 26–27.

21. Johnson MS, Van Cott CC. New radio service targets EMS communications. *Emerg Med Serv.* 1993;22(7):70–74.

22. Kuisma M, Holmstrom P, et al. Prehospital mortality in an EMS system using medical priority dispatching: a community based cohort study. *Resuscitation.* 2004;61(3):297–302.

23. Bailey ED, O'Connor RE, et al. The use of emergency medical dispatch protocols to reduce the number of inappropriate scene responses made by advanced life support personnel. *Prehosp Emerg Care.* 2000;4(2):186–189.

CHAPTER 19

DOCUMENTATION

KEY CONCEPTS:

Upon completion of this chapter, it is expected that the reader will understand these following concepts:

- The patient care report as an important medical, business, and legal document
- The patient care report as part of the quality assurance and performance—improvement program
- Different formats available for documentation that focus on a precise reflection of the events that occurred
- Special incidents, such as disasters, that require special reports

▶ CASE STUDY:

After all the excitement of the cardiac arrest was over, the new Paramedic realized she was faced with the tedium of documentation. Her senior Paramedic partner reminded her that documentation is important. He said, "The patient care report is a medical document that helps the physician determine the cause of the cardiac arrest. The patient care report is also used as a quality improvement tool, allowing our supervisor to ascertain whether we met certain performance goals, to identify weaknesses in our performance and to help establish training goals to correct those weaknesses. And," as he continued, "the patient care report is a legal record." Nodding acknowledgment she opened up the laptop and started to fill the fields.

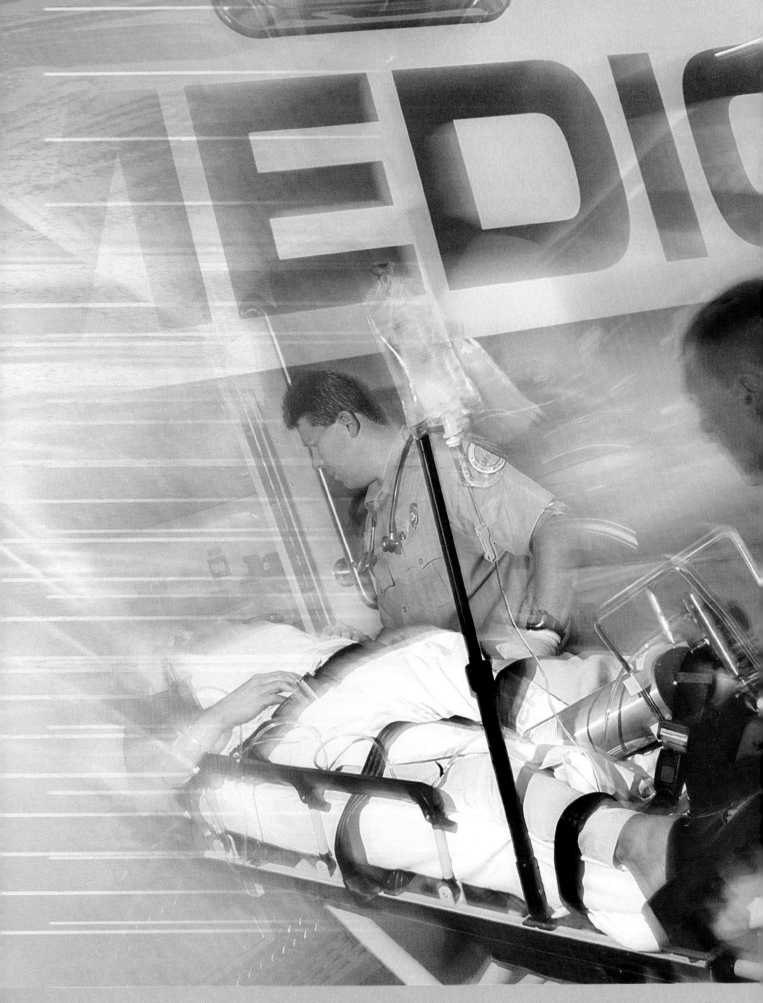

OVERVIEW

Documentation—whether it consists of patient care reports, special incident reports, affidavits, or triage tags—is an important responsibility for Paramedics. One study suggested that Paramedics spend as much as 28% of their patient contact time writing the patient care report (PCR), underscoring its importance.[1]

Some Paramedics, in order to focus on patient care, facilitate their report-writing by taking notes on 3 × 5 cards or notepads and then transcribe their notes to a more formal PCR later. It is also common to see a Paramedic writing critical patient information on a piece of tape affixed to a pant leg or on the corner of a sheet.

Purpose of EMS Documentation

Patient care documentation is a record of the pertinent findings and observations of the patient's health obtained through examination. It is also a log of the tests and treatments performed.

There are six-fold reasons for Paramedics to write an accurate patient care report. First and foremost, the PCR is a part of the patient's present medical care. Based upon the outcomes of treatments, noted on the PCR, the emergency department can make further treatment decisions. The PCR is a communication tool between the Paramedic, who has left the patient, and the emergency physician at the hospital still treating the patient. The PCR is therefore essential to the continuity of patient care. It emphasizes the Paramedic's role as a part of the healthcare team as well.

Second, the PCR is also a part of the **medical record**, which will be used in the future by other physicians and allied healthcare professionals for patient care. As a part of the medical record, the PCR often provides vital information to physicians about the origin of a condition or disease (Figure 19-1).

For example, a PCR written about a low-priority patient contact during a hazardous materials spill may be the evidence that links a minor exposure to a toxin to liver cancer 20 years later.

Third, the PCR is a tool for quality assurance and performance improvement programs. Through **PCR audits**—a careful review of the documentation for specific data—healthcare managers, EMS administrators, and EMS physicians can assure that the patient care provided out-of-hospital meets the established standard of care. PCR audits help to ensure that acceptable patient care is provided to all patients equally.

Analysis of the results of these PCR audits also helps to identify trends, such as increased patient contacts in a certain segment of a city or a consistent problem with patient care in a specific patient population. Identification of system issues in this manner provides EMS managers with an opportunity to remodel the system or educate the Paramedics.

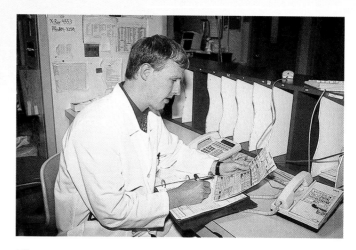

Figure 19-1 Physicians use prehospital patient care records to obtain information that might otherwise be unavailable.

Fourth, the PCR is a business record used for billing and operations. Careful and accurate documentation helps to ensure that insurance claims reviewers, during utilization review, will accept the patient care charges submitted.

Fifth, EMS researchers may also use the PCR as a research document. Following changes in EMS care documented on the PCR, researchers can publish either descriptive research findings or, using an experimental design, investigate new treatments in the field.

EMS educators often use selected PCRs for case presentation in a case of the utility of a practice. EMS physicians, in the course of a medical audit, often select illustrative cases documented on a PCR for individual instruction or an agency's continuing education. The PCR can also be utilized in a case-based method of teaching. These PCRs are often illustrative of a unique solution to an unusual problem or as a reinforcement to established methods.

Finally, the PCR is a legal record. The Paramedic can be subpoenaed to court with the PCR to testify during a trial (Figure 19-2). The PCR can be used as evidence in a trial. The trial may or may not even involve EMS as an issue. That

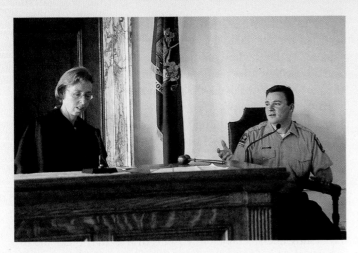

Figure 19-2 The prehospital patient care report is a legal document as well as a medical record.

PCR, exhibited to others in the legal system and the public, reflects upon its author and all other Paramedics.[2]

A PCR is an important tool for a Paramedic during a trial. With the number of lawsuits against Paramedics rising, Paramedics will depend on the PCR as a source of information to aid recall for activities on an EMS scene which may have occurred five or six years previously.[3]

Elements of a PCR

A PCR has many **fields**, which are places to enter data. Most of the fields are for patient care information, although some fields on a PCR are for administrative and/or business information.

In the past, documentation of patient care was imprecise and simply noted. For example, documentation may have stated that a person was transported and indicate very little else.

Physicians have entrusted a great deal of responsibility to Paramedics. However, physicians need to know how the patient was treated in the field. This reveals the need for thorough documentation. In addition, administrators (both public and private) who have interested "stakeholders," as well as the legal system, have mandated more thorough documentation of patient care.

Documentation Standards

At a minimum, a Paramedic should document the reason for the urgent transportation of a patient to an emergency department. The federal Center for Medicare and Medicaid Services (CMMS), in its definition of an emergency, states that an EMS call is medically necessary when the patient experiences a sudden onset of acute symptoms for which emergency medical intervention at a hospital would seem necessary. Medical necessity further requires that the absence of immediate medical attention could reasonably result in jeopardy to health, serious impairment of bodily function, or a serious dysfunction of a body organ or part.

The last statement is somewhat problematic as it assumes a foreknowledge of a determination yet to be made. Appreciating that the patient lacks this knowledge, and that the patient calls for EMS because of a belief that it is an emergency, the federal government has accepted the prudent layperson standard. The **prudent layperson standard** means that another person, not a physician, who was in the same or similar circumstances would think it is appropriate to call EMS; this is paraphrased from larger state and federal definitions.[4,5]

However, simply stating that there is a medical emergency, using the previous standard, is insufficient information for the purposes of the medical record, utilization review, and the courts. To fulfill the needs of these other parties, the Paramedic needs to provide complete documentation of care from the arrival on-scene to the transfer of care at the hospital.

Following a proscribed format the Paramedic should legibly write down his or her observations on the patient care record in black ink. If an action or observation is not documented, then that information is lost. While the loss of vital information can potentially harm the patient, it also calls into question the thoroughness of the Paramedic's exam and the justifications for treatment. The saying "If it wasn't written down, then it didn't happen," suggests that a treatment performed by the Paramedic is considered never to have happened, despite a Paramedic's protestations, if it wasn't recorded. As a result, there may be an appearance of dereliction of duty or possible negligence on the Paramedic's part.

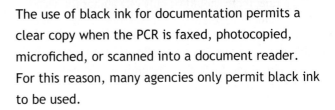

STREET SMART

The use of black ink for documentation permits a clear copy when the PCR is faxed, photocopied, microfiched, or scanned into a document reader. For this reason, many agencies only permit black ink to be used.

Legibility is another important issue in documentation. The purpose of the PCR is to transfer the information to, or communicate with, the physician and other patient care providers. If the writing is indecipherable, then the function of the document is lost. It is a good practice to have another Paramedic, one who was on-scene, read the PCR. Such proofreading serves several purposes. It helps to establish consensus regarding the observations and actions of the team, as well as ensures the readability of the PCR.

The use of slang and jargon in a PCR is inappropriate and unprofessional. Such terms do not add to the patient record and unnecessarily serve to distract the reader from the message. Similarly, bias and prejudice have no place on a PCR.

As a rule, Paramedics practice conservation with words and avoid excessive wordiness. While reading such technical writing may seem dry, its intention is to be precise and to convey a maximum amount of information in a short period of time.

Errors and Omissions

When an error is made on the PCR, the Paramedic should "strike-out" the mistake with a single line, leaving the content below the strike-out legible. Next to the strike-out, the Paramedic should place the date and initial the strike-out to indicate authorship. Heavy cross-outs give an appearance of deception, as does the use of erasure polishes such as White-out®, leaving the Paramedic open to questions about integrity.

It is common practice to place a single diagonal line across any open areas of the document, called "line-out," in order to prevent the addition of new content to a PCR by others after the Paramedic has completed the PCR.

Upon completion of the document, some Paramedics **sign-out** with time, date, and initial after the last entry. The line-out and the sign-out indicate that the PCR was written and completed by the person listed "in-charge" at the time and date listed.

Upon re-reading the PCR and determining an entire passage or entry is substantially in error, the passage should not be removed but instead "crossed out" with a single slash that is then dated and initialed. A revision should then be written on another page or on a continuation form with cross-reference made to the first entry (e.g., see PCR 123).

It is also permissible to add to the record after the call. In that instance, another page should be added. Additions should only be added when the entry will substantially clarify the record or document important patient information useful to the physician.

As a rule, there should be only one author for each PCR. Multiple authors generate concerns about the authenticity of the document and the accuracy of the events depicted. Discussion and collaboration with fellow EMS providers during the creation of the PCR should eliminate the need for multiple authors (Table 19-1).

Confidentiality

Some Paramedics use a **facsimile machine** to transmit documentation (e.g., to send the PCR from a base station to the hospital). The use of a facsimile machine (FAX) may be acceptable provided a few safeguards are in place.

Table 19-1 Documentation Standards

- Black ink is preferred.
- Legibility is important.
- Slang and jargon is not used.
- Errors noted with single strike-through and initialed.
- Empty space is lined out.
- Sign-out includes initials, date, and time.
- One author for each record.

The central question with facsimiles is confidentiality (i.e., did the PCR get to the intended recipient?). When "faxing" a PCR, the Paramedic should contact the receiver and advise that a facsimile will be transmitted shortly. When the facsimile is received, the recipient should respond with a verification of receipt.

If the PCR is inappropriately sent to the wrong address, the cover sheet should clearly indicate that the facsimile is confidential and ask the recipient to destroy the copy. If the Paramedic knows that the transmission was made in error, then the Paramedic should call the other party and request that the unintended recipient destroy the PCR.

Current regulations under the 1996 Health Insurance Portability and Accountability Act (HIPAA) may make the use of a facsimile machine inadvisable in the future (Figure 19-3). Also, such practices should be carefully scrutinized for compliance with regulations regarding confidentiality.[6]

Forms of Documentation

Electronic Documentation

Electronic documentation, although still in its infancy, is rapidly becoming state of the art. The use of **mobile data terminals (MDT)** on-board the ambulance or **personal digital assistants (PDA)** have replaced the pad and paper.

Electronic documents have several advantages over traditional documentation. Computers have built-in spell checker and grammar checker programs, increasing the readability of the PCR. Electronic documents can also have forced fields, mandatory fields which must be completed before submission. The use of forced fields helps to ensure that a minimum data set is completed. Data sets are discussed shortly.

Concerns about limited data entry has plagued electronic documentation programs in the past, but the addition of drop-down menus and handwriting recognition programs have helped eliminate some of those concerns.

To ensure patient confidentiality, all electronic documentation programs should be password protected and the

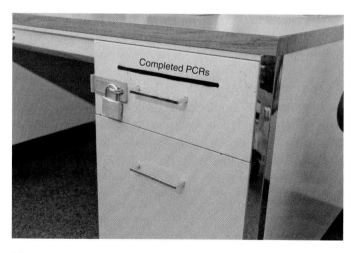

Figure 19-3 HIPAA regulations impact recordkeeping.

password changed as frequently as every 30 days. To further safeguard patient confidentiality, Paramedics should routinely shut down documentation programs when not in use to prevent uninvited intruders from entering the program and altering the record.

On-Scene Medical Records

The combination of mobile data terminals, secure satellite uplinks, and computer databases makes the possibility of obtaining patient medical records, while on-scene, not only possible but probable. The American Society of Testing and Materials (ASTM) has already produced standard F1652-95, Standard Guide for Providing Essential Data Needed in Advance for Prehospital Emergency Medical Service. The standard includes requirements for secure access and authorized use in order to protect patient confidentiality, as required under federal HIPAA regulations.

Problem-Oriented Medical Recordkeeping

In the past, physicians had private records for each patient that were stored in their offices. These were shared only with the patient and office staff whom the physician generally knew personally. Tracking the progression of a patient's disease in some cases was largely a function of the physician's memory.

With the advent of hospitals, medical specialties, and allied healthcare providers, all of whom need the same information, some order had to be brought to the massive collection of records generated for each patient by each provider. To help solve the dilemma, Dr. Lawrence Weed of the University of Vermont's Medical School advocated the concept of **problem-oriented medical recordkeeping (POMR)** information systems in 1969 to track and manage patient records.

In a POMR system, the **master problem list** of the record would list the medical conditions for which that patient had been, or currently was, receiving treatment.[7–10] Indexed as such, new entries in the medical record, called **progress notes**, would be placed into the patient's file under the problem listed. All healthcare professionals, from physicians to nurses to dieticians, would place their entries into the patient's record using the **SOAP notes** format.

The SOAP format may be one of the earliest standardized documentation formats. With POMR, any allied healthcare provider could open up the patient's record, called a chart, and read what other providers were planning to do, as well as review the patient's progress. With this knowledge in hand, the provider would make a patient assessment and then enter his or her SOAP note following the last entry.

The SOAP note would contain subjective (S) information obtained from the patient or the patient's family, objective (O) information obtained during physical examination, an assessment (A) of the patient's problem, and a plan (P) for action. SOAP notes proved to be invaluable for integrating information among a variety of healthcare professionals and ensuring the continuity of patient care.

EMS PCR Formats

Early EMS providers adopted the SOAP notes system for their documentation system. In some states, the progress note was virtually a blank sheet of paper, called an open form. The Paramedic was expected to document assessments and other information in SOAP format on the paper. While this approach permitted a great deal of freedom for documenting the patient's condition in a narrative manner, almost like telling a story, it made data gathering difficult for both the physician (who had to read the entire report to find one vital piece of information) and researchers (who looked at dozens of reports for one set of information).

In response to the need for standardized data collection, **minimum data sets** have been established. A minimum data set requires that the Paramedic complete certain fields with the requested information. The minimum data set permits the Paramedic and physician to track trends and note patient progress. A simple example of a data set would be response times. All EMS agencies strive to meet preset maximum response times (e.g., to be on-scene, or off the floor, in 10 minutes). Some agencies are obligated by contract to be on-scene in a minimum time. In both cases, the EMS agency wants to know its response times.

Every data set must also have a definition. In the previous example, does scene arrival mean when the ambulance is at the dispatched location or at the patient's side? The difference in these two interpretations of response times can mean minutes to a patient—minutes that make a difference in the patient's survival, such as with cardiac arrest.

The American Society of Testing and Materials (ASTM) has proposed a minimum data set for EMS, standard E1744. E1744-04 contains similar data sets as the Data Elements for Emergency Departments (DEEDS), a program distributed by the Centers for Disease Control and Prevention in 1979. Inclusion of DEEDS data sets into EMS data sets helps ensure a seamless documentation of care from the prehospital environment to the emergency department.

Using standardized data sets has tremendous research potential. With integrated standardized data sets, the efficiency of prehospital interventions can be measured against hospital patient outcomes and recommendations made for future practice.

To integrate patient information with minimum data sets, many EMS systems use a closed form method of documentation. Closed form documents use bubble forms, circles next to options, which the Paramedic fills in to provide information. These bubble forms can then easily be scanned by electronic readers to quickly obtain vast quantities of information.

Closed form documents assume most patients will have the same or similar complaints, symptoms, and so on, and are very restrictive. As a result, many Paramedics complain about their inability to document unique conditions or situations.

Many EMS systems use a combined form, one that has characteristics of a closed form and an open form. These combined forms allow rapid information gathering (the minimal data set), as well as the freedom to use some narrative, if needed.

CHEATED

Good patient care records paint an accurate picture of the patient's condition. For a time, SOAP notes were adequate. But as time progressed, Paramedics became increasingly dissatisfied with SOAP notes and started to modify the format to include elements unique to EMS.

Early EMS Documentation Formats

One of the first EMS documentation formats was the CHART (chief complaint, history, assessment, Rx [prescription], treatment) method. Rather quickly, Paramedics realized that CHART lacked some needed fields, such as an evaluation of the interventions. CHART was modified to become CHARTIE, adding I for intervention and E for evaluation to the previous information.

Another documentation format that was in common usage is NAP (narrative, assessment, plan of treatment). NAP is a short documentation format that is particularly well-adapted for first responder use. Narrative, the N in NAP, is a written description of the patient's complaints, current history, and any physical findings such as vital signs, which is written like a story. Assessment, the A in NAP, is typically complaint driven (e.g., shortness of breath). The plan of treatment, the P in NAP, includes disposition, or to whom the patient was turned over.

CHEATED Format

To help meet the Paramedic's needs for a more complete charting format, Valerie Conrad, EMS QI Coordinator in Traverse City, Michigan, developed an EMS-specific, user-friendly documentation method using the mnemonic **CHEATED**. The elements of CHEATED (chief concern/complaint, history, examination, assessment, treatment, evaluation, disposition) contain all of the additional fields needed by Paramedics and is inclusive of the SOAP notes previously used. This documentation method is a representation of one effective means of documenting an EMS event.

Chief Concern

The C in CHEATED, **chief complaint (CC)** or chief concern, is usually the reason that the patient called for EMS. If possible, the chief complaint should be stated in the patient's own words and placed within quotation marks.

If the patient is unable to speak, then the reason the patient is unable to speak (e.g., "unconscious") should be noted. The caller's words should then be noted. These are the words usually transmitted to the Paramedic by the dispatcher.

History

The H in CHEATED, history, contains the subjective information provided by he patient, the patient's family, and/or bystanders. The subjective information provided is called the patient's symptoms. The patient's history consists of an explanation of the symptoms (i.e., history of present illness) and the patient's past medical history.

History of Present Illness

The **history of present illness (HPI)** is a chronological description of the development of the patient's present illness, starting with the patient's chief complaint. If the patient is nonconversational (e.g., because the patient is unconscious), then family and/or bystander comments should be documented. Elements of an HPI typically include location, quality, severity, duration, timing, context, modifying factors, and any associated signs or symptoms of the illness.

The Paramedic's intent when gathering a history is to develop a **symptom pattern**. These symptom patterns (i.e., the list of symptoms) are then compared to the Paramedic's knowledge of other diseases, disorders, and syndromes. When the current symptom pattern matches a symptom pattern for one of these diseases, disorders, or syndromes, then a diagnosis can be made.

The mnemonic OPQRST (onset, provocation, quality of pain, radiation, severity, timing) is commonly used by Paramedics to help develop a symptom pattern (Table 19-2).[11] For example, the S in the OPQRST stands for severity. Using the anesthesiologists' pain scale, the patient is asked to rate the pain from 0, being no pain, to 10, being the worst pain the patient ever experienced. This line of questioning helps to establish the severity of the patient's pain as well as establish a baseline to gauge the effectiveness of pain relief.

While a patient history can be endless, the Paramedic focuses on those questions that will illuminate the cause of the patient's problem. It is helpful to have a more structured series of questions for a given problem.

Many EMS agencies have adopted the federal **Evaluation and Management Documentation Guidelines** created by the Health Care Finance Administration (HCFA), now called the Center for Medicare and Medicaid Services (CMS), and the American Medical Association (AMA). Standardized histories permit the Paramedic to identify diseases, disorders, and syndromes, vis-á-vis, through symptom pattern recognition, and document the medical necessity of the therapeutic services provided to the patient.

With the standardized history in hand, the Paramedic is now able to establish a diagnosis of the disease, disorder, or syndrome using the International Classification of Diseases (ICD-10) coding system.[12–14]

Table 19-2 OPQRST Mnemonic

O	Onset, the beginning of the symptoms
P	Provocation, what started or intensified the symptoms
Q	Quality of the pain
R	Radiation (Does the pain migrate to another body part?)
S	Severity, the intensity of the pain
T	Timing (Do the symptoms wax and wane?)

The ICD-10 is the latest edition of the international diagnostic classification system that first started in 1893 as the International List of Causes of Death. Since that time, the ICD coding system has evolved and become the standard for the description and classification of diseases.

With the diagnosis made, physicians and administrators can group patient populations with the same or similar diagnosis into **diagnosis-related groups (DRG)**. The original purpose of a DRG was to group patients who used similar resources together for reimbursement from Medicare. These DRG assignments are based on the ICD diagnosis. Currently the DRG, version 25, also takes into account procedures performed as well as the presence of significant comorbidities. In the case of EMS, a patient transport might be reimbursed for respiratory failure, as a DRG, if the patient was intubated. The patient may also be reimbursed for obesity, if the patient had that comorbidity.

For a high-priority patient, the Paramedic would obtain answers to a minimum of three elements among those listed. Elements of a history are listed according to body systems in the guidelines.

For a low-priority patient, the Paramedic would obtain a more detailed history that contains a minimum of six of the elements listed as well as some past medical history, and/or family and social history.

These minimum standards are used for all patients. The Paramedic's problem-focused history may elect, based on patient condition and clinical judgment, to expand on the history in order to more completely understand the patient's condition.

STREET SMART

Special notation should also be made if the patient threatens suicide. If possible, the patient's exact words and the context in which they were said should be noted. It may be the only utterance the patient makes about suicide.

Many Paramedics also document any **constitutional symptoms** noted. Constitutional symptoms are those general systemic reactions to illness that include fevers, unexplained weight loss, night sweats, chills, headaches, nausea, and vomiting. Constitutional symptoms can indicate that the patient may be infected and the Paramedic should reconsider the choice of personal protective equipment (PPE).

The HPI typically ends with the patient's **pertinent negatives**. Pertinent negatives are those symptoms which, if present, could indicate a more serious underlying problem. There could potentially be a large number of pertinent negatives, but Paramedics tend to limit the pertinent negatives specifically to those symptoms that imply pathology in a major organ system.

Starting in a head-to-toe progression, the traditional pertinent negatives are loss of consciousness, chest pain, shortness of breath, and abdominal pain. Other EMS systems may add other pertinent negatives as needed. These four pertinent negatives are ominous if, instead, they are positive. These conditions typically require advanced life support measures.

Past Medical History

Once the HPI is complete, the Paramedic would proceed to document the **past medical history (PMH)**. To aid with documentation of the PMH, the Paramedic often uses the mnemonic **AMPLE** (allergies, medications, past medical history, last meal, events).

The first element (A) of AMPLE is the patient's allergies, to both prescription and over-the-counter medications. If the patient has no allergies to drugs, then the acronym **NKDA** (no known drug allergies) is often used. If the patient has an allergy to a medication, and time permits, it may be helpful to get a history of the reaction to determine if it is a true allergy or an unpleasant side effect of the medication.

The next element (the M in AMPLE) stands for medications. The Paramedic should list all medications—including prescription, over-the-counter, botanicals, and illicit drugs—by name, dose, and frequency, if possible. It is appropriate for the Paramedic to use standard prescription shorthand to list the frequency (e.g., QD for once-a-day). These Latin terms are listed in the medical terminology chapter.

The next item (the P in AMPLE) stands for past medical history and should include the primary diseases recognized in each major body system (Table 19-3). Again, progressing in a head-to-toe fashion, a minimal past medical history would include questions about strokes and seizures (neurological), heart attack and hypertension (cardiovascular), asthma and chronic obstructive pulmonary diseases (COPD) (respiratory), diabetes (endocrine), and cancers (Ca). If the patient has a preexisting diagnosis for a disease, then that should also be listed.

Review of Systems

A more complete past medical history uses a **systems review** approach to history gathering. Using a head-to-toe approach, the following systems review represents a more complete

Table 19-3 Example of a Minimal Past Medical History

- Stroke
- Seizure
- Heart attack
- Hypertension
- COPD
- Asthma
- Diabetes
- Cancer

history gathering. The systems review can be used as a part of a comprehensive examination, or portions can be used to obtain a more complete focused examination.

Starting at the head, the patient should be asked if he has ever had a stroke, seizure, or traumatic brain injury (TBI). If the patient answers affirmatively to any of these stated conditions, then the Paramedic would use that opportunity to launch into a more extensive line of questioning. For example, if the patient admits to a history of seizures, then the Paramedic could inquire about the frequency of seizures, the date/time of the last seizure, what medications the patient is taking for the seizure condition, as well as compliance with those medications.

Proceeding to the cardiovascular system, the patient should be asked if he ever had angina (chest pain) or a diagnosis of acute myocardial infarction (AMI). If the patient answers yes, then the Paramedic might inquire which portion of the heart was affected. Next, the Paramedic would inquire about angioplasty, including the results and/or a coronary artery bypass graft (CABG). Some patients are so well educated about their condition that they can tell the Paramedic which vessel was involved, the percentage of blockage, and even their last ejection fraction.

A review of the respiratory system starts with documentation of any lung disease and often includes smoking history, listed in packs/years, and a diagnosis of emphysema.

The Paramedic should document any abdominal surgeries, including appendectomy, history of small bowel obstruction, and the presence of an abdominal aortic aneurysm, repaired or not repaired (Figure 19-4).

Proceeding to the genitourinary system, the Paramedic should document any history of sexually transmitted diseases. If the patient is a female, then a reproductive history—including the number of pregnancies and delivery of newborns—should be documented. A history of kidney stones may also explain flank/groin pain and should be documented.

If the patient has an extremity injury, then past medical history of injuries to the extremities, as well as the musculoskeletal system, should be documented. The history should include documentation of prior sprains, strains, and fractures, especially those that required surgical correction. Often Paramedics also take and document a pain history at this point, especially in regard to the prior use of morphine for similar injuries, in anticipation of orders for analgesia.

The Paramedic should document any endocrine disorders including diabetes, thyroid disorders, and thyroid surgeries. Similarly, any hematological disorders—such as leukemia, infections, blood transfusions, and overseas travel—should be documented.

If the patient has a behavioral disorder, then the Paramedic should document previous psychiatric admissions, any psychotropic medications, and use of alcohol or illicit drugs.

While the review of systems can be exhaustive, the intent is to discover preexisting medical conditions and then explore the medical treatments received for those conditions which might impact on current prehospital care. The previously listed questions in the review of systems merely cites some representative questions that could be used. More questions may be appropriate (Table 19-4).

The L in AMPLE has various interpretations. It typically stands for last meal. This is an important question if the patient may be destined for the operating room. Surgeons prefer patients who have not eaten prior to surgery (N.P.O.), thereby lowering the risk of aspiration. Some Paramedics also use the L to indicate last bowel movement (if the chief concern is abdominal pain) or last menses (if the patient could have a gynecological problem). Some Paramedics may use L to mean last time a medication was taken when the patient has a known history of epilepsy or diabetes.

The final element in AMPLE (E) refers to events and generally is aimed at previous events of the same or similar nature and/or other previous encounters with EMS.

Examination

The physical examination of the patient, the E in CHEATED, often starts with the position and condition in which the patient was found. For example, if the Paramedic finds the patient with shortness of breath in a tripod position, the Paramedic would note that as part of his general impression and document the same.

This type of "from the doorway" assessment is referred to as a **constitutional examination**. The constitutional examination

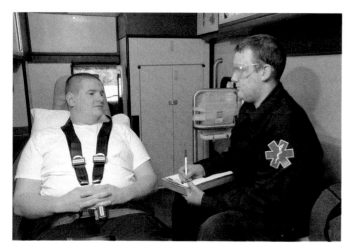

Figure 19-4 A Paramedic taking a history.

Table 19-4 Standard Review of Systems

- Neurological
- Cardiovascular
- Pulmonary
- Gastrointestinal
- Endocrine
- Genitourinary
- Integumentary
- Musculoskelal

assesses the patient's general appearance. Examples of the two extremes of appearance is the patient **in extremis**, or having great difficulty, and the patient in **no apparent distress (NAD)** (i.e., not appearing to be having difficulty). This "sick–not sick" impression can help the Paramedic establish the tempo of the call.

The constitutional examination may also contain objective observations about the patient's physical development such as "emaciated" or "obese." These descriptions speak to the patient's **body habitus**. For example, the morbidly obese patient typically has a list of medical conditions, such as heart failure and diabetes, associated with being obese. These descriptions of the patient are not slanderous or insulting, but are objective statements which are intended to make an inference about the patient's health.

Similarly, any overt deformities as well as personal grooming habits relate to the patient's health or the patient's ability to maintain health. The first sign of Alzheimer's disease, for example, may be the patient's inability to perform the activities of daily living, including personal grooming.

The Paramedic would then proceed to document the findings of the **initial assessment**, including the treatment of any life-threatening injury.

Next, the patient's **vital signs** are recorded. For blood pressure, it should be noted whether it was taken while the patient was supine, seated, or standing. For pulse, regularity (as well as rate, respirations, and temperature) should be recorded.

If the patient was high priority, then the Paramedic would document the problem-focused examination findings. The problem-focused examination, sometimes referred to as a vectored examination, is limited to the affected body area or organ system reflected in the chief complaint. The various body systems examined in a problem-focused examination include, from head-to-toe, the neurological system, the cardiovascular system, the respiratory system, the gastrointestinal system, the musculoskeletal system, and the psychiatric exam.

For example, a problem-focused physical examination for a patient with a complaint of substernal chest pain would include the cardiovascular system. Taking a look, listen, and feel approach to physical examination, the Paramedic would document the presence or absence of jugular venous distention and pedal edema. The auscultatory findings, including bilateral blood pressures and heart sounds, would be documented. Finally, findings assessed by palpation, such as pedal pulses and the location of the point of maximal intensity (PMI), might be documented.

It should be noted that any documentation of the abnormal without further elaboration is insufficient. The assumption is that the patient has normal findings unless otherwise noted.

If the patient is a low-priority patient, then a more **detailed physical examination** would be performed (Figure 19-5). Some Paramedics, especially in trauma cases, prefer a head-to-toe approach to the detailed physical examination, whereas others prefer a body systems approach to the examination.

If an ECG is attached to the documentation, it is important that the Paramedic standardize the notation of interpretation.

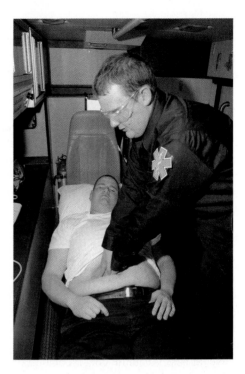

Figure 19-5 Paramedic performing a physical examination.

For example, all ECG criteria should be listed (QRS width, etc.) prior to noting an identification of the ECG rhythm. Many Paramedics will use a broad label, such as a narrow-complex tachycardia, and then note a presumptive interpretation, such as paroxysmal atrial tachycardia.

Assessment

While it is important for the Paramedic to accurately and completely describe the patient's condition, in order to arrive at a paramedical diagnosis, it is almost as important for the Paramedic to consider what is not seen. Documentation showing consideration of other possible etiologies demonstrates that the Paramedic has an open mind to other potential diagnoses and has considered them and then rejected them. This "head's up" attitude helps prevent the Paramedic from focusing too narrowly based on an assumption, without considering other possibilities. For example, the chest pain experienced by a patient could be due to pulmonary embolism secondary to a deep vein thrombus. If the Paramedic were to focus exclusively on a cardiac examination, he might miss the source of the pathology.

Following the discussions of various pathologies in subsequent chapters, the "rule out" or differential diagnosis for specific complaints will be discussed.

Paramedical Diagnosis

With the history and physical examination documented, the Paramedic would proceed to document the assessment. The assessment is, partly, a protocol-driven medical decision. Typically, for high-priority patients Paramedics use advanced life support (ALS) protocols, whereas for low-priority patients basic life support (BLS) protocols are used.

The documentation of the protocol-driven **field diagnosis** asserts and reinforces the Paramedic's medical control. If direct contact with medical control is made for purposes of consultation and specific orders, then that should be noted as well.

Treatment

The next section of the PCR is the treatment section. All interventions performed, both BLS and ALS, should be noted in the treatment section. If BLS first responders had already initiated patient care, then these treatments should also be noted in the treatment section, with the notation "performed by EMT Jones."

Evaluation

Following every treatment there should be an evaluation of the effectiveness of that treatment, or, at a minimum, a statement about the patient's ongoing condition. This is the evaluation phase of patient care.

Some have argued that Paramedic care is an unnecessary expense and that the majority of the Paramedic's treatments are ineffective, at best. Accurate documentation of the effect of prehospital care helps to demonstrate the value of early medical treatments performed by Paramedics.

Disposition

The last section of the CHEATED PCR is disposition. Some Paramedics refer to this as the patient report, a summary of the patient's condition and the status of treatments in progress when patient care was given over to another Paramedic or healthcare provider. It is imperative that the Paramedic document to whom the patient was **turned-over-to (TOT)** in order to avoid accusations of patient abandonment.

The disposition should also contain information about the patient's condition (i.e., changes and improvement), as well as the status of treatments. For example, a Paramedic might document that oxygen was continued, that the IV remained patent, and state the rate of infusion. The Paramedic might also want to document the volume of fluid infused as well as whether blood samples were turned over to the emergency department personnel. Finally, the Paramedic may document if the patient was left in the care of family, friends, or hospital personnel.

STREET SMART

After the patient is transferred from the ambulance gurney to the hospital stretcher, the side rails on the stretcher should be raised unless the patient is attended to by a hospital staff member. "Side rails up times two" is often the final line of documentation on the PCR.

Special Documentation

Several situations are not amenable to standard documentation procedures. These situations require special documentation or special notations, which will be discussed individually in the following section.

Refusal of Medical Assistance Documentation

The CHEATED format works well for documentation of refusal of medical assistance (RMA). Starting with the chief complaint, or chief concern, the Paramedic would document the history and the physical examination to the extent permitted by the patient.

In the assessment section, the Paramedic would address the issue of competence, including noting the patient's age. If the patient is of age, or is an emancipated minor, then the Paramedic would proceed and document the patient's mental status.

The key to capacity to consent, or to refuse, is the patient's mental status, discussed further in Chapter 6. Any physical or medical conditions that would prohibit the patient from consenting (e.g., intoxication or presumption of stroke) should be documented. Actions taken by the Paramedic to enlist the assistance of family, medical control, or law enforcement officers to convince the patient to seek medical attention should be documented as well.

In the treatment portion of the PCR, all treatments permitted by the patient, including those offered but refused, should be documented.

Instead of completing an evaluation, because treatment is being refused, the E in CHEATED means explanation of outcomes. The Paramedic should document that the patient was advised of foreseeable complications that are reasonably likely to arise, which could seriously jeopardize the patient's health and bodily functions or result in a serious dysfunction of an organ or body part if medical attention is refused.

The explanation of outcomes documented should include a list of the symptoms for which the patient should reconsider and recall EMS. Also, the encouragement to seek medical attention from a private physician should be noted.

Under the final disposition portion, the Paramedic should document with whom the patient was left and the patient's ability to summon aid or recontact 9-1-1.

The patient should then be asked to sign the completed PCR. A copy of the PCR should be left with the patient, if possible. Some EMS systems use special documentation forms for refusals of medical care. If the patient is unwilling to sign the PCR, the Paramedic should note the refusal and obtain the names, and signatures, of witnesses.

Hazardous Materials Operations Documentation

Key to hazardous materials operations documentation is an understanding that such documentation may be called into play in lawsuits and disability hearings years after the patient was seen by the Paramedic. Complicating matters, the average hazardous materials technician being assessed by EMS may not have any significant complaints and yet is given an on-scene physical examination as a part of the process of decontamination.

Using the CHEATED format in this venue, the Paramedic should document, under chief complaint, the exact potential chemical exposure, or exposures, if known. Under the history section, the Paramedic should explain the circumstances which caused the exposure.

A standard well-person physical examination, including vital signs, should be documented. Many EMS systems also perform a baseline cardio-thoracic examination for later comparison.

The patient's assessment and treatment are usually based upon prewritten protocols. The Paramedic should document if the patient's physiological condition meets or fails to meet those parameters and if treatment is indicated. In some instances, the treatment is limited to what is typically offered in a fire rehabilitation sector.

Finally, the patient's disposition, such as discharged to rehabilitation, discharged to home, or transported for further evaluation, should be documented.

Documentation of Multiple Casualties

Understandably, Paramedics cannot take the time to perform standard documentation during a mass casualty incident. In those circumstances, the **triage tag** is the only documentation that will be performed.

At the end of the incident, the Paramedics should complete an **event report** that details, like the hazardous materials incident report noted previously, the situation and conditions that occurred which led to the mass casualty incident. The event report should be as detailed as possible. The triage tags are then attached to the event report as a part of the permanent record.

In some cases, human error may have contributed to the incident and charges of negligence may be brought against those individuals who are believed to be responsible.[15–16] In that situation, the Paramedic may subsequently be called to testify about the conditions on-scene as well as the patient care provided.

Documentation of Pregnancy and Childbirth

Standard EMS documentation is designed to document the condition of an ill or injured person. The pregnant woman is neither ill nor injured. The wellness examination of the pregnant woman focuses on documenting the state of the pregnancy as well as identifying potential complications of childbirth.

Starting with a prenatal questionnaire, the Paramedic should document the answers to the questions about this pregnancy, such as date of last menstrual period (LMP) and/or the expected date of delivery (EDD). The Paramedic should then proceed to ask about inherited risk factors, personal habits (such as smoking or alcohol use), as well as document a systems review of the patient's health. When the prenatal questionnaire is completed, the Paramedic would document the patient's pregnancy history, including past difficulties with delivery.

Special Incident Report

Many Paramedics are asked to complete documentation that is not directly related to patient care. These documents, that can be broadly termed **special incident reports (SIR)**, are used for administrative purposes or as a part of a court proceeding.

One special incident report is an **exposure report**. The exposure report, separate from the patient care report that should be generated for each individual who was seen after exposure, details the circumstances that resulted in the Paramedic being exposed. The intention of an exposure report is to identify the problem and then correct the problem so that another exposure cannot occur. Therefore, names of exposed individuals may not be needed on the report. Under most circumstances, the designated officer (DO) for the agency receives the exposure report and would make recommendations for corrections to prevent problems in the future.

In most states, Paramedics are considered mandatory reporters of child abuse and are required to complete a standardized reporting form. This type of report would be considered a special incident report. Similar forms may also be available for reporting domestic violence or elder abuse.

Legal Proceedings

When a Paramedic has been a witness to a crime, or is a named party to a claim of negligence, the Paramedic may be called upon to provide special documentation.[17–20]

Some attorneys, or legally authorized persons, may only request that the Paramedic make a legal sworn statement, called an affidavit, about the events surrounding an incident. These statements are voluntary and typically witnessed by a notary public.

During the discovery phase of a trial, discussed in Chapter 6, the Paramedic may be requested to give a deposition. A deposition is the testimony of a witness (in this case, a Paramedic) in a setting outside of a court, where attorneys from both parties can interrogate the witness. The sworn testimony given by the witness is recorded by a stenographer. A transcript, a word-for-word account, is then produced for use in the lawsuit and may be submitted into evidence in a court of law. Often Paramedics rely on the PCR or a SIR to refresh recollection or for background information regarding the case.

In some cases, the attorney may elect to have the Paramedic answer questions in a written deposition, in a manner similar to an affidavit. This is discussed further in Chapter 6.

CONCLUSION

Documentation is an important aspect of EMS. The quality of patient care, and the Paramedic's professionalism, is often reflected in the patient care report. The beneficial nature of a patient care report is a function of its ability to communicate the message that the sender (the Paramedic) intended for the receiver (the emergency physician). By learning the correct medical terminology and abbreviations, and reporting thoroughly but concisely while utilizing a charting format consistently, the Paramedic can expect success with her documentation.

KEY POINTS:

- The first purpose of documentation is to use it as a medical record.

- The patient care report is also used for quality assurance and performance improvement.

- The PCR is also a business record used to bill federal and state governments as well as private insurance.

- The PCR is a legal document used in litigation.

- Documentation standards help to ensure that the standard of care was met.

- Specific protocols should be in place to resolve errors and omissions.

- In an electronic age, safeguards must be in place to ensure patient privacy from unwarranted invasion.

- While many documentation formats exist, Paramedics should choose the one that meets their agency's needs and provides the most complete documentation of the events that transpired.

- Special events, such as hazardous materials incidents or multiple casualty incidents, require a special incident report.

REVIEW QUESTIONS:

1. What are the six reasons cited for documenting patient care?
2. What is meant by the phrase "prudent layperson standard"?
3. What are the accepted practices for documenting errors and omissions?
4. How does the federal Health Insurance Portability and Accountability Act (HIPAA) affect documentation?
5. List three documentation formats and provide details for one of them.

6. Define "pertinent negatives."
7. What are the minimum elements required for a refusal of medical assistance?
8. What are the minimum elements required for documenting patient care for responders at the scene of hazardous materials operation?
9. What is the documentation tool used at a multiple casualty incident and what are the fields required?
10. What are the different legal instruments used at a legal proceeding?

CASE STUDY QUESTIONS:

Please refer to the Case Study at the beginning of the chapter and answer the questions below:

1. Why is accurate documentation of a cardiac arrest important?

2. How is the patient care report used for performance improvement?

3. Medically, what use does a physician have for a Paramedic's patient care report?

REFERENCES:

1. Shah R, Geisler CD, et al. A study of hospital based ambulance systems in Wisconsin. *J Clin Eng.* 1979;4(3):275–281.

2. Belding J. Patient refusal. What to do when medical treatment & transport are rejected. *Jems.* 2006;31(5):116–118.

3. Goldberg RJ, Zautcke JL, et al. A review of prehospital care litigation in a large metropolitan EMS system. *Ann Emerg Med.* 1990;19(5):557–561.

4. Stapczynski JS. Is the prudent layperson standard really a "standard"? *Ann Emerg Med.* 2004;43(2):163–165.

5. Johnson LA. Coverage disputes and the prudent layperson standard. *Ann Emerg Med.* 2004;44(4):426; author reply 426–427.

6. Davis, N, et al. Practice brief. Facsimile transmission of health information (updated). *J Ahima.* 2001;72(6):64E–64F.

7. Rakel RE. The problem-oriented medical record (POMR). *Am Fam Physician.* 1974;10(3):100–111.

8. Silfen E. Documentation and coding of ED patient encounters: an evaluation of the accuracy of an electronic medical record. *Am J Emerg Med.* 2006;24(6):664–678.

9. Bossen C. Evaluation of a computerized problem-oriented medical record in a hospital department: does it support daily clinical practice? *Int J Med Inform.* 2007;76(8):592–600.

10. Sandlow LJ, Bashook PG, et al. Gradual acceptance of POMR. *Internist.* 1980;21(3):6–7, 17.

11. Edgerly D. Assessing your assessment. *Journal of Emergency Medical Services* on-line. Available at: **http://www.jems.com/news_and_articles/columns/Edgerly/Assessing_Your_Assessment.html** Accessed May 16, 2009.

12. Cimino JJ. Review paper: coding systems in health care. *Methods Inf Med.* 1996;35(4-5):273–284.

13. Alexander S, Conner T, et al. Overview of inpatient coding. *Am J Health Syst Pharm.* 2003;60(21 Suppl 6):S11–S14.

14. Watzlaf VJ, Garvin JH, et al. The effectiveness of ICD-10-CM in capturing public health diseases. *Perspect Health Inf Manag.* 2007;4(6):6.

15. Zoraster RM, Chidester C, et al. Field triage and patient maldistribution in a mass-casualty incident. *Prehosp Disaster Med.* 2007;22(3):224–229.

16. Risavi BL, Salen PN, et al. A two-hour intervention using START improves prehospital triage of mass casualty incidents. *Prehosp Emerg Care.* 2001;5(2):197–199.

17. Nagorka FW, Becker C. Immunity statutes: how state laws protect EMS providers. *Emerg Med Serv.* 2005;34(6):93–94, 96–97.

18. Wiggins CO. Ambulance malpractice and immunity. Can a plaintiff ever prevail? *J Leg Med.* 2003;24(3):359–377.

19. Maguire BJ, Porco FV. An eight-year review of legal cases related to an urban 9-1-1 Paramedic service. *Prehosp Disaster Med.* 1997;12(2):154–157.

20. Colwell CB, Pons P, et al. Claims against a Paramedic ambulance service: A ten-year experience. *J Emerg Med.* 1999;17(6): 999–1002.

SECTION VI

CLINICAL ESSENTIALS

The final section of this volume includes the essential material in airway management, monitoring devices, intravenous access, pharmacology and ECG monitoring and acquisition that forms the basis for Paramedic assessment and treatment. This section provides the foundation for the clinical chapters in Volume II.

CHAPTER 20

AIRWAY ANATOMY AND PHYSIOLOGY

KEY CONCEPTS:

Upon completion of this chapter, it is expected that the reader will understand these following concepts:

- The route an oxygen molecule takes from the oral or nasal cavities to the alveolar capillaries
- Anatomy of airway structures as viewed with a laryngoscope
- Lung volumes/capacities and mechanisms for negative pressure ventilation
- Composition of air and the physiology of the internal and external exchange of respiratory gasses
- Key anatomical differences between the pediatric and adult airway and respiratory physiology

► CASE STUDY:

A Paramedic student is presented with a 120 kg patient who had a sudden onset of difficulty breathing while sleeping. The patient had a history of congestive heart failure and high blood pressure. The patient states he has had increased swelling in his legs over the past two days and sleeps with several pillows because of difficulty breathing while lying flat. The physical exam reveals increased work of breathing with diminished lung sounds in bases and diffuse rales. The student's treatment plan includes oxygen therapy, a breathing treatment, nitroglycerin, and furosemide. As the patient does not improve, the Paramedic student places the patient on continuous positive airway pressure (CPAP).

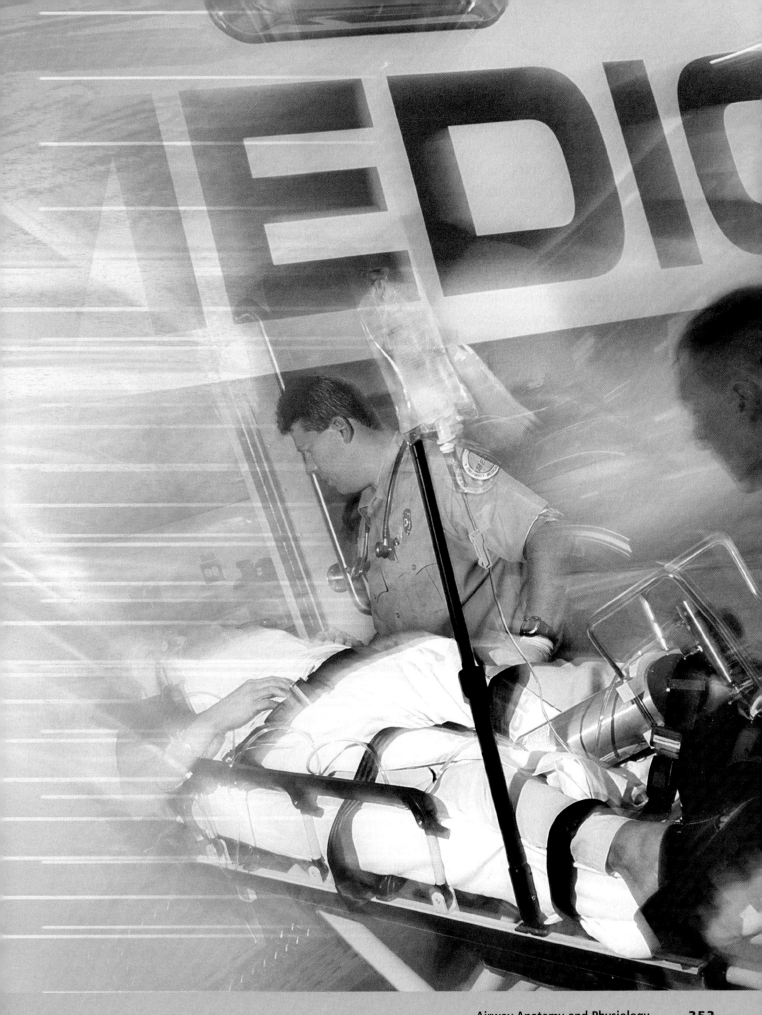

OVERVIEW

Assessing the patient's airway is a fundamental part of any initial patient assessment. Therefore, interventions may be needed to open and secure the airway or assist with ventilations. The act of breathing transports air entering the oral or nasal cavities to the alveolar sacs where gas exchange can occur. This chapter will examine the anatomy of the adult and pediatric airway and the physiology of each component. The Paramedic should have knowledge of how an oxygen molecule is transported from the oral or nasal cavities to the alveolar capillaries.

When performing advanced airway procedures, every Paramedic must possess an intimate knowledge of a patient's airway anatomy and respiratory physiology. Although minor individual anatomic variations exist, every patient will have a similar anatomic structure and respiratory physiology. If the Paramedic has a clear understanding of normal airway anatomy and ventilation, he can maximize his interventions and greatly improve his chances of successful airway management.

Airway Anatomy

The airway is divided into the upper and lower airway (Figure 20-1). The upper airway begins at the nares and mouth and extends to the glottis. The lower airway extends from the glottis to the alveoli. The respiratory system is composed of many other structures including a number of ligamentous, muscular, and bony structures in the neck and chest. The following section will look at each of these components and their role in both ventilation and airway management.

The Upper Airway

The openings of the mouth and nose define the beginning of the airway. From a functional perspective, the nose is the primary structure for air entrance. The nose provides an immunologic barrier (mucus), warms and humidifies air, and serves as a threat/food detection system (sense of smell). This compact unit allows an individual to simultaneously eat and breathe. In times of high ventilatory demand (e.g., exercise, fear, pulmonary disease) or instances when the nares are blocked, a person can also utilize the mouth for ventilation.

Air enters the nares and immediately passes along the turbinates (Figure 20-2). The nasal fossae are divided by the septum—a midline cartilaginous structure. In the average adult the fossae extend approximately 12 cm to the nasopharynx and, due to folds in the mucosa, each fossa provides approximately 60 cm² of surface area for filtration, warming, and humidification.[1] This heavily vascularized mucosa is composed primarily of ciliated columnar cells and goblet cells. Relatively minor trauma (e.g., insertion of a nasopharyngeal airway) can result in significant hemorrhage.

For an average-sized adult with normal ventilatory function, approximately 10,000 liters (L) of air pass through the nasal fossae each day. This air is humidified through the addition of 1 L of fluid produced by glandular secretion and transudation, or liquid diffusing across the mucous membrane into the nasal cavity. This fluid not only serves to humidify the air entering the lungs but also has significant antibacterial properties. In addition, large particulate matter is filtered via the nasal hairs and trapped in mucus. The area is also served by extensive lymphatic drainage.[1] Anatomically, the passage from the nare to the nasopharynx is a straight line parallel to the roof of the mouth. Knowing this anatomy is important prior to the placement of such devices as nasotracheal tubes, nasopharyngeal airways, and nasogastric tubes.

The nasopharynx lies posterior to the turbinates and superior to the soft palate. It terminates into the oropharynx inferior-posteriorly. The **pharynx** is the area of the airway composed of the spaces behind the nose (the nasopharynx) and the oral cavity (the oropharynx).

When the facial bones and the bones of the skull develop in the fetus, small air pockets called "sinuses" form. These sinuses are attached to the main airway passages and thus normally have an internal pressure equal to atmospheric pressure. The sinuses are lined with mucous membranes and may have a role in trapping bacteria. In addition, the weight savings of replacing bone with air make the skull significantly lighter. The walls of the sinuses are thin and easily fractured. Given their locations, fractures of certain sinuses may allow a direct connection from the inside of the skull to the exterior world, particularly in the case of a basilar skull fracture.

Despite occasionally serving as a passage for air, the mouth is much less suited for the processes of ventilation than is the nose. The mouth does not have the nose's ability to provide and maintain humidification and is not as well equipped to serve as a particulate/pathogen filter. Nonetheless, the Paramedic must be cognizant of the mouth's structures as the oropharyngeal route is the most common route for assisted airway management. The oral cavity is bound by

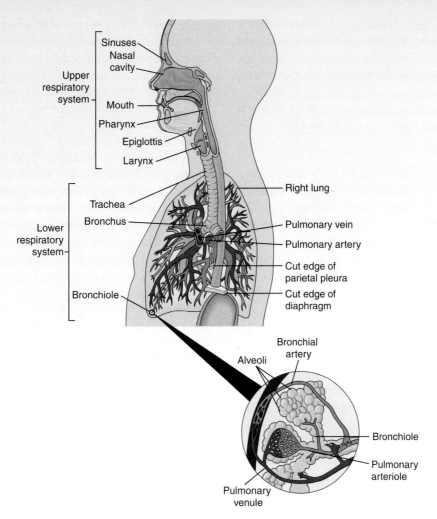

Figure 20-1   Overall respiratory system anatomy.

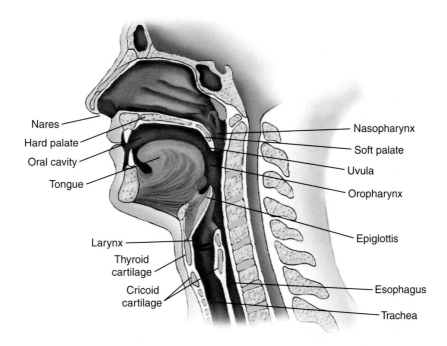

Figure 20-2   Upper airway anatomy.

the lips anteriorly, the buccal surfaces (cheeks) laterally, the tongue inferiorly, the hard palate superiorly, and the soft palate posteriorly (Figure 20-3). The tongue occupies much of the oral cavity and, as a muscular structure, can move freely throughout the cavity.

The lower jaw, or mandible, articulates with the temporal bones at the temporomandibular joints. The mandible is able to move inferiorly and superiorly (i.e., mouth opening and closing), laterally (i.e., moving side to side), and anteriorly (i.e., "jaw jutting"). The temporomandibular joint is relatively loose and the ball of the joint can move partially out of its socket to allow greater opening and anterior movement. Diseases that affect the temporomandibular joint decrease mouth opening and can make airway management more difficult.

The average adult has 32 teeth—16 upper and 16 lower. Through disease, wear, and trauma, the teeth may become loose or may be replaced by appliances. The teeth and these appliances (e.g., dentures, partials, etc.) give the lips and cheeks structure and help the Paramedic maintain an adequate face seal during ventilation. During intubation, however, teeth can impede the view of the lower airway structures. Thus, dental appliances should be removed before intubation.

The tonsillar pillars that form the walls of the oropharynx are composed of lymphatic tissue (the palatine tonsils) and the muscles used for swallowing. Along with a ring of other lymphoid tissue, these structures serve as an immunological barrier to pathogen entry in the pharynx. The palatine tonsils deserve special mention for the Paramedic. As with the rest of the upper airway, these structures are covered by a thin mucous membrane. The prominence of the palatine tonsils and the

vasculature of the mucous membrane make this a high-risk area for bleeding during airway management. In addition, during times of pharyngeal or oral infections, these tissues can swell and actually occlude the airway. Therefore, they may preclude standard orotracheal airway management practices.

The pharynx and hypopharynx are the areas of common passage for food and respiratory gasses (Figure 20-1). The area contains numerous structures including multiple constrictor and elevator muscles to aid in swallowing. The epiglottis also resides in this space. The **hyoid** bone, another structure of importance in this region, is the only bone in the body that does not directly articulate with another bone. Instead, it serves as a common point of attachment for a number of muscles and ligaments that function in swallowing and airway maintenance. The hyoepiglottic ligament is one such structure that will be discussed in more detail in the following text. Other attachment points include the mandible, the styloid process of the skull, the posterior skull, the sternum, the scapula, and the thyroid cartilage, making the hyoid a critical anchor point for many physiologic functions (Figure 20-4).

The **epiglottis** is one of the most important anatomic and physiologic structures of the upper airway. This "U" shaped structure composed of fibroelastic cartilage is attached to the anterior pharynx between the base of the tongue and the larynx. Although considered by some to be vestigial,[2] the epiglottis seems to serve a function in protecting the lower airway from foreign body aspiration. It is covered by a mucous membrane that is contiguous with the tongue. The space formed between the anterior-superior surface of the epiglottis and the posterior base of the tongue is the **valecula**. The epiglottis is attached to the midline of the thyroid cartilage by the thyroepiglottic ligament.

Given its size, contents, and multiple functions, the pharynx is a very common area for airway obstruction to occur. Traditional teaching has suggested that the tongue falls posteriorly in the obtunded patient and obstructs the airway. However, imaging work by Shorten et al.[3] has demonstrated that, in fact, the soft palate and epiglottis make contact with the posterior wall of the oropharynx and pharynx before the tongue does and that these structures cause airway obstruction. Thus, the action for opening an airway actually depends on the anterior traction on the epiglottis. This is accomplished through the hyoepiglottic ligament by the anterior displacement of the hyoid bone. The hyoid is lifted by anterior mandibular displacement (the hyoid has multiple muscular attachments to the mandible) that occurs with a head-tilt chin-lift or jaw thrust.

The Lower Airway

The visible structures of the lower airway (Figure 20-5a) can be seen by the Paramedic during orotracheal intubation. The **larynx,** also known as the "voice box," is the upper group of structures of the lower airway and opens with a number of cartilaginous structures. From anterior to posterior, these structures include the base of the epiglottis, the thyroid cartilage, and the aryepiglottic folds (Figure 20-5b and

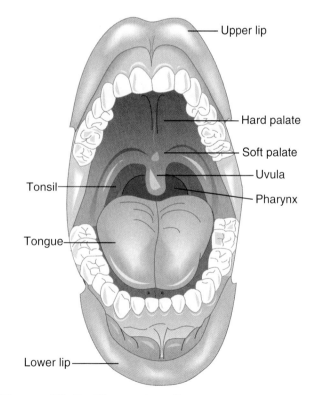

Upper lip

Hard palate

Soft palate

Uvula

Pharynx

Tonsil

Tongue

Lower lip

Figure 20-3 The oral cavity.

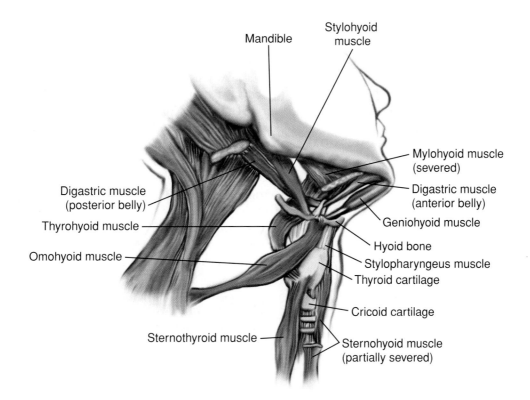

Figure 20-4 The hyoid bone and its muscular attachments.

Figure 20-5c). The aryepiglottic folds contain three separate cartilaginous structures: the cuneiform, corniculate, and **arytenoid** cartilages (from anterior to posterior). These structures are attached to each other and other structures by ligaments as well as the intrinsic and extrinsic muscles of the larynx. The whole complex is covered by mucosal folds.

STREET SMART

The arytenoids are the posterior-most structures of the laryngeal opening. Any endotracheal tube visualized passing anterior to the arytenoids is, by definition, passing into the larynx and trachea, even if the cords are not visualized. Any tube visualized passing posterior to the arytenoids is in the esophagus.

The thyroid cartilage is the large, anterior shield-like cartilage structure that forms the majority of the anterior portion of the larynx. It is attached superiorly to the hyoid via the thyrohyoid membrane and inferiorly to the cricoid ring by the cricothyroid membrane. From its anterior, superior midline notch, the thyroid cartilage extends laterally and posteriorly to form a "half-pipe" shape. In females, the thyroid cartilage is flatter than in males, resulting in a more prominent "Adam's

apple" in men as well as a lower pitched voice.[1] The posterior margins of the thyroid cartilage terminate in the superior and inferior thyroid horns or cornu.[4] The superior horns are attached to the hyoid via the thyrohyoid ligament and the inferior horns articulate with the cricoid cartilage via a true synovial ball and socket joint similar to the hip joint.

The open space below the laryngeal opening and superior to the vocal cords is called the vestibule. Small outpouchings in the mucosal folds that overlie the vestibular membrane of the quadrangular membrane form the false cords. The false cords, which do not serve in phonation (the production of speech and sound), are important because they can seal over the **glottis** to help protect the airway from aspiration of foreign materials.

The vocal cords are visible at the bottom of the vestibule. As with other structures of the larynx, the vocal cords are composed of mucosal folds overlying ligaments, cartilages, and muscles. The cricothyroid ligament starts anteriorly as the cricothyroid membrane that attaches the cricoid ring to the thyroid cartilage. The thickened central portion of the cricothyroid membrane, called the "conus elasticus," extends to the interior border of the thyroid cartilage and then turns posteriorly, splitting in half and attaching on the arytenoid cartilages. The medial edges of this portion of the cricothyroid ligament thicken and are called the vocal ligaments. With their associated mucosal folds, the vocal ligaments form the true vocal cords. These structures are typically found at the level of the 5th cervical vertebrae in an adult.

The vocal cords serve two main functions in the airway. The first is phonation. The extrinsic and intrinsic muscles of

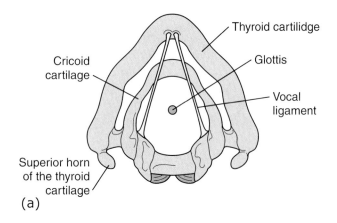

(a)

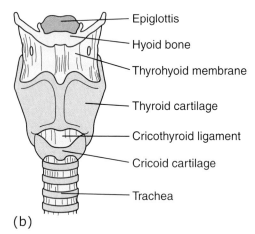

(b)

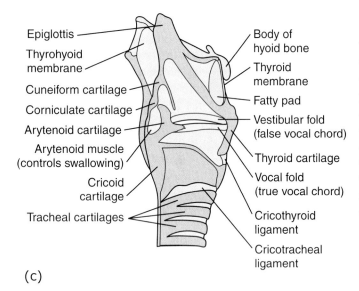

(c)

Figure 20-5 a-c Laryngeal anatomy. (a) As viewed during laryngoscopy. (b) From an anterior view. (c) From a lateral view.

the larynx move the various cartilages to change the shape and tension of the cords. The intrinsic muscles are most responsible for the modification of the cords. The changes in shape and tension allow the full vocal range. The innervation of the intrinsic muscles is primarily from the recurrent laryngeal nerve. On phonation, the vocal cords are adducted (brought together) to produce sound. On inspiration, the

vocal cords are abducted (moved away from each other) to maximize laminar (linear, nonturbulent) airflow. In the cadaver (and in paralyzed patients who have lost laryngeal muscular function), the resting position of the vocal cords is abducted and "loose" or "wavy" appearing.

The second function of the vocal cords (the glottis) is airway protection. The muscles that produce phonation can also adduct the glottis and the false cords to provide an impenetrable barrier to foreign material. The stimulation of nerve endings in the supraglottic region (the vestibule) triggers a short-lived involuntary reflex resulting in glottic closure. A number of stimuli including touch, temperature, and chemicals can trigger this reflex. If the glottis remains closed, it is called laryngeal spasm and can make airway management challenging.

STREET SMART

Most laryngospasms will resolve with positive pressure ventilation, timed with the patient's natural inspiration. If that does not succeed, then chemical paralysis or a rapid surgical airway may be required in order to oxygenate the patient.

The remaining cartilaginous structure of the larynx is the cricoid ring (Figure 20-5b). The cricoid ring, the only complete ring in the trachea, is located at the lowest portion of the larynx and the beginning of the trachea. The widest part of the ring is found posteriorly and rises toward the arytenoids. The cricoid ring supports the larynx above it and is attached by a number of ligaments; the tracheal rings are attached inferiorly by many muscles and ligaments. The complete nature of the ring makes it susceptible to fractures. Conversely, properly applied cricoid pressure allows the ring to compress the esophagus, essentially sealing off the esophagus and minimizing the risk of regurgitation.

STREET SMART

Many well-intentioned individuals, in attempting to apply "cricoid" pressure, actually go for the largest structure visible/palpable and apply "thyroid" (cartilage) pressure. Not only does this not necessarily occlude the esophagus, but pressure on the thyroid cartilage at its middle to inferior margin causes the vocal cords to rise anteriorly, making them more difficult to visualize during laryngoscopy.

Other important structures of the larynx include the intrinsic and extrinsic laryngeal muscles and their nerve supply. These muscles were previously described in terms of their function. Although knowledge of the individual muscles, their individual innervation, and their individual function is not critical to the Paramedic, understanding the overall function in terms of laryngeal movement, phonation, and airway protection is important. Of particular importance is the "gag reflex." This reflex arc depends on sensory nerves at the level of the oropharynx, the pharynx, and the larynx to trigger the response. The reflexive response is coughing and coordinated activity by the muscles of the hypopharynx, oropharynx, and pharynx to propel the offending stimulus into the mouth and out of the body.

There are a number of clinically significant structures external to the laryngeal airway (Figure 20-6). These structures are of importance to the Paramedic both because of their potential for injury during airway management and because, if injured, whether by the Paramedic or during a traumatic event, they can cause compromise of the airway.

The **thyroid gland** is a highly vascular "H" shaped structure that lies along the sides of the larynx and upper trachea. The crossbar of the "H" crosses the trachea just below the cricoid ring. A laceration of the thyroid will lead to significant bleeding. In addition, disease of the thyroid can result in swelling and deformation of the airway anatomy.

Two sets of major vascular structures—the common carotid arteries and the internal jugular veins—run parallel

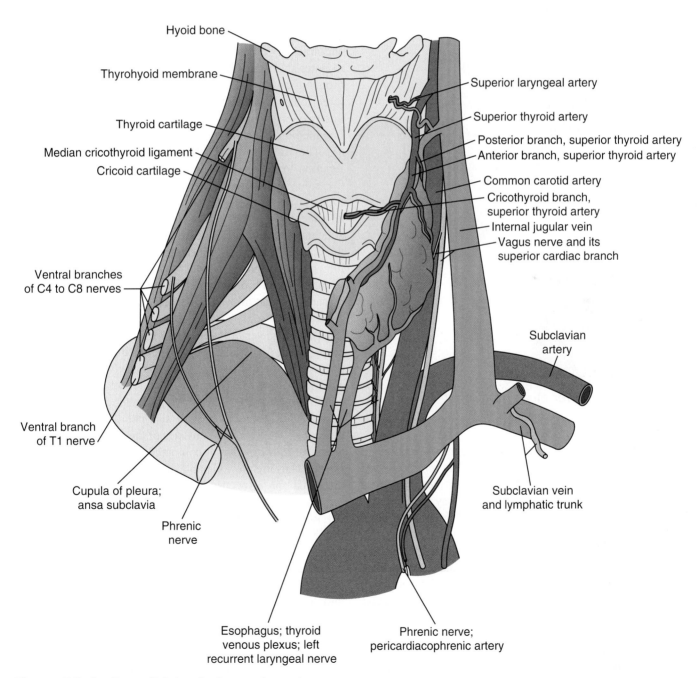

Figure 20-6 Superficial anterior neck anatomy.

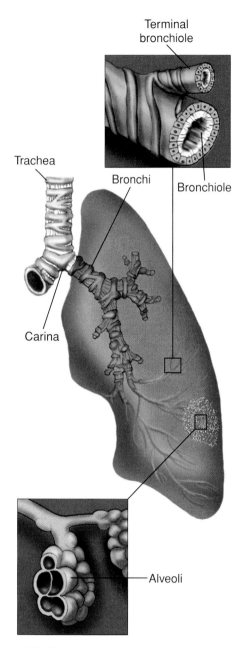

Figure 20-7 Lower airway anatomy.

to the pharynx. The carotid arteries are the major suppliers of blood to the brain while the internal jugulars return most of the cerebral blood to the heart. Bleeding from these structures can result in significant deformity of the airway. Additionally, injury to the carotids compromises blood flow to the brain and can result in cerebral hypoxia or anoxia.

The **trachea** is a conduit for respiratory gasses. In an adult, it is 10 to 20 cm long and 1 to 1.5 cm in diameter. Its superior attachment is the cricoid ring (level of the 6th cervical vertebrae) and it terminates at the **carina** (level of the 5th thoracic vertebrae) (Figure 20-7). The cartilage rings of the trachea are incomplete, with the posterior element void of cartilage and composed of muscle and elastic fibers.[5] The muscles of the trachea include an inner circular layer and an outer longitudinal layer. The walls of the trachea (and the bronchi) are composed

of an epithelial layer, mucous glands, lymphatic tissue, nerves, vascular structures, and structural cartilage. The most common cell in the large lower airways is the ciliated epithelial cell. The cilia (small hair-like projections) form the moving portion of the "mucociliary" escalator. The mucus secreted by goblet and serous cells traps small particles and pathogens. The cilia move the mucus up the airway into the hypopharynx where the secretions are swallowed and digested. The lymphatics also serve to move trapped pathogens to the lymph nodes so the immune system may deal with them. Mucous glands are seen through the lower airway to the level of the smallest bronchi; they are not seen in the alveoli.

At the level of the carina, the lower airway splits into the two mainstem **bronchi**—called the right mainstem bronchus and left mainstem bronchus. The two bronchi are angulated equally until age 3, when the right mainstem bronchus becomes more acutely angled. This acute angle predisposes endotracheal tubes, suction catheters, and foreign bodies to enter the right mainstem bronchus. The right mainstem bronchus is larger in diameter than the left and divides into three lobar bronchi. The left mainstem bronchus separates into two lobar bronchi. These lobar bronchi further subdivide into medium bronchi.

The walls of the bronchi are similar in structure and function to the walls of the trachea. They are composed of the same layers with equivalent functions. The posterior (non-cartilage containing) portion of the bronchial wall has its attachment points within the ring of cartilage rather than attaching the ends of the cartilage rings; during inspiration, the posterior wall of a bronchus will collapse further into the lumen than the posterior wall of the trachea does. At the level of the medium bronchi, the rings of cartilage become plates of cartilage that allow for a more symmetric contraction of the airway lumen.

At a diameter of less than 0.8 cm, the bronchi are called bronchioles. At less than 0.6 cm, the cartilage plates disappear as well, leaving structures held open only by elastic fibers and the muscles of the bronchial walls. Although the muscles continue to thin out as the airway diameter decreases, they do so at a slower rate than the rate at which the airway diameter decreases. Therefore, the muscles of the terminal bronchioles are proportionately larger compared with the diameter of the airway. They are more capable of closing off the airway when bronchial spasm occurs than are the muscles of the larger bronchioles or bronchi.

A terminal bronchiole ends in the acinus, or a sac-like part of the lung supplied by a single terminal bronchiole. Alveoli may branch off of the bronchiole at this level. However, the ends of the terminal bronchioles are the alveolar ducts that open into the alveolar air sacs. The alveolar sacs open into large collections of **alveoli** (single units being called alveolus). This large collection of smaller sacs provide a larger surface area for gas exchange than if the lung were made up of a single large sac (Figure 20-8). Although the trachea is the largest lower airway structure and the alveoli the smallest, each successive airway structural level (main

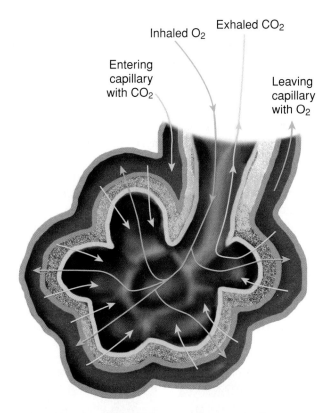

Figure 20-8 An acinus is composed of many alveoli and is surrounded by a capillary bed. This is where the exchange of oxygen and carbon dioxide occurs.

bronchi, lobar bronchi, etc.) increases the number of structures and, with it, the cross-sectional area of the airway. Therefore, with 500 million alveoli in the average adult lung, the cross-sectional area of the alveoli is 350 thousand times greater than the cross-sectional area of the trachea. This high cross-sectional area allows for massive gas exchange, which occurs by diffusion.

The surfaces of the alveoli are covered with **surfactant**, a fluid that decreases the alveoli's surface tension and prevents them from collapsing during expiration. The surfactant holds the alveoli open and prevents atelectasis (collapse of the alveoli and loss of gas exchange surface). Premature infants and drowning victims who aspirate water may have inadequate surfactant to prevent atelectasis, leading to significant hypoxia and ventilatory failure.

The remainder of the lungs not occupied by the airway structures and blood vessels (the lung parenchyma) is composed primarily of structural support and immune structures. The supporting structures are important during the mechanical act of respiration.

Bony Thorax Anatomy

The bony anatomy of the thorax not only provides protection to the thoracic organs and major blood vessels, but also produces the air pressure difference responsible for air movement in and out of the respiratory system. The bones of the thorax consist of the thoracic vertebrae, the rib cage, the sternum, the clavicles, and the scapulae (Figure 20-9). The clavicles and scapulae are not directly responsible for ventilation but serve as accessory anchoring points for either accessory muscles or for muscles that support the rib cage. The thoracic vertebrae are articulation points for the 12 ribs and form the posterior bony border of the thoracic cavity. The thoracic vertebrae typically do not move during respiration. The exception to this occurs during highly active breathing when an individual leans forward during expiration and then extends the spine and stands straight during inspiration. The ribs, however, do move and articulate with the transverse processes of the thoracic vertebrae. The sternum is a dagger-shaped bone that attaches to the clavicles and the ribs. It is the anterior-most bony structure of the thorax and provides structural support to the ribs during respiration.

The rib cage is the primary bony structure of respiration. Composed of 12 matched pairs of curved bones, the rib cage acts to protect the thoracic structures and serves as the fulcrum for the intercostal muscles of respiration. The ribs are numbered 1 through 12 and articulate posteriorly with their similarly numbered thoracic vertebrae. Anteriorly, the ribs are attached to the sternum by the costal cartilages. Ribs 1 to 7 are considered "true" ribs in that each has its own costal cartilage that attaches it to the sternum. Ribs 8 to 12 are considered "false" ribs. Ribs 8, 9, and 10 are attached to the sternum through a common costal cartilage; the cartilages from each of the rib tips merge into a single cartilage that is attached to the sternum. Ribs 11 and 12 are called "floating ribs" because, although they are attached to other ribs via the intercostal musculature and serve in respiration, they only articulate posteriorly on the thoracic vertebrae and are not directly attached to the sternum via a costal cartilage.[6]

The muscles of respiration can be divided into the principal and **accessory muscles** of inspiration and the active muscles of expiration. During quiet breathing, without pathologic

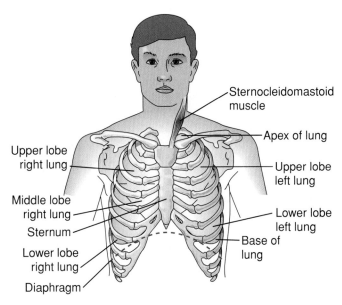

Figure 20-9 The bony thorax.

derangement, the principal muscles of inspiration drive inspiration while passive recoil of the chest wall and lungs drives expiration. During active breathing (e.g., with heavy activity or disease), the accessory muscles of inspiration are recruited, as are the active muscles of expiration. Knowledge of the normal muscles of quiet breathing is critical to understanding respiratory physiology (Figure 20-10).

One muscle and a major muscle group contribute to inspiration. The first and largest muscle involved in inspiration is the **diaphragm**. This large, thin, dome-shaped muscle divides the abdomen from the thorax. At rest, the diaphragm rises to the level of the 5th rib (approximately the level of the nipple). During inspiration, the diaphragm contracts and flattens. Since the margins of the diaphragm are fixed to the thoracoabdominal wall, contraction pulls the contents of the thorax inferiorly and pushes the abdominal contents inferiorly. Contraction of the diaphragm also assists the intercostal muscles to elevate the lower ribs.

The second major muscle group involved in inspiration is the intercostal group. The intercostal muscles are muscles that attach the ribs to each other. There are external and internal intercostals; the internal intercostals are further divided into interchondral (between ligaments) and intercostal (between bones) divisions. At rest, the ribs—attached anteriorly to the sternum and posteriorly to the thoracic vertebrae—tend to sag inferiorly and medially (Figure 20-11a). When the external intercostal muscles and the interchondral part of the internal intercostal muscles contract, they elevate the ribs in a motion similar to that of a bucket handle (Figure 20-11b). Functionally, when this happens in the rib cage, the volume of the rib cage increases.

The chest wall interacts with the lung parenchyma via the **pleura** (Figure 20-12). The easiest way to visualize the pleura is to think about standing a bottle up on a flat garbage bag. Since the bottle is on the outside of the bag, there are two layers of the bag underneath the bottom of the bottle. If the bag is then lifted up around the bottle, there will be two layers of garbage bag all around the bottle. Finally, the bag is collected at the neck of the bottle and attached with a rubber band. The end result is a bottle inside of a two-layered bag. The layer of the bag against the plastic bottle represents the visceral pleura and the outside layer of plastic represents the parietal pleura. The sealed area at the neck of bottle represents the way the pleura seals against the bronchi as they leave the lungs. In the body, the visceral and parietal pleura lie against each other with a small amount of fluid between them. This allows them to slide against each other but not to pull apart from each other.

Under normal physiological conditions, the two pleural layers are held together by the pleural fluid and expand and contract as a unit. The space between the pleura is a "potential" space because, under normal conditions, it does not exist. However, excessive fluid can build up between these spaces

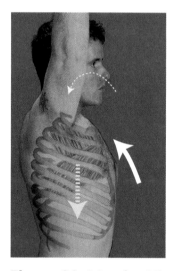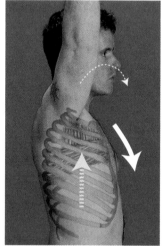

Figure 20-11 a-b Rib movement. (a) Full exhalation position. (b) Full inhalation.

Inhalation

Scalene muscles elevate 1st and 2nd ribs

Inferior part of sternum moves anteriorly

External intercostal muscles elevate ribs

Diaphragm moves inferiorly during contraction

Figure 20-10 Muscles of respiration.

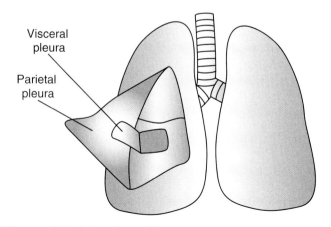

Visceral pleura

Parietal pleura

Figure 20-12 Pleural layers against the organs (visceral pleura) and chest wall (parietal pleura).

during various disease states (e.g., heart failure) and air can potentially enter the space (e.g., during chest trauma). When the pleural layers separate, they no longer function as a unit. This disrupts the pleural layers' ability to generate an adequate negative pressure during inspiration, thus reducing lung volumes and creating a sensation of difficulty breathing.

Respiratory Physiology

Understanding the anatomy of the airway and respiratory system only tells half of the story. Knowledge of the physiology, or the function, of the respiratory system allows the Paramedic to understand the effects disease has on the patient, the effects treatments have on the patient, and ways to troubleshoot the process when the patient does not respond as expected.

Lung Volumes and Capacities

Physiologically, the lung can be divided into several components. The measurements of lung volumes and capacities (Figure 20-13) are important to facilitate descriptions of the physiologic occurrences during respiration. The total lung volume is divided into a number of volume subsets. The first, and most important, volume is the **tidal volume**. This is the volume of a normal breath and is approximately 5 to 7 cc/kg of ideal body weight.[7] During exercise or certain pathological situations, a greater volume—the inspiratory reserve volume—is used. This is the maximum volume that can be inspired above the tidal volume. The maximum volume that can be expired beyond the tidal volume is the expiratory reserve volume. Any air left in the lungs after the expiratory reserve volume is exhaled is the residual volume and cannot be exhaled; it reflects the smallest possible airspace volume based on the anatomy of the lungs.

Alveolar volume is the volume of air in the alveoli. In the average adult male, this volume is 350 cc and reflects the volume of air available for gas exchange. The final volume is the anatomic dead space, which is the volume of the conducting airways. Gas exchange does not occur in the conducting airways, hence the term "dead space." The anatomic dead space is typically 150 mL in the average adult male. There is also a physiologic dead space, which is the volume of the lungs not eliminating carbon dioxide; in certain disease states (e.g., pneumonia, congestive heart failure (CHF), pulmonary embolus, chronic obstructive pulmonary disease (COPD), atelectasis, etc.) this volume may be greater than the anatomic dead space.[8]

Capacities are another way of describing the lungs' respiratory volumes. Total lung capacity is the sum of the residual volume, the expiratory reserve volume, the tidal volume, and the inspiratory reserve volume. It is a measure of all of the airspace volume in the lungs with the potential to exchange carbon dioxide. The total lung capacity can be broken down into smaller capacities. The vital capacity is a measure of the maximum volume that can move through the lungs in a single respiratory cycle and equals the inspiratory and expiratory reserve volumes plus the tidal volume. The **inspiratory capacity** equals the tidal volume plus the inspiratory reserve volume and is a measure of the maximum air that can be inspired. The air that remains in the lungs at the end of expiration of the tidal volume is the functional residual capacity and equals the expiratory reserve volume plus the residual volume.[9]

Minute ventilation measures the total volume of gas that passes through the lungs in a minute. It equals the respiratory rate (RR) times the volume per breath (Tidal Volume, or TV). Normally, the volume per breath is the tidal volume. Therefore, the standard formula for minute volume is RR × TV[9] (Figure 20-14). However, when other lung volume subsets are used (e.g., inspiratory and expiratory reserve volumes) or the patient is breathing breaths that are smaller than tidal volume breaths, the volume per breath will change and thus change the minute ventilation. Calculating minute ventilation becomes important when determining the rate and volume at which a patient should be ventilated.

Minute alveolar ventilation takes into account anatomic dead space (Figure 20-14). It is calculated by subtracting

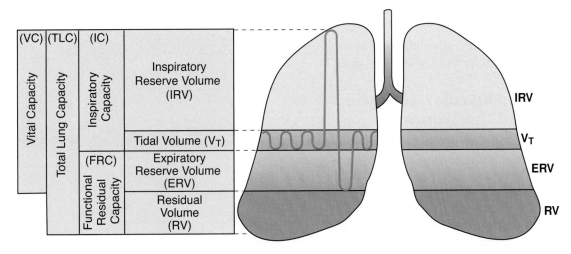

Figure 20-13 Lung volumes.

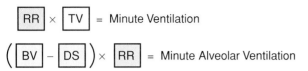

$$RR \times TV = \text{Minute Ventilation}$$

$$\left(BV - DS \right) \times RR = \text{Minute Alveolar Ventilation}$$

Figure 20-14 Minute ventilation and minute alveolar ventilation.

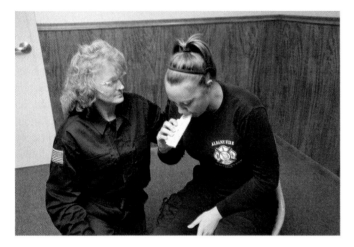

Figure 20-15 Paramedic measuring peak flow in a patient.

the dead space from the volume per breath and multiplying the result times the respiratory rate ([Breath Volume − Dead Space] × RR). This calculation becomes important as various devices such as endotracheal tubes, face masks, end-tidal carbon dioxide detectors, or ventilator circuits are added. These devices all increase the dead space.

While the capacities of the lungs and dead spaces are important, equally important is the flow of gasses through the structures. One of the most important flows is the **peak expiratory flow**, or maximum velocity of gas movement during exhalation (Figure 20-15 and **Skill 20-1**). Many diseases restrict the flow of gasses during exhalation. Peak flow measurement can be used in the prehospital environment in to assess an asthmatic patient's response to treatment.[10]

For a step-by-step demonstration of Peak Flow Measurement, please refer to Skill 20-1 on page 371.

The Bony and Muscular Thoracic Structures and the Pleura

Normal respiration occurs through a process of negative pressure, or vacuum, ventilation. Air moves into the lungs by the creation of a vacuum at the level of the alveoli. The structures responsible for this vacuum are the bony and muscular structures of the chest wall, the diaphragm, and the pleura.

At the end of expiration, the air pressure in the alveoli is essentially atmospheric pressure. When the principal muscles of inspiration contract, they increase the external volume of

the thorax. The parietal pleura is attached to the expanding structures and so increases in volume as well. Since the parietal and visceral pleura are functionally attached under normal conditions, the expanding parietal pleura pulls the visceral pleura along with it. Being attached to the exterior of the lung parenchyma, the expanding visceral pleura expands the parenchyma and, through the network of connective tissue structures, pulls open the alveoli. The alveoli are connected to the external atmosphere via the lower and upper airways. Just as increasing the volume inside a syringe by pulling back the plunger creates a suction which pulls in air or medication, air is also pulled into the alveoli when their volume increases. Air flows from a higher pressure to a lower pressure and fills the vacuum in the expanding alveoli with air. In this way, inspiration of fresh respiratory gasses occurs. The volume of gas inspired from contraction of the diaphragm (primarily) and the intercostal muscles during resting ventilation is the tidal volume.

As the lungs expand during inspiration, special sensory nerves called stretch receptors begin to fire and, via the vagus nerve, inhibit further inspiration. This action is called the Hering-Breuer reflex. Expiration during quiet breathing is the result of the passive recoil of the lung parenchyma and of the chest wall. As these structures collapse, air simply flows out of the airspaces until the interthoracic pressure equals the atmospheric pressure. This is similar to what happens to an inflated balloon when the neck is released; the elastic recoil of the balloon forces the air out into the environment. This elastic recoil is the expiratory component of the tidal volume and leaves the functional residual capacity in the lungs.

High volume, active respiration (e.g., during illness, exercise, or other periods of high respiratory drive) uses the accessory muscles of respiration. The accessory muscles include the sternocleidomastoid muscle and scalenes (Figure 20-16). The sternocleidomastoid muscle elevates the sternum and the scalenes elevate and hold in place the upper ribs.[11] Furthermore, the action of the intercostal

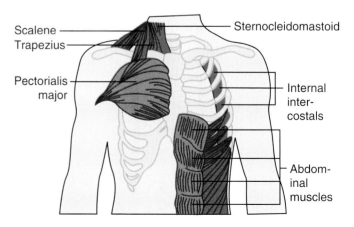

Figure 20-16 Accessory muscles of inspiration and expiration.

muscles becomes more pronounced, resulting in "intercostal retractions" in which the musculature pulls in and the ribs become more pronounced and visible. Although the use of accessory muscles is effective in increasing minute ventilation by increasing the volume of the thorax, involving the accessory muscles in respiration is very tiring. Patients with minimal reserve energy may rapidly decompensate.

Just as there are situations in which inspiratory reserve volume must be recruited, so too are there times in which active expiration must occur. During exercise or when expiratory airflow is obstructed (e.g., asthma, COPD exacerbation), the muscles of expiration may be recruited to increase the expiratory airflow above what can be accomplished through passive expiration. The muscles of expiration can be divided into two groups: the thoracic muscles of expiration and the abdominal muscles of expiration (Figure 20-16). The thoracic expiratory muscles are the intercostal parts of the internal intercostals. When the intercostal parts of the internal intercostals contract, they pull the ribs down and together, causing the rib cage to collapse. This decreases thoracic volume and forces air out of the lungs.[11]

The abdominal muscles are also important for active expiration. The rectus abdominis, external obliques, internal obliques, and transversus abdominus muscles perform two major expiratory functions. First, they depress and anchor the lower ribs, which assist the thoracic expiratory muscles to collapse the rib cage. Second, they compress the abdominal contents and lower the intraabdominal volume. This contraction causes the abdominal contents to push up on the diaphragm, further lowering the intrathoracic volume.[11] Although the muscles of expiration are used much less frequently than the muscles of inspiration, they are effective in improving expiratory airflow.

It is important to recognize that there are cardiac implications of **negative pressure ventilation**. When the intrathoracic pressure decreases, the pressure in the vena cava and right atrium decreases, increasing venous return. Therefore, during normal inspiration, venous return—and therefore preload—increases. When a patient receives **positive pressure ventilation,** either during intubation or bag-valve-mask ventilation, intrathoracic pressure remains positive during the entire respiratory cycle (Figure 20-17). As a result, venous return—and therefore preload—decreases, resulting in a loss of cardiac output and blood pressure. Air trapping and hyperventilation also cause an increase in intrathoracic pressure, producing a potential drop in blood pressure in patients with borderline or poor cardiac function. Additionally, the positive pressure in the lungs can increase pulmonary vascular resistance and right ventricular afterload, further exacerbating right heart failure. It is important to consider the hemodynamic effects of positive pressure ventilation when ventilating a patient. In general, patients should be ventilated at a slower rate and with a slightly smaller volume than physiologic respiration to avoid the hemodynamic effects of overventilation.

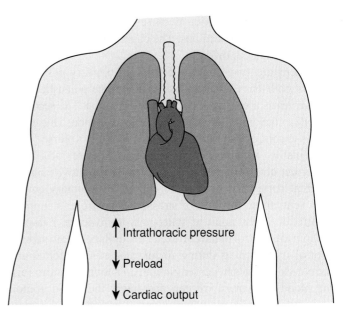

↑ Intrathoracic pressure

↓ Preload

↓ Cardiac output

Figure 20-17 Effects of normal and positive pressure ventilation on the circulatory system.

Neurological Control of Breathing

Although the process of breathing is essentially involuntary, there is a voluntary component as well. Differentiating between the two components assists the Paramedic in recognizing abnormal ventilation and considering possible causes.

Sensory information comes from stretch receptors in the lungs, the partial pressure of carbon dioxide in the bloodstream, the partial pressure of oxygen in the bloodstream, muscle spindle fibers, and proprioceptors (position sensors) and stretch sensors in the tendons and joints. Of these, increasing carbon dioxide is the greatest stimulus for ventilation in most patients. All of the signals are processed in the brainstem and modified by the cortex. Primitive, involuntary control occurs in the medullary respiratory center of the **medulla oblongata** (the brainstem) with major nerve input from the vagus nerve. There is an inspiratory center and an expiratory center of the medulla oblongata. The inspiratory center is responsible for inspiration and regular, rhythmic ventilation. There are a number of nerve inputs; output from this group is via the phrenic nerve (from the 3rd, 4th, and 5th cervical nerve roots) to the diaphragm.[9]

The expiratory center (the ventral respiratory group) is not normally active. It is responsible only for active expiration and therefore stimulates abdominal wall musculature and the intercostal parts of the internal intercostals.

Several chemicals act as stimuli for respiration. Carotid sinus and aortic arch chemoreceptors monitor carbon dioxide levels in the blood. Additionally, chemoreceptors monitor the cerebrospinal fluid for carbon dioxide, oxygen, and pH levels. Although carbon dioxide is the major determinant of respiratory drive, hypoxia is also a powerful stimulus to breathe. For some individuals with diseases that chronically increase the carbon dioxide levels (e.g., COPD), hypoxia may be the predominant stimulus. The chemoreceptors exert their effects through the medulla.

There are two other important involuntary respiratory centers, both located in the pons. The first is the apneustic center that serves as a backup stimulus for inspiration. The second is the pneumotaxic center, which inhibits inspiration. This center serves to control respiratory rate and inspiratory volume.[9]

Finally, as previously mentioned, there are other important contributions to respiration, particularly from the cerebral cortex. There is some degree of voluntary control over ventilation. In times of stress, it is possible to suppress respiration to the point of syncope from hypoxia. However, without the control of the cortex, the medullary centers resume control of breathing during unconsciousness. Additionally, the cortex controls hyperventilation, an activity that can raise the blood content of oxygen and lower the blood content of carbon dioxide, allowing extended periods of conscious apnea without a sensation of needing to breathe. In addition, strong emotions, fever, and pain will increase respiratory rate. The body's response to metabolic acidosis is to increase the respiratory rate and lower the carbon dioxide level (such as Kussmaul's respirations in diabetic ketoacidosis).

Pregnancy increases minute ventilation. Some medications and drugs of abuse increase respiratory rate while others (e.g., opioids) will decrease respiratory rate. Sleep also decreases the respiratory rate. For the vast majority of breathing, involuntary control by the medullary centers predominates (Figure 20-18).

Oxygen and Carbon Dioxide Metabolism

Respiration is the process of exchanging gasses, specifically oxygen and carbon dioxide, between an organism and its environment. The two major subtypes of respiration are

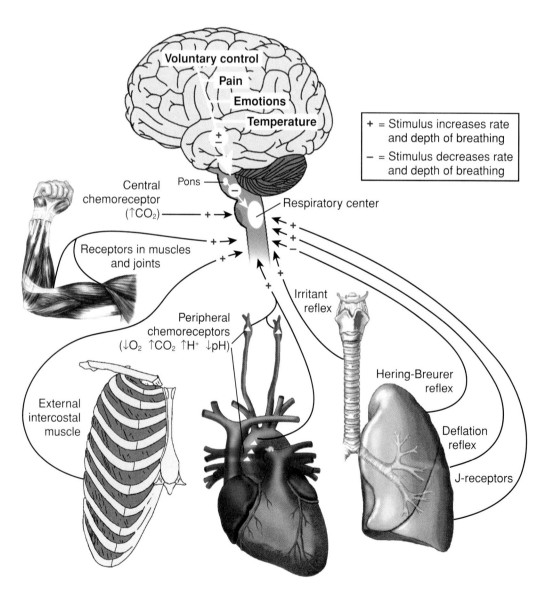

Figure 20-18   Neurologic control of respiration.

external respiration, which is the exchange of gasses between the lungs and the red blood cells, and internal respiration, which is the exchange of gasses between the red blood cells and cells that make up the various body tissues. The airway, lungs, respiratory structures, and circulatory system exist to assure adequate delivery of oxygen to the tissues and removal of carbon dioxide to the atmosphere.

The mechanisms described previously act to deliver oxygen to the alveoli and expel carbon dioxide out to the atmosphere. The amount of oxygen available at the alveoli, called the partial pressure of oxygen, depends on the total atmospheric pressure and fraction of inspired oxygen, abbreviated FiO_2. Room air, regardless of the atmospheric pressure, is made up of approximately 78% nitrogen, 21% oxygen, and 1% assorted other gasses. The concentrations of alveolar gasses, after dilution and humidification, are 75% nitrogen, 13% oxygen, 5% carbon dioxide, 6% water, and less than 1% other gasses. The inspired FiO_2 of room air is 21/100. Since FiO_2 is typically expressed as a decimal, room air FiO_2 is 0.21. Placing a patient on a high flow oxygen delivery device (e.g., a nonrebreather mask can increase the percentage of inspired oxygen to between 80% and 100%. If a person breathes 100% oxygen, then the FiO_2 is 100/100, or 1. A FiO_2 of 1 is the highest FiO_2 that can be delivered, because it means that all of the inspired air is composed of oxygen. The closer the FiO_2 is to 1, the more oxygen is available at the alveoli to diffuse into the blood.

The concept of partial pressure is another factor in determining the amount of oxygen available to the tissues. Normal atmospheric pressure at sea level is 760 torr (centimeters of water) and each gas in air makes up a percentage of that total amount, or total pressure. This is termed *partial pressure* (Figure 20-19) and is calculated by multiplying the air pressure by the fraction of that gas in the air. For example, to calculate the partial pressure of oxygen in room air at one atmosphere, multiply 0.21 (the FiO_2) by 760 torr (atmospheric pressure at sea level) to get a partial pressure of oxygen of 160 torr (Figure 20-19). Decreases in atmospheric pressure, such as could occur during an air medical transport, will decrease the partial pressures of a gas. Therefore, if the total pressure were decreased to one half atmospheric pressure (380 torr), the partial pressure of oxygen would be one half of what it was at sea level (21% × 380 torr = 80 torr) even if the percentage of oxygen remained the same (21%). This decreases oxygen delivery to the bloodstream. If the patient were placed on supplemental oxygen that increased the FiO_2 to 0.6 (60%) at sea level, the partial pressure of oxygen would increase to 456 torr, thus increasing the amount of oxygen delivered to the bloodstream. Partial pressures, therefore, are more important than percentages of the gas in determining how much oxygen will transfer from the alveoli to the bloodstream and, ultimately, to the tissues.

The pulmonary artery exits the right ventricle and divides into smaller and smaller subdivisions. Eventually, large capillary networks form over the surface of the alveoli. Small amounts of interstitial fluid and the very thin, highly permeable walls of the alveoli allow for rapid diffusion of respiratory gasses from areas of high concentration to areas of low concentration (Figure 20-20). In the case of carbon dioxide (a waste product of metabolism), the highest concentration is in the pulmonary artery and the blood arriving at the capillaries. The inspired air (and therefore the air in the alveoli) has a much lower concentration of carbon dioxide. Therefore, carbon dioxide diffuses from the bloodstream to the alveolar space. Conversely, oxygen is at its lowest concentration in the blood arriving from the pulmonary artery (having been used by the body during metabolism) and is at a much lower

Room Air at Sea Level		
atmospheric pressure	:	760 torr
FiO_2 21%	:	× 0.21
Partial Pressure Oxygen	=	160 torr

Room Air at Altitude		
atmospheric pressure	:	380 torr
FiO_2 21%	:	× 0.21
Partial Pressure Oxygen	=	80 torr

Supplemental Oxygen at Sea Level		
atmospheric pressure	:	760 torr
FiO_2 60%	:	× 0.60
Partial Pressure Oxygen	=	456 torr

Figure 20-19 Partial pressure of gasses.

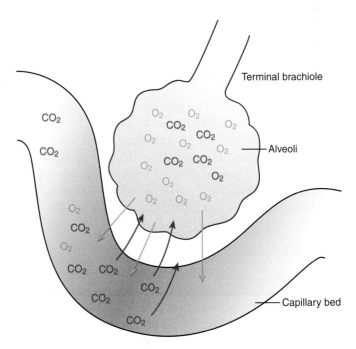

Figure 20-20 Diffusion of oxygen and carbon dioxide across the alveolar membrane occurs because of the concentration gradient across the membrane.

concentration than in the air in the alveoli. Therefore, oxygen will diffuse from the alveoli into the bloodstream. In this way, the major respiratory gasses are exchanged.

If oxygen simply dissolved into the blood, only small amounts of oxygen could be carried at a time. Therefore, a more efficient method of carrying oxygen is necessary. This method uses hemoglobin, a large molecule in red blood cells that is intended to carry oxygen from the alveoli to the tissues (and, to a lesser degree, to carry carbon dioxide back to the alveoli). Approximately 97% of the oxygen carried in the blood is bound to hemoglobin; the rest is dissolved directly into the plasma. Usually all of the systemic arterial hemoglobin is carrying oxygen and is therefore saturated with oxygen. Devices such as a pulse oximeter can measure the percentage of hemoglobin that is carrying oxygen. In healthy individuals, oxygen saturation is typically 98% or greater. Arterial pressure of oxygen, PaO_2, is a measurement of the amount (pressure) of oxygen in the blood. In a healthy adult breathing room air, the PaO_2 will be between 80 and 100 cm water.

Carbon dioxide (CO_2), produced by the tissues during metabolism, is returned to the alveoli for disposal. Approximately 33% of CO_2 is attached to hemoglobin. The rest is either dissolved in the blood or combines with water to form bicarbonate ions. These release the carbon dioxide when they reach the alveoli. The arterial pressure of carbon dioxide ($PaCO_2$) is the measure of carbon dioxide in the blood and is normally 35 to 45 mmHg.

Numerous disease states can affect the amounts of oxygen and carbon dioxide in the blood. Lowered atmospheric concentrations associated with partial pressures of oxygen and lowered hemoglobin concentrations both decrease the total amount of oxygen in the blood. Decreased surface area for exchange such as occurs in trauma (e.g., hemothorax, pneumothorax, pulmonary contusion) and medical diseases (e.g., COPD, pneumonia, effusions, atelectasis, CHF with pulmonary edema, etc.) will decrease the amount of oxygen reaching the tissues. Also, decreased mechanical effort—such as occurs with head injuries, strokes, overdoses, and pain—will decrease the available oxygen.

Carbon dioxide levels are primarily controlled by ventilation. Therefore, $PaCO_2$ will rise with hypoventilation and fall with hyperventilation. Although some metabolic processes can increase production of carbon dioxide, the lungs typically do an excellent job of compensating for these changes.

Pediatrics

Although there are significant differences between adult and pediatric patients—which are reflected in some changes in practice and equipment—the fundamental anatomy and physiology are the same. The same structures exist in both the adult and the pediatric airway and the ultimate purpose—exchange of respiratory gasses—remains the same. Therefore, with the previous discussion of adult anatomy and physiology in mind, this section will focus on the major differences between adult and pediatric patients.

Pediatric Anatomy

The most important differences between pediatric and adult airway anatomy are those of size and proportions. One of the most challenging differences between adult and pediatric airway management is that pediatric patients are simply smaller. Smaller spaces, smaller patients, and a requirement for more precision in action all combine to make the management of these patients potentially more difficult. The relative proportions of various structures are also important. These different proportions result in differences in management and technique between adult and pediatric patients. However, these differences do not necessarily make pediatric airway management more difficult; it is simply different. For the experienced Paramedic, the pediatric airway may be easier to manage than the adult airway; the key is the degree of familiarity with the structures, proportions, and equipment. Therefore, an understanding of the anatomical and proportional differences, as well as experience in pediatric airway management, is critical in making the provider comfortable with pediatric airway management. Table 20-1 summarizes the anatomical differences in pediatric patients.

The most obvious difference between pediatric and adult patients is size. However, it is probably the relative proportions that are most important. A pediatric patient's head, when compared to his body, is disproportionately larger than an adult's head. This is due to the more protuberant pediatric occiput.[12] Therefore, when a pediatric patient is in a supine position, the protuberant occiput will tend to flex the neck and compress airway structures, resulting in turbulence and increased resistance to airflow. As mentioned, the child's airway is smaller, so even a small degree of obstruction can significantly affect the pediatric patient's oxygenation and ventilation.

Advancing into the oropharynx, a child's tongue is disproportionately larger compared to the oral cavity than an adult's tongue. In addition, the tonsils and adenoids are disproportionately large and the mucosa over them and the entire pharynx is more friable, or fragile. When traumatized, these structures tend to bleed. Therefore, precision in blade

Table 20-1 Differences Between Pediatric Airway Anatomy and Adult Airway Anatomy

- More pronounced occiput, flexing head and neck when supine on a flat surface
- Proportionately smaller airway diameter
- Proportionally larger tongue, tonsils, and adenoids
- More friable mucosa
- Floppier and posterior sloping epiglottis
- Larynx position more anterior and toward head
- Vocal cords pinker and angled toward feet
- Airway smallest at level of cricoid cartilage
- Trachea angled anterior and shorter
- More susceptible to gastric distention

placement, care in movement of the devices and equipment in the mouth, gentle pressure, and control of the tongue are all critically important in the management of the pediatric airway.

Moving deeper into the hypopharynx, there is a much more acute angle from the pharynx to the epiglottis. The epiglottis is also "U" shaped and less rigid as the cartilage has not fully matured.[13] This immaturity also causes the epiglottis to slope more posteriorly, potentially obscuring the view of the glottis.

At the level of the larynx, the first recognizable difference is the position. At birth, the tracheal opening lies at the level of the first cervical vertebrae (C-1). By ages 5 to 7, relative differences in structural growth rates have moved the glottic opening to the C-3 to C-4 level, and by adulthood, the glottis rests at the C-5 level.[14] On laryngoscopic view, therefore, the glottis will be significantly closer to the oropharynx and will be in a relatively more anterior position than would be expected in an adult.

Examining the laryngeal opening, a number of differences are noted. The arytenoids are disproportionately large and are thus more prominent. The vocal cords are pinker and more difficult to differentiate from the surrounding tissue. In addition, the cords are angled toward the feet anteriorly and toward the top of the head posteriorly, sloping upward from the front of the child toward the back. This is different from adult vocal cords that tend to be on the same plane from front to back and creates the perception that the space is significantly smaller. These anatomic differences can be striking the first time a Paramedic visualizes the pediatric larynx.

At the level of the thyroid cartilage, another important difference is noted. The cricothyroid membrane is proportionately smaller in children and is almost nonexistent in infants. Up to age 10, it is difficult to identify the cricothyroid membrane by palpation. The cricoid ring is also different in the pediatric patient. In the adult airway, the vocal cords are the narrowest point in the upper airway. For the pediatric patient, the cricoid ring has the smallest cross-sectional area. This makes the larynx and trachea funnel-shaped. An endotracheal tube that is introduced into the airway, therefore, may pass the vocal cords without a problem but may have difficulty passing the cricoid ring. Aspirated foreign bodies may also lodge at this point.

There are also significant differences in the trachea itself. Compared to the adult trachea, the pediatric trachea is angled much more anteriorly as it travels inferiorly. In addition, the trachea is proportionately shorter and there is significantly less distance between the vocal cords and the carina. Minimal head movement in the pediatric patient can result in significant displacement of the tip of an endotracheal tube.

One other important anatomic difference related to management of the pediatric airway actually relates to the pediatric gastrointestinal tract. Pediatric patients are much more susceptible to gastric distention during positive pressure ventilation. Pediatric patients are less able to tolerate gastric distention due to their smaller lung volumes and their dependence on the diaphragm for respiration. Therefore, the pediatric patient should be ventilated with smaller pressures in an effort to minimize gastric inflation. Decompression of the distended stomach will significantly improve the respiratory mechanics and should routinely be performed on any child who has received positive pressure ventilation.

Physiology

Four major physiologic differences between adults and children are of significance to ventilation and airway management. The first of these relates to the nature of respiratory distress, respiratory failure, and cardiovascular collapse in pediatric patients. Multiple disease processes affect the basal metabolic rate and respiratory status of children. The common pathway to morbidity and mortality for many of these diseases is respiratory failure. Initially, pediatric patients are able to compensate for increasing respiratory demands. However, their dependence on the diaphragm for almost all inspiratory effort, their ability to recruit intercostal and accessory muscles, and the immaturity of the accessory musculature puts pediatric patients at risk to tire rapidly. Therefore, these patients decompensate quickly. By the time a pediatric patient goes into respiratory failure, most of his metabolic and oxygen reserves are depleted.[15] Secondary cardiovascular collapse, which is often irreversible, is likely to occur. This ability to initially compensate and then rapidly and irreversibly decompensate is a hallmark of pediatric respiratory failure. Table 20-2 summarizes the differences between pediatric respiratory physiology and adult respiratory physiology.

STREET SMART

By the time a pediatric patient is in respiratory failure and cardiovascular collapse, it may be very difficult to reverse the process. Early recognition of subtle signs (e.g., agitation, grunting, tripod positioning, retractions, etc.) of respiratory distress and rapid intervention are necessary to prevent respiratory failure and the ensuing cardiovascular collapse.

Table 20-2 Differences Between Pediatric Respiratory Physiology and Adult Respiratory Physiology

- Respiratory failure is primary cause of death in pediatric patients compared to cardiovascular failure in adults.
- Pediatric patients decompensate rapidly.
- Pediatric patients have proportionately higher oxygen consumption than adults.
- Pediatric patients have a smaller residual capacity than adults.
- Increased vagal tone in pediatric patients causes bradycardia.
- Hypoxia in pediatric patients causes bradycardia.

A second important metabolic difference between children and adults relates to oxygen consumption. For their size, pediatric patients consume more oxygen. Their basal metabolic rate is, by body surface area, significantly higher than an adult's and basal oxygen consumption per square meter can be twice as high as that of an adult.[16] Therefore, they become hypoxic rapidly during respiratory failure.

The third difference is that, for their size, pediatric patients have a disproportionately smaller functional residual capacity. Thus, in times of respiratory distress, children are less able to draw upon this capacity to provide supplemental ventilation. Furthermore, in times of apnea, the pediatric patient will become hypoxic up to twice as quickly as an adult.[17] Therefore, pediatric patients are more likely to progress to respiratory failure faster than an adult would in a similar clinical context and more likely to suffer early hypoxic injuries.

Finally, pediatric patients have the potential for high vagal tone. Minimal airway stimulation can result in excessively high vagal response including bradycardia and asystolic cardiac arrest. This includes stimulation from a laryngoscope blade. Pediatric patients tend to have copious secretions, increasing the risk for aspiration and difficulty maintaining an airway. Therefore, administration of appropriate vagolytic medications (e.g., atropine) before airway management is critical.

It is important to note, however, that pediatric patients will also become bradycardic when hypoxic. Therefore, rapid differentiation between hypoxia and excessive vagal tone is critical when a pediatric patient in respiratory distress becomes bradycardic.

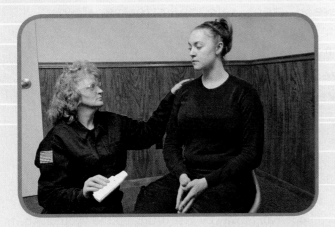

1 Position patient seated upright.

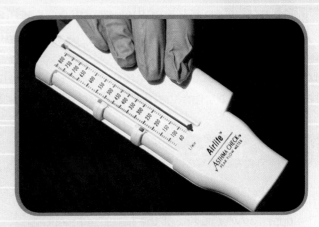

2 Reset indicator.

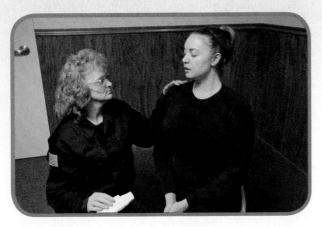

3 Instruct patient to inhale as deeply as possible.

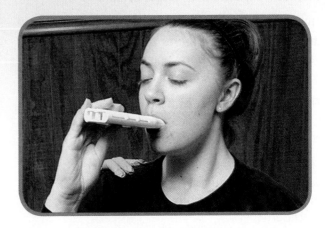

4 Instruct patient to tightly wrap mouth around mouthpiece.

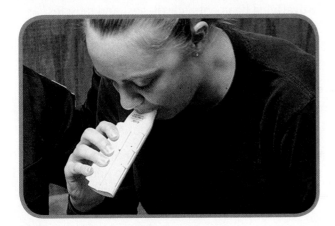

5 Instruct patient to exhale as fast as possible.

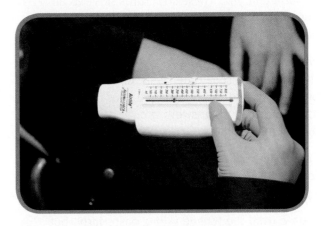

6 Read indicator.

CONCLUSION

The first step Paramedics require to achieve efficient, safe, and effective airway and ventilation management in their patients is to be familiar with normal airway anatomy and respiratory physiology. By being knowledgeable about these topics, the effective Paramedic can recognize abnormal findings and troubleshoot failures in the management of an airway or ventilation.

KEY POINTS:

- The airway is divided into upper and lower regions. The upper airway begins at the nares and mouth and extends to the glottis. The lower airway extends from the glottis to the alveoli.

- The mouth and nose both define the beginning of the airway. The nose serves as an immunological barrier, a source of warming and humidifying air, and a threat/food detection system.

- The pharynx is the area of the airway composed of the spaces behind the nose (nasopharynx) and the oral cavity (the oropharynx).

- The oral cavity is bound by the lips anteriorly, the buccal surfaces laterally, the tongue inferiorly, the hard palate superiorly, and the soft palate posteriorly.

- Food and respiratory gasses move through the oral cavity and tonsillar pillars that form the walls of the oral pharynx. These structures serve as an immunological barrier to pathogen entry in the pharynx.

- When performing airway management procedures the Paramedic should be aware of the high risk of bleeding due to vascularized mucous membranes as well as the risk of swelling or occlusion caused by oral infections.

- The epiglottis protects the lower airway from foreign body aspiration.

- Airway obstruction in the obtunded patient is not caused from the tongue falling posteriorly, but rather initially by the soft palate and the epiglottis making contact with the posterior wall of the oropharynx and pharynx.

- The head-tilt chin-lift or jaw thrust maneuvers open an airway by first lifting up the hyoid bone via anterior mandibular displacement.

- The larynx is made up of a number of cartilaginous structures including the thyroid cartilage and the aryepiglottic folds that contain the arytenoid cartilages.

- The "Adam's apple," formed by thyroid cartilage, is the large, anterior shield-like cartilage that forms the majority of the anterior portion of the larynx.

- The open space superior to the vocal cords is the vestibule. Folds in the vestibular membrane form the false cords that can seal over the glottis to help protect the airway from aspiration of foreign materials.

- The vocal cords are composed of mucosal folds overlying ligaments, cartilages, and muscles. As a part of the cricothyroid ligament, the vocal ligaments form the true vocal cords that are visible at the bottom of the vestibule.

- Vocal cords are responsible for the production of speech and sound as well as protection of the airway.

- A number of stimuli can trigger an involuntary reflex that causes the muscles to adduct the glottis and the false cords to provide an impenetrable barrier to foreign material.

- The cricoid ring, the only complete ring in the trachea, is located at the lowest portion of the larynx and the beginning of the trachea.

- The intrinsic and extrinsic laryngeal muscles and their nerve supply found in the larynx are responsible for the "gag reflex."

- The thyroid gland is a highly vascular, "H" shaped structure that lies along the side of the larynx and upper trachea.

- The common carotid artery and the internal jugular veins are two sets of major vascular structures that run parallel to the pharynx.

- The trachea is the portion of the airway from the cricoid ring to the carina.

- At the level of the carina, the lower airway splits into the two mainstem bronchi, the right and left. The right mainstem bronchus divides into three lobar bronchi and the left mainstem bronchus separates into two lobar bronchi. The right bronchus is more acutely angled and predisposes endotracheal tubes, suction catheters, and foreign bodies to enter more often than the left bronchus.

- As the bronchi decrease in diameter they become bronchioles. The muscles in the bronchi and bronchioles are capable of closing off the airway when bronchial spasms occur.

- The end of the terminal bronchioles have the alveolar ducts that open into the alveolar air sacs where gas exchange occurs.

- The fluid surfactant that holds the alveoli open by decreasing the surface tension of the alveoli prevents atelectasis (collapse of the alveoli).

- Determinations of lung volumes and capacities are important to facilitate descriptions of the physiologic occurrences during respiration. The most important measurement to the Paramedic is the volume of air moved at normal breath or tidal volume.

- Tidal volume multiplied by the respiratory rate is equal to the minute ventilation which is important in determining at what rate of volume a patient should be ventilated.

- The peak flow, or maximum velocity of gas movement, can be used to assess a patient's breathing, particularly in the assessment of asthmatic patients.

- Normal respiration occurs through a process of negative pressure ventilation.

- The muscles for inspiration can be divided into the principal and accessory muscles.

- Exhalation is normally passive; however, active muscles of expiration are utilized during periods of inadequate exhalation.

- Quiet breathing or normal inspiration is a function of principal muscles and passive exhalation. During active breathing, such as heavy activity, accessory muscles may be used for inspiration and active muscles used for expiration.

- The diaphragm is a large, thin, muscle that divides the abdomen for the thorax.

- The intercostal muscles attach the ribs to each other and are the major muscle group involved in inspiration.

- The chest wall is lined with the parietal pleura that lies against the outer lining of the lungs, the visceral pleura. A small amount of fluid between the two layers allows them to slide against each other but not pull apart.

- During inspiration, principal muscles increase the external volume of the thorax. The parietal pleura is attached to the expanding structures and, under normal conditions, pulls the visceral pleura along with it. The expanding visceral pleura expands the lung tissue, pulling open the alveoli.

- As the volume inside the alveoli increases, a lower pressure is created inside the alveoli.

- Lung expansion is controlled by stretch receptors that inhibit further inspiration. Expiration is the passive recoil of the lungs and chest wall that forces air out until interthoracic pressure equals that atmospheric pressure.

- Accessory muscles are used during high volume active respiration. Accessory muscles include the sternocleidomastoid muscles, the scalenes, and the intercostal muscles.

- Thoracic expiratory muscles and abdominal muscles may be used to decrease the thoracic volume and force air out of the lungs in times of exercise or when expired airflow is obstructed.

- During normal inspiration the decrease in intrathoracic pressure causes an increase in venous blood return or preload. When a patient receives positive pressure ventilations preload may decrease due to intrathoracic pressure remaining relatively the same.

Airway Anatomy and Physiology 373

- Increasing carbon dioxide is the greatest stimulus for ventilation in most patients, but sensory information comes from stretch receptors in the lungs.

- Involuntary control of respirations occurs in the respiratory center of the medulla oblongata. Sensory information is received from the vagus nerve and stimuli are sent out via the phrenic nerve. The inspiratory center of the medulla is responsible for inspiration and regular, rhythmic ventilation. The expiratory center is responsible only for active expiration when needed.

- Chemoreceptors monitor carbon dioxide levels in the blood and spinal fluid. For patients with diseases that chronically increase carbon dioxide levels, hypoxia (oxygen deficiency) may also be the predominant stimuli to breath.

- Located in the pons, the apneustic center serves as a backup stimulus for involuntary respiration and the pneumotaxic center inhibits inspiration. Although it is possible to suppress respirations, once the patient is unconscious medullary centers resume control.

- The two major subtypes of respiration are external respiration, which is the exchange of gasses between the lungs and the red blood cells, and internal respiration, which is the exchange of gasses between the red blood cells and cells that make up the various body tissues.

- Room air is made up of approximately 78% nitrogen, 21% oxygen, and 1% assorted other gasses. The FiO_2 of room air is expressed as a decimal, 0.21.

- Partial pressure of gasses is a factor in determining how much oxygen will transfer from the alveoli to the bloodstream and, ultimately, to the tissues.

- Diffusion of respiratory gasses from a high concentration to a low concentration occurs across the highly permeable wall of the alveoli.

- Diffusing from high to low concentrations, carbon dioxide diffuses out of the blood as oxygen diffuses from the alveoli to the bloodstream.

- Hemoglobin is a large molecule found in red blood cells that carries approximately 97% of oxygen from the alveoli to tissues. In addition, 33% of carbon dioxide is attached to hemoglobin as the blood returns from the tissues to the alveoli for disposal.

- Some oxygen and a large percentage of carbon dioxide are dissolved directly in the blood.

- Diseases that decrease the surface area for gas exchange can decrease the amount of oxygen in the blood, which decreases the amount of available oxygen reaching the tissues.

- Carbon dioxide levels are primarily controlled by ventilation in response to changes in $PaCO_2$. The lungs can compensate for changes in CO_2 through increasing or decreasing ventilatory rates.

- Differences between pediatric and adult airway anatomy are those of size and proportions:
  - A pediatric patient's head, when compared to his body, is disproportionately larger than an adult's.
  - In the oropharynx, a child's tongue is disproportionately larger than an adult's when compared to the oral cavity.
  - The structures of the oral cavity are also more fragile in pediatric patients than in adults.
  - In the hypopharynx of the pediatric patient, the epiglottis may obscure the view of the glottis due to the shape and acute angle of the pharynx.
  - The tracheal opening is relatively more anterior and significantly closer to the oropharynx.
  - Large arytenoids and pinker vocal cords that are set on an angle are further differences.
  - The narrowest point in the pediatric airway is not the vocal cords as found in adults, but the cricoid ring.
  - The pediatric airway is proportionally shorter and more anterior than the adult's.
  - Pediatric patients have smaller lung volumes than adults.
  - Pediatric patients depend on the diaphragm for respiration.

- Pediatric patients are able to compensate for increased respiratory demands but are at risk to tire rapidly and decompensate quickly.

- For their size, pediatric patients consume more oxygen than adults and may rapidly become hypoxic during respiratory failure.

- Consider hypoxia as the cause of bradycardia in a pediatric patient.

- Airway stimulation may also result in bradycardia due to the potential for high vagal tone found in pediatric patients.

REVIEW QUESTIONS:

1. Describe the route an oxygen molecule takes from the oral or nasal cavities to the alveolar capillaries.
2. List three functions of the nares.
3. Describe the anatomic "contents" of the oropharynx.
4. Diagram the anatomy of the epiglottis, glottis, vocal cords, and esophagus as viewed with a laryngoscope.
5. Describe the relationship of the hyoid bone to the tongue and epiglottis.
6. Name the most common cause of airway obstruction.
7. Differentiate between the "upper" and "lower" airway.
8. Diagram the relationship between the thyroid cartilage, the cricoid cartilage, the vocal cords, and their associated structures.
9. List the differences between the cricoid ring and lower tracheal rings.
10. List the airway structures of the lower airway.
11. Diagram the alveolar unit including the pulmonary capillaries.
12. List the cell types found in the walls of the lower airway structures.
13. Describe the bony and muscular structures of the chest wall.
14. Name the structure most responsible for the nervous system's control of ventilation.
15. Describe the two-layer nature of the pleura.
16. List two stimuli for breathing and identify which provides respiratory drive in most individuals.
17. Describe how positive pressure ventilation changes the normal intrathoracic pressure.
18. List key anatomic differences in the pediatric upper airway versus the adult upper airway.
19. List key anatomic differences in the pediatric lower airway versus the adult lower airway.
20. List differences in pediatric and adult respiratory physiology.

CASE STUDY QUESTIONS:

Please refer to the Case Study at the beginning of the chapter and answer the questions below:

1. What structures are kept open by continuous positive airway pressure (CPAP?)
2. Which of these structures exchange gasses?
3. How can changing the percentage of oxygen, or FiO_2, and the partial pressure of oxygen increase the overall exchange of respiratory gasses?
4. Describe "work of breathing."

REFERENCES:

1. Boerner TF, Ramanathan S. Functional anatomy of the airway. In: Benumof JL, ed. *Airway Management: Principles and Practice.* St. Louis: Mosby; 1996.

2. Williams P, Warwick R, Dyson M, et al. *Gray's anatomy* (37th ed.). New York: Churchill Livingston; 1989:1248–1286.

3. Shorten GD, Opie NJ, Graziotti P, et al. Assessment of upper airway anatomy in awake, sedated, and anesthetized patients using magnetic resonance imaging. *Anesths Intensive Care.* 1994;22:165.

4. Netter FH. *Atlas of Human Anatomy.* Summit: Ciga-Geigy; 1989:23–75.

5. Netter FH. *Atlas of Human Anatomy.* Summit: Ciga-Geigy; 1989:167–199.

6. Netter FH. *Atlas of Human Anatomy.* Summit: Ciga-Geigy; 1989:170–171.

7. Guyton AC, Hall JE. *Textbook of Medical Physiology* (9th ed.). Philadelphia: W.B. Saunders; 1996:481–485.

8. Costanzo LS. *Physiology.* Philadelphia: Williams and Wilkins; 1995:107.

9. Costanzo LS. *Physiology.* Philadelphia: Williams and Wilkins; 1995:108–124.

10. Richmond NJ, Silverman R, Kusick M, Matallana L, Winokur J. Out of hospital administration of albuterol for asthma by basic life support providers. *Academic Emergency Medicine.* 2005;12(5):396–403.

11. Netter FH. *Atlas of Human Anatomy.* Summit: Ciga-Geigy; 1989:183.

12. Luten RC. The pediatric patient. In: Walls RM, ed. *Manual of Emergency Airway Management.* Philadelphia: Williams and Wilkins; 2000:144.

13. Berens R, Day S. Airway management. In: Jaimovich D, Vidyasagar D, ed. *Handbook of Pediatric* and *Neonatal Transport Medicine* (2nd ed.). Philadelphia: Hanley and Belfus; 2002:174.

14. Luten RC. The pediatric patient. In: Walls RM, ed. *Manual of Emergency Airway Management.* Philadelphia: Williams and Wilkins; 2000:143.

15. Strange GR. (Ed.). *APLS: The Pediatric Emergency Medicine Course.* (3rd ed.). Dallas: ACEP; 2000:3–15.

16. Markenson DS. *Pediatric Prehospital Care.* Upper Saddle River: Prentice Hall; 2002:98.

17. Luten RC. The pediatric patient. In: Walls RM, ed. *Manual of Emergency Airway Management.* Philadelphia: Williams and Wilkins; 2000:143.

CHAPTER 21

THE ALGORITHMIC APPROACH TO AIRWAY MANAGEMENT

KEY CONCEPTS:

Upon completion of this chapter, it is expected that the reader will understand these following concepts:

- Algorithms that provide a specific planned set of actions and decisions where the if-then decisions are made in advance
- Ways the Paramedic utilizes an algorithmic approach to airway management
- The five criteria that determine how aggressive an approach to airway and respiratory management is needed
- Disease processes encountered in the prehospital environment that can cause a patient, the patient's airway, or the patient's respiratory status to deteriorate
- An algorithmic approach to patients who initially cannot be ventilated
- Airway management after a failed intubation attempt

▶ CASE STUDY:

The Paramedics were called to the intersection of Old State and Fish House Roads for a two-car MVC with significant injuries. The driver of a pickup truck was out of the vehicle and on the ground

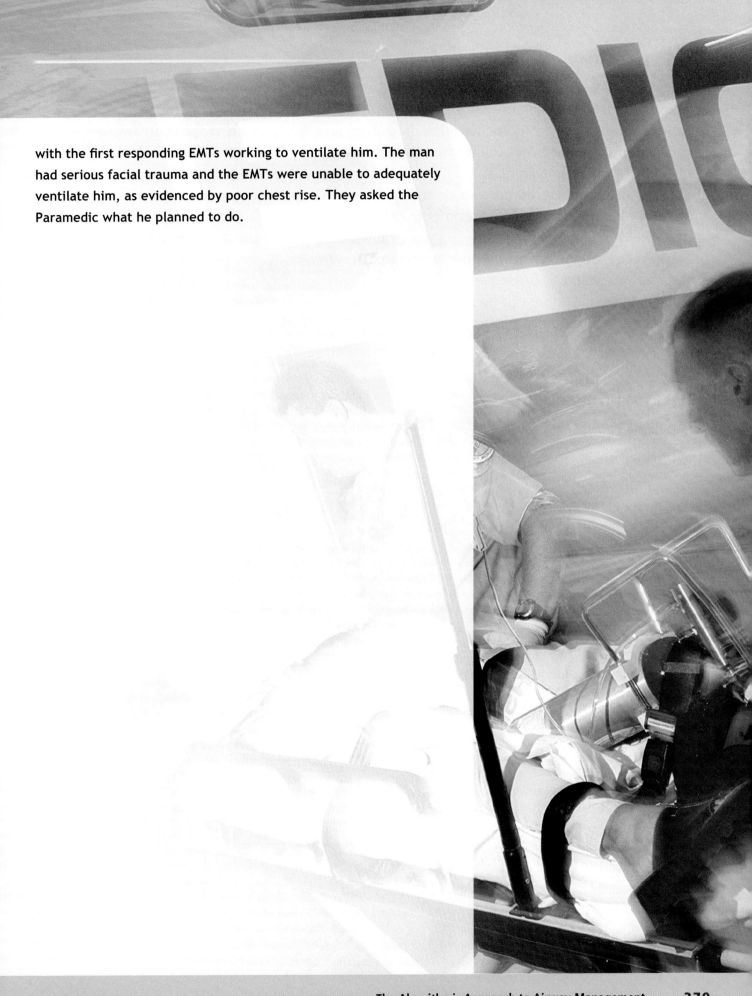

with the first responding EMTs working to ventilate him. The man had serious facial trauma and the EMTs were unable to adequately ventilate him, as evidenced by poor chest rise. They asked the Paramedic what he planned to do.

OVERVIEW

As part of the ABCs of primary assessment, airway management is a critical component in treating life-threatening conditions. As opposed to protocols that detail treatments for a specific working diagnosis, an algorithm provides the Paramedic with a specific planned set of actions and decisions where the if this–then that decisions are made in advance. The Paramedic can utilize an algorithmic approach to airway management based on criteria that determine a patient's need for airway and respiratory interventions. The Paramedic uses the airway management algorithm and knowledge of the many different disease processes that patients can present in the prehospital setting to identify and manage a patient's airway and respiratory status. When the Paramedic is presented with a patient who initially cannot be ventilated or whose airway is unable to be secured, the airway management algorithm offers a preplanned approach to ensure that the best patient care possible is provided.

Airway Management

Airway management is one of the most critical tasks a Paramedic performs. The consequences of an unmanaged or poorly managed airway are devastating and potentially fatal. For a Paramedic, however, the feeling of accomplishment that comes with properly managing the impossible airway can be its own reward. By definition, any emergency airway is considered difficult. Regardless of the patient's anatomy, the circumstances and urgency of managing the airway make it more difficult than in a non-emergency, in-hospital situation.[1-4] Preplanning becomes critical to prevent inaction, wrong action, and panic.

In patient care, the most common form of preplanning is the **algorithm**. This chapter examines the utility of algorithms and introduces the reader to three algorithms that can be utilized for the management of any prehospital emergency airway. Chapters 22 and 23 will examine each technique listed in the algorithms in depth. It is important to note that even if a Paramedic does not adopt a formal algorithm, the basic principle of preplanning remains the same. It is also important to emphasize that algorithms do not replace the Paramedic's critical thinking skills. By knowing what to do next if what is being done now doesn't work, the Paramedic can successfully negotiate any airway.

Algorithms

In every patient encounter, the Paramedic applies a group of patient care activities based on a presumptive conclusion called a **working diagnosis**. These activities have been previously planned and documented, usually in the form of a **protocol**.

Protocols are the fundamental guides to prehospital care. A protocol details a specific group of activities that are all to be accomplished for a given patient for a specific presumptive diagnosis. For example, a chest pain protocol may dictate that all patients with chest pain of possible cardiac origin must receive vital signs assessment, oxygen, aspirin, nitroglycerin, morphine, an IV, and cardiac monitoring.

Although there may be some specific order details within the protocol (e.g., "The first nitroglycerin may be given before an IV is established if the systolic blood pressure is greater than 120"), the actual order in which they are carried out is usually not critical to patient outcomes. It is expected that the Paramedic will perform all of the care specified in the protocol.

In certain emergency situations (e.g., cardiac arrest with ventricular fibrillation), specific tasks must be carried out the same way, in the same order, in a very limited time period. Furthermore, the care must be modified based on the patient's response to the interventions. In these cases, algorithms are applied. In essence, these are care guides based on "if-then" branch points. That is, a specific intervention is applied (e.g., defibrillation). *If* an event occurs (e.g., conversion to sinus rhythm) *then* another action is performed (e.g., administer an anti-arrhythmic medication). However, *if* a different event occurs (e.g., the patient remains in ventricular fibrillation), *then* a different action is performed (e.g., start CPR, intubate, insert an IV, and give epinephrine) (Figure 21-1).

The algorithm typically does not give wide latitude in decision making. By using a specific planned set of actions and decisions, the Paramedic, at the time of the emergency need only to perform the algorithm and monitor patient responses to ensure the best patient care is provided.

One of the greatest advantages of algorithms is that the if-then decisions are made in advance. Instead of having the Paramedic consider the advantages and disadvantages of a particular intervention while managing a critically ill patient, other individuals—in calmer and less pressured circumstances—have already considered the literature

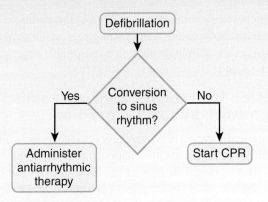

Figure 21-1 Example of an algorithm.

and anecdotal experience and have formed a consensus decision on treatment. Algorithms are developed in a low-stress environment where options can be discussed and fully evaluated as opposed to those decisions made at the patient's side, under high-stress and high-pressure circumstances.

In addition, algorithms provide an impetus for continuing action. In an emergency situation, the risk exists that a Paramedic can become so focused on a single task that, even in the face of failure of that task, the Paramedic repeatedly continues to perform that task. Use of an algorithm can prevent this from occurring.

For example, some scene management algorithms for critically ill trauma patients do not allow any attempts to initiate IV access on-scene before the patient is loaded and transported. These algorithms come from evidence that providers can become so fixated on inserting an IV that multiple attempts result in significant delays on-scene. By mandating that sequential tasks occur and that care "moves" and is not "stalled" on a single task, algorithms promote good care.

There are some important considerations in the use of an algorithm. Although the decisions about "what to do next" have already been made, they have not been made by the individual facing a particular airway at a particular time. Therefore, even the best algorithm can only serve as a guide; it is never a rigid absolute set of rules that must be mechanically followed. Deciding not to follow an algorithm, however, is not a decision to be made lightly.

The Paramedic should understand and routinely apply an airway management algorithm to the point that it is done automatically. This degree of familiarity implies that, when a radically different situation is encountered, the Paramedic can intelligently consider and reject the algorithm if it is inappropriate.

For example, a patient with a traumatic transection of the trachea is neither an appropriate candidate for repeated oral intubation attempts nor, when they fail, for the placement of a **blind insertion airway device**. In fact, this patient is a candidate for a technique not addressed in any airway algorithm: direct intubation of the trachea at the level of the transection.

However, without understanding standard algorithmic management and why it is inappropriate, the Paramedic

may be unable to make a good decision to try an alternative approach. Considering the use of an algorithm in every airway management event is completely appropriate. The algorithm, however, is just one of many tools used in airway and respiratory management. Appropriate equipment, education, practice, and a thorough knowledge base are also critically important tools. Therefore, the algorithm should be used in the context of excellent airway management skills and knowledge. It is the Paramedic's responsibility to maximize the quality of care.

Development of Algorithms

Currently, algorithms are the tools of choice for dictating care in critically unstable prehospital patients. Classes in which a Paramedic will be most familiar that rely on algorithms include Advanced Cardiac Life Support and Pediatric Advanced Life Support. In the airway management arena, the American Society of Anesthesiologists' "Difficult Airway Algorithm," the Advanced Trauma Life Support Trauma Airway Algorithm, and the National Emergency Airway Management Course Algorithm all represent various authors' and committees' approaches to addressing specific airway management issues. Of these, the ASA's "Difficult Airway Algorithm" has the most support in the literature.[5,6]

The ASA's "Difficult Airway Algorithm" resulted from the findings of a closed claims analysis of closed legal actions against anesthesiologists. The analysis found that three mechanisms (inadequate ventilation—38%, esophageal intubation—18%, and difficult airways—17%) accounted for almost three-quarters of all adverse outcomes. The Difficult Airway Algorithm was subsequently developed to address at least one of these three mechanisms.

In developing a systematic way to reduce the bad outcomes associated with difficult airways, the ASA Task Force on Management of the Difficult Airway looked to the literature for a valid methodology for guiding patient care activities in the setting of potentially critical illness. Two findings guided them in developing an algorithm. The first was the finding that certain specific management techniques had been clearly demonstrated to improve patient outcomes. The second finding was that, although there was no airway or anesthesia literature to demonstrate that linking the individual strategies to algorithms was beneficial, the cardiopulmonary resuscitation literature clearly demonstrated that algorithms were beneficial in the management of life-threatening cardiac events. Based on these two findings and expert consensus, an algorithmic approach to airway management was adopted.

Assessment of an Algorithm's Impact

The impact of airway management algorithms on patient outcomes, however, has not been clearly demonstrated. Assessing the impact of the ASA's Difficult Airway Algorithm is confounded by a number of variables.

Although this algorithm is almost universally used in the anesthesia setting, a repeat analysis of closed claims in 2000 that looked exclusively at difficult intubations was only able to find 98 cases from prior to implementation of the algorithm. The second difficulty in determining the algorithm's impact is the number of confounding factors. For example, the laryngeal mask airway was not commonly used before the algorithm was published; it is now very common in anesthesia practice and has been added to the algorithm. Changes in the number of non-physician anesthetists and their practice patterns all confound any analysis.

Finally, only historical control data is available to compare with new data; this increases the risk of unmeasured confounding factors impacting the outcome. In short, even with large numbers of patients and a strong monitoring system, using the largest database monitoring the impact of an airway algorithm may be inadequate to conclusively demonstrate that an algorithmic approach to emergency airway management is more effective than other approaches.

This limitation is true, however, only in the context of the ASA algorithm. Emergency airway algorithms have the advantage of starting with a single diagnosis: a patient in need of airway and ventilation management. Therefore, research into the efficacy of airway management algorithms in the prehospital environment may be possible if two similar EMS systems can be compared—one trained in and using an algorithm and one not. Until such research is completed, however, the debate between pro-algorithm and pro-point of care clinical decision making will continue.

Prehospital Airway Management Algorithms

Many algorithms are available for the prehospital provider to use. Some, such as the ASA Difficult Airway Algorithm, do not fit well in the prehospital environment since they are written for use in a relatively controlled environment of the operating room and may not be reasonable for the prehospital environment.[7–9]

Others may contain techniques in which the provider may not be trained. Still others may address only one aspect of airway management (e.g., intubation) while neglecting other aspects (i.e., non-intubated management, alternative devices).

Ultimately, it is the responsibility of the Paramedic, ALS agency, or medical director to select algorithms for use that are sufficiently comprehensive and reflect current practice. To this end, the following three algorithms are written to provide one method for an integrated approach to airway management developed by the author. There has been a traditional separation of "basic life support" and "advanced life support" airway skills. Although state rules and regulations dictate the scope of EMS practice at all levels, the lines distinguishing these skills have become progressively blurred.

For example, some EMT-Basics may be allowed to intubate while some EMT-Paramedics may not be allowed to place blind insertion airway devices such as the King LTS-D or laryngeal mask airways. Therefore, separating care into "BLS" and "ALS" algorithms is inappropriate. Instead,

dividing between intubating airway care (the ability to use an endotracheal tube or blind insertion airway device) and non-intubating airway management is a reasonable approach and the one taken in the following algorithms.

Decision to Intubate and/or Provide Respiratory Support Algorithm

The Paramedic's most important task is to recognize a patient's need for airway or respiratory support. Generally, this patient assessment is taught as part of the ABCs: Does the patient have a patent *airway*, is the patient *breathing*, and what is the patient's *circulatory status*? Parameters such as "respiratory rate < 10 or > 28" are used to guide interventions. However, using parameters fails to address the "why" aspect of airway management. By understanding why a patient may need airway and respiratory support, the Paramedic is better able to determine when and how to provide that support.

Every patient requires some degree of airway management and respiratory support. The question that must be answered is how much can the patient do on his own and how much support does he need from the Paramedic. For example, a healthy 23-year-old woman with an ankle fracture can probably completely support her own airway and respiratory status. The same patient, however, after high dose morphine may require active airway and respiratory support by the Paramedic. The key is recognizing the difference between these two scenarios.

There are five reasons why patients may require active airway or respiratory management (Table 21-1). By assessing each of these reasons in a systematic (algorithmic) fashion, the Paramedic will be able to determine how aggressive an approach to airway and respiratory management is needed. The Decision to Intubate and/or Provide Respiratory Support Algorithm (Figure 21-2) provides the algorithm for patient assessment of airway and respiratory status.

Although different from a typical algorithm in that each step is not necessarily an intervention but rather a question to be answered, this algorithm nonetheless systematically guides the Paramedic through the steps of assessing a patient's airway and respiratory status and is therefore considered to be an algorithm.

The algorithm is entered in the upper left-hand corner at the point indicated "Start Here." Looking at the left-most column, the five reasons for managing an airway are listed. As can be seen, they are listed in an order that allows for logical and rapid assessment. In each case, the Paramedic

Table 21-1 Indications for Definitive Airway Control

- Non-patent airway
- Inability to maintain a patent airway
- Failure to oxygenate
- Failure to ventilate
- Anticipated deterioration in the patient's status or the airway status

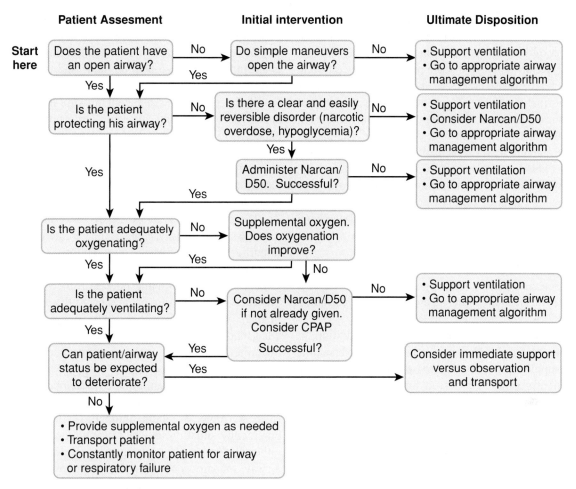

Figure 21-2 Decision to intubate and/or provide respiratory support algorithm.

asks a "Yes/No" question. If the factor (e.g., an occluded airway) will not have an impact on the patient's condition, then the Paramedic moves on to the next question.

If by the end of the question list there are no factors that would require active airway or respiratory intervention, the Paramedic simply monitors and continues to reassess the patient. By reaching the line of the algorithm that states "Provide supplemental oxygen as needed, transport patient, constantly monitor patient for airway or respiratory failure," the Paramedic can be assured that immediate airway or respiratory interventions are not needed.

Only when specific conditions exist that would compromise a patient's airway or respiratory status must the Paramedic perform interventions. The following evaluates the decision making required and actions to be taken given a specific condition.

If, on primary assessment, a patient does not have a patent airway, the first intervention is the use of simple maneuvers. These consist of head-tilt, chin-lift and jaw-thrust maneuvers to lift the epiglottis and soft palate from the posterior hypopharynx and pharynx. If these are successful at opening the airway, then the Paramedic should continue the assessment. Otherwise, the Paramedic should move on to the appropriate algorithm discussed in the following text.

Some patients may have patent airways on primary assessment or their airways can be opened with a simple intervention such as a jaw thrust. If the Paramedic determines that the patient has a patent airway but is unable to maintain that airway, then the provider's response is determined by the apparent cause of the disability. These are patients who are typically thought of as "unresponsive" but not in cardiac or respiratory arrest.

Therefore, hypoglycemia and narcotic overdose need to be considered as easily reversible causes of the mental status change. If one of these two causes is suspected, then the Paramedic should, if permitted by training and protocol, attempt to reverse these disease processes.

If 50% dextrose or naloxone successfully reverses the altered mental status, then the patient's airway maintenance issues will often also resolve. Even if hypoglycemia or narcotic overdose are not clearly the causes of a patient's mental status change, the provider should consider giving these medications prior to more invasive airway management if it seems clinically appropriate.

If the patient still is not able to maintain the airway, the Paramedic should proceed to the airway algorithm appropriate to his level of training.

If a patient has a patent airway and is maintaining that patent airway, it is possible that the patient may still not be effectively oxygenating (transferring oxygen to the tissues) or ventilating (removing carbon dioxide from the bloodstream).

A number of disease processes can affect oxygenation and ventilation. Typically, a single disease process will affect both. However, there are disease processes that may cause hypoxia in the face of normal ventilation. Conversely, a patient may have adequate tissue oxygenation while retaining carbon dioxide. An example of the first is a patient with pneumonia. The patient may be able to continue to exhale carbon dioxide at a normal rate but not be able to adequately deliver oxygen to tissues.

Rarely will hypoventilation occur without hypoxia. One example in which it does occur would be a patient with a morphine overdose. She may maintain a normal oxygen level if given high-flow oxygen but still be retaining carbon dioxide due to decreased respiratory rate or tidal volume.

By separating oxygenation from ventilation, the Paramedic can rapidly screen a patient for oxygenation status and, if it is normal, begin the more focused evaluation of ventilation status.

If a patient is found to be hypoxic, the addition of supplemental oxygen may be adequate to reverse the hypoxia. If supplemental oxygenation reverses the hypoxia, then the patient should be assessed for ventilation failure. If supplemental oxygen is inadequate, however, then the patient likely has oxygenation and ventilation failure and efforts should be made to reverse the ventilation failure. For the comatose patient with decreased respiratory rate or drive, Narcan or 50% dextrose may reverse the disease process. For the patient in congestive heart failure or COPD exacerbation, use of continuous positive airway pressure (CPAP) or bilevel positive airway pressure (BiPAP) may overcome the oxygenation or ventilation failure.[10,11] However, if the patient remains hypoxic or is hypoventilating in spite of these interventions, more aggressive interventions are needed. The Paramedic should move on to the appropriate airway management algorithm.

If a patient has a patent airway, is maintaining that airway, and is oxygenating and ventilating normally, then it is unlikely that an immediate, emergent intervention is necessary. However, the Paramedic must be knowledgeable concerning the natural progression of diseases. There are a number of disease processes encountered in the prehospital environment that can cause a patient, the patient's airway, or the patient's respiratory status to deteriorate. A few examples include airway burns, congestive heart failure, asthma exacerbation, and sepsis.

In each of these cases, the Paramedic must make an important decision as to whether to intervene immediately or to monitor the patient. Several conditions (e.g., airway and inhalation burns with dyspnea, stridor, or hoarseness) are almost absolutely guaranteed to progress to airway occlusion and mandate early intubation.

Patients in congestive heart failure, on the other hand, may improve dramatically after treatment even with hypoxia or hypoventilation during the primary assessment. The decision to perform early airway management is based on experience, knowledge of the disease process, ability of the provider, availability of equipment including medications, and often discussion with a medical control physician. This is an important decision to be made and must be done with careful consideration.

If the patient has a patent airway, is maintaining that airway, is oxygenating and ventilating normally, and is not expected to deteriorate, then the Paramedic has completely assessed the patient's airway and respiratory status. At this point, the Paramedic can continue with the remainder of the patient assessment. She should return to reassess the airway every few minutes, or sooner if the patient's status changes.

If a patient fails any of the five criteria for being able to manage his own airway, then it is the Paramedic's responsibility to perform more aggressive interventions. This is the premise of the Decision to Intubate and/or Provide Respiratory Support Algorithm. The right-hand column directs the Paramedic to provide ventilatory support and go to the appropriate airway management algorithm. In this case, appropriate refers not to what management would be most appropriate for the patient but rather to the algorithm that is appropriate to the Paramedic's practice level.

One other important point to remember is the Paramedic must perform excellent non-intubating airway skills prior to performing excellent intubating airway skills. In an emergency situation, the most experienced Paramedic must either perform airway management or directly supervise the airway management. The Paramedic who divides airway management tasks into ALS and BLS and believes that he is only responsible for ALS skills is mistaken and is providing poor patient care. Therefore, it is imperative that the Paramedic be comfortable with all aspects of airway management, including both the "non-intubating" and "intubating" airway management algorithms.

Non-Intubating Airway Management Algorithm

The "Non-Intubating Airway Management Algorithm" (Figure 21-3) is entered at the top with the assumption that an assessment is complete and the patient is in need of further airway or respiratory support and management. The next three interventions should all be automatic. The first and most important intervention is to minimize or prevent hypoxia. Hypoxic brain death occurs within 6 to 10 minutes of apnea or significant hypoxia.

Therefore, immediate application of high-flow oxygen is mandatory to provide as much of a time margin as is possible. Ideally, since the patient is at least in ventilatory failure and at worst is apneic, the oxygen will be applied through a bag-valve-mask (BVM) device or, if the patient is apneic, with an automatic transport ventilator (ATV). This may be delegated to another provider so the Paramedic can continue down the algorithm.

The second automatic task is to assemble airway management equipment. The equipment will depend on what

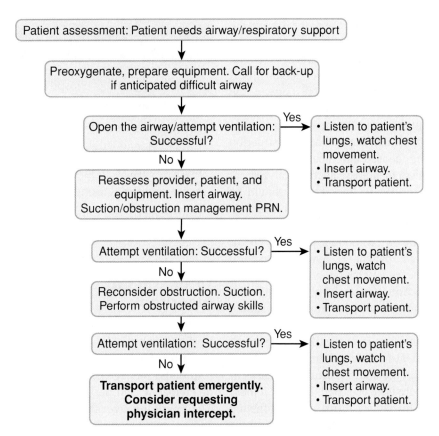

Figure 21-3 Non-intubating airway management algorithm.

skills the Paramedic is able to perform, but should ideally be available in a single bag or box and be organized, complete, and up-to-date.

Once these tasks have been accomplished, the next step is to begin supporting the patient. Opening the airway and providing ventilation is the first step in supporting the patient. If the patient is spontaneously but ineffectively breathing, then supported ventilations with a BVM is the most appropriate intervention.

If the patient is apneic, then either a BVM or an automatic transport ventilator attached to a mask can be used. If the Paramedic is successful at opening the airway and providing ventilation, then a rapid assessment of the intervention's adequacy is performed (auscultation, observation). Either an oropharyngeal or a nasopharyngeal airway is inserted depending on the absence or presence of a gag reflex, respectively. Finally, the patient is transported.

Note that in both the intubating and non-intubating algorithms, there are distinctions made between transport and transport emergently. These differences are based on a specific list of conditions (Table 21-2), which require emergent transport (the assumption being that for all other conditions, the risks of emergent transport may outweigh any benefits).

If a patient's vital signs are otherwise stable and the airway and ventilation adequately managed, the risk-to-benefit ratio

Table 21-2 Conditions Requiring Emergency Transportation

- Abnormal vital signs that cannot be corrected/do not respond to treatment
- Unmanageable airway
- Ischemic compromise of an extremity
- Complicated delivery
- Uncontrollable bleeding
- Cardiac arrest reversal with abnormal vital signs
- Cardiac arrest without defibrillation/medications available

for emergent transport may be too high. In that case, the Paramedic should consider non-emergency transport. If the patient's airway cannot be managed, however, then the patient should be transported emergently. This approach is taken by the "intubating" and "non-intubating" algorithms. In reality, the decision will be made based on local protocols, local standard of care, and medical direction.

There will be times when a patient's airway cannot be established or the patient cannot be ventilated on the first attempt. If this is the case, the Paramedic must quickly troubleshoot. Immediate actions should include repositioning the patient's head and, if needed, suctioning the airway and performing obstructed airway skills.

Once these interventions are performed, the Paramedic should make a second attempt to open the airway and ventilate the patient. If the second attempt is successful, then, as before, the Paramedic should assess the adequacy of ventilation, insert an oropharyngeal (OP) or nasopharyngeal (NP) airway, and transport the patient.

If, after the second attempt, the Paramedic is unable to establish a patent airway or ventilate the patient, an obstruction should be assumed. The appropriate obstructed airway management skills (Heimlich maneuver, unconscious patient abdominal thrusts, chest thrusts, or back blows) should be performed and another attempt should be made to ventilate the patient. If this attempt is successful, then the Paramedic should assess the adequacy of ventilation, place an OP or NP airway, and transport the patient. If, however, the third attempt at ventilation fails, then a change in tactics must be made. An analysis of the actions performed gives insight into why, after three ventilation attempts, the Paramedic should change tactics.

When the first attempt is made to ventilate the patient, it is assumed that the patient has normal anatomy and that "normal" (not including foreign body obstruction) causes of respiratory and airway failure have occurred. In most of these patients, a head-tilt, chin-lift or jaw thrust, in combination with BVM or ATV ventilation, will be adequate to open the airway and provide ventilation.

If these interventions fail, the next intervention is to rapidly troubleshoot and correct easily identifiable problems, including inadequate performance of skills, on the first ventilation attempt. Therefore, when the second attempt is made at ventilation, the Paramedic will still assume the patient has normal anatomy and "normal" causes of the airway and respiratory failure. In most of the remaining patients, these few corrections will open the airway and allow adequate assisted ventilation.

If the second attempt at ventilation fails, however, the Paramedic must consider abnormal conditions. Therefore, between the second and third ventilation attempts, the Paramedic performs all of his skills to correct or compensate for anatomical issues, airway obstruction, and physiological defects. The Paramedic corrects all the variables for which he is able to compensate. The third attempt at ventilation, therefore, is an optimized attempt.[12] If this attempt fails, there is little else the Paramedic can do. Therefore, after the third attempt, a different tactic must be taken.

The failure of the third ventilation attempt signifies that the Paramedic has no additional changes in care to offer. Therefore, the patient must be transported immediately to another provider capable of offering additional, advanced care. These are critically unstable patients and should be transported emergently. During that transport, the Paramedic should continue to perform obstructed airway skills and attempt to ventilate. If it will shorten the time to access advanced care, ALS providers should intercept the transport.

In some regions, prehospital physician intercepts are possible and, if available, should be requested at this time as well. If these intercepts will increase the time to definitive care (e.g., physician, emergency department, or operating room), then they should not occur and the patient should be emergently and safely transported. The Paramedic should not wait on-scene for an EMS Physician to arrive.

Intubating Airway Management Algorithm

As with the Non-Intubating Airway Management Algorithm, a patient enters the Intubating Airway Management Algorithm by virtue of having met one of the five criteria for airway and respiratory management and by having a Paramedic capable of intubating and performing other advanced airway skills. The top of the algorithm (Figure 21-4) is the entrance point and assumes that the patient needs to be intubated. As will be recalled, other non-intubated ventilatory support modalities should have been tried by this point. The algorithm directs the Paramedic toward a goal: a secure airway with adequate ventilation.

The Paramedic places the patient on high-flow oxygen or ventilates the patient with a BVM. At this point, if possible, the most experienced Paramedic should be performing or directly supervising the patient's care. While the Paramedic is doing this, the least experienced Paramedic on the scene, who is capable of preparing the intubation and airway management equipment, should be doing so. Having the most experienced providers directly managing the patient's care will optimize that care.

While there is some debate as to the definition of an intubation attempt, the National Association of EMS Physicians (NAEMSP) developed a standardized reporting tool (Table 21-3). As each unsuccessful intubation attempt will cause edema, bleeding, and patient deterioration, it is important that the first intubation attempt be the best intubation attempt.[13] Conditions must be optimized through proper, working equipment and, if used, drug selection. The patient must be correctly positioned, the Paramedic must be correctly positioned relative to the patient, and lighting should be controlled as much as possible. The proper route must be selected. In short, everything that can be controlled should be so as to make the first attempt most likely to succeed.

Once the equipment is prepared and conditions are optimized, the route must be selected. For a breathing patient, particularly one with a primary respiratory disease such as CHF or a COPD exacerbation, nasal intubation is an excellent choice.[14-18] These patients are likely to become hypoxic

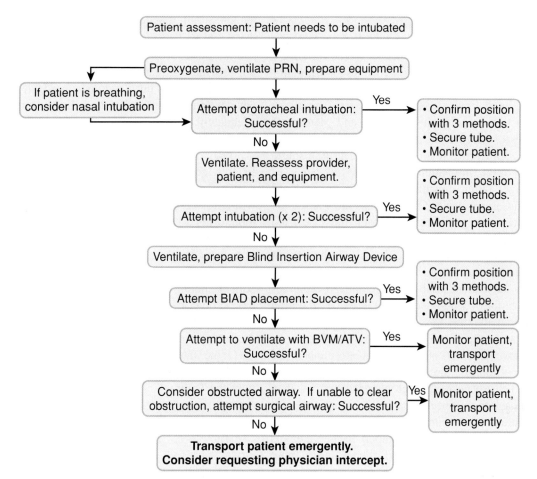

Figure 21-4 Intubating airway management algorithm.

Table 21-3 NAEMSP Definition of Intubation Attempt

1. Insertion of laryngoscope blade into mouth (for orotracheal methods)
2. Insertion of tube through nares of nose (for nasotracheal methods)
3. Insertion of rescue airway device into mouth (for Combitube, LMA, and other oral rescue airway devices)
4. Insertion of rescue airway devices through the neck (for cricothyroidotomy, needle jet ventilation, retrograde ETI, and other "surgical" methods of airway management)

H.E. Wang, R.M. Domeier, D.F. Kupas, M.J. Greenwood, R.E. O'Connor, "Recommended guidelines for uniform reporting of data from out-of-hospital airway management: position statement of the National Association of EMS Physicians," *Prehospital Emergency Care* 8, no.1 (2004): 58–72.

rapidly if medications are used to sedate or paralyze them as they have no reserve capacity. If the patient is not breathing, however, or has evidence of a basilar skull fracture, then an attempt at oral intubation is the next step.

After the endotracheal tube is passed, tube position is confirmed by auscultation and another confirmation device.

First, auscultate over the epigastrium while the patient is ventilated. If the endotracheal tube is correctly placed in the trachea, there should be an absence of gastric sounds. Next, auscultate over both the left and right lung fields for presence of equal breath sounds. If the right lung sounds are louder than the left, the endotracheal tube is likely in the right mainstem bronchus. Check depth of endotracheal tube placement and withdraw the tube by 1 or 2 cm, reinflate the balloon, and reassess lung sounds. If the lung sounds remain unequal, then assess the patient for a pneumothorax, as discussed in later chapters.

The two commonly accepted additional methods of confirming tube placement are esophageal detector devices and colorimic end-tidal carbon dioxide measurement.[19–21] Each of these methods has benefits and drawbacks. Using two or three tend to cancel out the problems inherent in each method.

Once the endotracheal tube is confirmed to be in a tracheal position, it must be secured using either a commercial device or tape. Additionally, the use of a cervical immobilization collar and cervical immobilization device (head blocks) will minimize tube movement and the potential for displacement. The use of waveform capnography in the intubated patient can provide an additional layer of safety as endotracheal tube dislodgement can be identified and corrected almost immediately. The Paramedic must continue to monitor the patient for changes in respiratory status and transport the patient.

If the first intubation attempt fails, however, then the Paramedic must reconsider his actions and determine the best course to increase the chances of success on the second attempt. Sometimes it is possible to identify a single item that caused the intubation attempt to fail, such as laryngoscope light failure, insufficient suction, or the need for sedation and/or paralysis. Other times, the Paramedic simply recognizes that a different approach must be tried without being completely sure why the first approach failed. Therefore, if the first intubation attempt failed, the patient must be ventilated as needed and the Paramedic must attempt to optimize the subsequent intubation attempt. The changes made to optimize the second attempt should be based on the findings of the first attempt.

Once the Paramedic is ready to reattempt intubation, no more than two more attempts should be made to intubate the patient. If, after a total of three attempts, the patient is not intubated and no clearly correctable problem is identified, then a different approach to the specific patient is required. By the time the third attempt has been made, the Paramedic should have maximized conditions. In all likelihood, further attempts will result only in more bleeding and edema and a more difficult airway to manage. The greater the number of attempts at endotracheal intubation, the lower the chance of success.[22]

If the second or third intubation attempt is successful, then the tube should be confirmed with three methods, it should be secured, and the patient should be monitored and transported. If these two additional attempts are not successful, however, then the airway manager must move on with his management plan. The patient should be ventilated as needed.

The next class of devices that are likely to succeed in at least partially securing the airway are devices designed for blind insertion into the upper portion of the airway above the glottis. Several terms have been used to describe these devices, including supraglottic airway devices, non-visualized airway devices, and blind insertion airway devices (BIADs). For the remainder of this discussion, we will use the term BIADs when referring to these airways. The BIADs commonly used include the King LTS-D airway, laryngeal mask airway (LMA), and the esophageal tracheal Combitube. Each of these devices has its strengths and weaknesses. In general, the esophageal obturator airway (EOA) and esophageal gastric tube airway (EGTA) should rarely be considered as they have a history of high complication rates and both require maintenance of a mask seal during use. Although they are still the BIADs of choice for some agencies, standard of care is moving away from the EOA and EGTA and toward one of the other devices.

It is rare that a blind insertion airway device will not provide at least some ability to effectively ventilate a patient. Although the airway may not be secure in the sense of having a tube beyond the vocal cords with direct access to the trachea, it is more secure than with simple face-mask ventilation. There will be occasions when these devices will not provide adequate ventilation. For example, in a patient with an inhalation burn and vocal cord edema, none of these devices can guarantee that air will pass through the cords to adequately ventilate the patient. However, as noted before, failure to provide some improvement in ventilation is rare.

Once the BIAD is in place, it needs to be confirmed. In this case, auscultation and end-tidal carbon dioxide measurement can be utilized. Esophageal detection devices will not necessarily work with any of the BIADs. Therefore, monitoring the patient's condition over time becomes the third method of confirming device placement. Once the placement has been confirmed, the BIAD must be secured in the manner recommended by the manufacturer and the patient should be monitored and transported. If the patient has no other concurrent issues and the BIAD is allowing for adequate oxygenation and ventilation, then a non-emergency mode transport may be appropriate.

If the BIAD will not pass (for anatomical reasons, injuries, etc.) or does not seem to be providing adequate ventilation, then the Paramedic must fall back on the fundamentals of airway management. The objective of airway management is to allow adequate oxygenation and ventilation.

Therefore, if all previous methods of securing the airway have failed, then face-mask ventilation with a BVM or ATV and an oropharyngeal or nasopharyngeal airway is appropriate. There will be patients whose airways cannot otherwise be managed due to injury or anatomy who will do well with face-mask ventilation. If the patient can be adequately ventilated by these interventions, then the patient should be monitored and transported. These patients with clearly difficult airways will usually qualify for emergent transport. If the patient improves and remains stable with face-mask ventilation alone, however, non-emergent transport can be considered.

If all other airway management modalities have failed and the patient still cannot be ventilated, then the Paramedic must assume that there is a pathological obstruction of the airway. This obstruction may be visualized during an intubation attempt or assumed from either the patient's disease process or simply from the failure to ventilate. If basic and advanced obstructed airway skills do not clear the airway, then the Paramedic is left to attempt to establish a surgical airway. If the pathology is at the level of the thyroid cartilage or above, a surgical airway will allow ventilation and oxygenation. If the obstruction is at or below the level of the trachea, however, a surgical cricothyrotomy will most likely fail.

If the surgical airway succeeds, the patient should be monitored and transported emergently. If, however, the surgical airway fails, then the patient must be transported emergently while the Paramedic attempts to oxygenate and ventilate the patient. If available, the Paramedic may consider a physician intercept or an intercept with a more experienced Paramedic while en route to the hospital.

CONCLUSION

Airway management can be one of the most life-saving tasks a Paramedic can perform for a patient. As has been demonstrated in the cardiopulmonary resuscitation arena, algorithms can greatly enhance consistent and correct task performance during life-threatening emergencies.

The value of an algorithmic approach to airway management has been recognized by professional organizations. Although the use of algorithms can greatly facilitate airway management, it is important to recognize that the algorithm is written for the majority of situations and that algorithms are not "one size fits all." Therefore, the Paramedic must recognize that an algorithm is simply one more tool to improve the quality of patient care. While it does not replace clinical judgment in a specific situation, it allows a systematic approach that will enhance patient care.

KEY POINTS:

- The algorithm is a form of preplanning in an emergency situation.

- Emergency airway algorithms all begin with a patient in need of airway and ventilation management.

- The Paramedic must determine what degree of airway management and respiratory support is needed for every patient.

- Active airway or respiratory management is required for each of the following:
  - Non-patent airway
  - Inability to maintain patient's own airway
  - Failure to oxygenate
  - Failure to ventilate
  - Anticipated deterioration of the patient's status or the airway status

- If, on primary assessment, a patient does not have a patent airway, the first intervention is the use of a head-tilt, chin-lift or jaw-thrust maneuver to open the airway. If the patient has a patent airway but is unable to maintain that airway, the Paramedic should determine the cause of the disability.

- Hypoglycemia or narcotic overdose should be considered when presented with patients who are typically thought of as "unresponsive" but not in cardiac or respiratory arrest.

- Despite having a patent airway, it is possible that the patient may still not be effectively oxygenating or ventilating.

- If the patient with a patent airway is maintaining that airway, is oxygenating and ventilating normally, and is not expected to deteriorate, then the Paramedic has completely assessed the patient's airway and respiratory status. She should continue monitoring for effect.

- The "Non-Intubating Airway Management Algorithm" addresses the need for airway or respiratory support and management, which is the first and most important automatic intervention to minimize or prevent hypoxia.

- The second automatic task is to assemble airway management equipment appropriate to the Paramedic's skill level.

- The Paramedic should support the patient with ineffective breathing or apnea by opening the airway and providing ventilation.

- The following conditions require emergent transport:
  - Abnormal vital signs that cannot be corrected/ do not respond to treatment
  - Unmanageable airway

- Ischemic compromise of an extremity
- Complicated delivery
- Uncontrollable bleeding
- Cardiac arrest reversal with abnormal vital signs
- Cardiac arrest without defibrillation/medications available

If the patient's airway cannot be managed, the patient should be transported emergently.

- The Paramedic should consider suctioning and repositioning the head as initial interventions for a patient who cannot be ventilated.

- If a second attempt is successful, the Paramedic should consider an OPA or NPA along with patient transport.

- If a second attempt is unsuccessful, an obstruction should be assumed. The Paramedic should perform the appropriate obstructed airway management skills (Heimlich maneuver, unconscious patient abdominal thrusts, chest thrusts, or back blows) and make another attempt to ventilate the patient.

- Continued failure to ventilate is an abnormal circumstance requiring all measures available to obtain a patent airway, including transporting the patient to a provider capable of offering an advanced level of airway care.

- Conditions prior to the first intubation attempt must be optimized by first selecting the proper provider, equipment, medications, and route. The Paramedic and patient must also be in proper positions with sufficient lighting.

- Nasal intubation is an excellent choice for the spontaneously breathing patient with a respiratory disease history.

- Oral intubation is a good choice for an apneic patient or one with a suspected basilar skull fracture.

- After the endotracheal tube is passed, tube position is confirmed by auscultating first over the epigastrium, then over the left and right lung fields for presence of equal breath sounds.

- The Paramedic confirms placement with at least one additional method. Waveform capnography is required in many EMS systems.

- The Paramedic should note the depth of the endotracheal tube placement and secure the endotracheal tube with tape or a commercial device.

- The Paramedic should use a cervical immobilization device to minimize tube movement and potential for displacement.

- The Paramedic should continue monitoring the patient for effect.

- If the first intubation attempt fails, the patient must be ventilated. No more than two more attempts should be made to intubate the patient.

- Blind insertion airway devices (BIADs) are likely to succeed in at least partially securing the airway and are designed for blind insertion into the upper portion of the airway above the glottis.

- Once the BIAD is in place, the Paramedic should confirm it by auscultation, end-tidal carbon dioxide measurement, or simply monitoring the patient's condition over time.

- An obstruction may be visualized during an intubation attempt or assumed from either the patient's disease process or the failure to ventilate.

- A surgical airway is often considered the last course of action that may allow ventilation and oxygenation.

REVIEW QUESTIONS:

1. Contrast the "if-then" approach of protocols with the methodology that algorithms offer.
2. What criteria are used to make a patient's transport decision?
3. What are two easily reversible conditions where the patient is thought of as "unresponsive" but not in cardiac or respiratory arrest?
4. Provide a disease process for each situation: a patient who is hypoxic with normal ventilation and a patient who has adequate tissue oxygenation but is retaining carbon dioxide due to ventilatory failure.
5. Why should the Paramedic have mastered the Non-Intubating Airway Management Algorithm before using the Intubating Airway Management Algorithm?
6. What are the automatic tasks the Paramedic should perform under the Non-Intubating Airway Management Algorithm?
7. What are the five reasons for which a patient may require active airway or respiratory management?
8. After the endotracheal tube is passed, how is tube position confirmed?
9. What should the Paramedic do if the first intubation attempt fails?
10. Describe the function of a blind insertion airway device.

CASE STUDY QUESTIONS:

Please refer to the Case Study at the beginning of the chapter and answer the questions below:

1. What early interventions can be performed to increase the likelihood of successful ventilation for this patient?
2. What airway device would you choose if the providers remained unable to adequately ventilate the patient? Explain your answer.
3. How would you assess the success of the placement?
4. What other devices/interventions are available for the provision of adequate airway/ventilation?

REFERENCES:

1. Combes X, Jabre P, Jbeili C, Leroux B, Bastuji-Garin S, Margenet A, et al. Prehospital standardization of medical airway management: incidence and risk factors of difficult airway. *Acad Emerg Med.* 2006;13(8):828–834.
2. Dorges V, Wenzel V, Knacke P, Gerlach K. Comparison of different airway management strategies to ventilate apneic, nonpreoxygenated patients. *Crit Care Med.* 2003;31(3):800–804.
3. Hoyle JD, Jr., Jones JS, Deibel M, Lock DT, Reischman D. Comparative study of airway management techniques with restricted access to patient airway. *Prehosp Emerg Care.* 2007;11(3):330–336.
4. Gerich TG, Schmidt U, Hubrich V, Lobenhoffer HP, Tscherne H. Prehospital airway management in the acutely injured patient: the role of surgical cricothyrotomy revisited. *J Trauma.* 1998;45(2):312–314.
5. Bishop MJ. Practice guidelines for airway care during resuscitation. *Respir Care.* 1995;40(4):393–401; discussion 401.
6. Candido KD, Saatee S, Appavu SK, Khorasani A. Revisiting the ASA guidelines for management of a difficult airway. *Anesthesiology.* 2000;93(1):295–298.
7. Timmermann A, Russo SG. Which airway should I use? *Curr Opin Anaesthesiol.* 2007;20(6):595–599.

8. Ezri T, Szmuk P, Warters RD, Katz J, Hagberg CA. Difficult airway management practice patterns among anesthesiologists practicing in the United States: have we made any progress? *J Clin Anesth.* 2003;15(6):418–422.

9. Ron M, Walls R, Michael F, Robert C, Robert E. *Manual of Emergency Airway Management.* Hagerstwon: Lippincott Williams & Wilkins; 2004.

10. Hunjadi D. From provider to patient. *Emerg Med Serv.* 2005;34(8):157–160.

11. Goss JF, Zygowiec J. Positive pressure: CPAP in the treatment of pulmonary edema & COPD. *Jems.* 2006;31(11):48, 50, 52–58 passim; quiz 64.

12. Wang HE, Yealy DM. How many attempts are required to accomplish out-of-hospital endotracheal intubation? *Acad Emerg Med.* 2006;13(4):372–377.

13. Butler KH, Clyne B. Management of the difficult airway: alternative airway techniques and adjuncts. *Emerg Med Clin North Am.* 2003;21(2):259–289.

14. Iserson KV. Blind nasotracheal intubation. *Ann Emerg Med.* 1981;10(9):468–471.

15. Danzl DF, Thomas DM. Nasotracheal intubations in the emergency department. *Crit Care Med.* 1980;8(11):677–682.

16. O'Brien DJ, Danzl DF, Hooker EA, Daniel LM, Dolan MC. Prehospital blind nasotracheal intubation by Paramedics. *Ann Emerg Med.* 1989;18(6):612–617.

17. Arora MK, Karamchandani K, Trikha A. Use of a gum elastic bougie to facilitate blind nasotracheal intubation in children: a series of three cases. *Anaesthesia.* 2006;61(3):291–294.

18. Butcher D. Pharmacological techniques for managing acute pain in emergency departments. *Emerg Nurse.* 2004;12(1):26–35; quiz 36.

19. Hayden SR, Sciammarella J, Viccellio P, Thode H, Delagi R. Colorimetric end-tidal CO_2 detector for verification of endotracheal tube placement in out-of-hospital cardiac arrest. *Acad Emerg Med.* 1995;2(6):499–502.

20. Cummins RO, Hazinski MF. Guidelines based on the principle "First, do no harm." New guidelines on tracheal tube confirmation and prevention of dislodgment. *Resuscitation.* 2000;46(1–3): 443–447.

21. Zaleski L, Abello D, Gold MI. The esophageal detector device. Does it work? *Anesthesiology.* 1993;79(2):244–247.

22. Wang HE, Domeier RM, Kupas DF, Greenwood MJ, O'Connor RE. Recommended guidelines for uniform reporting of data from out-of-hospital airway management: Position statement of the National Association of EMS Physicians. *Prehosp Emerg Care.* 2004;8(1):58–72.

CHAPTER 22

NON-INTUBATING AIRWAY MANAGEMENT

KEY CONCEPTS:

Upon completion of this chapter, it is expected that the reader will understand these following concepts:

- The benefits of preoxygenation for any patient in need of active airway management or ventilatory support
- The use of cricoid pressure during manual ventilation
- Simple airway maneuvers that can make all the difference
- Understanding ventilatory pressure and reducing gastric inflation
- Indications and application of continuous positive airway pressure (CPAP)
- Assessing the adult and pediatric patient for appropriate oxygenation and ventilation

CASE STUDY:

The Paramedics were called to the home of Mrs. Tedesco, an elderly woman with a lengthy history of congestive heart failure. When they arrived, Mrs. Tedesco's breathing appeared worse than usual. One Paramedic placed her on a nonrebreather mask but she continued to labor.

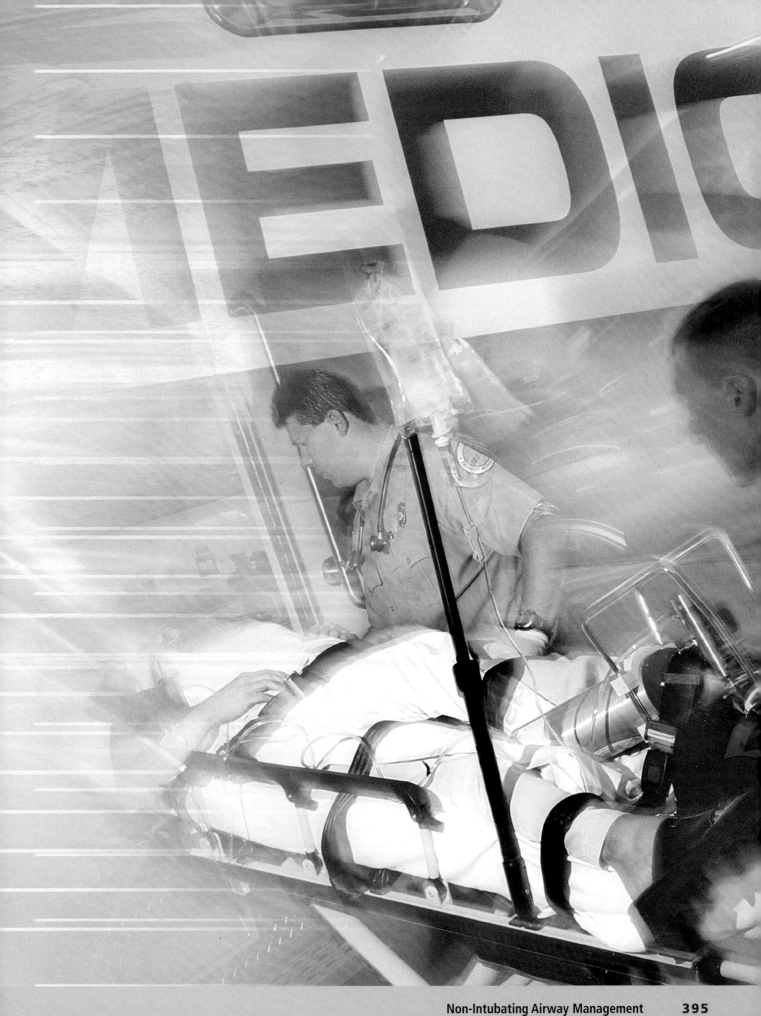

OVERVIEW

Knowledge and skill in basic airway management is mandatory. Often some of the most basic techniques are the most critical and fundamental airway management skills a Paramedic can perform. This chapter addresses a number of skills and simple devices the Paramedic can utilize to effectively ventilate patients through simple face-mask techniques. In addition, continuous positive airway pressure (CPAP) and other advances in airway technology allow critically ill patients to be managed without the need for intubation.

Basic Airway Management

Basic airway management is one of the most critical and fundamental skills an emergency medicine provider can possess.[1-3] Whether that provider is an EMT, a Paramedic, a nurse, or a physician, knowledge and skill in basic airway management is critical. As stated succinctly in the 1994 EMT national standard curriculum, "a patient without an airway is a dead patient." Although the knowledge and skill to perform intubations and other advanced airway maneuvers, as described in the next chapter, are a critical part of the Paramedic's practice, the non-invasive, basic skills are truly the most critical to master.

Using the Non-Intubating Airway Management Algorithm (Figure 22-1) as a guide, this chapter will review the fundamentals of basic airway skills. In addition, techniques to avoid intubation, such as CPAP and assisted ventilation, will be discussed.

STREET SMART

Correct positioning of the patient and the airway is the most basic airway maneuver.

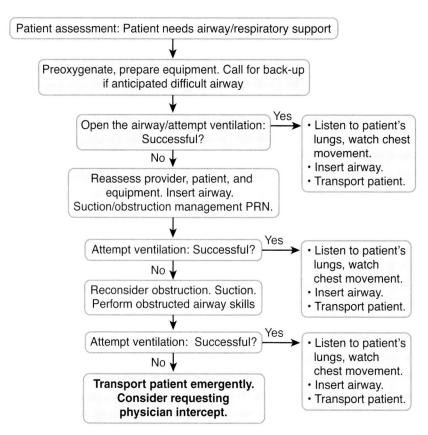

Patient assessment: Patient needs airway/respiratory support

↓

Preoxygenate, prepare equipment. Call for back-up if anticipated difficult airway

↓

Open the airway/attempt ventilation: Successful? — Yes →
- Listen to patient's lungs, watch chest movement.
- Insert airway.
- Transport patient.

No ↓

Reassess provider, patient, and equipment. Insert airway. Suction/obstruction management PRN.

↓

Attempt ventilation: Successful? — Yes →
- Listen to patient's lungs, watch chest movement.
- Insert airway.
- Transport patient.

No ↓

Reconsider obstruction. Suction. Perform obstructed airway skills

↓

Attempt ventilation: Successful? — Yes →
- Listen to patient's lungs, watch chest movement.
- Insert airway.
- Transport patient.

No ↓

Transport patient emergently. Consider requesting physician intercept.

Figure 22-1 Non-intubating airway management algorithm.

The Basic Airway Management Algorithm

By the time the Paramedic enters the basic algorithm, the decision has already been made to provide airway and ventilatory support to the patient. Once that decision has been made, the Paramedic must proceed in an orderly manner through the steps of care.

Preoxygenation

Any patient in need of active airway management or ventilatory support is in need of supplemental oxygen. Providing a patient with supplemental oxygen serves a number of purposes. Supplemental oxygen replaces nitrogen in the dead space of the lungs with oxygen, referred to as nitrogen washout. Not only does this increase the diffusion gradient, causing more oxygen to dissolve into the plasma, but it also provides a "reservoir" of oxygen in the lungs in the event the patient becomes apneic.[4,5] Oxygen can often decrease the patient's respiratory distress, in turn decreasing catecholamine release and myocardial oxygen demand.

Oxygen Delivery Devices

Oxygen equipment includes oxygen storage devices, regulators, and delivery devices (i.e., masks, nasal cannula). It is important that the Paramedic be skilled in the use of these devices.

Oxygen is stored as either a compressed gas, in steel or aluminum tanks, or as a liquid. Common compressed gas cylinders in the prehospital environment include D cylinders, which hold 400 L of oxygen when completely filled; E cylinders, which hold 660 L of oxygen; and M cylinders, which hold 3,450 L.[6,7] Since the cylinders contain oxygen at high pressure (1,800 PSI), it is important that they be handled with care to prevent damage to the valve.

Oxygen can also be chilled or compressed at high pressures and stored in a liquid form. Although **liquid oxygen (LOX)**, concentrated oxygen in liquid form, systems permit large volumes of oxygen to be stored in a relatively small space, there are several disadvantages to these systems. The tanks must be stored upright and special equipment is required for storage and cylinder transfer. Additionally, anecdotal reports suggest that, due to system leakage, unless the oxygen is used in a high volume agency, oxygen losses may exceed usage. Therefore, compressed oxygen cylinders are the most common method of storing oxygen in the prehospital environment.

Oxygen cannot safely be administered at the high pressure at which it is stored (500 to 1,800 PSI). Instead, a regulator is used to decrease the pressure to a tolerable level.

In addition, since oxygen is usually delivered in a continuous flow rather than on-demand, regulators are coupled with flow meters to deliver a fixed flow, measured in liters per minute (LPM). For portable regulators, the regulator and flow meter are integrated, while for fixed (on-board) oxygen systems, the flow meter is generally separate from the regulator. Oxygen flow rates range from 0.5 to 25 LPM. In addition, many regulators can deliver a 50 PSI source of oxygen for various devices (e.g., ventilators, continuous and bilevel positive airway pressure, and trans-tracheal jet ventilation equipment).

Oxygen is delivered to the patient from the regulator through a number of devices. The most commonly used devices are the nasal cannula, the simple face mask, and the nonrebreather mask. In addition, demand valve devices also provide a method for providing high concentration oxygen but are less commonly used.

The nasal cannula is a pronged device designed for nasal oxygen delivery (Figure 22-2). With oxygen flows from 0.5 to 6 LPM, these devices can deliver up to a 40% FiO_2. They are generally well tolerated and do not require a patient to breathe through his nose to be effective. Only complete bilateral nasopharyngeal obstruction would prevent oxygen delivery. Indications include the need for supplemental oxygen. Contraindications include severe hypoxia, apnea, and intolerance of the device.

The **high-flow nasal cannula (HFNC)** is an advance in nasal cannula technology. By humidifying and warming the oxygen, and using membrane technology, the device is able to comfortably deliver up to 40 LPM to the patient through a nasal cannula. Although this technology has not yet been applied in the prehospital environment, it does offer some promise.

The simple face mask is a low- to mid-concentration oxygen delivery device. The mask seals over the mouth and nose, delivering oxygen through an input port and drawing air through an open side port. At 10 LPM, a 40% to 60% FiO_2 is attained.[8] Unfortunately, increasing the oxygen flow above 10 LPM does not significantly increase FiO_2 since the same amount of room air will still be drawn through the side port on inspiration. Additionally, leaks around the mask will decrease the FiO_2. These masks are not used as commonly as the next class, the nonrebreather mask.

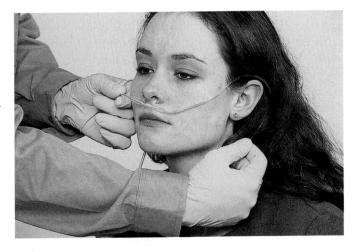

Figure 22-2 Nasal cannula.

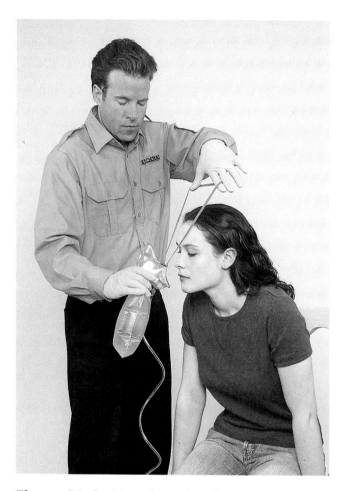

Figure 22-3 Nonrebreather face mask.

Nonrebreather face masks (Figure 22-3) are designed to overcome the issue of room air dilution by adding a reservoir to the oxygen supply system. While oxygen flows, it simultaneously supplies oxygen into the mask and into a reservoir bag. When the patient exhales, a one-way valve seals and the oxygen is directed into the reservoir. When the patient inhales, the one-way valve opens and the patient breathes the oxygen from the reservoir.

Although a normal adult male may have a minute ventilation of 6 to 8 LPM, this ventilation occurs during inhalation and airflow is not continuous. The flow during inhalation may approach 50 LPM![9] Oxygen delivery from a regulator, on the other hand, is continuous and limited to the liter flow settings on the regulator. The reservoir bag on the nonrebreather mask supplies the additional liter flow required during inhalation by storing oxygen during exhalation. This is why it is important that the liter flow is set high enough that the reservoir bag does not collapse during inhalation. Most nonrebreather face masks have two exhalation ports, at least one of which is left open. If the reservoir bag is collapsing during inhalation, room air is drawn through the side port to prevent rebreathing of carbon dioxide.

Nonrebreather face masks (NRFM), oxygen masks with an oxygen reservoir, can deliver up to 80% FiO_2; they do not deliver 100% FiO_2 because there will always be some room air mixing through the open side port.

A demand valve regulator is a device available that will provide 100% FiO_2 at appropriate liter flows. When attached to a 50 PSI oxygen source, this device delivers high LPM flows of 100% oxygen when the patient inhales. When the patient is exhaling, the valve closes and oxygen flow stops. This device is different from a manually triggered ventilation device in that it is the patient's inspiratory effort that triggers the device. Therefore, the risk of over pressurization injury is minimized. However, the device cannot be used in apneic patients.

Venturi masks, special masks with a restricted intake that permits an exact percentage of oxygen, can also be used to deliver oxygen, although their use in the prehospital environment is generally limited to specialty care services. These devices use a face mask connected to a specially designed adapter. These adapters have small holes in the sides and are designed so that when a specific oxygen liter flow is delivered to the adapter, a specific amount of room air is drawn into the adapter as well, called the venturi effect. This mixing provides a very specific oxygen concentration. Generally speaking, unless a patient is already using a venturi mask and is not hypoxic or is on a fixed FiO_2 during a specialty transport, there are no indications for the prehospital use of the venturi mask.

Generally speaking, patients can be thought of as being at minimal risk for hypoxia, at moderate risk for hypoxia, or hypoxic. Patients at minimal risk for hypoxia may benefit from a nasal cannula, depending on the patient's clinical condition. Patients at moderate risk for hypoxia or who are hypoxic should receive high-concentration oxygen (i.e., a nonrebreather mask). Any patient who requires active airway management should be preoxygenated with a nonrebreather mask. Once the patient is being oxygenated, the remainder of the basic airway management equipment should be prepared to address ventilations.

Equipment for Basic Airway Management

There are multiple methods for opening the airway and ventilating a patient who is in respiratory distress or respiratory arrest. A number of techniques can be used to manually open the airway. Devices, such as oropharyngeal and nasopharyngeal airways, can be used to help maintain an open airway. The most commonly used device for providing ventilatory assistance is the bag-valve-mask assembly. When used properly, these devices can effectively be used to ventilate most patients. Other devices such as the pocket mask, the manually triggered oxygen-powered ventilator, and the automatic transport ventilator are also available to provide ventilation. Furthermore, suction is an important and frequently overlooked adjunct to airway management.

Oropharyngeal and Nasopharyngeal Airways

Some of the most fundamental and easiest to use devices for airway management are the oropharyngeal and nasopharyngeal airways. As discussed in Chapter 20, the most

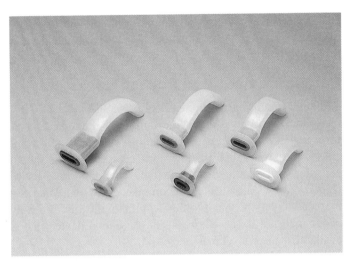

Figure 22-4 Oropharyngeal airway.

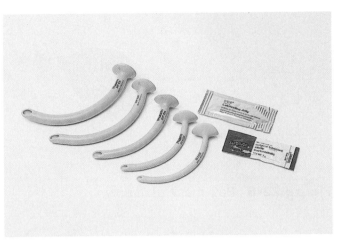

Figure 22-5 Nasopharyngeal airway.

common anatomic structures obstructing the airway are the soft palate and the epiglottis. Since the epiglottis is attached to the hyoid bone by the hyoepiglottic ligament, anterior displacement of the hyoid opens the airway. The hyoid is indirectly attached to the tongue, and anterior displacement of the tongue facilitates anterior displacement of the hyoid. Additionally, the tongue can increase airway turbulence by narrowing the upper airway. The oropharyngeal airway is designed to address this issue.[10,11] The nasopharyngeal airway helps to displace the soft palate anteriorly, improving airflow through the upper airway. Neither the oral airway nor the nasopharyngeal airway provide protection against aspiration.[12]

Oral airways come in a number of sizes, from neonatal to large adult (Figure 22-4). Preparation of an oropharyngeal airway involves measuring the appropriate size for the patient. Two common methods are used. The first is to measure the airway from the midline of the lips to the angle of the jaw. The second is to measure the airway from the corner of the mouth to the inferior tip of the ipsilateral earlobe. Either method is appropriate.

An airway that is too small will not displace the tongue and jaw anteriorly and is at risk of being lost in the airway. An oral airway that is too large will tend to rise out of the mouth and during ventilation, may actually displace the tongue posteriorly. Therefore, it is important to only use an oral airway if the appropriate size is available.

It is important to note that the oral airway may stimulate a gag reflex and should not be used in patients with an intact gag reflex.[13,14] If an oral airway is to be used, suction must be immediately available in the event that the patient vomits during placement.

While the oropharyngeal airway is made of hard plastic, the nasopharyngeal airway is made of soft silicone with a beveled tip (Figure 22-5). The nasopharyngeal airway is useful in patients with an altered mental status but with an intact gag reflex.

Although the nasopharyngeal airway is less likely to stimulate a gag reflex, patients may vomit or sneeze after nasopharyngeal airway placement. Therefore, suction must be immediately available when a nasopharyngeal airway is placed.

There are a number of advantages to the placement of the nasopharyngeal airway. These include the ability to place them in patients with trismus or in those who are otherwise unable to open their mouths. Nasopharyngeal airways can also be used in patients who have an intact gag reflex.

The only true contraindication to the placement of the nasopharyngeal airway is the patient's inability to tolerate the airway. Care must be taken if it is being used in someone with a head injury. Make sure that there is no evidence of a basilar skull fracture, as there is some risk, although very slight, of placing the airway into the cranium.[15–20] In addition, patients with bleeding disorders or who are on blood thinners are at risk of significant epistaxis from nasopharyngeal airway placement.

Like the oropharyngeal airway, the nasopharyngeal airway must be measured before placement to assure good sizing. The most common method for measuring the nasopharyngeal airway is to place the airway against the face, measuring from the nare to the ipsilateral inferior tip of the earlobe. Unlike the oral airway, the nasal airway should be lubricated before use. In addition, pretreatment of the nare with an inhaled vasoconstrictor (e.g., neosynephrine) and topical anesthetic (e.g., spray or viscous lidocaine) before placement may improve patient tolerance and decrease bleeding.

Bag-Mask Assembly

The bag-mask assembly is the most commonly used device for providing assisted ventilation. In the operating room, anesthesiologists use high-flow respiratory gasses that continuously flow through a bag to a mask and that are checked by a valve which the anesthesiologist controls; hence the name bag-valve-mask.

In the prehospital environment, self-inflating bags with a reservoir, or bag-mask assembly, are the most commonly

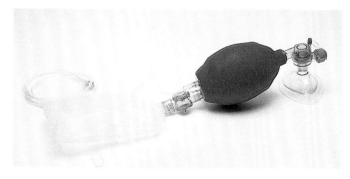

Figure 22-6 Bag-mask assembly.

used devices (Figure 22-6). The distal adapter of these bag-mask assemblies is designed to attach to a mask or to the 15 mm adapter of an endotracheal tube or an alternative airway device. They are available in adult and pediatric sizes. There are common features to all of the devices.

Every bag-mask assembly has a method of attachment to an oxygen source. This tubing runs into a self-inflating bag. Adult bags may be as large as 1,600 cc. Attached to the bag is a reservoir that serves the same function as the reservoir on the nonrebreather mask. The reservoir allows oxygen flows far above the flow from the regulator without entering room air. The oxygen passes through a one-way valve and out the distal port. On exhalation, expired gasses escape distal to the one-way valve, preventing remixing in the bag.

Although bag-mask assemblies are commonly used, they are not nearly as easy to use as they appear. As early as 1983, it was clearly demonstrated that use of the pocket mask proved to be far superior to the one-person bag-mask assembly technique. Although rescuers are able to deliver appropriate tidal volumes of 6 to 7 mL/kg, the excessively large volumes of adult bag-mask assembly ventilators are associated with over ventilation. In addition, technique can vary greatly, and overly rapid high-pressure ventilation typically results in gastric inflation. Excellent bag-valve-mask technique is therefore an important skill for the Paramedic to master.[21–23]

Preparation of the bag-mask assembly is simple. The device is removed from its packaging and attached to an oxygen source flowing at least 15 LPM. If a bag reservoir is attached, it should inflate. If the reservoir is made of collapsible tubing, it should be extended to its fullest length. The Paramedic attaches the mask to the ventilation adaptor. Some pediatric BVMs include a pressure relief pop-off valve between the bag and the mask. This pop-off valve should be closed to ensure adequate ventilation to the pediatric patient.

Although most bag-mask assemblies are packaged with a single mask, there are a number of different mask sizes and styles. Mask sizes vary from premature infant to large adult. Mask styles include masks with air-filled cuffs; masks without cuffs; soft, circular style masks; and gel-filled masks. The appropriate-sized mask is the mask that seats from the bridge of the nose to the chin.

Specific applications for different mask types will be discussed in the following text. In general, however, the air-filled

cuff style mask is the most commonly used. These various mask types can also be attached to the ventilation devices discussed later.

Barrier Devices and Pocket Masks

Although mouth-to-mouth ventilation is still taught in CPR, there should be no need for an on-duty Paramedic to perform this skill. If standard ventilation devices are not available to the prehospital provider during a response, he should consider carrying a disposable face shield barrier device (Figure 22-7). Although not recommended by the American Heart Association except to the lay public, they are probably better than no barrier device at all. A second device that is available is the pocket mask.

The pocket mask is a face-mask device that is powered by the lungs (Figure 22-8). Although devices without an oxygen inlet port are available, they should not be used in the emergency medical environment. Rather, a device with an oxygen inlet port should be used to provide enrichment to the 17% oxygen in an exhaled breath. The masks are equipped with a disposable one-way valve.

There are a number of limitations to the use of the pocket mask in the prehospital environment. Although they have been demonstrated to be superior to one-person bag-mask assembly

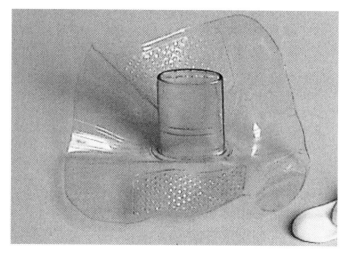

Figure 22-7 Barrier device.

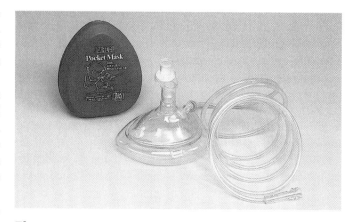

Figure 22-8 Pocket mask.

ventilation in regard to delivering appropriate tidal volumes, their inherent design makes them undesirable to use. They require a high degree of activity and respiratory fitness on the part of a rescuer to provide extended ventilation. Placing one's face so close to the patient's face increases the risk of blood, vomit, and body fluid exposure.[24–28] Also, the position for use is awkward. Nonetheless, these devices can be a good alternative to one-rescuer bag-mask assembly ventilation until assistance arrives.

The pocket mask is prepared by pushing the dome of the mask out of the cuff if the mask is stored in a collapsed position. The oxygen port is attached to an oxygen source at 15 LPM. An alternative is to place a nasal cannula on the rescuer at a high (10 LPM) flow. A one-way valve should be attached to the inhalation/exhalation port.

Manually Triggered Flow-Restricted, Oxygen-Powered Ventilation Devices

Manually triggered oxygen-powered ventilation devices have a long history in EMS. However, older models were neither flow nor pressure restricted and were prone to producing gastric inflation and barotrauma.[29,30] The more recent versions of these devices are flow restricted and the valve pressures are limited to less than 30 cm water, the commonly accepted cardiac sphincter opening pressure (Figure 22-9).

This pressure restriction limits gastric inflation, but does not eliminate it. Most of these devices can be both manually triggered or triggered in the same fashion as a demand valve device.

Flow-restricted oxygen-powered ventilation devices have the advantage of delivering high oxygen flow rates (40 LPM)

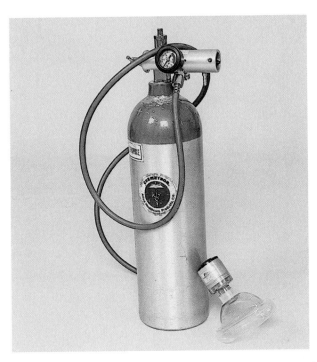

Figure 22-9 Flow-restricted, oxygen-powered ventilation device.

while using oxygen only during the "inhalation" phase of ventilation. They reliably deliver 100% oxygen. In addition, they can be used in patients who are awake to provide intermittent ventilatory support.

There are some limitations to these devices. These devices may still cause gastric inflation and barotrauma. Without a trigger extender, two rescuers are required to effectively use the devices. There are no studies that compare these devices to other ventilation devices. Nonetheless, they are still in use and may provide the Paramedic with a ventilatory alternative.

Preparation of a manually triggered flow-restricted, oxygen-powered ventilator is relatively straightforward. The device must be attached to a 50 PSI oxygen source. A mask is attached to the outlet port. Care must be taken to assure that the one-way valve unit is disassembled and cleaned after each use or that an in-line filter is used.

Automatic Transport Ventilators

Automatic transport ventilators (ATV), mechanical devices that deliver a specified volume of respiratory gas, have been used in the prehospital environment in Europe since the late 1970s. Although not used nearly as extensively in the United States, these devices are gaining increasing acceptance.[31,32] There are now several models of automatic transport ventilators that are designed specifically for use in the prehospital environment (Figure 22-10). Although most studies on these devices have focused on their use in the intubated patient, there has been some research into using automatic transport ventilators with a mask for face-mask ventilation.

The automatic transport ventilator has demonstrated a number of advantages compared to other methods of non-intubated ventilation. The ATV allows one rescuer to deliver consistent tidal volumes at a set rate. The automatic feature allows one rescuer to use both hands to seal the face mask. ATVs have demonstrated better lung inflation and less gastric inflation than bag-mask assemblies or oxygen-powered, manual-triggered devices. In addition, they consume significantly less oxygen than other devices.

There are disadvantages to the ventilators. They require an oxygen source to function and some even require an electrical source. They may be inappropriate for small

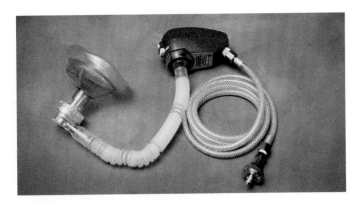

Figure 22-10 Automatic transport ventilator.

(<30 kg) patients. A bag-mask assembly must always be available for backup.

Although ventilators will vary widely by manufacturer, there are common features. All will have an oxygen input source that must usually be attached to a 50 PSI oxygen source. All will have a means of setting rate and volume. There is usually a method for providing various rates at different volumes and vice versa. Most will have a disposable circuit that attaches to the oxygen output, usually with an in-line filter and distal one-way valve. The distal end of the ventilation circuit will have a standard 15/22 mm coupling.

Beyond these features, however, the devices will vary widely. Most have a peak inspiratory pressure limit and an audible warning when that pressure is exceeded. Although most transport ventilators are volume cycled (deliver a specific volume regardless of pressure) or time cycled (deliver a set flow rate for a specific time period), there are pressure cycled (deliver to a specific pressure for a specific time) ATVs available. More sophisticated models will allow positive end expiratory pressure (PEEP) during ventilation as well as continuous positive airway pressure (CPAP). Finally, some devices may have a demand valve mechanism that allows patients to inspire on their own. These concepts in ventilation will be discussed in more detail in Chapter 25.

Suction

One of the most critically important pieces of airway management equipment is the suction unit. This device may

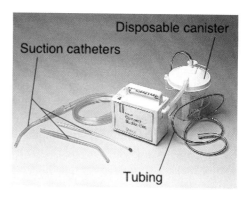

Figure 22-11 Portable suction unit.

convert an unmanageable airway into an easily managed airway through the removal of vomit, blood, and some foreign bodies. Prehospital suction units include portable devices (Figure 22-11) and fixed, wall-mounted units (Figure 22-12). Having these pieces of equipment immediately available during airway management is absolutely critical.

There are a number of different types of portable suction units. The least expensive are the hand-powered devices. Using the Paramedic's grip strength, these devices provide a lightweight, portable, and inexpensive alternative to portable suction. Unfortunately, they tend to have a low volume and are limited by the rescuer's hand strength and fatigue. Oxygen-powered suction units are another lightweight alternative.

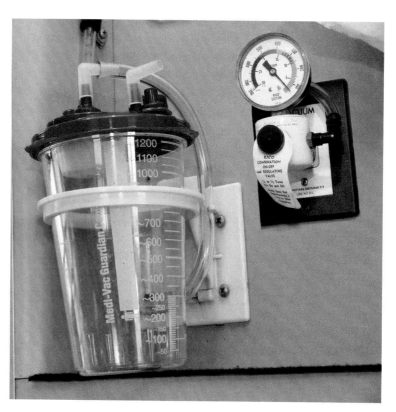

Figure 22-12 Wall-mounted suction unit.

They also have limited suction power and use large amounts of oxygen.

To provide more suction power, battery-powered suction units are often used. These devices, although more expensive, provide very strong suction and can suction large volumes. Their greatest limitation is that, in actual use, the batteries often loose their charge and integrity, resulting in loss of suction power after very short periods of suctioning. Some manufacturers have made devices that use interchangeable defibrillator batteries.

The strongest suction devices are the wall-mounted, vacuum-powered units. These units provide adjustable vacuum strength and completely disposable components. Although they provide the best suction, they are non-portable and can only be used in the ambulance. Nonetheless, they provide excellent suction.

Regardless of type, the suction unit should be able to generate an airflow at the tip of 40 LPM and a vacuum of 300 mmHg when the tubing is kinked closed. In addition, the collecting chambers and all parts of the device at high risk for contamination should either be disposable or easily disinfected.

In addition to the suction unit, the Paramedic will need suction tubing and suction catheters. The suction tubing should be thick walled and non-collapsible. The tubing should be large diameter, capable of handling large and highly viscous substances. In addition to the tubing, a selection of suction catheters will be needed including rigid and soft catheters.

The rigid pharyngeal suction catheters are known as Yankauer or tonsil tip catheters. They are designed to suction to the posterior pharynx and can handle large volumes of fluid rapidly.[33] Many of these catheters have a small side port that allows the Paramedic to apply suction only when desired. These devices are available in multiple sizes although they are most commonly grouped into the adult or pediatric size.

Multiple sizes of soft, sterile suction catheters should also be available to the Paramedic. These catheters come in a number of sizes and are flexible, allowing them to be passed through the mouth, the nose, an endotracheal tube, or a tracheostomy tube. These tubes, like the rigid pharyngeal suction tips, can become easily occluded with particulate matter. Therefore, it is important that water be available to flush the catheters. These catheters are often sized using the French catheter scale, which provides a measure of the outside diameter of the catheter. The smaller the number on the French scale, the smaller the outer diameter of the catheter.

There are side-port suction devices designed specifically to suction through endotracheal tubes. These devices feature a "T" or "Y" piece that allows the endotracheal tube to be attached to the ventilator circuit (or bag-mask assembly) without interrupting the gas flow. There is either an integrated soft suction catheter or a self-sealing port through which a soft catheter can be placed. These devices greatly facilitate endotracheal tube suctioning.

All suction devices should be routinely checked for function. Generally, suction tubing and sometimes even a rigid catheter are left attached to the suction device. If these are not attached, they should be stored on the device. Once the device has been turned on, the suction tubing should be kinked to test that adequate suction is generated.

Opening the Airway

Once the Paramedic has prepared his equipment, the next step is to open the airway and provide positive pressure ventilation. Using basic maneuvers is often the most important intervention a Paramedic can perform, particularly for the pediatric patient in respiratory distress or arrest but not yet in cardiac arrest.

As was discussed in Chapter 20, the most common anatomical cause of airway obstruction is the epiglottis along with the soft palate.[9] Since uvular manipulation is less important if the patient has a patent oral cavity and oropharynx, airway manipulation techniques are oriented toward establishing a patent hypopharynx. Although traditional teaching has focused on the tongue as the most common source of airway obstruction, head-tilt, chin-lift, modified jaw thrust, and jaw-thrust techniques apply equally well to epiglottis management. This is due to the ligaments and muscles that interconnect the epiglottis, the hyoid, the mandible, and the tongue.

For most non-trauma patients in respiratory arrest, the technique of choice for opening the airway is the head-tilt, chin lift. The maneuver extends the neck over the atlanto-occipital joint (the joint between the skull and the first vertebrae). In addition, the chin lift displaces the mandible anteriorly. This in turn pulls the hyoid anteriorly and via the hyoepiglottic ligament, the epiglottis.

The technique is performed by placing the palm of one hand on the forehead and either actively hooking the mandible with the fingers and lifting or griping the tip of the mentum (chin) between two fingers and pulling forward. A common error is to simply place the fingers on the mandible and push upward. This action closes the mouth without moving the hyoid anteriorly. The jaw must be actively displaced in an anterior and caudad direction. In addition, minimal pressure should be applied to the soft tissue under the mandible as this may push the hyoid posteriorly.

For the patient with suspected cervical spine injury, the head-tilt, chin lift can compromise the cerviocal spine; particularly in high cervical injuries involving the first and second cervical vertebrae.[34-37] Therefore, an alternative technique—the modified jaw thrust—must be used. This technique displaces the jaw anteriorly, pulling the hyoid and epiglottis anteriorly as well. There is minimal cervical spine movement if the jaw thrust is performed correctly.

The modified jaw thrust is usually performed from the top of the patient's head, although it can also be performed from an inferior position if needed. From above the patient's head, the right and left hand are placed palm-in on the right and left side of the patient's head. The thumbs are placed on the prominence of the cheekbones and the fingers are placed along the ramus and angle of the mandible. The fingers are then lifted anteriorly and caudally (toward the feet) while the thumbs push posteriorly. These opposing actions open the mouth and lift the hyoid and epiglottis. If the technique is performed from below the head, the only difference in hand position is that the airway manager's right hand will be on the left side of the patient's face and vice versa. The jaw will essentially be pulled toward the rescuer, again opening the airway.

The modified jaw thrust can be performed on any patient regardless of suspicion of C-spine injury. The hand positioning allows the Paramedic to both open the airway and form a mask seal at the same time. A sustained modified jaw thrust, however, can be very tiring and may require multiple rescuers to switch in and out of the role.

A third technique, the tongue-jaw lift, can also be used in limited circumstances. In this technique, the thumb is placed in the mouth and the fingers under the chin. The jaw is then pulled forward. Although this technique effectively opens the airway, it severely compromises the ability to ventilate the patient with a face-mask technique. In addition, it requires the Paramedic to keep his thumb in the patient's mouth. This technique puts the Paramedic at risk for losing a digit, something that should be avoided if at all possible. To avoid having the patient bite the Paramedic, a large oral airway can be lodged sideways in between the molars to act as a bite block. Even with the placement of an oral airway as a bite block, the tongue-jaw thrust is probably of limited practical use in the prehospital environment because it limits ventilation.

Cricoid Pressure

While opening the airway, the Paramedic should also consider the benefits of **cricoid pressure** (Figure 22-13). This technique, referred to as Sellick's maneuver, involves the identifying the cricoid ring and assigning an individual to gently apply approximately 10 pounds of pressure in a posterior direction throughout airway management; from the onset of ventilation until completion of intubation. Since the cricoid is a complete ring, the pressure is transferred directly to the esophagus and helps to keep the esophagus closed.[38-42]

Cricoid pressure has long been considered to prevent passive regurgitation and limit active emesis when properly applied. Additionally, cricoid pressure may decrease gastric inflation during positive pressure ventilation. It is a non-invasive technique and, as long as it is maintained continuously, can limit (although not eliminate) the risk of aspiration.

Cricoid pressure is not without its limitations. Cricoid pressure can actually worsen the view of the vocal cords

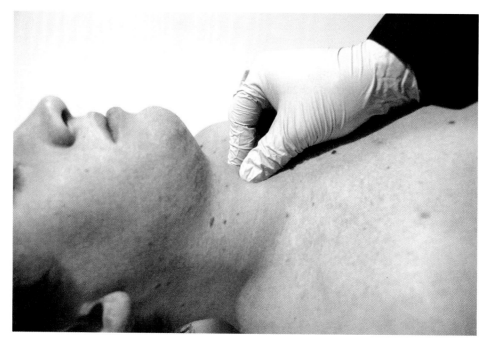

Figure 22-13 Cricoid pressure.

during laryngoscopy.[43] Even when properly applied, it does not completely eliminate the risk of aspiration. In addition, in vigorous emesis, it can lead to esophageal rupture; therefore cricoid pressure should be released if the patient actively vomits. Excessive posterior pressure can also compromise an unstable cervical spine injury, as the cricoid cartilage is juxtapositioned across from the fourth cervical vertebrae. Excessive posterior pressure may also cause laryngeal trauma if excessive force is applied. In pediatric patients, excessive force can actually occlude the trachea because the cartilage rings that maintain an open trachea have not fully formed in the younger pediatric patient.[44] Finally, cricoids pressure must be vigilantly maintained throughout airway management until large volume, high-capacity suction is available and, preferably, the patient is endotracheally intubated. Premature release of cricoid pressure can result in copious and explosive emesis.

Another significant limitation to cricoid pressure is that, unfortunately, pressure is often not on the cricoid at all but is applied to the thyroid cartilage. As will be discussed next, landmark recognition and appropriate identification of the cricoid ring can be difficult.[45] Often, pressure will be applied to the most prominent structure, usually the thyroid cartilage.

There are a number of untoward consequences of thyroid cartilage pressure. First, the thyroid cartilage is an incomplete structure, so posterior pressure will not achieve esophageal occlusion. Second, pressure on the thyroid cartilage may cause the opening of the larynx to tip anteriorly, making endotracheal intubation more difficult. Third, excessive pressure may cause laryngeal injury. Therefore, proper location of the cricoid ring is critical for effective and safe performance of this skill.

To overcome the challenges of locating the cricoid ring, the Paramedic should be familiar with the anatomy of the region, as described in Chapter 20. Although there are a number of methods for locating the cricoid ring, the easiest begins with locating the prominence of the thyroid cartilage. This is usually the most prominent anterior midline structure of the neck. Once this landmark is identified, the index finger should be placed on it and then moved inferiorly along the midline.

The next landmark is the cricothyroid membrane, the ligamentous band between the thyroid cartilage and the cricoid ring. The inferior border of the thyroid cartilage should be easily identified and a soft depression can be felt. The inferior border of this depression is a solid structure, the cricoid ring. Once the cricoid ring is identified, the thumb and index finger should be placed on it and pressure applied posteriorly.[46] This pressure should be maintained until the patient is intubated or, at a minimum, high-capacity suction is available.

Face-Mask Ventilation

Once the airway is opened, the patient may begin to breathe spontaneously. If this is not the case, the Paramedic must begin ventilation of the apneic patient. The skill of "assisted

ventilation" for the patient in respiratory distress, not arrest, will be discussed later. The technique for providing ventilation will depend on the device used.

The Mask/Face Interface

The most important task of bag-valve-mask ventilation is to form an effective mask seal while maintaining an open airway. Recalling that the mouth is kept open by caudad (footward) displacement of the mandible while the hypopharynx is kept open by the anterior displacement of the hyoid, any technique to form a mask seal must also displace the mandible correctly. Although much is made of the pressure on the mask in forming the seal, the most important component of a good mask seal is to actually bring the face anteriorly and into the mask.

The best mask seal which maintains an open airway is made with light downward pressure on the mask and more forceful upward displacement of the mandible. The lower face is, in essence, "gathered" into the mask to form the seal. This method of forming a mask seal maintains an open mouth, an anterior displacement of the hyoid and epiglottis, and a tight junction between the mask and the facial tissue. This is in contrast to strong posterior pressure on the mask that may close the mouth and will push the hyoid and epiglottis posteriorly.

The fundamental method of gripping the mandible and the mask is the "C" and "E" technique. The major difference between one-rescuer bag-mask assembly ventilation and other techniques (two-rescuer and three-rescuer bag-mask assembly, ATV, etc.) is that with one-rescuer bag-mask assembly ventilation, only one hand is used to make the seal while with the other techniques, one of the rescuers has both hands free for the procedure.[47–50]

The mask is gripped with the thumb at the nasal side of the mask and the index finger on the chin side of the mask. These two fingers are curved to make a "C" shape. The middle, ring, and little finger are extended along the mandible with the little finger pushing forward on the angle of the mandible. These three fingers are spread to make an "E" shape. Using the "C" and "E" technique, the Paramedic should be able to maintain a sufficient mask seal while bringing the lower face up into the mask. If a two-handed technique is used, both hands make mirror image "C's" and "E's."

Certain facial characteristics will also make forming a mask seal more difficult. These include a small jaw (**micrognathia**), a large tongue (**macroglossia**), facial hair and trauma, no teeth (**edentulous**), and patients with minimal subcutaneous fat.[9] Micrognathia and macroglossia require vigilance to anterior jaw displacement and maintaining the most open mouth possible. A better seal may be obtained on patients with facial hair if water-based lubricant is applied to the mask and the facial hair before ventilation. Patients with facial trauma present a significant challenge.

The best technique is to focus on gathering the face into the mask and suctioning frequently. Specific injuries such as penetrating objects or puncture wounds to the face may require stabilization and sealing of the wound with petroleum gauze to prevent air leakage. If a patient has dentures, these should be left in place to facilitate the mask seal.[51] Premature removal of the dentures will result in a poor mask seal. Patients with thin subcutaneous tissue or excessive subcutaneous fat will benefit from the use of a softer mask or one into which air can be added and removed.

Ventilation Volume and Airway Pressure

Once the Paramedic has opened and is maintaining the airway and has achieved a good mask seal, the next action is to ventilate the patient. When a patient is receiving ventilation from a face mask, ventilatory gasses have the opportunity to enter either the trachea or esophagus. Although the trachea usually offers the path of least resistance, the lungs have a limited volume beyond which they will not expand. Therefore, any excess volume will end up in the stomach.

The main determinant of esophageal resistance is the lower esophageal, or cardiac sphincter, opening pressure. Not an actual valve, the **lower esophageal sphincter (LES)** is a functional portion of the esophagus where the walls of the esophagus contract inwardly, forming a physical barrier to the reflux of stomach contents up the esophagus. Although probably somewhat lower in the prehospital patient, the accepted value for normal LES opening pressure in healthy individuals is 30 cm water. Upper airway pressures in excess of 30 cm water will cause the LES to open. Most likely, LES opening occurs over a range of pressures, with lower pressures causing small leaks and high pressures causing larger leaks.

In addition, there are a number of factors which relax the LES. Alcohol, mint, chocolate, and caffeine will all relax the LES. In addition, LES opening pressure drops in cardiac arrest to almost zero within a few minutes. If any of these factors are present, the LES will open at lower pressures, increasing the risk of gastric distention and vomiting. These are two consequences which can be minimized with thoughtful face-mask ventilation.

The tidal volume in a healthy individual is somewhere between 5 to 7 cc/kg of ideal body weight.[52–54] At a respiratory rate of 12, this results in a minute ventilation of 4 to 5 LPM. For an acutely ill patient (e.g., asthma), the minute ventilation demands may reach almost 20 LPM. In general, however, the ventilation demands of most prehospital patients do not exceed 7 cc/kg/breath. Therefore, the Paramedic should attempt to deliver a tidal volume of 6 to 8 cc/kg ideal body weight/breath.

The volume delivered can be thought of as depending on two variables: gas flow rate and duration of flow. That is, the same volume (i.e., 800 cc) can be delivered if the gas flow rate is 800 cc/second and the patient is ventilated for one second as is delivered if the gas flow rate is 400 cc/second and the patient is ventilated over two seconds.

This is important because the pressure is related to the flow rate of the gas. A higher pressure is needed to deliver a large volume in a short time period. On the other hand, less pressure is needed if that volume is delivered over a long time period. Since high airway pressure is the main cause for gastric inflation and barotrauma, it is important to maintain as low an airway pressure as possible during ventilation.

The gas flow/pressure/volume relationships are practical because oxygenated tidal volume delivery is probably the most important goal of bag-valve-mask ventilation. Since the same tidal volume (and same amount of oxygen) can be delivered at lower pressures if the inspiratory phase is longer, the Paramedic should focus on providing slower, longer duration, and lower pressure ventilations. In fact, ventilation that delivers less oxygen to the stomach and more to the lungs is better ventilation.

The practical consequences are that while the ventilatory rate (12 to 16 breaths per minute for an adult, 20 breaths per minute for a pediatric patient) remains the same, the ventilations themselves are given over a longer time period. The inspiratory phase of ventilation should occur over two seconds and the expiratory phase should take about the same amount of time. If a bag-mask assembly device is being used, the Paramedic should use a mental trigger like "squeeze, squeeze, release, release" while performing ventilations.

Bag-valve-mask ventilators are available with built-in and aftermarket add-on manometers that allow the Paramedic to know exactly how much airway pressure is being generated. In addition, most mechanical ventilation devices (manually triggered flow-restricted, oxygen-powered ventilators and automatic transport ventilators) have built-in pressure relief valves. Whenever possible, a manometer should be used to minimize the risks of overpressurization. If a manometer is not available, however, delivering the ventilations as previously described should provide the minimum pressures possible.

Bag-Mask Ventilation

The most commonly used device, as discussed previously, is the bag-mask assembly. The greatest limitation to this device is that it is difficult for a single rescuer to provide effective tidal volumes. The difficulty arises from the need to simultaneously form a mask seal, maintain an open airway, and squeeze the bag.

Effectively performing all three techniques single-handedly is almost impossible. Therefore, although one-rescuer bag-mask ventilation is commonly performed, two-rescuer ventilation is much preferred. In addition, there are three rescuer techniques that are also used, as will be discussed in the following text.

One key to proper performance of bag-valve-mask ventilation is maintaining a proper mask seal (Figure 22-14). The Paramedic's thumb and pointer finger form the letter "C" over the edge of the mask, applying pressure to hold the mask to the

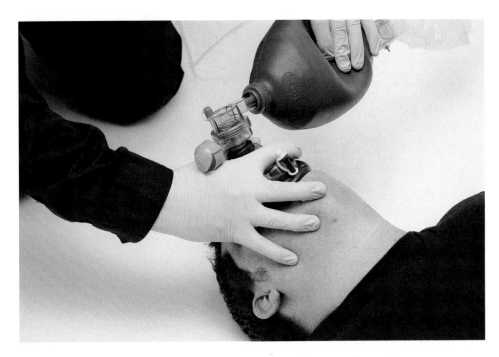

Figure 22-14 Proper hand positioning to maintain bag-valve-mask seal.

face. The other three fingers form the letter "E" firmly holding the mandible, allowing the provider to simultaneously provide either a jaw thrust or chin lift depending on the need to limit cervical spine movement.

Estimating the volume delivered can also be difficult. The Paramedic should take advantage of any opportunities to practice this skill when volume measuring is available. Several simple rules can assist the Paramedic in estimating the ventilation volume.

First, the volume should be sufficient to cause chest rise but not so much that the chest stops rising. The breath should enter with little resistance and abdominal distention should not be seen. There should, in fact, be almost no abdominal movement. In addition, the Paramedic should know the volume of the bag on the bag-mask assembly. The average adult bag is 1,600 mL. Therefore, for a 70 kg male, approximately one third of the volume of that bag should be delivered.

For Paramedics with small hands, there are techniques which may be employed as an alternative to squeezing the bag with two hands. Although no research has ever been performed to demonstrate the safety and efficacy of these techniques, there are anecdotal stories of effective ventilations being performed with their use. In the first technique, the bag is compressed between the rescuer's hand or forearm and a solid object, such as the rescuer's leg. In the second technique, the rescuer uses both hands to open the airway and form the mask seal while the bag mask is squeezed between the thighs. The major limitation of these techniques is the possibility of poor control of the delivered volume. If the Paramedic is unable to effectively estimate the delivered volume, then these techniques should not be used. In addition, since many larger muscle groups are being used, these techniques can be very tiring. These techniques are mentioned only because they have been described and used. However, they have not been validated. The Paramedic must decide what technique is safest and most effective for the patient.

Although the least recommended of the bag-mask assembly techniques, single-rescuer bag-mask assembly ventilation is probably the most common prehospital method of ventilation. There are several key points to remember in performing single-rescuer bag-mask assembly ventilation. The first is that maintaining an open airway while establishing a good mask seal with one hand is difficult and, in some patients, impossible. The Paramedic should recognize when a patient cannot be ventilated without a second rescuer and immediately call for assistance. The second key to performing good one-rescuer bag-mask assembly ventilation is to be able to provide appropriate one-handed tidal volumes.

The two-rescuer technique of bag-mask assembly ventilation (Figure 22-15) is a much more effective method of providing ventilatory support. The major difference between this and one-rescuer ventilation is that each rescuer can now focus on a specific component of the procedure. The Paramedic responsible for opening the airway and forming the mask seal can use both hands to do this while the Paramedic responsible for ventilation is better able to control the ventilatory volume and rate. The same techniques and volumes as mentioned for one-rescuer ventilation apply to two-rescuer ventilation. This is the recommended technique for performing bag-mask assembly ventilation.

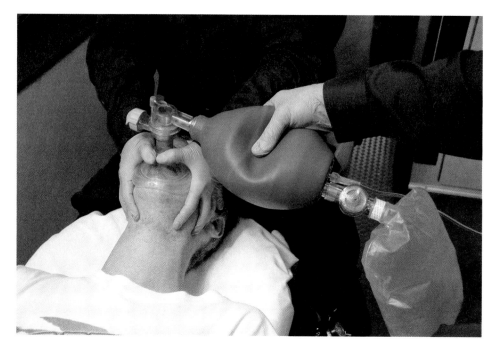

Figure 22-15 Two-rescuer bag-mask assembly ventilation.

There may be times when mask seal is difficult but additional rescuers are available. There are two forms of three-rescuer bag-mask assembly ventilation that can be performed.

In the first of the two techniques, the third rescuer assists in making a mask seal. Once the first two rescuers are in position, the third rescuer applies posterior pressure to the mask. Although there may be some merit to this technique if the mask seal is particularly difficult to obtain, it has a number of limitations.

As was discussed previously, the most effective mask seal is made by gathering the patient's face anteriorly into the mask, not by pushing the mask posteriorly. The posterior pressure increases the risk of occluding the airway. In addition, having three people this close to the head makes the airway very "crowded" and moving the patient or performing other techniques may become impossible.

The second technique for three-rescuer bag-mask assembly involves having the third rescuer apply posterior cricoid pressure, as discussed previously. This technique offers the advantage of having an extra hand available (the rescuer's hand not applying cricoid pressure) if needed to assist the two primary Paramedics without overcrowding the area around the patient's face. In addition, the benefits of cricoid pressure are also obtained.

Pocket Mask Ventilation

Using the pocket mask requires only two skills: forming a mask seal and not hyperventilating. The pocket mask is sealed to the face in the same manner as other masks. The Paramedic can use a two-handed technique to make the mask seal, improving the quality of the seal and allowing the

airway to be maintained open more easily. The key to preventing hyperventilation is for the Paramedic to take a slow deep breath during the patient's expiratory phase and then to deliver the ventilation slowly over two seconds.[55,56]

Manually Triggered Flow-Restricted, Oxygen-Powered Ventilation Devices

These devices offer a manual alternative for one-rescuer ventilation. The mask seal is made as described previously. If the ventilation device has a well-designed trigger, the mask seal can be made with two hands and the device still triggered without having to release the seal. If the trigger is poorly placed, however, it may be necessary to perform a one-handed seal while the other hand triggers the device. Otherwise, a two-rescuer approach may be needed. This second technique, unfortunately, negates most of the benefits that manually triggered flow-restricted, oxygen-powered ventilation devices offer over single-rescuer bag-mask assembly techniques.

Since the devices are manually triggered, it is important that the Paramedic provide no more than two seconds of ventilation at a time. Although the devices should have integrated overpressurization relief valves, a prolonged inspiratory phase without an expiratory phase may result in gastric inflation and the potential for barotrauma.

Automatic Transport Ventilators

The automatic transport ventilator is a relatively simple tool for face-mask ventilation. As was discussed previously, the ventilator is set at an appropriate rate and volume for the patient. The ventilator circuit is then attached to the mask

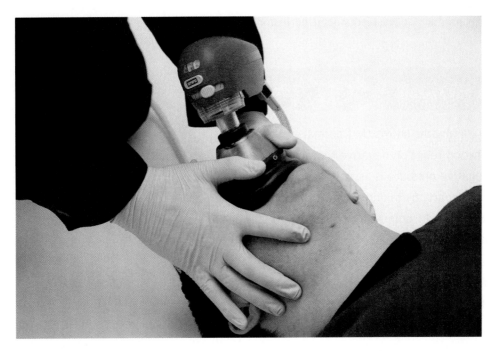

Figure 22-16 Assisting ventilations with an automatic transport ventilator.

and the mask seal obtained with a two-hand technique (Figure 22-16). The ventilator will automatically cycle at the preset rate, freeing the Paramedic to focus solely on maintaining the mask seal and keeping the airway patent. Shortly after ventilation is initiated, it is important to assess that the proper rate and volume have been selected. This is done through observation of the chest rise and fall. In addition, all ventilators should have an overpressurization relief valve and alarm. If the alarm sounds, it is important to immediately reduce the volume and check the rate to assure that "breath stacking" is not occurring. Breath stacking occurs when insufficient time is allowed for exhalation.

Continuing Ventilatory Care

If the Paramedic is able to successfully ventilate the patient, there are some immediate postventilation activities that must be performed. These include assessing the patient, inserting an oropharyngeal (if tolerated) or nasopharyngeal airway, and preparing the patient for transport. Each of these activities is important to assure that adequate ongoing care is being provided.

STREET SMART

The "look, listen, and feel" step of CPR is important for any patient who is being assisted in ventilation.

Patient Assessment for the Ventilated Patient

It is important for the Paramedic to assess all patients whom she believes are being adequately ventilated. The most important assessments are observation, auscultation, and physiologic monitoring. The most important task to complete immediately is to observe the patient. Chest rise and fall should be noted. The abdomen should be observed for signs of gastric inflation. In addition, unless the patient is in cardiac arrest, the signs of respiratory failure (pallor, cyanosis, and diaphoresis) should begin to improve. Immediate and ongoing observations of the patient and of the effectiveness of ventilation will provide early warning of ventilatory failure.

Once a general observation is complete, the Paramedic should auscultate lung sounds. Auscultation can give some idea of the adequacy of ventilation (e.g., are lung sounds heard over the lung bases?). In addition, diagnostic clues may be discovered including asymmetric lung sounds, adventitious lung sounds (wheezes, crackles, and rhonchi), or absent lung sounds. Auscultation over the epigastrium may also give the Paramedic a sense of how much gastric inflation is occurring. In addition, a complete reassessment of airway, breathing, and circulation, including lung field and epigastric auscultation, should be performed anytime a patient's status changes.

After observation and auscultation, the patient should have physiologic signs measured and monitored. These include pulse, blood pressure, EKG, and pulse oximetry. The pulse oximetry probe should be applied early. A good pulse oximetry signal at a finger or earlobe indicates a blood pressure sufficient to produce at least peripheral perfusion (Figure 22-17).

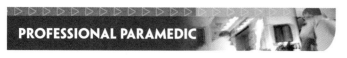

PROFESSIONAL PARAMEDIC

The professional Paramedic knows that normal pulmonary respiration relies on negative thoracic pressure. This negative pressure is assistive in allowing blood return to the heart. By taking over ventilation, the physiology is changed from negative pressure to positive pressure. The patient may experience signs of diminished cardiac output. This situation may be exacerbated by a ventilation rate that exceeds the suggested rate for age.

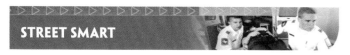

STREET SMART

Continuously monitored pulse oximetry allows the Paramedic to monitor oxygenation saturation during procedures such as suctioning and intubation. When the saturation begins to drop, stop the procedure and ventilate/oxygenate the patient.

In addition, the pulse oximetry will give a preliminary pulse rate and the hemoglobin oxygen saturation. The blood pressure and pulse rate should then be measured manually. An EKG (rhythm strip) should also be obtained to assess for arrhythmias. These parameters should be continuously monitored to assure that they remain stable or improve. Any deterioration (tachycardia, bradycardia, hyper- or hypotension, or hypoxia) should trigger an immediate search for a cause.

After assessment, the patient should be prepared for transport. Generally speaking, these patients are most easily transported on a long spine board. Care must be taken, particularly for pediatric patients, to assure that the positioning on the board does not cause the airway to obstruct. Unlike the intubated patient (discussed in Chapter 23), placement of a cervical collar for the non-trauma patient is not recommended as it will make maintaining a patent airway and mask seal more difficult.

Gastric Distention

Gastric inflation and subsequent vomiting and aspiration are significant risks associated with face-mask ventilation.[57–59] Although proper ventilation technique will minimize the risk of gastric inflation, the risk cannot be eliminated.

Therefore, the Paramedic must monitor for increasing abdominal girth, vomiting, and difficulty performing ventilation as signs of gastric inflation. If gastric inflation is detected, several interventions can be performed to minimize its impact.

At the first sign of gastric inflation, the airway manager should reassess the ventilation rate, volume, and airway pressures. These should be corrected if needed. In addition, suction should be prepared and made immediately available. If significant gastric inflation has occurred and is interfering with ventilation, it must be corrected by placing either a nasogastric or orogastric tube and attaching it to suction.

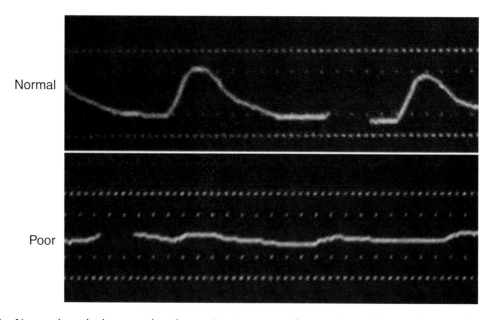

Figure 22-17 Normal and abnormal pulse oximetry waveform. A good waveform indicates adequate perfusion to produce an accurate numerical value.

Failed Ventilation

If the first attempt at ventilation is unsuccessful, the Paramedic must make an assessment of the causes of failure. This assessment should reevaluate the provider, the patient, and the equipment being used. Once this assessment is complete, further consideration of additional interventions and equipment must be made.

Reevaluation

In reevaluating the provider, the Paramedic must examine his own technique. Single-person bag-mask assembly ventilation, limited in the best of circumstances, may simply not be possible and another rescuer may be needed. All providers, however, should have sufficient skill and training to provide two-person bag-mask assembly ventilation.

The patient should also be reassessed. The most common cause of ventilatory failure is that the airway was not appropriately opened. Therefore, the airway opening technique and the patient positioning should be evaluated. Ideally, the airway opening maneuver should be performed again.[60] In addition, the patient should be reassessed to determine if anatomic or pathologic features are making ventilation difficult. Conditions which make forming a mask seal difficult were discussed earlier. The Paramedic must consider if any of these conditions are present.

The Paramedic must then assess the equipment. Equipment failure is not uncommon and can occur at highly inopportune times. Masks may leak and oxygen sources may be empty. Mechanical ventilators may suffer part fatigue or failure. If there is any suggestion of equipment malfunction, an alternative device should be considered and utilized.

Oropharyngeal and Nasophayngeal Airway Placement

Once the Paramedic has reassessed and repositioned the patient, he must consider the use of ancillary techniques and equipment. The insertion of an oropharyngeal or nasopharyngeal airway is therefore appropriate.

As discussed previously, oropharyngeal airways help to displace the tongue and, ultimately, the hyoid anteriorly. There are multiple methods for inserting oral airways. Personal preference, at least for the adult patient, is the best guide.

The ultimate position of the oral airway is with the flange resting at the lips and the curve of the oral airway matching the curve of the oropharynx. The airway can be inserted in one of three ways. For all three methods, the mouth must be opened using either a chin-lift technique or a crossed finger technique in which the thumb and index finger "cross" each other and push the teeth in opposite directions. Any visible foreign bodies should be removed.

In the first method, the tongue is controlled with a tongue depressor or by the Paramedic using a jaw-thrust technique. The oral airway is inserted with the curvature in the same direction as the curvature of the airway and the tip of the oral airway toward the glottis. The oral airway is advanced until the flange rests on the lips and the positioning is reassessed to assure that the tongue has not been pushed posteriorly. This method is recommended for pediatric patients.

The second and third methods are similar in that neither requires a tongue depressor and in both the tip of the airway is initially not pointing toward the glottis. Instead, the distal tip of the airway is either pointed toward the cheek (method 2) or toward the palate (method 3). The oral airway is advanced to approximately half its length and then rotated so that the distal tip points toward the glottis. The flange is again advanced to the lips and its position is confirmed.

Placement of the nasopharyngeal airway requires the Paramedic to assess which nostril is more likely to accommodate the airway. Evidence of nasal fracture or septal deviation should be noted. Once the nare has been chosen, the tip of the nose should be pushed superiorly so that the nares are closer to parallel with the face. With the bevel facing toward the septum, the nasopharyngeal airway is inserted parallel to the floor of the nasal cavity.

Due to the design of nasal airways, different initial orientation is required based on which nare is used. If the airway is inserted in the right nare, the curvature of the nasal airway should be in the same direction as the curvature of the nasopharynx. If the nasal airway is inserted into the left nare, however, the curvature is upside down. This is due to the way the bevel is designed. Once the bevel is entirely within the left side of the nasal cavity, the nasal airway is then rotated 180° and the airway advanced.

The airway is advanced until the flange rests against the opening of the nare. If resistance is met, the nasal airway should be gently rotated from side to side but should not be forced. The patient may gag and vomit; therefore, the Paramedic should be prepared to suction the patient if needed. If the patient is gagging excessively or appears to be having difficulty breathing, the Paramedic should remove the nasal airway and replace it with a shorter one.

Suctioning

While reevaluating the airway, it may become evident that vomit or fluids in the airway need to be suctioned. The suction unit should have already been prepared for just such an eventuality. Although the finger sweep (discussed later) or the use of the Magill forceps (discussed in Chapter 23) may be necessary to manage foreign bodies, blood and vomit can usually be handled with standard suctioning procedures. The primary goal of suctioning is to minimize the risk of aspiration and to prevent it, if possible. All suctioning efforts must be directed toward that end.

The rigid Yankauer or tonsil tip suction is the device of choice for suctioning the oral cavity and the oropharynx. If possible, the patient should be pre- and postoxygenated; however, this may not be possible if the patient is apneic and the Paramedic has not been able to ventilate the patient. The tip should be placed in the mouth and advanced to the posterior oropharynx. At no time should the distal end of the tip be completely out of sight. Suction is applied as the tip is withdrawn. The Paramedic should avoid applying suction to mucous membranes or other attached structures. No more than 15 seconds of suction should be applied continuously in order to avoid hypoxia.[61] After suctioning, the airway should be reassessed and, if appropriate, the patient should be ventilated and oxygenated. If on reassessment there remains a significant amount of material that interferes with ventilation, resuction the patient.

Obstructed Airway Management

If after the second ventilation attempt it is impossible to ventilate the patient, the patient should be assumed to have an airway obstruction. There are a number of causes of airway obstruction including the epiglottis, the soft palate, foreign bodies, laryngospasm, laryngeal edema, and airway trauma. If proper airway opening techniques were applied, then the epiglottis and soft palate should have been addressed. On the other hand, obstruction laryngospasm, laryngeal edema, and significant airway trauma cannot be dealt with at a basic airway management level. Efforts must focus on ventilating as best as possible and transporting the patient rapidly. Foreign body obstruction, however, can and should be addressed.

If the patient is conscious and has evidence of complete airway obstruction, then abdominal thrusts should be applied from behind. It is important, whenever possible, to treat an airway obstruction while the patient is conscious.[62-65] Once a patient with an airway obstruction becomes unconscious, mortality increases rapidly.[66] Therefore, aggressive management of the conscious patient with a possible airway obstruction is mandatory.

If, however, the patient becomes unconscious or is found unresponsive and has a foreign body airway obstruction, the techniques of abdominal thrusts described in the following text should be used.

For infants, back blows are the preferred method of clearing the airway (Figure 22-18). Otherwise, the sequence of back blows, airway assessment, and attempts at ventilation remain the same.

The finger sweep is a technique of limited value in the EMS environment. Suction and laryngoscopy perform the task of foreign body management much more effectively. Finger sweeps are probably most useful in the patient who is vomiting more than the suction can handle.

If the patient still cannot be ventilated after suctioning, repositioning, and obstructed airway skills have been applied,

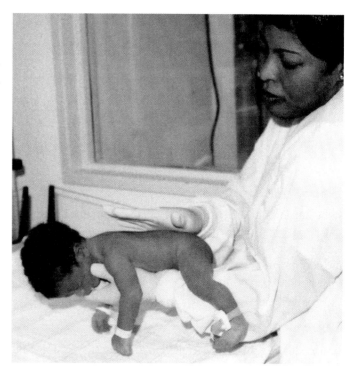

Figure 22-18 Infant back blows.

then the patient must be transported rapidly or turned over to a caregiver capable of performing advanced airway management procedures. No further value is gained by delaying on-scene.

Assisted Ventilation

Although most patients who receive face-mask ventilation in the prehospital environment are apneic, some breathing patients will benefit from ventilatory support. These patients may be tachypneic or bradypneic. The most important characteristic of these patients is that their ventilatory effort is insufficient to meet their metabolic demands.

Assisted ventilation is the process of augmenting the breaths a patient is taking to provide more effective respirations. The device most commonly used for this process is the BVM. The key to this technique is that the Paramedic must time ventilation with the patient's own inspiratory effort and assure a minimum minute ventilation. In the patient who is very bradypneic, it may be necessary to provide additional breaths between the assisted breaths to meet the minimum minute ventilation. On the other hand, for a patient who is tachypneic, it is not necessary to supplement every ventilation. The goal of assisted ventilation is to provide patients with approximately 12 to 20 breaths/minute that meet the patient's appropriate tidal volume (6 to 8 cc/kg).

If the patient remains responsive, it is important to explain what will be done and why it is being done. For the patient who is already hypoxic, the face mask may cause claustrophobia and a sense of suffocation. In addition, the patient may feel some resistance to inhalation. In addition, use of an anxiolytic such as diazepam or midazolam may make the patient more comfortable during assisted ventilation.[67]

An appropriate-sized mask is selected and the Paramedic makes a one-handed mask seal. The other hand gently compresses the bag and stops when the bag is slightly dimpled. The Paramedic waits until the patient begins to inhale before squeezing the bag to provide a full ventilation. When the patient begins to exhale, the bag is released. This process of supplementing the patient's own inspiration should occur 12 to 20 times/minute.

The most difficult part of this skill is the timing of the ventilation. If the ventilation is delivered while the patient is exhaling, not only will it be ineffective but also high airway pressures, barotrauma, and gastric inflation may occur. If the breath is delivered too early, the patient will feel suffocated and uncomfortable. Therefore, the timing of the assisted breath is critical. The Paramedic must be able to sense when the patient is beginning to inspire and deliver the assisted ventilation at that time. There are three ways in which the start of inspiration can be determined. The first is to simply observe the patient's chest. When the chest begins to expand, the patient is inspiring, and the breath should be delivered. Unfortunately, these patients will not usually tolerate being laid flat and the Paramedic will often stand behind the upright patient. Therefore, observation may be ineffective.

The two other methods of determining the start of inspiration do not require direct patient observation. The first involves placing a finger on the bag-mask assembly and mandibular soft tissues. When the patient begins to inspire, the mouth will usually open slightly and the larynx will pull superiorly. These movements can be palpated and recognized as the time to initiate ventilation. The other method involves dimpling the bag with the fingers before providing the ventilation. By applying a slight amount of pressure to the bag, the pressure within the mask can be monitored. When the bag begins to compress easily, the patient has begun to inspire and the bag should be squeezed to deliver the appropriate tidal volume. Although this technique requires some practice, it is a very effective method of determining when to ventilate.

The patient should be continuously assessed during assisted ventilation. While the increased tidal volume and adequate minute ventilation may cause the patient to improve, the patient's underlying disease process may cause him to decompensate. The Paramedic must be vigilant to assure that the patient is receiving adequate ventilatory support.

Continuous Positive Airway Pressure

With almost 70 years of use in the hospital and home setting, continuous positive airway pressure (CPAP) devices are slowly but surely making their way into the field of prehospital care.[68–72] Simple, more lightweight, and considerably less expensive technology has placed this mode of airway care into the reach of most EMS systems.

CPAP is essentially a way of assuring that in all phases of the respiratory cycle the airway pressure is above zero (zero being the atmospheric pressure). During the normal respiratory cycle, the intrathoracic pressure becomes negative during inspiration, zero at the end of inspiration, positive during expiration, and zero again at the end of expiration. These pressures are generated not by external forces but rather through the musculature and bony structures of the chest cavity. The mechanism for producing negative pressure was discussed in Chapter 20. Positive pressure is generated by the elastic recoil of the chest wall. The alveoli are held open via surfactant and their indirect attachment to the chest wall. At the zero pressure end of expiration, however, the alveoli can collapse, resulting in atelectasis. This is the issue that CPAP attempts to address.

In the healthy adult, sighing is a reflex mechanism that opens collapsed areas of the lung. Grunting against a closed glottis achieves the same end. These mechanisms become less effective during disease. For the patient with emphysema, the alveolar walls break down, decreasing effective oxygen exchange surface and increasing the risk of collapse. Patients with congestive heart failure (CHF) are also more susceptible to alveolar collapse. At the end of expiration, the surfactant in these patients may be insufficient to keep open the airways, allowing the alveoli to collapse during exhalation. These patients may not then have the ability to re-expand the collapsed alveoli, and so they have less gas exchange surface and become more hypoxic and hypercarbic.

CPAP uses a combination of gas flow and resistance to exhalation to increase the minimum airway pressure. High-flow gas (oxygen mixed with room air) is fed into the mask at 50 to 100 LPM. The mask is tightly sealed against the patient's face, only allowing exhaled gas to escape through an exhalation port and CPAP valve. The CPAP valve is a special valve designed to open at a set pressure (typically 5 to 15 cm water). If that pressure is not present, the valve will not open.

As respiratory gasses can only escape through the CPAP valve, gas will build up in the system, resulting in increased pressure. The whole connected system includes the CPAP generator, the large volume tubing, the face mask, the patient's airways, and the lungs. The pressure will eventually equalize throughout the system. Since the gas flow is so high, the pressure in the system quickly reaches the opening pressure of the CPAP valve. If the CPAP valve is set to open at 10 cm H_2O, then the pressure throughout the entire system, including the alveoli, will be at least 10 cm H_2O. This air pressure prevents alveoli from collapsing and helps to open alveoli that are already collapsed.[73,74]

A number of other physiologic benefits have also been found with CPAP. The continuous pressure results in more laminar (less turbulent) airflow. It has been associated with improved oxygenation and ventilation, mainly through improved diffusion and greater gas exchange surface area. There are a number of clinical benefits from these effects.

However, there are some limitations to CPAP. It does not provide positive pressure ventilation; there is no difference in gas flow between inhalation and exhalation. Furthermore, the effects of CPAP are limited to the alveoli and the small airways. Large airway diseases are not effectively treated.

CPAP has been used in a number of disease processes. The most common prehospital application has been for patients with congestive heart failure. Not only does CPAP address atelectasis, but it also helps to drive edema back into the circulatory system by decreasing preload and afterload via increased intrathoracic pressure. Several prehospital trials suggest that using CPAP decreases intubation rates, improves patient symptoms, and decreases myocardial damage during the acute phase of CHF.[75–80] No trial to date has demonstrated a long-term mortality difference. Nonetheless, there are more important markers of the effectiveness of the treatment of CHF than just mortality and CPAP has certainly been demonstrated to be effective in regards to these other markers.

CPAP has also been used in the treatment of COPD and asthma. There appear to be two main effects. First, turbulent airflow increases the work of breathing. The laminar airflow produced by CPAP, therefore, decreases the work of breathing. Additionally, inflammation plays an important role in asthma and chronic bronchitis. During acute exacerbations, CPAP may help to decrease the edema in the walls of the airways. Although CPAP has been studied extensively in COPD, there is minimal literature on its utility in acute asthma. Therefore, the two main prehospital indications for CPAP are COPD exacerbations and acute pulmonary edema.

CPAP devices have become smaller and much easier to use. Although nasal CPAP devices are used effectively in the sleep apnea populations and in some inpatient settings, full face-mask CPAP is the most commonly used modality in the prehospital and emergency department settings. The two main categories of CPAP devices for prehospital use are the fixed flow devices and the variable flow devices.

The fixed flow devices are typically the easiest to use. They have no moving parts and no adjustments. The device is designed to deliver a fixed flow of gas at a set oxygen percentage (usually 30% to 35%). The CPAP generator is attached to a 50 PSI oxygen source, the mask and tubing are attached, and a CPAP valve is selected. Some devices use a fixed level of CPAP, others allow the user to switch between different valves (typically 5, 7.5, and 10 cm H_2O), and some use an adjustable valve. Thus, although the gas flow and oxygen concentrations are preset with these devices, the level of CPAP can usually be adjusted.

In contrast, the variable flow devices allow the Paramedic some degree of choice in determining gas flow and oxygen concentration. In order to maintain the minimum CPAP pressure (the valve pressure) throughout the entire respiratory cycle, there must be sufficient gas flow to keep the CPAP valve slightly open at the point of most negative intrathoracic pressure. This point occurs during early inspiration. During the rest of the respiratory cycle, there will be a more significant gas leak through the CPAP valve. Although most patients will receive adequate gas flow from a fixed flow generator, there are some whose inspiratory effort and negative pressure will be in excess of the gas flow. When this happens, the CPAP valve closes and the pressure in the system drops below the level of the CPAP valve. For these patients, the variable flow generator allows the Paramedic to increase the gas flow to compensate for the patient's high demand. In addition, although the hypoxia these patients experience is usually due to a diffusion problem (not enough oxygen moving from the alveoli to the bloodstream), some patients do need higher oxygen concentrations. The variable flow generators usually allow the Paramedic to adjust the oxygen concentration as well. Therefore, although the variable flow generators are more complicated to use, they give the Paramedic flexibility for the occasional patient whose needs exceed the capabilities of the fixed flow generators.

CPAP is relatively simple to use (Skill 22-1). The CPAP generator is attached to a 50 PSI oxygen source. A filter is attached to the air intake valve and the high-volume tubing is attached to the generator output port. An appropriate-sized mask is selected, the high volume tubing is attached to the input port, and the head restraint is attached to the mask, leaving one side open if possible. If the mask uses interchangeable CPAP valves, the appropriate valve (usually 5 to 10 cm H_2O) is attached. If there is an adjustable valve, it is set to the lowest setting. If there is a built-in CPAP valve, no further preparation is necessary.

Next, the oxygen is turned on. If the generator has an on/off knob or switch, it should also be turned on. The system will begin flowing oxygen. The mask is handed to the patient, who should hold it to his face without sealing the mask. The patient should be allowed to exhale against the CPAP valve without the mask being completely sealed; this will reduce the feeling of suffocation the patient experiences. Once the patient begins to feel comfortable breathing against resistance, the mask should be firmly sealed against the face. The head strap should then be brought into place and the last leg attached. The mask and head strap should be adjusted so that the mask seals against the face and there are no leaks.

The patient should then be assessed for comfort and ability to breathe with the level of CPAP. If the patient cannot tolerate the CPAP, the level can be reduced (if not already at its lowest level) or the mask seal can be broken to slightly decrease the pressure in the system. If the patient is tolerating the CPAP he is on, it may be possible to increase the level. Usually a level of 5 to 10 cm H_2O is appropriate. Generally 15 cm H_2O is considered to be the upper limit. If a CPAP of 15 cm H_2O or greater is used, a nasogastric (NG) tube should be placed. There should always be a small air leak from the CPAP valve, even during inspiration. If there is no leak and a variable flow generator is being used, the flow can be increased until there is an air leak. In addition, the patient may benefit from an anxiolytic. However, care must be taken not to depress the respiratory drive.

The patient must be observed for tolerance, improvement, or decompensation.[81] Since the CPAP provides no ventilatory support, the patient must not be apneic. The patient is, however, at an increased risk for pneumothorax. Additionally, the patient may begin to fatigue and decompensate before atelectasis begins to resolve. If this happens, the patient may need to be intubated or the CPAP switched to assisted ventilation. The patient should be attached to a pulse oximeter, vital signs should be obtained, and the EKG (rhythm strip) should be monitored.

In addition, end-tidal carbon dioxide monitoring can be performed. This has never been formally studied but, anecdotally, a small but consistent waveform is seen. Therefore, the end-tidal CO_2 monitor may offer an apnea alarm.

If the patient is switched to positive pressure assisted ventilation, it may be possible to attach a positive end expiratory pressure valve to the exhalation port and, in essence, provide CPAP if the patient is also breathing on his own. There are no studies on using the PEEP valves this way, but they should serve the same function if a good mask seal is maintained.

CPAP has clearly been demonstrated to decrease intubation rates and to provide symptomatic improvement in prehospital patients with congestive heart failure. It is also effective for patients with COPD and may be effective with asthma as well. CPAP is easy to use and may free a provider who would otherwise need to provide assisted ventilation. Concurrent treatment for the underlying disease should also be performed: loop diuretics, morphine, nitrates, and oxygen for CHF and albuterol, ipratropium bromide, and steroids for COPD and asthma. When used appropriately, improved prehospital outcomes should be seen.

For a step-by-step demonstration of Application of Continuous Positive Airway Pressure, please refer to Skill 22-1 on page 416.

Pediatric Considerations in Basic Airway Management

In general, the techniques of basic adult and pediatric airway management are the same. However, there are a few important differences with which the Paramedic must be familiar. These relate to differences in anatomy and physiology.

The posterior occiput is significantly more prominent in the pediatric patient than in the adult.[82] Therefore, when the pediatric patient lays on a flat surface, the neck is flexed and the airway partially obstructed. To counter this, the Paramedic should place a folded towel beneath the shoulders so that the head rests in a neutral position. Conversely, the pediatric trachea is smaller and more susceptible to kinking. When the head is extended, there is a potential for the trachea to kink and become occluded. Therefore, head extension should be done carefully, again with the intent to keep the head in a relatively neutral position.

In addition, the nasal bridge of the pediatric patient is flatter than an adult's. The mask, therefore, is more difficult to seal. Due to the flexibility of the airway, however, increasing pressure on the mask puts the patient at increased risk for airway obstruction. Therefore, a two-rescuer approach to ventilation is often more successful.

Ventilating the pediatric patient requires care to prevent overpressurization. Causing a pneumothorax in a pediatric patient is relatively easy and may be difficult to diagnose in the prehospital environment. Additionally, pediatric patients are more susceptible to gastric inflation and are less able to tolerate it. Therefore, ventilation should be sufficient to just cause the chest to start to rise. Although cricoid pressure can be used to decrease the risk of gastric inflation and vomiting, the relatively malleable trachea puts the pediatric patient at risk for complete airway obstruction with excessive pressure.

Pediatric patients generally suffer cardiac arrest secondary to respiratory arrest, as opposed to adults who suffer primary cardiac arrest.[83–85] Once a pediatric patient goes into cardiac arrest, a grim prognosis is almost assured. Therefore, Paramedics must be more aggressive about providing early interventions and early respiratory support. As Gausche–Hill and her colleagues have demonstrated, the key to management of pediatric respiratory emergencies is not in the advanced skills, but rather in the basic airway manipulation and face-mask ventilation.[86] Therefore, constant retraining and practical experience are key elements to performing effective pediatric airway management.

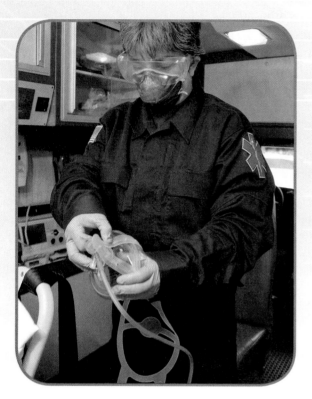

1 Assemble equipment.

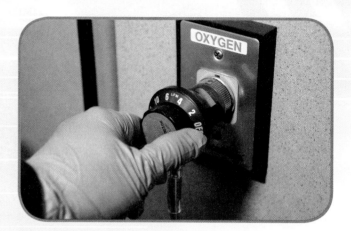

2 Set flow rate on device per manufacturer's recommendations and protocol.

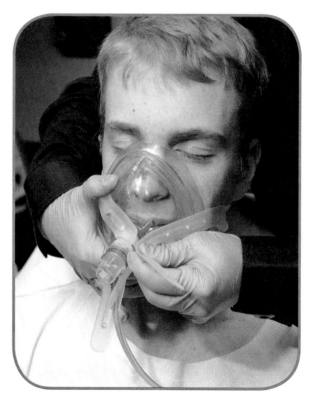

3 Apply face mask to patient and snug down straps.

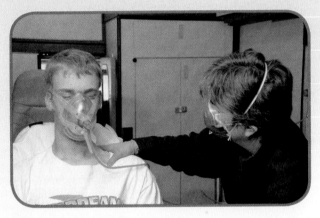

4 Coach patient to breathe with the mask.

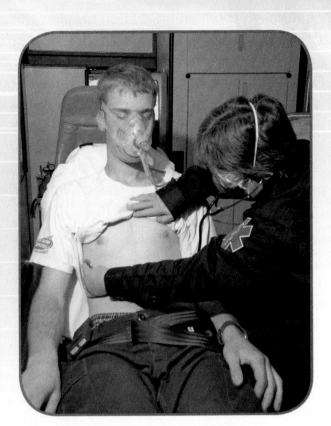

5 Monitor and reassess the patient.

CONCLUSION

Although tracheal intubation remains the "gold standard" of airway management, basic airway management is the most critical and fundamental airway management that the Paramedic can perform. Whether that provider is an EMT, a Paramedic, a nurse, or a physician, knowledge and skill in basic airway management is mandatory. Expertise with a number of skills and devices allows the Paramedic to ventilate patients through simple face-mask techniques. In addition, CPAP and other advances in airway technology allow critically ill patients to be managed without the need for intubation. The Paramedic should advocate for the best possible care for his patients and basic airway management is often just what the patient needs.

► KEY POINTS:

- Preoxygenation for any patient in need of active airway management or ventilatory support increases the diffusion gradient of oxygen into the plasma. It also provides a "reservoir" of oxygen in the lungs in the event the patient becomes apneic. Oxygen therapy can also decrease the patient's respiratory distress, in turn decreasing catecholamine release and myocardial oxygen demand.

- Compressed oxygen cylinders are the most common method of storing oxygen in the prehospital environment.

- A regulator is used to decrease the pressure from which oxygen is stored to a tolerable level suitable for patient use.

- The nasal cannula is a pronged device designed for nasal oxygen delivery at a rate of 0.5 to 6 LPM and can deliver up to a 40% FiO_2.

- The simple face mask seals over the mouth and nose and delivers oxygen and room air drawn in through an open side port. The mixture of room air and oxygen at 10 LPM can produce a FiO_2 of 40% to 60%.

- Oxygen delivered via a nonrebreather mask is not diluted by room air and uses a reservoir bag and one-way valve to ensure a continuous inspiratory flow of oxygen to the patient. The nonrebreather face mask can deliver up to 80% FiO_2.

- A demand valve regulator can provide 100% FiO_2 by delivering high LPM flows of 100% oxygen upon inspiration.

- The use of a venturi mask in the prehospital setting is generally limited to specialty care services.

- Oropharyngeal and nasopharyngeal airways facilitate displacement of the most common anatomic structures that obstruct the airway: the soft palate and the epiglottis.

- The bag-mask assembly is the most commonly used device for providing assisted ventilation and is available in adult and pediatric sizes.

- Excellent bag-valve-mask technique is important to prevent overventilation of the patient and gastric inflation. In addition to technique, the mask must be appropriately sized.

- Barrier devices and pocket masks can provide a good alternative to one-rescuer bag-mask assembly ventilation until assistance arrives.

- Manually triggered flow-regulated, oxygen-powered ventilation devices deliver high oxygen flow rates (40 LPM) while using oxygen only during the "inhalation" phase of ventilation.

- Manually triggered flow-regulated, oxygen-powered ventilation devices have a limited amount of research that compares these devices to other ventilation devices.

- Automatic transport ventilators (ATVs) are mechanical devices that deliver a specified volume of respiratory gas and allow one rescuer to deliver consistent tidal volumes at a set rate.

- The suction unit is used to remove vomit, blood, and some foreign bodies from a patient's airway.

- The patient should be pre- and postoxygenated and the Paramedic should suction for no more than 15 seconds while withdrawing the tip.

- A rigid pharyngeal suction catheter known as a Yankauer or a soft sterile suction catheter is useful in the prehospital environment.

- The most common anatomical cause of airway obstruction is the epiglottis and the soft palate, so airway management techniques are oriented toward establishing a patent hypopharynx.

- The modified jaw thrust must be used for patients with suspected cervical spine injury.

- Cricoid pressure is a non-invasive technique that, when maintained continuously, can limit the risk of aspiration and decrease gastric inflation during positive pressure ventilation.

- Limitations to cricoid pressure include excessive posterior pressure with patients with suspected C-spine injuries, possible laryngeal trauma or esophageal rupture, and in pediatric patients possible occlusion of the trachea.

- Bag-valve-mask ventilation requires an effective mask seal plus an open airway.

- When ventilating, the trachea usually offers the path of least resistance but excessive volumes of air will end up in the stomach.

- It is best to deliver a tidal volume of 6 to 8 cc/kg ideal body weight/breath.

- With ventilatory rates of 12 to 16 breaths per minute for adults and 20 breaths per minute for pediatric patients, the inspiratory phase of ventilation should occur over two seconds and the expiratory phase should take about the same amount of time.

- The average adult bag-valve-mask assembly holds 1,600 mL, and approximately one third of the volume of that bag would be delivered for a 70 kg patient.

- It is difficult for a single rescuer to provide effective tidal volumes while simultaneously forming a proper mask seal, maintaining an open airway, and squeezing the bag. Two-rescuer, and even three-rescuer, ventilation techniques are more commonly performed and preferred.

- While continuously monitoring the patient, the most important assessments are observation, auscultation, and physiologic monitoring.

- A complete reassessment of airway, breathing, and circulation, including lung fields and epigastric auscultation, should be performed anytime a patient's status changes. After observation and auscultation, the patient should have physiologic signs measured and monitored. These include pulse, blood pressure, EKG, and pulse oximetry.

- While reevaluating the airway, the Paramedic should be prepared to suction any foreign bodies, blood, or vomit from the airway.

- Some conscious and breathing patients may present with insufficient ventilatory efforts and will benefit from assisted ventilatory support commonly provided via a BVM.

- During the normal respiratory cycle, the intrathoracic pressure becomes negative during inspiration, zero at the end of inspiration, positive during expiration, and zero again at the end of expiration. The alveoli can collapse at zero pressure, resulting in atelectasis.

- Continuous positive airway pressure (CPAP) is used to re-expand collapsed alveoli caused by alveolar wall breakdown or insufficient surfactant that would otherwise decrease gas exchange surface area.

- Two main prehospital indications for CPAP are COPD exacerbations and acute pulmonary edema.

- CPAP delivery devices for prehospital use are either fixed flow devices or variable flow devices. Variable flow devices allow the Paramedic to increase gas flow to compensate for a patient's high demand or adjust the oxygen concentration, FiO_2.

- When using CPAP, the patient must be observed for tolerance, improvement, or decompensation.

- For pediatric patients, head flexion and extension may partially obstruct or occlude the airway when performing airway maneuvers and ventilations. The pediatric patient's head should rest in a relatively neutral position and a two-rescuer approach to ventilation is recommended.

- More successful outcomes of pediatric respiratory emergencies have been demonstrated not with advanced skills but rather with basic airway manipulation and face-mask ventilation.

▶ REVIEW QUESTIONS:

1. Why is preoxygenation important for any patient in need of active airway management or ventilatory support?
2. Compare and contrast the characteristics of, and indicated uses for, a nasal cannula and a nonrebreather face mask.
3. Describe the process measuring oropharyngeal and nasopharyngeal airways.
4. Before ventilating the patient with a bag-valve mask, how is the appropriate size selected for the patient?
5. Describe the proper technique for mask-to-face interface.
6. What is the significance of the 30 cm water when ventilating the patient?
7. When using an automatic transport ventilator, what should the Paramedic specifically monitor for while performing her ongoing assessment?
8. Why is it important to know how much air a bag valve device holds?
9. Describe one-, two-, and even three-rescuer ventilation techniques.
10. After opening the patient's airway and successfully ventilating him, what continuing ventilatory care should be carried out?
11. Name two indications for CPAP and explain how CPAP is beneficial to both.
12. How would one assess the adult and pediatric patients for appropriate ventilation?

▶ CASE STUDY QUESTIONS:

Please refer to the Case Study at the beginning of the chapter and answer the questions below:
1. How does CPAP decrease the work of breathing?
2. Describe how CPAP increases oxygenation.
3. What hemodynamic effects does CPAP cause?
4. What physiologic signs must the Paramedic assess when using CPAP?

REFERENCES:

1. Larmon B, Schriger DL, Snelling R, Morgan MT. Results of a 4-hour endotracheal intubation class for EMT-Basics. *Ann Emerg Med.* 1998;31(2):224–227.

2. Pratt JC, Hirshberg AJ. Endotracheal tube placement by EMT-Basics in a rural EMS system. *Prehosp Emerg Care.* 2005;9(2):172–175.

3. Lefrancois DP, Dufour DG. Use of the esophageal tracheal Combitube by basic emergency medical technicians. *Resuscitation.* 2002;52(1):77–83.

4. Nimmagadda U, Chiravuri SD, Salem MR, Joseph NJ, Wafai Y, Crystal GJ, et al. Preoxygenation with tidal volume and deep breathing techniques: the impact of duration of breathing and fresh gas flow. *Anesth Analg.* 2001;92(5):1337–1341.

5. Carmichael FJ, Cruise CJ, Crago RR, Paluck S. Preoxygenation: a study of denitrogenation. *Anesth Analg.* 1989;68(3):406–409.

6. Lutman D, Petros AJ. How many oxygen cylinders do you need to take on transport? A nomogram for cylinder size and duration. *Emerg Med J.* 2006;23(9):703–704.

7. Dobson MB. Oxygen concentrators and cylinders. *Int J Tuberc Lung Dis.* 2001;5(6):520–523.

8. Benner RW, Bledsoe BE. *Critical Care Paramedic.* Alexandria, VA: Prentice Hall; 2005.

9. Walls, R. et al. *Manual of Emergency Airway Management.* Philadelphia: Lippincott Williams & Wilkins; 2008.

10. Jevon P, Pooni JS. Cardiopulmonary resuscitation. Insertion of an oropharyngeal airway. *Nurs Times.* 2001;97(43):39–40.

11. McConnell EA. Inserting an oropharyngeal airway properly. *Nursing.* 1994;24(12):20.

12. Dulak SB. Placing an oropharyngeal airway. *Rn.* 2005;68(2):20ac21–20ac23.

13. Bajaj Y, Gadepalli C, Knight LC. Securing a nasopharyngeal airway. *J Laryngol Otol.* 2007;122(7):1–2.

14. Roberts K, Whalley H, Bleetman A. The nasopharyngeal airway: dispelling myths and establishing the facts. *Emerg Med J.* 2005;22(6):394–396.

15. Roberts K, Porter K. How do you size a nasopharyngeal airway. *Resuscitation.* 2003;56(1):19–23.

16. Muzzi DA, Losasso TJ, Cucchiara RF. Complication from a nasopharyngeal airway in a patient with a basilar skull fracture. *Anesthesiology.* 1991;74(2):366–368.

17. Fremstad JD, Martin SH. Lethal complication from insertion of nasogastric tube after severe basilar skull fracture. *J Trauma.* 1978;18(12):820–822.

18. Marlow TJ, Goltra DD, Jr., Schabel SI. Intracranial placement of a nasotracheal tube after facial fracture: a rare complication. *J Emerg Med.* 1997;15(2):187–191.

19. Walls RM. Blind nasotracheal intubation in the presence of facial trauma—is it safe? *J Emerg Med.* 1997;15(2):243–244.

20. Sacks AD. Intracranial placement of a nasogastric tube after complex craniofacial trauma. *Ear Nose Throat J.* 1993;72(12):800–802.

21. Taylor DM, Bernard SA, Masci K, Macbean CE, Kennedy MP. Prehospital noninvasive ventilation: a viable treatment option in the urban setting. *Prehosp Emerg Care.* 2008;12(1):42–45.

22. Davidovic L, LaCovey D, Pitetti RD. Comparison of 1- versus 2-person bag-valve-mask techniques for manikin ventilation of infants and children. *Ann Emerg Med.* 2005;46(1):37–42.

23. Updike G, Mosesso VN, Jr., Auble TE, Delgado E. Comparison of bag-valve-mask, manually triggered ventilator, and automated ventilator devices used while ventilating a nonintubated mannikin model. *Prehosp Emerg Care.* 1998;2(1):52–55.

24. Becker LB, Berg RA, Pepe PE, Idris AH, Aufderheide TP, Barnes TA, et al. A reappraisal of mouth-to-mouth ventilation during bystander-initiated cardiopulmonary resuscitation. A statement for healthcare professionals from the Ventilation Working Group of the Basic Life Support and Pediatric Life Support Subcommittees, American Heart Association. *Resuscitation.* 1997;35(3):189–201.

25. Mejicano GC, Maki DG. Infections acquired during cardiopulmonary resuscitation: estimating the risk and defining strategies for prevention. *Ann Intern Med.* 1998;129(10):813–828.

26. Blenkharn JI, Buckingham SE, Zideman DA. Prevention of transmission of infection during mouth-to-mouth resuscitation. *Resuscitation.* 1990;19(2):151–157.

27. Sun D, Bennett RB, Archibald DW. Risk of acquiring AIDS from salivary exchange through cardiopulmonary resuscitation courses and mouth-to-mouth resuscitation. *Semin Dermatol.* 1995;14(3):205–211.

28. Brenner B, Kauffman J, Sachter JJ. Comparison of the reluctance of house staff of metropolitan and suburban hospitals to perform mouth-to-mouth resuscitation. *Resuscitation.* 1996;32(1):5–12.

29. Barnes TA, Catino ME, Burns EC, Chan WK, Ghazarian G, Henneberg WR, et al. Comparison of an oxygen-powered flow-limited resuscitator to manual ventilation with an adult 1,000-ml self-inflating bag. *Respir Care.* 2005;50(11):1445–1450.

30. Zecha-Stallinger A, Wenzel V, Wagner-Berger HG, von Goedecke A, Lindner KH, Hormann C. A strategy to optimise the performance of the mouth-to-bag resuscitator using small tidal volumes: effects on lung and gastric ventilation in a bench model of an unprotected airway. *Resuscitation.* 2004;61(1):69–74.

31. Weiss SJ, Ernst AA, Jones R, Ong M, Filbrun T, Augustin C, et al. Automatic transport ventilator versus bag valve in the EMS setting: a prospective, randomized trial. *South Med J.* 2005;98(10):970–976.

32. Salas N, Wisor B, Agazio J, Branson R, Austin PN. Comparison of ventilation and cardiac compressions using the Impact Model 730 automatic transport ventilator compared to a conventional bag valve with a facemask in a model of adult cardiopulmonary arrest. *Resuscitation.* 2007;74(1):94–101.

33. Ahmad R. Problems with the Yankauer sucker for irrigating wounds. *Ann R Coll Surg Engl.* 2007;89(4):451; author reply 452.

34. Aprahamian C, Thompson BM, Finger WA, Darin JC. Experimental cervical spine injury model: evaluation of airway management and splinting techniques. *Ann Emerg Med.* 1984;13(8):584–587.

35. Gerling MC, Davis DP, Hamilton RS, Morris GF, Vilke GM, Garfin SR, et al. Effects of cervical spine immobilization technique and laryngoscope blade selection on an unstable cervical spine in a cadaver model of intubation. *Ann Emerg Med.* 2000;36(4):293–300.

36. Donaldson WF, 3rd, Towers JD, Doctor A, Brand A, Donaldson VP. A methodology to evaluate motion of the unstable spine during intubation techniques. *Spine.* 1993;18(14):2020–2023.

37. Lennarson PJ, Smith D, Todd MM, Carras D, Sawin PD, Brayton J, et al. Segmental cervical spine motion during orotracheal intubation of the intact and injured spine with and without external stabilization. *J Neurosurg.* 2000;92(2 Suppl):201–206.

38. Allman KG. The effect of cricoid pressure application on airway patency. *J Clin Anesth.* 1995;7(3):197–199.

39. Herman NL, Carter B, Van Decar TK. Cricoid pressure: teaching the recommended level. *Anesth Analg.* 1996;83(4):859–863.

40. Ewart L. The efficacy of cricoid pressure in preventing gastro-esophageal reflux in rapid sequence induction of anaesthesia. *J Periop Pract.* 2007;17(9):432–436.

41. Stanton J. Literature review of safe use of cricoid pressure. *J Periop Pract.* 2006;16(5):250–251, 253–257.

42. Butler J, Sen A. Best evidence topic report. Cricoid pressure in emergency rapid sequence induction. *Emerg Med J.* 2005;22(11):815–816.

43. Gobindram A, Clarke S. Cricoid pressure: should we lay off the pressure? *Anesthesia.* 2008;63(11):1258–1259.

44. Georgescu A, Miller JN, Lecklitner ML. The Sellick maneuver causing complete airway obstruction. *Anesth Analg.* 1992;74(3):457–459.

45. Haslam N, Parker L, Duggan JE. Effect of cricoid pressure on the view at laryngoscopy. *Anaesthesia.* 2005;60(1):41–47.

46. Sellick BA. Cricoid pressure to control regurgitation of stomach contents during induction of anaesthesia. *Lancet.* 1961;2:404–406.

47. Hackman BB, Kellermann AL, Everitt P, Carpenter L. Three-rescuer CPR: the method of choice for firefighter CPR? *Ann Emerg Med.* 1995;26(1):25–30.

48. Higdon TA, Heidenreich JW, Kern KB, Sanders AB, Berg RA, Hilwig RW, et al. Single rescuer cardiopulmonary resuscitation: can anyone perform to the guidelines 2000 recommendations? *Resuscitation.* 2006;71(1):34–39.

49. Srikantan SK, Berg RA, Cox T, Tice L, Nadkarni VM. Effect of one-rescuer compression/ventilation ratios on cardiopulmonary resuscitation in infant, pediatric, and adult manikins. *Pediatr Crit Care Med.* 2005;6(3):293–297.

50. Willis DH, Jr., Liberti JP. Post-receptor actions of somatomedin on chondrocyte collagen biosynthesis. *Biochim Biophys Acta.* 1985;844(1):72–80.

51. Conlon NP, Sullivan RP, Herbison PG, Zacharias M, Buggy DJ. The effect of leaving dentures in place on bag-mask ventilation at induction of general anesthesia. *Anesth Analg.* 2007;105(2): 370–373.

52. Putensen C, Wrigge H. Tidal volumes in patients with normal lungs: one for all or the less, the better? *Anesthesiology.* 2007;106(6):1085–1087.

53. Brower R, Thompson BT. Tidal volumes in acute respiratory distress syndrome—one size does not fit all. *Crit Care Med.* 2006;34(1):263–264; author reply 264–267.

54. The Acute Respiratory Distress Syndrome Network. Ventilation with lower tidal volumes as compared with traditional tidal volumes for acute lung injury and the acute respiratory distress syndrome. *N Engl J Med.* 2000;342(18):1301–1308.

55. von Goedecke A, Keller C, Wagner-Berger HG, Voelckel WG, Hormann C, Zecha-Stallinger A, et al. Developing a strategy to improve ventilation in an unprotected airway with a modified mouth-to-bag resuscitator in apneic patients. *Anesth Analg.* 2004;99(5):1516–1520; table of contents.

56. Hess D, Ness C, Oppel A, Rhoads K. Evaluation of mouth-to-mask ventilation devices. *Respir Care.* 1989;34(3):191–195.

57. Weiler N, Heinrichs W, Dick W. Assessment of pulmonary mechanics and gastric inflation pressure during mask ventilation. *Prehosp Disaster Med.* 1995;10(2):101–105.

58. Ho-Tai LM, Devitt JH, Noel AG, O'Donnell MP. Gas leak and gastric insufflation during controlled ventilation: face mask versus laryngeal mask airway. *Can J Anaesth.* 1998;45(3):206–211.

59. Vyas H, Milner AD, Hopkin IE. Face mask resuscitation: does it lead to gastric distension? *Arch Dis Child.* 1983;58(5):373–375.

60. American Heart Association. Part 4: adult basic life support. *Circulation.* 2005;112(24Supplement):IV-19–IV-34.

61. Butler KH, Clyne B. Management of the difficult airway: alternative airway techniques and adjuncts. *Emerg Med Clin North Am.* 2003;21(2):259–289.

62. Heimlich HJ, Patrick EA. The Heimlich maneuver. Best technique for saving any choking victim's life. *Postgrad Med.* 1990;87(6):38–48, 53.

63. du Toit DF. Heimlich manoeuvre: adjunctive emergency procedure to relieve choking and asphyxia. *Sadj.* 2004;59(1):18–21.

64. AMA Council on Scientific Affairs. Choking: the Heimlich maneuver (abdominal thrust) vs. back blows. *Conn Med.* 1984;48(9):609–612.

65. Dupre MW, Silva E, Brotman S. Traumatic rupture of the stomach secondary to Heimlich maneuver. *Am J Emerg Med.* 1993;11(6):611–612.

66. Kumar P, Athanasiou T, Sarkar PK. Inhaled foreign bodies in children: diagnosis and treatment. *Hosp Med.* 2003;64(4): 218–222.

67. Masip J. Non-invasive ventilation. *Heart Fail Rev.* 2007;12(2): 119–124.

68. Goss JF, Zygowiec J. Positive pressure: CPAP in the treatment of pulmonary edema & COPD. *Jems.* 2006;31(11):48, 50, 52–58 passim; quiz 64.

69. Sullivan R. Prehospital use of CPAP: positive pressure = positive patient outcomes. *Emerg Med Serv.* 2005;34(8):120, 122–124, 126.

70. Hubble MW, Richards ME, Jarvis R, Millikan T, Young D. Effectiveness of prehospital continuous positive airway pressure in the management of acute pulmonary edema. *Prehosp Emerg Care.* 2006;10(4):430–439.

71. Kosowsky JM, Gasaway MD, Stephanides SL, Ottaway M, Sayre MR. EMS transports for difficulty breathing: is there a potential role for CPAP in the prehospital setting? *Acad Emerg Med.* 2000;7(10):1165.

72. Hatlestad D. Calming the waters: noninvasive positive pressure ventilation in prehospital care. *Emerg Med Serv.* 2002;31(5): 67–71, 74.

73. Schreiter D, Reske A, Stichert B, Seiwerts M, Bohm SH, Kloeppel R, et al. Alveolar recruitment in combination with sufficient positive end-expiratory pressure increases oxygenation and lung aeration in patients with severe chest trauma. *Crit Care Med.* 2004;32(4):968–975.

74. Karmrodt J, Bletz C, Yuan S, David M, Heussel CP, Markstaller K. Quantification of atelectatic lung volumes in two different porcine models of ARDS. *Br J Anaesth.* 2006;97(6):883–895.

75. Moritz F, Brousse B, Gellee B, Chajara A, L'Her E, Hellot MF, et al. Continuous positive airway pressure versus bilevel noninvasive ventilation in acute cardiogenic pulmonary edema: a randomized multicenter trial. *Ann Emerg Med.* 2007;50(6): 666–675.

76. Ursella S, Mazzone M, Portale G, Conti G, Antonelli M, Gentiloni Silveri N. The use of non-invasive ventilation in the treatment of acute cardiogenic pulmonary edema. *Eur Rev Med Pharmacol Sci.* 2007;11(3):193–205.

77. Winck JC, Azevedo LF, Costa-Pereira A, Antonelli M, Wyatt JC. Efficacy and safety of non-invasive ventilation in the treatment of acute cardiogenic pulmonary edema—a systematic review and meta-analysis. *Crit Care.* 2006;10(2):R69.

78. Pang D, Keenan SP, Cook DJ, Sibbald WJ. The effect of positive pressure airway support on mortality and the need for intubation in cardiogenic pulmonary edema: a systematic review. *Chest.* 1998;114(4):1185–1192.

79. Park M, Sangean MC, Volpe Mde S, Feltrim MI, Nozawa E, Leite PF, et al. Randomized, prospective trial of oxygen, continuous positive airway pressure, and bilevel positive airway pressure by face mask in acute cardiogenic pulmonary edema. *Crit Care Med.* 2004;32(12):2407–2415.

80. Mehta S, Jay GD, Woolard RH, Hipona RA, Connolly EM, Cimini DM, et al. Randomized, prospective trial of bilevel versus continuous positive airway pressure in acute pulmonary edema. *Crit Care Med.* 1997;25(4):620–628.

81. Duncan AW, Oh TE, Hillman DR. PEEP and CPAP. *Anaesth Intensive Care.* 1986;14(3):236–250.

82. Gausche-Hill M. *Pediatric Airway Management for the Pre-Hospital Professional.* Sudbury: Jones and Bartlett Publishers, Inc.; 2005.

83. Bardella IJ. Pediatric advanced life support: a review of the AHA recommendations. American Heart Association. *Am Fam Physician.* 1999;60(6):1743–1750.

84. Wright JL, Patterson MD. Resuscitating the pediatric patient. *Emerg Med Clin North Am.* 1996;14(1):219–231.

85. Hickey RW, Cohen DM, Strausbaugh S, Dietrich AM. Pediatric patients requiring CPR in the prehospital setting. *Ann Emerg Med.* 1995;25(4):495–501.

86. Gausche M, Lewis RJ, Stratton SJ, Haynes BE, Gunter CS, Goodrich SM, et al. Effect of out-of-hospital pediatric endotracheal intubation on survival and neurological outcome: a controlled clinical trial. *Jama.* 2000;283(6):783–790.

INTUBATING AIRWAY MANAGEMENT

KEY CONCEPTS:

Upon completion of this chapter, it is expected that the reader will understand these following concepts:

- The implements of intubating airway management
- End-tidal carbon dioxide monitoring, the "gold standard" of proper placement
- Principles of patient airway assessment and how to make the first attempt at endotracheal intubation the best attempt
- A backup plan, using rescue devices when faced with a difficult airway
- Post-intubation care and special considerations in airway management

▶ CASE STUDY:

The patient was in cardiac arrest and emergency medical responders had been doing CPR before the arrival of the Paramedics. The patient's stomach was distended and she had vomited. Despite the best efforts of the responders, the airway could not be cleared with suctioning alone and the risk of aspiration was growing. "This patient will need to be intubated to protect that airway as soon as possible," thought the arriving Paramedic.

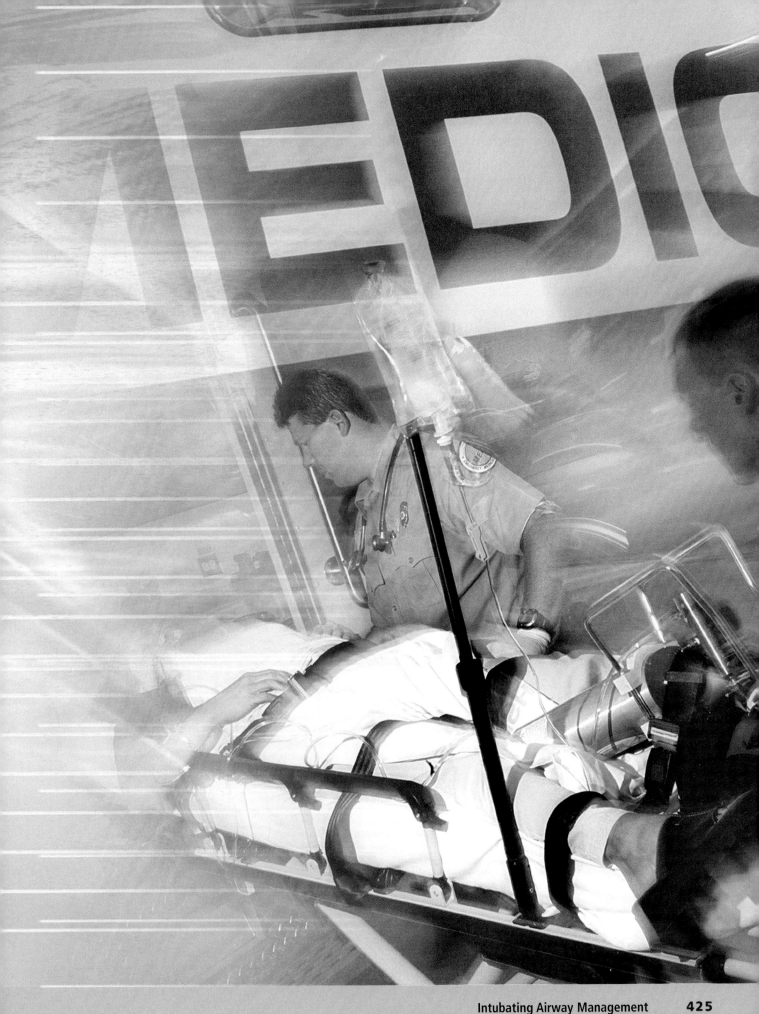

OVERVIEW

Endotracheal intubation remains the definitive airway management technique, even though it is a complex procedure which requires constant practice in order to remain proficient. Even under the best of circumstances, there are times when the Paramedic cannot intubate a patient. Therefore, it is important for the Paramedic to have a plan for that situation and alternative ways of managing the airway. The Paramedic must also provide continuous care for the intubated patient and be prepared for aberrant circumstances in airway management. The Advanced Airway Management Algorithm, together with the skills covered in this chapter and the last, should provide the Paramedic with the necessary tools to perform airway management and continuing supportive care. This chapter examines the use of intubating airway management and the principle of patient airway assessment to make the Paramedic's first attempt at endotracheal intubation the best attempt.

The Intubating Airway Management Algorithm

The Intubating Airway Management Algorithm (Figure 23-1) begins with the same assessment completed in Chapter 21: the patient is in need of active airway management. The Paramedic begins by preoxygenating the patient and, if necessary, ventilating the patient using the techniques discussed in Chapter 22. Once these interventions have been assured, the Paramedic must prepare his or her equipment.

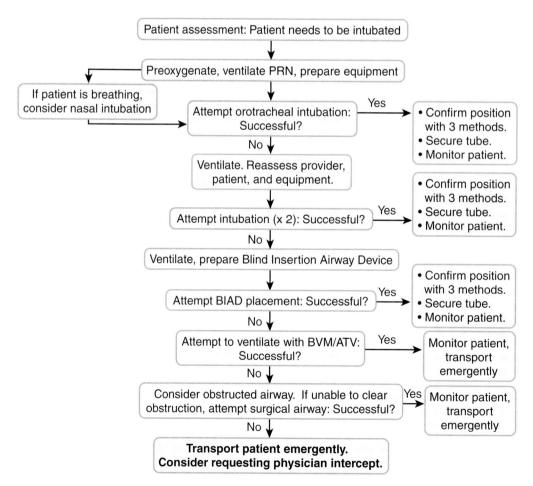

Figure 23-1 Intubating airway management algorithm.

Equipment for Intubating Airway Management

By far, the most common technique used to intubate patients is **orotracheal intubation** using direct laryngoscopy. A laryngoscope is used to visualize the larynx and the vocal cords, and an endotracheal tube is observed to pass through the vocal cords. Although simple in description, there are nuances to the equipment and procedure that can make intubation more or less easy. In addition, numerous other methods of intubation—such as nasotracheal intubation, digital intubation, fiberoptic assisted intubation, and lighted wand techniques—exist and are potentially important tools in the Paramedic's armamentarium.

Endotracheal intubation offers many advantages over other techniques. An endotracheal tube offers direct access to a patient's airway that is relatively protected. Intermittent positive pressure ventilation, tracheobronchial suctioning, and medication delivery are all possible. Although an endotracheal tube does not absolutely prevent aspiration, it significantly decreases the likelihood of aspiration. One of the greatest advantages of the endotracheal tube over non-intubated ventilation is that it does not cause gastric insufflation and the resulting distention, impingement on thoracic expansion, and vomiting.

However, there are some disadvantages to endotracheal intubation. Endotracheal intubation bypasses the natural functions of the upper airways including filtration, warming, and humidification. Complications of intubation include bleeding from the placement of the tube and from the manipulation of soft tissues with the laryngoscope. Laryngospasm, laryngeal swelling, mucosal necrosis and erosion, and vocal cord damage can all result from endotracheal intubation. In addition, the direct connection from the ventilation device to the lungs increases the risk of barotrauma and ventilator-associated pneumonia. Overventilation of the lungs can impede venous return by increasing intrathoracic pressure, which can decrease the systemic blood pressure. However, prehospital endotracheal intubation occurs in the setting of life-threatening diseases. If a patient requires intubation, then the benefits far outweigh the risks.

Although each different intubation technique necessitates the use of a specific set of equipment, there are some fundamental pieces of equipment which are standard tools of the Paramedic. These include endotracheal tubes, laryngoscope handles, laryngoscope blades, syringes, stylettes, endotracheal tube securing supplies, and Magill forceps (Figure 23-2, Table 23-1). In addition, endotracheal tube confirmation equipment (stethoscopes, end-tidal carbon dioxide monitors and detectors, and esophageal detection devices) and airway rescue devices (King airway, laryngeal mask airways, and esophageal tracheal Combitubes) should also be part of the Paramedic's standard airway management equipment. Finally, some specialty devices—such as direct fiberoptic intubation devices, direct visualization devices, the elastic

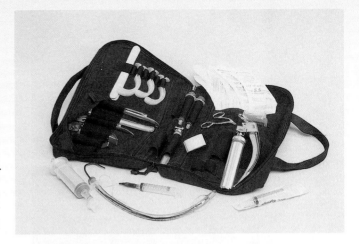

Figure 23-2 Endotracheal intubation equipment.

Table 23-1 List of Suggested Contents of an Airway Management Kit

- Laryngoscope handles (adult and pediatric)
- Miller blades (00 to 4)
- Macintosh blades (1 to 4)
- Full set oral airways
- Full set nasal airways
- Uncuffed endotracheal tubes (2.5 to 5.5)
- Cuffed endotracheal tubes (5.0 to 10)
- 10 cc syringe (2)
- Stylettes (adult and pediatric)
- Elastic gum bougie (adult and pediatric)
- Tape
- Rescue device (King airway, LMA, etc.)
- Magill forceps (adult and pediatric)
- Tube-securing device (adult and pediatric)
- Esophageal intubation detection device
- End-tidal carbon dioxide detector or adapters for capnometry/capnography
- Stethoscope
- Spare bulbs and batteries
- Extra PPE

gum bougie, continuous positive airway pressure (CPAP), and surgical airway management techniques—may also be part of a Paramedic's practice. Understanding the preparation and use of these devices is critical for excellent airway management.

Endotracheal Tubes

The basic tool of endotracheal intubation is the **endotracheal tube** (Figure 23-3). The endotracheal tube provides a conduit for oxygenation and ventilation between the

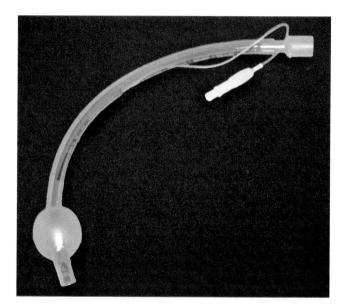

Figure 23-3 Endotracheal tubes.

patient's lungs and the ventilator (person or machine). The primary components of an endotracheal tube are the tube, the cuff (on cuffed tubes), and the 15 mm adapter. The tube acts as a gas conduit. The adapter allows the tube to be connected to a bag-valve-mask device or ventilator. The cuff (used on adult tubes) inflates to secure the tube and to form a tight seal below the level of the cords. Pediatric tubes are uncuffed because the pediatric trachea cones down in diameter below the cricoid ring, allowing the uncuffed tube to seal itself there. However, cuffed endotracheal tubes can be used in pediatric patients, particularly at the transition ages (ages 5 to 8).

There are some common features of all endotracheal tubes. The length of the tube is noted on the outside and is measured in centimeters. These markings allow the Paramedic to measure the depth to the end of the endotracheal tube. The distal end of an endotracheal tube is beveled. In addition, there is a "Murphy eye" on the distal right side of the tube. The Murphy eye improves ventilation to the right upper lobe and allows for some ventilation through the tube if the distal end becomes occluded.

Endotracheal tubes are sized based on their internal diameter (I.D.). The smallest tube commonly used is the 2.5 mm I.D. tube, while the largest is the 11.0 mm I.D. tube. Endotracheal tubes increase in half-millimeter steps from 2.5 to 11.0 mm. Selection of the size of the endotracheal tube for use with a given patient is made based on experience and the circumstances of the particular intubation. In general, an adult male will be able to accommodate an 8.0 to 8.5 mm tube while an adult female will accommodate a 7.5 to 8.0 mm tube. However, patients with airway edema or trauma may require a smaller endotracheal tube.

Sizing endotracheal tubes for pediatric patients can be done based on formulas that calculate an appropriate size based on age,[1] estimates based on the diameter of the

patient's small finger or nare, or length-based tapes that give the Paramedic all of the appropriate sizes of equipment and drug doses. Although there is some evidence to suggest that length-based tapes are superior to other methods,[2–4] it has been demonstrated that Paramedics can accurately determine weights of pediatric patients. Therefore, any method may be used as long as it is practiced and used consistently.

Nasotracheal intubation, placing an endotracheal tube through the patient's nostril and into the trachea, is another commonly used technique for managing a breathing patient's airway. Blind nasotracheal intubation can only be performed on a breathing patient. While a standard endotracheal tube can be used for nasotracheal intubation, special tubes for nasal intubation are different in many ways from a standard oral endotracheal tube (Figure 23-4). Nasal tubes are softer and more pliable than standard tubes to allow them to curve more easily along the posterior oropharynx. Endotrol® tubes also have a small ring or "trigger" that, when pulled, decreases the radius of the tube's curvature and curves the tip of the tube anteriorly. When compared to using standard endotracheal tubes for nasotracheal intubation, "trigger tubes" increase the rates of successful intubation.[5]

Once the Paramedic has selected the appropriate size and style of endotracheal tube, the next matter is to check and prepare the tube. The Paramedic opens the tube packaging and places a small amount of lubricant at the distal end of the tube. Although not a "sterile" technique, airway management should at least be a "clean" technique. Efforts should be made to minimize contamination of the endotracheal tube. If the tube is cuffed, the Paramedic should place 5 to 10 cc of air in the cuff with a syringe and gently squeeze the cuff to assure that it is not leaking.

The syringe should be removed from the inflation port to assure that the valve is working and then reattached to aspirate the air from the cuff. The syringe should be filled with 10 cc of air and left attached to the inflation port so that it is ready and easy to find at the time of intubation. The 15 mm adapter should be assessed to make sure it is snugly attached. For orotracheal intubation, a stylet (described in the following text) is placed and appropriately shaped, and the prepared tube (still in its package) is placed within reach of the Paramedic at the patient's side.

The well-prepared Paramedic recognizes that, although there are general size ETTs used for general "groups" (adult male, adult female, etc.), the availability of multiple sizes of endotracheal tubes (typically one smaller and one larger than the expected size) allows the Paramedic to quickly use an appropriately sized tube if the first attempt was not successful due to endotracheal tube size. Some endotracheal tubes are available preloaded with a stylet ("Slick Set®" Stylettes). Regardless of how the Paramedic prepares for an inappropriately sized tube, it is important that she at least be aware that the first ETT may not work and have a plan for what to do if that happens.

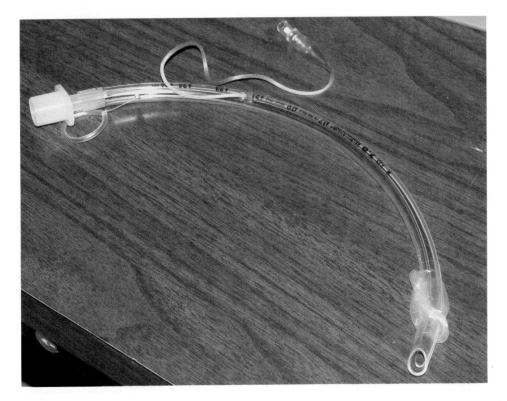

Figure 23-4 Endotrol "trigger" endotracheal tube.

The Laryngoscope

The **laryngoscope** is the primary device used to visualize the larynx. Since its original design, the laryngoscope has undergone a number of revisions to make it a more compact and self-contained device, affording improved visualization in some instances. Regardless of these changes, the basic principle remains the same: to allow direct visualization of the larynx.

There are two major components of the laryngoscope: the handle and the blade. The handle serves as a power source (or power and light source in the case of fiberoptic laryngoscopes) and grip point for the Paramedic. There are four common sizes of handles (Figure 23-5): large adult, adult, pediatric, and neonatal. One of the two adult sizes and a pediatric handle are the typical complement for an intubation kit. The neonatal handles may be seen in the obstetric and neonatal transport setting. Although the handles are labeled adult and pediatric, perhaps the more important differentiation is the Paramedic's hand size. A single laryngoscope system (standard versus fiberoptic and reusable versus disposable) should be used to prevent having incompatible blades and handles in a single kit. If this rule is followed, then all the handles should work with all of the blades in the set. A Paramedic with small hands may find that using the pediatric handle with an adult blade is the best for him.

Although there are multiple types of laryngoscopic blades available, the two most commonly used styles of blades are the Macintosh and Miller blades (Figure 23-6). Regardless of the type of blade, almost all blades in service are right

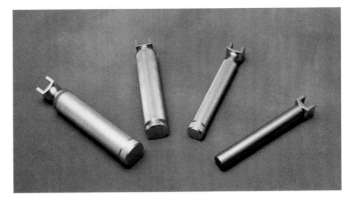

Figure 23-5 Variety of handle sizes.

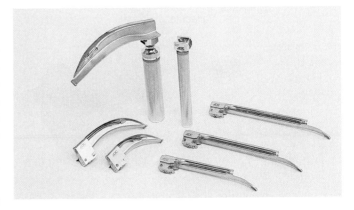

Figure 23-6 The two most common types of laryngoscope blades are the Macintosh on the left and the Miller on the right.

handed; that is, the laryngoscope is held in the left hand and the intubation is performed with the right hand. Although left-handed blades are available, unless the Paramedic plans to purchase his own set, it is best to learn to use right-handed blades. Blades are designed to provide a view of the laryngeal opening through control of the tongue and the epiglottis. The major differences between Macintosh and Miller blades, reflected in their design, are in the manner in which they control the tongue and epiglottis.

The **Macintosh** blade is a curved blade with common sizes from 1 to 4 (Figure 23-7). Its large flange and flat surfaces reflect a design to control the tongue. The tip of the blade is intended to fit into the vallecula (Figure 23-8) and elevate the epiglottis via the hyoepiglottic ligament. Although not intended to do so, some Paramedics use the tip to directly hook the epiglottis and control it in that manner.

Although small (size 1) Macintosh blades are available, they are typically not used in children under age 5. In children under 5, the epiglottis tends to be floppy and the vallecular placement of the Macintosh blade does not provide sufficient epiglottic control. The use of the Macintosh blade is described later.

The **Miller** blade is a straight blade with common sizes from 00 to 4. The small and curved flange is not designed to displace the tongue in the same manner as the Macintosh blade (Figure 23-9). Rather, the straight blade is designed to open a conduit to the larynx on the right side of the mouth and hold the tongue in the midline to the left side of the mouth. The tip of the blade is designed to capture and lift the epiglottis (Figure 23-10). This feature makes the Miller more desirable for the child under 5 years of age. The 00 Miller is designed for premature neonates. The use of the Miller blade is described later.

Selecting the appropriate size and type of blade depends on the patient's size and the clinical context. Commonly, a chart (or, in pediatric patients, a color-coded tape) is used

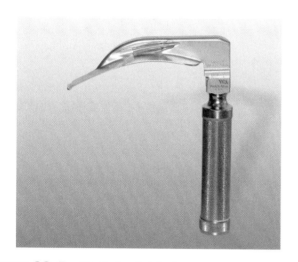

Figure 23-7 Macintosh blade.

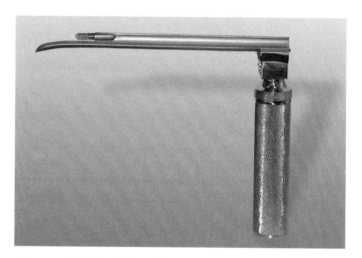

Figure 23-9 Miller blade.

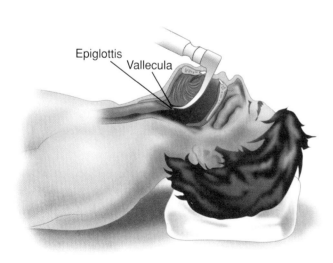

Figure 23-8 Proper placement of the Macintosh blade.

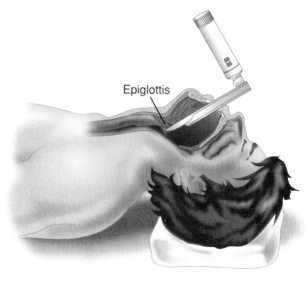

Figure 23-10 Proper placement of the Miller blade.

to select the appropriate-sized blade. As mentioned, Miller blades are typically used for children under 5 years of age. For patients older than 5, selection of the appropriate blade depends upon the provider's comfort level. There is a recommendation to use a Miller blade in trauma patients because it may provide a better view with less cervical spine manipulation. However, the Paramedic must select the blade with which he is most comfortable, as he will have to use that blade in high-stress situations.

Once the Paramedic has selected the correct blade, it is important to prepare and test the laryngoscope. The blade is attached to the crossbar of the laryngoscope's handle until it clicks into place. The blade is then rotated until the power points or fiberoptic channel are in contact with the opposite points on the handle and the blade locks into the top of the handle. At this point, the light should activate. The light should be "white, tight, and steady bright": white in color (clean blade), the bulb tightly screwed into the blade receptacle (not necessary in fiberoptic laryngoscopes), and steady and bright in intensity (good contact and good batteries). The laryngoscope should be turned with the blade down (the position of intubation) to assure that contact is maintained in that position. Finally, the blade should be folded back down on the handle to keep the batteries draining and the bulb from getting too hot (hot enough to burn the patient) or burning out.

Stylet

The **stylet**, a commonly used adjunct to oral intubation, provides rigidity to the endotracheal tube.

Made of a malleable material such as copper or aluminum, the stylet is a long, thin rod placed in the endotracheal tube to combat the inherent flexibility of the ETT. By straightening the proximal three quarters of the stylet and bending the lower quarter into a "hockey stick" shape (Figure 23-11), the tube can be shaped to maximize control of its distal tip and improve the chances of successful placement. It is important that the distal end of the stylet not extend beyond the

Murphy's eye on the endotracheal tube to decrease the risk of the stylet injuring the airway.

Although the use of a stylet is not mandatory, it is a useful adjunct that almost always makes intubation easier. There are adult and pediatric sizes as well. A technique of nasal intubation using a stylet has been described, although, generally speaking, nasal intubation is carried out without a stylet. However, for all oral intubations, the use of a stylet should be the rule, not the exception.

Securing Devices

Once an endotracheal tube is placed, it is important that it be secured to keep it from moving out of the trachea. Numerous devices, such as the Thomas tube holder (Figure 23-12), are available commercially. In addition, many other ties have been used and can be equally effective. Regardless of the device or technique used to secure the endotracheal tube, it is important that the endotracheal tube not be able to move. Although taping the endotracheal tube to a patient's face may be an acceptable practice in an operating room setting where the patient is not moved during the procedure, it is not sufficient for the prehospital environment. The risks of accidental tube dislodgment during patient movement are high. Not only is it important to secure the tube with an adequate device or technique, but it is also important to place a cervical collar to minimize neck extension and flexion.[6] However the Paramedic plans to secure the neck, it is important that the equipment be prepared prior to the intubation.

Secondary Confirmation Equipment

Although the process of confirming tube placement will be described later, it is important that the Paramedic prepare his equipment for tube placement confirmation prior to beginning intubation. The three most commonly accepted methods of confirming endotracheal tube placement in the prehospital environment are auscultation, esophageal detection devices (EDD), and end-tidal carbon

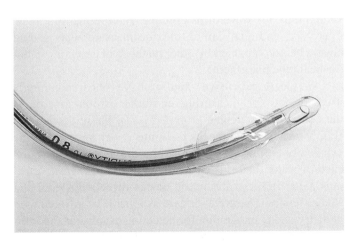

Figure 23-11 Stylet in place.

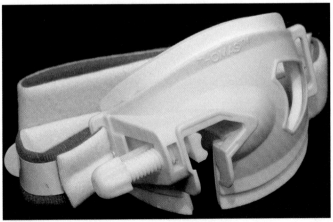

Figure 23-12 Thomas tube holder.

dioxide measurement. Visualization of the endotracheal tube passing through the vocal cords, although valuable and highly recommended, may not be possible due to other factors (e.g., traumatic airway, use of a elastic gum bougie, or nasotracheal intubation).

Auscultation of lung sounds, listening to the lung fields with a stethoscope, is a commonly accepted technique for assessing endotracheal tube placement. The only equipment necessary for this is a stethoscope. Therefore, a stethoscope should be immediately available. Although auscultation of the axilla alone to detect esophageal intubation is only 85% sensitive (and therefore misses 15% of esophageal intubations), the combination of auscultation over the epigastrium and in the axilla, when sounds can be well heard, has been shown to be 100% sensitive (detected all) for detecting esophageal intubation.[7]

Esophageal intubation detection devices should also be used to confirm endotracheal tube placement. Two major styles of these devices exist: self-inflating bulbs and syringe style aspirators (Figure 23-13). These devices operate on the principle that the esophagus is composed of soft, floppy musculature while the trachea is held open by rings of cartilage. Therefore, if suction is applied to an endotracheal tube placed in the esophagus, the walls of the esophagus will collapse on the tip and prevent inflation. Conversely, the trachea will be held open by cartilaginous rings. Therefore, the esophageal intubation detection device should inflate rapidly and completely with air.

A number of studies have been performed on both the syringe type and self-inflating bulb devices. The results are encouraging for its use. In several studies,[8–11] all of the esophageal intubations were detected. Although there are reports of the devices failing to detect esophageal intubations in patients with massive gastric insufflations,[12] this has not been seen universally. The greatest limitation seems to be that the devices will often indicate an esophageal intubation when, in fact, the tube is actually in the trachea. This can occur when the tip of the tube is on the carina or pushed against the trachea's wall. In addition, in patients with limited functional residual capacity—such as those in CHF, adult respiratory distress syndrome, or the morbidly obese—the devices may inflate slowly or with resistance.[11,13] Therefore, the devices must be used in conjunction with other methods. To prepare the equipment, the Paramedic needs only to open the packaging.

End-tidal carbon dioxide (ETCO$_2$) measurement and monitoring has become a standard method of both confirming endotracheal tube placement and monitoring patient status, ventilation, and continuing tube placement.[14] Carbon dioxide is a colorless, odorless gas that is produced during cellular metabolism. It is the primary exhaled waste product and its concentration in the exhaled respiratory gasses depends on adequacy of ventilation and circulation. End-tidal carbon dioxide measurement is used to assess endotracheal tube positioning and to monitor the adequacy of ventilation. The three classes of end-tidal carbon dioxide measurement are colorimetric measurement, capnometry, and capnography.

End-tidal carbon dioxide monitoring, in all of its forms, has been demonstrated to be a reliable and highly sensitive method for assessing endotracheal tube placement and monitoring tube placement over time.[15–19] End-tidal carbon dioxide monitoring has become the gold standard of confirming endotracheal tube placement. There are, however, conditions which can limit its reliability. Therefore, it is important to understand their impact on the use of these devices. Perhaps the most fundamental limit is that the patient must be producing carbon dioxide in order to exhale it. In patients in cardiac arrest, the lack of exhaled carbon dioxide may be mistaken for an esophageal intubation.[20] Of much more concern, however, is the risk of mistaking an esophageal intubation for a tracheal intubation. Bag-mask assembly ventilation with gastric insufflations,[21] ingestion of carbonated beverages and antacids,[22] and hypopharyngeal endotracheal tube placement[23] have all been shown to produce waveforms that would indicate tracheal intubation. However, with the exception of hypopharyngeal placement, after six ventilations (approximately 30 to 60 seconds of ventilation), the waveforms diminish and eventually vanish. Therefore, end-tidal carbon dioxide measurements should always be accompanied by other methods of assessing endotracheal tube placement.

The least expensive, and probably most commonly used, device for measuring end-tidal carbon dioxide is the **colorimetric device** (Figure 23-14). These devices are simply encapsulated pieces of litmus paper over which the exhaled breath flows. When carbon dioxide is in the presence of water, it forms carbonic acid; the pH sensitive litmus paper in the colorimetric device detects this acid and changes color. These devices are as reliable as infrared capnometry and capnography for detecting esophageal and tracheal intubations[20] and are reliable in infants and children larger than 15 kg.[24] The devices are designed to be attached

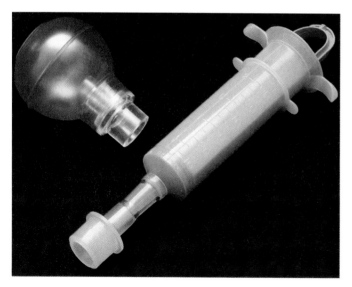

Figure 23-13 Esophageal detector devices.

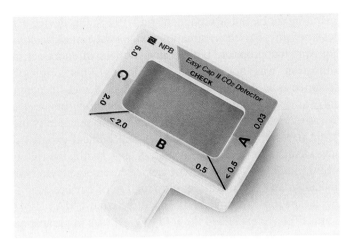

Figure 23-14 Colorimetric end-tidal carbon dioxide detector.

between the 15 mm adapter on the endotracheal tube or an alternative airway device and the BVM. Some manufacturers produce bag-mask assemblies with colorimetric ETCO$_2$ devices built into the exhalation valves. When CO$_2$ is < 0.5%, the paper is purple. When the CO$_2$ is between 0.5% and 2.0% of the exhaled gas, the paper becomes tan. Finally, when the exhaled CO$_2$ is > 2%, the paper turns yellow. Over time (approximately two hours for most in-line devices), the paper turns permanently yellow. Exposure to water, vomit, pulmonary secretions, medications, and so on, will hasten the deactivation of the device. Preparation of the colorimetric end-tidal CO$_2$ monitor involves simply opening the packaging.

The remaining two classes of monitoring—capnometry and capnography—are, outside of the operating room, based on infrared analysis of exhaled gasses. By shooting an infrared beam through a sample of exhaled gas, it is possible to measure the amount of CO$_2$ in the sample based on the absorption of light in the correct wavelength. The infrared beam and sensor can either be attached directly to the gas exhaust stream, called mainstream or in-line monitoring, or can be housed in a device that takes a small sample from the exhaled gasses, called sidestream or microstream monitoring.

Although mainstream measurements have the advantage of being instantaneous, the probes are more vulnerable to breakage and are more expensive. Sidestream devices protect the infrared sensors, but they have a delay in measuring due to the distance the gas sample must travel from the exhalation to the sample chamber.

Microstream devices have less of a delay than standard sidestream devices. Microstream devices may also be better suited for use in pediatric patients with very small tidal volumes than standard sidestream devices or bulky mainstream devices that can kink an endotracheal tube.[25] Regardless of the sampling system, however, the data interpretation and display methods differentiate between capnometry and capnography.

Devices that perform **capnometry** give a single, numeric peak reading of the exhaled CO$_2$. These monitors are usually considerably less expensive than capnography devices although they are also much more expensive than disposable colorimetric caps. Most of these devices have a numerical as well as a bar graph display. Although they do not display trends over time nor show a graph of the exhalation curve, if the Paramedic records the peak ETCO$_2$ over time it is possible to collect trending data. In addition, these devices are usually equipped with an apnea alarm and can alert the Paramedic to sudden changes in ventilatory function. Preparation of the equipment for use involves assuring that there is sufficient power. For a mainstream device, the probe must be attached to the monitor and an adapter that connects to the endotracheal tube (or alternative airway device) which should be attached to the probe. Sidestream and microstream monitors will have an adapter with a sampling tube that attaches to the exhalation stream.

End-tidal **capnography** gives the most information to the Paramedic. While numeric values for peak and trough ETCO$_2$ levels are displayed, the monitor also displays a graph of the exhalation curve (Figure 23-15). This graph allows for trending over time; demonstration of changes associated with complications such as displaced, kinked, and occluded tubes; and respiratory mechanics.[19] Capnography monitors are by far the most expensive, although they are often integrated into other multifunction devices such as cardiac monitors. Preparation of these devices for use, as with the capnometer, depends on whether the capnographer is a mainstream or sidestream/microstream device.

Rescue Devices

For a patient requiring airway and ventilatory assistance, the ideal situation is placement of an endotracheal tube. However, there will always be scenarios in which endotracheal intubation will not be possible. A review of the airway management algorithm clearly demonstrates that, after a third failed endotracheal intubation attempt, the Paramedic should strongly consider another approach to airway management. One class of **rescue devices** available are placed blindly and provide an airway that is superior to face-mask ventilation, yet not as protective as an endotracheal tube. These devices are collectively called supraglottic airway devices or blind insertion airway devices (BIADs). The most common supraglottic devices are the King LTS-D airway, the esophageal tracheal Combitube (ETC or Combitube), and the laryngeal mask airway (LMA). Although the esophageal obturator airway (EOA)

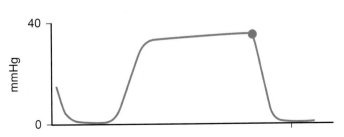

Figure 23-15 Capnography waveform.

and esophageal gastric tube airway (EGTA) were commonly used before the advent of the supraglottic airways, the need to maintain an adequate mask seal and inability to protect the trachea have decreased the use of the EOA and EGTA.

The King LTS-D airway (Figure 23-16) is one example of a supraglottic airway. It is designed to be placed in the esophagus and seal off the pharynx and esophagus with two balloons filled through a single port. A standard BVM adapter at the end of the device is used to ventilate the patient via small holes located between the balloons. A channel located in the anterior between the two balloons allows the use of an elastic gum bougie or endotracheal tube exchanger to replace the device with a standard endotracheal tube. Finally, a posterior lumen allows for passage of a nasogastric tube into the stomach once the King airway is in place, allowing stomach decompression. Due to the ease of use, this device is becoming popular in the prehospital community.

The **laryngeal mask airway** (Figure 23-17), a blind rescue airway device, was originally designed for use in the operating room. Introduced in the mid-1980s, this device was designed to be used in situations where face-mask ventilation was inappropriate but the invasiveness of endotracheal intubation was not necessary.[26] Although not originally designed as a "difficult airway" or "rescue" device, its potential was recognized early on. In the pilot study on its use, two of the patients were classified as having potentially difficult airways.[27] Subsequent studies and clinical experience have demonstrated that the LMA adequately fills the role of a blind insertion airway rescue device in emergency airway management.[28] Furthermore, introduction of devices such as the intubating LMA (ILMA) and disposable LMAs (LMA Unique®) have expanded the role of the LMA in prehospital airway management.[29,30]

The laryngeal mask airway, in essence, moves the mask of face-mask ventilation from the face to the opening of the larynx. The LMA is composed of a single lumen tube with a standard 15 mm adapter at the proximal end and an inflatable mask at the distal end. The mask is designed to cover the opening of the larynx and, with the mask inflated, provide a seal. The intubating LMA, in addition to placing the mask over the larynx, is designed to pass an endotracheal tube through the lumen and direct it into the trachea. The LMA Unique®, as a disposable device, is most likely to be used in the prehospital environment. The LMA does require some preparation before use. Once it is removed from the package, the mask should be inflated to assure that it holds air. The LMA mask must then be pressed against a firm surface and the air aspirated from the mask. This causes the rim of the mask to fold backwards and allows for easier placement. Finally, the distal tip of the mask should be lubricated to improve ease of placement.

The design of the **esophageal-tracheal Combitube (ETC)** (Figure 23-18) reflects a response to the complications associated with the esophageal obturator airway (EOA) and the esophageal-gastric tube airway (EGTA). Like the

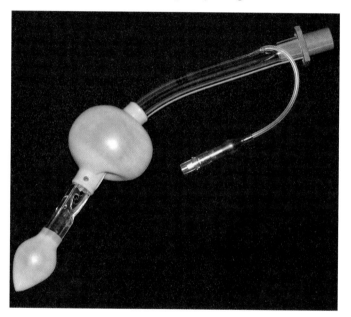

Figure 23-16 King LTS-D airway.

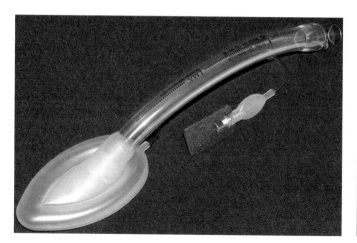

Figure 23-17 Larnygeal mask airway.

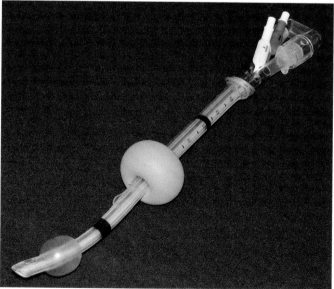

Figure 23-18 Esophageal-tracheal Combitube.

EOA and EGTA, the ETC is placed into the esophagus; however, tracheal placement of the ETC is possible. The double-lumen design allows for endotracheal as well as esophageal intubation.

The Combitube is a double-lumen device with two separate and distinct lumens, a proximal and distal lumen named by where they exit from the tube. Each lumen has a standard 15 mm connector at the proximal end to allow attachment to a ventilation device. Each has two cuffs: a large proximal cuff designed to seal the hypopharyngeal portion of the airway and a smaller distal cuff designed to seal the esophagus or trachea, depending on the placement.

There are several advantages and disadvantages to the use of supraglottic airway devices. Since they can be passed blindly, no special equipment is needed other than the device itself. The Combitube has been demonstrated to cause less C-spine movement than conventional endotracheal intubation,[31] which may be clinically significant in the patient with known or suspected C-spine injury. The devices are easy to place and have success rates of almost 100%.[32] Placement is easier with these devices than with standard intubation when patients are in unusual positions.[33] There are, however, multiple disadvantages to these devices. The King airway and Combitube are currently only available for adult patients. They must be inserted orally and, when placed in the esophagus, are difficult to intubate around, owing to their large size and rigidity. Furthermore, caustic ingestions and known esophageal trauma or disease are contraindications to use of these devices. Finally, they are considerably more expensive than standard endotracheal tubes.

Both devices are intended for esophageal placement, which occurs approximately 90% to 99% of the time. In the esophageal position, the distal cuff seals the esophagus while the proximal cuff seals the hypopharynx. The proximal lumen ventilates through a number of small holes between these two cuffs. Since the opening to the larynx lies between these cuffs, ventilatory gasses passing through the proximal lumen can only go into the larynx and subsequently to the lungs. There are some limitations to the esophageal placement. Most importantly, epiglottic, perilaryngeal, and laryngeal injury or deformity (burns, trauma, edema, etc.) can prevent effective ventilation. Furthermore, respiratory secretions and bleeding between the two cuffs will be aspirated. Finally, medication administration and deep suctioning of the lungs are not possible with esophageal placement.

It is possible to obtain endotracheal placement of the Combitube. Anecdotally, increased rates of tracheal placement occur with well-performed cricoid pressure. When the devices are placed in the trachea, the distal cuff serves to seal the trachea (like the cuff of an endotracheal tube) while the proximal cuff helps stabilize the device. Ventilation is performed through the distal lumen that opens at the end of the tube, distal to the smaller cuff. Tracheal placement allows the device to function as an endotracheal tube and all procedures and medications normally performed with an endotracheal tube can be performed with the Combitube. In contrast, the King airway is not designed to be used if placed in the trachea. If tracheal placement of the King airway is suspected, immediately remove the device.

Preparation of these devices is similar to that of an endotracheal tube. They must be removed from their packages and the cuffs inflated to test their integrity and the functioning of the valves. For the King airway and Combitube, this is done with the syringes that are prepackaged with the device. The distal end of the tube should be lubricated with a water-soluble lubricant and the devices returned to the packaging.

Elastic Gum Bougie

In those situations where intubation is difficult due to patient anatomy, often it is only possible to visualize the posterior arytenoids. Although any tube that passes anterior to the arytenoids will be passing through the larynx, it is often difficult to physically place the tube in that location. A small diameter, semi-rigid device that would be easier to place would assist with intubation. The **elastic gum bougie** and several similar devices meet that need.

First introduced in 1949, the elastic gum bougie, or simply gum bougie, appears at first glance to simply be a very long stylet[34] (Figure 23-19). However, it is somewhat larger in diameter, is made entirely of wound gum rubber, and has a hard, smooth, and round plastic tip. The device is directed through the vocal cords and into the trachea to serve as a guide for an endotracheal tube. The distal end is designed to minimize the chance of trauma to the larynx. Furthermore, the small plastic "button" at the end "clicks" as it passes over tracheal rings, giving the user feedback about placement. Once the device has been placed, the endotracheal tube is threaded over the proximal end and advanced into the trachea. It has been shown to improve intubation rates in difficult airway situations.[35–37]

There are multiple variants on the elastic gum bougie including plastic bougies,[38] large-diameter feeding tubes, and endotracheal tube exchanges. This last class is of interest because some manufacturers make devices

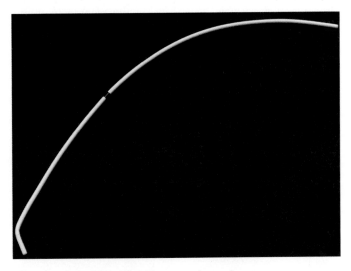

Figure 23-19 Elastic gum bougie.

through which a patient can be ventilated. All of these devices are used similarly to the elastic gum bougie. There is no preparation of the devices other than to remove them from their packaging. If a disposable tube exchanger is packaged in a bent-in-half position, the bend should be straightened as this will improve control of the device and help thread the tube.

Lighted Stylettes/Translaryngeal Illumination Intubation

Due to the close proximity of the trachea to the anterior surface of the neck, it is possible to visualize light on the anterior neck if a bright light source is placed on the trachea. **Lighted stylettes** (Figure 23-20) are, essentially, malleable stylettes with a bright light source at the distal end and a power source at the proximal end. When placed in the trachea, a bright, well-circumscribed light is seen in the midline of the trachea. Placement in either pyriform fossa results in a light off the midline while esophageal placement results in a diffuse, dim glow.

There are advantages and disadvantages to the use of lighted stylettes. Although the lighted stylettes were designed for use as adjuncts to standard orotracheal intubation,[39] subsequent work has demonstrated their efficacy as an alternative to laryngoscopic intubation.[40,41] Lighted stylettes can be placed while the Paramedic is positioned either above a patient's head or while the Paramedic is positioned alongside the patient. They minimize C-spine movement and are therefore excellent devices for management of trauma airways.

There are a few disadvantages to the use of lighted stylettes. If a patient has a very large neck, it may be impossible to differentiate between esophageal and tracheal placement. Bright lighting or sunlight may make visualization of the neck on the anterior neck difficult. Finally, there is some evidence that lighted stylettes may cause laryngeal injury.[42]

The lighted stylet should be removed from its package. Preparation for use is dependent on the manufacturer, but there are some universal preparations. The device should be turned on to test the batteries and the stylet portion should

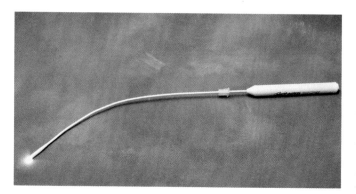

Figure 23-20 Lighted stylet.

be placed in the endotracheal tube with the distal end of the stylet 1 to 2 cm inside the distal end of the endotracheal tube. The stylet is then bent into a "J" and the whole device placed aside for use.

Surgical Airways

One of the other advantages of the trachea's close proximity to the anterior neck is that surgical airway management can be achieved rapidly and effectively. There are three common variants on the technique. The first is the classical **surgical cricothyroidotomy**, a surgical procedure to gain entry to the trachea through the anterior neck. The other two techniques are the needle and percutaneous cricothyrotomy techniques. Many manufacturers produce **percutaneous cricothyrotomy** kits that enable the placement of a single lumen tube either similar to a large IV catheter or to a tracheostomy tube. The preparation and use of these kits is highly specific to the manufacturer and will only be discussed in general terms. It is important to note that a surgical airway should be performed only if that patient cannot be intubated, a rescue device cannot be placed, and the patient cannot be ventilated with standard face-mask techniques. The only exception to the last requirement is if a patient can be ventilated with a face-mask technique but the situation (prolonged transport, difficult extrication, or circumstances that would make surgical airway placement difficult at a later time) requires a more secure airway.

Opening a true or classical surgical airway is a relatively simple process that involves the identification of the cricothyroid membrane, cutting a hole through the cricothyroid membrane, and placing an endotracheal tube or cuffed tracheostomy through that hole. The process has been used successfully in a number of prehospital systems and provides an effective method of obtaining airway control when standard orotracheal intubation and rescue device utilization have failed.[43] There are complications associated with the procedure. These include bleeding, carotid artery and jugular vein injury, thyroid injury, accidental tracheostomy, pneumothorax, mediastinal intubation, and esophageal perforation and intubation.[44] The procedure is contraindicated in patients under the age of 12, with needle cricothyroidotomy being the procedure of choice for these patients, and in patients without recognizable anatomic landmarks. Extreme caution is needed in patients with neck injuries; if a hematoma has formed from a vascular injury, accidental decompression of the hematoma can make airway and bleeding control impossible. The hematoma may also obscure landmarks or deviate the trachea to one side, increasing the difficulty of the procedure.

Little equipment is needed for a surgical airway. A scalpel, a tracheal hook, and a 6.0 or 6.5 endotracheal tube or tracheostomy tube are all that are needed. The endotracheal tube should be prepared as described previously and the scalpel and hemostats should be removed from their packaging.

Needle cricothyrotomy, also known as translaryngeal cannula ventilation and/or **transtracheal jet ventilation (TTJV)**—ventilation of the lungs using special high-pressure devices—is a commonly taught and performed technique for emergent oxygenation.[45] In this technique, a large bore IV catheter (12 to 16 gauge) is placed through the cricothyroid membrane and a high pressure (50 PSI) oxygen source delivers oxygen to the lungs. As with the other surgical techniques, translaryngeal cannula ventilation is only indicated if less invasive techniques have failed.

There are some important contraindications to this technique. The equipment and technique rely on high pressure to move a large volume of oxygen through a small device. Exhaust valves are not built into the device and therefore all exhalation must occur through the patient's own upper airway. If the patient has a complete airway obstruction (inspiratory and expiratory), high-pressure ventilation without escape of gasses results in overpressurization injuries.

Past teaching stated that this technique provides only a method of oxygenation and that there is no ventilation (carbon dioxide exhalation). However, a number of animal studies[46,47] and human studies[48,49] have demonstrated normal, and even low (overventilation), carbon dioxide levels if a flow rate of 1,600 mL/sec (the flow rate through a 21 gauge catheter with a 50 PSI oxygen source) is used. Therefore, transtracheal jet ventilation with appropriate equipment is a valid method of oxygenating and ventilating a patient in whom an airway cannot otherwise be established.

The equipment for needle cricothyrotomy consists of a large bore IV catheter (12 to 16 gauge), a 5 to 10 cc syringe, and a high pressure (50 PSI) oxygen source. Although various methods of ventilating through a needle catheter have been described, including syringe to BVM adapters[44] and oxygen tubing with a small hole cut in the side to control "on" and "off",[45] many commercial TTJV devices are available and are the best choice for this technique (Figure 23-21).

These devices attach to the high pressure output ports of standard oxygen regulators either by screwing onto the regulator or via a previously attached quick-connect device. To prepare for a needle cricothyrotomy, the IV catheter should be removed from its packaging and attached to the syringe. This will not work with safety catheters. If a safety catheter is being used, the syringe is not used. The TTJV device should be attached to the oxygen regulator if it is not already. The oxygen should then be turned on and the device activated to assure that the control valve works properly and does not stick.

There are a number of different manufacturers of percutaneous cricothyrotomy kits. Each device and technique has advantages and disadvantages, so it is important to obtain samples of each device and test them before adopting any specific device. Many have multiple parts that are easily lost in the uncontrolled prehospital environment. Others require fine motor dexterity to utilize.

It is best to choose a device that is simple to use, has a minimal number of parts that can be lost, and is easily stored and adapted to equipment already being used.

Patient Preparation

Once the decision to intubate has been made and the appropriate equipment has been prepared, the next step is to prepare the patient for intubation. Preparing the patient occurs in three ways: assessment of the patient, positioning of the patient, and, if needed, medication administration.

It is important to assess all patients before undertaking an intubation (or any airway management). There are a number of anatomic features that may suggest difficulty will be encountered during the airway management. Although the presence or absence of the characteristics will not change the need to manage the airway, they do influence decisions such as the use of medications for sedation and paralysis as well as optimal patient positioning and equipment selection. Therefore, the Paramedic should assess all patients before attempting airway management.

Several studies have looked at the problem of anticipated and unanticipated difficult airways.[50–54] Several factors have been identified as predictors for difficult airway management and/or difficult tracheal intubation (Table 23-2).

Although some of these characteristics cannot be easily identified before the intubation (i.e., a floppy epiglottis), others can and have led to mnemonics and memory aids for anticipating a difficult airway. Two of the most useful are the **3-3-2 rule** and the **LEMON law**, both developed as part of the National Emergency Airway Course.[55]

The 3-3-2 rule is a simple method for rapidly evaluating a patient's anatomy. In an "easy" airway, the Paramedic should be able to:

- Place three fingers between the tip of the chin and the hyoid bone
- Place three fingers between the upper and lower teeth at the maximal mouth opening
- Place two fingers between the thyroid notch and the floor of the mouth

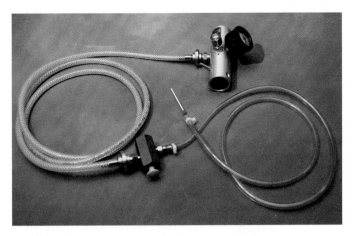

Figure 23-21 Transtracheal jet ventilation.

Table 23-2 Difficult Intubation Conditions

- Male gender
- Obesity
- Age between 40 to 59
- Decreased mouth opening
- Shortened thyromental distance
- Poor visualization of the hypopharynx
- Limited neck extension
- Receding chin
- Abnormal dentition
- Large tongue
- Beards
- Supraglottic mass
- Floppy epiglottis
- Trauma patient
- Pregnant patient
- Mallampati score > 2 (Figure 23-22)

The LEMON law similarly provides a rapid mnemonic for evaluating a patient. The elements of the LEMON law are to:

- L—Look externally for anything that will hinder ventilation or intubation
- E—Evaluate the 3-3-2 rule to assess the airway anatomy
- M—Mallampati classification (Figure 23-22)
- O—Obstruction, either new or chronic, should be evaluated
- N—Neck mobility should be determined if not contraindicated (contraindicated in suspected C-spine injury)

These two rules, if applied to every patient, should help to predict a difficult airway and help the Paramedic to prepare accordingly. Of these guidelines, the Mallampati score is the most difficult to determine in the field. The score is most accurate when the patient is assessed in a seated position, opens her mouth, and sticks out her tongue. This is not practical for most patients requiring prehospital airway management.

Positioning the patient is one of the most critical steps in improving the rates of successful first intubation attempts. Although every intubation attempt should be a best attempt, in the emergent setting of prehospital intubations the first attempt is often made from the position in which a patient is found. Unfortunately, each attempt at intubation increases edema and bleeding in the airway, making subsequent attempts more difficult. Therefore, although the temptation exists to "just get a tube in," the reality is that without forethought, a difficult airway can be made into an impossible-to-intubate-or-ventilate airway.

Although intrinsic issues such as suspected cervical spine trauma may preclude optimal patient positioning, in most other cases some simple interventions can properly position a patient for intubation. The ideal position, described by Chevalier Jackson in 1913, is the "sniffing" position[56] (Figure 23-23).

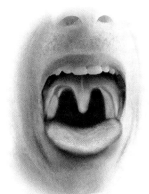
Class I: soft palate, uvula, fauces, pillars visible
No difficulty

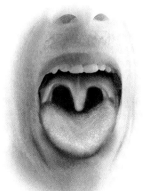
Class II: soft palate, uvula, fauces visible
No difficulty

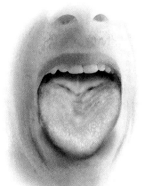
Class III: soft palate, base of uvula visible
Moderate difficulty

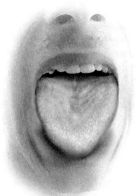
Class IV: hard palate only visible
Severe difficulty

Figure 23-22 Mallampati classification.

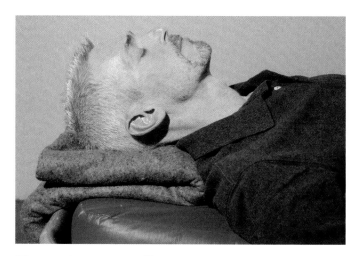
Figure 23-23 Sniffing position.

Bannister and MacBeth, in 1944, clarified the position as one in which the oral axis, the pharyngeal axis, and the laryngeal axis are all aligned through flexion of the neck to 30 degrees and extension of the head on the atlanto-occipital joint.[57]

Although there is some research to suggest that simple head extension, which is obtained in a "head-tilt, chin-lift" maneuver (Figure 23-24), may be as effective as the sniffing position in providing a good laryngoscopic view,[58] this has not been validated.[59] Therefore, for anatomical and theoretical reasons, the sniffing position is considered to be the position of choice for patient positioning during intubation.[60]

At the time of intubation, most patients will already be in the "head-tilt, chin-lift position" commonly used for face-mask ventilation. This position places the head in extension along the atlanto-occipital joints, bringing the pharyngeal and laryngeal axes—but not the oral axis—into alignment. By lifting the head anteriorly approximately 7 cm, the neck is flexed to 30 degrees and the oral, pharyngeal, and laryngeal axes are brought into alignment. This alignment allows for the best view during intubation.

It is important to note that it may be difficult to obtain neck flexion in obese patients or patients with very short necks. Sitting these patients upright can "create" a neck and change a difficult intubation into a relatively easy intubation. This position can be obtained by sitting the patient upright on a chair, packing multiple blankets underneath his shoulders and back, or positioning the stretcher at a 50 to 70 degree angle and placing a folded blanket or towel behind the head.

The **head elevated laryngoscopic position (HELP)** is a patient position that places the head in extension along the atlanto-occipital joints, bringing the pharyngeal, laryngeal, and oral axes into alignment using an elevation pillow. It can also be used in patients who are unable to lay flat (i.e., CHF patients or morbidly obese patients) or to help clear secretions. In addition, patients in the HELP position require less force for glottic visualization.[61] The use of this position is contraindicated in suspected cervical spine or back injuries.

In trauma patients, the issue of positioning becomes more difficult. Clearly, neck flexion and head extension are contraindicated. However, anterior displacement of the jaw via a modified jaw thrust partially mimics head extension. In addition, proper application of backward, upward, and rightward pressure (the BURP technique discussed later in this chapter) may improve the view. Finally, having an assistant open the cervical collar and provide in-line stabilization from the inferior direction will allow greater mobility of the jaw. All of these techniques substitute for ideal positioning in the trauma patient.

The final step in patient preparation is the appropriate use of sedatives and paralytic agents. A full discussion of these agents, as well as the techniques of medication facilitated and rapid sequence intubation, can be found in Chapter 24.

Oral Endotracheal Intubation

Once the equipment and patient have been prepared, it is time to perform the intubation. The vast majority of intubations are performed via the oral route and it is therefore likely to be the first technique the Paramedic performs on a given patient. The process can be broken down into four important steps: visualizing the vocal cords, passing the endotracheal tube, confirming endotracheal tube placement, and securing the endotracheal tube. Mastery of each of these steps increases the chances of a successful intubation.

It is important to note that endotracheal intubation is a team activity. Although Paramedics often find themselves with minimal assistance, it is important that all available resources be used effectively. There should be at least two team members performing the intubation—the Paramedic and an assistant. It is the assistant's job to check and assemble equipment, assist in preparing the patient, and then provide extra hands during the intubation. The two common tasks of the assistant are handing equipment to the intubator and providing digital pressure to the upper airway during the intubation.

There are three ways in which the assistant can provide digital airway pressure. The first technique, cricoid pressure maneuver, applies 10 pounds of backward pressure on the cricoid ring. This pressure minimizes the risk of passive regurgitation. Unfortunately, cricoid pressure maneuver may worsen the laryngoscopic view of the tracheal opening. In addition, often the pressure is mistakenly applied to the thyroid cartilage. Thyroid pressure not only does not seal the esophagus (the thyroid cartilage is an incomplete ring posteriorly) but it does not improve the laryngoscopic view; in fact, it often tips the vocal cords even more anteriorly, making them more difficult to see.

A superior method to improve laryngoscopic view is backward, upward, and rightward pressure (the **BURP technique**[62]). Finally, if the Paramedic is performing two-handed

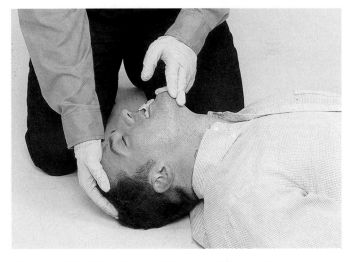

Figure 23-24 Head-tilt, chin-lift position.

laryngoscopy or external laryngeal manipulation, the assistant may be asked to hold the larynx in the position that provides the Paramedic the best view of the vocal cords.

Visualizing the Vocal Cords

To visualize the vocal cords, the Paramedic must use the laryngoscope to provide lighting and a direct line of sight through the mouth to the larynx. Although there are differences in technique between the two most commonly used blades—the Macintosh (curved) and Miller (straight) blade—there are many similarities as well.

The patient's mouth must first be opened. If the patient was already receiving face-mask ventilation, an oropharyngeal airway will probably already be in place. If this is the case, it should be removed while the head and jaw are held still to maintain an open airway. If the mouth has not already been opened, a crossed finger technique using the thumb on the lower teeth and the index finger on the upper teeth should be used. Once the airway is opened, the laryngoscope, held in the left hand, is inserted in the right side of the mouth, lateral to the tongue. The laryngoscope should be held with the tips of the fingers and the thumb as the procedure is one of skill and finesse, not brute force. The laryngoscope is swept to the midline. In the case of the Macintosh blade, the large flange should completely displace the tongue to the left and the blade can be moved slightly past the midline. The Miller blade will not completely displace the tongue and should therefore be swept no further than the midline. Once this has been done, the Paramedic should have a clear view of the oropharynx.

The tip of the laryngoscope is advanced under direct visualization. Once the epiglottis is identified, the blade tip is appropriately placed and the whole laryngoscope is pushed anteriorly and laterally, essentially lifting the mandible away from the pharynx and larynx at a 45-degree angle to the body. The direction of movement should be like aiming for the junction of the ceiling and wall on the opposite side of the room. This anterior and lateral lifting prevents the Paramedic from tilting the handle superiorly and damaging the upper teeth. At this point, the laryngeal structures should be visible.

The **paraglossal approach** to intubation involves inserting the entire length of the laryngoscope blade blindly into the esophagus and then slowly withdrawing the blade under direct visualization.[63,64] When using this method, both curved and straight blades are used to capture and lift the epiglottis. Although there is no evidence to support this method or the methods described in the following text, there is anecdotal evidence that this method can be performed consistently and is less traumatic than other methods.

The tip of the Macintosh blade is designed to fit into the vallecula. Therefore, the Paramedic should see the tip of the blade slip between the tongue anteriorly and the epiglottis posteriorly. When the blade is lifted anteriorly and laterally, the tip pulls on the hyoepiglottic ligament, which in turn pulls the epiglottis anteriorly and reveals the vocal cords. It is also possible for the tip of the Macintosh blade to capture the epiglottis in the same manner as the Miller blade. If this happens and the vocal cords are visualized, do not move the blade. If, however, the blade obscures the view of the vocal cords then it needs to be repositioned in the vallecula.

The Miller blade is designed to pin the epiglottis against the base of the tongue anteriorly and provide a straight-on view of the vocal cords. The Paramedic should therefore see the tip of the blade slide posteriorly to the epiglottis and, when the blade is lifted anteriorly and inferiorly, the tip should lift up the epiglottis to reveal the vocal cords. It is important to note that since the Miller blade provides less displacement of the tongue, the view is more likely to be down the right side of the mouth as opposed to down the midline, as is the case with a Macintosh blade.

Obtaining a view of the vocal cords is often the most difficult part of the intubation. Once the Paramedic has begun the intubation, it is important to assess the degree of difficulty in seeing the cords. Although a simple "easy" or "difficult" system can be used, there are quantitative measures. The most commonly used is the **Cormack-Lehane grading system** (Figure 23-25).

The system grades the view of the glottic opening by how much is occluded by the tongue—Grade I is a clear view of the entire glottic opening whereas IV is visualization of the tongue or soft palate only. Proper patient position and external laryngeal manipulation, described later, can improve the view by one to two grades.

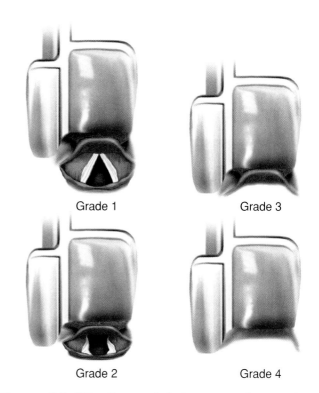

Grade 1   Grade 3

Grade 2   Grade 4

Figure 23-25 Cormack-Lehane grading system.

Aside from patient positioning there are several techniques that can be performed once the laryngoscope is in place. Two of the most effective are **external laryngeal manipulation** ("two-handed laryngoscopy") and retraction of the right corner of the mouth. These two techniques improve visualization of the glottic opening. External laryngeal manipulation has been well described in the ear-nose-and-throat[65,66] and airway management literature.[67, 68] In this technique, the Paramedic performs direct laryngoscopy with his left hand while manipulating the larynx with his right hand (Figure 23-26). Once he has an improved view of the glottic opening, the Paramedic has an assistant take over the external laryngeal manipulation, holding the larynx absolutely still.

Alternately, the assistant may place his hand on the cricoid cartilage while the Paramedic grasps and guides the assistant's hand with his right hand. In this variant, once the proper positioning is attained, the assistant already has his hand in the correct position. External laryngeal manipulation greatly improves successful glottic visualization.

Often it is difficult to see past the lips. Having an assistant hook the right corner of the mouth with a finger and retract the corner of the mouth may provide a sufficient opening to allow visualization of the glottic opening. It is important that the assistant's finger not be placed between the teeth in the event the patient has a seizure, suffers a muscle spasm, or decides to bite. This technique is particularly useful in the patient with large cheeks, lips, or a large, difficult-to-control tongue.

Foreign bodies and body fluids such as mucus or vomit can make visualization of the glottic opening difficult. If suctioning is required, a rigid suction catheter should be used. No more than 15 seconds of suction should be applied and the suctioning should be performed under direct laryngoscopy. By suctioning with visualization, airway and soft-tissue trauma is minimized. If a large foreign body is encountered, the Paramedic should attempt to move it with Magill forceps (Figure 23-27). The attempts should be made under direct visualization to avoid pushing the foreign body further into the airway. If the foreign body is subglottic and cannot be grasped with the Magill forceps, it should be pushed into a mainstem bronchus with an endotracheal tube and the tube withdrawn to above the carina to allow at least one lung to be ventilated.

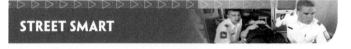

STREET SMART

The tips of the Magill forceps, due to their shape, grip best on smaller and irregularly shaped objects. Large, smooth objects are almost impossible to grasp and may require pinning the object between the Magill forceps and the suction catheter to lift it.

Ambient light may also make visualization of the glottis difficult. Very bright light can "wash out" the structures and cause reflections off of secretions that make landmark identification impossible. Turning lights down or off while inside a building or in the back of an ambulance can make visualization much easier. If it is impossible to decrease the ambient light, placing a large sheet or blanket—or flipping a coat—over the Paramedic's and patient's heads should prove adequate shade to allow better visualization.

Passing the Endotracheal Tube

Once the glottis has been visualized, the next step is passing the endotracheal tube through the vocal cords. The tube should either be in a location where the Paramedic can find

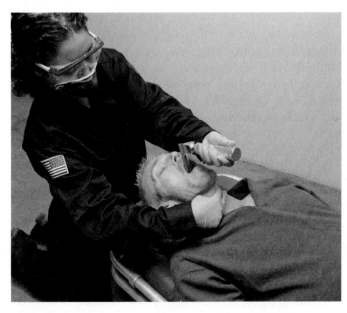

Figure 23-26 External laryngeal manipulation.

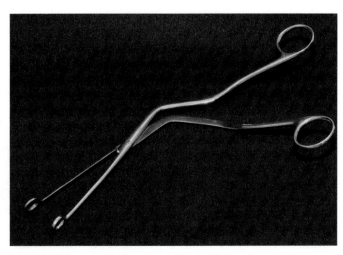

Figure 23-27 Magill forceps.

it without looking away from the vocal cords, or the assistant should hand the tube to the Paramedic, since looking away increases the risk of movement and the need to revisualize the glottic opening. The tube is grasped in the right hand and introduced from the right side of the mouth. It is often easiest to place the tube in the mouth sideways with the inside of the curve toward the right side of the mouth so the Paramedic can watch the tip move toward the cords without the rest of the tube obstructing his view. Once the tip of the tube is at the level of the vocal cords, the tube should be rotated counterclockwise 90 degrees so that the curve of the tube is in the same direction as the curve of the airway. The tube is advanced through the cords under direct visualization until the cuff is 2 to 3 cm below the cords or, in pediatrics, the cords lie between the two black rings.

If the cords are closed, as occurs with laryngospasm, or only partially open, it will be difficult to advance the tube. In the case of laryngospasm, gentle pressure of the lip of the tube bevel between the cords may cause them to relax sufficiently to pass the tube. The Paramedic should not "force" the tube or the stylet between the cords. If this does not work, alternative approaches (e.g., a surgical airway) may be necessary. If the cords are partially open, placing the tip of the tube into the space between the cords and applying gentle pressure may allow the tube to advance. Again, the Paramedic should not force the tube. Gently turning the tube clockwise and counterclockwise may also allow it to advance. Finally, having the assistant remove the stylet while the tip of the tube gently presses against the vocal cords may give the tube enough flexibility to advance.

Once the endotracheal tube has passed between the cords, the Paramedic should look at the depth of the tube as measured by the centimeter marking at the lip line and not let go of the tube until it has been secured in place. The depth will typically be 22 to 24 cm in the average sized adult patient. However, if the cuff was advanced 2 cm below the vocal cords, then the endotracheal tube is in the correct position. The stylet should be removed and the cuff inflated. The tube position should be confirmed and the tube secured. At this time, the Paramedic may release the tube.

Confirming Endotracheal Tube Placement

Once the tube has been placed, a bag-mask assembly device or automatic transport ventilator should be attached to ventilate the patient. Ideally, an end-tidal carbon dioxide detector or measuring device should be in-line from the first ventilation. When the first breath is delivered, the epigastrium should be auscultated (Figure 23-28a). Loud noises over the epigastrium with abdominal distention and no chest movement strongly suggest esophageal placement. The tube should be removed immediately while cricoid pressure is maintained. If no sounds are heard at the epigastrium, auscultation at the mid-axillary lines at the level of the nipple line should be performed bilaterally (Figure 23-28b).

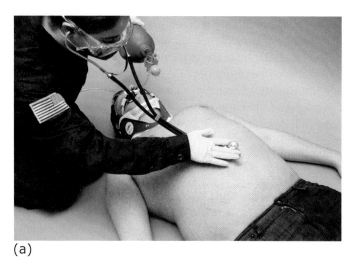

(a)

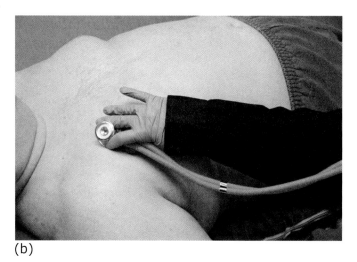

(b)

Figure 23-28 (a) Auscultation of epigastric and (b) breath sounds.

Equal sounds heard bilaterally strongly suggest proper tube placement. Due to the anatomy of the carina and the mainstem bronchi (see Chapter 20), an endotracheal tube that is inserted too deeply will more often advance into the right mainstem bronchus. If this occurs, lung sounds will be heard on the right but will be diminished or absent on the left. If this occurs, the cuff of the endotracheal tube should be deflated and the tube withdrawn 1 to 2 cm. After tube movement, the cuff should be reinflated and the lungs reauscultated. This procedure is repeated until equal breath sounds are heard or the tube is pulled from the larynx. The second situation implies left lung pathology or a pneumothorax, depending on the clinical context. It is important to recognize that left mainstem intubations can occur and should be treated in the same manner as right mainstem intubations.

Once the tube position is assessed by auscultation, the Paramedic should assess placement using end-tidal carbon dioxide measurement. Although $ETCO_2$ measurement does have some limitations as previously described, it is considered by many to be the gold standard of endotracheal tube placement assessment in the patient with spontaneous circulation.

If a disposable colorimetric capnometer is used, the appropriate size (adult or pediatric) should be selected and placed between the ventilation device and the 15 mm adapter on the endotracheal tube. Six breaths should be delivered to wash out carbon dioxide from the stomach in case an esophageal placement has occurred. The device will originally be purple. If the tube is properly placed, the color will change to yellow with each breath and fade back to a yellow-purple color during inspiration. If the color change is intermediate between purple and yellow, tube placement must be confirmed by other methods.

If a continuous monitoring device is used, the sampler adapter is attached between the ventilation device and the 15 mm adapter on the endotracheal tube. If a mainstream device is being used, the infrared device must also be attached. The Paramedic should watch the numerical readings (capnometry) or the waveform (capnography). Although readings of 30 to 40 are considered normal, the more important information is that the numbers or the wave rises and falls appropriately with ventilation, that the waveforms are consistent in shape, and that no abrupt changes occur. It is important to realize that while different waveforms have different implications, the presence or absence of a waveform (or consistent numerical trends with a capnometer) is the most valuable piece of information for confirming tube placement. It is also important to note that end-tidal carbon dioxide detectors will not assess for mainstem intubation or for hypopharyngeal placement of the endotracheal tube.

The limitations of end-tidal carbon dioxide detectors in patients without spontaneous circulation are clear: a patient who is not producing carbon dioxide nor circulating it to the lungs will not exhale carbon dioxide. Therefore, using an esophageal detector device for confirmation of endotracheal tube placement is appropriate. If a squeeze bulb is used, it should be squeezed and attached to the 15 mm endotracheal tube adapter. Immediate (less than 4 seconds) silent inflation confirms tracheal placement while noisy, flatus-like sound or delayed inflation suggest esophageal intubation. If a syringe-type device is used, 40 mL of air in adults and 10 mL of air in children older than 2, that is withdrawn without resistance, confirms tracheal placement. Resistance or inability to withdraw air suggests esophageal placement. It is important that the syringe plunger be all the way down and that the bulb be squeezed before attachment to the endotracheal tube.

If an esophageal intubation occurs, the Paramedic must make a choice. If the patient is still well-oxygenated, a second intubation attempt can be made with the esophageal tube in place. This method has the advantage of the esophagus already being occupied by the misplaced endotracheal tube. The second endotracheal tube is placed in the only remaining opening, the larynx. The disadvantage of this technique is that it can be difficult to intubate around a tube that is already in place. Additionally, the patient is at increased risk for hypoxia.

If the patient is hypoxic or it is impossible to intubate around the esophageal tube, several steps must be taken.

Suction must be prepared. The misplaced tube is removed carefully. The patient is ventilated until the hypoxia resolves while the tube is re-prepared or a second tube is prepared. Further steps to be taken before the repeat intubation attempt are discussed in the following text.

A mnemonic that can help the Paramedic remember the causes of problem intubations is **DOPE**. The D in dope stands for displaced endotracheal tube; the O stands for obstructions of the endotracheal tube, such as a mucous plug; the P suggests the possibility of a pneumothorax; and the last letter, E, indicates equipment failure.

Securing the Endotracheal Tube

Once endotracheal tube position is confirmed, the tube must be secured to prevent movement. The most common way to do this is through the use of a commercial or homemade tube tie. If a commercial device is used, be sure to confirm endotracheal tube depth before placing the device as many prevent visualization of the tube at the lips. If a homemade tie is used, the Paramedic must confirm that the tube cannot slip or move once the tie is complete. Taping the endotracheal tube to the face, although appropriate in the operating room, is not appropriate in the prehospital setting due to the amount of patient movement that will occur.

There is growing evidence that many endotracheal tubes found in the esophagus or the hypopharynx once the patient reaches the emergency department are not misplaced tubes, but rather are displaced tubes. That is, the tube was originally in the trachea, but during patient movement it became displaced. Therefore, it is important that the tube position be assessed after each move. In addition, the biggest determinant of tube movement is neck flexion and extension. It has been demonstrated that placement of a cervical collar and cervical immobilization device (head blocks and backboard) on all intubated patients decreased the rates of displaced tubes.[69] Therefore, all intubated medical and trauma patients should have a cervical collar placed and be immobilized on a long spine board, if possible (**Skill 23–1** and Figure 23-29).

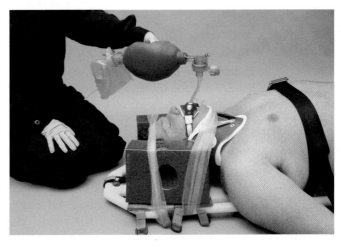

Figure 23-29 Intubated patient immobilized to prevent dislodgement of the endotracheal tube.

For a step-by-step demonstration of
Orotracheal Intubation, please refer to Skill 23-1
on page 455.

Nasotracheal Intubation

If the patient is breathing, the Paramedic has the choice of performing a nasotracheal intubation. Nasotracheal intubation is particularly well suited for patients who, due to their disease process (e.g., COPD exacerbation, CHF), are likely to experience rapid decompensation if they lay flat. In addition, patients who are difficult to access (e.g., entrapped patients) may be easier to nasotracheally intubate than to orotracheally intubate. Contraindications to nasotracheal intubation include apnea, evidence of basilar skull fracture, or inability to pass the tube through a nare (e.g., from a deviated septum).

Patient Preparation

If the decision is made to nasotracheally intubate a patient, the patient must be prepared. The optimal position is the "sniffing position" with the patient sitting upright. The neck is flexed and the head slightly extended across the atlanto-occipital joint. The nose must be prepared with anesthesia and lubricant. The patient should be asked for a history of nasal fracture, surgery, or septal deviation. Although the larger nostril is most likely to provide the greatest success, once the nose is anesthetized, internal palpation with the small finger may provide a good deal of information about obstructions and anatomy.

Once the patient is properly positioned, the nose should be premedicated with a mixture of a nasal decongestant containing neosynephrine and viscous lidocaine or lidocaine jelly (if the patient is not allergic to lidocaine). If possible, the patient should inhale as these medications are administered to maximize the area reached. Use of the nasal decongestant decreases the risk of bleeding while the topical anesthetic improves patient comfort. Placing a nasopharyngeal airway coated with lidocaine jelly also helps anesthetize the mucosa and prepares the patient for the sensation of a device in the nose.

Intubation

If possible, an endotracheal tube designed for nasal intubation should be used. The tube should be placed in the most patent nare with the tip of the tube parallel to the floor of the nose. The tube is advanced until breath sounds are audible through the tube. A Beck Airway Airflow Monitor (BAAM) should be used, if available. This device changes the sound of airflow to a whistle. The tube is rotated until breath sounds or the whistle is at its loudest. The tube is then advanced through the cords during inspiration. The patient may cough as the endotracheal tube passes through the cords; the Paramedic should continue to advance the tube. The tube should be advanced until approximately 2 cm protrude from the nose. If the tube is advanced to the hub, it is at risk for becoming detached from the adapter and the patient aspirating the endotracheal tube.

Confirming Placement

The endotracheal tube placement is confirmed in the same manner as in an orotracheal intubation. Lung sounds should be auscultated, an esophageal intubation detection device should be attached, and end-tidal carbon dioxide should be measured. One important difference is that patients who are nasally intubated are breathing spontaneously. Therefore, auscultation may be misleading. Additionally, if the patient's status does not improve after the intubation, reassessment for tube placement is necessary as the patient may appear to be tracheally intubated but in fact be esophageally intubated.

Securing the Endotracheal Tube

Most commercial devices designed for securing an oral endotracheal tube are not suited for securing nasal intubations. Folded tape, ties, or IV tubing is much better suited for securing the tube. The tie should go the whole way around the head to provide maximum security. Again, the patient's head and neck should be secured with a cervical collar and cervical immobilization device if the patient is able to tolerate these devices (Skill 23-2).

For a step-by-step demonstration of
Nasotracheal Intubation, please refer to Skill 23-2
on page 456.

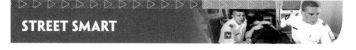

STREET SMART

The phrase "the hose follows the nose" describes the behavior of an endotracheal tube. When the neck is extended (nose moves up), the endotracheal tube is displaced superiorly. When the neck is flexed (nose moves "down") the ETT is displaced inferiorly. This rule predicts the effects of head movement.

Failed Intubation

If the intubation fails, the Paramedic must perform a rapid assessment of why the failure occurred. If the first attempt failed, performing the exact same techniques with the exact same equipment almost guarantees a second failure. Therefore, it is important that the Paramedic understand why the failure occurred and what remedies will correct the failure.

The assessment of a failed intubation should focus on operator failure, patient preparation failure, and equipment failure or incorrect selection. Operator failure is an honest assessment of the Paramedic's ability to perform the intubation. The best

Paramedics are the ones who recognize when they are faced with an airway that is beyond their abilities to manage. This recognition in no way implies that the Paramedic is incompetent. Some patients' anatomy is not compatible with oral or nasal endotracheal intubation without adjunctive devices such as intubating LMAs or fiberoptic devices. If the Paramedic is sure that ability is not the issue, then the next step is to assess patient positioning failure.

Once the laryngoscope is in the patient's mouth, it is often possible to recognize that a different position would allow for optimal oral, pharyngeal, and laryngeal axis alignment. If this is the case, repositioning the patient, adding or subtracting padding behind the head, or changing to a HELP position are all acceptable actions. Often times the first intubation attempt is made in an "as found" position. This should be corrected for any subsequent intubation attempts.

The final area of assessment is of equipment. The most basic question is whether or not the equipment is functioning correctly. A burnt-out laryngoscope bulb makes airway visualization impossible. The second question is the appropriateness of the equipment. If the incorrect blade or blade size has been chosen, an appropriate substitution should be made. The final decision is the appropriateness of the technique and adjunctive devices.

There are several intubation techniques and adjuncts that can be used to facilitate endotracheal intubation on the second and third intubation attempts. These include digital intubation, use of the elastic gum bougie, translaryngeal illumination, and use of a fiberoptic stylet or bronchoscope. It is important to note that the Paramedic should not use these techniques for the first time during an emergency situation. Instead, they should be practiced in controlled circumstances, for example in an OR or simulation lab.

Digital Intubation

Digital intubation is an endotracheal intubation technique that uses the Paramedic's hand to identify laryngeal structures and to guide tube placement. It should only be used for patients who are at no risk of biting the Paramedic. Like nasal intubation, it is a blind technique. Therefore, multiple techniques of tube placement confirmation are critical. One advantage of digital intubation is that the patient's head remains in a neutral position without movement. In addition, digital intubation can be performed on a patient in a sitting position and from below the head, which is useful for patients for whom access to the head is limited.

The Paramedic prepares the endotracheal tube in the standard manner. The patient's tongue is grasped with gauze and retracted out of the mouth by an assistant. The Paramedic's hand is then advanced to the posterior oropharynx. The index finger is used to palpate and lift the epiglottis while the middle finger palpates the arytenoid cartilages (Skill 23-3 and Figure 23-30). The dominant hand is used to advance the tube between the epiglottis and the arytenoids. Once the tube is in place, it is confirmed and secured in the standard manner.

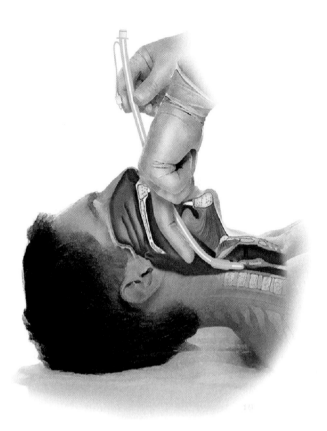

Figure 23-30 Digital intubation.

For a step-by-step demonstration of Digital Intubation, please refer to Skill 23-3 on page 458.

The Elastic Gum Bougie

The elastic gum bougie is a useful adjunctive device for the management of the difficult airway. It is placed under direct visualization with a laryngoscope. It is most useful when the only anatomy that can be visualized are the posterior arytenoids. The tip of the bougie is advanced anterior to the posterior arytenoids until the tip "clicks" along the tracheal rings. An endotracheal tube is threaded over the external end of the bougie and advanced into the trachea. The external end of the bougie should be stabilized to prevent it from becoming displaced. The cuff is inflated and the gum bougie is withdrawn. The tube is confirmed and secured in the usual fashion (Skill 23-4).

For a step-by-step demonstration of Elastic Gum Bougie, please refer to Skill 23-4 on page 459.

Translaryngeal Illumination

Translaryngeal illumination, using a lighted stylet, takes advantage of the larynx's proximity to the anterior surface of the neck for endotracheal intubation. The patient should be placed into a neutral position for the intubation. If possible, the scene should be made as dark as possible. Placing a blanket over the Paramedic and the patient may make it possible to perform the technique during daylight conditions. Turn the stylet on and advance it into the midline of the pharynx, following the mouth's curvature. The stylet is advanced until a focal, bright midline glow is visible at the level of the larynx. It is advanced another 1 to 2 cm and then the stylet is removed. The cuff of the endotracheal tube is inflated and the tube confirmed and secured.

Fiberoptic Stylettes/Bronchoscope

In some circumstances, obtaining a view from the distal end of the endotracheal tube can improve the chances of successful intubation. Although expensive, these devices may turn an unobtainable airway into an obtainable one. It is unlikely that they will be commonly used in most EMS systems, but they may have a place in specialty systems. Two classes of devices—bronchoscopes (in which the tip can be controlled by the operator) and fiberoptic viewing stylettes (in which the stylet is molded into shape before the intubation but cannot be moved during the intubation)—are used. The second class of devices is less expensive. Both are limited in their utility if there is blood or vomit in the airway; the view through the scope is rapidly degraded by these substances.

The devices should be prepared according to the manufacturer's specifications. The endotracheal tube is loaded onto the scope and the viewing tip of the scope treated with antifog solution. If a fiberoptic viewing stylet is used, it should be molded into a hockey stick shape before insertion. The scope and tube are advanced under direct visualization until the tip of the scope passes through the cords. If a bronchoscope is used, the tip can be manipulated to direct the scope into the larynx. The endotracheal tube is then advanced through the cords, the scope is withdrawn, and the cuff is inflated. Usual methods of confirming tube placement and securing the tube are used.

Fiberoptic devices can also be used to confirm endotracheal tube placement in difficult intubations. Once the endotracheal tube has been placed, the scope can be passed through the tube under direct visualization. Once the scope advances beyond the tip of the endotracheal tube, the Paramedic can identify the trachea by the presence of tracheal rings or the esophagus by the lack of rings and the collapsing walls. Although other methods, such as end-tidal carbon dioxide monitoring and the esophageal intubation detection devices, are generally reliable, direct visualization of tracheal rings is another way of confirming tube placement.

The Paramedic should make the most of each intubation attempt. He should make no more than three attempts to intubate the patient. There are two main reasons for establishing a clear limit to the number of intubation attempts. The first is that each intubation attempt causes airway trauma and makes each subsequent intubation attempt more difficult. In addition, each intubation attempt decreases the success of other methods of securing the airway and of being able to face-mask ventilate the patient. Continuing attempts could potentially lead to a completely unmanageable airway.

The second reason for setting a limit to the number of airway attempts is that it drives the Paramedic to abandon a technique (endotracheal intubation) that is not working. By having a set limit on intubation attempts, the Paramedic must move on to other, more productive techniques. This limit prevents the "I'll get it on the next attempt" syndrome that can only hinder patient care. Therefore, after three failed intubations, the Paramedic should move on to other techniques.

Supraglottic Airway Devices

Once conventional endotracheal intubation has failed, the next step is to use a supraglottic airway device. These devices provide a method of at least partially securing the airway in the difficult-to-intubate patient. The three most commonly used devices, as described earlier, are the King LTS-D airway, the laryngeal mask airway, and the esophageal-tracheal Combitube.

King LTS-D Airway

Prepare the patient as previously described for endotracheal intubation, including preoxygenation, monitoring, and supine position. With the left hand, grasp the tongue and jaw and lift toward the ceiling. With the right hand, insert the King airway from the right side of the mouth and direct it toward the oropharynx. As the King airway is advanced, rotate the airway counterclockwise as it seats in the proper position. Advance the airway until the orogastric port is approximately at the level of the front teeth. Inflate the balloons and ventilate the patient. Auscultate breath sounds while gently pulling back on the airway until the sounds are the loudest. Secure the King airway in position after confirming placement (**Skill 23-5**).

> For a step-by-step demonstration of King Airway Placement, please refer to Skill 23-5 on page 461.

The Laryngeal Mask Airway

The laryngeal mask airway transfers the seal of the face mask from the patient's face to his larynx. The prepared device, as previously described, has the cuff mask deflated and the tip lubricated. The mask should be picked up with the thumb in the space between the tube and the mask. The mask is placed in the oropharynx with the tip against the hard palate. It is advanced into the hypopharynx with gentle pressure from the thumb. The mask is pushed until resistance is met. If the appropriate-sized mask is used, it will sit with the tip in the proximal esophagus and automatically position the mask. The pilot balloon will indicate the correct volume of inflation for the mask. When the mask is inflated, the tube should "lift" slightly out of the mouth as it seals (Figure 23-31).

Laryngeal mask airway placement is confirmed by auscultation, end-tidal carbon dioxide measurement, and assessment of patient status. The esophageal intubation detector device does not function with the LMA. Even when the epiglottis is folded over, the LMA provides highly effective ventilation.[70] The LMA is secured with the tube curved toward the feet with a wrap of tape.

The Esophageal-Tracheal Combitube

The Combitube offers an effective method of securing the airway in either esophageal placement or tracheal placement. Once the equipment is prepared as previously described, the jaw is grasped and lifted anteriorly with the thumb in the mouth and the fingers under the mandible. The device is inserted following the curvature of the oro- and hypopharynx

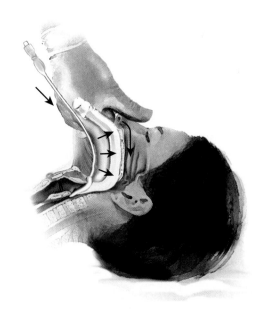

Figure 23-31 LMA placement.

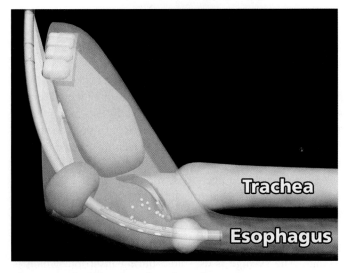

Figure 23-32 Combitube placement.

until it rests securely at its appropriate depth (depth markers on the tube should be at the level of the teeth). If resistance is met, the device should not be forced. A small amount of cricoid pressure may increase the chances of a tracheal placement, and should be avoided.

Once the Combitube has been inserted, the pharyngeal cuff is inflated first with 100 cc of air. Then, the distal cuff is inflated with 10 to 15 cc. The patient is ventilated through the pharyngeal lumen. Chest rise and lung sounds indicate esophageal placement and ventilation is continued through this tube. If no lung sounds are appreciated and the chest does not move, the patient is ventilated through the tracheal lumen; the patient should now have lung sounds and chest rise (Figure 23-32).

Device placement is confirmed with auscultation and end-tidal carbon dioxide monitoring. The esophageal intubation device will not work on the pharyngeal lumens and has not been confirmed as reliable for use on the tracheal lumens; it should therefore not be used. The patient's status must be continuously monitored. Although the pharyngeal balloon contributes greatly to tube security, the device must still be secured with a tie and the patient should have a C-collar and cervical immobilization.

Despite their ease of use, both devices do have complications associated with them. Excessive force during insertion can cause tracheal and esophageal injury. The devices can become dislodged and misidentification of tube position has been reported in some cases. Therefore, careful monitoring and frequent patient reassessment is necessary. If a blind insertion airway device does not successfully secure the airway, the Paramedic must move on to other options.

Bag-Valve Mask and Automatic Transport Ventilator Face-Mask Ventilation

If the Paramedic has attempted to intubate and to place a blind insertion airway device without success, he is faced with a "can't intubate" situation and his options are limited. Two alternatives remain, either manual ventilation or a surgical airway. If it is possible to face-mask ventilate the patient, then no further interventions are needed (Figure 23-33).

Constant vigilance and frequent patient reassessment is the key to good, high-quality non-intubated face-mask ventilation and airway management. An oropharyngeal or nasopharyngeal airway should be inserted in these patients.

It is possible that a patient who cannot be intubated can also not be ventilated (a "can't intubate, can't ventilate" situation). Trauma, facial hair, burns, or anatomic distortion may lead to this condition. If this is the case, the patient must be prepared for a surgical airway.

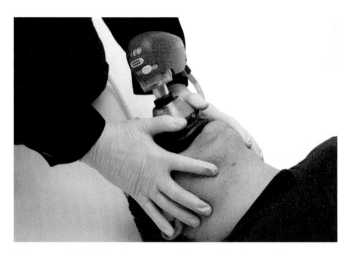

Figure 23-33 Face-mask ventilation using an automatic transport ventilator.

Surgical Airway

In the patient that can neither be intubated nor ventilated, emergency access of the trachea via a surgical technique is mandatory. This technique can be life-saving for the patient who has an otherwise unmanageable airway. The three most common methods of obtaining this type of airway access are the surgical cricothyroidotomy, needle cricothyroidotomy, and placement of a percutaneous cricothyrotomy device.

Surgical Cricothyroidotomy

The surgical cricothyroidotomy is a conceptually simple procedure that involves cutting through the cricothyroid membrane and placing an endotracheal tube through that hole. In practice, it is a difficult procedure in that it is done under emergency situations and the factors that make intubation and ventilation difficult (trauma, anatomical distortion, or anomalies) also make performing a surgical cricothyroidotomy difficult. Like all airway procedures, it is best practiced before it is needed.

The equipment needs, discussed previously, include a scalpel, a tracheal hook, and a 6.0 to 6.5 mm ID endotracheal tube. The patient should be placed in a supine position and, if possible, the neck prepped with an iodine-containing solution or alcohol.

Although there are a number of ways to perform a surgical cricothyroidotomy, the rapid four-step cricothyroidotomy method[71] is simple, relatively safe for the Paramedic, and an easy-to-perform procedure. The four steps to this procedure include identification, incision, traction, and intubation. Each of these steps will be reviewed individually.

First, stand or kneel to the left of the patient. Using the left hand, palpate the cricothyroid membrane with the index finger. If difficulty is experienced in locating the cricothyroid membrane, begin palpating at the sternal notch and move toward the head until the uppermost tracheal ring is felt. This is the cricoid cartilage. Use the thumb and middle fingers to palpate—but not occlude—the patient's carotid pulses and stabilize the trachea. Once the landmarks have been identified and stabilized, hold a #20 scalpel low in the right hand at a 90-degree angle to the membrane. Make a stab incision in a horizontal plane through the skin and membrane and hold the scalpel in place. The left hand can now release the trachea, grasp the tracheal hook, and place the hook into the incision. Gently pull against the cricoid ring toward the patient's feet to again stabilize the trachea. Once the cricoid ring is stabilized by the tracheal hook, remove the scalpel. Now, using the right hand, pick up the tracheostomy tube or endotracheal tube and place it into the trachea through the incision. If you are using an endotracheal tube, take care not to insert the tube too far into the trachea. A mainstem bronchus can easily be intubated with this procedure due to the relatively long length of the endotracheal tube.

It is important to note that the patient will bleed during this procedure; it is to be expected. Even if the patient is bleeding heavily, the Paramedic's first priority must be to secure the airway. Once a tube is safely in place, the issues of bleeding can be addressed.

Endotracheal tube placement should be assessed in the usual manner. The tube should be secured with a strap which ties completely around the neck. The endotracheal tube should be trimmed to the shortest length possible without damaging the cuff inflation system. If a C-collar with an opening on the anterior surface is available, this should be placed as well. However, the Paramedic must be able to constantly reassess the neck for signs of air infiltration (swelling or crepitus) (**Skill 23-6**).

For a step-by-step demonstration of Rapid Four-Step Surgical Cricothyrotomy, please refer to Skill 23-6 on page 462.

Needle Cricothyroidotomy

The technique of **needle cricothyroidotomy** is a simple, fast, and efficient method of turning an "emergency" (no airway or ventilation) into an "urgency" (definitive airway still needed but patient now oxygenating). The keys to the technique are good landmark identification and care in ventilation to prevent overpressurization.

The patient is positioned supine with the neck in a neutral position. The non-dominant hand is used to stabilize the larynx while the dominant hand locates the cricothyroid membrane. If a safety catheter is being used, it is inserted through the cricothyroid membrane directed toward the feet in the same manner as the insertion into a vein (Figure 23-34).

When resistance decreases, the IV is in the trachea and the catheter should be advanced to the hub while the needle is slowly withdrawn. Once the IV catheter has been advanced to the hub, the safety mechanism on the IV is activated. If a non-safety IV catheter is used, the device is attached to a 5 to 10 cc syringe. The syringe is aspirated during insertion, which is also toward the feet. When air returns, the whole device is

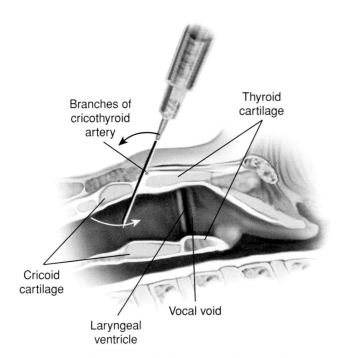

Figure 23-34 Needle insertion for needle cricothyroidotomy.

advanced 5 mm and then the needle is carefully withdrawn while the catheter is advanced to the hub.

The catheter is stabilized in place while the high-pressure oxygen source and flow control device are attached (they attach with a standard threaded adapter). Although the catheter should be secured with tape, it should also be stabilized by hand throughout the entire management so that high pressures and movement do not dislodge the catheter. The gas flow through a 21 gauge catheter with a 50 PSI source is 1,600 mL/sec.[72] Therefore, ventilation time is 0.5 to 1 second with 3 to 5 seconds (an inspiration to expiration ratio of 1 to 3) between each ventilation to allow adequate expiration.

One variant of the needle cricothyroidotomy is the use of an Arrow Rapid Infusion Catheter (RIC) set (Figure 23-35) to increase the size of the catheter. Once a 21 or 16 gauge catheter is in place, a small wire is inserted through that catheter until the distal end of the wire is in the trachea. The original IV catheter is removed, a small nick is made in the skin, and the RIC catheter and dilator are threaded over the wire and inserted through the skin to the hub. The dilator and the wire are then removed and the larger RIC catheter remains in place.

Percutaneous Devices

There are a number of manufacturers of percutaneous airway management kits. As each manufacturer's device and insertion technique is different and new kits are being introduced, it is not practical to examine each specific device. Instead, it is important to recognize that there are three general techniques and most devices use a variant of one of these techniques. The three techniques are direct insertion of a larger device

with a removable trochar, insertion of a small device with subsequent dilators, or a Seldinger (over the wire) technique.

The first class of devices (Figure 23-36) uses a relatively large catheter to puncture the cricothyroid membrane. Once in the trachea, the needle is removed and the catheter advanced to its maximum depth. It is secured in place and attached to a BVM with a built-in 15 mm adapter. These devices have a minimum of parts and are easy to use.

The second class of devices (Figure 23-37) is placed through the use of a smaller needle for puncture. Once a small needle is introduced into the airway, serial dilation or placement of a through-the-needle larger catheter allows the size of the original catheter to be increased. Once the largest device is in place, the trochar is removed and the device is secured. There is an adapter on the largest cannula that allows a BVM or ventilator to be attached. These devices are also

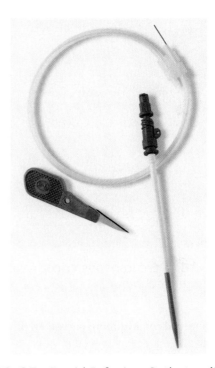

Figure 23-35 Rapid Infusion Catheter (RIC) set.
(Courtesy of Teleflex Medical/Arrow International)

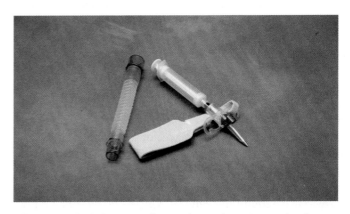

Figure 23-36 Needle and trochar-type device.

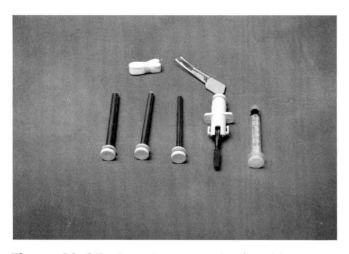

Figure 23-37 Percutaneous cricothyroidotomy using dilators.

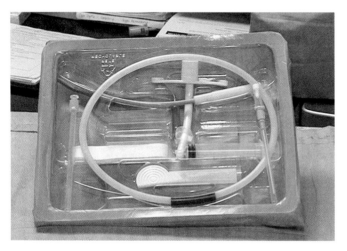

Figure 23-38 Percutaneous cricothyroidotomy using Seldinger technique.

easy to use but tend to have more parts than direct insertion devices.

The third class of devices (Figure 23-38) uses a Seldinger, or over the wire, method of placing a tracheostomy-like tube. A small catheter is used to cannulate the airway and a wire is placed through that catheter. The original catheter is removed and progressively larger catheters are placed until a final, large tube is placed. The wire is then removed and the device secured. Although these devices allow for the placement of a large final airway, they have many parts and require some degree of dexterity to use. Therefore, their application in the prehospital environment is somewhat limited.

Regardless of the percutaneous technique used, there are some important rules. Landmark recognition is a critical component of correct performance of this skill. Furthermore, bleeding is expected. As with other techniques, the Paramedic must first secure the airway and then focus on bleeding control. Finally, all of these techniques should be practiced regularly as they require some motor skill and familiarity with the equipment.

Post-Intubation Care

Once a patient has been intubated, the tube placement confirmed, and the tube secured, there are some procedures that may need to be performed to maximize the patient's respiratory care. Although ongoing ventilation is the most obvious of these procedures, other care should also be considered. Other procedures include placement of a nasogastric or orogastric tube and tracheobronchial suctioning.

Post-Intubation Ventilation

It is important for the Paramedic to recognize that the major goal of emergency airway management is to oxygenate the patient. Therefore, proper post-intubation ventilation is critical to minimize hypoxia.

Most providers will use the bag-valve-mask device as their standard "ventilator." Although adequate ventilation can be obtained with the BVM, the finer details of its use are not intuitive. The volume of an adult-sized BVM device will range based on the manufacturer but will usually be between 1,500 and 2,000 mL. For an intubated patient, ventilation volumes of 7 cc/kg ideal body weight (3 to 3.5 cc/lb ideal body weight) are usually adequate. At a ventilatory rate of 12 breaths per minute, a 70 kg adult will have a minute ventilation of approximately 6 liters. This is adequate for most patients; those with asthma or other pulmonary disease, however, may require minute ventilations of up to 20 LPM. Therefore, ventilation must be adjusted to suit the patient's clinical condition. Unfortunately, it may be difficult to adequately gauge minute ventilation when using a BVM as it is difficult to determine exactly what volume is being delivered. Furthermore, using a BVM requires a provider to squeeze the bag, thereby tying up someone who could be providing other care.

Many services, particularly those performing critical care transports, have begun to use more and more sophisticated ventilators to provide ventilation to intubated patients. These devices may range from selecting preset volume/rate combinations to being able to independently control volume, rate, and end-expiratory pressures to being able to select between pressure control modes, volume control modes, and support modes. The most basic parameters to be set are the rate and volume (or peak pressure); these two parameters establish the minute ventilation. By being able to set the minute ventilation, the patient will receive consistent ventilation without factors such as human fatigue playing a role.

Every manufacturer has special features and characteristics of its ventilators. Therefore, it is important that all Paramedics familiarize themselves with the ventilator that they will be using. The manufacturer should be able to provide training and reference materials for the use of its equipment and special features of that particular type of ventilation.

There are a number of advantages and disadvantages to automatic transport ventilators. Most importantly, they provide consistent and predictable ventilation. They also free a provider from the task of squeezing a BVM device. They are lightweight, relatively inexpensive, and most are oxygen powered. Many have high-pressure alarms and other alerts that notify the Paramedic of changes in the airway or of the patient's condition. Disadvantages include an inability to detect sudden changes in compliance (e.g., displaced tube, pneumothorax), the start-up costs of the devices, the need to have disposable ventilator circuits available, and the dependence on an oxygen source to provide ventilation. Nonetheless, many agencies find the overall convenience and utility of ventilators offset their disadvantages.

Orogastric and Nasogastric Tube Placement

All patients who receive positive pressure ventilation before intubation have some degree of gastric inflation. In adults, this gastric distention increases the risk for vomiting and aspiration and, to some degree, compromises respiratory mechanics. In the pediatric patient, the same concerns for vomiting and aspiration exist. However, the ventilatory compromise that occurs with gastric inflation can make ventilation completely ineffective. Therefore, the placement of an **orogastric tube**, a single-lumen tube passed through the mouth into the stomach to evacuate air from the stomach, in all patients who have received non-intubated bag-valve-mask ventilation should be considered mandatory. In addition, conscious patients with bowel obstruction or toxic ingestions may benefit from the placement of a **nasogastric tube**, a single-lumen tube passed through the nose into the stomach to evacuate air from the stomach.

There are contraindications to the placement of gastric tubes. Patients with esophageal obstruction cannot have a gastric tube placed. In addition, caution must be used in placing a gastric tube in a patient with a history of esophageal disease (varices or caustic ingestion) and, in the case of nasogastric tubes, in patients at risk for basilar skull fractures.

Gastric tubes are long, thin tubes of various internal diameters designed to be blindly placed into the stomach. The tube is sized based on its purpose (decompression of the stomach or evacuation of contents), the size of the patient, and if nasogastric (smaller tube) or orogastric (larger tube) placement is planned. A gastric tube, a catheter tip syringe, and some form of lubricant (Figure 23-39) are needed to place the tube.

Placement of a nasogastric tube is typically done in an awake patient who will not tolerate an orogastric tube. The patient and equipment must be prepared. Unless contraindicated, use of a nasal decongestant (e.g., Afrin®) and a topical anesthetic (e.g., viscous lidocaine or lidocaine jelly) to premedicate the patient is advised. The patient should be examined for nasal pathology (e.g., tumors, trauma, and septal deviation) which would preclude use of the nostril. The patient should then sit in a neutral position.

If possible, prewarming the gastric tube will make it pass more easily. The tube must be measured for size. For a nasogastric tube, the tip of the tube is placed just inferior to the xyphoid. The tube is then measured to the ear and bent anteriorly where it is measured to the tip of the nose. This distance

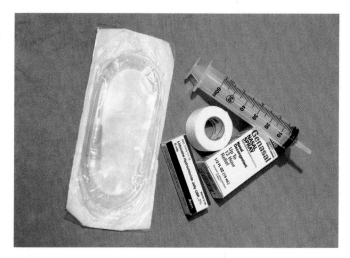

Figure 23-39 Nasogastric tube.

should be marked or otherwise noted as this is the proper depth of insertion for the tube.

The tip of the tube is then lubricated and inserted into the nare parallel to the floor of the nose. A common mistake is to angle the tube superiorly during insertion. This tendency can be eliminated by putting the index finger of the non-dominant hand on the tip of the nose and lifting up to pull the nostrils upward. The tube is then advanced until it strikes the posterior nasopharynx. Gentle pressure and rotation will make it turn downward. It should be advanced to the previously noted insertion depth. Although the patient may gag with correct placement, coughing or loss of the ability to speak suggest placement of the gastric tube through the vocal cords. In that case, the tube should be partially withdrawn. Having the patient swallow while the tube is being advanced will increase the chances of successful placement.

Once the tube is at its proper insertion depth, immediate return of stomach contents indicates a gastric placement. Even if nothing returns, 500 cc of air should be injected into the tube while the Paramedic auscultates over the epigastrium. Loud sounds confirm proper tube placement. The tube is then secured to the nose and face with tape and the stomach either suctioned or allowed to equilibrate with the outside pressure (Skill 23-7).

For a step-by-step demonstration of Nasogastric Tube Placement, please refer to Skill 23-7 on page 463.

Orogastric tube placement is generally performed in the unresponsive, apneic patient after intubation. The patient will typically be supine. The tube is measured from the point just below the tip of the xyphoid to the angle of the jaw and then to the lips. The patient is prepared by performing a jaw lift. The gastric tube, already lubricated, is inserted into the mouth and advanced until it strikes the posterior oropharynx. Gentle manipulation should cause it to turn inferiorly. It is advanced to its proper depth and position is confirmed in the same way as for the nasogastric tube. Generally the

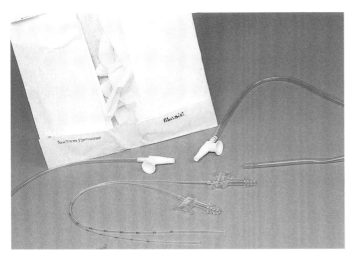

Figure 23-40 Flexible French suction catheters.

gastric tube is secured separately from the endotracheal tube to prevent a mishap with one from affecting the other.

Gastric tubes are not without their complications. Complications associated with both oral and nasal placement include supragastric placement, curling in the oropharynx, endotracheal placement, and tube obstruction. Endotracheal placement can even occur in the patient who is already endotracheally intubated, particularly if a smaller diameter gastric tube is used. For nasogastric (NG) placement, nasal trauma can lead to extensive bleeding. The patient with an orogastric (OG) tube is at risk of biting the OG tube if some type of bite block protection is not used. Excessive force during placement can cause airway injury, laryngeal injury, and esophageal injury.

Tracheobronchial Suctioning

Many patients who require intubation have some degree of lung pathology. This can range from aspiration to thick mucus plugging to blood. Once a patient has been intubated, the Paramedic has access to the trachea and bronchial tree for suctioning in a way that is not possible without intubation. Therefore, the technique of deep tracheal or **tracheobronchial suctioning**, direct suctioning of the secretions in the bronchial tree, is an important skill to master.

Soft, long, and thin suction catheters (Figure 23-40) are used for tracheobronchial suctioning. These catheters can either be single-use catheters or can be designed as a preassembled component of a ventilator circuit. This second type of catheter offers the advantage of not requiring that the ventilator be unhooked from the endotracheal tube before suctioning. These devices do, however, add more dead air space to the ventilator circuit.

The patient should be prepared for deep tracheal suctioning with aggressive preoxygenation. If the patient has copious or thick secretions, a 3 to 5 cc saline flush down the endotracheal tube followed by two to three quick ventilations may help. The catheter should be advanced carefully and inserted until resistance is met. The catheter is then withdrawn with a total time of no more than 15 seconds. The patient is then oxygenated and ventilated before another suction attempt is made (**Skill 23-8**).

For a step-by-step demonstration of Tracheobronchial Suctioning, please refer to Skill 23-8 on page 465.

Special Circumstances

Although the Advanced Airway Management Algorithm will provide guidance for most airway management issues, there are a few circumstances that are not easy to predict and do not fall into a single category of action. It is therefore important for the Paramedic to be well versed in the management of special circumstances. These circumstances include patients with stomas, trauma patients, and pediatric patients.

Stoma Management

Patients may have stomas for any number of reasons. For the Paramedic, it is important to recognize whether the patient only has a tracheostomy (where the airway is otherwise intact) or if the patient has had a laryngectomy as well (where the trachea is rerouted to the skin and there is no connection between the upper airway and the trachea). Patients with complete laryngectomies are completely dependent on the patency of their tracheostomy to ventilate. Patients may also have a well-healed stoma or may still have a tracheostomy tube in place. If there is a tube in place, it is at risk for occlusion and displacement with subsequent obstruction.

Tracheostomy tubes and stomas may become occluded with mucus or other substances. Often, simple suction maneuvers are sufficient to clear these orifices. Suctioning is performed by preoxygenating the patient and injecting 2 to 3 cc of normal saline into the stoma. The patient exhales and a soft-tip catheter is inserted until resistance is met. The site is then gently suctioned. If there is an inner cannula to the tracheostomy tube, it can be removed and either replaced or cleaned and returned.

Over time, a stoma may undergo stenosis or narrowing. This can be a life-threatening condition if stoma stenosis prevents ventilation and the patient can acutely decompensate. The patient should have an endotracheal tube placed through the stoma immediately to relieve the obstruction.

Tube replacement is accomplished through the use of a tracheostomy tube or an endotracheal tube. In addition, critically ill patients with stomas who need to be ventilated should have a tube placed to facilitate ventilation. The tracheostomy tube or cuffed endotracheal tube is lubricated. It is advanced through the stoma until the cuff is in approximately 2 cm. The cuff is then inflated, the position confirmed, and the tube secured to the neck. Care must be taken to avoid excessive movement of the tube as there is only a small amount of the tube in the airway.

The Trauma Patient

Airway management of the trauma patient is not fundamentally different from airway management of any patient. There are some important considerations, however. These include concerns about airway injuries, cervical spine movement, the need for early interventions for respiratory compromise from chest wall or pulmonary injuries, and consideration for the early and aggressive use of sedation and paralysis.

Any patient experiencing a traumatic injury is at risk for trauma to the airway itself. When assessing a trauma patient, the Paramedic must quickly evaluate the impact of all injuries on the airway and how they will affect his decisions and techniques. Burns tend to produce early and significant airway damage requiring rapid intubation. Laryngeal trauma can distort anatomy, obstruct the airway, and produce copious airway bleeding. Tracheal transection makes successful orotracheal intubation unlikely. An open tracheal transection, however, invites intubation through the wound. When managing a traumatized airway, suction and good tube placement confirmation skills are critical.

All trauma patients with an altered level of consciousness or an appropriate mechanism must be considered to have a cervical spine injury. Therefore, all of these intubations must be performed with the patient's head in a neutral position. One provider should be assigned the task of maintaining C-spine immobilization and the C-collar should be opened anteriorly to facilitate jaw movement. Always remember that apnea in an otherwise apparently uninjured patient may represent a spinal cord transection.

Trauma to the chest can cause considerable injury. Two important injury processes—flail chest and tension pneumothorax—will have an impact on airway and ventilation management. In flail chest, two or more fractures of two or more consecutive ribs disrupt the stability to the rib cage, resulting in paradoxical collapse inward of that section of the chest wall during inspiration. This results in underinflation of the affected lung. In addition, the trauma necessary to produce a flail segment will also usually injure the underlying lung. Therefore, early stabilization of the flail segment is important to maximize the patient's ventilatory function.

A pneumothorax may also cause significant respiratory compromise. Although there is emerging evidence that prehospital needle decompression does not have a significant impact on patient outcome,[73] few would argue that a patient with respiratory compromise, unilateral diminished or absent lung sounds, and shock should not receive the benefit of a needle decompression. Early recognition and rapid diagnosis of the injury is absolutely necessary.

Trauma patients, particularly multi-trauma patients, often are sufficiently ill to have lost their airway reflexes and to be combative, but not to be obtunded. This is particularly true if the patient has a head injury. Early and aggressive use of medication-facilitated and rapid sequence intubation techniques to secure these patient's airway is warranted. The issue will be discussed in greater detail in Chapter 24.

The Pediatric Patient

Pediatric patients present the Paramedic with a special set of issues and problems. Although the fundamental equipment and techniques are the same, the anatomic and physiologic differences discussed in Chapter 20 result in differences in the airway management of these patients. As was discussed in Chapter 22, good face-mask ventilatory skills are mandatory for pediatric airway management.

Best Practice

Traditionally, it has been accepted that prehospital intubation of pediatric patients is good care. Studies have demonstrated that Paramedics can perform pediatric endotracheal intubation[74] although usually with higher complication rates and lower success rates than for adults.[75-77] Most of these studies have been retrospective in nature and therefore are somewhat limited by study design and data collection. The only major prospective trial on prehospital pediatric endotracheal intubation demonstrated a trend toward worse outcomes with intubation.[78]

Although no single trial should completely change practice, the findings of this study should cause all Paramedics and medical directors to give strong consideration to reviewing system pediatric intubation success rates and outcomes. At present, there is no recommendation for or against pediatric intubation. What is clear, however, is that excellent non-intubated face-mask ventilation skills are important in the management of critically ill children.

The Advanced Airway Management Algorithm

There are significant anatomical and physiological differences between adult and pediatric patients. Earlier in this chapter, differences in the size of equipment were noted, although the equipment itself is fundamentally the same. In addition, the Advanced Airway Management Algorithm can be applied to adults and pediatric patients. There are some important differences, however, in the techniques that should be applied.

Patient Preparation

The anatomic differences of the pediatric head make positioning much more important. Laying a child supine without padding will result in neck flexion with "crimping off" of the airway (Figure 23-41). However, excessive head extension can also "crimp off" the airway. Therefore, neutral positioning is much more ideal.

Airway manipulation of children under age 8 increases vagal tone and may become a major concern during airway management. These children can rapidly become bradycardic and asystolic. Therefore, premedication with atropine (0.02 mg/kg, minimum 0.1 mg, maximum 0.5 mg) is mandatory in all of these children. Use of atropine or glycopyrrolate will also help to minimize secretions.

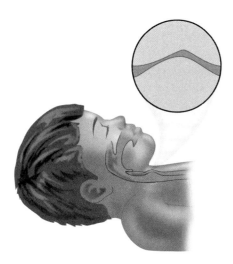

Figure 23-41 Overextension can cause obstruction in a pediatric airway.

Pediatric Intubation

Techniques for selecting the proper-sized blade and endotracheal tube were discussed previously. In most children under 4 to 5 years of age, a straight blade is the most appropriate blade to use. For older children, the Paramedic should use the blade type with which she is most comfortable.

When intubating, the redundant and loose oral mucosa has the potential to compromise visualization of the vocal cords. Therefore, purposeful precise movement to control as much tissue as is possible is mandatory. In addition, care must be taken to minimize bleeding from these very friable tissues. Suction, if used, should be applied judiciously and never directly to the tissue.

The pediatric patient has minimal respiratory reserve. Therefore, hypoxia occurs early and prolonged intubation attempts put the patient at risk for rapid desaturation. Failed intubation attempts should be abandoned early in favor of face-mask ventilation. In addition, as face-mask ventilation may result in better outcomes than intubation anyway, a single failed intubation attempt should cause the Paramedic to consider whether further attempts are warranted or if face-mask ventilation is the better choice.

When passing the endotracheal tube, the smallest diameter of the pediatric airway is at the cricoid ring. Therefore, if the tube passes through the vocal cords but does not advance any further, a smaller tube may be needed. A small air leak around the tube is acceptable and, if airway pressure manometry is being performed, the leak should occur at around 10 cm H_2O. This leak acts as a "safety valve" for preventing acute barotrauma.

The pediatric endotracheal tube has a pair of black lines at the distal end of the endotracheal tube. These lines are depth markers and should be positioned on either side of the vocal cords. Although ultimately the tube may need to be moved due to findings on patient examination, these markers generally do an excellent job of placing the tip of the endotracheal tube at about the middle of the trachea.

Tube Placement Confirmation

Confirming the endotracheal tube placement in pediatric patients can be challenging. Due to the smaller body size, lung sounds and epigastric sounds may be hard to distinguish. The esophageal intubation detector device may report an esophageal intubation despite placement in the trachea due to low lung volumes. However, in a patient with a pulse, an appropriately sized colorimetric end-tidal carbon dioxide detector or capnography device will work. Therefore, constant reassessment of the end-tidal carbon dioxide and vigilant monitoring of the patient's status is critical.

Once the tube position is confirmed, continuous monitoring for a displaced endotracheal tube is also critical. The smaller size of pediatric patients puts them at high risk for tube dislodgment. Any changes in the patient status should make one consider the "DOPE" mnemonic: displaced endotracheal tube, obstructed tube, pneumothorax, or equipment failure. Immobilization of the patient is an important preventative measure against tube dislodgement.

Airway Rescue Devices

The major difference between adult and pediatric patients regarding rescue devices is that the King airway and the Combitube are not sized for pediatric patients. However, there is evidence that the laryngeal mask airway (LMA) is an excellent rescue device for children.[79, 80] The LMA is sized for infants and children and is easily placed. Therefore, the LMA should be the rescue airway of choice for pediatric patients in whom orotracheal intubation cannot be performed.

Surgical Airway Options

The small size of the pediatric airway and the significant risk of airway scarring contraindicates all surgical airway management techniques with the exception of the needle cricothyroidotomy. This technique can be performed on children of all ages. Catheter placement should be performed in the same manner as the placement of an IV in a vein. Although the ideal location is through the cricothyroid membrane, it is often impossible to locate this structure in very small infants. Therefore, a general location of the thyroid cartilage should be determined and the catheter placed in the midline just inferior to the thyroid cartilage. Short inhalation times and a smaller catheter should also be used to minimize peak pressures, to deliver appropriate volumes, and to minimize the risk of acute barotrauma.

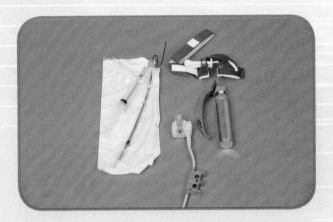

1 Prepare equipment.

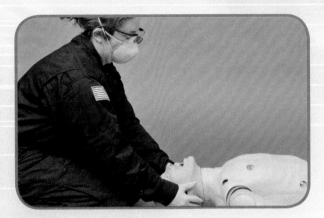

2 Position patient.

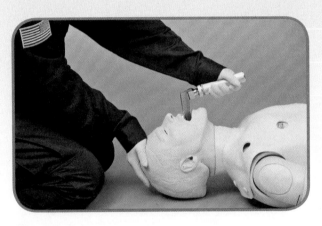

3 Holding laryngoscope in the left hand, place it in the right side of the mouth and sweep to the left.

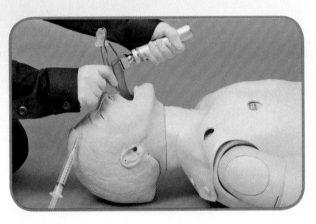

4 Pass endotracheal tube.

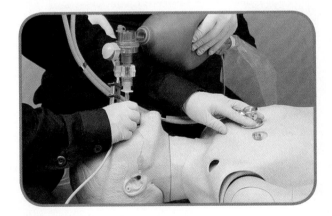

5 Confirm placement.

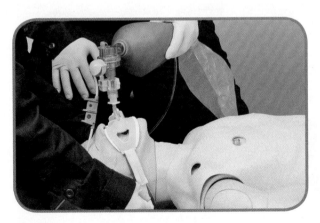

6 Secure the endotracheal tube.

Skill 23-2 Nasotracheal Intubation

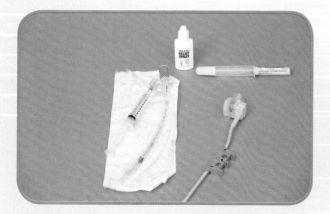

1 Prepare equipment.

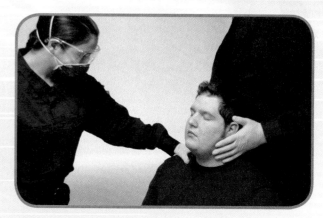

2 Position patient.

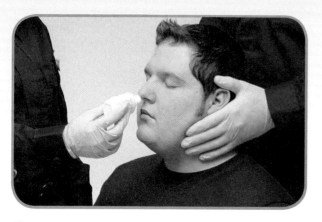

3 Use afrin and lidocaine jelly to prepare nostril.

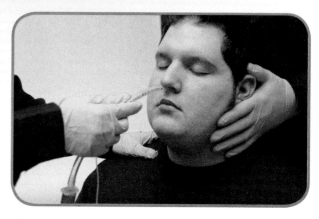

4 Insert right nostril.

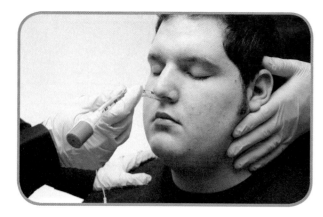

5 Pass into nasopharynx.

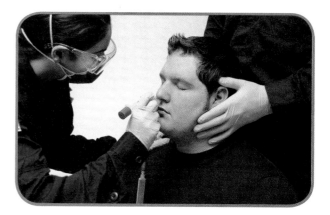

6 Listen for loudest breath sounds.

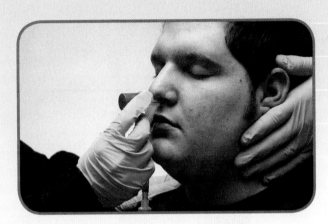

7 Advance during inhalation.

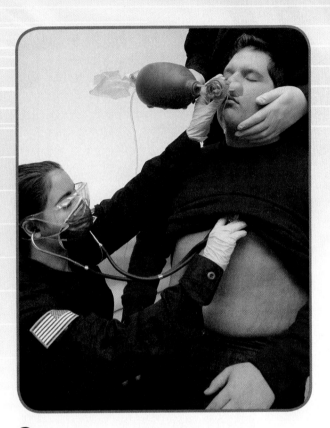

8 Confirm placement.

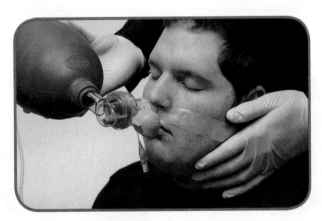

9 Secure nasotracheal tube.

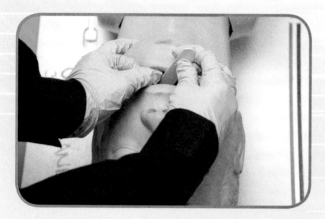

1 Prepare equipment and confirm absence of gag reflex.

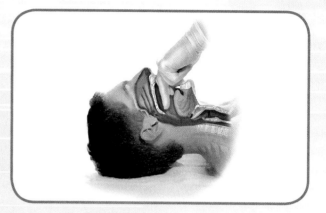

2 Insert hand into mouth and walk fingers down tongue.

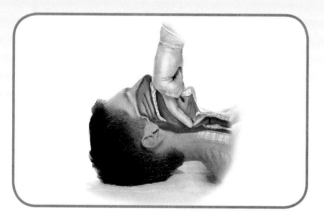

3 Lift epiglottis with middle finger.

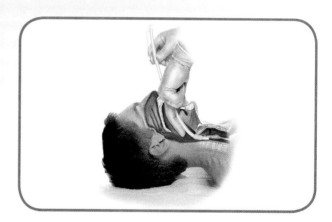

4 Guide endotracheal tube into trachea.

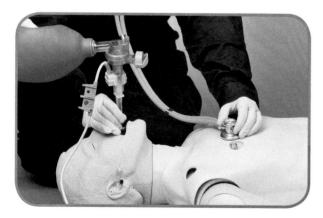

5 Confirm placement.

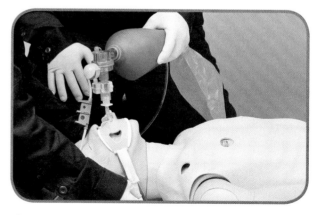

6 Secure endotracheal tube.

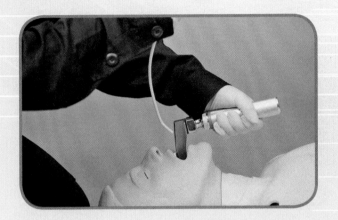

1 Perform laryngoscopy in the usual fashion.

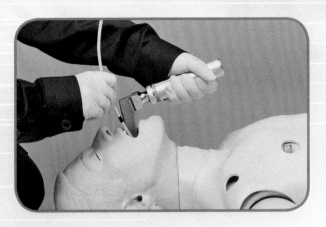

2 Place bougie by aiming the tip midline and anterior.

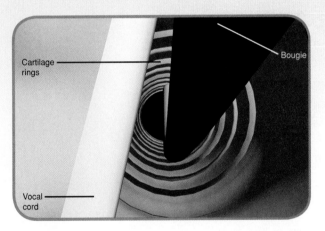

Cartilage rings

Bougie

Vocal cord

3 The bent tip will click as it passes across the cartilage rings and advance until the black band is at the corner of the mouth.

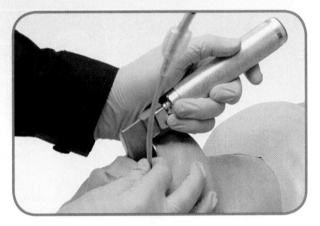

4 Assistant passes endotracheal tube over bougie while keeping the tissues out of the way with the laryngoscope.

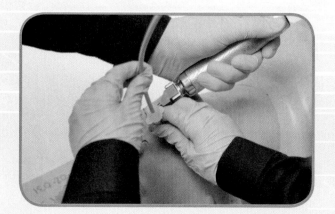

5 Insert endotracheal tube.

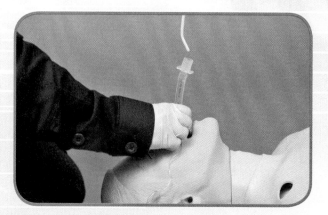

6 Remove bougie.

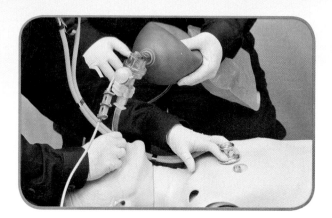

7 Confirm placement and secure endotracheal tube.

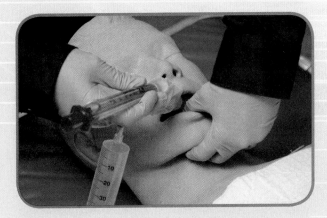

1 Grasp tongue and jaw, lifting toward ceiling. Place tip of tube toward oropharynx, approaching from the patient's right.

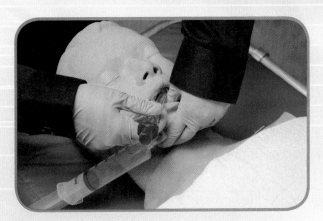

2 Rotate the airway counterclockwise as it is advanced.

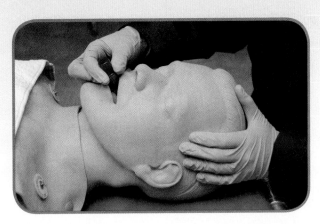

3 Advance until the orogastric port is at the level of the teeth.

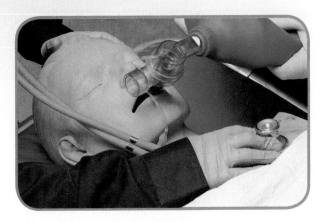

4 Inflate balloon, bag-ventilate the patient, and auscultate breath sounds.

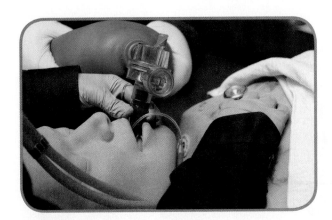

5 Slowly withdraw while listening until breath sounds are the loudest.

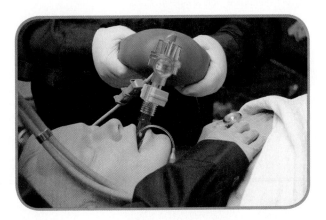

6 Confirm placement and secure airway.

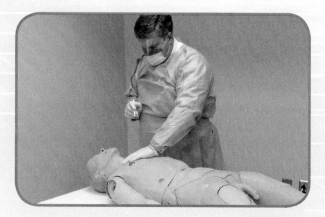

1 Position to the patient's left side.

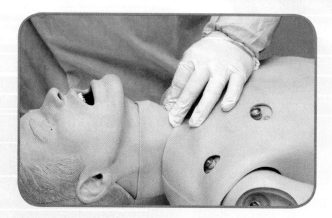

2 Palpate landmarks and stabilize cricoid ring with left hand.

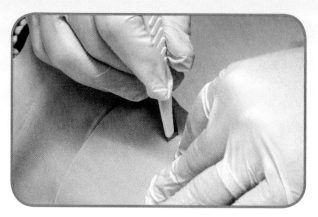

3 Make stab incision with scalpel over the cricothyroid membrane. In obese patients, make a vertical incision and use the handle to bluntly dissect the tissue until you visualize the cricothyroid membrane. Hold scalpel in space.

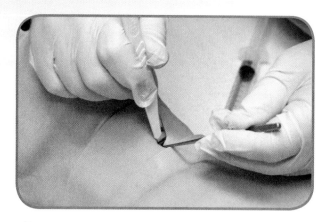

4 With the left hand, place tracheal hook around the cricoid cartilage and gently pull toward the patient's feet.

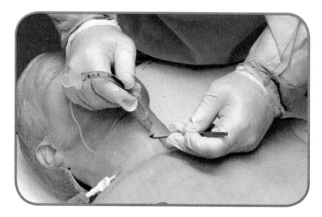

5 Place endotracheal or tracheostomy tube.

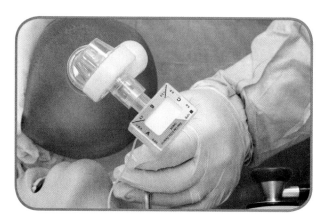

6 Confirm placement, control bleeding, and secure tube.

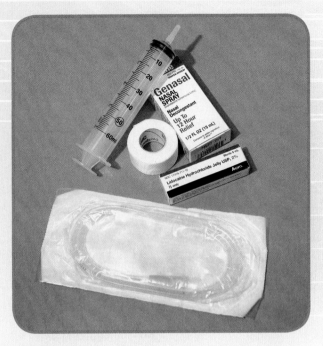

1 Prepare equipment.

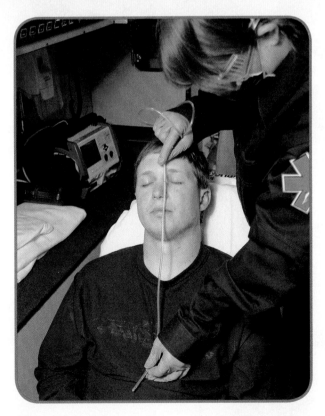

2 Position and premedicate if possible.

3 Measure for length.

4 Insert lubricated tube in nostril.

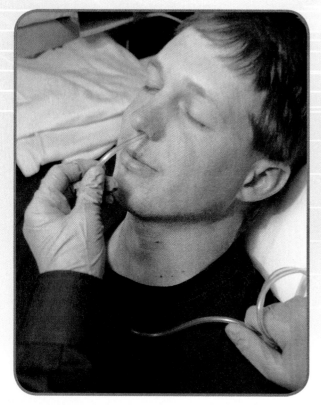

5 Ask patient to swallow as tube is advanced.

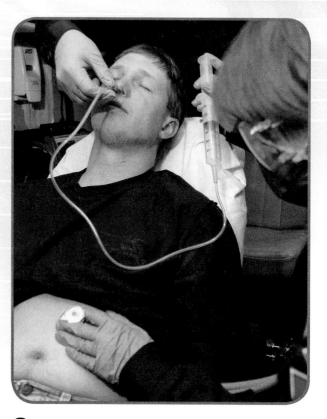

6 When tube is at length, confirm placement by instilling 60 cc of air with a Toomey syringe while auscultating the epigastrium.

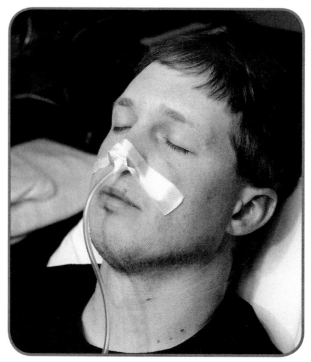

7 Secure the tube with tape.

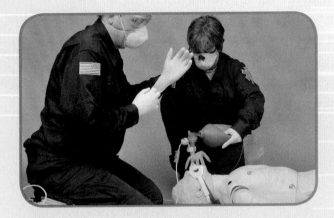

1 Prepare equipment and don sterile gloves.

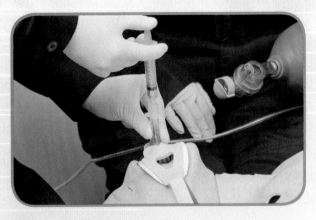

2 Place 3 to 5 cc of saline down endotracheal tube as a flush.

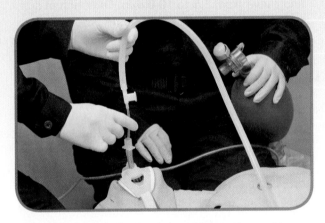

3 Advance suction catheter until resistance is met.

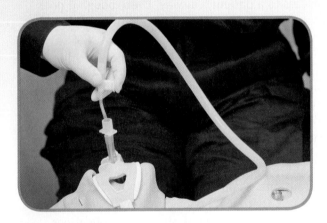

4 Apply suction.

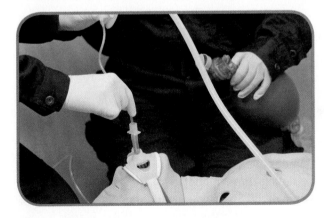

5 Twist the catheter while withdrawing with suction on.

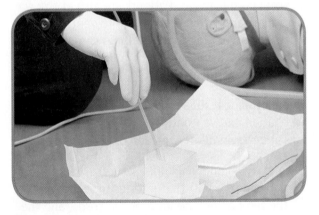

6 Suction sterile saline to clear suction catheter.

CONCLUSION

It is critically important that the Paramedic master basic, non-intubating airway management. However, the definitive management of the airway involves endotracheal intubation. Even under the best of circumstances, however, there are times when the Paramedic cannot intubate a patient. Therefore, it is important for the Paramedic to have a plan and alternatives. The Advanced Airway Management Algorithm, used along with the Paramedic's skills, should provide the Paramedic with the tools necessary to perform definitive advanced airway management.

KEY POINTS:

- An endotracheal tube (ET tube) offers direct access to a patient's airway. Even though it does not absolutely prevent aspiration, it significantly decreases the rates of aspiration.

- The endotracheal tube also allows the Paramedic to perform intermittent positive pressure ventilation, tracheobronchial suctioning, and medication delivery. Perhaps the greatest advantage over non-intubated ventilation is that it does not cause gastric insufflation.

- Disadvantages of endotracheal intubation include the fact that air is no longer filtered, warmed, or humidified by the upper airway. Complications of intubation include bleeding, laryngospasm, laryngeal swelling, mucosal necrosis and erosion, and vocal cord damage. Patients are also at risk for barotrauma and infections related to ventilation devices. Overventilation of the lungs can increase intrathoracic pressures, causing a decrease in systemic blood pressures.

- The endotracheal tube provides a conduit for oxygenation and ventilation between the patient's lungs and the ventilator (person or machine).

- The primary components of an endotracheal tube are the tube, the cuff that inflates to secure and seal the tube below the level of the cords, and the 15 mm adapter that can be connected to a BVM or ventilator. Pediatric tubes are often uncuffed.

- Common features of the endotracheal tube include length markings in centimeters and a beveled distal end with a "Murphy eye."

- ET tubes are sized based on their internal diameter and range from 2.5 to 10.0 mm. Selection of size for pediatric patients can be done based on age, estimating the diameter of the patient's small finger or nare or using length-based tapes.

- Nasotracheal intubation is the placement of an endotracheal tube through the patient's nostril and into the trachea. Blind nasotracheal intubation can only be performed on a breathing patient. Nasal tubes are softer and more pliable than standard tubes to allow them to curve more easily along the posterior oropharynx. They may have a small ring or "trigger" that is used to curve the tip of the tube anteriorly.

- Although not a "sterile" technique, airway management should at least be a "clean" technique and efforts should be made to minimize contamination of the endotracheal tube.

- Preparation of the endotracheal tube includes applying lubricant, checking the cuff for leaks, and placing a stylet. Several other sizes of ET tubes should also be available.

- The laryngoscope is the primary device used to visualize the larynx. The handle serves as a power source and grip point for the Paramedic and the blades are designed to provide a view of laryngeal opening through control of the tongue and the epiglottis. The two most commonly used styles of blades are the Macintosh and Miller blades.

- The Macintosh blade is a curved blade with a large flange and flat surfaces. Common sizes range from 1 to 4. The tip of the blade is intended to fit into the vallecula and elevate the epiglottis via the hyoepiglottic ligament.

- The Miller blade is a straight blade with common sizes from 00 to 4. The straight blade is designed to open a conduit to the larynx on the right side of the mouth and hold the tongue in the midline to the left side of the mouth. The tip of the blade is designed to capture and lift the epiglottis.

- Selecting the appropriate size and type blade depends on the size of the patient and the clinical context. Miller blades are typically used for children under 5 years of age and for trauma patients.

- The blade is attached to the crossbar of the handle until it clicks into place. Once the blade is rotated in place, the light should activate. The Paramedic should make sure the light is white in color, the bulb is tightly screwed into the blade, and the light is steady and bright in intensity.

- The stylet is placed inside an endotracheal tube to provide rigidity and can be shaped to maximize control of its distal tip and improve the chances of successful placement. It is important that the distal end of the stylet not extend beyond the Murphy's eye on the endotracheal tube. A stylet is generally not used for nasotracheal intubations.

- There are numerous devices for securing the endotracheal tube. Regardless of the device, it is important that the endotracheal tube not be able to move. Because the risks of accidental tube dislodgment during patient movement are high, a cervical collar can be applied to the patient to minimize neck extension and flexion.

- To confirm the proper placement of an ET tube, the Paramedic should have a stethoscope immediately available for the auscultation of lung sounds. An esophageal detection device should also be available to use to confirm endotracheal tube placement.

- End-tidal carbon dioxide ($ETCO_2$) measurement and monitoring has become the gold standard for both confirming endotracheal tube placement and monitoring patient status, ventilation, and continuing tube placement. A limit to $ETCO_2$ is that, in patients in cardiac arrest, the lack of carbon dioxide may be mistaken for an esophageal intubation. Conversely, an esophageal intubation may be mistaken for an endotracheal intubation with gastric insufflation, leading to ingestion of carbonated beverages and antacids.

- The least expensive, and probably most commonly used, device for measuring end-tidal carbon dioxide is the colorimetric device. These devices are simply encapsulated pieces of litmus paper over which the exhaled breath flows. A color change indicates CO_2 is being exhaled and the ET tube is properly placed.

- Capnometry devices give a single, numeric peak reading of the exhaled CO_2. End-tidal capnography provides the Paramedic with the numeric values for both the peak and trough $ETCO_2$ levels and displays a graph of the exhalation curve.

- Supraglottic airway devices or blind insertion airway devices (BIADs) include the King LTS-D airway, the esophageal-tracheal Combitube (ETC or Combitube), and the laryngeal mask airway (LMA). The laryngeal mask airway, in essence, moves the mask of face-mask ventilation from the face to the opening of the larynx. The mask should be inflated to assure that it holds air and the distal tips of the mask should be lubricated to improve ease of placement.

- The esophageal-tracheal Combitube (ETC) is a double-lumen device with two separate and distinct lumens that are placed in the esophagus (90% to 99% of the time). However, tracheal placement of the ETC is possible. Each has two cuffs: a large proximal cuff designed to seal the hypopharyngeal portion of the airway and a smaller distal cuff designed to seal the esophagus or trachea, depending on the placement.

- No special equipment is needed for supraglottic airway devices. It has been demonstrated to cause less C-spine movement than conventional endotracheal intubation. The devices are easy to place and may be a useful alternative when patients are in unusual positions. Disadvantages include the inability of medication administration and deep suctioning of the lungs. An elastic gum bougie is a small diameter, semi-rigid device that is directed through the vocal cords and into the trachea to serve as a guide for an endotracheal tube. The endotracheal tube is then threaded over the proximal end and advanced into the trachea.

- Lighted stylettes are essentially malleable stylettes with a bright light source. When placed in the trachea, provide a bright, well-circumscribed light that can be seen in the midline of the trachea.

- One of the other advantages, besides illumination, of the close proximity of the trachea to the anterior neck is that surgical airway management can be achieved rapidly and effectively. A true or classical surgical airway is a relatively simple process that involves the identification of the cricothyroid membrane, cutting a hole through the cricothyroid membrane, and placing an endotracheal tube or cuffed tracheostomy through that hole.

- It is important to note that a surgical airway should be performed only if that patient cannot be intubated, a rescue device cannot be placed, and the patient cannot be ventilated with standard face-mask techniques.

- Needle cricothyrotomy ventilates the lungs using special high-pressure devices after a needle device is used to introduce a catheter or tracheostomy tube.

- To prepare the patient for intubation, the Paramedic should first assess the level of difficulty before attempting airway management. The 3-3-2 rule and the "LEMON" law are two methods for assessing a patient's airway along with the Paramedic assigning a Mallampati score.

- When positioning the patient for endotracheal intubation, the sniffing position is considered to be the intubation position of choice. Both the sniffing position and head-tilt, chin-lift maneuvers help to align the oral, pharyngeal, and laryngeal axes, allowing for the best view during intubation.

- For patients who are unable to lie flat, the Head Elevated Laryngoscopic Position (HELP) may be used.

- Neck flexion and head extension are contraindicated in trauma patients. While providing in-line stabilization from the inferior direction, the

Paramedic can utilize the modified jaw-thrust maneuver or BURP technique to create ideal positioning.

- The final step in patient preparation is the appropriate use of sedatives and paralytic agents.

- The process for intubation can be broken down into four steps:
  1. Visualizing the vocal cords
  2. Passing the endotracheal tube
  3. Confirming endotracheal tube placement
  4. Securing the endotracheal tube

- Endotracheal intubation is a team activity, and the Paramedic may ask other EMS personnel to provide cricoid pressure, BURP technique, or external laryngeal manipulation.

- The tip of the MacIntosh blade is designed to fit into the vallecula. When lifted anteriorly and inferiorly, the blade lifts the hyoepiglottic ligament, which pulls the epiglottis anteriorly and reveals the vocal cords.

- The Miller blade is designed to pin the epiglottis against the base of the tongue anteriorly and provide a straight-on view of the vocal cords. The tip of the blade lifts up the epiglottis to reveal the vocal cords.

- The Cormack-Lehane grading system grades the view of the glottic opening by how much is occluded by the tongue. Grade I is a clear view of the entire glottic opening while IV is visualization of the tongue or soft palate only.

- To assist the Paramedic in visualizing the cords, an assistant can use a finger or rigid suction catheter to hook and retract the corner of the patient's mouth.

- Suctioning itself may be used to improve visualization and minimize airway and soft tissue trauma.

- Magill forceps are used to remove large foreign bodies occluding the airway. If the foreign body is subglottic and cannot be grasped with the Magill forceps, it should be pushed into a mainstem bronchus with an endotracheal tube. The tube is then withdrawn to above the carina to allow at least one lung to be ventilated.

- If the cords are closed due to laryngospasm or only partially open, the Paramedic should apply gentle pressure to the lip of the tube bevel between the cords, which may cause them to relax sufficiently to pass the tube. The tube or the stylet should not be "forced" between the cords.

- When the first breath is delivered, the epigastrium should be auscultated. Loud noises over the epigastrium with abdominal distention and no chest movement strongly suggest esophageal placement.

- Diminished or absent lung sounds on the left are often due to the endotracheal tube being placed in the right mainstem bronchus.

- Once the tube position is assessed by auscultation, the Paramedic should assess placement using end-tidal carbon dioxide measurement. The Paramedic should look for readings of 30 to 40 with a wave that rises and falls appropriately with ventilation and has a consistent shape.

- For patients without spontaneous circulation, the Paramedic should use an esophageal detector device for confirmation of endotracheal tube placement.

- The mnemonic DOPE can help the Paramedic remember the causes of problem intubations.

- It is important that the tube position be assessed after each move.

- Nasal intubation is indicated for patients who are difficult to access or, due to their disease process, are likely to experience rapid decompensation if they lay flat.

- Contraindications to nasotracheal intubation include apnea, evidence of basilar skull fracture, or inability to pass the tube through a nare.

- The tube should be placed in the most patent nare with the tip of the tube parallel to the floor of the nose. A Beck Airway Airflow Monitor (BAAM) should be used to detect breath sounds. The tube is then advanced through the cords during inspiration until approximately 2 cm protrude from the nose.

- The endotracheal tube placement is confirmed in the same manner as in an orotracheal intubation.

- If the intubation fails, the Paramedic should assess reasons why it failed and make attempts to correct it before attempting intubation a second time.

- A digital intubation is a blind technique that is useful not only for supine patients, but patients who are in a sitting position or for whom access to the head is limited.

- The elastic gum bougie is placed under direct visualization with a laryngoscope. The tip of the bougie is advanced anterior to the posterior arytenoids until the tip "clicks" along the tracheal rings. An endotracheal tube is threaded over the external end of the bougie and advanced into the trachea.

- When the Paramedic is performing translaryngeal illumination with a lighted stylet, the stylet is advanced until a focal, bright midline glow is visible at the level of the larynx.

- Supraglottic airway devices provide a method of at least partially securing the airway in the difficult-to-intubate patient. The three most commonly used devices, as described earlier, are the
  1. King LTS-D airway
  2. The laryngeal mask airway
  3. The esophageal-tracheal Combitube

- When performing a needle cricothyroidotomy, proper technique requires good landmark identification and care in ventilation to prevent overpressurization.

- Percutaneous devices include the direct insertion of a larger device with a removable trochar, insertion of a small device with subsequent dilators, or use of a Seldinger (over the wire) technique.

- Post-intubation care involves ventilating, monitoring the airway, placing a nasogastric or orogastric tube, and performing tracheobronchial suctioning.

- Automatic transport ventilators can provide the Paramedic consistent and predictable ventilation; control over volume, rate, and expiratory pressures;

and high-pressure alarms. Disadvantages include its dependence on an oxygen source to provide ventilation.

- To reduce the risk of vomiting or aspiration caused by gastric inflation, the Paramedic should place an orogastric or nasogastric tube.

- Soft, long, and thin suction catheters are used for tracheobronchial suctioning.

- Any patient experiencing a traumatic injury is at risk for trauma to the airway itself.

- With the assessment findings of a flail chest injury or tension pneumothorax, the conditions should be treated during airway and ventilatory management.

- Early and aggressive use of medication-facilitated and rapid sequence intubation techniques to secure these patients' airways is warranted with trauma patients who have lost their airway reflexes and are combative, but not to be obtunded.

- Face-mask ventilation skills are important in the management of critically ill children.

- The Paramedic should note that the pediatric patient has minimal respiratory reserve. Prolonged intubation attempts put the patient at risk for rapid desaturation.

- The LMA should be the rescue airway of choice for pediatric patients in whom orotracheal intubation cannot be performed.

- Needle cricothyroidotomy can also be performed on children of all ages.

- To minimize peak pressures, short inhalation times and a smaller catheter should be used to deliver appropriate volumes, and to minimize the risk of acute barotrauma.

▶ REVIEW QUESTIONS:

1. Weigh the advantages and disadvantages of endotracheal intubation.
2. Describe the components of an endotracheal and nasotracheal tube.
3. Create a chart that compares and contrasts the Miller blade with the Macintosh blade.
4. A Paramedic is presented with a patient in severe respiratory distress who is decompensating quickly. How would the Paramedic quickly and efficiently assess the patient's airway?
5. The Paramedic decides that the patient requires endotracheal intubation. While the team members are performing bag-valve-mask ventilations with cricoid pressure, what equipment must the Paramedic have prepared, checked, and ready before breaking the mask seal?

6. What does continuous end-tidal capnography offer the Paramedic?
7. For each of the following blind insertion airway devices, describe the preparation and technique for insertion: King LTS-D airway, the esophageal-tracheal Combitube (ETC or Combitube), and the laryngeal mask airway (LMA).
8. How can the use of an elastic gum bougie make the first attempt at endotracheal intubation the best attempt?
9. The process for intubation can be broken down into four steps. Describe each step.
10. Why is it important for the Paramedic to reassess tube position each time the patient is moved? What are some causes of tube displacement, and how would the Paramedic know that it is out of place?

11. If attempts to intubate and place a BIAD fail, what two alternatives remain for the Paramedic?

12. Describe the technique for landmark identification for a needle cricothyroidotomy.

13. After intubation, the Paramedic notices copious thick secretions, decreased O_2 saturation, and poor ventilatory compliance. What can be done to remedy this situation and improve the patient's oxygenation and ventilation?

14. Who should receive an orogastric or nasogastric tube? How is each prepared for placement in the patient?

15. What considerations must be made for intubating the pediatric patient?

CASE STUDY QUESTIONS:

Please refer to the Case Study at the beginning of the chapter and answer the questions below:

1. Why were the emergency medical responders experiencing problems with the patient vomiting?

2. What could they have done to help prevent the patient's vomiting?

3. What indications did the Paramedic have to intubate the patient?

REFERENCES:

1. Hazinski MF, eds. *PALS Provider Manual*. Dallas: AHA; 2001:100.

2. Vilke GM. Estimation of pediatric patient weight by EMT-Ps. *J Emerg Med*. 2001;21(2):125–128.

3. Hofer CK. How reliable is length-based determination of body weight and tracheal tube size in the paediatric age group? The Broselow tape reconsidered. *Br J Anesthesia*. 2002;88(2):283–285.

4. Luten R. Error and time delay in pediatric trauma resuscitation. Addressing the problem with color-coded resuscitation aids. *Surg Clin N.A* 2002;82(2):303–321.

5. Vilke GM, O'Connor RE, Megargel RE, Schnyder ME, Madden JF, Bitner M, Ross R. Paramedic success rate for blind nasotracheal intubation is improved with the use of an endotracheal tube with directional tip control. *Annals Emerg Med*. 2000;36(2):328–332.

6. Grove P. Endotracheal tube stability in the resuscitation environment. *Australian Critical Care*. 2000;13(1):6–8.

7. Andersen KH, Hald A. Assessing the position of the tracheal tube: the reliability of different methods. *Anesthesia*. 1989;44(12):984–985.

8. Donahue PL. The oesophageal detector device: an assessment of accuracy and ease of use by Paramedics. *Anesthesia*. 1994;49(10):465–467.

9. Salem MR, Wafai Y, Joseph NJ, et al. Efficacy of the self-inflating bulb in detecting esophageal intubation: does the presence of a nasogastric tube or cuff deflation make a difference? *Anesthesiology*. 1994;80(1):42–48.

10. Zaleski L, Abello D, Gold MI. The esophageal detector device: does it work? *Anesthesiology*. 1993;79(2):244–247.

11. Tanigawa K, Takeda T, Goto E, Tanaka K. Accuracy and reliability of the self-inflating bulb to verify tracheal intubation in out-of-hospital cardiac arrest patients. *Anesthesiology*. 2000;93(6):1432–1436.

12. Andres AH, Langstein H. The esophageal detector device is unreliable when the stomach has been ventilated. *Anesthesiology*. 1999;91(2):566–568.

13. Lang DJ, Wafai Y, Salem MR, et al. Efficacy of the self inflating bulb in confirming tracheal intubations in the morbidly obese. *Anesthesiology*. 1996;85(2):246–253.

14. Salem MR. Verification of endotracheal tube position. *Anes Clin North America*. 2001;19(4):813–839.

15. Denman WT, Hayes M, Higins D, et al. The Fenem CO_2 detector device: an apparatus to prevent unnoticed oesophageal intubation. *Anaesthesia*. 1990;45(6):465–467.

16. Goldberg JS, Rawle PP, Zehnder IL, et al. Colorimetric end-tidal carbon dioxide monitoring for tracheal intubation. *Anesth Analg*. 1990;70(2):191–194.

17. Bhavani-Shankar K, Moseley H, Kumar AY, Delph Y. Capnometry and anesthesia. *Can J Anes*. 1992;39(6):617–632.

18. Knapp S, Kofler J, Stosier B, et al. The assessment of four different methods to verify tracheal tube placement in the critical care setting. *Anesth Analg*. 1999;88(4):766–770.

19. Frakes MA. Measuring end-tidal carbon dioxide: clinical applications and usefulness. *Crit Care Nurse*. 2001;21(5):23–35.

20. MacLeod BA, Heller MB, Gerard J, Yealy DM, Menegazzi JJ. Verification of endotracheal tube placement with colorimetric end-tidal CO_2 detection. *Ann Emerg Med*. 1991;20(3):267–270.

21. Sum Ping ST, Mehta MP, Anderton JM. A comparative study of methods of detection of esophageal intubation. *Anesth Analg*. 1989;69(5):627–632.

22. Sum Ping ST, Mehta MP, Symreng T. Reliability of capnography in identifying esophageal intubations with carbonated beverages or antacid in the stomach. *Anesth Analg*. 1991;73(3):333–337.

23. Werman HA, Falcone RE. Glottic positioning of the endotracheal tube tip: a diagnostic dilemma. *Ann Emerg Med*. 1998;31(5): 643–646.

24. Bhende MS, Thompson AE, Cook DR, Seville A. Validity of a disposable end-tidal CO_2 detector in verifying endotracheal tube placement in infants and children. *Ann Emerg Med*. 1992;21(2):212–245.

25. Singh S, Venkataraman ST, Saville A, Bhende MS. NPB-75: a portable quantitative microstream capnometer. *Am J Emerg Med*. 2001;19(3):208–210.

26. Campo SL, Denman WT. The laryngeal mask airway: its role in the difficult airway. *International Anes Clin*. 2000;38(3):29–45.

27. Brain AJJ. The laryngeal mask airway—a new concept in airway management. *Br J Anes*. 1983;55(8):801–806.

28. Benumof JL. Laryngeal mask airway and the ASA Difficult Airway Algorithm. *Anesthesiology*. 1996;84(3):686–699.

29. Reinhart DJ, Simmons G. Comparison of placement of the laryngeal mask airway with endotracheal tube by Paramedics and respiratory therapists. *Ann Emerg Med*. 1994;24(2):260–263.

30. Levitan RM, Ochroch EA, Stuart S, Hollander JE. Use of the intubating laryngeal mask airway by medical and nonmedical personnel. *Am J Emerg Med*. 2000;18(1):12–16.

31. Agro F, Frass M, Benumof JL, Krafft P. Current status of the Combitube™: A review of the literature. *J Clin Anesth*. 2002;14(4):307–321.

32. Gaitini LA, Vaida SJ, Mostafa S, et al. The Combitube in elective surgery: a report of 200 cases. *Anesthesiology*. 2001;94(1):79–82.

33. Frass M, Rodler S, Frenzer R, et al. Esophageal tracheal Combitube, endotracheal airway, and mask: comparison of ventilatory pressure curves. *J Trauma*. 1989;29(11):1476–1479.

34. MacIntosh RR. An aid to oral intubation. *BMJ*. 1949;1(4591):28.

35. McGill JW, Vogel EC, Rodgerson JD. Use of the gum elastic bougie as an adjunct for orotracheal intubation in the emergency department [Abstract]. *Acad Emerg Med*. 2000;7(5):526.

36. Dogra S, Falconer R, Latto IP. Successful difficult intubation. Tracheal tube placement over a gum elastic bougie. *Anesthesia*. 1990;45(9):774–776.

37. Gataure PS, Vaughan RS, Latto IP. Simulated difficult intubation. Comparison of the gum elastic bougie and the stylet. *Anesthesia*. 1996;51(10):935–938.

38. Moscati R, Jehle D, Christiansen G, et al. Endotracheal tube introducer for failed intubations: a variant of the gum elastic bougie. *Annals Emerg Med*. 2000;36(1):52–56.

39. MacIntosh R, Richards H. Illuminated introducer for endotracheal tubes. *Anesthesia*. 1957;12(2):223–225.

40. Raj P, Forestner J, Watson TD, Forris RE, Jenkins MT. Techniques for fiberoptic laryngoscopy in anesthesia. *Anesth Analg*. 1974;53(5):708–714.

41. Vollmer TP, Stewart RD, Paris PM, Ellis D, Berkebile PE. Use of a lighted stylet for guided orotracheal intubation in the prehospital setting. *Ann Emerg Med*. 1985;14(4):324–328.

42. Aoyama K, Takenaka I, Nagaoka E, et al. Potential damage to the larynx associated with light guided intubation: a case and series of fiberoptic examinations. *Anesthesiology*. 2001;94(1):165–167.

43. Calkins MD. Combat trauma airway management: endotracheal intubation versus laryngeal mask airway versus Combitube use by Navy SEAL and reconnaissance combat corpsman. *J Trauma*. 1999;46(5):927–932.

44. Gens DR. Surgical airway management. In: Tintinalli, JE, Kelen, GD, Stapczynski JS. *Emergency Medicine: A Comprehensive Study Guide* (5th ed.). New York: McGraw-Hill; 2000:97–101.

45. American College of Surgeons Committee on Trauma. Airway and ventilatory management. In: *Advanced Trauma Life Support for Doctors* (8th ed.). Chicago: American College of Surgeons; 2008:38, 51–53.

46. Klain M, Smith RB. High frequency percutaneous transtracheal jet ventilation. *Crit Care Med*. 1977;5(10):280–287.

47. Thomas T, Zornow M, Scheller MS, et al. The efficacy of three different modes of transtracheal ventilation in hypoxic hypercarbic swine. *Can J Anaesth*. 1989;36(6):624–628.

48. Jacobs HB. Transtracheal catheter ventilation: clinical experience in 36 patients. *Chest*. 1974;37(6):36–40.

49. Weymuller EA, Paugh D, Pavlin EG, et al. Management of the difficult airway problems with percutaneous transtracheal ventilation. *Ann Oto Rhino Laryngol*. 1987;96(6):34.

50. Koay CK. Difficult airway management—analysis and management in 37 cases. *Singapore Medical Journal*. 1998;39(33):112–114.

51. Rose DK, Cohen MM. The airway: problems and predictions in 18,500 patients. *Can J Anaesth*. 1994;41(5):372–383.

52. McIntyre JRW. The difficult intubation. *Can J Anesth*. 1987;34(2):204–213.

53. Jones AEP, Pelton DA. An index of syndromes and their anesthetic implications. *Can Anaesth Soc J*. 1976;23(6):207–226.

54. Mathew M, Hanna LS, Aldrete JA. Preoperative indices to anticipate a difficult tracheal intubation. *Anaesth Analg*. 1989;68(2 Supplement):S187.

55. Murphy MF, Walls RM. The difficult and failed airway. In: Walls RM, Luten RC, Murphy MF, Schneider RE, eds. *Manual of Emergency Airway Management*. Philadelphia: Lippincott Williams and Wilkins; 2000:31–39.

56. Adnet F, Borron S, Lapostolle F, Lapandry C. The three axis alignment theory and the "sniffing position": Perpetuation of an anatomic myth? *Anesthesiology*. 1999;91(6):1964.

57. Bannister FB, MacBeth RG. Direct laryngoscope and tracheal intubation. *Lancet*. 1944;55(2):651–654.

58. Adnet F, Baillard C, Borron SW, et al. Randomized study comparing the "sniffing position" with simple head extension for laryngoscopic view in elective surgery patients. *Anesthesiology.* 2001;95(6):836–841.

59. Benumof JL. Comparison of intubating positions: the end point should be measured. *Anesthesiology.* 2002;97(3):750.

60. Benumof JL. Patient in "sniffing position." *Anesthesiology.* 2000;93(5):1365–1366.

61. Hochman II, Zeitels SM, Heaton JT. Analysis of forces and position required for direct laryngoscopic exposure of the anterior vocal folds. *Ann Oto Rhino Laryn.* 1999;108(8):715–724.

62. Takahata O, Kubota M, Mamiya K, et al. The efficacy of the "BURP" maneuver during difficult laryngoscopy. *Anesthesia and Analgesia.* 1997;84(2):419–421.

63. Henderson JJ. The use of paraglossal straight blade laryngoscopy in difficult tracheal intubation. *Anaesthesia.* 1997;52(6):552–560.

64. Schneider RE. Basic airway management. In: Walls RM, Luten RC, Murphy MF, Schneider RE, eds. *Manual of Emergency Airway Management.* Philadelphia: Lippincott Williams and Wilkins; 2000:43–57.

65. Brunnings W. Autoscopy by counterpressure. In: Phillips W, ed. *Direct Laryngoscopy, Bronchoscopy, and Esophagoscopy.* London: Balliere, Tindall, and Cox; 1912:110–115.

66. Zeitels SM, Vaughn CW. "External counterpressure" and "internal distention" for optimal laryngoscopic exposure of the anterior glottic commissure. *Ann of Oto, Rhino, and Laryn.* 1994;108(8):669–675.

67. Ochroch AE, Levitan RM. A videographic analysis of laryngeal exposure comparing the McCoy levering laryngoscope blade and external laryngeal manipulation. *Anesthesia and Analgesia.* 2001;92(1):267–270.

68. Benumof JL, Cooper SD. Qualitative improvement in laryngoscopic view by optimal external laryngeal manipulation. *J Clin Anesth.* 1996;8(2):136–140.

69. Grove P. Endotracheal tube stability in the resuscitation environment. *Aust Crit Care.* 2000;13(1):6–8.

70. Landsman IS. The laryngeal mask airway. *Int Anesthes Clin.* 1997;35(3):49–65.

71. Brofeldt BT, Panacek EA, Richards JR. An easy cricothyrotomy approach: the rapid four-step technique. *Academic Emergency Medicine.* 1996;3(11):1060–1063.

72. Gaughan SD, Ozaki GT, Benumof JL. Comparison in a lung model of low and high flow regulators for transtracheal jet ventilation. *Anesthesiology.* 1992;77(1):189–199.

73. Sullivan DM. Myths in trauma. In: Ferrera PC, Colucciello SA, Marx JA, Verdile VP, Gibbs MA, eds. *Trauma Management: An Emergency Medicine Approach.* St. Louis: Mosby; 2001:702–709.

74. Brownstein D, Shugerman R, Cummings P, Rivara F, Copass M. Prehospital endotracheal intubation of children by Paramedics. *Ann Emerg Med.* 1996;28(1):34–39.

75. Aijian P, Tsai A, Knopp R, et al. Endotracheal intubation of pediatric patients by Paramedics. *Ann Emerg Med.* 1989;18(5):489–494.

76. Stratton SJ, Underwood LA, Whalen S. et al. Prehospital pediatric intubation: a survey of the United States. *Prehospital and Disaster Medicine.* 1993;8(4):323–326.

77. Pointer JE. Clinical characteristics of Paramedics' performance of pediatric endotracheal intubation. *Am J Emerg Med.* 1989;7(4):364–366.

78. Gauche M, Lewis RJ, Stratton SJ, et al. Effect of out-of-hospital pediatric endotracheal intubation on survival and neurological outcome: a controlled clinical trial. *JAMA.* 2000;283(6):783–790.

79. Mason DG, Bingham RM. The laryngeal mask airway in children. *Anesthesia.* 1990;45(9):760–763.

80. McGinn G, Haynes SR, Morton NS. An evaluation of the laryngeal mask airway during routine paediatric anaesthesia. *Paediatr Aneasth.* 1993;3(1):23–28.

CHAPTER 24

MEDICATION-FACILITATED INTUBATION

KEY CONCEPTS:

Upon completion of this chapter, it is expected that the reader will understand these following concepts:

- Differentiating between medication-facilitated and rapid sequence intubation
- Physiology of neuromuscular blockers including differentiation between depolarizing and non-depolarizing neuromuscular blocking agents
- Patients who are candidates for paralytic agents
- The protective effect of preoxygentaion
- Knowing the "Nine P's of RSI"

▶ CASE STUDY:

It was prom night. Although many police agencies presented material regarding the dangers inherent in partying, the young people in the Honda Civic didn't get the message. Their car hit a pole at a fast speed and the driver had head and chest injuries from the impact. His breathing was impaired and he was combative. The closest trauma center was 35 minutes away by air. The Paramedics made the decision to intubate the driver prior to the helicopter's arrival.

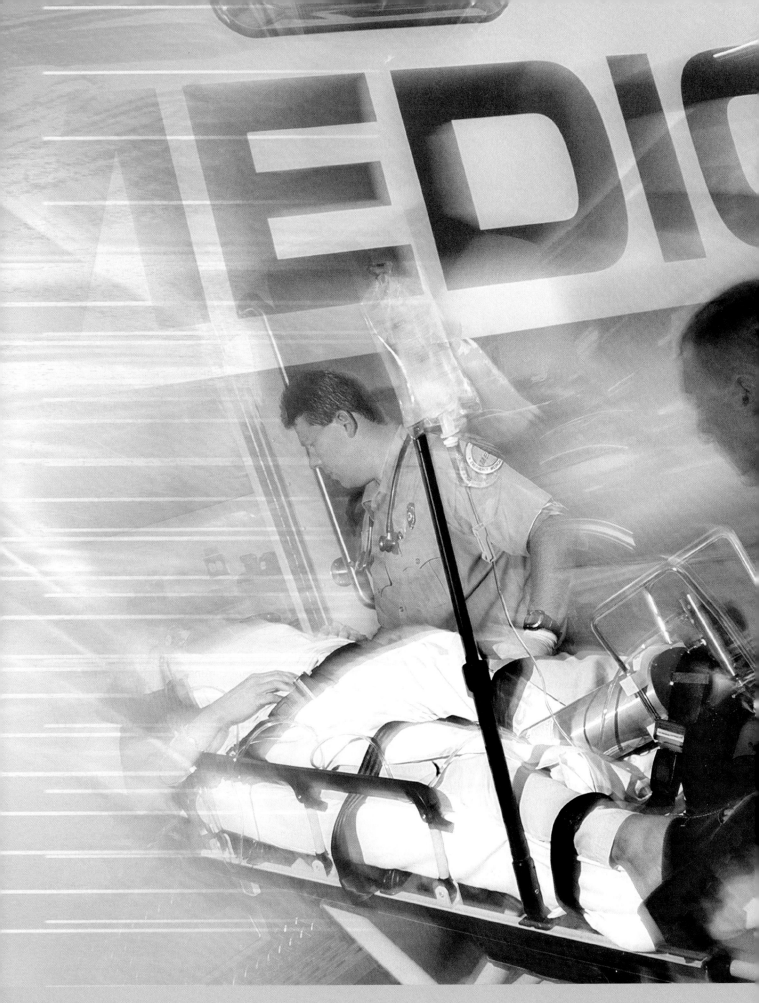

OVERVIEW

Although medication-facilitated and rapid sequence intubation have been relative newcomers to paramedicine, they have become very useful tools in airway management. This chapter outlines the key differences in sedative agents used for intubation and the mechanisms of action for both depolarizing and non-depolarizing neuromuscular blockers. Not all patients should receive paralytic agents.

This chapter will examine the issue of whether or not paralytics should be used in the prehospital environment. This review will then be followed by a discussion of the medications used for medication-facilitated and rapid sequence intubation. The "Nine P's of RSI" will be reviewed, as well as patient assessment and the decision to administer paralytics.

Medication-Facilitated Intubation

Paramedics have always done an excellent job of taking procedures and techniques developed for the in-hospital setting and adapting them for use in the prehospital environment. In addition, many medications have been validated in the prehospital setting, sometimes before being validated in the hospital environment. It is therefore no surprise that in the arena of airway management, the techniques of medication-facilitated and rapid sequence intubation have been trialed and applied in the prehospital setting. As with some other techniques, however, the question of whether Paramedics *should* perform these skills was not nearly as well researched as whether EMS providers *could* perform them. Only recently has that question been addressed.

Medication-facilitated intubation is not a new technique. In fact, it has been used for decades in the operating room and emergency department settings. The use of adjunctive medications, like any other adjunct to intubation, has been (and should be) seen as one more tool to protect patients and improve their quality of care. Broadly speaking, medications for airway management can be divided into those that provide sedation and those that cause muscular paralysis.

In general, many more intubations are performed with sedatives alone. Many EMS agencies and medical directors are more comfortable with sedative-facilitated intubation than with the use of paralytics. Using a variety of sedative agents, Paramedics are able to make patients more comfortable, less anxious, and amnestic to the events of the intubation. Some newer agents such as etomidate are able to provide sufficient sedation to often eliminate the need for paralytics.[1] Sedative-facilitated intubation is therefore becoming a common approach to intubation of the non-cardiac arrest patient.

Paralytic agents can be some of the most dangerous medications Paramedics can administer. By providing and performing the emergency care which causes paralysis, the Paramedic takes a patient with an ability to maintain his airway and ventilate and then eliminates those abilities. Extraordinary clinical judgment is necessary for anyone in the position to paralyze a patient. Nonetheless, there is clear evidence that patients who receive paralytics have better outcomes than those who receive only sedatives.[2] When used properly, sedation and paralysis enable otherwise impossible intubations and eliminate the need for face-mask ventilation and its associated complications (aspiration, gastric distention, etc.). Paralytics, therefore, play an important role in managing patients' airways.

It is important to recognize that if a Paramedic is going to perform rapid sequence intubation with paralytics, then he or she must be properly trained and proficient in adequate alternative airway techniques. Although proper patient selection should minimize the risk of paralyzing a patient who can neither be intubated nor ventilated, the risk exists that this situation might occur. If it does, an alternative is mandatory to prevent hypoxic complications. Although the question of whether or not Paramedics should be using paralytics may not be clearly answered, the fact remains that many providers are using paralytics and therefore it is incumbent on the Paramedic to be familiar with this tool.

Prehospital Provider Use of Paralytics

The use of paralytic agents to facilitate intubation is a long-standing source of controversy among Paramedics and medical directors. The research for and against the use of paralytics has not clearly demonstrated that paralytics have a definitive role in daily EMS practice. Conversely, there is strong evidence that paralytics can be used safely by selected groups of Paramedics providing that they have adequate training, good medical direction and medication utilization review, and a rescue device.

One of the largest studies in support of prehospital use of succinylcholine is a 20-year retrospective study by Wayne and Friedland.[3] Spanning 20 years of practice, this retrospective review evaluated 1,657 consecutive intubations. Overall, a 95.5% successful intubation rate was found. There was a 0.3% unrecognized esophageal intubation rate that was almost eliminated with the addition of capnography and esophageal detector device use. The remaining patients who could not be intubated were successfully managed with alternative methods. This study provides strong support for the prehospital use of paralytics. Similarly, a retrospective study by Hedges et al.[4] conducted 10 years before Wayne and Friedland's study had suggested a similar efficacy and safety profile for succinylcholine-assisted intubation. Several other small studies have also addressed the issue, each demonstrating that out-of-hospital providers can successfully perform rapid sequence intubation.[5–7]

A more recent study by Ochs et al.[8] has clarified some questions concerning the utility of paralytic-assisted intubations. Their study, which focused on head injured patients with otherwise unmanageable airways, demonstrated an 84% successful intubation rate. Of the remaining patients, all but one were successfully managed with a Combitube. The last patient was successfully managed with BVM ventilation. Although this study certainly indicates that prehospital use of succinylcholine will result in some degree of airway management in the vast majority of patients, the intubation failure rate of 16% raises concerns about whether or not field EMS providers get enough experience with routine intubations to expertly manage every airway with which they are faced. Nonetheless, the study population is certainly one in whom airway management has been demonstrated to be critical.[9,10] Furthermore, the use of a supraglottic airway device (discussed in Chapter 23) is a clearly recognized and appropriate alternative to airway management in the patient with an otherwise unmanageable airway. This study, therefore, provides support for the prehospital use of paralytics for critically ill trauma patients.

Consistently, the most important factors in the success of RSI programs have been the involvement of an active medical director, review of each intubation, and strong educational components. If the decision is made to add RSI to an agency's airway management options, it must be made with an effective monitoring program in place and with the recognition that, if the program is not performing well, it must be stopped and evaluated.

Medication-Facilitated and Rapid Sequence Intubation

The use of medication-facilitated and rapid sequence intubation has the potential to greatly increase a Paramedic's ability to successfully intubate a patient. To use these tools effectively, it is important to understand the medications, how they function, and their indications and contraindications. The following covers the most important points of the medications from the Paramedic's perspective.

Pharmacological Adjuncts for Intubation

As was discussed previously, the pharmacological agents that facilitate intubation can be divided into those that provide sedation and those that cause paralysis. In addition, adjunctive medications that are often used in RSI include vagolytics (atropine) and lidocaine. It is important to be familiar with all of these medications as they are used in the setting of intubation.

Sedatives

Sedative agents are medications that are used to decrease a patient's level of consciousness, cause muscular relaxation, and cause amnesia to the intubation. There are a number of different sedatives with varying hemodynamic effects, respiratory effects, and side effects. It is important that the Paramedic be an expert on the agents that he or she will use. It is important to recognize that no one agent is ideal for all patients. Therefore, familiarity with a number of agents and their characteristics allows for an educated decision about which agent to use. Four of the most commonly used agents (and representative of the major classes of prehospital agents) are midazolam (a benzodiazepine), etomidate, ketamine, and fentanyl (a narcotic). Understanding these medications and others in their respective classes will allow the Paramedic to select the most appropriate medication for a patient.

Midazolam

As a class, **benzodiazepines** are probably the most commonly used medications for sedation in the emergency airway management arena. This use comes from familiarity and a history of safe and effective utilization. Midazolam is chosen as a representative of this class because it is short acting, shares the characteristics of the other benzodiazepines, and has been studied in the prehospital environment as a sole agent to facilitate intubation.[2,11] Other benzodiazepines that are used for intubation include diazepam and lorazepam.

The benzodiazepines are best known for their ability to provide excellent amnesia. Other effects include sedation, muscular relaxation, CNS relaxation, treatment of active seizures, and anxiolysis. Midazolam may also decrease intracranial pressure. They work directly on a benzodiazepine receptor in the brain. The onset of action relates to how quickly the agents pass into the brain, with midazolam having an onset of action of 30 to 60 seconds. The benzodiazepines are metabolized by the liver; the half-life for midazolam is 1.5 to 2.5 hours.

The greatest difficulty in using midazolam for sedation is the wide variability in patient response to the agent. Doses as low as 1 mg have caused apnea in some patients while others require up to 0.3 mg/kg to achieve adequate sedation. In general, male patients and elderly patients require the smallest doses.

The most significant complication associated with midazolam is a dose-related vasodilation and myocardial depression. Therefore, although midazolam has been routinely used in trauma patients and others with potential for hypotension and hypovolemia, it does pose a risk for converting a patient in compensated shock to a state of decompensated shock.

Indications for midazolam, therefore, are broad, although it must be used with caution in the elderly and in patients at risk for significant cardiovascular decompensation. Glaucoma has been identified as a contraindication to benzodiazepine use.

The dosing for midazolam, because of the difficulty in predicting response, requires some degree of titration. The standard dose is 0.2 mg/kg, although this varies from 0.05 to 0.3 mg/kg. A dose of 0.1 mg/kg, followed by additional doses as needed, will result in a relatively safe side effect profile. The onset of action is about 2 minutes. The variability in dose response, however, may result in a patient who is under-sedated during paralysis. This is manifested by hypertension and tachycardia. If these hemodynamic changes are noted, the patient should be given additional sedation.

Midazolam is also useful as a post-intubation sedative. Repeated doses of 20% to 50% of the original dose every 30 to 60 minutes as dictated by the patient's level of consciousness and cardiovascular parameters should provide excellent sedation.

Etomidate

Etomidate is a newer agent that functions primarily as a hypnotic, although it also is an excellent amnestic. Its increasing popularity in the emergency airway management setting is because it has minimal hemodynamic effects and only moderate respiratory depression at induction doses. In addition, it provides excellent relaxation and often does not require the addition of a paralytic to achieve an intubation, thus making it a good agent when paralysis is contraindicated.[1,12]

Although the hemodynamic stability associated with etomidate is perhaps its greatest asset, it also has a cerebroprotective effect. It both attenuates an increased ICP and decreases the negative effects of laryngoscopy.[13]

Etomidate is not without side effects, however. Transient muscle jerks are common and trismus has been reported.[14] In addition, many patients experience nausea and vomiting, although this more often occurs on awakening and is therefore less important in the airway management setting.[15] Finally, patients may experience burning at the site of infusion; this can be decreased by using a large vein and a rapid IV fluid rate. Etomidate, when used as a continuous drip, can cause adrenal suppression. This has not been reported in the single-dose setting of airway management.

It is important to recognize that the hypnotic effects of etomidate end approximately 20 to 30 minutes after administration. When used with a long-acting paralytic such as vecuronium, it is critical that additional sedation (usually in the form of a benzodiazepine) be administered after the intubation to assure that the patient is not awake and remains paralyzed.

Other than drug allergy, there are no true contraindications to the use of etomidate. It is not routinely used in children under 10 years of age. It should be used with caution in the elderly (as should any sedative agent), and the dose can be titrated to effect in hemodynamically unstable patients.

Etomidate is generally dosed at 0.2 to 0.3 mg/kg in the adult patient. A standard intubating dose in an average-sized adult is 20 mg. A dose of 0.1 mg/kg is often used for procedural sedation and is a good starting point for elderly patients. Because there is minimal drug accumulation, it can be redosed if needed. Typical time to onset is 1 to 2 minutes.

The lack of hemodynamic effects, the cerebroprotective effect, and the relative ease of use have made etomidate the first choice of many Paramedics for trauma airway management. It is also an excellent choice for the unstable medical patient. It must always be used in conjunction with a second sedative agent once the intubation is complete.

Ketamine

Ketamine is a dissociative anesthetic with several unique properties. A derivative of PCP, ketamine provides excellent amnesia, analgesia, and anesthesia during procedures and intubation. Most notably, however, it has minimal respiratory depression even at very high doses. In addition, it increases heart rate and blood pressure through the release of catecholamines. Finally, it has the pulmonary effect of reducing bronchospasm through smooth muscle relaxation.[13]

Ketamine's properties have made it an excellent "specialty" sedative in airway management. Its bronchodilatory properties make it an excellent choice for the asthmatic patient. In addition, hypotensive patients without evidence of head injury benefit from the catecholamines that are released. Its efficacy in the pediatric population is also clearly established.[16] Although an IV would clearly be preferable in the emergency airway management setting, ketamine can be given IM as well.

There are patients in whom ketamine is not a good agent for induction. Research in the early 1970s reported an increase in intracranial pressure associated with the use of ketamine.[17] Although recent research brings this finding into question,[18] the current standard is to avoid the use of ketamine in patients with head injuries or those at risk of increased intracranial pressure. In addition, the catecholamines released during ketamine administration increase myocardial oxygen demand, making this a poor sedative for the patient with known or suspected coronary artery disease. Drug allergy, as always, is also a contraindication.

Ketamine has a number of side effects, only a few of which are relevant to airway management. Increased salivation is associated with ketamine use, particularly in pediatric patients. Prior administration of atropine can minimize this effect. Although patients usually experience relaxation after ketamine administration, some will become restless and move purposelessly. Finally, ketamine is associated with "emergence reactions" or hallucinations. These occur more commonly in adults than in children and should not be an issue in emergency airway management as the patient will be sedated, usually with a benzodiazepine, after the intubation is complete.

Ketamine is given in doses of 1 to 2 mg/kg IV or, if given IM, 2 to 4 mg/kg. The onset of action is typically 30 seconds to a minute and can be recognized by the roving eye movements called nystagmus and the awake but unaware appearance of the patient. The effect of ketamine typically lasts up to 10 minutes for intravenous administration and up to 25 minutes for intramuscular administration.

Although somewhat of a specialized drug, ketamine is an important drug in the airway management of selected patients. Its minimal respiratory effects, bronchodilation, and positive hemodynamics make it a useful medication for sedation.

Fentanyl

Narcotics, a class of drugs known for their ability to induce a profound state of sedation, as a general rule, are rarely used as the sole sedative agents in emergency airway management. Nonetheless, they may be the only agent a prehospital provider has available. In addition, they are often used adjunctively in airway management, making them important medications with which to be familiar. Narcotics provide analgesia and hypnosis as well as some degree of amnesia. In addition, they attenuate the increased ICP that is a reflexive response to laryngoscopy.[13] Although fentanyl is used as a sole indication agent at very high doses (22 to 30 μg/kg) in the operating room, lower doses of narcotics can be used in emergency airway management to achieve some degree of patient sedation.

Fentanyl is a synthetic opioid that is highly potent. It is known for not causing histamine release, unlike morphine. Therefore, the patient exhibits minimal hypotension when used in small (1 to 4 μg/kg) doses. Like other narcotics, fentanyl causes respiratory depression and therefore places patients at risk for hypoxia and hypercarbia; this should not be a problem during airway management as the patient will be continuously monitored.

Fentanyl, at high doses and rapid administration rates, is associated with chest and abdominal wall muscular rigidity. This is an idiosyncratic reaction and results in the patient's inability to breathe or to be ventilated. Generally speaking, this effect is not reversible and the patient must be paralyzed immediately. Other common effects of narcotics include nausea and vomiting. Fentanyl is often associated with an itchy nose sensation.

Fentanyl is indicated in the patient who may experience significant harm if there is a large catecholamine release. Patients with acute MI, increased intracranial pressure, or vascular disease such as aortic dissection or aneurysm fall into this classification. In addition, any patient may benefit from the analgesia and hypnosis associated with narcotics during airway management, particularly if a narcotic (usually morphine) is the only agent that the Paramedic has available to her.

Fentanyl is given in doses of 1 to 3 μg/kg slow IV push. Morphine can be given in doses of 0.05 to 0.1 mg/kg slow IV push for sedation. If morphine is used, the Paramedic should expect a greater hemodynamic response (e.g., hypotension). The onset of action is usually rapid (30 to 60 seconds) and the duration of fentanyl is typically 22 to 30 minutes. Narcotics may be redosed in 22 to 30 minutes as needed. They may be used for short-term sedation after an intubation, although longer-acting agents such as benzodiazepines are preferred.

Neuromuscular Blocking Agents (Paralytics)

Neuromuscular blocking agents (NMBAs) are medications that block transmission of nerve impulses to skeletal muscle at the neuromuscular junction. When a nerve impulse reaches the neuromuscular junction, the molecule **acetylcholine**, a neurotransmitter, is released into the synapse from the presynaptic membrane of the nerve. The acetylcholine moves across the synapse to the postsynaptic membrane of the muscle. There it binds to receptors and causes the muscle to contract (Figure 24-1). Normally, the contraction stops when the acetylcholine is broken down by **acetylcholinesterase**.

Skeletal muscle paralytics block the binding of acetylcholine to the receptors on the postsynaptic membrane. There are two major classes of neuromuscular blockers: depolarizing agents and non-depolarizing agents. The main difference between the two is whether the medication binds to the receptor and causes a muscular contraction (a depolarizing agent) or simply blocks acetylcholine from binding to the receptor without causing the receptor to activate (a non-depolarizing agent). There is only one depolarizing agent that is commonly used (succinylcholine) while there are multiple non-depolarizing agents.

Depolarizing Neuromuscular Blockers

Succinylcholine is the most commonly used **depolarizing neuromuscular blocker**. It is called a depolarizing agent because, when it binds to the acetylcholine receptor on the muscle, it causes the muscle to depolarize or contract. This contraction is limited in duration and is recognized by the Paramedic as fasciculations that occur shortly after the succinylcholine is administered (Figure 24-2). Molecularly, succinylcholine is composed of two acetylcholine molecules hooked back to back. It is metabolized by pseudocholinesterase, an enzyme found throughout the body (but not actually in the neuromuscular junction).

Succinylcholine is the most commonly used neuromuscular blocker for rapid sequence intubation. It offers a number of advantages over the non-depolarizing agents. The two greatest assets are a rapid onset of action (30 to 60 seconds) and rapid termination of effect (3 to 12 minutes)[19] with return of sufficient ventilation to sustain life in 8 to 10 minutes.[20] Although the duration of action is sufficiently long that a patient receiving no ventilatory support would become hypoxic,[21] the short duration means that assisted ventilation will be needed for a much shorter time than with non-depolarizing agents.

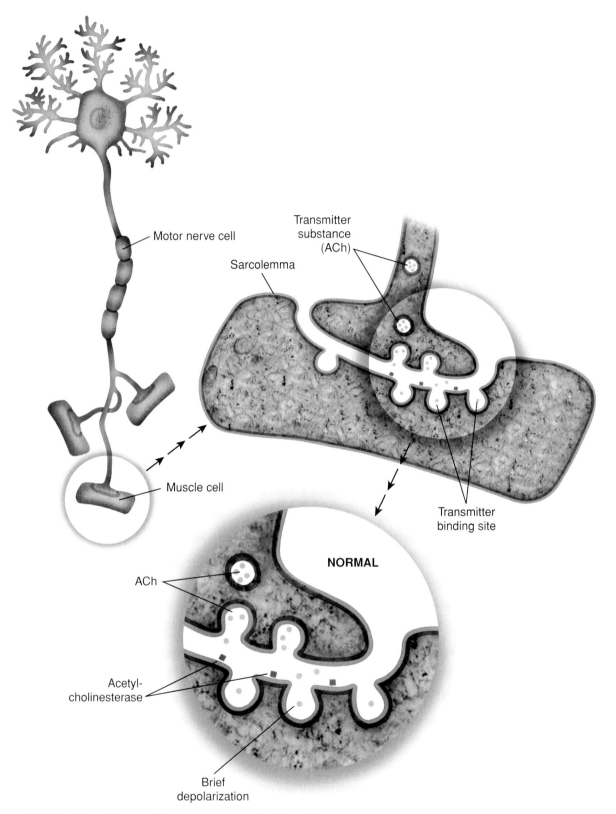

Figure 24-1 Physiology of a neuromuscular junction.

Despite its possession of very desirable pharmacokinetic properties, succinylcholine does have a significant side effect profile. Side effects of greatest importance in the prehospital environment include fasciculations, hyperkalemia, and bradycardia.

Since succinylcholine causes muscular contraction when it initially binds to the acetylcholine receptor, the Paramedic will see transient muscular fasciculations approximately 22 seconds after the medication is administered. These fasciculations are associated with an increase in intragastric

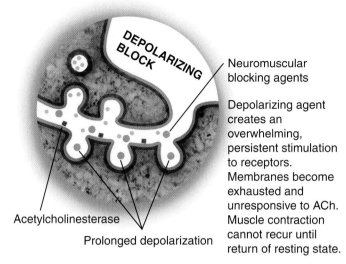

Acetylcholinesterase

Prolonged depolarization

Figure 24-2 Depolarization of the neuromuscular junction.

DEPOLARIZING BLOCK

Neuromuscular blocking agents

Depolarizing agent creates an overwhelming, persistent stimulation to receptors. Membranes become exhausted and unresponsive to ACh. Muscle contraction cannot recur until return of resting state.

pressure, intraocular pressure, and intracranial pressure. The increase in intragastric pressure may put the patient at risk for regurgitation and aspiration; cricoid pressure is mandatory as soon as pretreatment medications are administered (sedatives, etc.). In theory, the increase in intraocular pressure could cause globe contents to herniate in the case of traumatic eye injury. It is enlightening to note that many anesthesiologists still use succinylcholine without a defasciculating dose of a non-depolarizing agent (discussed in the following text) in the setting of open globe injuries.[20] The rise in intracranial pressure of approximately 5 mmHg is of no known clinical significance[22] but can be blunted through pretreatment, as will be discussed later.

Succinylcholine administration has also been associated with an increase in serum potassium levels. This tends to happen in patients with a precipitating event (burns, neuromuscular disease, pre-existing hyperkalemia, crush injuries, and muscle denervation). In addition, for those patients with traumatic causes, the effect is not seen for two to seven days from the event. Therefore, although the Paramedic must consider whether a patient is at risk for hyperkalemia, there are few prehospital situations (other than in patients with known hyperkalemia, neuromuscular disease, or in the critical care transport environment) where the risk for hyperkalemia will be important.

There is increased vagal tone that occurs with the administration of succinylcholine. Although the clinical significance is low for adults after a single dose of succinylcholine, the effect can be dramatic in children, leading to bradycardia and even asystole. The effect is easily mitigated with pretreatment with atropine.

There are a few absolute contraindications to the administration of succinylcholine. These include a personal or family history of **malignant hyperthermia** (a skeletal muscle disease that leads to a life-threatening reaction to succinylcholine and some other inhaled anesthetics), burns more than 24 hours old, or degenerative muscle disease. Patients with recent traumatic muscle denervation or crush injuries more than seven days prior should also not be given succinylcholine. Finally, paralytics are contraindicated in all patients who cannot be face-mask ventilated in case the Paramedic is unable to intubate the patient.

Succinylcholine dosing is based on the fact that very little succinylcholine actually travels to the neuromuscular junction. Since incomplete paralysis makes intubation much more difficult, a general rule is to use larger (rather than smaller) doses. For an adult patient, 1.5 mg/kg of succinylcholine is administered via rapid IV push. It can also be administered IM at a dose of 3 mg/kg, although it is not as predictable in efficacy. For children under 10, a dose of 2 mg/kg IV is appropriate, and for infants and neonates, 3 mg/kg rapid IV push should be used.

Despite its significant side effect profile, succinylcholine remains the neuromuscular blocker of choice for emergency airway management. Some thought should be given to the contraindications and side effects of the medication, but multiple studies have demonstrated its safety and efficacy in the emergency airway management arena.

Non-Depolarizing (Competitive) Neuromuscular Blockers

Non-depolarizing neuromuscular blockers also cause paralysis through blocking acetylcholine, although through a somewhat different mechanism than succinylcholine. These agents compete with acetylcholine for the acetylcholine receptor on the postsynaptic membrane (Figure 24-3), but do not cause the receptor to fire. Therefore, there are no fasciculations. The molecular model for non-depolarizing neuromuscular blockers is curare.

There are a number of non-depolarizing neuromuscular blockers available for the Paramedic, all of which are of the aminosteroid class of NMBAs. The most commonly used

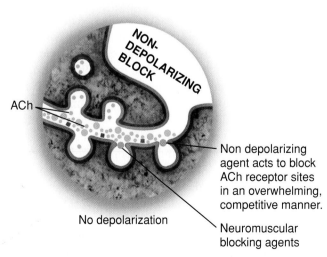

ACh

NON-DEPOLARIZING BLOCK

Non depolarizing agent acts to block ACh receptor sites in an overwhelming, competitive manner.

Neuromuscular blocking agents

No depolarization

Figure 24-3 Neuromuscular blockade.

agent in the prehospital environment is **vecuronium**; other agents of this class include rocuronium, pancuronium, and rapacuronium. Although these agents have a much less significant side effect profile than succinylcholine, they generally have a longer time to onset at standard doses and they all have a prolonged duration of action. Two agents, rocuronium and rapacuronium, have onset of action in about 60 seconds and rapacuronium has a duration of action that is almost the same as succinylcholine.[23,24] Therefore, these agents offer the potential to replace succinylcholine in the emergency airway management setting.

Unfortunately, rapacuronium, the most promising of the agents (30- to 60-second onset, 20-minute paralysis without reversal, 10-minute paralysis with reversal agent), also has the most significant side effect profile.

Fasciculations, hyperkalemia, and increased intracranial pressure are not seen with the use of non-depolarizing NMBAs. Therefore, in patients at risk for adverse outcomes from those side effects of succinylcholine, a non-depolarizing NMBA is the paralytic agent of choice.

In most other cases, the delay in onset of paralysis and the prolonged paralysis make these agents less desirable. Pancuronium and rapacuronium have both been associated with tachycardia, and rapacuronium has also been associated with transient hypotension and bronchospasm. vecuronium and rocuronium have relatively few side effects.

Neostigmine, an acetylcholinesterase inhibitor, can be used to reverse the effects of the competitive (non-depolarizing) NMBAs. They do this by inhibiting acetylcholinesterase, the enzyme that breaks down acetylcholine. With acetylcholinesterase blocker, more acetylcholine builds up in the synapse, displacing the NMBA and decreasing recovery time. Although neostigmine does not instantly reverse the NMBA, it can cut the recovery time in half.

There are three primary indications for the use of a non-depolarizing neuromuscular blocking agent. The first is a paralytic patient with a contraindication to the use of succinylcholine. The only true contraindication that succinylcholine and the non-depolarizing NMBAs share is the one against their use in patients who cannot be effectively face-mask ventilated. Paralyzing a patient who can neither be intubated nor ventilated is truly the worst case scenario in airway management using RSI. It is important to note that if vecuronium is used for paralysis, the patient will usually become apneic before adequate paralysis occurs and the patient will need face-mask ventilation. This problem can be mitigated if a large (0.3 mg/kg) dose of vecuronium is used or a priming (0.01 mg/kg 2 to 3) dose of vecuronium is administered two to three minutes before the intubating dose is administered.

Non-depolarizing NMBAs possess the unique ability to block fasciculations. In doses of one tenth its intubating dose (e.g., 0.01 mg/kg), vecuronium given two to three minutes before succinylcholine will prevent fasciculations and the side effects associated with fasciculations (increased ICP, etc.).

The use of a **defasciculating dose** of a non-depolarizing agent is most often used in the setting of the head-injured patient. A defasiculating dose is a small dose of a non-depolarizing paralytic which, when administered before administering succinylcholine, prevents the fasciculations associated with succinylcholine.

The only risk associated with this technique is that the patient may occasionally become apneic and fully paralyzed with the defasciculating dose. The Paramedic must therefore be prepared to administer the full paralytic dose and intubate the patient.

Non-depolarizing agents are also commonly used for post-intubation care. In the prehospital environment, it is usually more important that an intubated patient be protected from himself and the risk of accidental self-extubation than it is to perform serial neurological exams. This is particularly important in the air medical environment where re-intubation can be extraordinarily difficult. Therefore, most prehospital patients who are rapid sequence intubated are given a full paralyzing dose of vecuronium to minimize patient movement and the risks of extubation.

Since the duration of action of the vecuronium (30 to 60 minutes) will typically be longer than the duration of action of most sedatives, it is important to monitor for tachycardia and hypertension, both of which suggest that the patient is paralyzed but not sedated.

As noted, vecuronium is the most commonly used non-depolarizing neuromuscular blocker used in the prehospital setting. The usual dose is 0.1 mg/kg. As mentioned, doses of 0.3 mg/kg can be given to attain paralysis in 60 to 90 seconds, but the patient will be paralyzed for up to 100 minutes. This is a problem if the patient cannot be intubated and must be face-mask ventilated. At a dose of 0.1 mg/kg, the usual onset of action is in two to three minutes. Since most sedative agents have an earlier onset of action, administering the vecuronium and awaiting signs of muscular weakness before administering the sedative may decrease the incidence of apnea before adequate paralysis occurs.

The non-depolarizing neuromuscular blocking agents offer many advantages over succinylcholine in terms of their side effect profile. Unfortunately, they are limited in their use by their delayed onset of action and prolonged paralysis. Currently, they are used primarily for defasciculation and post-intubation paralysis. Newer agents with more rapid paralysis and short duration of action may offer a reasonable alternative to succinylcholine in the future.

Adjunctive Medications

Lidocaine and atropine are two agents that are commonly used as adjuncts to emergency rapid sequence intubation. Both of these drugs are used to counter the effects of paralytics and of airway manipulation.

Lidocaine

Lidocaine, a drug thought to offer some neuroprotection, is commonly used during the RSI of patients with head trauma, evidence of increased intracranial pressure, and bronchospastic airway disease.[25] Although there is controversy about the clinical significance of the effects of lidocaine, when used, it is most often used for patients with head trauma.

Through a combination of deepened sedation and multiple cerebral hemodynamic effects, lidocaine is thought to provide some cerebral protection for patients undergoing airway manipulation and may be protective against the effects of succinylcholine. In addition, lidocaine may blunt the sympathetic response to laryngoscopy, although this has not been definitively demonstrated. When used, IV lidocaine at a dose of 1.5 mg/kg is administered at least three minutes before administration of succylcholine.

Atropine

Airway management, particularly in pediatric patients under 10 years old, can cause excessive vagal stimulation. Furthermore, large or multiple doses of succinylcholine put patients at risk of increased vagal tone. Therefore, **atropine**, a parasympathetic blocker that decreases vagal response, must be available for the treatment of these patients. In addition, atropine decreases oral secretions, an effect that is useful for patients sedated with ketamine or with excessive secretions.[19]

All patients under 5 years of age should be pretreated (two to three minutes before paralysis) with 0.2 mg/kg of IV atropine (0.1 mg < dose < 0.5 mg). In addition, any adult patient receiving a second dose of succinylcholine should either be pretreated with 0.5 mg IV or atropine should be immediately available if the patient becomes bradycardic.

The 9 P's for Medication Facilitated Intubation and Rapid Sequence Intubation

The most commonly used tool to guide safe and effective intubation is the rule of the "Nine P's of RSI." The nine "P's" are:

1. Preparation
2. Predict the degree of difficulty
3. Preoxygenate
4. Pretreat
5. Pressure on the cricoid
6. Paralyze
7. Pass the tube
8. Position (confirm) and secure
9. Post-intubation care

Correctly applying each of these "P's" greatly enhances the safety and efficacy of the intubation.

Preparation

Preparation for medication-facilitated or rapid sequence intubation involves assuring that all necessary equipment is properly assembled and ready for use (Table 24-1).

The Paramedic should also verify the last oral intake, if possible.

Predict the Degree of Difficulty

Prediction is the most important step in making the decision to perform a medication-facilitated or rapid sequence intubation. The actual skill of intubating a person who is chemically paralyzed is no more difficult than if that person were completely comatose with no muscle tone (i.e., a patient in cardiac arrest). The difference lies in the fact that a person who is alive, breathing, and protecting his airway enough to prevent intubation without medications is still alive. If the Paramedic proceeds to paralyze this patient, he takes full responsibility for the consequences of removing the patient's (limited) ability to care for himself. Therefore, extraordinary judgment must be exercised before deciding to sedate and, more importantly, chemically paralyze a patient. The most critical deciding factor is whether or not the Paramedic will be able to intubate the patient and, if not, provide face-mask ventilation. The guiding principle of all medical care is *Primum non nocere* or "first, do no harm." Chemical paralysis provides the opportunity to do grave and irreparable harm to a patient.

Table 24-1 Equipment List for MFI

- Continuous cardiac monitoring
- Continuous pulse-ox
- BVM attached to 100% O_2
- Oral airway
- Suction set-up
- $ETCO_2$ detector/continuous monitoring $ETCO_2$
- Ventilator attached and ready (if using)
- RSI medications drawn up
- IV established
- Intubation equipment

The need to perform an airway evaluation on all patients before and during airway management is self-evident. Two tools—the LEMON law and the 3-3-2 rule—were introduced in Chapter 23. It is important to apply the LEMON law before any rapid sequence intubation. The Paramedic must recognize when conditions exist which will prevent him or her from being able to intubate the patient after paralysis. If the patient's airway is simply too difficult for a Paramedic's skill level, then the patient should not be paralyzed.

In addition to assessing the difficulty of the intubation, however, it is also important to assess how difficult it will be to perform face-mask ventilation. Facial hair, facial trauma, micrognathia (small jaw), and other anatomic anomalies may make face-mask ventilation difficult or impossible. Any patient who cannot be face-mask ventilated should not receive paralytic agents or sedatives in doses that could cause apnea. Although this may be a difficult decision, medication-facilitated intubation is as much about deciding not to give the medications as it is about giving the medications.

Preoxygenate

It is possible to extend the time allowed for an intubation attempt by adequately preoxygenating a patient. Administration of high flow oxygen for three to five minutes or for 10 to 22 deep breaths removes nitrogen from the lungs and replaces it with oxygen. Respiratory gasses at the level of alveoli include 75% nitrogen for the patient breathing room air. By "washing out" the nitrogen through preoxygenation, a much larger reserve of alveolar oxygen is created. Patients can therefore be apneic for prolonged periods (two to five minutes) before oxygen desaturation occurs. Since hypoxia is so potentially damaging, this safety reserve can protect a patient during the prolonged apnea that can be associated with the use of sedatives and paralytics.

Pretreat

Once the decision has been made to perform sedation-aided or rapid sequence intubation and the patient is preoxygenated, it is important to administer any pretreatment medications that will be used. Sedatives are considered "pretreatment" since they are used to prepare a patient for paralytics. Lidocaine, atropine, and defasciculation doses of non-depolarizing neuromuscular blockers are the other commonly used pretreatment medications.

There is no evidence that routine use of pretreatment medications (other than sedatives) in patients without specific indications (i.e., increased ICP, pediatric patients.) improves patient outcomes. Therefore, atropine, lidocaine, and defasciculating drugs (e.g., vecuronium 0.01 mg/kg IV) should only be used if an indication exists. If they are going to be given, they should be administered two to three minutes before the paralytic agent.

The timing of the sedative's administration will depend on its onset of action and the paralytic that will be used. For example, succinylcholine and etomidate have almost the same time of onset and therefore are administered almost simultaneously. Midazolam, on the other hand, has a two to three minute time of onset and must be administered well in advance of succinylcholine. As was discussed previously, if vecuronium is going to be used, it should probably be administered before the sedative to minimize the risk of apnea.

The Paramedic must be alert during the pretreatment phase. Some patients, particularly those who already have a significantly altered mental status, may become apneic after receiving pretreatment medications. Therefore, all equipment for the intubation must be ready for immediate use and the patient closely monitored.

Cricoid Pressure

While sedative or defasciculating medications are being administered, an assistant should be assigned to apply cricoid pressure to minimize the risk of aspiration. A patient who has received sedatives will have decreased airway reflexes and may have a decreased lower esophageal pressure. These two factors put the patient at risk for vomiting and aspirating.

If the Paramedic is performing a sedation-aided intubation, the intubation attempt is made now (see the "Pass the Tube" section later). In addition, many providers will make an attempt at intubation before paralytics are administered if the patient appears to be sufficiently sedated. If the patient is successfully intubated with sedation alone, many of the risks of paralysis can be avoided.

Paralyze

Once the patient has been pretreated and an appropriate time interval has passed, the paralytic agent should be given. One of the most significant mistakes a Paramedic can make is to attempt to intubate the patient too quickly after the paralytic is given. If an intubation attempt is made before the patient is completely paralyzed, not only will the patient fight the attempt but the risk of aspiration is also greatly increased. Therefore, either a clock/watch should be used or the Paramedic should count out 45 seconds once succinylcholine is administered. No attempts to intubate should be made before then and, unless the patient desaturates, no face-mask ventilation should be applied. If a non-depolarizing agent is used, a similar approach of waiting for complete paralysis should be followed.

Pass the Tube

Once the patient is completely paralyzed, standard methods of oral endotracheal intubation should be used. Suction must be immediately available in the event the patient vomits. External laryngeal manipulation and/or the BURP maneuver should be used to optimize visualization.

Position (Confirm) and Secure

Once the patient has been intubated, the tube position must be confirmed with at least three methods. The paralyzed patient is completely dependent on being ventilated. If the patient is esophageally intubated, he cannot continue to breathe around the tube the way a non-paralyzed, non-apneic patient can. Therefore, confirmation must be rapid and accurate. The paralyzed patient is also at risk for complications from a displaced tube, particularly after receiving post-intubation sedation and paralysis. Use of continuous end-tidal carbon dioxide monitoring decreases the risk of a missed displaced tube.

Properly securing the endotracheal tube also decreases the risk of tube dislodgment. Any method is acceptable as long as it prevents the endotracheal tube from moving. The depth of the endotracheal tube at the lips should be noted and recorded to verify that there is no tube movement. The neck should be secured with a cervical collar to prevent flexion and extension and the patient should be secured to a long-spine board for transport.

Post-Intubation Care

Once the patient has been successfully intubated and the tube is secured, there are several important post-intubation tasks to be performed. All patients who are intubated should have a nasogastric or orogastric tube placed to allow active or passive decompression of the stomach. This is particularly true for pediatric patients who can suffer significant respiratory compromise from gastric inflation.

There are also two important post-intubation medications that should be administered. The first important medication to administer is a long-acting non-depolarizing neuromuscular blocker, generally vecuronium. As was discussed previously, post-intubation paralysis decreases the risk of accidental extubation. If vecuronium was used to perform the intubation, it is not necessary to administer a second dose.

The second important medication is a long-acting sedative (e.g., midazolam). If etomidate is used for the intubation, it will begin to wear off in 10 to 20 minutes after administration. Although other sedatives (e.g., midazolam, ketamine) may have a longer duration of action, their duration will still be less than that of vecuronium. Therefore, the patient should be monitored for signs (tachycardia and hypertension) of inadequate sedation.

STREET SMART

The Paramedic will recognize that induced paralysis does not alter sensation. The patient is acutely aware of noise, lights, odors, pain, and other sensations such as pressure. These stimuli should be reduced or eliminated by altering the environment or administering appropriate medications.

The Paramedic should be aware and monitor for signs of malignant hyperthermia. This is a genetic muscular disease that affects some people after receiving inhaled anesthetics or succinylcholine. Signs of malignant hyperthermia include fever, muscular rigidity (as opposed to being flaccid), tachycardia, and tachypnea. Although most EMS providers will not have access to Dantrolene, the medication used to treat malignant hyperthermia, the patient can be cooled with cold packs and exposure. In addition, the receiving facility should be notified of the patient's condition.

CONCLUSION

Medication-facilitated and rapid sequence intubation offer the Paramedic an expanded range of tools for patient care. Patients who could not previously be intubated can receive the benefits of translaryngeal endotracheal intubation. These medications, however, are not without side effects and their use is associated with complications. The actual acts of administering the medications and performing the intubation are no different than in any other patient. The most critical difference, particularly for the use of paralytics, is the judgment required to make the initial decision to paralyze the patient. Chemical paralysis cannot be done lightly or without forethought; it is an intervention with the potential to kill a patient. Nonetheless, there are clear benefits to performing rapid sequence intubation and therefore the Paramedic should be familiar with the procedure.

KEY POINTS:

- The most important factors in the success of RSI programs have been the involvement of an active medical director, review of each intubation, strong educational components, and an overall effective monitoring system.

- The use of pharmacological agents to facilitate intubation can be thought of as those that provide sedation and those that cause muscular paralysis. In addition, adjunctive medications that are often used in RSI include vagolytics (atropine) and lidocaine.

- Sedative agents are medications that are used to decrease a patient's level of consciousness, effect muscular relaxation, and cause amnesia to the intubation. Four of the most commonly used agents are midazolam (a benzodiazepine), etomidate, ketamine, and fentanyl (a narcotic).

- Midazolam, a short-acting benzodiazepine, has an onset of action of 30 to 60 seconds and a half-life of 1.5 to 2.5 hours.

- Response to midazolam varies widely. In general, male patients and elderly patients require the smallest doses. The most significant complication associated with midazolam is the development of shock.

- Etomidate is a newer agent that functions primarily as a hypnotic and amnestic. It has minimal hemodynamic effects and only moderate respiratory depression at induction doses. Etomidate also attenuates an increased ICP and decreases the negative effects of laryngoscopy. Side effects may include transient muscle jerks and trismus. Many patients experience nausea and vomiting upon awakening.

- Ketamine is a dissociative anesthetic that provides excellent amnesia, analgesia, and anesthesia during procedures and intubation. Ketamine also has minimal respiratory depression; it increases heart rate and blood pressure through the release of catecholamines and has the pulmonary effect of reducing bronchospasm through smooth muscle relaxation. It should be avoided in the head-injured patient.

- Narcotics provide analgesia and hypnosis as well as some degree of amnesia. In addition, they attenuate the increased ICP that is a reflexive response to laryngoscopy. Lower doses of narcotics can be used in emergency airway management to achieve some degree of patient sedation.

- Fentanyl is a synthetic opioid that is highly potent and has minimal hemodynamic effects. Like other narcotics, it causes respiratory depression. It may be indicated in the patient who may experience significant harm if there is a large catecholamine release.

- Neuromuscular blockers prevent transmission of nerve impulses to skeletal muscle at the neuromuscular junction by either binding to the receptor, causing a muscular contraction (a depolarizing agent), or simply blocking acetylcholine from binding to the receptor without causing the receptor to activate (a non-depolarizing agent).

- Succinylcholine is a depolarizing agent. It binds to the acetylcholine which binds to the receptor, causing the muscle to contract, and then prevents further contractions.

- Contraindications for succinylcholine include a personal or family history of malignant hyperthermia, burns more than 24 hours old, degenerative muscle disease, and crush injuries more than seven days prior.

- Paralytics are contraindicated in all patients who cannot be face-mask ventilated in case the Paramedic is unable to intubate the patient.

- Vecuronium, rocuronium, pancuronium, and rapacuronium are non-depolarizing agents that do not cause fasciculations. These agents generally have a longer time to onset at standard doses and they all have a prolonged duration of action.

- Neostigmine inhibits acetylcholinesterase, allowing more acetylcholine to build up in the synapse, displacing the NMBA and decreasing recovery time.

- A non-depolarizing neuromuscular blocking agent is commonly used to block fasciculations through a low dose administration called a defasciculating dose.

- Lidocaine and atropine are used to counter the effects of paralytics and of airway manipulation.

- Airway management, particularly in pediatric patients under 5 years old, can cause excessive vagal stimulation, primarily bradycardia.

- The most commonly used tool to guide safe and effective intubation is the rule of the "Nine P's of RSI." The nine "P's" are (1) preparation, (2) predict the degree of difficulty, (3) preoxygenate, (4) pretreat, (5) pressure on the cricoid, (6) paralyze, (7) pass the tube, (8) position (confirm) and secure, and (9) post-intubation care.

- To prepare for medication-facilitated or rapid sequence intubation, and to assure the "first attempt is the best attempt," the Paramedic should ensure all necessary equipment is properly assembled and ready to use.

- Predicting the degree of difficulty is the most important step in making the decision to perform a medication-facilitated or rapid sequence intubation.

- Preoxygenation of the patient is performed by administering high flow oxygen for three to five minutes or for 10 to 22 deep breaths. This removes nitrogen from the lungs and replaces it with oxygen which can extend the time allowed for an intubation attempt.

- Pretreatment medications—lidocaine, atropine, and defasciculating doses of non-depolarizing neuromuscular blockers—should be given two to three minutes before the paralytic agent.

- While sedative or defasciculating medications are being administered, a patient care provider should apply cricoid pressure to minimize the risk of aspiration.

- Once the patient has been pretreated and an appropriate time interval has passed, the paralytic agent should be given. Once succinylcholine is administered, no face-mask ventilation should be applied and the Paramedic should count out 45 seconds before attempting to intubate.

- After paralysis is achieved, standard methods of oral endotracheal intubation should be used.

- Following intubation, tube position must be confirmed rapidly and accurately with at least three methods. Standard methods for securing the tube are then performed, and continuous end-tidal carbon dioxide monitoring is used to monitor for tube displacement.

1. What two general categories of medications exist for airway management?
2. What are the key differences between the following sedative agents: midazolam, etomidate, ketamine, and fentanyl?
3. What is the mechanism of action of a depolarizing neuromuscular blocking agent (NMBA)?
4. What is the mechanism of action of a non-depolarizing NMBA?
5. How does neostigmine affect neuromuscular blockade?
6. Describe four side effects of succinylcholine.
7. Explain the difference between a "defasciculating" and a "paralytic" dose of a non-depolarizing NMBA.

8. List two reasons why succinylcholine is used preferentially to non-depolarizing NMBAs.
9. Name two adjunctive medications for RSI and give their indications.
10. What are the "Nine P's of RSI"?
11. How should the Paramedic assess the airway for medication-facilitated and rapid sequence intubation?
12. Explain the protective effect of preoxygenation.
13. Identify two post-intubation medications and explain why they are used.

▶ CASE STUDY QUESTIONS:

Please refer to the Case Study at the beginning of the chapter and answer the questions below:

1. List at least three reasons for using medications during intubation of this patient.
2. What adjunctive medications are indicated for this patient? Why?

3. Approximately 15 minutes into the flight, the flight medic observes an increase in heart rate and blood pressure. What might cause this response? What actions are indicated?

REFERENCES:

1. Bozeman WP, Young S. Etomidate as a sole agent for endotracheal intubation in the prehospital air medical setting. *Air Med.* 2002;21(4):32–36.

2. Wang HE, O'Connor RE, Megargel RE, et al. The utilization of midazolam as a pharmacologic adjunct to endotracheal intubation by Paramedics. *Prehosp Emerg Care.* 2002;4(1):14–18.

3. Wayne MA, Friedland E. Prehospital use of succinylcholine: a 20-year review. *Prehosp Emerg Care.* 1999;3(2):107–109.

4. Hedges JR, Dronen SC, Feero S, Hawkins S, Syverud SA, Shultz B. Succinylcholine-assisted intubations in prehospital care. *Ann Emerg Med.* 1988;17(5):469–472.

5. Vilke GM, Hoyt DB, Epperson M. et al. Intubation techniques in the helicopter. *J Emerg Med.* 1994;12(2):217–224.

6. Syverud SA, Borron SW, Storer DL, et al. Prehospital use of neuromuscular blocking agents in a helicopter ambulance program. *Ann Emerg Med.* 1988;17(3):236–242.

7. Sing RF, Reilly PM, Rotondo MF, et al. Out-of-hospital rapid-sequence induction for intubation of the pediatric patient. *Acad Emerg Med.* 1996;3(1):41–45.

8. Ochs M, Davis D, Hoyt D, Bailey D, Marshall L, Rosen P. Paramedic-performed rapid sequence intubation of patients with severe head injuries. *Ann Emerg Med.* 2002;40(2):159–167.

9. Winchall RJ, Hoyt DB. Endotracheal intubation in the field improves survival in patients with severe head injury. Trauma Research and Education Foundation of San Diego. *Arch Surg.* 1997;132(6):592–597.

10. Karch SB, Lewis T, Young S, et al. Field intubation of trauma patients: complications, indications, and outcomes. *Am J Emerg Med.* 1996;14(7):617–619.

11. Dickinson ET, Cohen JE, Mechem CC. The effectiveness of midazolam as a single pharmacologic agent to facilitate endotracheal intubation by Paramedics. *Prehosp Emerg Care.* 1999;3(3):191–193.

12. Reed DB. Regional EMS experience with etomidate for facilitated intubation. *Prehosp Emerg Care.* 2002;6(1):50–53.

13. Schneider R. Sedatives and induction agents. In: Walls R, et al., eds. *Manual of Emergency Airway Management.* Philadelphia: Lippincott, Williams, and Wilkins; 2000:129–139.

14. Chohan N, ed. *Physician's Drug Handbook* (8th ed.). Philadelphia, Lippincott, Williams and Wilkens; 1999:424–425.

15. O'Connor RE, Levine BJ. Airway management in the trauma setting. In: Ferrera PC, Colucciello SA, Marx JA, et al. *Trauma Management: An Emergency Medicine Approach.* St. Louis: Mosby; 2001:52–74.

16. Chohan N, ed. *Physician's Drug Handbook* (8th ed.). Springhouse: Philadelphia, Lippincott, Williams and Wilkens; 1999:593–594.

17. Gibbs JM. The effect of intravenous ketamine on cerebrospinal fluid pressure. *Br. J. Anesth.* 1972;44(12):1298–1302.

18. Sloan T. Anesthetics and the brain. *Anesthiol Clin North America.* 2002;20(2):265–292.

19. Yamamoto LG. Rapid sequence anesthesia induction and advanced airway management in pediatric patients. *Emerg Med Clin North America.* 1991;9(3):611–638.

20. Schneider R. Muscle relaxants. In: Walls R et al., eds. *Manual of Emergency Airway Management.* Philadelphia: Lippincott, Williams, and Wilkins; 2000:122–128.

21. Benumof JL. Succinylcholine duration and critical hemoglobin desaturation in the healthy adult. *Anesthesiology.* 1998;88(6):1686–1688.

22. Storer DL. The pharmacology of airway control. *Emerg Care Q.* 1991;7(1):64.

23. DeMay JC, Debrock M, Rolly G. Evaluation of the onset and intubation conditions of rocuronium bromide. *Eur J Anesthesiol Suppl.* 1994;9 (Suppl):37–40.

24. Fleming NW, Chung F, Glass PS, et al. Comparison of the intubation conditions provided by rapacuronium (ORG9487) or succinylcholine in humans during anesthesia with fentanyl and propofol. *Anesthesiology.* 1999;91(5):1311–1317.

25. Schneider R. Drugs for special clinical circumstances. In: Walls R, et al., eds. *Manual of Emergency Airway Management.* Philadelphia: Lippincott, Williams, and Wilkins; 2000: 135–139.

CHAPTER 25

VENTILATION

KEY CONCEPTS:

Upon completion of this chapter, it is expected that the reader will understand these following concepts:

- The formation of acid from respiratory and metabolic mechanisms and physiological pH
- Three important chemical buffers found in the bloodstream
- Respiratory and renal compensation by deriving the acid-bicarbonate formula
- Acidosis as an imbalance

▶ CASE STUDY:

The Paramedics were called to the local community college for an instructor suffering an acute asthma attack. Mr. Byrnes had a lengthy history of asthma beginning in high school. His last attack, four months ago, had required intubation and two days on ventilatory support.

The nurse in the health office had placed Mr. Byrnes on oxygen along with monitoring pulse oximetry. He had tried to use his rescue inhaler but could not take deep enough breaths. Even though his pulse oximetry reading was at 97%, one look indicated that he was laboring, tachypneic, and fearful.

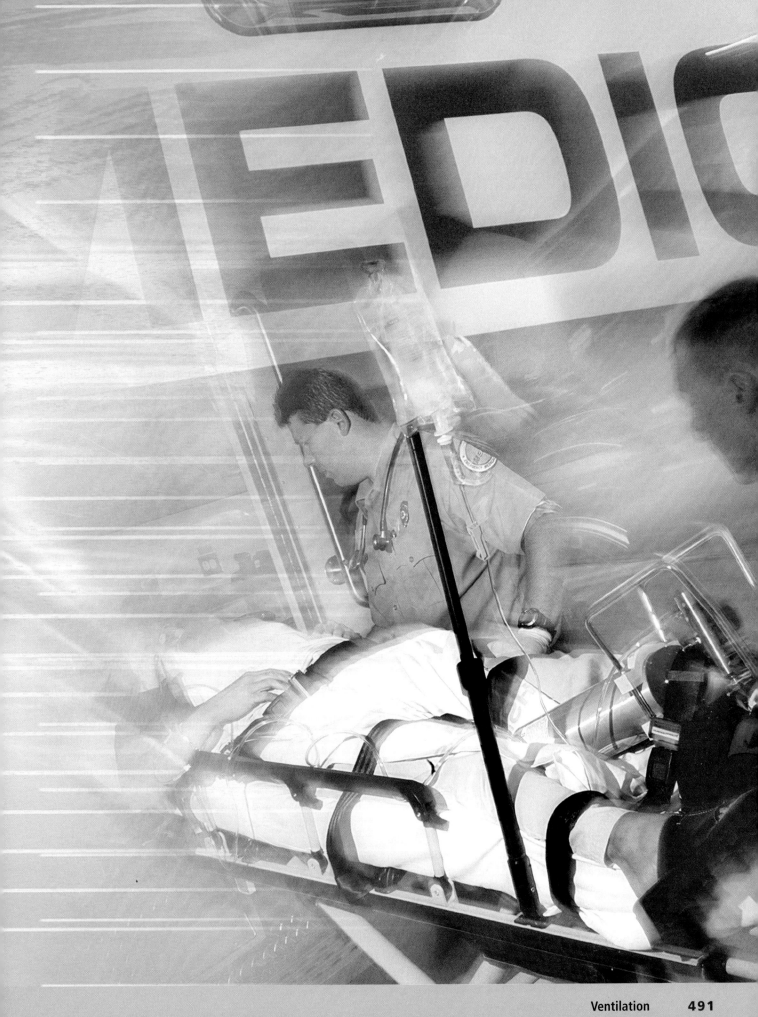

OVERVIEW

Ventilation is more than just the movement of air in and out the lungs. For the Paramedic, examining ventilation involves understanding the physiology of gas exchange and the different ways the body maintains a balanced pH. Metabolically, the body's organs work together to maintain an acid–base balance. This chapter examines the basic chemistry of pH, the chemical buffers, and how ventilation provides a first line of defense from acid imbalance. Respiratory and renal mechanisms also play an important role by driving the acid-bicarbonate formula, which works to regulate pH. Respiratory acidosis is seen as an imbalance that the Paramedic can recognize and treat.

Respiration and Oxygen Transportation

The term "respiration" has several definitions applicable to Paramedic practice.[1] The first definition of respiration is the movement of respiratory gasses in and out of the lungs. As discussed in Chapter 16, one respiration is the cycle of inspiration and expiration which moves air in and out of the lungs. On a cellular level, respiration is defined as "the chemical processes by which an organism supplies its cells and tissues with the oxygen needed for metabolism and relieves them of the carbon dioxide formed in energy-producing reactions." Respiration includes everything from inspiration, movement of oxygen into the bloodstream, absorption of oxygen into the cells, utilization of oxygen to make energy, the movement of carbon dioxide to the bloodstream and ultimately across into the air in the alveoli, and the exhalation of carbon dioxide into the atmosphere (Figure 25-1). Through this process, the human body is able to live and function.

The components of this process that the Paramedic can affect during the breathing step in the resuscitation involve several actions that improve oxygenation and ventilation. Before we can assess those components, let's review how the body transports oxygen and carbon dioxide.

Oxygen Transport

Oxygen comprises 21% of room air. As discussed in Chapter 20, the fraction of inspired oxygen, FiO_2, can be increased by providing supplemental oxygen to the patient through one of several oxygen delivery devices. Inspiration fills the lungs with oxygen-rich air. Oxygen diffuses across the alveoli and capillary wall because of the higher concentration of oxygen in the alveoli compared with the lower concentration of oxygen in the blood surrounding the alveoli (Figure 25-2).

Oxygen is transported to the tissues by two different mechanisms. Approximately 3% of oxygen that enters the bloodstream is dissolved into the plasma, or liquid portion of the blood, similar to the way carbon dioxide is dissolved into liquid to produce the fizz in carbonated beverages. This is an ineffective method for carrying oxygen to the tissues because oxygen does not easily dissolve into liquid and only a small amount of oxygen can be delivered. A more effective mechanism for oxygen transport involves binding the oxygen molecules directly to a compound or structure within the blood for transportation to the tissues. This transport mechanism is responsible for the other 97% of oxygen transported to the tissues and involves red blood cells and the hemoglobin molecule that makes up the majority of the red blood cell.

Each red blood cell contains approximately 270 million hemoglobin molecules. Each hemoglobin molecule can normally bind up to four oxygen molecules (Figure 25-3). When the hemoglobin molecule attaches at least one oxygen molecule, it is called oxyhemoglobin. The hemoglobin molecule that is not attached to any oxygen molecules is called deoxyhemoglobin. As oxygen attaches to each of the binding sites, the shape of the hemoglobin molecule opens up around the other oxygen-binding sites, making it easier to bind oxygen to the next site. Due to this property, it takes a smaller increase in partial pressure of oxygen (see the discussion on partial pressures in Chapter 20) to saturate the hemoglobin molecules with oxygen when hemoglobin is in the deoxyhemoglobin state. As hemoglobin nears complete saturation, it then takes a larger change in partial pressure of oxygen to fully saturate all oxygen-binding sites. Figure 25-4 demonstrates this relationship between partial pressure of oxygen and hemoglobin saturation. It should be noted that arterial blood typically has a saturation of approximately 97%, whereas venous blood will typically have a oxygen saturation of approximately 75%.[2]

There are several factors that affect oxygen's ability to bind to hemoglobin. Some of these factors are used by the body to enhance the release of oxygen as part of normal transport, whereas others occur when the body is ill or injured (Table 25-1). The factors that increase oxygen binding in effect shift the curve in Figure 25-4 to the left. By shifting the curve to the left, it takes a smaller change in partial pressure of oxygen to increase the saturation of the hemoglobin. Conversely, the factors that decrease oxygen binding move the

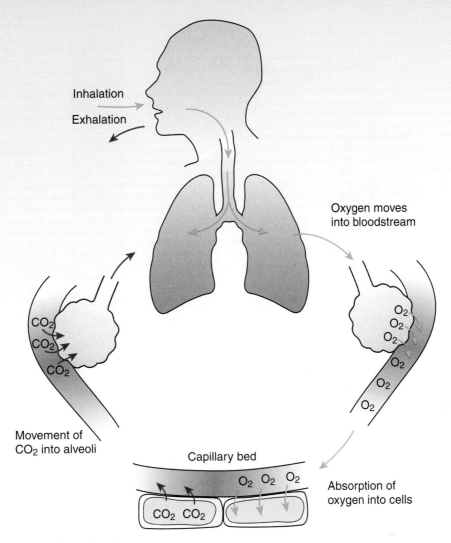

Figure 25-1 The process of respiration.

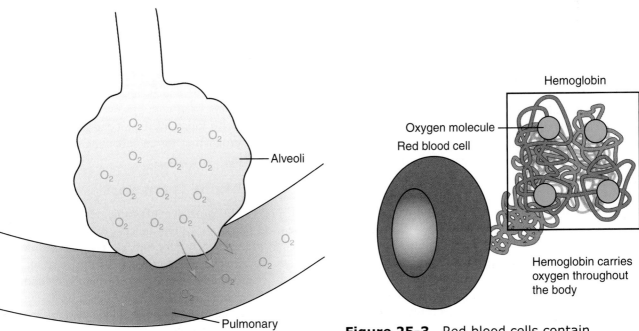

Figure 25-2 Oxygen movement across the alveoli–capillary membrane.

Figure 25-3 Red blood cells contain hemoglobin, the oxygen-carrying portion of the blood, which can transport up to four oxygen molecules per hemoglobin molecule.

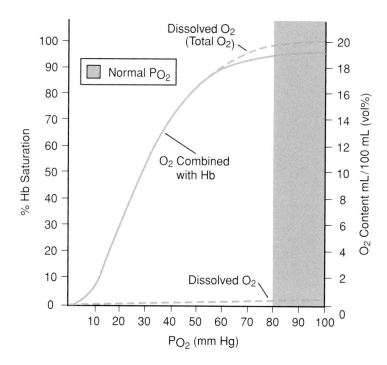

Figure 25-4 The oxygen–hemoglobin dissociation curve. In the lower portion of the curve, it takes a small increase in partial pressure of oxygen to produce a large increase in oxygen saturation.

Table 25-1 Factors That Affect the Ability to Bind Oxygen to Hemoglobin

Increased	Decreased
• Alkalosis	• Acidosis
• Decreased CO_2	• Increased CO_2
• Decreased temperature	• Increased temperature
• Decreased 2,3-BPG	• Increased 2,3-BPG

curve to the right, requiring a larger change in partial pressure of oxygen to saturate the hemoglobin molecules.

Both alkalosis and acidosis will be discussed later in this chapter. Alkalosis will cause a shift in the curve to the left, increasing the affinity of hemoglobin to oxygen, and acidosis will cause a shift in the curve to the right, decreasing the affinity of hemoglobin for oxygen. This change in affinity helps the hemoglobin either hold on to the oxygen molecules or enhances the release of oxygen molecules from hemoglobin.

A second way the body enhances release of oxygen from hemoglobin is through a compound called 2,3-BPG. 2,3-BPG occurs naturally in the hemoglobin, enhancing the release of oxygen from hemoglobin at the tissues to provide oxygen for the energy production process at the cellular level. This compound can be found in higher concentration in situations where the amount of oxygen inhaled into the lungs is decreased or in conditions where there is chronic tissue hypoxia. This is a way for the body to compensate for less available oxygen at high altitudes or for advanced chronic respiratory conditions. Increased production of 2,3-BPG helps to prevent hypoxia in the tissues.

Temperature also affects hemoglobin's ability to off-load oxygen at the tissues. Decreased temperatures shift the curve to the left while increased temperatures will shift the curve to the right. This is why patients who have sustained traumatic injury, who are often cold from exposure, even in warmer climates, should be kept warm and provided with supplemental oxygen to compensate for the difficulty in off-loading oxygen as a result of decreased body temperature.

Once the hemoglobin circulates to the tissues, some of the oxygen bound to hemoglobin dissociates, or is released, from the hemoglobin into the blood and taken into the cells. The environment in the capillary blood has a lot of the factors that enhance oxygen release from hemoglobin, including increased carbon dioxide and increased levels of 2,3-BPG. In the cell, oxygen is used with glucose to produce energy to carry out the cell's functions (e.g., contraction for muscle cells, chemical production for an endocrine cell, or to fight bacterial invaders).

Carbon Dioxide Transport

Carbon dioxide is a by-product of cellular respiration. During the chemical processes within the cell, oxygen and glucose are used to produce energy for the cell. Carbon dioxide and water are produced as waste products of this reaction. The carbon dioxide diffuses across the cell membrane and into the blood. Once in the blood, some carbon dioxide is taken up and carried to the lungs in the red blood cells while some stays dissolved in the plasma.

Carbon dioxide is 20 times more soluble than oxygen in the blood at the same partial pressure, and much of the carbon dioxide transported by the blood is dissolved within the plasma. Some of the dissolved carbon dioxide is then absorbed into the red blood cells and then released back into the blood as bicarbonate, which is then transported to the lungs. A small amount of carbon dioxide travels back to the lungs attached to the hemoglobin molecules, at a different site from the oxygen molecules, and some carbon dioxide molecules combine with other compounds in the blood. Therefore, carbon dioxide is transported to the lungs in one of three ways: dissolved in the blood plasma, attached to hemoglobin, or contained with bicarbonate.

At the lungs, the bicarbonate is changed back to carbon dioxide and water. The dissolved carbon dioxide off-gasses and the hemoglobin releases its carbon dioxide. The carbon dioxide then diffuses across the alveolar membrane and into the alveolar air, ready for exhalation. The transport of carbon dioxide is affected by many factors including both the amount of carbon dioxide produced by the cells (metabolism rate) and the amount of blood volume circulated through the lungs. If the patient is hypotensive, there is less blood circulating through the lungs and reduced transportation of carbon dioxide to the lungs. Similarly, if the patient has hemorrhaged than there are fewer red blood cells, which means less hemoglobin to bind oxygen and plasma to carry the carbon dioxide.

These factors culminate to increase carbon dioxide levels in the tissues. Carbon dioxide, together with water, forms a weak acid called carbonic acid (H_2CO_3). The level of carbonic acid in the body is referred to as the "acid load."

During any form of shock there is an increase in the body's acid load. An increased acid level in the body can have devastating effects to the normal metabolic functions of the body if not corrected.

Acid–Base Balance

Acids are created in the course of both aerobic (with oxygen) and anaerobic (without oxygen) metabolism. The majority of acid in the body is formed when excess carbon dioxide reacts with water to form carbonic acid (H_2CO_3) before conversion into bicarbonate. It is called the **respiratory acid** as it is the intermediary step in carbon dioxide transport. Other acids (e.g., lactic acid and pyruvic acid formed during anaerobic metabolism, and amino acids formed by the breakdown/oxidation of proteins) are called the **metabolic acids**. Regardless of the source, an overabundance of acid can interfere with the normal enzyme action within the cells. Acid levels must be controlled by the body.

An **acid**, by definition, is a molecule that has a proton (a positively charged atomic particle) that is not orbited by a paired negatively charged atomic particle called an electron. The particle that exists in nature with one proton is the hydrogen particle and thus hydrogen is considered a primary acid. And acids are chemical compounds with positively charged hydrogen (H+) particles or **ions** attached; ions being charged particles. Being positively charged, these hydrogen ions are extremely reactive, meaning that the hydrogen ion wants to

couple with other molecules, even if it means uncoupling one chemical molecule from another and bringing about the destruction of the molecule compound in order to allow the hydrogen to attach, or bond, with another chemical.

In some cases, a molecule may be negatively charged, such as the hydroxyl molecule (−OH). These chemicals are called **bases** and bases lack a proton and want to accept the protons from acid in order to become electrically balanced. For example, if an acid (H+) was to join with a base (−OH), the result would be water (H_2O). The acid is then said to be **buffered**, or rendered neutral (i.e., not having an electrical charge) once it combined with a base to form water.

Trying to describe the different amounts of acidity or alkalinity in a solution can be difficult, since there can be as much as a thousand-fold difference from one extreme to the other. Practically speaking, using such a range is difficult. To ease the process of describing the strengths of acids and bases, the **pH scale** (abbreviated for potential hydrogen) was developed to describe the differing degrees of acidity or alkalinity. Mathematically, pH is the negative logarithm of the hydrogen ion concentration ($pH = -\log 10[H+]$). The range of pH is from 0 to 14, with 7 being neutral; pure distilled water is neutral. A weak acid has a pH closer to 7, somewhere in the range of 5 to 7, whereas a weak base has a pH somewhere in the 7 to 9 range. Human blood has a pH of 7.35 to 7.45, and is slightly alkaline. When the concentration of hydrogen ions increases, the solution becomes more acidic, and the pH decreases. When the concentration of hydrogen ions decreases, the solution becomes more basic, and the pH increases (Figure 25-5).

Excessive amounts of acid in the tissues, in sum total called an **acid load**, can be devastating to proteins within the cells. Excess acid can eventually break down (i.e., denature) proteins in the cells and eventually lead to cell death or necrosis.

Acid is eliminated from the interstitial space when the acid dilates the capillary beds. The acid passes into the capillary bed and the acid is washed out in the blood. Upon entering the bloodstream, the acid can now be acted upon by the body's buffering mechanisms.

Buffering Systems

Any acid, whether metabolic or respiratory, entering the bloodstream immediately encounters the three chemical buffers that circulate throughout the body in the bloodstream. Bicarbonate (HCO_3^-), the most common chemical buffer, almost instantaneously couples and neutralizes the acid (H+), releasing heat in the process. The result is carbonic acid (H_2O_3). Carbonic acid then reverts into water (H_2O) and carbon dioxide (CO_2) in the lungs. The water (H_2O) is then either absorbed or excreted by the kidneys and the carbon dioxide (CO_2) is exhaled in the breath.

While bicarbonate is a powerful buffer, the amount of bicarbonate in the bloodstream is limited and only provides approximately one half of the blood buffering capacity.

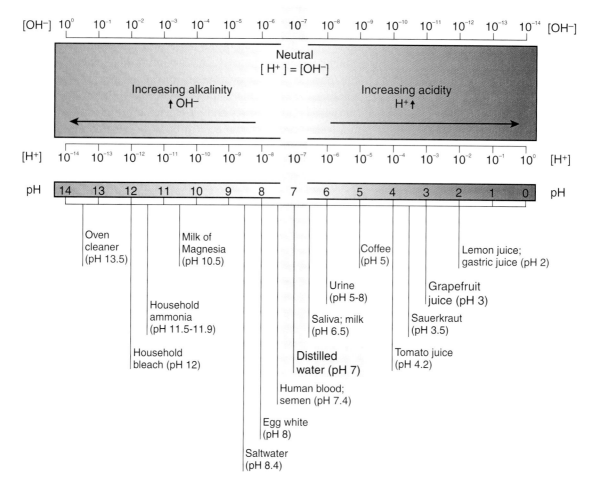

Figure 25-5 pH scale with common acids and bases shown.

Another chemical buffer, phosphate (PO_4), also helps to buffer acids. Phosphate buffers bind with acid and carry the acid to the kidneys to be excreted, thus making urine acidic.

Finally, the proteins in the blood have a limited ability to buffer acid. All blood proteins, including albumin the most abundant blood protein, are made of chains of amino acids. These amino acids became neutralized when bonded in chains, but these proteins are capable of accepting more acids. Therefore, albumin is important to helping maintain an acid–base balance. Albumin is so important that patients who have liver disease, and subsequently reduced albumin, are more likely to have problems with maintaining acid–base balance.

Blood proteins also include the hemoglobin molecules contained within the red blood cells (erythrocytes). Hemoglobin can preferentially bind to either oxygen (O_2) or acid (H+), and therefore it releases its oxygen at the capillary level and picks up acid at the venous side for removal in the lungs or kidneys. Patients who have lost large volumes of blood will have difficulty with maintaining an acid–base balance because they have lost hemoglobin.

In addition to the chemical buffering that occurs to handle the day-to-day production of acids in response to

metabolism, there are two other ways the body can compensate for increased acid production. Both respiratory compensation and renal compensation kick in during times when the body is producing additional acids, whether through increased metabolic load, disease, or lack of oxygen. The three means of buffering—chemical, respiratory, and renal—are interlinked and any weakness in one is compensated for by the others.

Respiratory Compensation

The lungs also have an ability to help rid the body of acid by driving the acid–bicarbonate formula. The acid–bicarbonate reaction is easily reversible, releasing acid back into the bloodstream in the form of carbonic acid (H_2CO_3) (Figure 25-6). Sensitive central chemoreceptors monitor cerebrospinal fluid (CSF) for an increase in carbonic acid, the respiratory acid, and stimulate the medulla to increase respirations. Increased respirations increase removal of carbon dioxide and drive the formula to the left, forcing the conversion of acids into bicarbonate, then carbon dioxide and water, which are removed through ventilation and urination. This process of increasing the respiratory rate in response to increased acidity of the cerebral spinal fluid occurs rapidly, within several minutes.

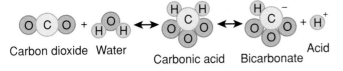

Carbon dioxide   Water   Carbonic acid   Bicarbonate   Acid

Figure 25-6 The acid–bicarbonate reaction. Increased ventilation forces this chemical equation to move to the left, increasing production of carbon dioxide and water, which are then removed from the body.

Renal Compensation

In the triad of buffering systems, the kidneys are the last line of defense. When carbonic acid reaches the kidneys, an enzyme called carbonic anhydrase (an- – "without", hydra – "water", -ase – "enzyme") breaks the carbonic acid down into bicarbonate (HCO_3^-) and acid ($H+$). The acid is excreted in the urine. In the process, the bicarbonate (HCO_3^-) is regenerated for use in the bloodstream. The kidneys also can create ammonia from the breakdown of the amino acid glutamine by the enzyme glutaminase, an enzyme that works best in an acidic environment. Ammonia (NH_3) then couples with acid ($H+$) to become ammonium (NH_4) and is excreted in the urine. Ammonium is a volatile acid, meaning that it off-gasses into the atmosphere and gives urine its distinctive odor.

This process of enzyme activation, reabsorption of bicarbonate, and excretion of acids can take up to 49 hours to fully activate. For this reason, compensation by the kidneys is ineffective during an acute emergency. Renal compensation only comes into action in patients who are chronically ill or who have been acutely ill for several days.

Effects of an Acidic Environment

The efficiency of all of the body's chemical processes, whether in the bloodstream, within the cells, or in the space between the cells, depends on the local pH where the process takes place. If the local environment becomes too acidic or too basic, the chemical process may not occur at all. Transport of materials across cell membranes may also not occur if the pH of the blood is too far outside the normal range. This can affect important body functions (e.g., produce cardiac dysrhythmias, affect oxygen transport, and affect muscle strength). Two important areas pertaining to Paramedic practice are oxygen transport and the effect of medications.

Acidosis and Oxygen Transport

As discussed earlier in this chapter, oxygen is picked up by the hemoglobin in the red blood cells and transported to the tissues where it is released and used to produce energy. Hemoglobin's attraction, or affinity, for oxygen is due to the iron molecules that make up the hemoglobin. However, acids have a greater affinity for oxygen. When acid is present, it will cause oxygen to separate (dissociate) from the hemoglobin. This phenomenon, called the Bohr effect, is responsible for oxygen entering the tissues at the cellular level in the interstitial space, where

the environment is slightly more acidic than in the central circulation. The process of cellular respiration starts with metabolically active cells. These cells produce acid as one of the by-products of metabolism. These cells also need more oxygen to sustain their aerobic (with oxygen) metabolism. The acid causes the capillary beds to dilate, permitting more oxygen-carrying hemoglobin red blood cells in the blood to enter the capillary. Once the blood is in the capillary bed, and in the presence of the acid, the oxygen is released from the hemoglobin and moved into the cells. The use of oxygen in the cell is a process called cellular respiration.

A problem occurs when the blood in the central circulation becomes acidotic from a large "acid load" developing within the body. Under normal conditions the acid in the blood, as carbonic acid, changes to carbon dioxide, diffuses in the alveoli, and is exhaled. With the acid eliminated from the blood, the oxygen in the alveoli can be attached to hemoglobin and carried out to the capillary beds. If the acid load in the central circulation is too great (e.g., secondary to hypoventilation or an increase in metabolic acids), then the oxygen will not be released into the tissues and the patient may experience hypoxemia. Due to the effect of acid and temperature on the oxyhemoglobin curve described in Figure 25-4, the oxygen saturation of a patient who has a fever or who has a large acid load, as is the case with a septic patient from a severe infection, will be lower than expected. The oxygen saturation may remain lower than expected despite the presence of high-flow oxygen via nonrebreather face mask until the underlying metabolic cause—in this case, the infection—is treated.

Acidosis and Medication

Acidosis, excessive acid in the system, can have a profound effect upon the body's uptake, distribution, and the effectiveness of medications administered by the Paramedic as well. Once a medication is in the bloodstream and enters the interstitial space it must cross the cell wall, a lipid–protein matrix. This semipermeable membrane readily accepts those medications that are not ionized (i.e., did not dissolve in solution). These "lipid-soluble" medications easily diffuse across the lipid–protein cell membrane (i.e., "like dissolves like"). The problem occurs when a medication enters the bloodstream and is dissolved, meaning the medication becomes divided into two charged or "ionized" portions. Some medications start as a salt and then dissolve in solution to become ionized as either a weak acid or weak base. These ionized (charged) medications are repelled by the cell membrane and are called lipophobic (lipo- – "fat", phobic – "fear") medications. Lipophobic medications require carriers or other compounds (e.g., bicarbonate or an amino acid) to carry the medication into the cell. When the surrounding tissues are acidotic, the medication is not dissolved normally and absorption is reduced, thus reducing the drug's efficiency.

Acid–Base Disorders

Changes in the acid–base balance in the body can have dramatic effects on the patient's signs, symptoms, physiology, and the effects of medications on the patient. Even in the brief patient contact time as part of many EMS calls, the Paramedic can detect subtle signs of these derangements and initiate treatment that can prevent or slow catastrophic deterioration in the patient's condition. These disorders are typically identified through either an arterial blood gas or a venous blood gas, where a blood sample from either an artery or a vein is analyzed for the pH, the partial pressures of carbon dioxide and oxygen (pCO_2 and PO_2), the bicarbonate, and the oxygen saturation. These parameters are examined to assess for an acid–base disorder. While the interpretation of arterial and venous blood gas is outside the scope of the typical street Paramedic, there are several causes for each and associated signs and symptoms.

The blood can either become acidotic if the pH falls below 7.35 or alkalemic if the pH rises above 7.45. Each of these main disorders has respiratory causes and metabolic causes for the acidosis and alkalosis. Therefore, the four main acid–base disorders, in order of most common to least common for Paramedics, are respiratory acidosis, metabolic acidosis, metabolic alkalosis, and respiratory alkalosis.

Acidosis

The blood becomes acidotic if the pH falls below 7.35. As previously discussed, the blood in the capillaries is slightly more acidotic than the blood in the central circulation, which assists in the off-loading of oxygen and removal of carbon dioxide from the tissues. Acidosis can occur as a result of either problems with the respiratory acids or the metabolic acids. It is possible to have a mixed respiratory and metabolic cause for a patient's acidosis when a chronically ill patient has an acute exacerbation of her disease or when more than one active disease process is present.

Respiratory Acidosis

The problem of respiratory acidosis can be further subdivided into two categories: either too much carbonic acid production or too little ventilation. The classic case of too much carbonic acid production is the patient with a fever, **pyrexia**, whose body is hypermetabolic. The acute nature of fever causes the body's metabolism to increase, producing additional carbon dioxide and other by-products.

The more traditional cause of respiratory acidosis is hypoventilation. Conditions such as strokes, brain trauma, and drug intoxication—especially with opiates—can depress the respiratory drive at the respiratory center in the medulla. Spinal cord trauma and diseases that affect the nerves or the muscles can cause either the respiratory muscles or the nerves controlling the respiratory muscles to provide inadequate ventilation, which in turn causes hypoventilation. Illness and injury to the lungs themselves can result in hypoventilation. Any condition, either traumatic or medical, that impairs gas exchange reduces the lungs' ability to exchange oxygen and carbon dioxide, producing a respiratory acidosis.

Treatments for the patient experiencing respiratory acidosis focus on ensuring the patient has adequate oxygenation and ventilation. This may include administration of supplemental oxygen or invasive airway management maneuvers as discussed in previous chapters.

Metabolic Acidosis

During metabolism, the body makes acids other than carbon dioxide. These metabolic acids can cause systemic acidosis as well. The quintessential example of metabolic acidosis is the patient experiencing diabetic ketoacidosis. During hypoglycemic conditions, the body breaks down fats for energy and produces ketonic acids in the process, leading to ketoacidosis, or ketonic acids in the blood. Other causes of metabolic acidosis include cyanide poisoning and carbon monoxide poisoning. Both of these conditions deprive the cells of oxygen and force anaerobic (without oxygen) respiration.

While too much lactic acid, pyruvic acid, or ketonic acid can produce metabolic acidosis, the absence of bicarbonate can also result in a relative metabolic acidosis. Under normal conditions, the kidneys and the bowels reabsorb bicarbonate, making it available for reuse. Therefore, any gastrointestinal or urinary disease can cause serious problems with maintaining acid–base balance. For example, the gallbladder secretes bicarbonate to neutralize the acid created by the stomach. This bicarbonate is then reabsorbed in the intestines. When massive or persistent diarrhea occurs, then the intestines cannot reabsorb the bicarbonate. When a patient experiences renal failure, the kidneys cannot absorb the bicarbonate that is excreted into the urine. The patient may become acidotic from the lack of the bicarbonate buffer.

Metabolic acidosis can also be caused by ingestion of substances that are toxic or in toxic doses. Certain alcohols cannot be metabolized by the body and produce metabolic acids as a result of this incomplete metabolism.

Aspirin is another medication that can lead to acidosis. Aspirin is a medication that many people take to decrease the risk of a heart attack, whereas some people take it as an analgesic. Aspirin is the active ingredient in many over the counter (OTC) medications. In high doses, aspirin, (chemical name: acetylsalicylic acid and abbreviated as ASA) can cause metabolic acidosis. In severe cases of aspirin overdose aspirin inhibits the respiratory center in the medulla, leading to hypoventilation and compounding the metabolic acidosis with a respiratory acidosis.

Treatment of acidosis from a metabolic cause typically involves first ensuring adequate circulation. This may include administering intravenous fluids, administering medications to increase the patient's blood pressure, administering antibiotics to treat infection, or performing chest compressions during cardiac arrest. These supportive measures help the body resolve the acidosis naturally. Sodium bicarbonate is sometimes administered intravenously in an attempt to correct a severe metabolic acidosis by providing additional bicarbonate to buffer the acid.

As acidotic patients tend to hyperventilate as a way of compensating for the metabolic acidosis, if the Paramedic needs to secure the airway, the Paramedic must remember to either ventilate the patient at a higher rate or set the respiratory rate on the ventilator to a higher-than-normal rate in order to maintain an adequate ventilatory rate for that compensation. If too low of a respiratory rate is provided, and the underlying metabolic process is not corrected, the patient will continue to become more acidotic until the patient goes into a cardiac arrest. Cardiac arrest in these cases often does not respond to treatment because of the severe acidosis.

Alkalosis

The blood becomes alkalotic if the pH rises above 7.45. As with acidosis, this can be due to either a respiratory or metabolic cause. Alkalosis from a metabolic cause occurs more often than from respiratory etiologies.

Metabolic Alkalosis

Metabolic alkalosis is caused by an increase in the production of bicarbonate in the blood. This can be due to a metabolic process in the body and can also be due to increased kidney reabsorption of bicarbonate from the urine. Common causes of metabolic alkalosis include severe volume depletion and acid loss, as occurs in dehydration from vomiting, and electrolyte disturbances (e.g., low potassium), which triggers reabsorption of bicarbonate by the kidneys. Certain endocrine disorders can also produce a metabolic alkalosis by decreasing the serum potassium level. The use of some diuretics, specifically those that spill potassium into the urine (e.g., potassium wasting diuretics), can cause a metabolic alkalosis because they cause an increase in reabsorption of bicarbonate.

Treatment of metabolic alkalosis depends upon the cause. In the case of volume depletion (e.g., from vomiting, diarrhea, or overdiuresis), administering normal saline will help correct the volume loss. It is important to monitor the patient's oxygenation, as the body's primary means of compensating for a metabolic alkalosis is to hypoventilate, producing a mild respiratory acidosis to compensate for the metabolic alkalosis. In patients with normal respiratory function, the effect of the hypoventilation is minimal. However, in patients who have a significant respiratory condition (e.g., chronic obstructive pulmonary disease (COPD)), hypoventilation may not be tolerated well and the patient may become hypoxic. Supplemental oxygen may be required to treat the hypoxia. In patients who are paralyzed and on a ventilator, the respiratory rate can be decreased to help treat the metabolic alkalosis.

Respiratory Alkalosis

Respiratory alkalosis occurs when ventilation is greater than the body's CO_2 production. As previously discussed, the CO_2 generated by the body is primarily removed by the respiratory system. Changes in the respiratory rate occur very rapidly in response to an increase or decrease in the circulating CO_2 level. When the metabolic rate increases quickly (e.g., when a person jumps up from a resting position and runs a quarter mile sprint), the respiratory rate increases rapidly in response to the increased metabolic CO_2 production. At the end of the race, when the metabolic production of CO_2 decreases, the respiratory rate will decrease to the baseline rate over the course of several minutes. In some conditions, however, there is a mismatch between the respiratory rate and CO_2 production, with the patient breathing at a faster rate than required to handle the production of CO_2. This increased minute ventilation lowers the CO_2 level, producing the alkalosis. When a patient has a condition that causes metabolic acidosis, this mechanism compensates for the acidosis and helps move the pH back toward the normal range. However, when the patient does not have an existing metabolic acidosis, this increased ventilation stimulus produces the respiratory alkalosis.

There are several causes for the increased stimulation. Normally, if hypoxemia occurs in the central circulation, receptors in the aorta and carotid arteries will signal the respiratory center to increase the respiratory rate in order to compensate for the decreased oxygenation. However, in some situations, the central circulation is not hypoxemic. However, the tissues are hypoxic, and cause an increase in respiratory rate. Any condition that decreases the off-loading of oxygen at the tissue level (e.g., shock or anemia) can cause an increase in the respiratory rate.

A second abnormal stimulus for increased ventilation can occur with abnormal stimulation of the stretch receptors located in the alveoli and smaller air passages in the lungs. Normally, the stretch receptors help signal the start and stop of ventilation. However, in the case of irritation of the alveoli from pneumonia, pleural effusion (abnormal liquid in-between the pleural layers), or congestion in the pulmonary capillaries, the stretch receptors can trigger increased ventilation, producing a respiratory alkalosis.

The respiratory center can be directly stimulated by a variety of conditions and produce increased ventilation. Certain toxins, either ingested or produced by other conditions (e.g., liver failure or renal failure) can trigger increased ventilation. Fever or the toxins in sepsis can also increase ventilation and produce a respiratory alkalosis. Certain hormones can also stimulate increased ventilation. This occurs as a normal part of pregnancy to increase respiratory rate late in pregnancy to compensate for difficulty in fully expanding the lungs due to the growing fetus. Changes in blood chemistry that occur when at altitude also produce a mild hyperventilation to compensate for the lower partial pressure of oxygen at high altitude.

Finally, psychologically induced hyperventilation can occur as a response to fear, anxiety, pain, or any number of emotional stressors. This increased respiratory rate can be either involuntary or voluntary and often responds to calming and reassurance. With severe hyperventilation, the decrease in blood CO_2 causes vasoconstriction of cerebral blood vessels, reducing blood flow. In some cases, this can cause light-headedness or even syncope.

It is very easy to blame hyperventilation on a psychological cause. Be aware that many other conditions can produce hyperventilation, including hypoxia, shock, and sepsis. Search for these causes during your patient assessment and treat them appropriately. Do not allow the patient to breathe into a paper bag or an oxygen mask that is disconnected from supplemental oxygen! This rebreathing will produce an abnormal increase in CO_2. For the patient that is hyperventilating in response to a pathologic cause, this increase in CO_2 may produce unconsciousness, profound metabolic derangements, and cardiac arrest.

Treatment of respiratory alkalosis depends on the cause. If the patient is hypoxic or there is a reason for tissue hypoxia (e.g., shock), then providing supplemental oxygen or treatment of shock may improve the alkalosis. If psychogenic causes are present, attempt to calm the patient, provide reassurance, and appropriately treat pain and anxiety. Consider other respiratory or central causes when developing a paramedical diagnosis, ensure the patient's ABCs, and provide supportive care.

Mixed Disorders

The four acid–base disturbances should not be thought of as isolated entities. In reality, the body is complex and will respond both acutely and chronically to compensate for these dysfunctions. Some disease processes, or combination of disease processes, may cause a mixed acid–base disorder, where a primary disorder (e.g., respiratory acidosis) is partially compensated by the body by another disorder (e.g., a metabolic alkalosis). In some cases, the acidosis and alkalosis can have both a respiratory and metabolic cause (e.g., a respiratory and metabolic acidosis that can occur with some conditions). These disorders can be challenging to sort out. When in doubt, fall back to the ABCs and ensure the patient has a patent airway, is well ventilated and oxygenated, and is not in shock. This can be easily summarized as supporting the ABCs. This initial attempt at resuscitation and stabilization can go a long way in improving the patient's condition.

Assessment of Oxygenation and Ventilation

The Paramedic has several tools at her disposal to help assess oxygenation and ventilation in the critical patient. Clinical assessment of oxygenation and ventilation was discussed

in Chapter 16 and during the airway management chapters (Chapters 22 and 23). In this section, we will discuss some of the objective measures of oxygenation and ventilation, including pulse oximetry, capnography, co-oximetry, and arterial blood gas sampling.

Pulse Oximetry

Pulse oximetry is a non-invasive measure of the percentage of hemoglobin sites in the red blood cells that are bound to oxygen, or oxyhemoglobin. This percentage of oxyhemoglobin is called oxygen saturation and is abbreviated as SpO_2. A normal SpO_2 is between 95% and 100%. An SpO_2 reading between 90% and 95% indicates mild hypoxemia, and a reading between 85% and 90% indicates moderate hypoxemia. A reading below 85% indicates severe hypoxemia requiring intervention by the Paramedic. There are two ways to report oxygen saturation: One is displaying a quantitative measure of the oxygen saturation and the other is displaying the oxygen saturation as a waveform over time. For oximeters that only display a numerical value, there is an indication of signal strength that provides the Paramedic with an indication of the strength of the blood flow across the sensor. For oximeters that provide a waveform display in addition to the numerical value, the shape of the waveform provides the Paramedic with a visual indication of the strength of the blood flow across the sensor (Figure 25-7).

Technology

Measurement of the SpO_2 involves beaming a light wave across the patient's capillary bed and detecting the wavelength on the opposite side of the capillary bed. The light

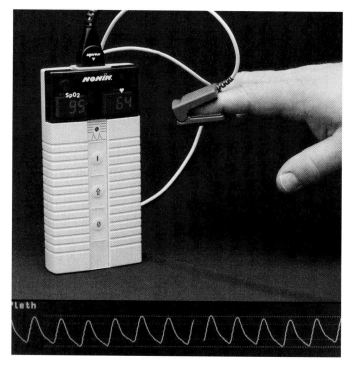

Figure 25-7 Pulse oximeters may display a numerical indication of SpO_2 or waveform display of SpO_2.

wave is combined red and infrared frequencies. As the wave passes through the capillary bed, the light is absorbed by the hemoglobin differently depending on if it is in the oxyhemoglobin form or the deoxyhemoglobin form. The oxyhemoglobin form absorbs more infrared light than red (therefore explaining the bright red color of oxygenated blood) and deoxyhemoglobin absorbs more red light than infrared. The wavelengths at the light source are known and compared to the wavelengths detected at the sensor. The ratio between the wavelengths transmitted and received is compared with a database of known values and is used to calculate the SpO_2. These known values are only available in the range of 70% to 100% saturation as this information was derived from actual patients.

The most common source used to measure SpO_2 is the tip of a finger. Light travels easily through the fingertip and the capillary bed is relatively superficial to the skin surface. Alternatively, the earlobe can also be used for a similar reason. Two other sites include tip of the toes, useful in children, and the skin on the forehead, useful in hypothermic patients.

The strength of the signal detected by the pulse oximeter is reported as the perfusion index on oximeters that do not display a waveform. The perfusion index is measured from 0.02% to 20%, with the larger number indicating a stronger signal. The higher the perfusion index, the more accurate the reading. Therefore, when using device pulse oximeter, the Paramedic can use the perfusion index indicator to know if the pulse SpO_2 reading displayed is an accurate reading. In some cases, the Paramedic will need to try several different sites before obtaining an accurate SpO_2 reading. The pulse rate is calculated from the time between peaks of the fluctuating pulse oximetry wave.

For devices that display a waveform, the shape of the waveform can be used to determine the accuracy of the SpO_2 reading (Figure 25-8). The waveform amplitude fluctuates normally, corresponding to the flow of blood through the capillary bed. If the Paramedic encounters a poor quality waveform (Figure 25-9), the Paramedic will need to place the sensor on a different site.

Clinical Application

There are several factors that affect the accuracy of the waveform or the perfusion index. In low blood flow states (e.g., hypotension from shock or cardiac arrest), there may not be a sufficient movement of blood through the capillary bed to provide an accurate reading. Decreased capillary blood flow can also occur when the sensor site is cold and the blood vessels are constricted. Vasoconstriction is a normal response to cold, shunting warm blood toward the core to maintain a normal body temperature; however, it can be problematic when attempting to obtain an accurate SpO_2 reading. Vibration from shivering and motion artifact during transport may also affect the quality of the waveform, although this is not as much of an issue with the later models of pulse oximeters. Nail polish may affect the ability of the light to pass through the fingertip and may need to be removed if a poor waveform or inadequate perfusion index is noted. Finally, the pulse oximeter is inaccurate below an SpO_2 of 70% because the reference database in the machine does not contain information below 70%.

A normal SpO_2 reading doesn't mean the patient does not require supplemental oxygen. While anemia, or decreased hemoglobin, does not affect the SpO_2, total blood oxygen content—and therefore the delivery of oxygen to the tissues—is decreased. Total blood oxygen content depends on the amount of hemoglobin in the blood and the amount of oxygen diffused into the blood. The total amount of dissolved oxygen in the blood can be increased by administering

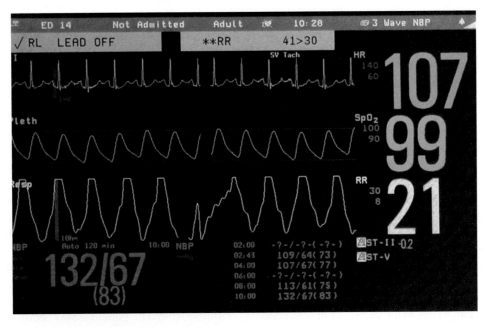

Figure 25-8 Normal pulse oximetry waveform.

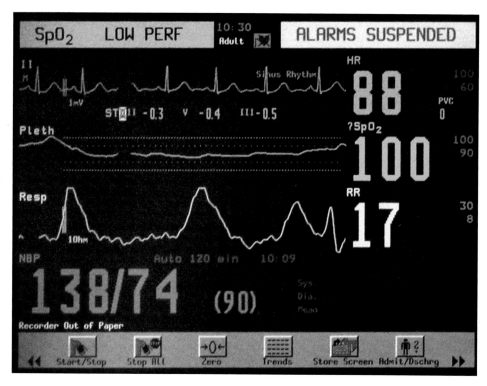

Figure 25-9 Poor waveform that affects the accuracy of the SpO$_2$ reading.

supplemental oxygen to patients suspected of anemia from acute blood loss, and may help prevent tissue hypoxia from inadequate oxygen transport. Patients in respiratory distress or shock often increase their respiratory rate and pulse rate in order to move more oxygen into the blood and circulate more oxygen to the tissues in response to a lack of oxygen at the tissues. In many cases, a patient in respiratory distress will be able to improve his SpO$_2$ by increasing his respiratory rate and compensating for his hypoxemia. The use of supplemental oxygen should not be based on SpO$_2$ alone, but also on other clinical assessment of respiratory distress as discussed in Chapter 16.

Certain conditions will also affect the SpO$_2$ reading. Carbon monoxide also attaches to hemoglobin; because, it has a significantly higher affinity than oxygen. This means that carbon monoxide is 200 times more likely to attach to the hemoglobin molecule than oxygen, creating carboxyhemoglobin. Though the hemoglobin is bound to carbon monoxide rather than oxygen, the wavelengths of light used in first generation pulse oximeters are not capable of differentiating the two hemoglobins. A patient who has had carbon monoxide poisoning may demonstrate a normal SpO$_2$. Other forms of hemoglobin (more specifically, one form called methemoglobin) will also provide a false SpO$_2$ reading. Methemoglobin is a form of hemoglobin that is chemically different from hemoglobin and cannot carry oxygen. This is often the form hemoglobin takes as it reaches the end of its useful life. A small amount of methemoglobin is present in the blood at all times. However, the level can be markedly increased in some conditions, decreasing oxygen transport. Fortunately, co-oximeters

are available that can detect the presence of these two conditions. This will be discussed later in this chapter.

Pulse oximetry also does not provide an indication or measure of the patient's ventilatory status. This is especially true when the patient is on high-flow supplemental oxygen. The supplemental oxygen can replace the other gasses in the lungs, increasing the oxygen gradient between the alveoli and the pulmonary capillary blood. This encourages transport of oxygen into the blood, even when there is insufficient airflow in and out of the lungs. That airflow in and out of the lungs (ventilation) is required to remove carbon dioxide from the system. With inadequate airflow, the carbon dioxide levels increase in the alveoli, decreasing the gradient from the blood to the alveoli, reducing carbon dioxide transport and therefore increasing blood carbon dioxide levels. Pulse oximetry alone would not detect this hypoventilation. This is well illustrated in a case report from 1993, approximately 5 to 10 years after pulse oximetry's introduction into regular clinical use.[3] In this case report, an elderly woman was monitored after a surgical procedure with blood pressure, ECG, and pulse oximetry on supplemental oxygen after her procedure. The patient became less and less responsive. Finally, the nurses could not wake the patient up. The patient was seen by the anesthesiologist, was noted to be ventilating very poorly, and was intubated and placed in the ICU until she woke up. The pCO$_2$ on her blood gas was 280 mmHg, with a normal pCO$_2$ at 40 mmHg. Most patients who acutely develop a pCO$_2$ over 80 or 90 mmHg become minimally responsive or unresponsive. The patient's SpO$_2$ never fell below 96%. The take-home message from this case is while pulse oximetry is an excellent tool to help assess a patient's oxygenation and ability to oxygenate a patient, it cannot detect hypercapnea, or a rise in CO_2, from inadequate ventilation. This is where capnography can help.

Capnography

Capnography, the measurement of the amount of carbon dioxide exhaled from the lungs, is a newer technology that can help guide the Paramedic with treatment in several clinical situations. Several different methods of capnography are available to measure exhaled carbon dioxide. The measurement often cited is the end-tidal carbon dioxide, which is the amount of carbon dioxide in the air at the end of exhalation. End-tidal carbon dioxide is abbreviated as $EtCO_2$. The three methods of measuring $EtCO_2$ include colorimetric capnometry, quantitative (numerical) capnometry, and waveform capnography.

Colorimetric capnometry is a familiar form of $EtCO_2$ for many Paramedics. This device consists of a piece of litmus paper within the sensor's body. This paper is impregnated with a chemical that changes color when exposed to exhaled carbon dioxide (Figure 25-10). This device is placed in-line with the endotracheal tube immediately after endotracheal intubation to help confirm that the the endotracheal tube is in the trachea. If the endotracheal tube is in the trachea the capnometer should change color from purple up to yellow depending on the amount of carbon dioxide in the exhaled air. One exception is when a patient has been in cardiac arrest for a prolonged period of time. In this situation, very little CO_2 is transported to the lungs because of circulatory collapse, therefore there is little in the lungs and a low level in exhaled gas.

The colorimetric capnometer is a qualitative device, meaning it gives gross estimations of the presence or absence of carbon dioxide and not specific levels of carbon dioxide. This, and other limitations, give colorimetric capnometry limited utility in the prehospital setting. Some Paramedics only use colorimetric capnometer as an initial method of endotracheal confirmation then utilize continuous waveform capnography or capnometers.

Quantitative capnometers provide a numerical value for the $EtCO_2$, reporting the CO_2 measurement at the end of exhalation. In contrast, waveform capnography records the values of exhaled carbon dioxide throughout the inspiration–expiration cycle and graphs that value over time, producing a waveform that can be clinically useful to interpret.

Technology

As previously described, the colorimetric capnometers utilize a paper impregnated with a chemical that changes color depending upon the amount of carbon dioxide in the exhaled air. For quantitative capnometry and waveform capnography, the amount of carbon dioxide in exhaled air is found by shining a beam of infrared light through a sample of the exhaled breath. The intensity of the light is then compared to a measurement taken from an air sample that does not contain carbon dioxide. The certain wavelengths of infrared light are absorbed by the presence of carbon dioxide compared to the air that does not contain carbon dioxide. This is converted into a numerical measure of the carbon dioxide.

Exhaled air for use in capnography or capnometer is sampled in one of two different methods. Mainstream capnography involves placing the sensor in-line with the exhaled air stream and can only be used in intubated patients (Figure 25-11a). The sensor is placed between the endotracheal tube and the ventilation device (e.g., bag-valve mask assembly).

The second method is called sidestream sampling. Sidestream capnography involves taking a sample of the exhaled air by aspirating a small amount of it from the exhaled air stream, either from the endotracheal tube or through the use of a modified nasal cannula (Figure 25-11b). Sidestream technology allows capnography to be used in patients who are not intubated.

One disadvantage to sidestream capnography/capnometer is that there is some loss of carbon dioxide from the air sample that occurs between the patient and the monitor. This is overcome in many capnography/capnometer devices by calibrating the EtCO2 monitor whenever the monitor switches measurement methods from endotracheal measurements to nasal cannula.

A second disadvantage of nasal cannula sidestream capnography/capnometer is if the patient is receiving high-flow oxygen (e.g., using a nonrebreather or CPAP mask) at the time of sampling, the result will be artificially low because the high-flow oxygen blowing past the sampling port will wash out much of the carbon dioxide in the exhaled air.

The sampled exhaled air is taken to a chamber where a beam of infrared light is directed through the sample. The carbon dioxide present in the air absorbs some of the infrared light, changing the wavelength of the light that continues through to the sensor. This change in wavelength varies with the amount of carbon dioxide present in the sample. The sample taken from exhaled air is compared with infrared light

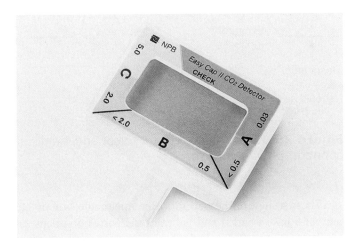

Figure 25-10 The EasyCap® colorimetric capnometer. The color changes from purple when exposed to > 4 mmHg CO_2, to tan, and then to yellow when exposed to > 15 mmHg CO_2.

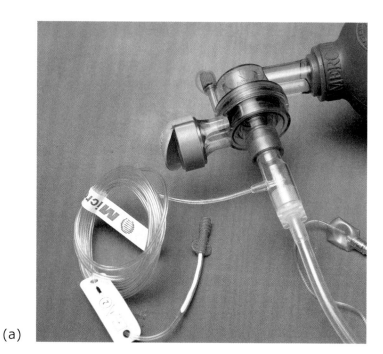

(a)

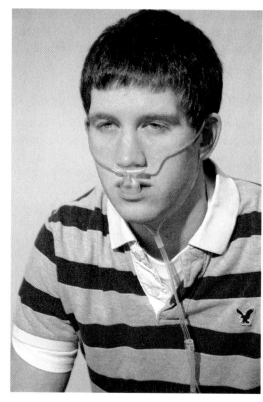

(b)

Figure 25-11 Mainstream versus sidestream sampling. (a) In mainstream capnography, the sensor is located between the endotracheal tube and the bag-mask assembly. (b) A modified nasal cannula is used to sample carbon dioxide from exhaled air.

beamed through a sample with a known concentration of carbon dioxide. This comparison determines the level of exhaled carbon dioxide in the patient's breath. In the absence of respiratory disease, this measure of exhaled carbon dioxide should be within 5 mmHg of the partial pressure of carbon dioxide ($PaCO_2$) of the patient's arterial blood.

Capnography: Waveform Interpretation

Unlike capnometers which either provide a visible color change or a numeric readout, a capnography provides a graph of the $EtCO_2$ measurement as it changes during inspiration and expiration (Figure 25-12), The capnography waveform has several components, each representing a phase.

Phase I is the respiratory baseline and occurs at the time between inhalation and exhalation. It should be at zero, as it represents the carbon dioxide in free air, that is found in the anatomical dead space in the lungs.[4] The next part of the waveform, Phase II, is also called the expiratory upstroke and represents the beginning of exhalation of air from the lungs that contains carbon dioxide. The third part of the waveform, known as Phase III or the alveolar plateau, represents exhalation of alveolar air during exhalation. The peak of this plateau at the end of exhalation is the $EtCO_2$ measurement displayed on the monitor. The final portion of the waveform is the inspiratory downstroke or Phase 0, and represents the patient's inspiration. During the inspiratory downstroke, the $EtCO_2$ falls rapidly to zero, as the inspired air should contain little carbon dioxide.

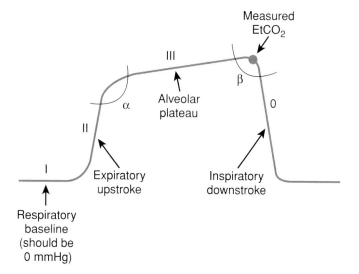

Figure 25-12 Anatomy of a typical end-tidal capnography waveform.

The first angle on the waveform, the alpha angle, is the angle between Phase I and II and indicates the correlation between ventilation and perfusion in the lung (i.e., the movement of air in and out versus the flow of blood through the lungs). The second angle, the beta angle, the angle between Phase III and 0, is usually close to a 90-degree angle. However, it will increase if the patient is rebreathing exhaled carbon dioxide, as can occur if the oxygen flow rate on a nonrebreather is inadequate and the reservoir bag does not refill between breaths.

Clinical Application

The earliest clinical use of capnometry in the prehospital setting was using colorimetric capnometer to confirm proper placement of the endotracheal tube after orotracheal or nasotracheal intubation. After intubation, and auscultation of breath and epigastric sounds, the colorimetric capnometer is placed between the bag-valve mask assembly and the endotracheal tube and the bag is squeezed several times. If the endotracheal tube is located within the trachea, then carbon dioxide should be present in the exhaled air. If the endotracheal tube is located in the esophagus, there should be no carbon dioxide in the exhaled air. If the endotracheal tube is located in the trachea, the capnometer should turn from a purple color during inhalation to a yellow color during patient exhalation.

The Paramedic should provide at least six ventilations before relying on the colorimetric capnometer's color change to indicate proper position. In patients who have ingested carbonated beverages, such as beer, just prior to intubation, it is possible for the carbon dioxide in the stomach from the beverage to provide a false indication of the presence of carbon dioxide.[5] While this is clinically an uncommon event, the Paramedic should be aware of this potential pitfall. Regardless of whether colorimetric capnometry or waveform capnography are used, the level of carbon dioxide present in the stomach in that situation will rapidly decrease to zero during ventilation, thus confirming the endotracheal tube is in the esophagus.

Continuous waveform capnography can provide the Paramedic with an assurance that the properly placed endotracheal tube remains in the trachea during transport. The prehospital environment is full of situations wherein patient care can easily dislodge the properly placed endotracheal tube, from log-rolling the patient onto a backboard at the scene to moving the patient from the EMS stretcher to the emergency department gurney. When the patient is monitored with continuous waveform capnography, dislodgement of the endotracheal tube is immediately indicated by a loss of capnography waveform (Figure 25-13). As discussed in Chapter 24, a well-oxygenated patient without significant respiratory disease can endure nearly eight minutes of apnea time before her SpO_2 falls below 90%. With the loss of exhalation waveform from continuous waveform capnography, the Paramedic immediately recognizes endotracheal tube dislodgement. This was well demonstrated clinically in a study that examined the rate of misplaced endotracheal tubes in intubated patients transported to their trauma center by various EMS services.[6] Some EMS services had implemented endotracheal tube placement monitoring with continuous waveform capnography while others had not. In the group of patients that were monitored with continuous waveform capnography, zero patients arrived with an endotracheal tube in the esophagus compared with 23% of the patients in the group that was not monitored using continuous waveform capnography. Continuous monitoring with waveform capnography

not only represents a significant means of improving patient safety but also is a risk management tool used to protect Paramedics from allegations of malpractice..

Changes in the shape of the capnography waveform can also provide valuable information to the Paramedic regarding the patient's respiratory disease, circulatory status, and equipment failure. For example, with severe bronchospasm, the patient will have difficulty exhaling. This is reflected in a sloping of the alveolar plateau (often referred to as a "shark fin shape") and a longer alveolar plateau (Figure 25-14) representing the prolonged expiration that occurs in patients with bronchospasm. As the patient is treated with medications that reduce the bronchospasm, the waveform should return to a normal or near normal shape.

For intubated and paralyzed patients, waveform capnography can indicate when the paralytic medication is wearing off. As the paralytic medication wears off, the patient will start attempting to breathe. The Paramedic will first notice this by observing a dip in the alveolar plateau as the patient attempts to take a shallow breath; an increasing carbon dioxide level stimulates the patient to breath (Figure 25-15). This will often precede muscular movement and provide an early indication of

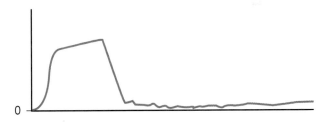

Figure 25-13 A sudden loss of the capnography waveform often signals dislodgement of the endotracheal tube from the trachea.

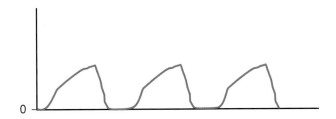

Figure 25-14 Characteristic shape of the waveform for a patient with bronchospasm.

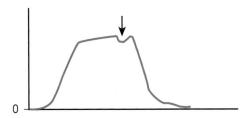

Figure 25-15 The "curare cleft" in the alveolar plateau is the first sign that the paralytic medication is wearing off.

the need to administer additional paralytic medication before the patient begins to resist positive pressure ventilation by coughing against inhalation, called "bucking" the ventilator.

Waveform capnography can also alert the Paramedic to technical or equipment problems. From failure of valves in the bag-valve-mask assembly to kinking of the endotracheal tube, equipment failure can reduce airflow both in inspiration and expiration and cause changes in the waveform (Figure 25-16). This pattern is also seen in partial obstruction of the endotracheal tube which can occur with excessive mucus or other material in the airway. A raising baseline suggests that the patient may need deep endotracheal suctioning.

A gradual rise in the Phase I baseline often indicates contamination of the sensor when using mainstream capnography (Figure 25-17). This can occur from either foreign material or a buildup of condensation on the sensor that changes the infrared light transmission across the exhaled air. Disconnecting and cleaning the sensor generally resolves this problem.

Capnography can also detect hyper- and hypoventilation, both in spontaneously breathing patients and ventilated patients. A gradual decrease in the height of the waveform indicates hyperventilation (Figure 25-18a). This occurs as the increased alveolar minute volume removes additional carbon dioxide, decreasing the amount of carbon dioxide in subsequent breaths. This can be used during bag-valve ventilation to maintain a constant rate and depth to prevent hyperventilating the patient. Conversely, a gradual increase in the height of the waveform with a constant baseline indicates hypoventilation (Figure 25-18b) and may indicate to the Paramedic that he needs to intervene to improve the patient's ventilation.

Another use for capnography is to predict the likelihood of survival in cardiac arrest. The initial $EtCO_2$ readings in a patient in cardiac arrest are near zero, not because of the lack of carbon dioxide in the blood or in the lungs, but because of the lack of carbon dioxide diffusion secondary to lack of circulation due to cardiac arrest. Capnography or capnometry alone may not be sufficient to confirm proper placement of the endotracheal tube in a patient who has been in cardiac arrest for a prolonged period of time due to the lack of circulation. Once adequate chest compressions begin, the $EtCO_2$ rises as there is generally enough circulation to produce a noticeable level of exhaled carbon dioxide. If the $EtCO_2$ level remains below 10 mmHg after 20 minutes of the usual resuscitation efforts, there is a 0% chance of survival.[7,8]

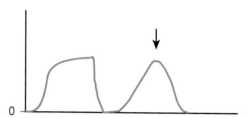

Figure 25-16 Abnormalities in both the Phase III and 0 parts of the waveform may indicate kinking or partial obstruction of the endotracheal tube.

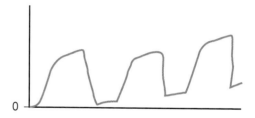

Figure 25-17 The gradual increase in respiratory baseline often indicates a problem with the mainstream capnography sensor.

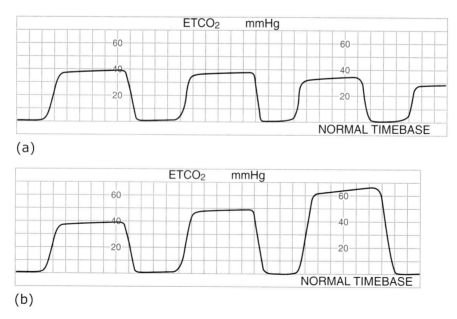

(a)

(b)

Figure 25-18 Gradual changes in the waveform height while maintaining a zero baseline can indicate (a) hyperventilation or (b) hypoventilation.

Upon return of spontaneous circulation, the $EtCO_2$ level will sharply rise, often before the pulse is palpable.[9,10] Capnography has also been suggested to help guide the effectiveness of chest compressions in cardiac arrest. However, it is not known whether this translates into improved survival from cardiac arrest.[11]

End-tidal carbon dioxide level will change with changes in the patient's hemodynamics and may be a useful tool in guiding trauma resuscitation.[12] It is important to note that while specific $EtCO_2$ levels do not correspond to specific levels of shock, sudden changes or trends can assist the Paramedic in guiding treatment. As previously discussed, $EtCO_2$ will change with changes in blood flow due to decreased perfusion and carbon dioxide transport to the lungs. The issue with using $EtCO_2$ in guiding trauma is the reading is not only dependent on circulatory flow, but also dependent on carbon dioxide transport from the blood into the alveoli and constant alveolar minute volume, which varies based on the tidal volume and ventilation rate. Changes in $EtCO_2$ levels should reflect changes in circulation if the alveolar minute volume is held constant. For trauma patients who have sustained a chest or respiratory system injury significant enough to impede gas exchange, changes in the $EtCO_2$ reading may reflect worsening pulmonary condition rather than circulatory status. Sublingual capnometry using a non-invasive probe that sits underneath the tongue showed some promise in more accurately detecting tissue perfusion without relying on maintaining a constant ventilation minute volume. However, the manufacturer recalled the probes and the device is not currently available.[13]

Finally, capnography can be used during procedural sedation as a way of monitoring the patient's respiratory rate and ventilation status during the sedation. The most common use for procedural sedation in the prehospital setting is for cardioversion, which involves applying an electric shock across the chest to stop a fast heart rhythm, or when electrically pacing the patient, which involves periodically applying electricity across the chest to produce a mechanical cardiac contraction. Both of these procedures are painful. Medications that are used for sedation also have the side effect of depressing respiration and decreasing ventilation. As discussed in the case study described in the pulse oximetry section, it is possible to have a well-oxygenated and poorly ventilated patient who can progress to respiratory failure. Capnography adds a level of safety by providing a graphical representation of the patient's respiratory rate, depth of respiration, and $EtCO_2$. As the patient becomes more sedated, and ventilation deteriorates, the $EtCO_2$ will rise, providing an alert to the Paramedic that she may need to intervene by either assisting ventilations or reducing the level of sedation before the patient suffers respiratory failure.

Co-oximetry

As discussed under the section on pulse oximetry, one of the pitfalls of pulse oximetry is that other forms of hemoglobin can change the wavelength of the light beam in such a way that it mimics oxyhemoglobin. Two situations where this can occur are when a patient has carbon monoxide poisoning and

when the patient has developed methemoglobinemia. Carbon monoxide differs from carbon dioxide in that carbon monoxide only has one oxygen atom in the molecule. Carbon monoxide attaches to the same site as oxygen on the hemoglobin molecule, only it attaches 200 times stronger than oxygen. This displaces oxygen and decreases the overall ability to transport oxygen to the tissues. A pulse oximeter, however, will still see the hemoglobin as saturated, and report a normal SpO_2. Methemoglobinemia occurs when the hemoglobin molecule undergoes a change in its form that removes one electron from the atom. This form of hemoglobin cannot carry oxygen. The pulse oximeter will often read falsely low SpO_2 in patients with a low level of methemoglobinemia and falsely high SpO_2 in higher percentages of methemoglobinemia.[14]

Carboxyhemoglobin (COHgb) and methemoglobin (MetHgb) levels are often obtained in the hospital using a sample of either arterial or venous blood and requiring a special co-oximeter. More recently, a non-invasive co-oximeter was developed to non-invasively measure SpO_2, COHb, and MetHB.

Technology

The Masimo® RAD-57 was introduced as the first handheld non-invasive co-oximeter. Eight different wavelengths of light are transmitted through the capillary bed.[15] Changes in the wavelength of these eight different beams are used to compute a percentage of SpO_2, COHgb, and MetHgb in the blood in the capillary bed. This particular co-oximeter also reports the perfusion index, which is helpful in determining signal strength, and ultimately the accuracy of the patient's SpO_2.

Clinical Applications

The Masimo® RAD-57 may show some promise in the prehospital environment in helping to triage a large number of patients who may have been exposed to carbon monoxide, thus minimizing transports.[16] The Paramedic's ability to non-invasively monitor COHgb levels in firefighters during fireground operations may detect elevated COHgb in interior firefighters during both fire suppression and overhaul operations.[17,18] This may impact firefighter health by keeping firefighters out of the rotation while treating mildly elevated levels of COHgb, as it has been established that carbon monoxide exposure can cause long-term cardiac effects.[19]

Arterial Blood Gas

The gold standard measurement of oxygenation and ventilation in medicine before the advent of pulse oximetry and capnography was the arterial blood gas (ABG). Even today, in the emergency department and critical care setting, the ABG provides a lot of useful information about not only the patient's oxygenation and ventilation, but also data used to assess the patient for acid–base disorders. While the ABG is the most accurate measure and provides a significant amount of information, the process to obtain the ABG can be a painful procedure for most patients. While ABG sampling is often not an EMS procedure, Paramedics working in a critical care transport environment will be exposed to blood gas analysis and may need to use this information to guide therapy during transport. For Paramedics working in the traditional street EMS environment, conceptual knowledge of ABG analysis will help them understand the underlying pathophysiology present in their patient.

What Is Measured?

The ABG sample is taken from a superficial artery and is rapidly analyzed using a blood gas analyzer. The most common location for sampling is the radial artery at the wrist; however, the brachial artery near the elbow or the femoral artery in the groin can also be used to obtain a sample. Critical patients who are undergoing transport may have an arterial line (Figure 25-19) placed by the sending hospital to continuously monitor the patient's blood pressure and serve as a means of painlessly acquiring multiple ABG samples in an unstable patient.

The ABG sample is measured for the pH, pCO_2, PO_2, bicarbonate (HCO_3^-), and oxygen saturation. The ABG analyzer may also include serum electrolytes, lactate, glucose, hemoglobin, and base excess or deficit (Table 25-2). The values from the ABG sample can be used to determine if the patient has an acid–base disorder and, if a disorder is present, identify the acid–base disorder.

Interpretation of Arterial Blood Gasses

This section uses a simple method to identify the primary acid–base disorder (Figure 25-20). The primary acid–base disorder is the disorder that is the primary cause of the academia or alkalemia. As previously discussed, the body will work to compensate for the primary disorder in an attempt to bring the arterial blood pH back toward normal. In reviewing the algorithm, notice that if the pH and bicarbonate move in

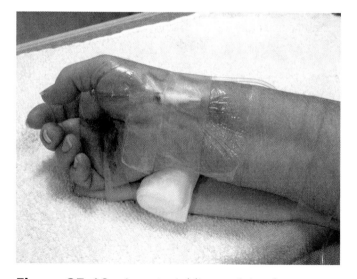

Figure 25-19 An arterial line painlessly allows multiple ABG samples as well as invasive monitoring of the patient's blood pressure during transport. (Photo courtesy of Keith D. Lamb, RRT)

Table 25-2 Components of the Arterial Blood Gas

Component	What Is Measured	Normal Range
pH	Amount of hydrogen atoms in the blood sample Below 7.35 is **academia** and above 7.45 is **alkalemia**	7.35–7.45
pCO_2	Partial pressure of carbon dioxide dissolved in the blood sample Less than 35 is **hypocapnea** and greater than 45 is **hypercapnea**	35–45 mmHg
PO_2	Partial pressure of oxygen dissolved in the blood sample Less than 70 is **hypoxia** and greater than 100 is **hyperoxia**	70–100 mmHg
HCO_3^-	Amount of bicarbonate ions in the blood sample Less than 22 is **hypocarbia** and greater than 30 is **hypercarbia**	22–30 mmol/L

Algorithm structure:

pH
- <7.35 → Acidosis
  - HCO_3^-<24 → Metabolic Acidosis
  - pCO_2>40 → Respiratory Acidosis
- >7.45 → Alkalosis
  - HCO_3^-<24 → Metabolic Alkalosis
  - pCO_2<40 → Respiratory Alkalosis

Figure 25-20 Algorithm for interpreting arterial blood gas.[20]

the same direction (e.g., both increase or both decrease), then the primary disorder is a metabolic disorder. If the pH and the pCO_2 move in opposite directions (e.g., pH decreases and the pCO_2 increases), then the primary disorder is respiratory.

An ABG sample taken from a patient returns with a pH of 7.25, a pCO_2 of 60 mmHg, and an HCO_3^- of 25 mmol/L. Starting at the top, the pH is below 7.35, which moves toward the acidosis arm. Looking at the pCO_2 of 60 mmHg, this is greater than 45, indicating a primary respiratory acidosis. As previously discussed, this would likely be due to hypoventilation.

Mixed disorders have a component of two primary acid–base disorders. In order to detect the presence of a mixed disorder, the Paramedic needs to determine the degree of compensation by the body for the primary disorder. If the degree of compensation is not as expected, this suggests a mixed disorder is present.

There are two ways to determine the degree of compensation. The first is to use formulas to compare the measured values in the ABG with the expected values (Table 25-3). With this method, the Paramedic first uses the algorithm in Figure 25-20 to determine the primary disorder. Next, the

Table 25-3 Formulas used to Determine if the Patient Is Compensating for His Primary Disorder[21]

Primary Disorder	Expected Change
Metabolic acidosis	$pCO_2 = 1.5 \times [HCO_3^-] + 8$ (range of ± 2)
Metabolic alkalosis	$pCO_2 = 0.7 \times [HCO_3^-] + 20$ (range of ± 5)
Respiratory acidosis	Acute: $HCO_3^- = 24 + ((pCO_2 - 40)/10)$ Chronic: $HCO_3^- = 24 + 4 \times ((pCO_2 - 40)/10)$
Respiratory alkalosis	Acute: $HCO_3^- = 24 - 2 \times ((40 - pCO_2)/10)$ Chronic: $HCO_3^- = 24 - 5 \times ((40 - pCO_2)/10)$ (Range of ± 2)

Paramedic looks in Table 25-3 to determine what formula to apply to determine compensation. For example, a Paramedic determines that her patient has a respiratory acidosis. Under respiratory acidosis in Table 25-3, the Paramedic computes the expected bicarbonate using the formula for acute respiratory acidosis. If the actual bicarbonate on the blood gas is different, then the Paramedic computes the expected bicarbonate using the formula for chronic respiratory acidosis. If the expected value still is not close to the measured value, this suggests that a mixed acid–base disorder is present.

A second method of determining the degree of compensation is to use a nomogram (Figure 25-21) after using the algorithm in Figure 25-20 to identify the primary disorder.

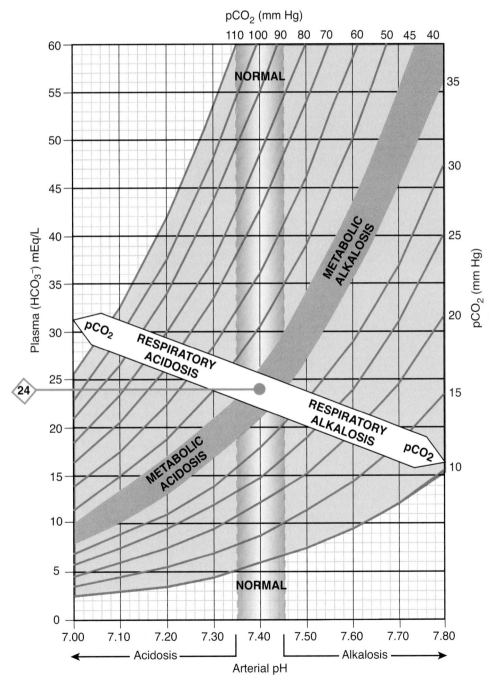

Figure 25-21 Acid–base interpretation nomogram.

The pH is listed across the bottom of the chart, the HCO_3^- is listed along the left side, and the curved lines are the values for the pCO_2. The three values for the pH, HCO_3^-, and pCO_2 are plotted on the chart. Depending on where the intersection of those three values falls on the chart, the shaded areas on the nomogram will indicate the type of disorder present. If the point falls outside the shaded area, this indicates a mixed disorder is present.

Venous Blood Gas

A venous blood gas is analyzed in the same way as an arterial blood gas. The difference between the arterial blood gas and venous blood gas in the venous blood gas sample is taken from a peripheral vein instead of an artery. This is much less painful for the patient and can often be drawn from an existing intravenous line. While the PO_2 is drastically different between an arterial and venous sample, the pH is approximately 0.04 less than the arterial sample, pCO_2 is within 6 mmHg of the arterial sample, and HCO_3^- is within 1.5 mmol/L.[22] While in some patients this may not adequately reflect their acid–base status, in many patients this will provide sufficient information to detect the presence of, and determine, the primary acid–base disorder with less patient discomfort.

CONCLUSION

This chapter has discussed several methods to objectively assess a patient's oxygenation and ventilation through the use of pulse oximetry, capnography, co-oximetry, and arterial blood gas analysis. The technology and clinical applications of each of these devices were discussed as well as their limitations. The physiology of acid-base disorders and their effects was also discussed. As with all technology, it is important to remember to treat the patient as a whole and not rely solely on one device or technology in determining the paramedical diagnosis and developing an appropriate patient treatment plan.

KEY POINTS:

- Acids are produced by either respiratory or metabolic processes. Although highly necessary for human survival, a superfluous amount of acid can be dangerous to the cells.

- An acid is a molecule that has a proton without a paired negatively charged atom. This molecule, when exposed to nature, takes the form of a positively charged hydrogen (H+) ion with one proton. Bases are negatively charged molecules, sometimes called hydroxyl molecules (−OH), which accept the positively charged molecules of an acid to create a more neutral or buffered molecule.

- A pH scale was developed in order to describe the differing degrees of acidity or alkalinity. This scale ranges from 0 to 14. The lower the number, the more acidotic a molecule, whereas the higher the number, the more alkaline a molecule. A value of 7 is considered neutral.

- An acid that enters the bloodstream encounters three chemical buffers: bicarbonate (HCO_3^-), phosphate (PO_4) and blood proteins. Bicarbonate binds with an acid to eventually create water and CO_2 that is eventually exhaled. Phosphate binds with acid, which in turn gets excreted into the kidneys. This leads to the acidity of urine. Blood proteins, including molecules like hemoglobin, bind with acid from the veins and eventually are removed in the lungs or kidneys.

- The lungs also have the ability to help rid the body of acid. They do this by driving the acid-bicarbonate formula to the left by exhaling additional CO_2. To do so, the lungs can increase ventilation, which converts more carbonic acid to CO_2 and water. Chemoreceptors monitor cerebrospinal fluid for an increase in carbonic acid, followed by a stimulation of the medulla to increase respirations.

- The kidneys are the last line of defense when the three interlinked buffering systems are unable to suffice. The kidneys perform two processes: They break down excess carbonic acid into bicarbonate, which is reabsorbed into the bloodstream, and excrete excess acids and ammonium in the urine. Kidney compensation is seen in chronically ill patients and not acute emergencies due to the fact that these processes take a long time to activate.

- Hemoglobin, which is found in the blood, has a high attraction to oxygen. It binds to oxygen and transports it to the body's tissues, where it is released.

- Active cells need oxygen to survive. These cells produce acid, which in turn dilates the capillaries and allows more oxygen bound to hemoglobin to enter. The acid then causes the oxygen to separate from its hemoglobin.

- If the acid in the blood is not released from the body as CO_2, oxygen will not attach to its hemoglobin again and be carried out to the capillaries. This will cause a patient to become hypoxic.

- Acidosis, excessive acid in the body, can also hinder the effects of a drug upon the body. If the tissues are acidotic, it causes a decrease in drug absorption into the cell, thus reducing the drug's effectiveness.

- Acidosis can be caused by either respiratory or metabolic acids. In terms of respiratory acidosis, a patient can either produce too much carbonic acid, which may cause the metabolism to race, or cause a patient to hypoventilate. Hypoventilation is, in part, due to certain damage caused by drug abuse, strokes, and brain injuries.

- During metabolism, the body makes a variety of acids. The production of too many acids can cause metabolic acidosis (i.e., diabetic ketoacidosis). The body's organs work together to maintain an acid-base balance. Any illness or problem with the organs can deter this process.

▶ REVIEW QUESTIONS:

1. What two types of acid are products of aerobic and anaerobic metabolism and what are they formed from?
2. By definition, what defines a substance as an acid or a base? What happens when an acid is joined with a base?
3. Create a pH scale and label it with the following terms: weak acid, strong acid, neutral, weak base, and strong base.
4. Explain how carbon dioxide is transported from the cells through the bloodstream and released into the exhaled air.
5. Describe the three chemical buffers found in the blood and how they help regulate pH.
6. How do the lungs compensate for an increase in carbonic acid?
7. Using an oxyhemoglobin curve, define the relationship between oxygen saturation and acid load.
8. What are two causes of acidosis and how can the Paramedic recognize them?

▶ CASE STUDY QUESTIONS:

Please refer to the Case Study at the beginning of the chapter and answer the questions below:

1. How could Mr. Byrnes be having respiratory difficulty and still have a 97% oximetry reading?
2. If Mr. Byrnes requires intubation, what methods exist to confirm placement of the endotracheal tube in a spontaneously breathing patient?
3. The Paramedic observes that Mr. Byrnes' capnography exhibits a shark fin pattern. Explain this finding.

REFERENCES:

1. Merriam-Webster on-line medical dictionary. Available at: **http://www2.merriam-webster.com/cgi-bin/mwmednlm?book=Medical&va=respiration.** Accessed December 16, 2007.

2. Ganong WF. *Review of Medical Physiology* (21st ed.). New York: McGraw-Hill; 2003:670.

3. Davidson JAH, Hosie HE. Limitations of pulse oximetry: respiratory insufficiency—a failure of detection. *BMJ.* 1993;307(6900):372–373.

4. Ward KR, Yealy DM. End-tidal carbon dioxide monitoring in emergency medicine, part 1: basic principles. *Academic Emergency Medicine.* 1998;5(6):628–636.

5. Garnett AR, Gervin CA, Gervin AS. Capnographic waveforms in esophageal intubation: effect of carbonated beverages. *Annals of Emergency Medicine.* 1989;18(4):387–390.

6. Silvestri S, Ralls GA, Krauss B, et al. The effectiveness of out-of-hospital use of continuous end-tidal carbon dioxide monitoring on the rate of unrecognized misplaced intubation within a regional emergency medical services system. *Annals of Emergency Medicine.* 2005;45(5):497–503.

7. Levine LR, Wayne MA, Miller CC. End tidal carbon dioxide and outcome of out of hospital cardiac arrest. *N Engl J Med.* 1997;337(23):1694–1695.

8. Grmec S, Klemen P. Does the end-tidal carbon dioxide concentration have prognostic value during out of hospital cardiac arrest? *European Journal of Emergency Medicine.* 2001;8(4):263–269.

9. Hatlestad D. Capnography as a predictor of the return of spontaneous circulation. *Emergency Medical Services.* 2004;33(8):75–80.

10. Kraus B. Capnography in EMS. *Journal of Emergency Medical Services.* 2003;28(1): 29–41.

11. Anderson CT, Breen PH. Carbon dioxide kinetics and capnography during critical care. *Critical Care.* 2000;4(4):207–215.

12. Kupnik D, Skok P. Capnometry in the prehospital setting: are we using its potential? *Emergency Medicine Journal.* 2007;24(9):614–617.

13. Creteur J. Gastric and sublingual capnometry. *Current Opinion in Critical Care.* 2006;12(3):272–277.

14. Lee DC, Fergusen KL. Methemoglobinemia. Available at: **http://www.emedicine.com/emerg/topic313.htm.** Accessed January 18, 2008.

15. Masimo product website. Available at: **http://www.masimo.com/Rainbow/rb-overview.htm.** Accessed January 18, 2008.

16. Hampson NB, Weaver LK. Noninvasive carbon monoxide measurement by first responders: a suggested management algorithm. *JEMS.* 2006;31(5):S10–12.

17. Cone DC, MacMillin DS, Van Gelder C, et al. Noninvasive fireground assessment of carboxyhemoglobin levels in firefighters. *Prehospital Emergency Care.* 2005;9(1):8–13.

18. Dickinson ET, Mechem CC, Thom SR, et al. Noninvasive carboxyhemoglobin monitoring of firefighters engaged in fire suppression and overhaul operations. *Prehospital Emergency Care.* 2008;12(1):96–97.

19. Henry CR, Satran D, Lindgren B, et al. Myocardial injury and long term mortality following moderate to severe carbon monoxide poisoning. *JAMA.* 2006;295(4):398–402.

20. Abelow, B. *Understanding Acid Base.* Baltimore, Williams & Wilkins; 1998.

21. Acid Base Physiology. Bedside rules for assessment of compensation. Available at: **http://www.anaesthesiamcq.com/AcidBaseBook/ab9_3.php.** Accessed January 16, 2008.

22. Rang LCF, Murray HE, Wells GA, MacGougan CK. Can peripheral venous blood gases replace arterial blood gases in emergency department patients? *CJEM.* 2002;4(1): pp. 7–15.

26

PRINCIPLES OF MEDICATION ADMINISTRATION

KEY CONCEPTS:

Upon completion of this chapter, it is expected that the reader will understand these following concepts:

- The metric system of measurement
- Basic drug calculations including weight-dependent drugs and intravenous infusion rates
- The six rights of medication administration
- Routes for medication administration
- Topical anatomy and proper technique for injections

► CASE STUDY:

Mr. Whittendam was a pleasant and proper gentleman with a lengthy cardiac history. He had the new Paramedic enthralled with his recall of previous heart attacks and all of the treatments that he had received in the tiny country hospital many years prior. He said that he had once needed two doses of morphine 1/6gr for severe pain. The senior Paramedic smiled and said he hadn't thought about grains in a long time. Their current protocols were written in metric measurement.

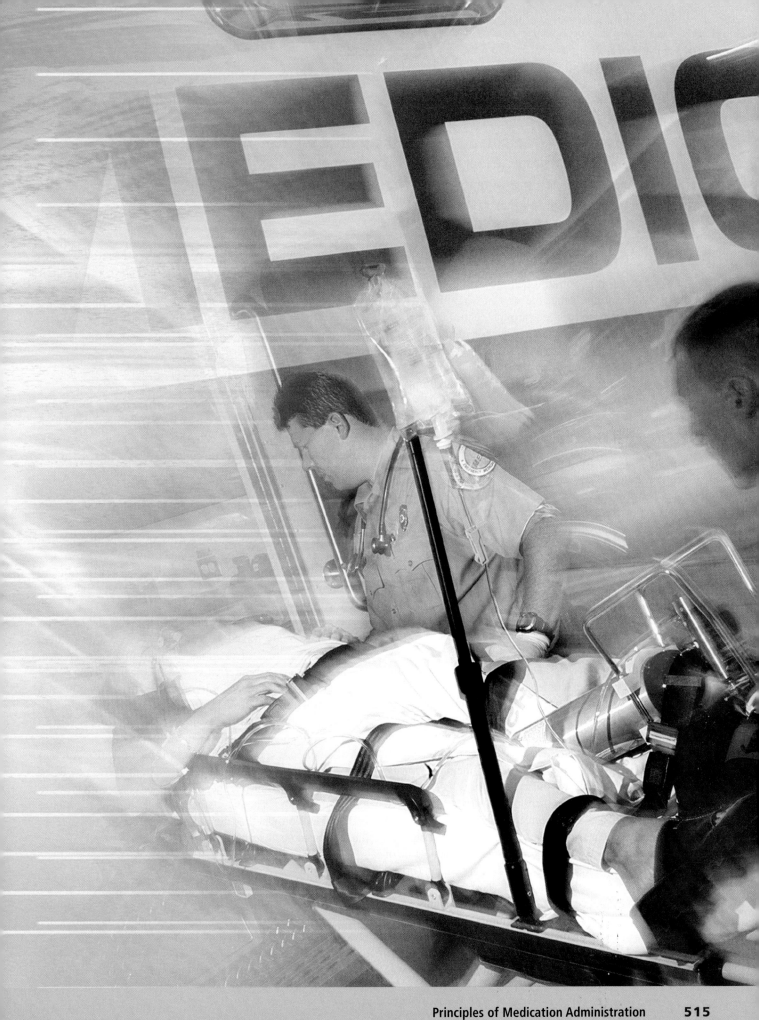

OVERVIEW

The Paramedic has many responsibilities before administering any medication to a patient. These tasks include the six rights of medication administration as well as an ability to carry out calculations using the metric system. This chapter discusses techniques for proper medication administration for the various enteral and parenteral medication routes. Each medication route has pros and cons that will be explored to ensure safety and effectiveness.

Medication Administration

In some instances, it is not so much the medicine administered that is crucial but rather the way in which it is given. A medicine that is not absorbed into the central circulation, where it can be carried to the target organ, is ineffectual. It is a Paramedic's responsibility to choose the right drug and the right dose for the patient, as well as to administer it by the right route at the right time in order to achieve the optimal therapeutic effect.

Forms of Medication

The statement "form follows function" holds true for medications. For the untrained layperson, an easy-to-swallow pill may appear to be the best carrier for a medication. However, for the very old, the very young, and the infirmed, who have difficulty swallowing, a liquid medicine may be better accepted.

Numerous forms of medicine have been created over the centuries. These forms can be grossly categorized into liquids, solids, and injectable liquids.

Liquid Medication Forms

The earliest liquid medications were called spirits. **Spirits**, brewed from various materials, are liquids which have a volatile oil that evaporates at room temperature and leaves a distinctive odor in the air. For example, spirit of ammonia has a distinctive pungent smell that makes it easily distinguishable from other spirits. An ancient spirit thought to cure a large variety of maladies is the "spiritus fermenti." The modern term for the spiritus fermenti is whiskey. Alcoholic beverages, including spirits, have long been recognized for their medicinal value.

Tinctures are medicinal substances that are dissolved in alcohol. Alcohol has long been used in pharmacy, in part because of its excellent solvent properties and, in part, because of its ready availability. Examples of tinctures include tincture of merthiolate, an early antiseptic, and tincture of benzoin (Friar's balsam), a combination of balsamic acids whose aromatic vapors are used to relieve nasal congestion and soothe bronchitis.

Laudanum, a simple tincture of opium, is highly effective in relieving a number of maladies including pain and constipation. However, its unpleasant aftertaste made it highly objectionable. To improve its palatability, laudanum was flavored with camphor, aniseed, and benzoic acid. Sweetening any tincture makes it into an **elixir**. The resulting elixir in this case is called paregoric, Greek for something that soothes. Paregoric is very effective against diarrhea, a common malady in developing countries plagued with dysentery and cholera. Paregoric is still listed in the United States Pharmacopoeia as camphorated opium tincture.

Liquid oral medications commonly face the problem of tasting badly. The old adage that "a teaspoon of sugar makes the medicine go down" shows yet another attempt at making the taking of medicine more pleasant. Medicines mixed with sugar and water are called **syrups**. Many cough formulas, some with the opiate codeine, contain sugar water (syrup).

Some medications will not dissolve in a solvent and thus remain as finely pulverized particles floating in the liquid. This medication form is called a **suspension**. It is important that a suspension be shaken before being administered. Forgetting to shake the suspension leaves an uneven distribution of medicine in the solution. Subsequently, the first dose may completely lack the medication if the drug has settled out and therefore may be impotent, whereas the last dose will be saturated with medication and very potent.

Powdered drugs with particles so large that they are visible when they are mixed, or suspended, in water are called **magmas**. Examples of magmas include milk of magnesia. Oil is also used as an alternative to water as a carrier. Finely pulverized particles placed into oils, such as cod liver oil, are called **emulsions**. The oil in these emulsions also acts as a nutritional supplement; for example, cod liver oil is rich in omega-3 fatty acids as well as vitamins A and D.

Medications meant for the skin (i.e., **topical** medicine) placed in water are called **lotions**, whereas those placed in either lanolin, an oil from sheep's wool, or petroleum jelly are called **ointments**. The choice of oil, water, or chemical base is dependent on whether the medicine is too dry to place on the skin or to be absorbed into the skin.

Solid Medication Forms

During manufacturing, many medicines can be either extracted chemically or synthesized and then reduced to a dry powder. The advantage to dry powders is that they are easier to store, they can be stored for a longer period of time without gross deterioration, and they are generally easier to handle.

Use of dried medicine makes sense as most medicines are reconstituted in the water within the body, and water is a universal solvent. When the patient swallows the powder, the body's water dissolves the medicine. It is then absorbed into the digestive tract and passes through the portal circulation.

Some dry medicines still come in a loose powder, usually placed in a waterproof envelope made of wax paper. Goody's headache powder® is an example of a loose powder medication. However, most powdered medications are processed into a convenient shape for easy swallowing. A dry medicinal powder that is compressed into a pill shape is called a **tablet**. Tablets are often **scored**, adding a depression across the middle that makes dividing the tablet in half easier. Some tablets also have a number or letter code embossed across the tablet's face for easy identification.

Medicinal powder placed within a gelatin casing is called a **capsule**. Capsules are generally easier to swallow and, perhaps more importantly, do not dissolve in the water-based saliva of the mouth very easily.

Some medicines are altered by the acids in the stomach, making them impotent, whereas some medicines, specifically those that are acid-based, can irritate the stomach lining, leading to ulcerations. To protect the medicine and/or the stomach, pharmacists have covered tablets in a protective **enteric coating**. Enteric coating permits the tablet to travel, unaltered, through the stomach and into the intestine for absorption.

The elderly, the infant, and the infirmed often have difficulty swallowing tablets and capsules. In some cases, it is acceptable to crush the tablet, with a mortar and pestle, or open the capsule and place the medicine in another carrier, such as apple sauce. However, not all medicines can be administered in this way. A clear example would be any enteric-coated tablet. It is important to refer to the manufacturer's recommendations and the information available from a pharmacist before altering the form of the medicine.

In some instances, it is desirable to have the medicine dissolve in the mouth. Such medicines exert a local or topical effect (e.g., they may be used to treat sore throats). Medicines intended to dissolve in the mouth are called **lozenges**. The lozenge, also called **troches**, owes its origins to the traditional French anise candy, called pastilles, popular in the eighteenth century. Like elixirs, medicine mixed in a sweet medium is more palatable, which makes patient compliance with the prescription more likely. Troches dissolve and are absorbed in the mouth through the oral mucosa.

Medication absorbed into the oral mucosa also enters the central circulation, bypassing first pass metabolism within the liver.[1-3] **First pass metabolism** is a chemical degradation of the drug by the liver that markedly reduces the drug's bioavailability. For this reason, it is sometimes advantageous to administer a medication orally (i.e., sublingual or in the buccal pocket). An example of a drug administered in this fashion would be nitroglycerin.

Some antibiotics and natural hormone replacements (NHR) are now carried in a troches. This method of medication administration results in drug levels that are comparable to injected drug levels, without the annoyance of a needle. Troches come in more than a dozen flavors, including blueberry, butterscotch, caramel, chocolate, peanut butter, and watermelon, and are conveniently packaged in a molded plastic container which can be carried in a pocket or purse.

Other forms of medication that are typically given internally for a local effect are **suppositories**. Suppositories contain the medicine within a wax carrier which melts at body temperature. There are vaginal suppositories, used for yeast infections, urethral suppositories, and rectal suppositories. Some rectal suppositories contain chemicals that irritate the bowel lining, triggering defecation and elimination of feces.

Rectal suppositories can also carry medications meant for systemic effect. The hemorrhoidal venous network in the rectum readily absorbs medications, at levels comparable to venous injection, into the central circulation.[4-6] Use of rectally inserted diazepam, available in a gel, is an acceptable means of administering this life-saving medication during status epilepticus when ordinary venous access is unobtainable.

Injected Medications

Injectable medications come in either ampoules, generally reserved for single patient use, or vials, intended for multiple patients. Glass ampoules were originally used to store a medication that was volatile and would easily evaporate. A beer bottle might be an example of an ampoule to carry a spirit. In some instances, the medicine was very valuable, or very dangerous, and an ampoule was used to preserve the security of the medication. To obtain the medicine from the ampoule in those cases, one had to break the neck of the ampoule, making pilferage obvious. Morphine was originally stored in a tear-shaped cobalt-blue ampoule, in part for this reason.

In a sense, vials are resealable ampoules. Typically, the glass container, and now a plastic bottle, has a rubber stopper which can be breached with a needle and syringe, or a needleless system, and a volume of medicine withdrawn. A concern with vials is sterility. Whenever the integrity of a container has been breached there is a concern about bacterial contamination. For this reason, many intravenous medications are manufactured in single-use ampoules. More discussion regarding the use of ampoules and vials is contained further in this chapter.

STREET SMART

Generally all drugs used in emergencies are clear, except diazepam. Diazepam is yellow. Any discoloration of any drug should alert the Paramedic that the drug is potentially contaminated and should be discarded.

Drug Measurement and Dosing

As drugs become more refined and newer, more potent compounds are developed, the importance of precise measurements becomes increasingly important. In the past, medicines were prescribed in teaspoons and grains, and as a result inaccuracies abounded. Today medicines are prescribed in micrograms, a unit so small as to be barely visible with the naked eye.

The correct measurement of drug quantity can make the difference between a therapeutic dose and a toxic dose, between better health and iatrogenic death. Needless to say, it is every Paramedic's responsibility to try and administer the correct therapeutic dose of drug to the patient.

Systems of Measurement

The ancient Egyptians measured length in a cubit, the distance from one's elbow to the outstretched thumb. As one might imagine, this led to a great number of inaccuracies, However, precision was not as important then. As time went on three systems of standardized measurement would be developed; in order, they were the apothecary, the common household, and the metric system. Each took generations to accept and each took generations to unlearn when the newer system was introduced. In each case, the previous system was phased out in favor of the more precise new system.

Apothecary System

In medieval times, apothecaries would dispense medications. The root of the word "apothecary" is the Greek "apotheke," which means storing place. Apothecaries were storing places for different substances (some mineral and some animal) and compounds that would be mixed by the apothecary on the order of a physician. These apothecaries developed a system of measuring small quantities of medication. An apothecary is somewhat analogous to the modern pharmacist.

Apothecary measurements included the grain (gr), which equaled the weight of one grain of wheat, and the minim, the weight of water equal to a grain. Needless to say, the weight of a grain of wheat could vary dramatically, influenced by such factors during the growing season as drought and flood.

However, without a satisfactory alternative, the apothecary system flourished for centuries. Notations in the apothecary system included the use of a Roman numeral representing the quantity after the unit of measurement. This arrangement of notation still persists in the prescriptions of some physicians who might note ii, meaning two, indicating the number of tablets. This would be preceded by the letters "ap" meaning apothecary.

Common Household System

The common household system, also referred to as the United States customary system, contains such units of measurement as the foot, the ounce, and the teaspoon. Some measurements (e.g., the yard, which equals the distance from the king's nose to the tip of his outstretched thumb) were widely accepted despite their obvious inadequacies.

One of the earliest attempts at standardization was the development of the Troy system. These efforts at standardization have also led to a great deal of confusion. For example, a pound apothecary equals 12 ounces, whereas a pound Troy equals 16 ounces (avdp). Avdp is the abbreviation for *avoir de pois*, a French term meaning "goods sold by weight" and is placed after a notation to indicate that it is *avoir de pois*.

A constant in using systems of measurement was business community needs.[7,8] For commerce to occur, industry needed a common system to count, with accuracy, the goods sold and bartered in trade. Despite its apparent inaccuracies, the common household system remains the predominant system of measurement in the United States and Canada.

Metric System

Advances in science demanded a more accurate system of measurement, and so the metric system was born out of necessity. The metric system, from the Greek word *metron*, translated to mean "to measure," was advanced by the Frenchman Msr. Gabriel Mouton in 1670. His system of measurement depended on a universal standard from which other measurements could be obtained in units of 10. This system of measurement made scientific measurements easier to calculate.

The French quickly adopted the metric system and called for its international adoption. Many countries followed suit, and *Le Systeme Internationale d'unites*, the international system of units (noted as SI following the number), became widely accepted in both the scientific as well as the business community. A comparison of metric standard measurements to household common measurements shows their differences (Table 26-1).

The standard for length measurement adopted was the meter. The meter, originally defined as one ten millionth of the distance from the north pole and the equator, was later redefined to be the distance that light, in a specified spectrum, travels over in 1/299,792,458 of a second (light-second) while in a perfect vacuum.

Interestingly, the SI unit of volume is not the liter but the cubic meter, the amount of water that could be contained within one cubic meter. However, the liter has become widely accepted in both the Americas as well as Europe. A cubic

Table 26-1 Metric Equivalents of Household Common Measurements

Metric	Household	
0.06 mL	1 drop	
1 mL	15 drops	
5 mL	1 teaspoon	60 gtt
15 mL	1 tablespoon	180 gtt
30 mL	2 tablespoons	1 ounce
180 mL	1 teacup	6 ounces
240 mL	1 cup	8 ounces
500 mL	1 pint	16 ounces
1,000 mL	1 quart	32 ounces

centimeter (cc) of water equals 1 milliliter (mL) of water; therefore, the two are often used interchangeably.

By convention, all abbreviations of SI units are in lowercase. For example, 1 meter is abbreviated 1 m. To recognize that liters are not SI units, the abbreviations for liters are abbreviated in capital letters. For example, 1 milliliter, a thousandth of a liter, would be properly abbreviated 1 mL.

Also by convention, all quantities of the measurement are placed in front of the unit of measurement and noted in Arabic numerals, not Greek. For example, 10 liters would be noted as 10 L and not L 10. Finally, to decrease confusion, a space is always placed between the number and the unit, indicating that the metric system is being used.

STREET SMART

While most Paramedics can access preprinted tables and personal digital assistant (PDA) devices for many drug calculations, every Paramedic should be knowledgeable about how to perform these rudimentary calculations in case the battery in the PDA dies or the drug sheets are lost.

Special Units

The dose of some medications has to be determined by biological assay or bioassay, a method of determining the relative strength of a substance by testing it on an organism. To standardize these bioassay measurements, scientists have created the **international unit (IU)**. Examples of medications that are measured and administered in international units include insulin and penicillin.

Insulin is frequently self-administered by the patient. To decrease errors in converting from metric to international units, and thus improve patient compliance, special insulin syringes are manufactured which are marked in international units. Confusion can occur when a Paramedic tries to use a standard syringe for insulin administration and mistakenly thinks that the measurements on the barrel of the syringe are international units when in fact they are minims, an old apothecary measure.

Measurement Devices

The timeless medicine glass is the quintessential example of a medicine measurement device. Marked with metric units on one side and apothecary units on the other, pharmacists and families alike have used the medicine glass to measure all forms of medicine, from cough syrup to antiseptics.

Another traditional measurement device is the medicine dropper. The medicine dropper draws up a precise volume into its stem and the medicine is then dispensed, drop by drop, into a substance such as juice or water.

Mathematical Conversions

Conversions of metric measurements from one unit to another are relatively simple because all units are based on a factor of 10, either 10 times greater or 10 times lesser. For example, a kilogram is 1,000 times greater than a gram and a milligram is 1,000 times less than a gram. Therefore, to change a gram to kilograms, the Paramedic only need move the decimal three spaces to the right: 1 gram equals 0.0001 kilogram.

Conversely, to change a gram to a milligram, the Paramedic need only move the decimal three spaces to the left: 1 gram equals 1,000 milligrams.

The key in understanding these conversions is to understand the prefixes that precede the unit. All multiplications above 1 gram are noted in the Greek prefixes kilo-, hector-, and deca-, whereas all divisions of a gram are noted by the Latin prefixes deci-, centi-, milli-, and micro- (Table 26-2).

STREET SMART

The abbreviation in the laboratory for micro- (for example, in the measurement micrograms) is the Greek symbol μg. However, this notation is impractical in keyboard-based documentation and potentially confused with mg (milligram). Necessarily, healthcare providers have adopted the abbreviation mc to indicate micro- (for example, mcg equals microgram).

The importance of accurate drug calculations is reinforced by the most recent MedMAX data. MedMAX is an anonymous national database of medication errors. Of 40,936 medication errors reported in 2000, 23% were errors in the quantity of the dose of the medication given. These errors could be, in part, due to miscalculation.[9–11]

The more difficult calculations are the conversions of household common measurements to the metric system. While common conversion factors are available (Table 26-3),

Table 26-2 Metric Prefixes

Standard Weight: Gram	
Multiply (Greek)	
Deca-	× 10
Hecto-	× 100
Kilo-	× 1,000
Divide (Latin)	
Deci-	÷10
Centi-	÷100
Milli-	÷1,000
Micro-	÷1,000,000

Table 26-3 Conversion of Measurements in the Common Household and International Metric System

Unit US	Conversion	Unit Metric
Inch	26.4	Millimeter (mm)
Ounce	28.3	Gram (gm)
Pound	0.453	Kilogram (kg)
Gallon	3.79	Liter (L)

Metric	Conversion	Unit US
Millimeter	39.6 (1/25.4)	Inch (in.)
Gram	0.035 (1/28.3)	Ounce (oz)
Kilogram	2.25 (1/0.453)	Pound (lb)
Liter	0.264 (1/3.79)	Gallon (gal)

Note: The symbol for a pound = lb comes from the Latin *libria* meaning scales.
Note: The term "mile" comes from the Latin *mille passus*, meaning a thousand paces.

these conversions are not exact and errors of 10% are not uncommon.

The conversion of household common to metric standard measurements in the field is rare. The medical community in the United States has adopted metric measurements as the standard and all medications come with metric notation.

Conversion of Weight

The exception to the rule regarding mathematical conversions is the calculation of the patient's weight. Patients usually know their weight in pounds, not kilograms, forcing the Paramedic to translate pounds into kilograms.

The most accurate method of converting a patient's weight from pounds to kilograms is dividing the patient's weight in pounds by 2.26. For example, a 185-pound patient would weigh approximately 83.71 kilograms.

While this is the most accurate method, it is not the most convenient. Many Paramedics prefer to divide the patient's weight, in pounds, in one-half, then subtract 10% off from the result. For example, half of 185 pounds would be roughly 92 +/− 0.5, then subtract 9 from 92 for an approximate weight of 83 kilograms. Such gross estimates of a patient's weight while in the field are acceptable, provided the estimated weight is within 10% of the actual weight.

STREET SMART

The Paramedic should use the more accurate method of determining weight in any child under the age of 8.

Concentration

A common first step in any drug calculation is determining the amount of drug on hand. This is typically referred to as the drug's concentration. For simplicity of calculation, and in order to establish a common denominator, concentrations are described as the amount of drug in 1 milliliter (mL) of a solution. For example, if the drug on hand is 5 mg of diazepam in a 2 mL prefilled syringe, then the concentration of the drug would be 2.5 mg per mL. To make drug calculations easier during an emergency, many pharmaceutical companies now provide the concentration in notations on the sides of the drug box and/or on the prefilled syringe.

Dilution

Some medications (e.g., Solumedrol) lose potency when in solution for a prolonged period of time. These medications are necessarily mixed at the patient's side in order to ensure maximum effectiveness. A medication being mixed is called the solute and the liquid that the medication is being mixed into is called the solvent. When combined, the solute and solvent make a solution. If the mixture is a one-to-one, one part solvent to one part solution, then the resulting drug is said to be at 100% strength.

In some cases, it is desirable to weaken a drug by dilution. For example, 50% dextrose in sterile water (D50) is too hypertonic for a child's blood but may be all that is available and on hand. The D50 would then be called the **stock solution**. To decrease its tonicity, D50 can be cut in half, to make D25, by adding an equal volume of sterile water. The resulting mixture would be half-strength, yet have a dilution of 1 to 3—one part dextrose in three parts of solution (Table 26-4).

Weight in a Volume

In some instances, it is necessary for a Paramedic to know the amount of a drug in a volume of solution. For example, how much dextrose is in a 500 mL bag of Dextrose 5% in sterile water (D_5W)?

A percent weight/volume is defined as 1 gram of solute dissolved in 100 mL of solvent to obtain a 1% solution. Therefore, 5 grams of solute is dissolved in 100 mL of solvent to make a 5% solution. If the total volume of the solution is 500 mL, and there are 5 grams per 100 mL, then there are 25 grams in 500 mL of D_5W.

Table 26-4 Drug Dilutions

C_1V_1 =	c_2v_2
Concentration of stock (C1) =	50%
Volume of stock (V1) =	50 mL
Concentration desired (c2) =	25%
Volume of new solution (v2) =	x mL
(50)*(50) =	(25)*(x)
(2,500) =	(25x)
x =	2,500/25
v2 = x =	100 mL

Therefore, to obtain D25, add 50 mL of sterile water to 50 mL of stock solution to obtain a volume of 100 mL of D25.

Elements of a Drug Order

A standard drug order, whether written in a standing order or given verbally to the Paramedic, will contain the following elements: the amount of the drug, the name of the drug, and the route that is to be administered.

It is important that the Paramedic listen carefully to, and note (preferably on paper), the specifications within the drug order. The order has essential information regarding the necessary calculations which must be performed in order to administer the correct dose to the patient.

For example, if the physician gives an order of x mg of a drug to be given in y number of mg per unit weight over z minutes, then the Paramedic must calculate the amount on hand, the patient's weight, and the flow rate of this infusion to obtain the correct dose of drug.

As related earlier, a drug's concentration must be known before it can be administered in almost every case. Therefore, it is common practice for Paramedics to obtain this value immediately, either by consulting the drug packaging or by calculating the concentration mentally and making a notation.

Similarly, many drugs are weight-dependent, especially pediatric medications. Therefore, it is common practice for the Paramedic to immediately obtain, either directly from the patient or by estimation, the patient's weight and then convert that weight from pounds into kilograms.

Once those basic values have been obtained, the Paramedic can then review the order at hand. If the order contains the term "per kilogram" then the patient's weight must be included in the calculation.

If the term "per minute" is included in the order, then the drug must be a solution that is to be infused intravenously and the drip factor of the intravenous administration set must be included in the calculation. By convention, all drug infusions are administered via a micro-drip administration set. All micro-drip administration sets, regardless of manufacturer, produce 1 mL per every 60 drops of solution.

STREET SMART

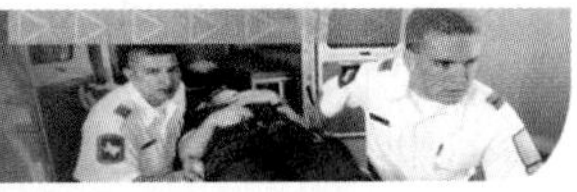

Medications can have two names: proprietary and generic. If this was not confusing enough, some generic names sound alike as well. To decrease confusion, and a possible medication error, the Paramedic should always confirm orders after receiving them, using a communications technique referred to as echo technique. If the drug name is in doubt, ask the physician to spell it out.

Standard Drug Order

A standard drug order would mean x amount of drug is to be given to the patient. The manner in which it is given

---

Physician orders 20 mg furosemide IV bolus. In the drug box is 40 mg of furosemide (i.e., a concentration of 10 mg per mL).

$$\frac{10\text{ mg}}{1\text{ mL}} = \frac{20\text{ mg}}{x\text{ mL}}$$
$$(10) \times (x) = (20) \times (1)$$
$$10x = 20$$
$$x = \frac{20}{10}$$
$$x = 2\text{ mL}$$

Figure 26-1 Proportional method of drug calculation.

(i.e., injection, tablet, etc.) is a function of the medication. The issue for the Paramedic is determining if there is sufficient drug on hand to administer to the patient. One simple method, referred to as the proportional/ratio method, exists for calculating this value. On one side of the equation the Paramedic lists the order (i.e., what is desired; for example, 10 mg given intravenously). On the other side of the equation the Paramedic lists what is on hand. The problem the Paramedic is solving is the x (i.e., the volume that needs to be given). Through a process of cross-multiplication, the value is obtained (Figure 26-1).

Weight-Dependent Drug Order

Calculation of weight-dependent drug doses is simple if the Paramedic follows the order of calculation in a disciplined, step-wise fashion. Whenever an order is received for a drug to be given (so many milligrams per kilogram), then the Paramedic must calculate the patient's weight first, using one of the two methods previously described. Having obtained the patient's weight in kilograms, the Paramedic proceeds to the next step, multiplying the patient's weight times the dose ordered. The result is the amount of drug that must be administered. The final step for the Paramedic would be to compare the amount of drug on hand to the dose ordered to ensure that a sufficient quantity is available. Then, the Paramedic proceeds to administer that dose.

STREET SMART

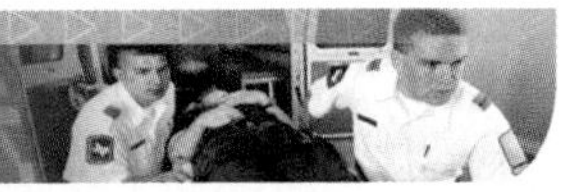

Since many of the drugs a Paramedic uses are administered during an emergency, prefilled ampoules are standardized to contain the dose that an average 70-kg patient would need. Therefore, if after a drug calculation the result appears to require 10 ampoules, then the calculations should be rechecked. Typically, a misplaced decimal explains the error.

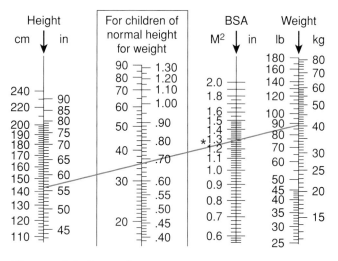

Example for a child who is 52 inches tall and weighs 90 pounds

Height	For children of normal height for weight	BSA	Weight

Figure 26-2 Pediatric nomogram.

Pediatric Dosing

The vast majority of pediatric medications are adjusted for the child's weight. In many cases, the order is given as a weight-dependent dose. When an adult dose must be adjusted to a pediatric dose, and the pediatric dosing is not available, then the child's total body surface area (BSA) is divided against the adult's total body surface area (approximately 1.73 meters squared for a six-foot tall, 150-pound adult). The resulting percentage is then taken from the adult dose and is roughly equal to the pediatric dose.

Calculation of a child's BSA is easy when a pediatric nomogram is used. The Paramedic would obtain the child's height and weight, then cross-reference on the nomogram to the child's BSA (Figure 26-2).

Intravenous Infusions

Continuous infusion of intravenous fluids is frequently required in the out-of-hospital care of an ill or injured patient. When the patient's condition requires that a large fluid bolus be infused (e.g., in order to increase a blood pressure for perfusion), then the intravenous fluid is usually infused rapidly, or **wide open (WO)**. The number of liters of volume-expanding fluid—traditionally lactated Ringer's solution (LR) or normal saline solution (NSS)—infused should be adequate to ensure a minimally acceptable blood pressure in the range of 80 to 90 mmHg systolic is maintained.

At other times, the aggressive fluid resuscitation just described would be inappropriate. However, constant venous access (e.g., for purposes of medication administration) would be desirable. Without any fluids infusing, the IV catheter could become occluded by a blood clot. To prevent occlusion, a minimal infusion of solution is continued, typically at an infusion rate equaling 30 mL per hour. The primary purpose of this slow infusion is to **keep the vein open (KVO)** in the IV catheter

Table 26-5 Calculation of a Continuous Infusion

Order	= 126 mL per hour
Administration set drip factor	= 60 gtts/mL
Step 1: x gtts/min	= 126 mL $\times$ 60 gtts/mL/60 minutes
Step 2: x gtts/min	= 7,500/60
Step 3: x	= 126 gtts/min

* By convention, all microdrop administration sets provide 1 mL for every 60 drops.

Table 26-6 Drip Factors and Ratios for Common Administration Sets

Drip Factor		Ratio
Micro-drip	60 drops equals 1 mL	1:1
Macro-drip	10 drops equals 1 mL	6:1
	15 drops equals 1 mL	4:1
	20 drops equals 1 mL	3:1

patient. Some Paramedics use the abbreviation TKO, meaning **to keep open**, to indicate this minimal infusion.

In certain circumstances, the patient's condition requires an infusion of a specific volume. If the volume is infused rapidly over several seconds or minutes, then the infusion is called a **bolus**. If the volume is to be evenly administered over the course of an hour, then the infusion is called a **continuous infusion**.

Continuous Infusion

The task facing the Paramedic, once the order for a continuous infusion is given, is to determine how many drips per minute must occur. There are two methods of determining the drip rate for a continuous infusion.

The formula method enlists all of the necessary information into the calculation and the result is a defined drip rate. To obtain this number, the Paramedic multiples the drip factor of the tubing (every tubing has a drip factor; for example, so many drops equals 1 mL), then divides the total by the number of minutes that the infusion is to last (Table 26-5).

The other method is the ratio/factor method. Understanding that there are 60 minutes in one hour and that a micro-drip administration set provides 1 mL for every 60 drops of fluid, then a 1:1 relationship has been established between minutes to drops and time to volume. It is apparent that, because of the 1:1 relationship, the number of milliliters per hour is always going to be equal to the number of drops per minute (Table 26-6). This 1:1 relationship is only true in the case where a micro-drip administration set is used. However, by understanding this 1:1 relationship, similar ratios can be established for other intravenous administration sets.

For example, if the drip factor of a macro-drip administration set is 15 drops equals 1 milliliter, or one-fourth less drops than a micro-drip administration set, then a 4:1 ratio has been established between this macro-drip administration set infusion rate and a standard micro-drip administration set infusion rate.

To use an example, if the order is for 200 mL per hour, then the drip rate with a micro-drip administration set would be 200 gtts per min. However, if a 15 drop macro-drip administration set was used, then the order, 200 mL/hr, would be divided by a factor of 4. The resulting drip rate would be 50 drops per minute.

Intravenous Drug Infusion

Intravenous drug infusions require precise control (i.e., titration) of the drug in order to provide the intended effect. Errors, plus or minus the ordered drug infusion, can result in undesirable effects. Before an order for an intravenous drug infusion can begin to be administered, the Paramedic must first prepare the solution, or access a premixed solution, then determine the number of drops per minute to be infused.

There are two methods of determining the drop rate. The first method, the formula method, requires the Paramedic to multiply the dose in the order given times the drip factor, then times the solution in order to obtain the desired drip rate (Table 26-7).

Alternatively, Paramedics can use the **clock method** to determine the infusion rate. By observing a few fundamental conditions, the clock method of drug infusion permits the Paramedic to mentally visualize a clock with a sweep hand pointing out the drug infusion rate. When the sweep hand is at the 15 second point, that represents 1 milligram of drug at 15 drops per minute or 15 milliliters an hour. When the sweep hand is at the 30 second position, it represents 2 milligrams of the drug infusing at 30 drops per minute, and so forth.

Foundational to the clock method is the condition that the drug's concentration is 4 to 1. Regardless of the amount of drug on-hand (1 gram or 200 mg), if a 4:1 mixture can be made (i.e., 250 mL or 50 mL), then the clock method can be used (Table 26-8).

Weight-Dependent Intravenous Drug Infusion

Some drugs are so potent that it is important to precisely infuse (i.e., titrate) the drug to the patient's weight. As complicated as the process sounds, a weight-dependent intravenous drug infusion only adds the patient's weight to the standard drug infusion calculations (Table 26-9).

Table 26-7 Calculation of Intravenous Drug Infusion Rate Using a Formula

Order	=	3 mg per minute (3 mg/min)
Administration set	=	60 drops per mL
Solution on-hand	=	500 mL physiologic saline
Drug on hand	=	1 gram
Drip rate	=	X
Formula	=	Order × Solution × Administration set

Step 1: Calculate the concentration

1 gram in 500 mL	=	2 milligrams per 1 milliliter
1,000 gram/500 mL	=	2 mg/mL

(Conversion to common units makes calculations easier)

Step 2: Set up the formula

Order × Drip factor/Drug concentration	
3 mg/min × 60 gtt/mL/2 mg/mL = X	

Step 3: Eliminate like units

3 min	× 60 gtt/2	= X
180 gtt/min/2	= X	
90 gtt/min	= X	

Table 26-8 Calculation of Intravenous Drug Infusion Rate Using the Clock Method

Order	=	3 mg per minute (3 mg/min)
Administration set	=	60 drops per mL
Solution on-hand	=	250 mL physiologic saline
Drug on-hand	=	1 gram
Drip rate	=	X

Step 1: Calculate the concentration

1 gram in 250 mL	=	2 milligrams per 1 milliliter
1,000 gram/250 mL	=	2 mg/mL

(Conversion to common units makes calculations easier)

Step 2: Step up the clock

1 mg = 15 drops per min	=	30 mL/hour
2 mg = 30 gtt/min	=	30 mL/hr
3 mg = 45 gtt/min	=	45 mL/hr
4 mg = 60 gtt/min	=	60 mL/hr

Table 26-9 Weight Dependent Drug Infusion

Order	=	5 microgram per kilogram per minute (5 mcg/kg/min)
Administration set	=	60 drops per mL
Solution on-hand	=	500 mL physiologic saline
Drug on-hand	=	1 gram
Drip rate	=	X
Patient weight	=	70 kg

Formula = Order × Solution × Patient's weight (kilograms) × Drip rate of administration set ÷ Concentration of the drug

Step One: Calculate the concentration

1 gram in 500 mL	=	2 milligrams per 1 milliliter
1,000 gram/500 mL	=	2 mg/mL = 2,000 mcg/mL

Step Two: Set up the formula

Order × Drip factor × Patient weight ÷ Drug concentration	
5 mcg/kg/min × 60 gtt/mL × 70 kg/2,000 mcg/mL = X	

Step Three: Eliminate like units

5 × 60 gtt × 70 min/2,000	= X	
25,000 gtt/min/2,000	= X	
10.5 gtt/min	= X	

The Paramedic's failure to convert a patient's weight from pounds (household common) to kilograms (metric) is a source of error in some calculations. It is essential that all Paramedics convert all units to a common system before performing drug calculations.

Temperature Measurement

A patient's body temperature has come to be regarded as a key indicator of a patient's health or illness (i.e., a vital sign). A fever greater than 101°F, might indicate the presence of an infectious process inside a patient's body or that the patient's body has undergone a significant heat stress. A fever greater than 100.4°F but less than 101°F, may indicate an inflammatory response. Regardless of the source of a patient's elevated (or depressed) temperature, the body can only tolerate a very narrow range of temperature change from its baseline and still function. Core temperatures above or below this range can lead to cessation of essential metabolic processes and chemical reactions critical to all organ function. Understanding the importance of body temperature as a vital sign, Paramedics often obtain a temperature using a red-dyed alcohol thermometer or, more recently, a tympanic membrane thermometer.

While Galileo Galilei invented the water thermometer in 1593, then called a thermoscope, the invention of the first accurate and functional mercury thermometer was attributed to a meteorologist named Daniel Gabriel Fahrenheit in 1714. Using a water and salt solution as a standard, he established a freezing point for the solution, at 0°F, then established the freezing of water alone (30°F) and temperature of the human body (90°F). These values (later adjusted to 32°F and 98.6°F, respectively), when obtained by thermometer, established a rapid and objective means of assessing a person's body temperature.

Shortly after establishing the **Fahrenheit scale**, Anders Celsius, a Swedish astronomer, replaced the previously used salt solution with pure water and again froze and then boiled the pure water at sea level (standard atmospheric pressure). Using these measurements as a baseline, he evenly divided the difference into 100 increments, or a centigrade scale, with zero being frozen water and 100 being boiling water. This centigrade scale, also called the **Celsius scale**, was adopted by an international conference on weights and measures, held in 1948, as the official temperature scale.

Analogous to the duality of household common and metric measurement systems, the public (particularly in English-speaking countries) adopted the Fahrenheit scale whereas the scientific community adopted the Celsius scale.

While many thermometers produced have both Celsius and Fahrenheit scales imprinted on the glass cylinder, in some instances a Paramedic may be asked to convert Fahrenheit to Celsius or vice versa. The most apparent difference between these two scales is that one is based upon 180 even divisions between freezing and boiling, whereas the other is based upon 100 even divisions. Therefore, any conversions will necessarily involve a 9/5 or a 5/9 adjustment to make the scales equal.

Similarly, the Fahrenheit scale does not have water freezing at zero degrees but at 32 degrees. Therefore, to balance the two scales 32 must be either added or subtracted from the result. To convert Fahrenheit to Celsius (medical standard temperature measurement) the EMS provider must first subtract 32 from the number and then multiply the Fahrenheit temperature by 5/9. For example, for a temperature of 103°F, subtract 32 and multiply the result by 5/9 to get the temperature on the Celsius scale—$(103 - 32) \, 5/9 = (71)5/9 = 39.4°C$. The opposite would be true to convert Celsius to Fahrenheit.

Administration of Medication

The administration of medications may be one of the greatest responsibilities that a Paramedic has to perform. Because of the nature of a medical emergency, Paramedics are permitted to administer powerful and potentially lethal drugs. When given correctly, these medications can help to improve a patient's condition or relieve some suffering. Given incorrectly, the Paramedic may make a bad situation worse. Therefore, Paramedics are ever mindful of their responsibilities whenever drugs are being administered. Like nurses, Paramedics practice the five rights of medication administration (right person, medication, dose, route, and time). The five rights simply represent an intelligence, a way of thinking, that decreases the potential for medication errors.

The first right refers to the right patient. Although this is an infrequent request, the Paramedic may be asked to assist in giving medications to patients with whom he is not familiar, such as during a mass casualty incident, while practicing in an expanded role, or while acting within an emergency department as part of the staff. In those instances, the Paramedic would be expected to identify the patient. If the patient is awake, alert, and able to communicate, then a personal identification may be attempted. If the patient is part of a system where personal identification, usually in the form of an identification band, is provided, then the Paramedic may check the band to verify the patient's identity as well as identify the patient personally.

The remaining rights refer to the actual administration of the medication. At the beginning, the Paramedic will check to be sure that the right medication is being given. Generic medications can have names that either sound alike or are spelled similarly. Careful attention to detail, such as the spelling in the order and the spelling on the medicine container, will prevent a medication error.

It is good practice to verify a medication's name when it is obtained from stock (whether that is a drug box or medicine cart), when it is being measured, and then finally when it is being administered. This triple check of the medication's identity is expanded to include verification of the drug's expiration as well as the clarity of the medication in the container. If there is any suspicion of potential contamination, then the drug should be immediately and safely discarded and a new supply of the drug obtained from stock.

As a drug is being prepared for administration, the Paramedic should be attentive to the next right, the right dose. While measuring a dose of medicine, the Paramedic may be at greatest risk of committing an error.

As previously mentioned, most emergency drugs are prepared so that one prefilled ampoule will be the correct dose for the average 70-kg patient. Unfortunately, patients do not always weigh 70 kg, so adjustments must be made. Furthermore, almost all pediatric medications, a large number of medications for the elderly, and an ever-increasing number of adult medications require weight specific dosing.

Calculating a weight-dependent dose, described earlier in this chapter, is often difficult in the out-of-hospital setting. Poor lighting as well as patient urgency can lead to unintended errors. The creation of drug charts and use of personal digital assistants (PDA) have helped alleviate some of the difficulty of calculating the correct dose. Nevertheless, responsible Paramedics typically confirm—and then re-confirm—a drug calculation with another Paramedic. If another provider is not immediately available, then communication with the hospital emergency department is advocated. A colleague, such as a registered nurse or physician's assistant, seated in a well-lit room with abundant resources at hand (including a calculator) can offer reassurance to a Paramedic who is alone calculating a critical medication dose.

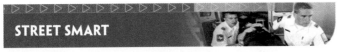

STREET SMART

To decrease confusion and errors, medication orders of fractions of a whole are documented as 0.X instead of .X (e.g., 0.5 instead of .5). When given orally, they are said as "zero point X." By adhering to this practice, when an order for a one-half milligram dose of a drug is heard, it will not be mistaken for 5 milligrams of the drug. Similarly, whole numbers are listed as the digit (i.e., 1 is 1, not 1.0) and thereby prevent the accidental administration of 10 mg of a drug.

The next right, the right route, may seem at first blush to be obvious, as Paramedics usually administer drugs intravenously. Even when a drug is given intravenously, however, if the drug is not followed by a bolus to clear it from the intravenous administration set, or external chest compressions are not performed to circulate the drug, then the drug will not get to the target organ. In other instances, medications administered subcutaneously to a hypoperfused patient will not be absorbed and the patient will not benefit from the medication. The Paramedic should give heed to the warning (right route) and consider the method of which he is about to administer a medication in terms of its efficiency and effectiveness.

The final right, the right time, speaks to the administration of drugs on a repetitive schedule. At first blush, this might seem inapplicable to EMS. However, some drugs are given repeatedly in the field in order to obtain and maintain a certain therapeutic effect. For example, epinephrine is usually repeated every three to five minutes during a cardiac arrest until there is a return of spontaneous circulation (ROSC).[12–14] In other situations, medications need to be given in a specific order (i.e., at the right time). For example, during a cardiac arrest, vasopressin or epinephrine always precedes an antidysrhythmic and paralytic drugs follow pre-induction medications.

After being given a drug, the patient is re-evaluated to see if the drug was effective. No exceptions should be made. Even the benefit of a seemingly innocent drug such as oxygen must be followed up with a re-evaluation of the patient's condition. This re-evaluation, and subsequent documentation of patient response to medication, is so important that some Paramedics refer to it as the sixth right, the right documentation.

The initials DARE, a simple mnemonic, can help Paramedics remember the elements of documentation for every medication administration. First, what was the data (D) that was obtained and what action (A) was taken in response to that data? The documentation of the action, if it was a medication administration, should include the drug's name, the exact dose of the drug, and the administration route, as well as the time of administration. After an appropriate interval, usually determined by the drug's onset of action and peak effect, the patient's response (R) to the drugs is assessed, both subjective and objective information obtained, and an evaluation (E) of the efficiency made. In some instances, the drug may be effective and further treatment is not indicated, while in other cases the drug has to be repeated.

Medication Routes

Practical necessity generally determines the route that a medication is given. If time is of the essence and it is important to get a precise dose to a target organ, without risk of first pass metabolism, then the intravenous route is preferred. If a local effect (e.g., skin preparation for a large bore intravenous needle) is needed, then a topically applied cream or subcutaneous injection would be appropriate. Each medication route offers specific advantages as well as disadvantages over other medication routes. Therefore, the route of medication administration is chosen with an express advantage or specific purpose in mind.

Preparation for Medication Administration

Regardless of the route of medication administration, whether it is a local route or a systemic route, the Paramedic must prepare both the patient and himself. The patient has the right to know what is being done and what medications are being given. A review of the discussion on informed consent is advised if the Paramedic is unsure of whether—and under what conditions—a patient can give informed consent.

The process of obtaining an informed consent from a competent patient can be summarized by the mnemonic AIR. First, the Paramedic must ask the patient if he has any allergies (A), particularly to the medication that is to be given. Then the patient should be advised of the intended (I) effect of the medication. Finally, the patient must be advised of reasonable (R) risks associated with the procedure and the medication. After obtaining the patient's consent, the Paramedic should practice medical asepsis, including hand washing and donning gloves.

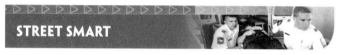
STREET SMART

When asking about allergies, the Paramedic should specifically ask the patient about allergies to latex, since a significant number of patients with chronic medical illnesses or healthcare workers have developed an allergy to latex. The Paramedic may find it difficult to differentiate whether the patient's allergic symptoms were from the medication itself or the latex within products used to administer that medication. If the patient advises the Paramedic that he is latex-sensitive/allergic, then non-latex products must be used during care. Manufacturers are increasingly removing latex from their products for this reason.

Local Routes

Local routes of medication administration are intended to target a specific organ or function and confine the effects of the medication used to that area. For example, medications topically applied to the eyes are called **optic** medications. Paramedics occasionally apply a local anesthetic (e.g., pilocaine) to the eyeball to anesthetize it in preparation for irrigation. The eye is an important sense organ and administration errors can lead to blindness. Strict adherence to medical asepsis can decrease the potential for this complication.

When a medication is an ointment or gel, then a ribbon of the medicine is placed along the inside of the lower lid. To gain access to the inside of the lower lid, the Paramedic should first withdraw the eyelid from the eyeball and then roll the eyelid over a cotton swab, inverting the eyelid in the process. The ribbon of medication should then be applied from the inner canthus, proximal to the bridge of the nose, outward.

To avoid the risk of cross-contamination and infection, optic drops, ointments, and disks are single-patient use only. After use, the medication should be immediately discarded to avoid any opportunity for re-use.

Otic Medication

Medications applied into the ear are called **otic** medications. While it is rare for a Paramedic to instill medications into a patient's ear, if the occasion should arise the patient should be instructed to tilt the head so that the affected ear is facing upward. After the correct volume of medicine has been drawn into the medicine dropper, the Paramedic would approach the patient. With the ear canal exposed and no visible drainage or obstruction noted, the Paramedic would place the dorsum of the dominant hand on the patient's temple with the ear dropper firmly held in the hand and poised over the ear opening. This position prevents the ear dropper from being inadvertently dropped into the patient's ear if the patient should startle and jerk. Grasping the pinna of the ear with the nondominant hand and pulling upward and outward, the medicine can be safely instilled into the ear. If the patient is incapable of cooperating with care, then consider placing the patient in the lateral recumbent position. If drainage is desired afterward, simply have the patient roll over to the opposite side.

Local Nasal Medication

The inner mucosa of the nostrils has a rich capillary bed that is an excellent route for the administration of systemic medications, discussed later in this chapter. However, this same quality also makes the nose prone to bleeding (a nosebleed is called an epistaxis).

Epistaxis is an all-too-common event whenever a nasal pharyngeal airway or an endotracheal tube is introduced into the nostril. Subsequent bleeding can drain back into the hypopharynx and into the stomach, inducing nausea and possible regurgitation. To decrease the incidence of epistaxis, many Paramedics prepare the nostril with a topically applied vasoconstrictor, such as phenylephrine (Neosynephrine®). Placing the tip of an atomizer into the intended nostril, the atomizer bulb is given one or two squeezes, propelling the medicine against the mucosa.

Following this application of a local vasoconstrictor, some Paramedics lubricate the patient's nares with a topical anesthetic, such as lidocaine gel. Using a nasal pharyngeal airway as an introducer, the Paramedic would liberally coat the airway and then insert the airway as usual. It is important that the Paramedic ascertain if the patient has any allergies to these medications before use. Alternatively, a water-based gel can be used to lubricate the nare. Under no conditions should a petroleum-based gel, such as Vaseline®, be used to lubricate the nostril prior to introduction of the airway device.

Phenylephrine and epinephrine (1:10,000) are also used in the treatment of severe epistaxis prior to packing. Approximately 90% of nosebleeds are anterior nosebleeds. Topical application of these potent vasoconstrictors provides local vasoconstriction that helps to decrease bleeding.

Local Oral Medications

Like the nose, the mouth has a capillary-rich mucosa that will rapidly absorb any medicine and distribute it systemically. Systemic medications are typically placed in the buccal pocket of the cheek or underneath the tongue in the sublingual space. This route of medication administration is discussed in further detail later in the chapter. However, the implication is clear. Large doses of topical oral medication can have a systemic effect and the patient should always be monitored carefully for untoward effects.

Various forms of topical oral medications are available. Gargles, such as a salt-water gargle, can be used to cleanse the mouth of contaminations, such as a blood splash, as well as dilute any potential pathogens. Hard lozenges and troches are designed to dissolve in the mouth, extending the duration of contact that the medicine has with the mucosa, perhaps to sooth ulceration.

Topical Medications

While a variety of options are used to apply medicine to the skin, such as liniments and lotions, and for a wide variety of purposes, from muscle aches to sunburn, Paramedics typically do not apply many topical medications. The exception may be the application of a topical antibiotic at the insertion site of an intravenous catheter. The benefits of topically applied antibiotic ointment are discussed in Chapter 27.

Other Local Routes

For completeness, both douches and enemas should be mentioned. Paramedics rarely perform either of these procedures unless they are acting in an extended role. Both douches (solutions introduced into the vagina via an apparatus) and enemas (solutions similarly introduced into the anus via an apparatus) instill these solutions into those body cavities. Adding a medication to these solutions can provide a local therapeutic effect, such as when treating a yeast infection.

Routes for Systemic Medications

Medications can have a local effect or they can have a **systemic** effect (i.e., an impact on more than one internal organ system). Medications that are intended to have a systemic effect may be given via the gastrointestinal tract or via an injection. The first route, also referred to as the **enteral** route, is more common and includes taking oral medications, in the form of pills, as well as suppositories. The second route bypasses the gastrointestinal system and is called the **parenteral** route. The parenteral route is preferred during an emergency because of the rapidity of onset of the medication's action as well as predictability of the drug levels.

The next section reviews the enteral route of drug administration, from head to toe, followed by a discussion of the parenteral routes of medication administration by inhalation and injection.

Enteral Drug Administration

Sublingual Route

The first enteral route to be discussed is the sublingual route. The lingual space is an area inferior to the tongue. The floor of the sublingual space has abundant capillaries which can rapidly absorb medications. It drains into the lingual vein and then into the systemic circulation, sometimes at levels comparable to intravenous injection.

A distinctive advantage of sublingual medication administration is that it bypasses the liver and thus avoids hepatic first pass metabolism.[15] Some medications are extremely sensitive to this first pass metabolism; for example, a healthy liver inactivates approximately 90% of oral nitroglycerine.[16] Furthermore, variations in blood flow, including hypotension-induced shock-liver, as well as variations in hepatic enzyme activity, secondary to competition, make the drug's metabolism in the liver unpredictable.

Sublingual medication can be given as either a liquid or a solid (pill). The Paramedic starts by lifting the tongue (assistance with a tongue blade is helpful) and depositing the medicine into the sublingual space. If the medication is a tablet or pill, it must dissolve to be effective. If the patient lacks saliva, a squirt from a pearl of sterile water can provide the needed solvent to accomplish liquefaction of the medication.

Patients who have received sublingual medication should be discouraged from smoking immediately afterward. Nicotine present in the smoke will produce vasoconstriction, hindering the absorption of the medication.

Buccal Route

Administering medications using the buccal route is similar to administering medications sublingually. In cases in which the patient has difficulty with lifting the tongue to the roof of the mouth (e.g., following a stroke), then the medication can be placed in the buccal pocket created by the cheek. Placing drugs in the buccal pocket has been a common practice since antiquity. Peruvian Indians used to stuff chewed coca leaves into their buccal pockets, thus absorbing the stimulant directly into the bloodstream. Tobacco has also been placed in the buccal pocket, as tobacco chew, and the nicotine absorbed into the central circulation.

Oral Route

Clearly, the vast majority of medications that are self-administered are swallowed. The medication—solid pill, capsule, or liquid—is then absorbed into the gastrointestinal tract where it is passed, via the portal circulation, through the liver and on into the central circulation. The image of a nurse passing pills in a paper medicine cup, also called a soufflé cup, leaps to mind when one thinks of hospital care. However, Paramedics seldom use this route to administer medicine.

First, the absorption of medications via the gastrointestinal route can be protracted and erratic. Local conditions such as the presence or absence of food, stomach acidity, gastric motility, and mesenteric blood flow all influence drug absorption. Perhaps more importantly from an EMS perspective, the patient must be able to maintain the airway independently and swallow the medication. Paramedics are often called to the scene of a patient who is semiconscious, making this route impractical.

Gastric Tubes

One means of passing medication to an obtunded or comatose patient is via a gastric tube. Gastric tubes have been used for decades to administer medications and treatments, and for a variety of other purposes, but have only recently seen use in the field.

John Hunter was credited with inventing the first gastric tube in 1869, using the skin of an eel to pass liquids into the stomach of a patient who had difficulty swallowing (dysphagia). Subsequently, Matas and Meyer used gastric tubes to treat paralytic ileus, a common post-operative complication.

The purposes of a gastric tube are numerous. Gastric tubes can be placed to instill feedings (either intermittently or continuously), as well as instill medications (either liquid or solid drug that is pulverized and then mixed in a liquid carrier). One of the earliest gastric tubes, called the Levin tube, is a simple red rubber catheter that is often placed for this purpose.

Gastric tubes can also be used to remove air; decompressing the stomach. Insufflation of the stomach during ventilation of the unconscious patient frequently requires the placement of a gastric tube to decompress the stomach and permit more effective ventilation. Decompression of the stomach with an orogastric tube is important for ventilation of children. Over-inflation of the stomach in a child decreases diaphragmatic excursion, increases resistance to ventilation, and decreases compliance, culminating in decreased efficiency in ventilation of the child. For this reason, it is routine practice to insert an orogastric tube during pediatric intubation.

Gastric tubes can also be used to remove liquid and small bits of solid matter from the stomach, such as pill fragments.[17] Evacuation of the stomach using a large diameter tube, such as an Ewald tube, may be a part of decontamination after a potentially lethal ingestion.

In addition, gastric tubes can be used to compress the inside of the stomach and the esophagus. Bleeding from esophageal varices or gastric ulcers can be significant and potentially life-threatening. Use of a special gastric tube, called a Sengstaken-Blakemore tube, permits the Paramedic to apply direct pressure, internally, to the source of bleeding.[18,19]

A gastric tube may be inserted either orally or nasally. Nasogastric tubes are typically inserted into patients who are awake, those with an intact gag reflex, or those for whom the gastric tube is expected to be long-term. However, application of a local anesthetic (e.g., Hurricane spray®) can deaden the gag reflex and permit passage of the gastric tube orally in an awake patient. Alternatively, a gastric tube may also be passed orally in the obtunded or unconscious patient. This is the most common route and the preferred route for EMS providers.

As in all procedures, the Paramedic should first discuss the procedure with the patient, inquiring about allergies, advising the patient of the intended effect, and warning the patient about reasonably expected side effects.

The process of orogastric tube insertion includes selection, preparation, and measurement of the tube; tube

placement, verification of placement, and either evacuation of the stomach or instillation of medications.

A rudimentary understanding of fluid dynamics is needed before the Paramedic selects the appropriate tube. Fluids tend to flow from areas of higher pressure to areas of lower pressure, measurable as milliliters per hour (mL/hr). Naturally, the thicker the fluid, the more pressure is needed to cause flow. The viscosity of the fluid, and the resultant friction, plays a large role in the selection of the proper tube. The speed of the flow is a function of the pressure that is being exerted upon it. Pressure is measured as the height that a column of water or mercury would raise under the same pressure and is labeled either cm H_2O or mmHg.

The diameter of the inner portion of the tube (the lumen) also contributes to the friction loss. The smaller the tube, the greater the friction loss. Therefore, greater pressure will be needed to create flow. Gastric tube lumens are measured in the French scale, where a smaller number means a smaller lumen. The length of a gastric tube also contributes to friction loss. However, since the lengths tend to vary marginally, the contribution of length of the gastric tube is often discounted.

Most Paramedics insert an orogastric tube in order to evacuate or decompress the stomach. The application of suction to the end of an orogastric tube can effectively accomplish this function. Suction, a pressure that is less than atmospheric (a negative pressure), creates a flow in a fluid, either gas or liquid. Most ambulances and portable suction units can provide substantial continuous suction, greater than 180 mmHg.

However, continuous suction will cause a single-lumen gastric tube, such as a Levin tube, to adhere to the gastric mucosa, leading to local irritation and bleeding. To prevent this predictable complication, dual-lumen tubes (such as the Salem sump) were invented. Dual-lumen gastric tubes always have one port open, a port that entrains air into the stomach and prevents suction from adhering to the stomach wall.

If a dual-lumen tube is not available, then intermittent suction can be accomplished by periodically turning the suction off, allowing the gastric tube to dislodge. Healthcare facilities frequently have wall-mounted suction devices which permit intermittent suction for this purpose.

If the blue atmosphere port of a dual-lumen gastric tube is lower than the stomach, stomach contents will drain through the atmosphere port by gravity. As happens on occasion, the Paramedic may unwittingly allow the tube to fall to the patient's side. Subsequently the tube drains the stomach contents onto the Paramedic's shoes and/or the floor. To prevent this complication, the tube should be plugged and the tail of the tube pinned to the patient's clothing near the collar.

Initially, preparation for gastric tube insertion entails collecting the necessary equipment first. Either a single-lumen gastric tube (such as a red rubber Levin or an Ewald tube), or a dual-lumen gastric tube (such as a Salem sump) should be chosen. All gastric tubes are approximately 50 inches (127 cm) long and come in sizes 12 to 18 French. An average adult will accept a 16 French gastric tube.

If the nasogastric route is to be attempted, a tube of water-soluble lubricant should be available, as well as towels, emesis basin, soft-tip or covered clamps, a large syringe (30 mL), and a stethoscope.

After obtaining the necessary consent, the patient is placed in the high-Fowler's position. If the patient is unable to be placed in the high-Fowler's position, then the patient can be placed in the left lateral recumbent position.

If a nasogastric tube is to be inserted, then the Paramedic should first visualize the external nare and choose the largest nostril, avoiding nasal polyps or a deviated septum. Premedication with phenylephrine and lidocaine gel, as previously described for nasopharyngeal airway insertion, will reduce the trauma associated with this approach.

Next, the gastric tube must be premeasured. A nasogastric (NG) tube is measured from the bridge of the nose to an earlobe, then from the earlobe to the xiphoid process. An orogastric (OG) tube is measured from the corner of the lips to the xiphoid process instead. Once measured, the Paramedic should make note of the measurement. Most gastric tubes have incremental markings, consisting of black bands placed every so many centimeters.

Once the tube is measured and the patient prepared, the Paramedic then lubricates the last 6 inches of the gastric tube with a water-soluble gel, and proceeds to pass the tube. An NG tube is advanced perpendicular to the plane of the face and directly into the nares. If resistance is felt, then the tube should be slightly withdrawn, approximately 1 inch, and then rotated in the fingers 90 degrees. Then another attempt should be made. A twisting action with the tip of the tube will help the tube pass over the turbinates in the nose.

Alternatively, an OG tube is directly advanced over the midline of the tongue until the posterior pharynx is reached. Care should be taken to not strike the posterior pharynx as it might elicit a gag reflex.

The gastric tube, now in the proximity of the posterior pharynx, is ready to be passed. If the patient is willing and able to cooperate, then ask the patient to sip a glass of water through a straw. This facilitates the passage of the gastric tube into the esophagus by closing the glottis over the trachea, thereby preventing accidental tracheal intubation.

If the patient has persistent paroxysms of gagging and retching, then visualize the posterior oropharynx with a penlight. It is not uncommon to find the gastric tube coiled in the posterior pharynx. In that case, withdraw the gastric tube until it is unfurled and then proceed once more.

Once the gastric tube is in the esophagus, approximately one-half the length of the measurement, then the gastric tube should be advanced briskly. If the patient begins to cough, then the gastric tube may be in the trachea and pressing against the carina. Withdraw the tube approximately 6 inches and retry.

After the gastric tube has been completely passed, then its placement must be confirmed. The Paramedic would first draw up 10 to 20 mL of air in a slip-tip syringe and place it at the distal opening. The Paramedic would then place a stethoscope firmly against the epigastrium and instill the air into the tube. If the gastric tube is properly placed, then a swooshing sound will be heard over the epigastrium.[20-22]

The same sound will not be heard over the lungs; therefore, auscultating the lungs may not be a reliable indicator of misplacement. Instead, the Paramedic should ask the patient to speak. A gastric tube misplaced into the lungs will separate the vocal cords and the patient will have difficulty speaking (dysphonia).

Finally, the Paramedic should aspirate the gastric tube. The presence of gastric contents is proof positive that the gastric tube is in the right place. Other signs of a misplaced tube include condensation in the tube as well as dropping pulse oximetry readings, indicating desaturation of the blood.

The gastric tube can then be attached to wall suction and low suction can be applied, approximately 90 mmHg. The patient should be continually monitored throughout this procedure. Signs of hypoxia, such as premature ventricular contractions (PVC), and altered level of responsiveness may indicate that the gastric tube is misplaced into the trachea, or has migrated from its original position into the trachea, and the suction is drawing air out of the lungs.

Once placement of the gastric tube has been confirmed, the Paramedic should proceed to secure the gastric tube to prevent accidental displacement. An approximately 6-inch piece of 1-inch tape placed in a chevron fashion over the nose will secure the NG tube. An OG tube can be secured to the corner of the mouth with a tie-wrap, similar to an endotracheal tube. Alternatively, if an endotracheal tube is in place, then the OG tube can be secured to the endotracheal tube itself.

On occasion, the flow from the gastric tube may stop, suggesting that the gastric tube is not functioning. Under those conditions, the Paramedic should disconnect the suction and reassess placement to eliminate the possibility of displacement. If the gastric tube is not displaced, then the Paramedic should assess the gastric tube for obstructions. To accomplish this, the Paramedic irrigates the gastric tube. To irrigate a gastric tube, approximately 30 mL of saline or sterile water is instilled into the tube via a syringe. If a great deal of resistance is met, then the Paramedic should clamp the gastric tube closed.

For ease during transfer, the patient can be disconnected from the suction and the gastric tube clamped. The atmosphere port of a dual-lumen gastric tube (the blue pigtail on a Salem sump) can be connected with the other port, making a closed circuit. Soft-tip clamps can be used for single-lumen gastric tubes, but care should be taken to ensure that the teeth of the clamp do not perforate the wall of the gastric tube.

Rectal Route

Although Paramedics rarely use the rectal route for a medication administration, the rectal route has a number of distinctive advantages that make it a desirable site for medication administration. The rectum has a rich blood supply via the hemorrhoidal venous plexus. Drugs that are absorbed from the rectum avoid inactivation by stomach acids and intestinal enzymes. In fact, 50% of the absorbed drug bypasses the portal circulation, minimizing the impacts of first pass metabolism and biotransformation. These factors, in combination, allow for comparable drug levels between intravenous administration and rectal administration. The rectal administration route is also useful when the patient is unable to accept oral medications, such as in the case of infants or if the patient has persistent vomiting.

Before administering medication using the rectal route, and after obtaining consent, the patient must be properly positioned. The Paramedic should ask the patient to assume a left lateral recumbent position. Once in that position, the patient is asked to bring her right knee to the chest as far as practical. The Paramedic should then take care to only expose what is necessary to accomplish the task at hand, while leaving the remainder of the body covered. This modified left lateral position, called the **Sim's position**, provides optimal access to the anus while minimally compromising the patient's dignity.

With the patient in position, the Paramedic would then take a well-lubricated suppository, or rectal medication administration device, and insert the device into the rectum approximately 4 inches in adults and 2 inches in children. The Paramedic should ask the patient to breathe through her open mouth to help her relax during medication administration. Once the medication administration device is in place, the medication is deposited in close proximity to the hemorrhoidal venous plexus.

On occasion, as the medication administration device is advanced, the Paramedic may feel resistance from a stool that is within the rectal vault. In that case, the device should be withdrawn and an alternative route considered.

Parenteral Drug Administration

When a rapid onset of drug action is required (e.g., during an emergency), the most direct route to the target organs sidesteps the gastrointestinal system (enteral administration) and enters drugs directly through the central circulation. This administration route is called the parenteral route because it goes around the gastrointestinal, or enteral, system.

Parenteral drug administration has several distinct advantages over enteral drug administration. Enterally administered drugs have to be absorbed from the lumen of the intestines where absorption can be erratic. Gastrointestinal drug absorption can also be adversely affected by a number of factors, including the presence of gastric secretions, mesenteric circulation, gastrointestinal motility, co-ingested foodstuffs, and a host of other variables.[25–27] Drugs deposited into the intestines are also acted upon by a number of enzymes which can immediately deactivate certain drugs. Conversely, drugs administered via the parenteral route circumvent all of these factors, plus they avoid the liver's first pass metabolism. Therefore, parenterally administered serum drug levels are more predictable than enterally administered serum drug levels for these reasons.

Finally, drugs administered parenterally can be given to patients who are uncooperative or incapable of cooperation (i.e., unconscious). These several advantages combine to make parenteral drug administration routes the preferred drug route in an emergency.

Intranasal Route

A medication administration route recently adopted by Paramedics, is the intranasal route. The intranasal route takes advantage of the nasal passages. These nasal passages are lined with very vascular mucous membranes which can absorb medications quickly and have a shared connection with the brain. This allows these medications to go directly to the brain, without the risk of first pass metabolism associated with enteral routes of drug administration.[28-30] This factor makes intranasal medication administration desirable for Paramedics under certain conditions.

For example, the combination of a patient with altered mental status, especially one who is combative, and/or a moving ambulance can make obtaining intravenous access difficult. The intranasal medication route, which is both quick and easy, makes success under these trying conditions more likely. However, the clear advantage of intranasal administration of drugs is the decreased risk of accidental needle injury. The federal Centers for Disease Control and Prevention (CDC) estimates that as many as 600,000 needlestick injuries may occur annually in the United States. With minimal training, a Paramedic can effectively and safely administer medications while avoiding needlestick injury. In some cases, newer Paramedics can be trained just before use (called "just in time training").

The use of intranasal medication administration technology, a truly needleless system, is an example of an "engineered control." Engineered controls are means of preventing exposure to potentially infectious materials (PIM). In this case, the risk of exposure is through accidental needlestick. Prevention methods are mandated by OSHA and intranasal medication administration is consistent with the intent of the Needlestick Safety and Prevention Act of 2000.[31]

One drug that shows promise for Paramedic practice is naxolone (Narcan®). A study in Denver's EMS demonstrated that naxolone can be safely and effectively administered to patients who are suspected of opioid overdose.[32] Paramedics in Denver administered 1 mg in 1 mL per nostril of naxolone to patients who met the criteria. For those with suspected opioid overdose, the mean response time was 3.9 minutes. As a result, the Denver Paramedics started 29% fewer IV lines in that patient population.

However, the use of intranasal naxolone is considered an off-label use. The term "off-label use" implies that using the drug in that manner has not been approved by the federal Food and Drug Administration (FDA), which requires experimental studies to approve a drug or the use of a drug in another manner. In some cases, pharmaceutical companies are not willing to underwrite the expenses of experimental studies for non-patent drugs. This should not be construed to mean that a drug cannot be used in this manner. Physicians, during the practice of medicine, can order drugs administered in an off-label use. Some drugs can be given intranasally, some off-label (Table 26-10).

The volume administered intranasally should be no more than 1 mL of liquid and the drug should be atomized to a particle size of between 10 mcg and 50 mcg, the optimal particle size for absorption. Currently several different devices are available that can meet these operational criteria. Contraindications for use of intranasal atomizers for medication administration include epistaxis, septal wall defects, and intranasal cocaine use.

Table 26-10 Intranasal Medications

Drug	Use
Atropine	Organophosphate poisoning
Epinephrine	Cardiac arrest
Fentanyl	Pain management
Glucagon	Hypoglycemia
Influenza	Flu prophylaxis
Insulin	Hyperglycemia/Crush injury
Lidocaine	Cardiac arrest
Midazolam	Seizure control
Naloxone	Opiate overdose
Nitroglycerin	Hypertensive crisis/acute coronary syndrome
Steroids	Reactive airway disease

CULTURAL/REGIONAL DIFFERENCES

In some regions, a common street practice is to mix cocaine (an upper) with heroin (a downer), a practice called speedballing, snowballing, or smack and crack. The intended effect is to first get high, then "coast" down with the heroin. Some "double" inject the two drugs, whereas others inject the heroin and inhale, or snort, the cocaine through the nostrils. When the heroin, or co-ingested substances like alcohol, depress the respiratory system, the Paramedic could consider the use of intranasal naxolone to reverse the opioid-induced respiratory depression. However, if the cocaine was snorted, then the vasoconstrictive effects of the cocaine may prevent the absorption of the naxolone.

Obtaining intravenous access while a patient is having an unremitting seizure, a condition called status epilepticus, can be difficult. Intranasal administration of anticonvulsants, such as midazolam, would be advantageous in controlling the seizure. One study of intranasal midazolam showed that it had a 73% bioavailability when compared to intravenous administration[33] and that it had the added advantage of rapid onset.

Respiratory Route

Inhalation of medications has several distinct advantages over other means of medication administration. Inhalation of a drug-laden vapor can quickly lead to therapeutic drug levels in the bloodstream via absorption through the capillary-covered alveoli. Inhalation also avoids first pass metabolism in the liver, allowing a rapid buildup of the drug in the systemic circulation. This method avoids the use of needles, thus lessening the threat of blood-borne pathogens for the Paramedic.

Inhalation therapy also has several drawbacks which tend to reduce its efficiency. Inhalation therapy requires that the patient be able to assist with treatment (i.e., perform inhalation). A lack of coordination is the most frequent cause of ineffectual breathing treatments. Inhalation therapy is also dependent upon the patient's breathing pattern, particularly upon the period of holding one's breath during inspiration.

Pulmonary Treatments

To a large extent, the treatment of pulmonary disorders from asthma to emphysema is focused on the delivery of respiratory agents directly into the pulmonary tree. These bronchodilators, such as albuterol (Ventolin®), and anticholinergics, such as ipratropium bromide (Atrovent®), are inhaled using one of the several respiratory therapy devices discussed later to provide immediate relief from bronchospasm. Other respiratory drugs, such as the anti-inflammatory drug cromolyn sodium, and even antibiotics, such as tobramycin, can be inhaled to treat respiratory disease.

In the past, the majority of inhaled medications were designed to exert a local pulmonary effect and to treat reactive airway disease. Currently, research is underway to administer vaccines and other antimicrobial treatments which would have a more systemic impact via the pulmonary system. There is even development and study of an inhaled insulin (Exubera®) which uses the capillary-rich lung fields to absorb powdered insulin instead of requiring subcutaneous injection.[34,35]

Personal Protective Equipment

Drug-ladened exhaust from the various respiratory treatment platforms present the Paramedic with a potential threat. To minimize that threat, the federal Centers for Disease Control and Prevention (CDC) recommends that Paramedics use a mask and gloves while administering these medications. EMS vehicles should also be designed so that stale air in the patient compartment is expelled and fresh air circulated frequently. In some cases, where vapor is visible, it may be reasonable for a Paramedic to wear eye protection, such as a splatter shield or goggles, while in close proximity to the patient.

Fluid Dynamics

Air, like water, is fluid and is subject to laws of fluid dynamics. For example, the more resistance air encounters (e.g., in a narrowed airway), the more turbulent the airflow. Turbulent airflow is slower. The structure of the lungs takes this fact into account and the airways divide some 23 times before they reach the alveoli, allowing nearly non-existent airflow at the alveolar level. This dead air in turn permits easier diffusion of gasses such as oxygen and carbon dioxide.

The slowing of air in the airways also serves another purpose—it encourages **fallout**. Fallout occurs whenever large particles carried in the air current settle out as airflow velocity is lost. An example of this is dust settling out. Turbulence and

a reduction in the velocity of airflow cause particles between 6 and 20 microns to "fall out" in the nose and particles greater than 6 microns to fall out in the trachea. As the pulmonary tree divides further, more fallout occurs; particles greater than 2 microns fall out in the bronchi and 2 micron particles fall out in the bronchioles. The result is that nearly particulate-free air enters the alveoli.[36,37]

While fallout generally serves a protective function, acting as a particle trap to keep contagions and pollution out of the lungs, it also tends to keep large droplets of aerosolized medications from penetrating the terminal bronchioles and distal alveoli. This dramatically reduces the effectiveness of many respiratory drugs.

To complicate matters further, the propellants used to deliver these medications use cold gasses (room temperature gasses) to deliver these medications into the bronchi. Upon contact with cold air, the bronchi and bronchioles reflexively spasm air to protect the sensitive alveoli. Paradoxically, the respiratory medications which are given to treat bronchospasm can induce more bronchospasm.

Metered Dose Inhaler

The **metered dose inhaler (MDI)** remains the gold standard for respiratory therapy. Portable and simple to operate, the MDI enjoys a high degree of patient acceptance. This is due in part because it does not require extraordinary breathing maneuvers. Also important to the Paramedic is that the sealed pressurized unit is tamper-proof and its contents are protected from degradation by light and water.

While the MDI is a preferred personal respiratory treatment platform for many, it is relatively ineffective, depositing less than 20% in the distal lung fields. To improve efficiency, as well as to assist those patients with abnormal breathing patterns, a **spacer** device can be utilized.[38-40] The spacer allows a more controlled inhalation of smaller, ideal-sized drug particles suspended in the vapor within the chamber (see Figure 26-3).

Dry Powder Inhalers

Dry powder inhalers (DPI), such as the Diskhaler®, use a solid drug which is pulverized into micro-fine particles for inhalation. The DPI, while an effective platform for the delivery of pulmonary medications, depends upon the patient's inspiration for uptake of the drug and proper dispersal of the drug across the lung fields. If the patient has a reduced inspiratory flow, less than 60 L/min, then the drug will not reach the distal alveoli.

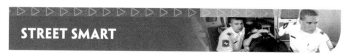

STREET SMART

Healthcare providers have complained of headaches, bronchospasm, and conjunctivitis from secondhand exposure to the dust exhausted from a DPI. Use of PPE can help to reduce the incidence of passive exposure to the droplets.

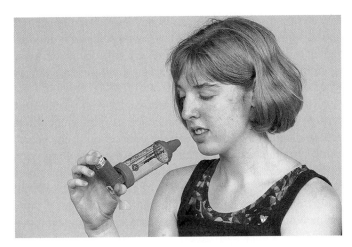

Figure 26-3 Use of an MDI with spacer.

Small Volume Nebulizer

The **small volume nebulizer (SVN)** is an alternative platform for the delivery of inhaled medications. More difficult to set up and operate, it is thought to produce a better particle size for inhalation. Hypothetically, more of the drug is deposited in the patient's alveoli.

The medication is suspended in a stream of air which is then smashed against a round surface in the SVN. The resulting liquid shear creates micro-fine particles, in the 1 to 3 micron range, which are ideal for inhalation. Three factors combine to alter the efficiency of this mechanism: jet design, gas pressure, and fluid dynamics.

It is critical that the gas-emitting jet of the SVN has the ideal orifice diameter, as well as distance to the baffle, for atomization. For an SVN to function properly, the gas pressure must be adequate, but not excessive. In addition, the surface tension of the aqueous solution, usually a function of the liquid's viscosity, must be within acceptable limits. These factors being equal, the SVN is a good platform for the delivery of pulmonary medications to the patient in respiratory distress.

Prior to using an SVN, the Paramedic should obtain a history from, and perform a physical on, the patient. A demonstrated history of responsiveness to MDI bronchodilators indicates a greater likelihood of success with the SVN (Figure 26-4). The physical examination should include auscultation for wheezes or, more ominously, absent breath sounds, as well as pulse oximetry. Some Paramedics obtain a baseline peak flow meter reading as well. Key to assessing the effectiveness of any SVN treatment is the patient's subjective judgment regarding her own dyspnea.

Use of an In-Line Small Volume Nebulizer in Bag-Valve-Mask Assembly

In special circumstances, an intubated patient could benefit from a respiratory treatment. In those cases, an SVN may be attached in-line with the bag-valve-mask assembly. This

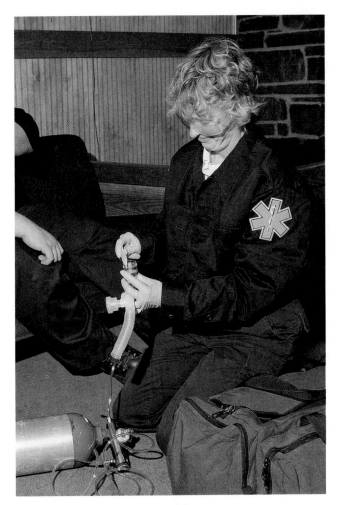

Figure 26-4 Assembly and operation of the SVN.

assembly, SVN-BVM-ET, changes the conditions under which an SVN normally operates.

First, an average 26 cm long, 8 mm internal diameter (ID) endotracheal tube decreases dead space from an average of 75 mL in the trachea to approximately 60 mL, but does so at a cost. The smaller dead space is owed to a smaller airway lumen. A smaller airway lumen immediately results in greater airway resistance. Greater airway resistance produces greater fallout of the inspired vapor. Decreasing the lumen of the airway (e.g., from an oral endotracheal tube size of 8 mm to a nasal endotracheal tube size of 6 mm) increases the airway resistance exponentially, in this case 4.2 times more resistance.

Resistance is also increased with the higher ventilatory flow rates, typically seen in manual or mechanical ventilation. The combination of increased airway resistance, and airway turbulence, combine to generally cause less medication disposition in the alveoli, from a normal of 20% to less than 15%.[41]

To defeat these disadvantages, the American Association of Respiratory Therapists recommends that intubated adult patients, who are receiving respiratory treatments, should be ventilated with a smaller tidal volume (< 500 mL). Gentle ventilation with reduced flow, as well as the addition of an inspiratory pause at the height of each positive pressure ventilation, should be employed.

Topical Route

For sustained systemic delivery of a medication, an alternative administration is the topical route. Medication, contained within a cream carrier, is applied to the skin and is then absorbed directly into the subcutaneous capillary beds, where it passes on to the central circulation. The rate of absorption is variable and dependent upon several circumstances.

Factors affecting topical medication absorption, also called **transdermal** medicine, include the skin's vascularity and perfusion, as evidenced by capillary refill and temperature (warmth). Furthermore, skin conditions such as rashes, eczema, and open lesions can also affect absorption.

A number of medications are available in transdermal patches including nicotine, hormone replacement, opiate analgesics, and nitroglycerine. An example of a topical medication applied by Paramedics in the field is nitroglycerine paste. A Paramedic takes a ribbon of paste, measured in inches, and applies it to an impermeable paper barrier which is then applied onto the skin. Assuming that the patient is not hypoperfused and/or hypothermic, the medication-laden nitroglycerine cream melts, is absorbed through the epidermis, and enters the subcutaneous capillary beds underneath. Nitroglycerine can have a profound effect on blood pressure, inducing almost immediate hypotension. Therefore, the location of the paste/patch should be in an easy-to-reach place such as the upper arm or posterior shoulder. To remove the nitroglycerine paste quickly and effectively, a tongue blade can be scraped across the skin in the direction of hair growth.

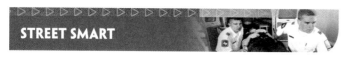

STREET SMART

The cream used in the manufacture of nitroglycerine paste is similar to the conductive medium used for manual defibrillation. It is prudent to remove any nitroglycerine patch or paste prior to defibrillation/cardioversion.[42] Failure to remove a patch/paste may result in arcing and a loss of defibrillation energy.

Injections

Tools for Injections

The quintessential tool for parenteral drug injection is the hypodermic syringe. Whether it is used for a subcutaneous injection, an intramuscular injection, or to gain intravenous access, a syringe is a key component of the assembly.

In the past, glass syringes with calibrations carefully etched on their sides were used in the hospital and sterilized between repeated patient uses. Today, most Paramedics use plastic syringes, prepacked in sterile wrappers, for individual patient use. However, glass syringes are still available for use in circumstances in which the drug would adversely react with the plastic syringe.

The components of a hypodermic syringe include the syringe and the needle. The connection of the syringe to the needle is called the adaptor and the connection of the needle to the syringe is called the hub. Some needle adaptors attach to the syringe hub by use of a twist connection, called a **luer lock**, where the adaptor on the syringe is grooved and will mate with a flange on the needle hub. This provides a more secure connection, decreasing the chances of accidental disconnection. Other syringe adaptors simply slide inside the needle hub and are called **slip-tip** adaptors.

The shaft of the syringe is called the **barrel**. Syringes are labeled according to the volume within the barrel (i.e., 1, 3, 5 mL) and the calibrations on the side of the barrel. Traditional hypodermic syringes are marked in divisions of a milliliter, and those would be called a 1 mL syringe, 3 mL syringe, and so on. Many hypodermic needles have dual calibration: tenths of milliliter on one side (metric) and minims (common household) on the other. Paramedics should be cautious and not confuse 0.10 mL with 10 minims, as they are not equivalent measures.

An insulin syringe is an exception to the rule of syringe marking. Insulin is not administered in milligrams per milliliter (mg/mL), as most standard medications are, but in international units (IU) determined by bioassay. Therefore, a special syringe, marked in units, is manufactured for insulin injection. The insulin syringe looks similar to the 1 mL syringe frequently used for tuberculosis testing. Paramedics should look at the syringe carefully to avoid confusing a tuberculin syringe with an insulin syringe.

The purpose of a syringe is to either inject a liquid medication out of the barrel or to withdraw blood into the barrel. In both cases, the barrel of the syringe is filled with a liquid. When the horizontal surface of a liquid interfaces with the vertical wall of the barrel, cohesive forces (i.e., surface tension) tend to pull it away from the wall while adhesive forces between the syringe's wall and the liquid tend to pull it toward the wall of the barrel. As a result, the liquid moves upward. These two forces—surface tension and wall adhesion—cause the liquid's surface to form into a concave-curved shape called a **meniscus**. As a matter of practice, Paramedics compare the bottom of the meniscus with the calibrations on the barrel in order to determine the volume of drug in the syringe.

To facilitate injecting drugs, or withdrawing blood, a plunger is placed inside the barrel. The head of the plunger is fitted tightly inside the barrel, thus preventing liquid from seeping past the plunger. However, on occasion, an imperfect match will occur. If this happens, liquid will seep past the plunger and drip the drug onto the Paramedic's hands. For this reason, Paramedics are advised to always wear gloves whenever a syringe is used.

At the apex of the plunger's head is a convex head. The head's shape is intended to offset the meniscus, leaving a flat surface that is easier to measure. In the past, nurses would draw up approximately 0.1 mL of air, an air bubble, into the syringe to offset the effect of the meniscus. However, the convex head of the plunger corrects this problem, making the practice unnecessary. If the plunger head is convex, then the Paramedic should measure the volume of drug from where the plunger touches the barrel of the syringe.

To administer a liquid drug, the Paramedic merely has to push down on the shaft of the plunger to push the drug out of the syringe. However, the pressure applied to push the drug out can cause the patient some discomfort. To ease the patient's pain and to give the Paramedic added control of the syringe, most syringes have a flange at the top. By placing her first and second finger under the flange and pushing upward on the flanges while simultaneously pushing downward with her thumb on the plunger, the Paramedic can control both the rate of administration as well as the pressure applied to the patient's skin.

Hypodermic Needle

The heart of the hypodermic syringe is the needle. Needles are generally made of surgical-quality stainless steel and may be either pre-assembled with the syringe or individually packaged in a sterile wrap. The parts of the needle include the hub and the shaft. The hub, generally made of plastic, has an external flange designed to mate with the syringe adaptor.

Like syringes, needles come in a variety of sizes and lengths, each according to their intended purpose. Needles are measured in gauges—the smaller the number means the larger the diameter of the needle (e.g., 14 gauge > 20 gauge).

The decision of which gauge to choose is largely a function of two factors. The first factor is the viscosity of the fluid. The thicker the fluid to be injected or withdrawn through the needle, the larger the needle that will have to be used.

> **STREET SMART**
>
> Paramedics seldom use less than an 18 gauge needle when drawing blood, either through an intravenous catheter or via direct needle insertion. Smaller catheters tend to break the red blood cells apart in the turbulence, called lysing of the red blood cells. Lysed red blood cells spill the cell's contents, including potassium, into the plasma. The result is false plasma values obtained from the laboratory.

The other factor in needle selection is the speed of delivery. A smaller diameter needle creates greater resistance to flow (i.e., friction loss) and requires higher pressures to push a given volume of liquid at a faster rate. To reduce the pressure being applied, the Paramedic may alternatively choose a larger diameter (smaller gauge) needle.

The length of a needle, the other physical characteristic of a needle, is also typically a function of the task at hand. A shorter needle, approximately 1 inch, is used when injecting a drug into the medication port of an intravenous set. By using a longer needle, the Paramedic would risk bypassing the protection afforded by the hard plastic of the medication port and piercing the tubing's soft sidewalls.

A longer needle is used when an intramuscular injection of medication is given to an obese patient. In some cases, a needle as long as 4 inches is needed so that the medication reaches the muscular layer.

A needle is essentially a hollow wire which is cut to length. The end of the wire is often cut obliquely, in such a fashion that a sharp leading edge is created, called the **point**. The sharper the point, the easier the needle will enter into the patient's skin or the stopper in a vial.

The needle now has an angled surface called the **bevel**. The bevel, the angle of the needle point, is calculated for a specific purpose. A regular bevel is designed to quickly pierce the skin with a minimum of pain. A **Huber** bevel is intended to pierce a stopper without coring it, preventing leakage of the contents within the catheter from leaking out of the stopper when the needle is withdrawn. Blunt bevels, used for intradermal injections, are designed to deposit the medication just below the skin without penetrating deeper layers of skin below.

Needle Safety

The majority of exposures healthcare workers, including Paramedics, experience to blood-borne pathogens are the result of accidental puncture of the skin with a hollow-bore needle. The United States Centers for Disease Control and Prevention estimates that over 600,000 needlesticks will occur annually. Many of them are preventable. Infection control expert Kathrine West, RN, estimates that each needlestick injury will cost employers approximately $1,200 in emergency care, lost hours and wages, and medical follow-up for a case with a non-infectious exposure.[43]

In response to this occupational hazard, the U.S. Congress strengthened the Occupational Safety and Health Administration (OSHA) blood-borne pathogens rule, enacted in 1991, with the Needlestick Safety and Prevention Act of 2000, effective the April 18, 2001. The Needlestick Safety and Prevention Act requires wider use of engineering controls which can prevent needlestick injury.[44] Examples of engineering controls which can help prevent needlestick injury include retractable needles, needles that are withdrawn into the syringe barrel by a spring-action mechanism, self-sheathing needles, needles that have a retractable hard case that is advanced over the needle as the needle is withdrawn, and hooded needles that have a protective covering over the needle.

Manufacturers, in an effort to eliminate the needle entirely, have created needleless medication systems which use non-needle connections at the medication ports. They also have created jet injection systems that use high-pressure air to open the skin temporarily while medicine is deposited beneath the skin. However, there are still circumstances in which a needle will be used. Therefore, the Paramedic must be familiar with its use.

Every Paramedic is responsible for safely disposing of used/contaminated needles into a safe sharps container. The sharps container should be close at hand, within arm's reach, and be easy to access. Under no circumstances should a needle be bent or cut. Cutting a needle can create a microspray of drug and/or blood in the air, which can be inhaled or settle into the eyes.

Medication Containers

Medications are packaged in either vials or ampoules. The Paramedic must withdraw the drug from its container, into a needle and syringe, before use. Ampoules, a single-use, single-patient drug container, is manufactured alone or as a part of an ampoule with syringe delivery system, sometimes called a "preloaded ampoule." In the emergency setting, where time is of the essence, these prefilled ampoule/syringe systems are commonplace. They are generally filled with the amount of drug needed to treat a 70-kg patient.

When using one of these ampoule systems, the Bristo-jet®, the Paramedic removes the two end caps which protect the ampoule and the syringe. With the caps removed, the Paramedic would mate the two pieces, twisting them together so that a recessed needle within the syringe portion would penetrate the stopper. When this step is completed, the Paramedic would discard any extra drug and air which may be contained within the ampoule and proceed to introduce the syringe's preset needle into the medication port of the administration set or to inject the drug into the patient (Figure 26-5).

The Paramedic should use caution when discarding excess drug so as to avoid accidental injury. Drugs, carelessly discarded into the air, can splash onto the ambulance ceiling and fall back into the eyes of unsuspecting occupants in the patient compartment, including the patient.

Some ampoules still have to be broken before the medication can be withdrawn (Figure 26-6). The Paramedic should first shake the medicine down out of the ampoule's neck and into its body. Once accomplished, the Paramedic would then place the ampoule on a flat firm surface and grasp the ampoule's body with the thumb and forefinger of the nondominant hand. Using either a commercially available ampoule breaker (which is preferred) or a 2-inch gauze pad, the Paramedic would grasp the ampoule's head and, while holding it in a direction away from him, smartly snap the ampoule's neck. The Paramedic should avoid the sharp shards of glass from flying into the eye. The Paramedic is advised to wear protective eyewear, as splinters of glass can fly from the ampoule into the eye. Having accessed the ampoule, the

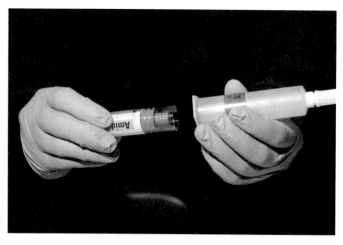

Figure 26-5 Preparing a prefilled medication syringe.

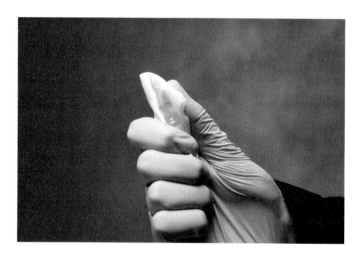

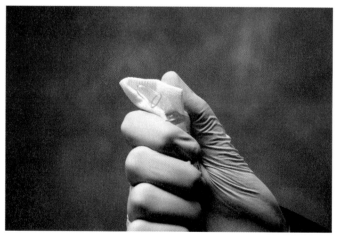

Figure 26-6 Safely break the glass stem of the ampoule before inverting the ampoule and withdrawing the medication.

Paramedic would introduce the syringe, with a glass-filtering needle, into the medication just below the meniscus.

In some cases, the Paramedic may elect to invert the ampoule and withdraw the medication. The medication will remain in the ampoule, provided the needle does not touch the walls of the ampoule and break the liquid surface tension. However, most Paramedics, particularly when in the back of a moving ambulance, prefer to keep the ampoule on a firm surface with the bottom down in order to aspirate the drug into the syringe. When the medication has been withdrawn, and the ampoule is useless, then the glass ampoule should be discarded like any other sharp, into an approved sharps container.

Vials are intended for multiple use and therefore are more likely to become contaminated. Some EMS organizations and healthcare institutions require that the vial's contents be used within a specific period of time (e.g., 24 hours) and then discarded in order to avoid possible contamination. Many Paramedics discard vials after use and do not use vials on multiple patients.

The risk of contamination is higher when a Paramedic is in the high-pressured, time-limited environment of an emergency. Innocent errors in medical asepsis are frequent enough that single-patient ampoules, and individually packaged patient supplies, are routinely used by Paramedics to avoid these problems.

When a vial is used, the Paramedic should first remove the plastic cover, then take a moment and clean the stopper with an alcohol-soaked pad or gauze, commonly called a prep pad, to remove gross surface contaminants.

After calculating the proper volume for the dose, based on the drug's concentration, the Paramedic would then draw up an equal volume of air. Vials are a closed system, and withdrawing a volume from the vial without replacing it with an equal volume would create a vacuum, one that could draw in any surface contamination. Furthermore, the Paramedic will encounter difficulty withdrawing the medication if the pressures are not equalized. Therefore, it is essential that the Paramedic first inject air, in equal volume, into the vial before withdrawing the medicine.

Conversely, overpressurizing the vial, with additional volume of injected air from the syringe may make the drug withdrawal quicker and easier. However, as the needle is withdrawn a fine mist of medicine will escape into the air. Some commonly used medications which are packaged in a multidose vial (e.g., epinephrine) can be very caustic to the Paramedic's unprotected eyes when aerosolized in this fashion.

To withdraw medicine from the vial, the vial should be placed on a firm flat surface and held in place by the thumb and forefinger of the nondominant hand. As the Paramedic introduces the needle into the vial's stopper, the bevel should be facing upward and a slight downward pressure exerted. The downward pressure will ensure that the needle's bevel slices the stopper and does not core it. With the needle in place, visible just beyond the stopper, the Paramedic would invert the vial, inject the premeasured volume of air into the vial, and then withdraw the medicine from the vial.

Once the syringe is filled, the Paramedic would then invert the vial again and place it back onto the flat surface. With the vial stabilized between the thumb and forefinger of

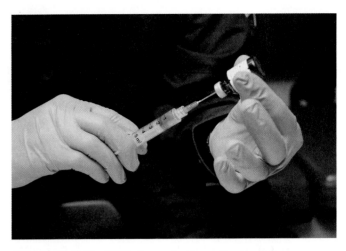

Figure 26-7 Withdrawal of medication from a vial.

the nondominant hand, the needle is then withdrawn quickly (Figure 26-7).

Inserting a needle into a dime-sized stopper held over the Paramedic's head, especially while in a moving ambulance, is dangerous and places the Paramedic at risk for a needlestick injury.

On occasion, air bubbles will inadvertently arise, typically if the medication is withdrawn too fast. If the air bubbles are visible in the barrel of the syringe, a smart tap with the forefinger will generally dislodge them, allowing them to rise to the top of the syringe. The air can then be expressed from the syringe.

STREET SMART

Some Paramedics use a large-bore "mixing" needle to draw the medication up quickly from a vial, then replace it with the smaller needle used for injection. This helps decrease potential contamination as well as speeding up the process of medication administration.

Routes of Injection

Hypothetically, the best means to get a drug directly into a target organ is to inject the organ directly. Intrathecal (within the spinal column), intrapleural (between the lung's pleura), intra-articular (within a joint), and intracardiac (within the heart) injections are just some examples of medication injections into target organs.

With the exception of intracardiac injections performed by early Paramedics before the advent of current intravenous techniques, Paramedics generally have injected drugs into the peripheral circulation and depended on the circulatory system to get the medication to the target organ. Even drugs injected into the endotracheal tube depend on absorption from the alveolar capillary beds.

The greatest drawback of indirect parenteral injection may be its dependence on adequate circulation to reach the target organ. In many cases, the patient presents to the Paramedic with inadequate circulation (these patients are hypoperfused). Subsequently, insufficient quantities of drug get to the target organs when injected via an indirect parenteral route.

Preparation for Parenteral Injection

As in all procedures performed, the Paramedic would identify the patient, introduce oneself, inquire about the patient's allergies, advise the patient about the procedure's intended effects, and then explain what reasonable and foreseeable risks could be experienced.

After obtaining informed consent, the Paramedic should practice medical asepsis, starting with hand washing with soap and water or an acceptable hand sanitizer and then don gloves. Generally, non-sterile gloves are adequate for the tasks at hand.

Success in many of these injection techniques can be improved if the Paramedic takes the time to first position the patient. With the patient resting comfortably, the Paramedic would proceed by selecting a site, chosen in accordance with commonly accepted sites used for that particular injection technique. When assessing the various sites for injection, before choosing one, care should be taken to ensure that the selected site is not hard, swollen, or tender and is free of rashes, moles, birthmarks, burns, scars, or broken skin.

After identifying the intended injection site, the Paramedic would place an isopropyl-soaked pad on the site and, working outward in ever-expanding circles, prepare an area approximately twice the length of the needle. The purpose of the alcohol bath is to remove any gross contaminates from the skin's surface as well as oils that would prevent the bandage from adhering to the skin. The alcohol bath itself does not render the skin sterile, just clean. Incidental surface contamination (bacteria and the like), which may be dragged into the wound created by the injection is dealt with by the body's defenses.

Iodine-based solutions, such as Betadine®, are generally not used because iodine seeping into the stab wound created by the injection can be irritating. It may also delay new cell growth and damage sensitive tissues in the vicinity of the injection.

With the patient prepared and the area prepped, the Paramedic would then pick up the prefilled syringe in the dominant hand and remove the needle guard. The Paramedic must then stabilize the skin with the nondominant hand. With the needle and syringe firmly in hand, the Paramedic would then proceed to firmly, and with authority, insert the needle under the skin. Studies have shown that the speed of insertion does not decrease the pain which the patient may experience.[45] However, hesitation on the Paramedic's part is telegraphed to the patient, which may cause the patient's anxiety may increase. Patient anxiety has been shown to have a positive correlation to the perception of pain.

With the needle in place, the Paramedic would gently aspirate to ensure that the needle was not inadvertently placed into a vein. If a blood flash is witnessed, then the needle should immediately be withdrawn, the medication pulled back into the syringe, and new equipment prepared. The bloody medication solution should not be injected. Instead, a new dose of medication should be drawn up in a new syringe.

Intradermal Injection

Paramedics perform **intradermal** injections under a limited set of circumstances. Intradermal injection is used when preparing an intravenous site with a local anesthetic. Intradermal injection is also used for tuberculosis testing. The objective of an intradermal injection is to place a small quantity of medicine just under the epidermis and in close proximity of the subcutaneous tissue. Because the space within the skin is very small, no more than 0.5 mL should be injected into one site.

The tools that the Paramedic needs to assemble for an intradermal injection include a 1 mL syringe and a short needle about 3/8 inch to 1/2 inch that is either 26 or 27 gauge. Sites for intradermal injection include the anterior forearm, the upper chest, and the posterior shoulders. After drawing up a small quantity of the medication (typically 0.01 to 0.1 mL), the patient is prepared as previously described.

Grasping the syringe as one would a sewing needle, the Paramedic would place the needle gently on the surface of the skin, with the needle at a 15-degree angle, and advance the needle under the skin. With the length of the needle under the skin, a small 1 cm blister is created by injecting the medication. This blister, called a **bleb**, is about the size of a mosquito bite. The needle should remain visible just under the skin the entire time.

When the task is completed, the needle is withdrawn in the same direction as it was advanced and immediately placed in a sharps container. If capillary bleeding is evident, then an adhesive bandage can be placed loosely over the site.

Capillary Blood Draw

Paramedics are increasingly requested to perform capillary blood sampling in the field. The capillary blood can then be used for blood glucose analysis or field Troponin levels. These **point of care** blood tests enhance the Paramedic's ability to provide immediate emergency services while still in the field and to transmit critical information to the emergency department.

The most common capillary blood draw is the finger stick. However, a heel stick may be preferred for small infants or children. With the limb in the dependent position, encouraging peripheral vascular congestion, the Paramedic would proceed with the routine battery of questions in order to obtain consent.

Once consent is given, the side of the finger tip proximal to the pad of the finger tip is cleansed with an alcohol prep pad (wipe). While the alcohol is drying, the lancet is picked

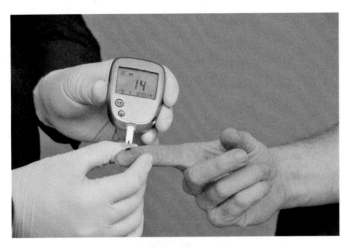

Figure 26-8 Capillary blood draw.

up by the dominant hand and prepared. In some cases, a protective cover must be removed from the lancet. In other cases, the lancet is spring-loaded and retracts back into a protective sheath. In those cases, the lancet may have to be activated (armed) before use.

Grasping the patient's finger with the gloved nondominant hand, the Paramedic would place the lancet over the site and either pierce the skin in a quick darting motion or depress the actuator of the spring-loaded lancet. Once the skin is pierced, it should bleed freely. In some cases, it may be necessary to gently milk the tip of the finger to get a hanging drop of blood. Vigorous or forceful pressure on the tip of the finger may damage local tissue. It might also introduce new fluids into the sample, possibly causing any subsequent blood test results to be invalid.

After immediately disposing of the lancet in an approved sharps container, the Paramedic would collect the droplet sample and then apply a gauze pad or self-adhesive bandage to the fingertip. The patient should be encouraged to elevate the arm above the heart (Figure 26-8).

Subcutaneous Injections

Subcutaneous injection of medication is the slowest and least dependable means of obtaining therapeutic drug levels in the bloodstream. Local conditions in the skin, such as capillary perfusion and adipose tissue, combine to make drug absorption slower and more erratic than intravenous injection.[46-48] Yet for some medications, such as heparin and insulin, the subcutaneous route is acceptable.

After providing the appropriate information and obtaining consent, an acceptable site is prepared. A variety of sites are acceptable for subcutaneous injections including the abdomen, the lateral aspects of the upper arm, and the anterior thigh, as well as the ventrodorsal gluteal area. Studies have shown that the subcutaneously injected medication is absorbed quickest from the abdomen, followed by the upper arm and then the anterior thigh. There is no data comparing the gluteal injections to the other sites.

A complication of frequent subcutaneous injections at one site, such as may occur with repeated insulin injections, is tissue fibrosis. Tissue fibrosis occurs when phagocytes infiltrate the area and attempt to remove the irritating foreign matter (the medication) and create a sterile abscess. Drugs injected into fibrotic tissues cannot be absorbed readily and will adversely affect the patient's response to the medication.

Generally, a 1 mL to 3 mL syringe is used for subcutaneous injections. The syringe is tipped with a 1/2-inch 26 to 30 gauge needle. With the syringe loaded with no more than 1.5 mL of medication for one injection and held in the dominant hand, the Paramedic would gently grasp the skin around the site with the nondominant hand. With the skin tented approximately 1 inch between the fingers, the Paramedic would insert the needle into the skin at a 45-degree angle. If the skin is tented approximately 2 inches, then it is acceptable to insert the needle at a 90-degree angle. Once the needle is inserted into the skin, the Paramedic would gently aspirate for blood and then inject into the subcutaneous pocket which has been created by pinching the skin.

Intramuscular Injections

Intramuscular injection is a common method of medication administration. Once the drug is deposited between the layers of the muscle, and below the subcutaneous tissue, it can escape into the surrounding capillary beds within the muscles and provide rapid systemic action. Intramuscular injection is frequently used for the uncooperative patient who is in need of sedation/chemical restraint to prevent harm to himself or others. Antipsychotic agents, such as haloperidol, can be given in this manner during a psychiatric or behavioral emergency. However, not all medications should, or can, be given via intramuscular injection. Digoxin, diazepam, and phenytoin are just some of the medications that are poorly absorbed via intramuscular injection.

Intramuscular injection has an advantage over intravenous injection in the elderly and immunocompromised patient. Intravenous injection bypasses the majority of the body's defenses against infection, whereas intramuscular injection preserves several of those defenses.

Intramuscular injections depend on adequate peripheral circulation. Intramuscular injections, and intramuscular injections in certain sites, may be contraindicated in patients with peripheral vascular disease and disease states which create Hypoperfusion (e.g., anaphylactic shock). Intramuscular injections also create trauma during the injection, creating a puncture wound. Some patients with coagulation disorders, such as the patient with hemophilia or one who is status-post fibrinolysis, may experience significant bleeding (a hematoma) at the injection site.

The slow distribution of intramuscular medications makes intramuscular injection a preferred route for so-called depot medications. Depot medications are medications deposited under the skin which produce sustained therapeutic levels over a longer period of time.

The intramuscular needle range is between 18 to 24 gauge and the selection of the length of the needle is more important than the gauge. If the patient is less than 110 pounds (50 kg), a 1-inch needle will generally reach the muscle below the skin. If the patient weighs between 110 and 220 pounds (50 to 100 kg), then a ½- to 2-inch needle is appropriate. For patients over 220 pounds, a needle longer than 2 inches may be needed. In the case of the morbidly obese patient, it may be necessary to use a 4-inch needle.[49] It is important that the Paramedic carefully assess the injection site. Variations in muscle development can alter the Paramedic's decision regarding needle length.

Because of the barrel's diameter, a 3 mL syringe is generally used for intramuscular injections as it provides better control. However, the syringe chosen is dependent on the volume to be administered per injection which is, in turn, dependent upon the site selected.

After the patient has consented and is properly prepared, the site is selected. There are four common intramuscular injection sites to choose from, and each site has specific advantages over the other sites.

The first site, the **ventrogluteal (VG)**, is located on the lateral thigh proximal to the hip.[50–52] The muscles underlying the VG are the gluteus medius and the gluteus minimus. What may be more important is that no large veins, arteries, or nerves underlie the area. Beyea and Nicoll reported that the ventrogluteal site had the lowest risk of nerve damage, muscle spasm, gangrene, and pain of any of the other injection sites.

To locate the site, the patient is placed in a side-lying position (lateral recumbent). The Paramedic would then palpate the bony prominence where the femur inserts into the pelvis. Placing the palm of the hand over the insertion, the Paramedic would grasp the anterior superior iliac crest with the fingers. The injection site is between the first finger and the thumb (Figure 26-9).

An alternative intramuscular injection site is the **vastus lateralis (VL)** (Figure 26-10). After positioning the patient in the supine or semi-Fowler's position, the anterior thigh is exposed. The Paramedic mentally divides the vastus lateralis muscle into three equal portions. Choosing the middle section of the VL, the Paramedic prepares the intended injection site with an alcohol-soaked pad. Next, the Paramedic draws

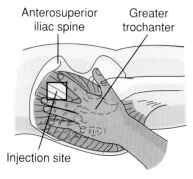

Figure 26-9 Ventrogluteal injection site.

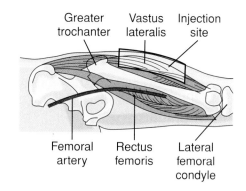

Figure 26-10 Vastus lateralis injection site.

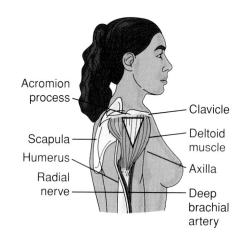

Figure 26-11 Deltoid injection site.

up the medication in the syringe and prepares the patient for the injection. Up to 2 mL of medication can be injected in the vastus lateralis without causing the patient significant discomfort.

Paramedics generally prefer to use the **deltoid** muscle (Figure 26-11) because it requires less patient exposure and is easier to access. The deltoid muscle overlays the shoulder and extends downward toward the elbow, forming an inverted triangle in the process. With the patient in high-Fowler's position, the Paramedic would instruct the patient to bend the arm at the elbow, thus relaxing the deltoid muscle. The Paramedic would then palpate the bony prominence where the humerus inserts into the shoulder. Locating the humerus, the Paramedic would measure approximately three finger-breadths down to the middle, or belly, of the deltoid muscle and prepare the site with an alcohol-soaked pad. Approximately 1 mL of medication can be given into each deltoid. The deltoid site should not be used for children who lack the muscle development in the shoulders appropriate for the injection.

The most common intramuscular injection site is the **dorsogluteal (DG)** (Figure 26-12). A large muscle, the gluteus medius, underlies the injection site and provides an excellent location for a depot of medicine. The patient is typically in the prone position (an uncommon position for patients to be transported by EMS) and then the patient's buttocks exposed. Alternatively, the patient can be placed in the side-lying

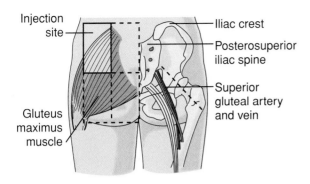

Figure 26-12 Dorsogluteal injection site.

position, or lateral recumbent position, and only the upper portion of the buttocks and the patient's flank is exposed. It should be noted that the gluteus is not synonymous with the buttock. The gluteus is located proximal to the inferior portion of the patient's flank.

As the gluteus medius is relatively large, compared to the muscles underlying the other injection sites, use of the DG site is advantageous during a restraint situation. In those situations where the patient needs sedation and/or chemical restraint for a behavioral emergency, the DG offers a large "target" and thus a greater chance of success. After the patient has been given sedatives, he should be placed in the supine, face-up position as soon as possible in order to monitor respirations and avoid positional asphyxia.

To ascertain the location of the DG injection site, the entire one buttock is mentally divided into four quadrants. The uppermost and outermost quadrant, proximate to the iliac crest, is prepared. Great care should be taken estimating the injection site as the sciatic nerve transverses two of the other three quadrants. Unintended injection into the sciatic nerve can lead to paresthesia, paralysis, and permanent nerve damage. Alternatively, the Paramedic can draw an imaginary line from the height of the iliac crest to the insertion of the femur and choose the midpoint of that line.

Generally, the DG injection site is reserved for adults. Children must be walking before a DG injection site should be considered. In the adult patient, a maximum of 5 mL can be injected into each DG site. However, the Paramedic should consider splitting the dose and doubling the sites for injection to increase patient comfort.

Painless Injections

Patients complain, sometimes bitterly, about the discomfort which can accompany an intramuscular injection. This discomfort can be related to the needle puncture and the tearing/shearing of the dermis and muscle as the needle passes through the tissue layers, as well as the presence of the medication within the tissue.

Several products are available that help to reduce the pain of needle insertion. The first, a **eutectic mixture of local anesthetics (EMLA)**, is a cream of lidocaine 2.5% and prilocaine 2.5%. EMLA is available as a self-adhesive anesthetic

disk or a cream that is applied to the intended injection site and left in place for a minimum of 60 minutes. Following removal of the dollop of cream, or the patch, the skin should be anesthetized.[53,54] While EMLA cream may not be convenient for use in the field, it should be considered in cases where repeated injections of medicine may be needed.

Alternatively, **fluori-methane** has great potential for use in the field.[55–57] Fluori-methane, a topical refrigerant, numbs the skin at the injection site in as little as 15 seconds. Fluori-methane, also referred to as a **vapocoolant spray**, can be either applied directly to the skin, though some patients complain of transient sharp discomfort, or onto a cotton ball for topical application. One study suggested that a vapocoolant spray was equally as effective as EMLA cream. Another study indicated that placing ice alone on the skin, for 30 seconds, was not effective in reducing pain during injection.

The next potential source of injection pain is the trauma created by the needle's insertion. One study suggests that the biomechanics of injection (i.e., proper injection technique) is important to the patient's comfort.[58–61] A needle held and inserted in a linear manner, perpendicular to the plane of the skin, reduces the "path width" compared to the path width seen with a curved (arcing) needle path. Tissue shearing is minimized and therefore patient discomfort lessened.

Finally, there is the matter of the medication deposited within the muscle. This discomfort is, in large part, due to the leakage of the caustic and irritating drugs into the pain receptors of the subcutaneous tissues. The deeper muscle layers are relatively free of pain receptors. The application of a few easy to perform techniques which "lock" the drugs into the muscle will decrease the patient's discomfort and improve the Paramedic's confidence with injection skills.

Two techniques have been developed by nurses to decrease this leakage and the accompanying discomfort. Both techniques involve careful attention to the particulars of the injection technique. The first technique, the **airlock**, is performed while preparing the drug in the syringe for injection. The second technique, the **Z-track**, involves manipulation of the injection site during the injection.

The airlock technique has the Paramedic injecting a small bubble of air into the injection, essentially sealing off the drug below from leaking out to the subcutaneous tissues above. To create an airlock, the Paramedic fills the syringe with the medication as usual. With the syringe clear of the ampoule, the Paramedic would then withdraw the plunger further, clearing the drug from the needle and entraining about 0.1 mL of air into the syringe. It is important that the Paramedic verify that the correct volume of drug remains in the syringe (Figure 26-13).

Quickly inverting the syringe should cause an air bubble to be created at the apex of the plunger. With the air bubble in place, the Paramedic would proceed to the injection. For the airlock technique to work, it is essential that the syringe remain at an upright 90-degree plane from the injection surface. This ensures that the air bubble is injected at the end of the injection. The ventrogluteal (VG) site and the dorsal gluteal (DG) site are conducive to this technique.

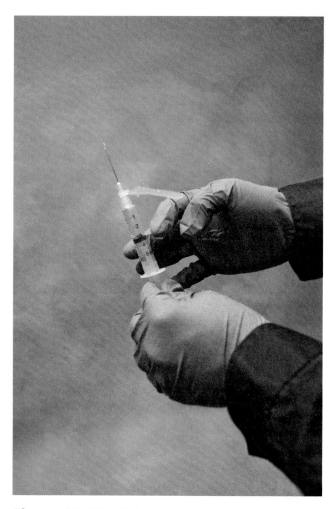

Figure 26-13 Airlock technique.

Another technique that can help prevent drug leakage into the subcutaneous tissue is the Z-track technique. The Z-track technique creates an offset injection pathway, using subcutaneous tissue to block leakage.[62]

To create a Z-track, the Paramedic with the drug-filled syringe in the dominant hand, bevel up, would pull gentle traction on the injection site with the nondominant hand. Frequently, Paramedics will grasp the upper arm, if the deltoid is used, and pull traction with the thumb of the nondominant hand. With a smart flick of the wrist, as if one was throwing a dart, the needle is inserted into the skin. After aspiration confirms proper placement, the drug is injected in a deliberate fashion. Injecting the drug too quickly can create discomfort as stretch receptors are stimulated by the presence of the space-occupying depot of medicine. Alternatively, injecting, or "pushing," the drug too slowly can cause increased patient apprehension. Practice establishes the best rate of administration.

The next actions taken by the Paramedic are critical to the success of the Z-track technique (Figure 26-14). Before the needle is withdrawn from the skin, the Paramedic must release the traction on the skin. Thus, when the needle is completely withdrawn the skin overlying the muscle will slide over the medication depot, closing it off to the surface.

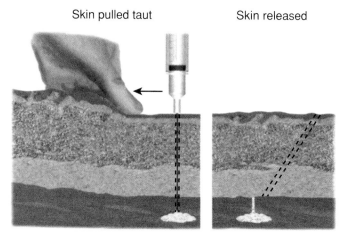

Figure 26-14 Z-track injection technique.

Injection Site Massage

Some controversy surrounds the common practice of massaging the area surrounding the injection site immediately after the injection. In some cases, it is acceptable to gently massage the area surrounding the injection. Gentle pressure applied to the area dissipates the impact of the sharp pain receptors through competition with various pain fibers. However, some medications are caustic to the muscle tissue. With these medications, massaging the area distributes the medication over a larger area, creating more discomfort for the patient.

The Paramedic should be knowledgeable about the medication before just routinely proceeding with massaging all injection sites. For example, it is acceptable to massage the site following an injection of morphine sulfate in order to decrease the patient's discomfort, but massaging the site after an injection of diazepam would only serve to increase the patient's discomfort.

Also at issue with the routine practice of massaging an injection site is its impact on absorption. While intramuscular injection of insulin is uncommon, its rate of absorption is quicker via intramuscular injection than subcutaneous injection. This quality makes intramuscularly injected insulin attractive during a diabetic emergency. However, massage of the injection site can dissipate the insulin even further, making its uptake more rapid and creating a risk of unanticipated hypoglycemia. If the Paramedic is unsure if massaging the injection site is acceptable, then the maxim of "do no harm" should be followed and the injection site should not be massaged.

Special Populations

The two extremes of age—elderly and children—each present a special challenge for the Paramedic who must perform an injection. Both the patient and the provider alike are anxious during a pediatric injection. To develop strategies to improve success, the Paramedic must take into account the child's developmental stage and adjust the approach accordingly.

In many cases, the infant is unaware of the events surrounding him or her, but is acutely aware of the discomfort that follows. In those cases, it may be acceptable to have the infant held in the mother's arms to be comforted after the procedure.

The greatest challenge may be the toddler. The toddler is keenly aware of his or her environment, is able to comprehend the situation, and receives a great deal of emotional feedback from parents as well as caregivers. Typically, a toddler must be temporarily restrained during the injection. One technique is to place the toddler on the parent's lap, chest to chest, with the parent's arms entrapping the child. The toddler's legs would then be aside and behind the parent. The Paramedic would approach the parent from behind, grasp the outstretched leg, and perform the injection.

The elderly patient presents a challenge of another kind. The combination of age and poor nutrition reduces muscle mass, limiting available injection sites. These emaciated patients, with less muscle mass and loss of the capillary beds, tend to absorb medications less readily.

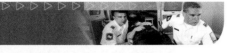

STREET SMART

Uninformed Paramedics mistakenly think it is preferable to inject medications below the level of injury of a paraplegia patient, eliminating the pain which can accompany an injection. The drug absorption below the level of the spinal injury is erratic and unpredictable.

CONCLUSION

The large number of medication administration routes and techniques represent a substantial portion of the universe of skills that a Paramedic must master. Each medication route has its advantages and its drawbacks, its indications and its contraindications. It is the Paramedic's responsibility to ensure that the patient's medication needs and the preferred medication route are compatible.

KEY POINTS:

- It is a Paramedic's responsibility to choose the right drug and the right dose for the patient, and to administer it by the right route at the right time in order to achieve the optimal therapeutic effect.

- Forms of medication can be grossly categorized into liquids, solids, and injectable liquids.

- Injectable forms of medication come in either ampoules or vials. Vials are essentially resealable ampoules and may be used for multiple patients.

- The apothecary system of measurements includes units of grain (gr) and is rarely used today by physicians.

- The common household system or United States customary system contains such units as the ounce and the teaspoon and remains the predominant system of measurement in the United States and Canada.

- The metric system is based in units of 10.

- Insulin and penicillin are examples of medications that are measured in international units (IU). This unit represents the relative strength of the substance after it has been tested on an organism.

- Conversions of metric measurements are based on a factor of 10. All multiplications above 1 gram are noted in the Greek prefixes kilo-, hecto-, and deca-, whereas all divisions of a gram are noted by the Latin prefixes deci-, centi-, milli-, and micro-.

- The most accurate method of converting a patient's weight from pounds to kilograms is dividing the patient's weight in pounds by 2.26 and obtaining the weight in kilograms. However, the Paramedic may also divide the patient's weight, in pounds, in half, then subtract 10% off from the result for an approximate weight.

- A drug concentration is described as the amount of drug in 1 milliliter (mL) of a solution.

- Some prehospital medications must be mixed just before use to ensure maximum effectiveness.

- A standard drug order states the amount of the drug, the name of the drug, and the route that is to be administered.

- When an adult dose must be adjusted to a pediatric dose, and the pediatric dosing is not available, then the child's total body surface area (BSA) is divided against the total body surface area of an adult— approximately 1.73 meters squared for a 6-foot tall, 150-pound adult. The resulting percentage is then taken from the adult dose and is roughly equal to the pediatric dose.

- Intravenous fluids may be infused at a "wide open" rate to administer a large volume of fluid quickly, at a prescribed rate per hour or minute, or at a KVO rate of 50 mL per hour to keep the catheter patent.

- Methods for determining an intravenous drug infusion rate include the formula method and the clock method.

- Weight-dependent intravenous drug infusions include the patient's weight in the standard drug infusion calculation.

- To convert Fahrenheit to Celsius (medical standard temperature measurement), the EMS provider subtracts 32 from the Fahrenheit result and then multiplies by 5/9.

- Paramedics practice the five rights of medication administration.

- After being given any drug, the patient is re-evaluated to see if the drug was effective. This re-evaluation, and subsequent documentation of patient response to medication, is so important that some Paramedics refer to it as the sixth right, the right documentation.

- The initials DARE, a simple mnemonic, can help Paramedics remember the elements of documentation for every medication administration.

- The Paramedic can use the mnemonic AIR to obtain an informed consent from a competent patient.

- Local routes of medication administration are intended to target a specific organ or function. Optic medications are applied directly to the eye, and otic medications are applied to the ear.

- The inner mucosa of the nostrils has a rich capillary bed that is an excellent route for the administration of systemic medications. Local nasal medications can be applied via an atomizer into the intended nostril, propelling the medicine against the mucosa. Like the nose, the mouth has a capillary-rich mucosa that will rapidly absorb any medicine and distribute it systemically.

- Though not widely used, local topical medications may include the application of a topical antibiotic at the insertion site of an intravenous catheter. Other local medications can be douches (solutions introduced into the vagina via an apparatus) or enemas (solutions introduced into the anus via an apparatus).

- The enteral route of systemic drug administration refers to medications given via the gastrointestinal tract (e.g., oral medications). Parenteral routes of medication administration include inhalation and injection.

- The sublingual route is an enteral route whereby medication, in a liquid or solid form, is placed in the space inferior to the tongue, where it is rapidly absorbed. The distinct advantage to the sublingual route is that it bypasses the liver and thus avoids hepatic first pass metabolism. Using the buccal route, or cheek, is similar to administering medications sublingually.

- The vast majority of self-administered medications are swallowed. The solid pill, capsule, or liquid is then absorbed in the gastrointestinal tract, where it is passed (via the portal circulation) through the liver and on into the central circulation. From an EMS perspective, the patient must be able to maintain the airway independently and swallow the medication.

- Gastric tubes can be placed to instill feedings as well as medications in the form of liquids or suspensions. Most Paramedics insert an orogastric tube in order to evacuate or decompress the stomach. Use of a special gastric tube, called a Sengstaken-Blakemore tube, permits the Paramedic to apply direct pressure inside the stomach or esophagus to the source of bleeding.

- Intermittent suction or the placement of a dual-lumen gastric tube helps prevent a gastric tube from adhering to the gastric mucosa, leading to local irritation and bleeding. After the placement of a gastric tube, the patient should be monitored for signs of hypoxia, such as premature ventricular contractions (PVC), and altered level of responsiveness. If the gastric tube is obstructed, the Paramedic can irrigate the tube with saline or sterile water instilled into the tube via syringe.

- Drugs that are absorbed from the rectum avoid inactivation by stomach acids and intestinal enzymes. Around 50% of the absorbed drug bypasses the portal circulation, minimizing the impacts of first pass metabolism and biotransformation. To administer the medication, the patient is placed in a modified left lateral position, called the Sim's position. The rectal administration route is useful when the patient is unable to accept oral medications, such as in the case of persistent vomiting or continuous seizures in children.

- When a rapid onset of drug action is required (e.g., during an emergency), the parenteral route offers the most direct route to the target organs, sidestepping the gastrointestinal system (enteral administration) and delivering drugs directly to the central circulation. Advantages of these routes include circumventing the GI absorption process, maintaining more predictable serum drug levels, and using them with patients who are uncooperative or incapable of cooperation (e.g., unconscious).

- Intranasal administration takes advantage of the nasal passages. They are lined with very vascular mucous membranes that can absorb medications quickly and without the risk of first pass metabolism associated with enteral routes of drug administration. The intranasal route works well with patients with altered mental status or combativeness, and/or when the Paramedic is in a moving ambulance. Several drugs can be administered intranasally. The clear advantage of intranasal administration of drugs is the decreased risk of accidental needle injury.

- Naxolone is a drug used for suspected opioid overdoses. The use of naxolone intranasally is considered "off-label use," meaning the FDA has not approved the drug for use in this manner. The volume administered intranasally should be no more than 1 mL of liquid, and the drug should be atomized to a particle size of between 10 mcg and 50 mcg, the optimal particle size for absorption.

- The inhalation of medications is the inhalation of drug-laden vapors into the bloodstream via the respiratory route. Pulmonary treatments focus on the delivery of respiratory agents directly into the pulmonary tree. The common drawback to both these methods is the dependence on the patient's respiratory function.

- As air enters the lungs, it meets resistance as the structures narrow. The resistance slows the air down; by the time it reaches the alveoli, it is nearly still. This encourages fallout, as large particles carried in the air settle out as the velocity is lost. The result is that nearly particulate-free air enters the alveoli. This works against large droplets of aerosolized medications and reduces the effectiveness of many respiratory drugs.

- The metered dose inhaler (MDI) is a portable and well-accepted respiratory treatment platform. However, it is relatively ineffective, depositing less than 20% of the medication in the distal lung fields. A spacer device can be used to increase MDI's effectiveness. Dry powder inhalers (DPI) use a pulverized solid drug for inhalation with a delivery device similar to an MDI. Again, the effectiveness of

the medication depends on the patient's inspiratory effort.

- By suspending the medication in a stream of air, the small volume nebulizer (SVN) is thought to produce a better particle size for inhalation (about 1 to 3 microns). Prior to using an SVN, the Paramedic should conduct a history to determine the patient's responsiveness to MDI bronchodilators. He should also perform a physical, auscultating for wheezes or absent breath sounds. Key to assessing the effectiveness of any SVN treatment is the patient's subjective judgment regarding her own dyspnea. For intubated patients, a SVN may be attached in-line with the bag-valve-mask assembly.

- Topical medication absorption into the subcutaneous capillary beds, or transdermal medicine, offers a drug administration route that can have sustained systemic delivery of a medication. Medications given via a transdermal patch can include nicotine, hormone replacement, opiate analgesics, and nitroglycerine.

- The components of a hypodermic syringe include the syringe and the needle, often connected via a luer lock or slip-tip adaptor. Syringes are labeled according to the volume within the barrel (e.g., 1, 3, 5 mL) and the calibrations on the side of the barrel. The exception is insulin syringes, which are labeled in international units (IU). Surface tension and adhesion of water to the walls of the syringe form a meniscus. The volume of the drug in the syringe is determined by comparing the bottom of the meniscus with the calibration on the barrel.

- The needle is the second component of the hypodermic syringe. Measured in gauges, the smaller the number means the larger the diameter of the needle (e.g., 14 gauge > 20 gauge). The Paramedic should choose a needle size dependent on the viscosity of the fluid and speed of delivery. Injecting a drug into a medication port of an intravenous set, or performing an intramuscular, subcutaneous, or intradermal injection, all require a specific size and length needle.

- Retractable needles, self-sheathing needles, needles that have a retractable hard case that is advanced over the needle as the needle is withdrawn, and hooded needles that have a protective covering over the needle are all efforts made through engineering controls to help prevent needlestick injury.

- It is every Paramedic's responsibility to safely dispose of used/contaminated needles into a safe sharps container. The sharps container should be close at hand, within arm's reach, and be easy to access.

- Medications are packaged in either vials or ampoules. There are prefilled ampoules/syringe systems as well as glass ampoules that have to be broken before the medication can be withdrawn. When withdrawing air from a vial, it is essential that the Paramedic first inject air, in equal volume, into the vial before withdrawing the medicine to prevent a vacuum.

- There are many routes of injection that deliver a drug directly into the target organ. Indirect parenteral injections are also effective means of delivering medications. However, the greatest drawback is its dependence on adequate circulation to reach the target organ.

- Positioning the patient is the first step in preparation for an injection. The injection site selected should not be hard, swollen, or tender and must be free of rashes, moles, birthmarks, burns, scars, or broken skin. The Paramedic should place an isopropyl-soaked pad on the site and, working outward in ever-expanding circles, prepare an area approximately twice the length of the needle. The skin is stabilized with the Paramedic's nondominant hand and, with the needle in the dominant hand, the needle is inserted under the skin. With the needle in place, the Paramedic would gently aspirate to ensure that the needle was not inadvertently placed into a vein.

- Intradermal injections may be used when preparing an intravenous site with a local anesthetic or for tuberculosis testing. The objective of an intradermal injection is to place a small quantity of medicine just under the epidermis and in close proximity of the subcutaneous tissue. Point of care blood testing can be performed with blood glucose analysis or field troponin levels. A finger stick or, for pediatric patients, a heel stick is performed to obtain a small sample of blood for analysis.

- Subcutaneous injection of medication is the slowest and least dependable means of obtaining therapeutic drug levels in the bloodstream. Acceptable sites for subcutaneous injections including the abdomen, the lateral aspects of the upper arm, and the anterior thigh, as well as the ventrodorsal gluteal area. Frequent subcutaneous injections at one site, such as may occur with repeated insulin injections, result in tissue fibrosis.

- Intramuscular injection deposits the drug between the layers of the muscle, and below the subcutaneous tissue, providing rapid systemic action. Intramuscular injections are contraindicated in patients with peripheral vascular disease and disease states which create hypoperfusion (e.g., anaphylactic shock). Intramuscular injection is a preferred route for so-called depot medications deposited under the skin to produce sustained therapeutic levels over a longer period of time.

- There are four common sites for intramuscular injection. The first site, the ventrogluteal (VG) muscle, is located on the lateral thigh proximal to the hip. A more anterior injection site is the middle portion of the vastus lateralis (VL) muscle of the thigh. Requiring less exposure and easier access is the deltoid muscle. The most common intramuscular injection site is the dorsogluteal (DG) muscle. The gluteus is located proximal to the inferior portion of the patient's flank.

- EMLA cream, a topical anesthetic, can be used to reduce the pain of needle insertion. Fluori-methane and vapocoolant spray are also applied directly to the skin for anesthetic effects. The deeper muscle layers are relatively free of pain receptors, although irritation may occur from a drug if leaked into subcutaneous tissues. To prevent this, the airlock and Z-track techniques may be used by the Paramedic for intramuscular injections.

- The elderly and children each present a special challenge to the Paramedic who must perform an injection. To develop strategies to improve success of a pediatric injection, the Paramedic must take into account the child's developmental stage and adjust the approach accordingly. For the elderly, the combination of age and poor nutrition reduces muscle mass, limiting available injection sites.

REVIEW QUESTIONS:

1. Before administering any medication, what are the six rights a Paramedic is responsible for confirming?

2. Explain how medication levels comparable to venous injection can be provided using rectally inserted medications (e.g., suppositories).

3. Define what the international unit (IU) represents and give two examples of medications that are administered using this system of measurement.

4. The Paramedic is presented with a patient who weighs 260 pounds. Medical control has ordered that the Paramedic administer dopamine 5 mcg/kg/min using a 60 drop administration set. The Paramedic has one vial of dopamine 400 mg in 4 mL and a 250 cc bag of normal saline. Write out the formula and calculate the number of drops per minute that should be administered.

5. Identify and describe the characteristics of solid and liquid forms of medication.

6. Explain why the metric system or SI is used for medication calculation as opposed to household measurements.

7. What is the relationship between cubic centimeters of water and milliliters of water?

8. What complications exist when treating a patient with either an inhaler or nebulized medication? What can the Paramedic do to overcome these challenges?

9. Using proper anatomical terminology, describe the four locations for intramuscular injections.

10. Describe the two techniques that have been developed to decrease the leakage and discomfort of IM injections.

CASE STUDY QUESTIONS:

Please refer to the Case Study at the beginning of the chapter and answer the questions below:

1. What systems of measurement exist? Why are protocols written in metric measurements?

2. What are the standard metric units for length, volume, and weight?

3. What are two measures of temperature?

4. You have contacted medical control, given report, and have now been given an order for a medication. What are the elements of a drug order that should be performed when receiving a medication order?

REFERENCES:

1. Pond SM, Tozer TN. First-pass elimination. Basic concepts and clinical consequences. *Clin Pharmacokinet.* 1984;9(1):1–25.

2. Foulkes J, Wallace DM. Haemorrhage from stomal varices in an ileal conduit. *Br J Urol.* 1975;47(6):630.

3. Flomenbaum N, Goldfrank L, Hoffman R, Howland M, Lewin N, Nelson L. *Goldfrank's Toxicologic Emergencies.* New York: McGraw-Hill Professional; 2006.

4. de Boer AG, Moolenaar F, et al. Rectal drug administration: clinical pharmacokinetic considerations. *Clin Pharmacokinet.* 1982;7(4):285–311.

5. Lee C, Gnanasegaram D, et al. Best evidence topic report. Rectal or intravenous non-steroidal anti-inflammatory drugs in acute renal colic. *Emerg Med J.* 2005;22(9):653–654.

6. Appleton R, Martland T, et al. Drug management for acute tonic-clonic convulsions including convulsive status epilepticus in children. *Cochrane Database Syst Rev.* 2002;4:CD001905.

7. Bergeson PS, Smith EI. The international system of units (SI) and medicine. *West J Med.* 1981;135(6):526–529.

8. Barclay WR. Medicine, metrication, and SI units. *JAMA.* 1980;244(3):241–242.

9. Brunetti L. Abbreviations formally linked to medication errors. *Healthcare Benchmarks Qual Improv.* 2007;14(11):126–128.

10. Hicks RW, Becker SC. An overview of intravenous-related medication administration errors as reported to MEDMARX, a national medication error-reporting program. *J Infus Nurs.* 2006;29(1):20–27.

11. Hicks RW, Cousins DD, et al. Selected medication-error data from USP's MEDMARX program for 2002. *Am J Health Syst Pharm.* 2004;61(10):993–1000.

12. Angelos MG, Butke RL, et al. Cardiovascular response to epinephrine varies with increasing duration of cardiac arrest. *Resuscitation. 2007;77*(1):101–110.

13. Reynolds JC, Rittenberger JC, et al. Drug administration in animal studies of cardiac arrest does not reflect human clinical experience. *Resuscitation.* 2007;74(1):13–26.

14. Ong ME, Lim SH, et al. Intravenous adrenaline or vasopressin in sudden cardiac arrest: a literature review. *Ann Acad Med Singapore.* 2002;31(6):785–792.

15. Zhang H, Zhang J, et al. Oral mucosal drug delivery: clinical pharmacokinetics and therapeutic applications. *Clin Pharmacokinet.* 2002;41(9):661–680.

16. Kirsten R, Nelson K, et al. Clinical pharmacokinetics of vasodilators. Part II. *Clin Pharmacokinet.* 1998;35(1):9–36.

17. Vale JA, Kulig K. Position paper: Gastric lavage. *J Toxicol Clin Toxicol.* 2004;42(7):933–943.

18. Christensen T. The treatment of oesophageal varices using a Sengstaken-Blakemore tube: considerations for nursing practice. *Nurs Crit Care.* 2004;9(2):58–63.

19. Pasquale MD, Cerra FB. Sengstaken-Blakemore tube placement. Use of balloon tamponade to control bleeding varices. *Crit Care Clin.* 1992;8(4):743–753.

20. Brimacomb J, Keller C, et al. Reliability of epigastric auscultation to detect gastric insufflation. *Br J Anaesth.* 2002;88(1):127–129.

21. Neumann MJ, Meyer CT, et al. Hold that x-ray: aspirate pH and auscultation prove enteral tube placement. *J Clin Gastroenterol.* 1995;20(4):293–295.

22. Elpern EH, Killeen K, et al. Capnometry and air insufflation for assessing initial placement of gastric tubes. *Am J Crit Care.* 2007;16(6):544–549; quiz 550.

23. O'Dell C, Shinnar S, et al. Rectal diazepam gel in the home management of seizures in children. *Pediatr Neurol.* 2005;33(3):166–172.

24. Dreifuss FE, Rosman NP, et al. A comparison of rectal diazepam gel and placebo for acute repetitive seizures. *N Engl J Med.* 1998;338(26):1869–1875.

25. Welling PG. Influence of food and diet on gastrointestinal drug absorption: a review. *J Pharmacokinet Biopharm.* 1977;5(4):291–334.

26. Williams L, Hill DP, Jr., et al. The influence of food on the absorption and metabolism of drugs: an update. *Eur J Drug Metab Pharmacokinet.* 1996;21(3):201–211.

27. Fagerholm U. Prediction of human pharmacokinetics—gastrointestinal absorption. *J Pharm Pharmacol.* 2007;59(7):905–916.

28. Costantino HR, Illum L, et al. Intranasal delivery: physicochemical and therapeutic aspects. *Int J Pharm.* 2007;337(1-2):1–24.

29. Salinas E. Abbott LF. Transfer of coded information from sensory to motor networks. *J Neurosci.* 1995;15(10):6461–6474.

30. Song Y, Wang Y, et al. Mucosal drug delivery: membranes, methodologies, and applications. *Crit Rev Ther Drug Carrier Syst.* 2004;21(3):195–256.

31. United States Department of Labor, Occupational Safety and Health Administration. Bloodborne pathogens 29 CFR – 1910.1030. Available at: http://www.osha.gov/pls/oshaweb/owadisp.show_document?p_table=STANDARDS&p_id=10051. Accessed May 28, 2009.

32. Barton ED, Ramos J, Colwell C, et al. Intranasal administration of naloxone by paramedics. *Prehospital Emergency Care.* January-March 2002;6(1):54–58.

33. Gudmundsdottir H, Sigurjonsdottir JF, Masson M, et al. Intranasal administration of midazolam in a cyclodextrin based formulation: bioavailability and clinical evaluation in humans. *Die Pharmazie.* December 2001;56(12):963–966.

34. Silverman BL, Barnes CJ, et al. Inhaled insulin for controlling blood glucose in patients with diabetes. *Vasc Health Risk Manag.* 2007;3(6):947–958.

35. Hollander PA. Evolution of a pulmonary insulin delivery system (Exubera) for patients with diabetes. *MedGenMed.* 2007;9(1):45.

36. Dolovich MA. Influence of inspiratory flow rate, particle size, and airway caliber on aerosolized drug delivery to the lung. *Respir Care*. 2000;45(6):597–608.

37. Thompson PJ. Drug delivery to the small airways. *Am J Respir Crit Care Med*. 1998;157(5 Pt 2):S199–S202.

38. Geller DE. Comparing clinical features of the nebulizer, metered-dose inhaler, and dry powder inhaler. *Respir Care*. 2005;50(10):1313–1321; discussion 1321–1322.

39. Buxton LJ, Baldwin JH, et al. The efficacy of metered-dose inhalers with a spacer device in the pediatric setting. *J Am Acad Nurse Pract*. 2002;14(9):390–397.

40. De Benedictis FM, Selvaggio D. Use of inhaler devices in pediatric asthma. *Paediatr Drugs*. 2003;5(9):629–638.

41. MacIntyre NR, Cheng KC, et al. Applied PEEP during pressure support reduces the inspiratory threshold load of intrinsic PEEP. *Chest*. 1997;111(1):188–193.

42. Wrenn K. The hazards of defibrillation through nitroglycerin patches. *Ann Emerg Med*. 1990;19(11):1327–1328.

43. West K. Infection-control basics. A common sense review for EMS personnel. *Jems*. 2002;27(5):115–118, 120, 122–125.

44. Tatelbaum MF. Needlestick safety and prevention act. *Pain Physician*. 2001;4(2):193–195.

45. Redd DA, Boudreaux AM, et al. Towards less painful local anesthesia. *Ala Med*. 1990;60(4):18–19.

46. Hildebrandt P. Subcutaneous absorption of insulin in insulin-dependent diabetic patients. Influence of species, physico-chemical properties of insulin and physiological factors. *Dan Med Bull*. 1991;38(4):337–346.

47. Hildebrandt P, Birch K. Basal rate subcutaneous insulin infusion: absorption kinetics and relation to local blood flow. *Diabet Med*. 1988;5(5):434–440.

48. Hildebrandt PR, Vaag AA. Local skin-fold thickness as a clinical predictor of depot size during basal rate infusion of insulin. *Diabetes Care*. 1993;16(1):1–3.

49. Zaybak A, Gunes UY, et al. Does obesity prevent the needle from reaching muscle in intramuscular injections? *J Adv Nurs*. 2007;58(6):552–556.

50. Donaldson C, Green J. Using the ventrogluteal site for intramuscular injections. *Nurs Times*. 2005;101(16):36–38.

51. Small SP. Preventing sciatic nerve injury from intramuscular injections: literature review. *J Adv Nurs*. 2004;47(3):287–296.

52. Greenway K. Using the ventrologluteal site for intramuscular injection. *Nurs Stand*. 2004;18(25):39–42.

53. Zempsky WT, Cravero JP. Relief of pain and anxiety in pediatric patients in emergency medical systems. *Pediatrics*. 2004;114(5):1348–1356.

54. Blouin A, Molez S, et al. A novel procedure for daily measurements of hemodynamical, hematological, and biochemical parameters in conscious unrestrained rats. *J Pharmacol Toxicol Methods*. 2000;44(3):489–505.

55. Yoon WY, Chung SP, et al. Analgesic pretreatment for antibiotic skin test: vapocoolant spray vs ice cube. *Am J Emerg Med*. 2008;26(1):59–61.

56. Cohen Reis E, Holubkov R. Vapocoolant spray is equally effective as EMLA cream in reducing immunization pain in school-aged children. *Pediatrics*. 1997;100(6):E5.

57. Williams RH, Nollert MU. Platelet-derived NO slows thrombus growth on a collagen type III surface. *Thromb J*. 2004;2(1):11.

58. Warren BL. Intramuscular injection angle: evidence for practice? *Nurs Prax N Z*. 2002;18(2):42–51.

59. Katsma DL, Katsma R. The myth of the 90 degrees-angle intramuscular injection. *Nurse Educ*. 2000;25(1):34–37.

60. Petousis-Harris H. Needle angle when giving i.m. vaccinations. *Nurs Prax N Z*. 2002;18(2):52–53.

61. Chung JW, Ng WM, et al. An experimental study on the use of manual pressure to reduce pain in intramuscular injections. *J Clin Nurs*. 2002;11(4):457–461.

62. Rodger M.A. King L. Drawing up and administering intramuscular injections: a review of the literature. *J Adv Nurs*. 2000;31(3):574–582.

CHAPTER 27

INTRAVENOUS ACCESS

KEY CONCEPTS:

Upon completion of this chapter, it is expected that the reader will understand these following concepts:

- Fluid balance
- Indications for intravenous access
- Method for venipuncture
- Complications of intravenous access
- Techniques and strategies for pediatric phlebotomy and intravenous access
- Alternative access points and central venous access devices

▶ CASE STUDY:

As the second unit rolled up onto the scene of a two-car MVC, the Paramedics heard from the first unit that they should set up a trauma line for the driver of car #2. She was being extricated now and had significant injuries. Oh, and by the way, the driver was Mrs. Gorino.

Everyone knew Mrs. Gorino. She was a pleasant woman who had battled back from breast cancer but needed frequent hospitalizations for a myriad of medical problems. Only the best of the best Paramedics could find IV access on her.

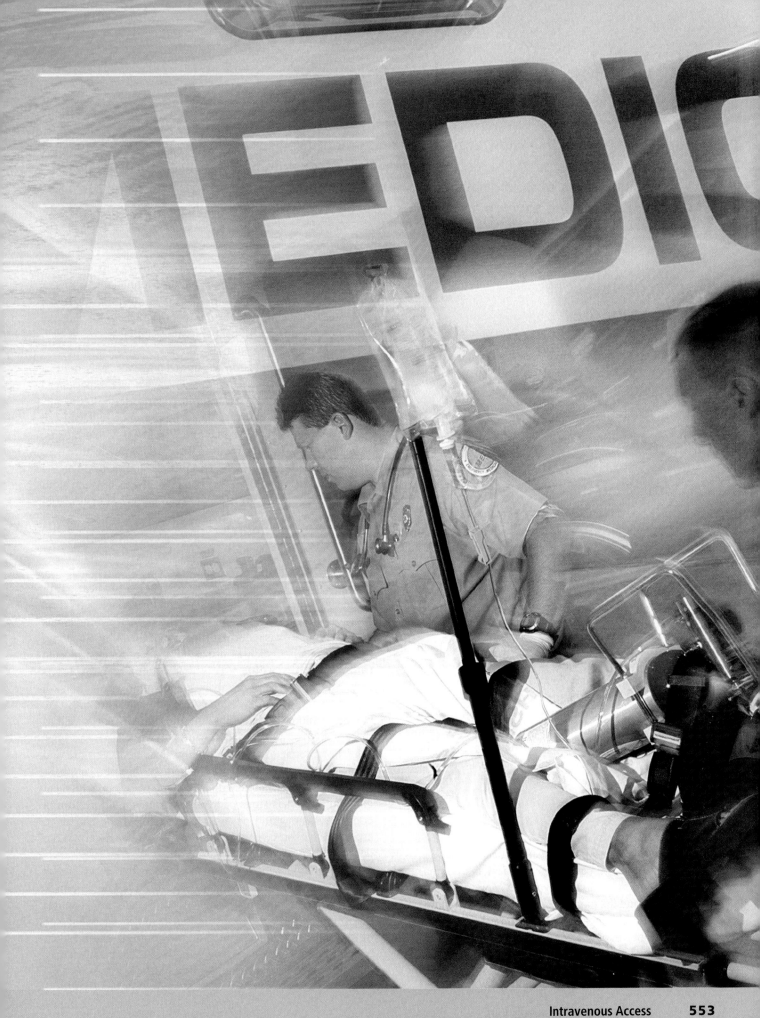

OVERVIEW

Intravenous access allows the Paramedic to administer medications and manage a patient's intravascular volume. To effectively care for the patient, the Paramedic must have a commanding knowledge of the equipment used for intravenous access, as well as complete assessment skills and techniques. By examining the sources of fluid loss and clinical signs of fluid displacement, the Paramedic can determine the need for intravenous access and develop an appropriate treatment plan. Needs and skills vary according to age and clinical condition.

Intravenous Access and Paramedics

The public distinguishes the Paramedic from basic life support providers by the Paramedic's ability to start intravenous access (IV). The public knows that an IV permits the Paramedic to give pain medicine and other life-saving drugs. Perhaps no other ALS skill is practiced as often as intravenous access. Therefore, the Paramedic should be an expert at establishing intravenous access.

Physiology Review

The human body is primarily made up of water, about 30 liters of water, which is distributed across three compartments. When thinking of body fluids, the first compartment generally considered is the intravascular space in which the blood volume is contained within the arterial, capillary, and venous vessels. However, the bulk of the water is contained within the second compartment, the intracellular compartment (ICF), while the remaining volume is contained in the third compartment, the extracellular fluid (ECF). The extracellular fluid (ECF) bathes the cells as interstitial fluid.

The constant ebb and flow of these fluids across these three compartments, exchanging gasses, hormones, glucose, fatty acids, and wastes, is the basis for nutritional flow. Using this nutritional flow to an advantage, Paramedics can inject a concentrated quantity of medication, called a **bolus**, into the intravascular space and reasonably expect that the medication will make it into the cells of the target organ.

Medical vs Trauma

The rationale for obtaining intravenous access can be grossly broken down into two categories: medical and trauma. Both patient populations undoubtedly need venous access in cases of emergency, and the risk/benefit of obtaining an intravenous line leans so decidedly toward providing benefit that Paramedics attempt venous access almost all emergent patients and most urgent patients. What remains undecided is the use of intravenous infusions in specific cases.

Medical lines, sometimes called lifelines, are a means of giving medications directly into the circulation. A number of methods have been devised to gain venous access, yet one constant remains for all of them—intravenous access is necessary for medication administration.

The second indication for intravenous access is trauma. Blood losses can make the patient who has experienced trauma hypovolemic. A **trauma line** is inserted into the vascular space so that intravascular volume can be replaced and homeostasis restored. In some cases, a patient with traumatic injury may need medications. Conversely, a medical patient may experience a significant loss of fluid and require volume replacement, though there has been no trauma. It is apparent that the divisions are not clean and each type of line is sometimes used for the other purpose.

Sources of Fluid Loss

Fluid loss, due to either illness or injury, is an indication for intravenous access. By understanding the sources of fluid loss, the Paramedic can anticipate the need for intravenous access. Fluid loss is a normal function of the body. Such loss may be apparent, such as urination, or may be unsuspected (insensible). **Insensible loss** is that volume of fluid that is lost from the body in the form of perspiration off the skin (1.1 liters/daily) and the vapor in the breath. Normally, the patient would replace this loss through fluid intake as well as the water contained in the foodstuffs ingested.

The amount of fluids normally lost, both sensible and insensible losses, can be accelerated by disease. Paramedics who are confronted with a patient who has a medical complaint and has signs of hypoperfusion should perform a complete history and physical assessment of the patient to ascertain the source of the fluid loss as well as ascertain the degree of hypovolemia.

A common cause of increased insensible fluid loss is increased perspiration secondary to fevers due to infection.[1,2] This loss, combined with the anorexia (lack of appetite) that often accompanies a fever, can result in an imbalance of fluid intake versus output. Add the vomiting and diarrhea which often accompanies many illnesses, and the patient may quickly develop a significant fluid imbalance.

During a 24-hour period, the average person will excrete—and then reabsorb—approximately one-half of her intravascular volume into the lumen of the intestines. This process of excretion and reabsorption of nutrient ladened fluids constitutes **nutritional flow** and is essential to the body's sustenance. Any process which interferes with that flow can create fluid imbalances.

Beyond the fluid loss that accompanies vomiting and diarrhea, other gastrointestinal problems can create hypovolemia secondary to the fluid loss. For example, a patient with a small bowel obstruction will not be able to reabsorb the fluids in the large bowel as the patient normally would. Subsequently, the fluids excreted into the small bowel are sequestered behind the obstruction, leading to a distended abdomen. The volume of fluids is not returned to the central circulation as would normally occur.

Draining abdominal fistula, ileostomy, colostomy, and aggressive nasogastric tube suctioning, as well as overuse or misuse of renal diuretics, are other examples of important sources of fluid loss.

However, it is trauma, with its problematic hemorrhage, that can cause the quickest fluid loss. Rupture of solid organs, such as the spleen and liver, following either blunt or penetrating trauma can quickly create profound hypovolemia. The Paramedic is well-advised to consider occult trauma whenever confronted with hypoperfusion of unknown origin.

Past Medical History

A number of pre-existing medical conditions can also contribute to increased fluid loss. The following short list of medical conditions can lead to increased and/or excessive fluid loss leading to hypovolemia; this list not all inclusive of medical conditions that can lead to fluid loss.

Diabetes insipidus, secondary to brain tumor or any other space-occupying lesion, can cause life-threatening dehydration within hours. Diabetes insipidus causes the kidneys to pass the filtrate from the plasma almost unchanged. Normally 99% of this filtrate is reabsorbed.

Emphysema, with its accompanying persistent tachypnea, can lead to significant insensible fluid loss through rapid respiration. Coupled with the diuretic action of many respiratory drugs such as aminophylline, and without adequate fluid replacement, the patient can become markedly dehydrated.

Initially, the thought of congestive heart failure summons thoughts of fluid overload, and during an acute exacerbation this may be the case. However, the combination of forward failure and subsequent inadequate renal perfusion, coupled with overuse of prescribed diuretics and a constant shifting of fluid volumes across all three fluid compartments, can culminate in a complicated clinical picture which can include cellular dehydration, vascular volume depletion, and electrolyte imbalances. Heart faiulure, therefore, is a problem of fluid maldistribution coupled with interstitial dehydration.

Despite an apparent constant intake of fluids, the alcoholic patient is prone to fluid deficits as well. While alcohol itself is a diuretic, the impact of liver cirrhosis is probably greater upon the patient's fluid volume state. When the liver is not producing sufficient blood proteins, such as albumin, secondary to cirrhosis, the colloidal osmotic pressure (COP) within the blood falls, and with it the patient's intravascular volume.

Hyperglycemia can be another cause of acute fluid loss. Hyperglycemia, the hallmark of new onset diabetes mellitus, acts as an osmotic diuretic and draws fluid from the interstitial space into the central circulation. As this volume increases, the kidneys increase urine output to excrete the excess volume. The patient, whose tissues are now dehydrated, craves water. Despite drinking steadily (polydipsia), the patient cannot take in enough fluids to offset the excessive output from urination (polyuria).

Physical Examination for Dehydration

The patient who has lost significant intravascular volume, secondary to dehydration, may manifest signs of hypoperfusion which will be evident during the initial assessment. These signs include decreased level of responsiveness, tachypnea, tachycardia, hypotension, or postural hypotension. When these signs culminate to present a clinical picture of hypoperfusion, the Paramedic may decide to institute fluid replacement immediately.

A number of other signs may precede this presentation and suggest dehydration and impending hypoperfusion. These signs, in a head-to-toe fashion, are lackluster eyes, eyes that are sunken into their sockets and appear dull. The absence of tears in a child's eyes should alert the Paramedic to the presence of dehydration.

Dry and cracked lips along with pale mucous membranes in the oropharynx are signs of dehydration. The tongue may be the best external measure of the patient's hydration. Normally, a tongue is plump, and moistened with saliva. However, when a patient is dehydrated the tongue becomes dry and furrowed (furrows being long fissures in the tongue).

Next, the Paramedic should examine the neck, particularly the jugular veins. Some Paramedics regard the jugular veins as the "dipstick" of the heart. Under normal conditions when a patient is lying flat, the external jugular veins are at least minimally distended and clearly visible, indicating a sufficient blood volume. In the case of the patient who is dehydrated, the jugular veins will lie flat against the neck when the patient lies flat.

The next indicator of hydration is the urine output. While not practical in the field, unless the patient has an indwelling urinary catheter, measuring a patient's hourly urinary output is an excellent indicator of vascular volume. When urine output drops below 20 mL per hour (**oliguria**), then the patient is experiencing significant hypoperfusion of the kidneys, an early indicator of shock.

In the hospital setting, the gold standard for fluid balance is the patient's weight. Even with constant monitoring and recording of intake and output, many critical care units weigh their patients regularly, in some cases daily, in order to monitor fluid balance. Long-term care facilities also regularly weigh their patients.

The Paramedic who looks for these early signs of dehydration and fluid deficits will not be surprised when the patient becomes hypotensive. Perhaps more importantly, the Paramedic may be able to intervene early and prevent hypotension.

Intravenous Fluids

Intravenous fluids used for medical patients are intended to be either intravenous routes for therapeutic medications, or to be therapeutic in and of themselves. Intravenous fluids used for trauma patients are more often intended to replace lost volume and therefore are therapeutic.

In the case of trauma, the optimal fluid replacement for lost blood would be blood. However, current blood storage requirements and inadequate prehospital equipment make blood replacement in the field impractical. In an effort to overcome these obstacles, physicians and scientists are trying to create a variety of blood substitute. To date, trials of these blood substitutes are falling short of expectations, but more blood substitutes are being researched.

These blood substitutes contain proteins, and are thus called a **colloid**. These colloidial fluids are capable of both pulling fluids from within the interstitial space into the circulation, to help augment the circulating volume, and remaining within the blood stream for a prolonged period of time, helping to maintain the circulating volume.

In the interim, and until these solutions are available, Paramedics must use electrolyte-containing fluids during trauma resuscitation. These electrolyte solutions, when dehydrated, create crystals. Thus, these electrolyte-containing fluids are referred to as **crystalloids**.[3-6]

The electrolytes commonly found in crystalloid solutions—sodium, chloride, and potassium—are the same electrolytes found within the blood. In fact, several crystalloid solutions were created in an effort to reproduce a "blood-like" mixture. British physicist Sidney Ringer was made famous when he tried to create a "balanced solution" in 1873, the solution which still bears his name, but was unable to bottle the solution because of its effervescence. Improving on Dr. Ringer's solution, and solving the problem of effervescence, Dr. Hartmann added lactate, resulting in lactated Ringer's solution (LR). Lactated Ringer's solution remains the solution of choice of trauma surgeons (advanced trauma life support, or ATLS) and in the treatment of burn patients (American Burn Foundation or ABF).[7-10]

When caring for a medical patient, a number of additives may be added to the solution to provide a therapeutic benefit. The most common additive is dextrose, a simple sugar which can be quickly metabolized to meet the ill patient's higher energy demands. Other additives include antibiotics, vasopressors, antidysrhythmics, and a host of other medications. Many of these therapeutic solutions are run intermittently, as a secondary intravenous solution, through a primary infusion line containing either 0.9% sodium chloride in sterile water (0.9% NaCl) or 5% dextrose in sterile water (D_5W).

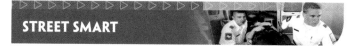

Tonicity

A solution is considered balanced if it has the same concentration of solutes to solvent as there are solutes to solvent present in the blood. Any imbalance of this solute concentration would cause an osmotic effect to be created when administered intravenously, potentially overhydrating or dehydrating a cell. In other words, **tonicity** could be thought of as the solution's ability to alter a cell's internal fluid balance through osmotic force created by the imbalance between the tonicity of the solution outside of the cell versus the tonicity of the fluid within the cell. When the percentage solute in the solution is similar to the percentage solute in the blood, such as is the case with a balanced solution, the solution is said to be **isotonic**. Examples of nearly isotonic fluids include D_5W, LR, and NSS. When additional substances or additives are added, thus increasing the concentration of the solutes compared to blood, then the solution is said to be **hypertonic**. Hypertonic solutions will, by osmotic force, draw water out of the cell, causing the cell to dehydrate and collapse or **crenate**. Conversely, if pure sterile water, or a solution which has fewer solutes than blood, was injected, then the solution would be referred to as a **hypotonic** solution. Cells would then, by osmotic force, draw water into themselves, expanding in the process to the point where the cell would burst. Various changes occur when isotonic, hypotonic, and hypertonic solutions are mixed with red blood cells as shown in the following figure (Figure 27-1).

Intravenous Fluid Administration

Once a solution has been selected, the Paramedic turns his attention to the administration of that fluid. Intravenous solutions come in either plastic containers or, more rarely, glass bottles and in volumes ranging from 25 mL to 3,000 mL. Paramedics typically use 250 mL, 500 mL, and 1 L solutions. Glass containers are noncollapsible and must be open to air, or vented, to prevent the creation of a vacuum. While plastic

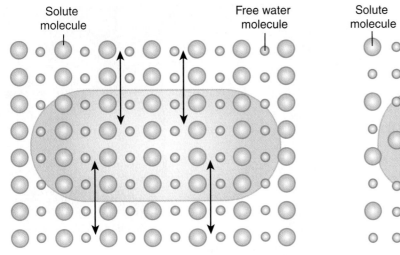

Isotonic environment:
The solute concentration and the
free water concentration are the same
inside and outside the cell.
Water flows in and out of the cell at an equal rate.

A

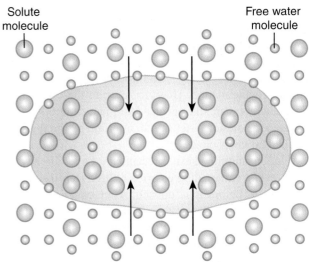

Hypotonic solution:
The solute concentration is greater
inside the cell; the free water
concentration is greater outside.
Free water flows into the cell.

B

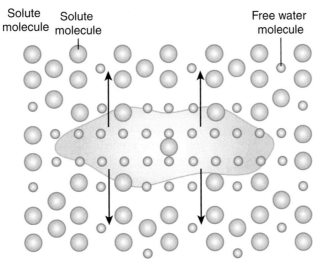

Hypertonic solution:
The solute concentration is greater
outside the cell;
the free water concentration is greater inside.
Free water flows out of the cell.

C

Figure 27-1 (a) Isotonic solution. (b) Hypertonic solution. (c) Hypotonic solution.

containers are increasingly more common, glass containers are still used for medications which react with or are absorbed into the plastic. **IV bags** are soft plastic solution containers which collapse as the solution is withdrawn, eliminating the need for venting, and create a closed system which helps to decrease the risk of outside contamination.

A careless infusion of intravenous fluids can lead to serious systemic complications. For example, contaminated intravenous fluid can lead to septic shock. An intravenous infusion bypasses many of the body's defenses against infection. Without these protections, the patient's blood could become infected, a condition called septicemia, and the patient could develop a potentially life-threatening sepsis. When a Paramedic starts an intravenous access, it is understood that the Paramedic has the responsibility to take all reasonable precautions to prevent such an occurrence.

There are a number of occasions when the intravenous fluid can become contaminated. The intravenous solution could have become contaminated before the Paramedic handled the solution. The container could have been accidentally punctured, or contaminants accidentally introduced along with the additives during the manufacturing process. Understanding this risk, every manufacturer takes precautions to prevent contamination. However, despite these precautions, contamination can still occur. Most manufacturers will only guarantee a solution's sterility for a certain period time, a date stamped on the package.

Understanding these precautions have already been taken, every Paramedic performs a three-step inspection of the solution before it is opened. After confirming that the correct solution has been chosen, the Paramedic verifies that the solution is not expired. The expiration date, stamped or printed on the container, is evidence that the solution is less likely to be contaminated.

Next, the Paramedic examines the solution for clarity. Intravenous solutions are generally clear, with some notable exceptions being medications like diazepam (pale yellow). With the solution held up to a light, the Paramedic should inspect the solution for any discoloration or any particulate matter. If contamination is suspected, then the solution should be discarded immediately.

Finally, the Paramedic should test the container to see if it is intact and without microscopic holes that could be portals for contamination. A firm twist of the bag should reveal any leaks. If the bag does leak, it should be discarded and another solution chosen.

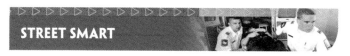

STREET SMART

Some intravenous solutions come with a second protective outer wrap around the bag. Due to differences in humidity from the site of manufacture and the present location, condensation may have occurred. The Paramedic should first wipe the bag down and then test the container's integrity. Follow this rule, however: "If in doubt, throw it out."

Administration Sets

The next step in preparing to administer an intravenous solution is connecting an administration set to the solution. During this procedure, the greatest risk of contamination may occur. Careful attention to detail is important to prevent sterile components from contacting nonsterile surfaces. The purpose of an intravenous administration set is to provide a sterile pathway for the intravenous fluid from the container into the patient.

The selection of an administration set is largely dependent upon the patient's condition. When volume replacement is needed (e.g., during a trauma resuscitation), then a short,

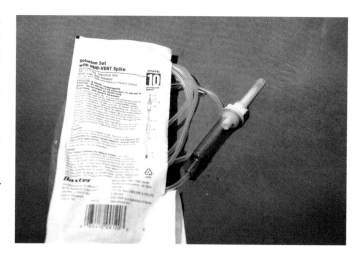

Figure 27-2 Macro-drop intravenous administration set.

straight line with the fewest obstructions, such as filters or medication portals, is desirable. These administration sets are referred to as **macro-drop** administration sets (Figure 27-2).

When careful titration of medicated fluid is desired (e.g., when a medical patient needs a slow infusion of a drug), then fine control of the infusion stream is needed. These administration sets are referred to as **micro-drop** administration sets.

Anatomy of an Administration Set

Every administration set has a **spike**, sometimes called a bayonet, which is used to pierce the fluid container. As the name implies, the spike is very sharp and is as capable of cutting flesh as easily as it is capable of piercing a plastic seal in a bag of intravenous solution. Caution should be observed when mating the spike of the administration set to the solution bag to prevent inadvertent puncture of the side of the solution bag, which can result in a puncture of the Paramedic's finger as well.

Below the spike is the drip chamber. Hanging drops are formed inside the drip chamber. These drops can be counted, as drops (gtt) per minute (gtt/min), and the rate of flow established. If the chamber has a thin, or needle, dropper, then the administration set is called a micro-drop set. By convention, all manufacturers have set 60 drops from a micro-drop set to equal 1 mL. The needle dropper is visible within the drip chamber (Figure 27-3).

If the drip chamber does not have a needle dropper, then the set is called a macro-drop set. Unlike the micro-drop set, macro-drops can vary in size. The variation in the size of the drop directly relates to the number of drops per 1 mL. To determine the drip rate for a particular macro-drop administration set, the Paramedic should refer to the labeling on the packaging. In some cases, the drip rate is embossed directly into the plastic on the spike as well.

Further down the length of the tubing is a drip rate control device. The drip rate control device allows the Paramedic to regulate the flow (i.e., the rate of drop formation) so that

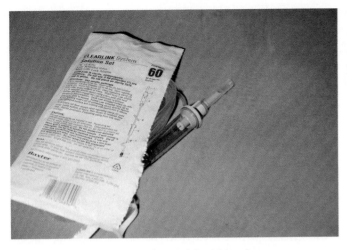

Figure 27-3 Micro-drop drip chamber.

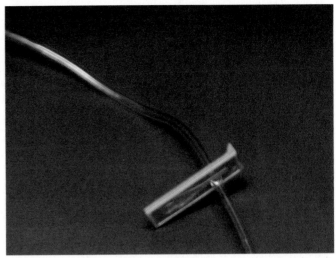

Figure 27-5 Intravenous administration slide clamp.

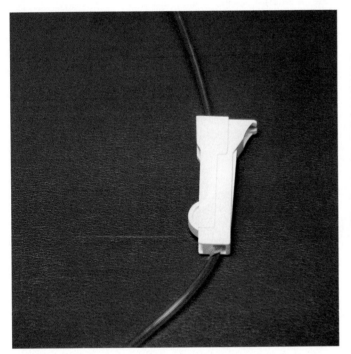

Figure 27-4 Control devices: Roller clamp type.

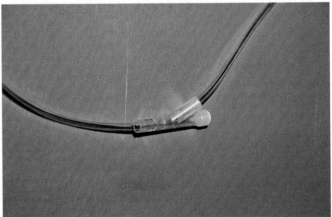

Figure 27-6 In-line medication port.

precise volumes can be administered (drops per minute being equated to mL per hour). Most control devices have either a roller clamp (Figure 27-4) or screw-type device, both of which function by compressing the tubing. The roller clamp, a common control device, has a thumb wheel which compresses the tubing against a hard plastic back and thus limits flow.

Another control device, the slide clamp (Figure 27-5), is used to cut off flow entirely. This is necessary during intravenous drug boluses to prevent retrograde infusion of the medication into the intravenous tubing rather than into the patient. By sliding the tubing into the groove, flow is stopped. Similar to a slide clamp, some administration sets have a squeeze-clamp which can cut off solution flow.

Some administration sets come with a mid-line, in-line check valve designed to prevent the administration set from running dry. If an administration set does run dry, there is a

risk that the venous catheter will become clogged by a blood-clot, rendering it useless. To prevent the catheter from clogging, the check valve leaves a standing column of solution in the line.

Hard plastic in-line medication ports (Figure 27-6) provide access for injection of drugs into the solution stream. These ports can be either capped with a self-sealing membrane, into which a needle would be inserted, or a needleless check-valve system designed to accept a syringe's luer lock tip.

Some intravenous administration sets have a device called a flash bulb. The flash bulb is a soft in-line pyramid-shaped device. When the tubing is clamped and the flash bulb is squeezed, a show of blood can be seen in the distal tubing. This blood "flash" is an indicator that the venous access is still patent. Some flash bulbs are made of self-sealing materials which permit insert of a needle for injection of medications, thus making the flash bulb the most proximal medication port to the venous access.

Some intravenous administration sets also have an in-line filter. The in-line filter is designed to strain the solution for large particles of undissolved medication, solution crystals,

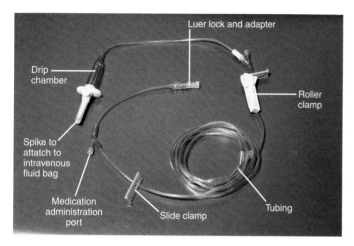

Figure 27-7 Anatomy of an intravenous administration set.

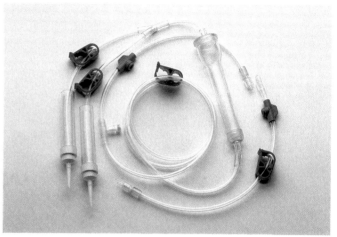

Figure 27-8 Trauma tubing. (Courtesy of Arrow International)

contaminants, and the like. Disk-like in appearance, these in-line filters are usually found proximal to the drip chamber but distal to any medication ports.

The place where the administration set inserts into the hub of the venous catheter is called the adaptor. The adaptor is sterile where it couples with the catheter hub and a cap is in place over the adaptor to prevent contamination. In some cases, the impervious hard plastic adaptor must be removed in order to allow the solution to be run through the administration set prior to insertion. In those cases, the cap must be retained to re-cover the sterile adaptor once the solution has been run out in order to maintain the sterility of the adaptor. Other adaptors have a semi-porous cap which permits fluid to run out through the cap without compromising sterility (Figure 27-7).

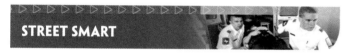

STREET SMART

When the adaptor's cap is misplaced, the administration set can be capped with a spare covered sterile needle. The diameter of the hub and a needle are the same. When the administration set is to be attached to the hub of the venous catheter, the needle is then discarded into a sharps container.

Trauma Tubing

Factors that influence the rate of flow for an administration set are the length of the tubing, the height of the solution bag, and the diameter of the tubing.[11–14] Tubing length may have the greatest impact on flow rates. Whenever fluids run down a tube, the fluid strikes the walls of the tubing, creating turbulence, and the turbulence slows the speed of the fluid. This phenomenon is called friction loss. The longer the tubing, the greater the friction loss, and the slower the flow of the solution. For this reason, trauma tubing is generally short in order to facilitate a rapid flow of solution into the patient.

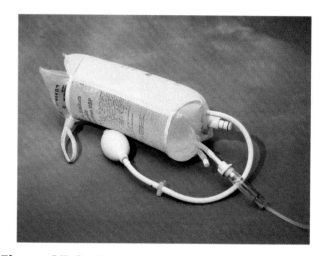

Figure 27-9 Pressure bag.

Trauma tubing generally has a larger internal diameter, or bore, than standard tubing (Figure 27-8). The combination of a short length and large bore allows the rapid administration of large volumes of solution.[15,16] This administration is so rapid, in fact, that some trauma tubing sets are also Y-sets, meaning that they have two fluid connections, each with a spike. This allows two bags of solution to be hung at one time.

The addition of a pressure bag can also increase the rate of flow and decrease the time to infuse a liter of solution. A pressure bag is a sleeve with a bladder device. The solution is placed within the sleeve and the bladder exerts direct pressure onto the solution bag. The increased pressure subsequently increases the rate of flow. Inflated in the same manner as a blood pressure cuff using a bulb with relief screw, a pressure bag is inflated to a preset pressure, visible on the gauge, or until a pressure relief valve activates (Figure 27-9).

Whenever there is a large volume of fluid to be administered, there is the concomitant risk of inducing hypothermia via infusion of less-than-body-temperature solutions. To prevent this predictable complication, special warmth-preserving solution sleeves are available (Figure 27-10). These sleeves have one pocket for a hot pack and another for the solution. There is insulation around both to prevent heat loss.

Blood Transfusion Sets

Blood's viscous nature makes it difficult to flow and thus special large-bore tubing has been created for the transfusion of blood. Blood tubing also has a large drip chamber with a sieve-like filter at the bottom which prevents clots from being transfused (Figure 27-11). Frequently, an infusion of NSS is also co-administered with the blood. The NSS helps to thin the blood and keep the blood running freely.

In special cases, it is desirable to add another drug port for concomitant drug infusions, or an additional length of tubing to the administration set. Optional extension sets are available for this purpose. The extension set connects with the adaptor of the administration set and is connected to the venous catheter.

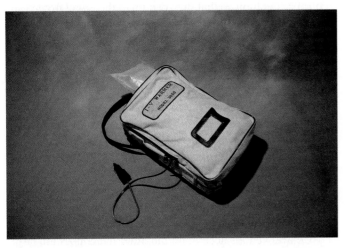

Figure 27-10 Intravenous solution warming sleeve.

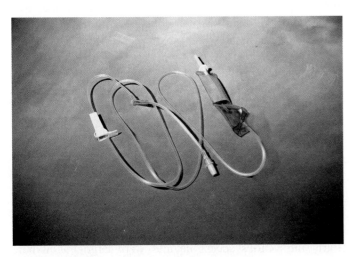

Figure 27-11 Blood transfusion set.

The volume to be infused in children must be carefully controlled to prevent any incidence of fluid overload. For pediatric infusions, a special in-line burette may be added. A burette has another fluid chamber above the micro-drop drip chamber. The first chamber is prefilled with a specified volume of fluid from the solution bag and then the infusion rate is adjusted. The solution chamber of the burette is rigid; for this reason, it has a vent to equalize pressures. Burettes also have a built-in check valve to prevent the administration set from running dry.

When it is necessary to infuse a second bag of solution (e.g., a medicated solution) and only one venous access is available, a secondary set can be set up to run through the primary administration set. This arrangement has several advantages. It prevents the need to establish a second venous access, which is especially important in venous-impoverished patients. It permits continuous hydration between intermittent drug infusions, such as antibiotics. Finally, it permits a secondary drug infusion (e.g., an antidysrhythmia drug) to be temporarily discontinued so that a potentially incompatible drug can be injected through the primary administration set after the tubing is cleared of drug by a fluid bolus. A description of the preparation and use of a secondary set follows later in this chapter.

Preparing the Intravenous Administration Set

Preparation of an intravenous administration set is done in a deliberate stepwise fashion and after practice becomes almost second nature. However, a moment of inattention to the details can set up a situation that is problematic later.

After removing the chosen intravenous administration set from the packaging, taking care to not let any part of the set to drop onto the ground, the Paramedic should inspect the set for all of the needed components. For example, if it is anticipated that a medication will be given by injection, then a medication port as well as a clamp should be available. Administration sets vary and not all components are present on every set.

In the next step in the preparation of an administration set, the Paramedic would slide the flow rate control device proximal to the drip chamber and clamp the tubing closed. Clamping the tubing shut prevents premature drainage of the drip chamber. It also places the roller clamp at eye level when the solution is suspended, or hung, and thus permits better eye-to-hand control when adjusting the flow rate later.

The Paramedic would then set the intravenous administration set aside so that the solution can be prepared. After the Paramedic has ensured that the chosen solution is the correct solution, the solution is not expired, the solution is not contaminated, and the container is intact, the protective covering over the solution's administration set port can be removed. Some intravenous solutions come with a medication administration port, used to inject medications into the solution, which is adjacent to the administration set port. If the self-sealing membrane covering the medication administration port is inadvertently removed, the entire contents of the intravenous bag will flow out. Therefore the Paramedic should carefully choose the correct port.

The Paramedic would then pick up the intravenous administration set and remove the protective cover from the spike. Carefully aligning the administration set's spike in line with the administration set port, the Paramedic would carefully slide the spike into the port. When the Paramedic feels resistance to the spike, a one-half twist of the spike will effectively open the administration set port by coring the membrane sealing the solution and will seat the spike firmly into the administration set port. Caution should be observed when connecting the intravenous solution to the administration set. First, the administration set's spike is sterile. Contact with the outside of the solution's administration port, the Paramedic's fingers, or any other nonsterile surface will contaminate the administration set. If this occurs, then another administration set must be used. Second, the spike is capable of breaching the sidewall of the administration port and piercing the Paramedic's gloved hand. Firm control and deliberate action can usually avert this problem.

With the administration set in place and the solution held upright so that the drip chamber is at eye level, the Paramedic would then squeeze the drip chamber and release. If the spike is properly set, fluid will start to flow. If there is no flow, then the Paramedic should advance the spike further into the solution bag and re-attempt the maneuver until successful. A one-half-full drip chamber is optimal. The Paramedic should continue to squeeze the drip chamber until it is one-half full.

An overfull drip chamber is not acceptable, as it does not allow the Paramedic to see the drops as they form on the needle. If the drip chamber is inadvertently overfilled, the Paramedic would invert the solution bag and squeeze the drip chamber again, replacing the solution back into the bag.

Failure to fill the drip chamber is also problematic. If the drip chamber is open when the solution starts to flow, the stream will entrain air into the solution and the entrained air be seen along the length of the tubing. While a small number of air bubbles is generally not harmful to the patient, a larger volume of air could potentially create an air embolism. If air should accidentally get into the solution stream, as evidenced by bubbles along the length of the tubing, the Paramedic should pull the tubing taut and gently snap the tubing to dislodge the bubbles, which should then float upward into the drip chamber.

With the drip chamber one-half full, the Paramedic releases the clamp and allows solution to fill the tubing. If the stream is too fast, then turbulence in the drip chamber will entrain air into the tubing where it will adhere to the tubing walls. A slow steady stream of solution clears the tubing of air and prevents air bubbles from forming along the tubing's walls.

If after releasing the clamp there is no flow, then the Paramedic should examine the length of the tubing, starting at the drip chamber, for a closed slide clamp or other signs of obstruction of the tubing.

In many cases, there is an impervious cap over the administration set adaptor which must be removed before flow will begin. The Paramedic should carefully place the cap aside, remembering where it was placed, so it can be replaced later.

After the intravenous administration tubing is cleared of any air and fluid runs freely from the end, a process called **running the line out**, the tubing is clamped and set aside until after the venous access has been obtained. The Paramedic should ensure that the sterility of the solution is maintained by recapping the end of the administration set and keeping the tubing from touching the ground. To help ensure the sterility of the administration set and solution, some roller clamps have a built-in clip on the roller clamp. The adaptor is simply slipped into the clip and clamped into place (Skill 27-1).

For a step-by-step demonstration of Preparation of an Intravenous Adminsitration Set, please refer to Skill 27-1 on page 586.

Intravenous Access

Venous access is an assured means of getting drugs into the central circulation so that they can go to the target organs and exert their intended therapeutic effect. The speed at which a drug can be delivered to the target and confidence that the dose delivered will attain the therapeutic window has made venous access the preferred route for medication administration during an emergency.

Emergency venous access can be divided into two types: peripheral venous access and central venous access. Peripheral venous access has the advantage of ready availability. Peripheral venous access is also compressible in the event that the venous cannulation attempt is unsuccessful and bleeding occurs. Unfortunately, a number of circumstances, such as cardiovascular collapse during a cardiac arrest, can make peripheral venous access more difficult to obtain.

Central venous access, on the other hand, uses the larger veins located deep inside the body. The high rate of blood flow in these veins permits drugs that are normally incompatible to be given sequentially and nearly simultaneously. Perhaps more importantly, these large veins are still accessible, even during times of cardiovascular collapse. Unfortunately, these veins often run parallel and proximal to arteries and nerves, as well as adjunct to several major organs. Inadvertent arterial access, nerve damage, and organ damage are attendant risks with central venous access.[17–19] For example, a pneumothorax is a predictable complication of central venous cannulation of the subclavian vein. While central venous access is practiced in the field by some Paramedics, the majority of venous access obtained by Paramedics is peripheral venous access. The following sections discuss the details of obtaining peripheral venous access and accessing central venous devices.

Peripheral Venous Access Devices

Early intravenous access devices were large hollow-bore straight needles which were placed, whole-length, into a vein. These early needles had to be sharpened by hand on a stone and then sterilized overnight in an autoclave for surgery the next day. Current venous access devices can be either metal or plastic and are sterilized when they are packaged. Manufactured with precision machines to exacting standards, these catheters are extremely sharp and come in a variety of sizes.

The size of an intravenous needle is measured as a gauge—the smaller the gauge, then the larger the needle. Typical intravenous needles start at 12 gauge and go down to 24 gauge. The selection of the gauge, as well as the selection of the intravenous administration set, depends on its intended use. A larger needle is preferred for trauma patients in that it can be anticipated that either viscous blood or large volumes of crystalloids will be infused. Blood transfused through a smaller gauge needle (less than 18 gauge) can cause physical destruction (lysis) of red blood cells.[20,21]

Smaller gauge needles (e.g., a 20 gauge needle) are preferable if the Paramedic anticipates the venous access will be maintained for a longer period of time. A smaller gauge needle decreases the incidence of thrombophlebitis. Thrombophlebitis occurs more readily in veins cannulated with a large-bore needle than a small-bore needle because the large-bore needle occupies more of the lumen of the vein, slowing blood flow, and creating optimal conditions for platelet aggregation, the nadir for a thrombus.

Categories of Venous Access Devices

The most widely used intravenous (IV) access devices are the catheter over the needle devices (Figure 27-12). Individually packaged, with a large number of gauges and lengths available for selection, these IV devices are easy to insert.

The heart of a catheter-over-the-needle IV device is the needle. The hollow-bored needle acts as a rigid introducer into the vein and allows blood to backup into the needle to become visible to the Paramedic. The catheter-over-the-needle device allows the Paramedic to thread the plastic catheter over the needle and into the vein. When the insertion is complete, the metal needle is withdrawn—all that remains inside the vein is the plastic catheter.

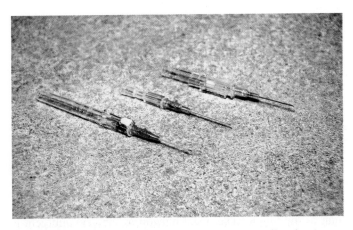

Figure 27-12 Catheter-over-the-needle devices.

The tip of the needle (small portion lies exposed at the end of the plastic catheter) has a short bevel tip which permits easy penetration of the skin while lessening the chance of accidental puncture of the distal wall of the vein. The length of the needle and catheter, like the hypodermic needle, is dependent on the size of the patient. Pediatric IVs may be 1/2 to 1 inch long, while the average adult IV is 1 1/2 inches long. Extra long needles, 3 to 4 inches long, are used for special populations of patients such as the patient with severe burns (where subcutaneous swelling can literally pull an IV out) and obese patients.

Butterfly IV catheters, a throwback to the days of steel needles, are still used for pediatric patients. These shorter steel needles are embedded into a plastic anchor device which has wings, like a butterfly. Grasping the wings permits the Paramedic better control of the needle during insertion, as well as a firm surface to anchor the device against the skin when securing the device in place. This makes them popular for use in the pediatric population.

The third venous access device is the needle-over-the-catheter device. These devices are used almost exclusively for central venous access, in part because there are more steps to perform during insertion; the Seldinger technique. Use of the needle-over-the-catheter device is discussed further in a later section on central venous access.

Needle Safety

Accidental needlestick injuries present the Paramedic with the greatest risk for an occupational exposure to HIV and other blood-borne pathogens.[22] IV catheter manufacturers have developed a number of "engineered" safety features which appear in newer IV catheters, in an effort to decrease the incidence of preventable needlestick injuries. Paramedics should make use of this available safety technology (Figure 27-13). Whenever an intravenous access is attempted, a sharps container should be immediately available (i.e., within arm's reach of the Paramedic).

STREET SMART

The phrase "Use and drop" refers to the process of using a needle (IV catheter, IM or SQ needle) and being able to immediately drop it into the sharps container without taking a step away from the patient or turning away from the patient.

Peripheral Site Selection

While any vein in an extremity is considered a peripheral vein, certain veins have more desirable qualities than others. These veins are preferred by Paramedics for venous access.

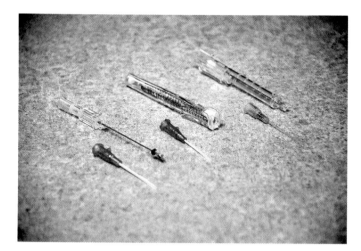

Figure 27-13 Engineered safety catheter.

The following text describes the steps taken to obtain intravenous access.

While it is easy to see some surface veins, deeper and less visible veins may be more desirable. These deeper veins are anchored in subcutaneous fat, helping to stabilize them and prevent them from moving, or rolling, away from the needle. They are also generally larger in diameter. To distend these veins, making them easier to either visualize or palpate, a venous tourniquet is applied.[23] A venous tourniquet is made of a soft, wide material which can apply a constricting force around the circumference of a limb. Examples of materials used for a tourniquet include leather straps, blood pressure cuffs, and rubber strips. A popular tourniquet is a length of penrose drain. A penrose drain is a tubular rubber hose which lies flat and provides a wide band of compression.

The tourniquet is typically placed around the arm, either above the elbow or above the wrist, and then tied into a slip knot, with the knot on the medial surface. Next, the distal pulse is palpated. A distal arterial pulse should remain palpable at all times and the limb should not become cyanotic. If the pulse is obliterated and/or the patient's limb becomes cyanotic, then the tourniquet should be immediately removed. As a general rule, a venous tourniquet should not remain in place for more than a few minutes. In most cases, the Paramedic can accomplish all of the tasks needed to obtain venous access within that time period.

After a moment, the veins will start to distend and become more visible. Starting proximal and moving distal, the Paramedic should be able to identify the following veins: axillary, basilic, cephalic, and dorsal arch.

The axillary vein (Figure 27-14) runs from the shoulder over the biceps toward the elbow. This vein is more prominent in thin people and those who do considerable lifting for a living. The advantage of the axillary vein is two-fold. One is its proximity to the trunk. This is particularly advantageous when administering certain medications, such as adenosine. The axillary vein also has fewer valves than other more distal veins, making it easier to cannulate.

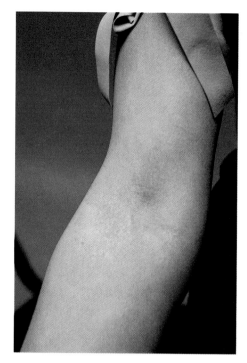

Figure 27-14 Gaining access in the axillary vein.

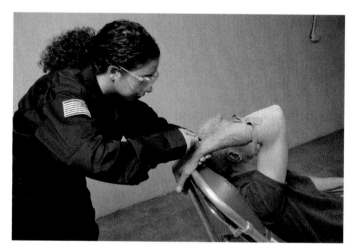

Figure 27-15 Gaining IV access in a potentially violent patient using the basilic vein.

The next vein, the basilic vein, runs down the dorsal aspect of the arm and ends at the medial wrist. The basilic vein is particularly advantageous when trying to start an IV on a confused or combative patient. The Paramedic would position himself at the head of the stretcher and pull the patient's arm toward him. With the arm bent at the elbow, the arm can essentially be locked into position, permitting unimpeded access to the vein (Figure 27-15).

The vein running down the forearm, immediately opposite the basilic, is the cephalic vein. The cephalic vein runs down the lateral aspect of the forearm and terminates proximal to the thumb. The distal portion of the cephalic vein is most commonly used by Paramedics (Figure 27-16).

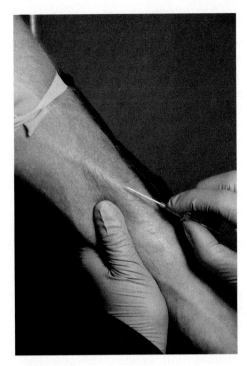

Figure 27-16 Gaining IV access in the cephalic vein.

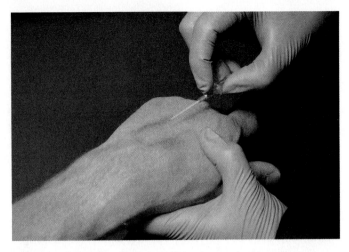

Figure 27-17 Gaining IV access in the dorsal arch.

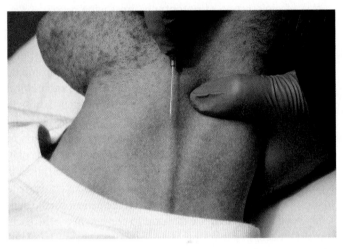

Figure 27-18 Gaining IV access in the external jugular vein.

To stabilize the cephalic vein, the Paramedic takes the patient's hand as if shaking hands. With a firm grasp of the hand, the Paramedic palpates for a void at the distal forearm called the autonomic sniff box. The cephalic vein generally lies within the autonomic sniff box.

The most distal peripheral veins of the arm are part of the dorsal venous plexus, a group of veins that originate between each digit and from an arch across the dorsum of the hand. While the veins of the dorsal arch are generally the most visible, making them appear attractive to Paramedics, they contain a number of valves and tend to be somewhat torturous. If an IV is to be attempted here, a short 1-inch needle is preferred.

To start an IV in the dorsal arch of the hand, the Paramedic should first grasp the fingers and bend them inward toward the palm. With the fingers stabilized by the thumb, the Paramedic can proceed with insertion of the IV (Figure 27-17). Generally, the plane of the insertion of the needle is sharper as the veins of the hand are more superficial.

Although the external jugular vein (EJV), strictly speaking, is not a peripheral venous access, it is treated as such by many Paramedics because it can be easily visualized, readily palpated, and more importantly, it is compressible if extravasation should occur. Because of its location, the actual method of preparing the site for insertion of an IV device is slightly different. To identify the external jugular vein, the patient should be placed in a supine position to maximize venous return.[24,25]

While it would be impractical to apply a tourniquet around a patient's neck, it is possible to compress (**tamponade**) the vein by applying a thumb to the distal portion of the external jugular vein just superior to the clavicle, at the mid-clavicular line. By turning the patient's head away from the intended insertion side, the external jugular vein should be clearly visible. The EJV starts proximal to the angle of the jaw and inferior to the ear and then takes a relatively straight course toward the mid-clavicular line (Figure 27-18).

The saphenous vein, often overlooked by Paramedics, provides an excellent point for venous access when the upper extremities are not available, perhaps due to burns or fractures, for example.[26,27] The long saphenous vein, one of two superficial veins in the leg, is the longest vein in the body, stretching from the groin to the foot. The short saphenous vein extends from the top of the foot, proximal to the outer or lateral malleolus, then runs alongside it, then crosses the Achilles tendon to end in the middle of the back of the knee and connects with the popliteal vein. Both saphenous veins communicate with deeper veins via bridging veins called perforators, which literally perforate the fascia of the muscle bundles to connect with the deeper veins. This unique aspect of the saphenous vein permits drugs given via this route to gain rapid access to the larger veins of the legs.

Some patients, particularly patients with diabetes, have poor circulation in the lower extremities. This poor circulation tends to retard healing of a wound. Therefore, Paramedics generally avoid starting an IV in the foot if the patient is known to have diabetes or poor circulation in the extremities (peripheral vascular insufficiency). Other signs of poor circulation in the feet include misshapen toenails and distal cyanosis of the toes when dependent.

The basilic vein, the cephalic vein, and several bridging veins between the basilic and the cephalic veins, including the cubital vein, exist in the area of the anterior elbow, called the **antecubital fossa (AC)**. Some Paramedics prefer to obtain venous access in this area, perhaps because of their experience of having observed test blood drawn (**phlebotomy**) from the area. The decision to attempt an IV access in the antecubital fossa should be made only after careful considerations of the risks. The antecubital fossa is a part of the elbow joint. Intravenous access obtained proximate to the elbow joint risks being dislodged if the patient should suddenly bend the joint or move the arm. To prevent this occurrence, it may be necessary to restrict the patient's movements by securing the arm to a rigid armboard.

To complicate matters, the median nerve, the brachial artery, the radial bone, the ulna bone, the humerus bone, the basilic vein, and the cephalic vein, plus numerous muscles, tendons, and ligaments, cross through or terminate in the elbow.[28,29] Accidental infiltration of an IV that contains hyperosmolar or caustic chemicals (e.g., dextrose 50% or dopamine) for example, can create tissue ischemia and necrosis of structures within the elbow, possibly leading to permanent disability.

Difficult Venous Access

Patients who are elderly, who have undergone chemotherapy, who have a poor nutritional status, or who are obese, plus a number of other medical conditions, may have a poverty of visible peripheral veins. These patients present a special challenge to the Paramedic.

To improve venous filling of the peripheral veins, it is important to maintain the limb in the dependent position, below the heart. Elevating the limb to "eye level," instead of kneeling next to the patient, will quickly drain the limb and the venous distention will be gone.

Some Paramedics advocate applying a warm wrap around the dependent limb approximately 10 minutes before the IV access is to be attempted. This technique is acceptable, but caution is advised when applying heat to the skin of the elderly patient or those with impaired sensation. Unintentional burns can occur due to the application of heat pads.

Indirect (tangential) lighting from a flashlight held to the side of the patient's arm may also improve venous visibility. However, the best results are obtained when the Paramedic has an understanding of peripheral venous anatomy combined with gentle palpation of the forearm to detect deeper veins. When a vein is palpated under the skin, it should rebound (i.e., feel spongy). If the Paramedic is unsure if the structure palpated is a tendon or vein, then she should ask the patient to move the extremity through a slight range of motion while palpating. Tendons will move with the motion whereas the vein will not.

Every vein should be palpated to ensure that the vein is not an artery. In low output states (i.e., hypoperfusion), it may be difficult to distinguish an artery from a vein. To complicate matters, some arteries, nerves, and veins run together as a bundle deeper in the extremity and proximal to bone. In the circumstance that an artery is accidentally cannulated, blood may rapidly back up the administration set and pulsations may be visible in the column of blood. In those cases, the catheter should be removed immediately and a direct pressure applied to the arterial puncture site (Skill 27-2).

For a step-by-step demonstration of Venous Cannulation Using a Catheter-Over-the-Needle Device, please refer to Skill 27-2 on pages 587–588.

Venous Site Precautions

During an emergency, any venous access is acceptable, however, when time permits, and under special circumstances, the Paramedic should carefully consider the alternative IV access sites. For example, if the patient is suspected of having an acute myocardial infarction, then attempts to obtain IV access in the right antecubital fossa are reserved until last. The right AC is a preferred access site for interventional cardiac procedures, such as angiocatheterization and angioplasty.

As a courtesy to the patient, it is preferred that the IV site selected be on the nondominant arm. This allows the patient greater flexibility and movement, including the ability to attend to the activities of daily living (ADL) such as signing admission papers. To quickly ascertain the nondominant hand, the Paramedic should look for a wristwatch. In most cases, the patient will wear the watch on the nondominant hand. If the watch must be removed to obtain an IV access or to prevent damage to the watch, the Paramedic should make a notation on the patient care report (PCR) including a notation as to whom the watch was given.

Several medical conditions, such as long bone fractures, burns, and breast cancer, preclude the Paramedic from starting an IV on an affected limb, except under extraordinary circumstances. The Paramedic should make careful note of these conditions and avoid starting an IV on the affected limb if at all possible.

The presence of an armboard to stabilize a fracture may be seen as an invitation to start an IV on the immobilized limb. However, the circulation surrounding a bone fracture may be disrupted and infiltration of intravenous solutions into the injury may further complicate the patient's care. Therefore, IVs are generally not started on injured limbs.

Burns represent another relative contraindication to an IV access. Whenever alternative access sites are available, the Paramedic is encouraged to use them. However, if the patient has sustained massive burns, and no other sites are available, some burn authorities advocate starting the IV through the burn tissue.

When an intravenous solution is infused, it remains in the circulation until a number of factors, such as decreased colloidal osmotic pressure, combine to create a mismatch between the actual tonicity of the patient's blood and the tonicity of the intravenous solution and cause it to shift into the third space, the interstitial fluid. For example, it has been estimated that NSS only remains in the bloodstream for about 20 to 30 minutes before it "leaks" into the tissues.[30,31] Thus intravenous infusions can create an increase in interstitial fluid. Normally, the body's lymphatic system would help to drain the excess interstitial fluid out of the tissues, and back in the central circulation, bringing the body's fluids back into balance. However, patients with breast cancer frequently undergo a procedure called an axillary lymph node dissection, as a part of a diagnostic or therapeutic intervention for the cancer. These patients may no longer be able to drain the excess fluid from the affected limb, and a condition called **lymphedema** sets into the affected limb. Lymphedema, unchecked, can cause swelling of the limb, compression of nerves, and paralysis. For this reason, Paramedics avoid starting an IV on the same side as the axillary lymph node dissection.[32–34] Frequently, these patients have been educated to warn Paramedics about starting an IV, or taking blood pressures, on the affected side, and many wear medical alert bracelets warning that the patient has lymphedema. If the patient is unconscious and has had a mastectomy, or is wearing a compression stocking on the arm, or there is surgical scar in the axilla, then the Paramedic should assume that an axillary lymph node dissection has taken place and choose another site for venous access.

Site Preparation and Disinfection

Properly preparing the patient prior to placement of the peripheral catheter will help to ensure success. The patient should be assisted to a comfortable position (such as semi-Fowler's, if possible) and an informed consent obtained for the IV insertion using the AIR mnemonic. The patient's arm should be removed from his shirt sleeve, or, if practical, the patient should be instructed to put on a gown. A moment of preparation prevents having to "string" the IV solution and administration set through the patient's clothing in order to put on a hospital gown upon arrival at the emergency department and risk accidentally dislodging the IV access in the process.

Next, the Paramedic should apply the tourniquet. After applying the tourniquet, the Paramedic should carefully consider potential sites for IV access and select a primary site as well as a secondary site. Then, with the necessary supplies assembled, including a padded arm splint if the IV access is going to be near a joint, the Paramedic is ready to prepare the area. The following procedure is recommended; however, different systems have different approaches to IV site preparation, so local/regional procedures should be followed.

After opening an isopropyl alcohol-soaked gauze (i.e., a prep pad), the Paramedic liberally swabs the area, removing gross surface contaminates and skin oils. The prep pad is placed exactly where the IV access will be attempted and moved outward in ever-widening circles. The purpose of this first wash is to remove sweat, dirt, and oils that could undermine the dressing. Therefore, the area cleansed should be liberal, approximately the same area to be covered by the dressing, bandage, and tape.

It is difficult to get tape to adhere to the grossly diaphoretic patient. One tactic is to apply **tincture of benzoin** to help the dressing remain fast. After placing a small quantity of tincture of benzoin on a gauze pad, the Paramedic swabs the area around the perimeter of the IV insertion site. It is important to not swab the insertion site directly, as benzoin is not an astringent. After the benzoin has dried, the tape/dressing can be applied.

PROFESSIONAL PARAMEDIC

Some jurisdictions allow Paramedics to draw a blood alcohol sample for law enforcement officers (LEO), provided there is patient consent. In this situation, the Paramedic should use povidone only to prepare the venipuncture site to avoid claims of contamination of the sample with the isopropyl alcohol used in the wipes. The Paramedic should document the use of povidone only on his chart.

A germicidal wash follows, such as povidone-iodine-based solutions (Betadine®), and is applied in the same fashion as the previous wash, starting at the intended insertion site and sweeping outward in expanding and ever-widening circles. Regardless of whether the Paramedic is using a prep pad or a swab for the germicidal wash, the wipe should never re-cross an already washed area. The Paramedic is attempting to create a mini-sterile field. The area of the circular sterile field should minimally be twice the length of the IV needle—one length under the IV needle as it approaches the insertion site and another length for the distance under the skin where the IV needle will be lodged. The germicidal solution should be allowed to dry. This will allow for the maximum germicidal effect.

Paramedics can gently palpate the site before the site preparation, to help identify a viable vein. However, the Paramedic should not re-palpate the intended IV access site once the site preparation has begun. Placing a gloved finger on a sterile field contaminates the field, forcing the Paramedic to re-cleanse the area.

STREET SMART

If the patient is sensitive, or allergic, to povidone-iodine-based solutions, then the Paramedic should only use an isopropyl alcohol-soaked gauze to cleanse the site. When practical, alcohol-soaked gauze should be placed on the site and allowed to remain in place until the Paramedic is ready to insert the IV needle.

PROFESSIONAL PARAMEDIC

Many hospital IV teams use a chlorhexidine + isopropyl alcohol-soaked swab for IV access preparation. These are more expensive than plain alcohol and povidone-iodine but may offer improved bacteriocidal effects. The professional Paramedic will monitor the literature in order to promote evidence-based practice for his/her agency.

Using a new alcohol prep pad for this final step, the Paramedic sets the alcohol prep pad on the insertion site and swipes distally, removing some of the dried povidone-iodine solution from the skin; if an alternative germicidal solution was used then this step is unnecessary. The vein should now be visible underneath the skin. The entire process of site selection and preparation should take approximately one minute.

Venipuncture

After careful consideration, the Paramedic would select the preferred IV device, remove it from the packaging, and uncap the IV needle. The IV needle and catheter should be examined for any burrs which could cause the patient pain. Under no circumstances should the catheter be slid up and down the needle. Sliding the catheter over the needle in this fashion risks shearing the end of the catheter and creating a catheter embolism. However, it is not uncommon to rotate the catheter around the shaft of the needle to ensure its easy removal from the needle. Satisfied that the IV needle and catheter are acceptable, the Paramedic would grasp the IV needle between the thumb and forefinger and approach the selected site.

Some Paramedics use the nondominant hand to grasp the skin below the IV site, applying gentle stabilization to the vein with the thumb. This helps to prevent the vein from moving under the skin (i.e., rolling). Rolling veins are more common in the elderly who have less subcutaneous fat and collagen to help stabilize the vein. Other Paramedics prefer to use the nondominant hand to stabilize the limb, encircling the limb with the Paramedic's own hand below the site. If the patient should suddenly try to pull the limb away, once the IV needle has been inserted, the Paramedic can help hold the limb in place while trying to calm the patient. This approach is particularly useful in children.

With the IV needle poised above the intended venous access point, the Paramedic can take one of two approaches for **venous cannulation**, the process of threading a catheter into a vein. The first approach is a direct in-line approach in which the IV needle immediately enters the vein. The alternative approach is the indirect approach.

With the indirect approach, the Paramedic inserts the IV needle under the skin and next to the vein. Once the needle is under the skin and next to the vein, the Paramedic changes the line of approach and enters the vein. The indirect approach is useful in people with thicker skin as well as children who are likely to flinch. After the needle has pierced the skin, the Paramedic can pause, allowing the patient to recover from the pain before proceeding. The indirect approach also helps decrease the incidence of "overdrive," an accidental through and through venous puncture. The indirect approach is sometimes preferred by less-experienced Paramedics who are trying to gain practice experience.

With the direct approach, the IV needle is placed immediately atop the vein. With the bevel of the IV needle facing up, the IV needle is inserted at an approximately 45-degree angle. When the IV needle is in contact with the vein, the Paramedic may feel a slight resistance to forward motion. When this resistance is overcome, some Paramedics refer to this as the "pop." This indicates the needle is in the lumen of the vein and a blood flash should be observed distal to the needle hub. Absence of blood in the needle and catheter (the flash) implies that the IV is not in the vein.

With the IV needle assumed to be in the lumen of the vein, the Paramedic should decrease the angle of approach to parallel the vein and then advance the IV needle approximately ¼ to ½ inch to ensure that the IV needle and catheter are clearly inside the vein. By failing to perform this maneuver, the Paramedic risks losing the IV access. The purpose of this maneuver is not just to ensure that the IV needle is inside the vein, but also that the IV catheter (which is approximately 1/4 inch behind the tip of the needle) is also inside the vein.

Once the IV needle and catheter are within the lumen, the catheter is threaded off the needle and into the vein. It is important to realize that the needle is not withdrawn from the vein, but rather the catheter is threaded into the vein. The needle remains in place to help maintain the patency of the incision.

If the nondominant hand is available and not holding stabilization, it can be used to advance the catheter into the vein. Otherwise, the first two fingers can grasp the hub of the catheter, in a pincer-like maneuver, and advance the catheter. With the complete length of the IV catheter in place, the needle can be withdrawn slightly. Leaving the IV needle inside the IV hub blocks the catheter's lumen and prevents bleeding through the catheter until the Paramedic can tamponade the vein.

In anticipation of either attaching the IV administration set adaptor or a blood sampling device, the Paramedic should manually tamponade the vein. To tamponade a vein, the Paramedic applies pressure above the end of the catheter in the vein, which should be just above the sterile field. Some Paramedics also elect to place a small gauze pad under the hub to catch any bleeding at this time.

When the needle is completely withdrawn, it must be immediately rendered safe. Some IV needles are self-sheaving whereas others are not. Regardless of the presence of any engineered safety devices, all IV needles should be immediately placed in a sharps container.

The entire time for insertion should be approximately two minutes, from the time the tourniquet was applied to the time the tourniquet was released. Proper preparation of supplies, pre-assembled as necessary, helps to improve overall efficiency.

Cannulation of the External Jugular Vein

The insertion of an IV into an external jugular vein (EJV) requires a few modifications in technique, but the procedure is largely the same as for inserting any peripheral IV. To distend the vein, the patient should be placed supine, preferably with legs slightly elevated about 6 to 12 inches off the floor in modified Trendelenburg position. Standing or sitting at the patient's head and facing the patient, the Paramedic would then place the thumb and forefinger of the nondominant hand on the EJV. The thumb should tamponade the blood flow, causing the vein to distend, and the forefinger should stabilize the EJV in the supraclavicular space. From this stance, the Paramedic would place the IV needle directly over the prepared EJV site. The angle of insertion for an EJV cannulation is more parallel to the skin, approximately 30 degrees, than the angle of insertion for other peripheral IVs. The IV needle is then advanced until a flash is witnessed.

The insertion of an IV needle into the external jugular vein creates a neck wound. The concern with neck wounds is that room air can be drawn into the wound, creating an air embolism. To minimize this risk, the Paramedic should wait until the patient exhales before attaching the IV administration set adaptor.[35,36] Once the EJV IV is in place, precautions should be taken to protect the site. The patient's head should remain in a neutral in-line position. Some Paramedics apply a cervical collar or use a cervical immobilization device to help protect the site.

Blood Samples

Obtaining, or drawing, blood samples from an IV site is easy and could potentially prevent an additional needlestick, saving the patient from avoidable pain and other healthcare providers from a potential needle exposure. The most commonly used blood drawing system is the vacuum-tube system. To use this system, the Paramedic preassembles the vacuum tube collection device and sets it aside for use after the IV access is obtained.

With the catheter in place, the Paramedic would withdraw the needle and attach the needleless adaptor to the hub of the IV catheter. With the adaptor in place, the Paramedic inserts a blood tube into the barrel. Grasping the flange of the device stabilizes the assembly. The blood tube is now pushed down, by the thumb, over the covered needle inside the barrel. The needle pierces the rubber stopper and the vacuum draws blood into the tube.

This process is repeated until all of the blood tubes are filled. Then the device is removed and replaced with the adaptor of the administration set. More information regarding types and uses of blood sampling tubes is found later in this chapter.

Continuous or Intermittent Infusion

Once IV access has been obtained, the Paramedic has the choice between instituting a continuous infusion or an intermittent infusion. To establish a continuous infusion, the Paramedic would take the adaptor from the intravenous administration set, remove the protective cap, withdraw the needle completely from the catheter while maintaining tamponade, and attach the adaptor to the hub. Once the intravenous administration set is attached, the Paramedic would then release the roller clamp and allow the fluid to flow freely for a moment.

If the fluid does not run, it may be a sign of a misplaced or dislodged IV catheter. To troubleshoot the problem, the Paramedic should check to see if the tourniquet has been removed. One of the more common reasons that the fluid is not running freely is that the tourniquet may have inadvertently been left in place (e.g., covered by a falling sleeve) and out of the Paramedic's sight. Next, the Paramedic would start at the solution and methodically examine down the length of the administration set for possible mechanical obstructions to flow. A gentle squeeze of the drip chamber should indicate if there is a passage between the solution and the spike. Continuing down the length of the tubing, the Paramedic would check all clamps and control devices to ensure that they are open. Inspection of the tubing may reveal that a tiny obstruction, such as a plug from the IV solution bag, has lodged in the filter, or that the tubing is kinked. Barring any obstructions in the administration set, which should have run freely before it was attached, the Paramedic would next observe the insertion site.

The difficulty may lie with the catheter itself. Sometimes a catheter will become lodged against the posterior wall of a vein or against a valve. To unblock the catheter, it merely has to be withdrawn slightly and the flow reattempted. If all these measures fail, then it can be assumed that the IV catheter is not in the vein and the IV catheter should be withdrawn.

If the fluid is running freely, then the Paramedic would observe the insertion site for any swelling, a sign of infiltration. If swelling is observed, then it can be assumed that either the catheter slipped out of the insertion site or that the needle, when inserted, was driven through the posterior wall of the vein, creating a hole in the vein. Regardless, the IV site is no longer usable, the IV is "blown," and the catheter must be removed. A description of how to remove an IV catheter follows shortly.

Alternatively, if intermittent infusion is indicated then the IV catheter can be "capped" with a plug-like device that appears and functions like the medication port on the administration set. In the past, an intermittent infusion device was filled with heparin, and described as a **heparin well**. Research has indicated that the use of heparin to prevent thrombus formation at the distal catheter tip was unnecessary. Simply filling the intermittent infusion device with saline would seal, or lock, the device and prevent thrombus formation. Subsequently, **saline locks** have been used almost exclusively (Figure 27-19).

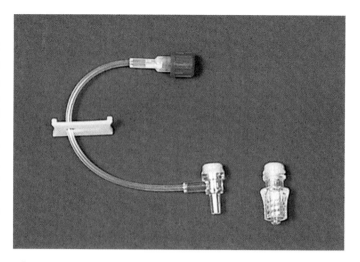

Figure 27-19 Saline lock.

Securing the Intravenous Catheter

With either the administration set attached or the saline lock in place, the entire apparatus needs to be protected from accidental displacement. Many Paramedics elect to secure the IV hub in place with tape, even if a commercial IV dressing is to be used later. There are various kinds of tape available and each has its advantages.

Standard 1/2-inch "silk" tape, adhesive applied to a woven nylon backing, is ideal in most circumstances. If 1/2-inch tape is not available, then larger sizes, such as 1 inch, can be divided into two 1/2-inch strips.

The adhesive of standard tape may be too strong for fragile skin (e.g., on the elderly patient or the neonate). Removing standard tape from their skin can cause a skin tear. For those patient populations, a paper-backed tape may be more appropriate. While paper tape is gentler on the skin, it does not adhere as well. The IV dressing should be constantly monitored.

With two approximately 6-inch lengths of tape prepared, the Paramedic may elect to use one of two methods to secure the hub. The first method, called the **chevron** method, involves slipping the inverted tape, sticky side up, under the hub until it adheres to the hub, then crossing it over the hub. When completed and in place, the tails of the tape extend at an approximately 90-degree angle from the site, forming a V shape. When the tape chevron is in place, the tape should not be directly in contact with the catheter or cover the insertion site (Figure 27-20). In some cases, it is advantageous to place two chevrons, each opposite the other. Once the chevron is secured, another length of tape can be placed directly over the hub.

An alternative to the chevron method is called a "squared out" method. Like the chevron method, a length of tape is slid under the hub of the needle. But instead of immediately turning the ends, an approximately 1-inch span of tape is left exposed under the hub and the ends turned out at a 90-degree angle. With the first tape in place, another strip of tape is

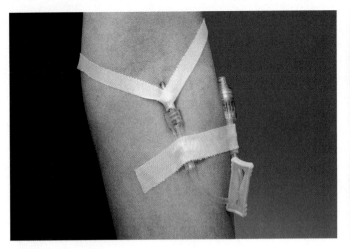

Figure 27-20 Tape chevron.

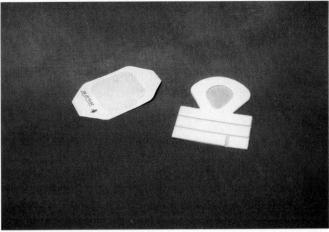

Figure 27-21 Transparent membrane dressing.

placed directly across the first piece and the hub of the catheter. The hub of the catheter, now encircled by tape, is secure as long as the tape adheres to the skin.

To protect the insertion site, which is a puncture wound, either a dry sterile dressing (DSD), such as a gauze pad, or a self-adhesive bandage may be applied. Many Paramedics apply a small quantity of antibiotic ointment to the insertion site before applying the dressing. Commercially available antibiotic creams (e.g., Neosporin®) applied at the insertion site create a physical barrier to bacteria and prevent capillary action from wicking contaminated oils from the skin into the wound.

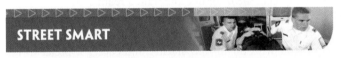

STREET SMART

If a povidone-iodine-based solution was not used to wash the site prior to IV insertion, then the application of a dab of antibiotic cream to the site can help decrease the incidence of infection. Only a small amount is necessary. Too much antibiotic cream can undermine the dressing, causing it to fall off.

Many Paramedics choose to use commercially available transparent membrane dressings (Figure 27-21). These transparent membrane dressings have several advantages which make them attractive for field use. Since they are prepackaged in individual sterile packets, transparent membrane dressings are convenient to use. Once a transparent dressing is applied, the moisture under the dressing can pass through the semipermeable membrane while microorganisms, such as bacteria, cannot pass under the dressing and into the wound. Furthermore, transparent membrane dressings allow the Paramedic the opportunity to continuously monitor the insertion site for signs of inflammation and infiltration without breaking down the dressing. This is an advantage when injecting medications.

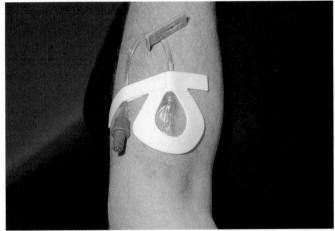

Figure 27-22 Omega loop.

The final step in securing an intravenous infusion is to tape the intravenous administration set tubing to the patient. Initially, a strip of tape is laid across the adaptor and against the skin. Then a loop of tubing is taped across the first strip of tape. This creates a stress loop, called an **omega loop**, which will absorb any tension on the tubing and potentially prevent the IV catheter from being displaced (Figure 27-22).

Adjusting the Infusion Rate

Before starting any infusion, it is important that the Paramedic review the indications for the infusion as well as the contraindications. A reassessment of the patient's vital signs, jugular venous distention, and lung sounds should be made. Then the Paramedic should check for signs of pulmonary edema to establish a baseline.

The selection of an intravenous administration, in part, determines the rate of infusion. For example, a micro-drop administration set cannot produce the same volume of flow in mL per hour, even when the fluid is running as a straight stream, that a macro-drip administration set can.

Conversely, it is more difficult to dispense a precise volume for infusion using a macro-drop intravenous administration set. For this reason, Paramedics use micro-drop intravenous administration sets as a standard practice for medication infusions to help ensure that the exact dose is administered. When a precise volume of infusion is needed, the Paramedic would suspend the solution ("**hanging the bag**") from a hook-like device called a **hanger**. The Paramedic gradually releases the roller clamp, counting the drops in one minute to equal the desired flow rate. EMS drug infusion rates are influenced by a number of physical factors which are part of the reality of practice in the field and can alter the drip rate.

To control the drip rate, the roller clamp or screw clamp applies pressure against the tubing to offset the pressure within the tubing, thus increasing or decreasing flow accordingly. The pressure within the tubing is a function of the height of the column of fluid and the diameter of the tubing.

Many factors can influence the rate of flow, such as the friction loss within the tubing, the diameter of the tubing, the viscosity of the fluid within the tubing, and the length of the tubing. Assuming that all these variables remain constant, the lone act of raising or lowering an intravenous bag—for example, to go through a door or enter an ambulance—will alter the height of the column of fluid. Therefore, the pressure within the tubing is affected, and that will in turn change the drip rate. This all happens without adjusting the roller clamp. Once a drip rate has been established, it is important to try to constantly maintain the intravenous bag at the same height.

Even with the best efforts of the Paramedics involved in a patient's care, other factors that cannot be as easily controlled will influence a drip rate. For example, cold fluids run through an IV access tend to cause vasospasm in the affected vessel. Efforts to warm fluids can help prevent this occurrence. However, warming an intravenous fluid to room temperature still means that chilled (less than body temperature) fluid is being infused.

Temperature changes, which are not common in the hospital setting, are a fact of life for the Paramedic. Intravenous tubing exposed to cold temperatures, such as occurs when transferring a patient to the ambulance in sub-zero degree weather, will stiffen the IV tubing and alter the tension applied by the roller clamp, as well as change the viscosity of the fluid within the tubing. Even when the patient is safely secured within the ambulance's temperature-controlled patient compartment, other factors (such as turbulence at the end of a catheter or slack in an armboard) can cause the IV catheter to migrate up against a valve or the wall of the vein, occluding the flow.

With all of these variables in mind, it is important that a Paramedic regularly confirm, and then re-confirm, the drip rate, particularly if a medicated solution is being infused. Minimally, a drip rate should be rechecked after the patient is placed in the ambulance and then upon arrival at the hospital. Preferably, the drip should be checked with every set of vital signs. Out-of-control drip infusions, called **runaway infusions**, can have serious implications. A runaway infusion of a medicated solution results in the patient being overmedicated. As is the

case with any overdose, a runaway infusion must be reported to medical control so that appropriate measures can be taken to mitigate the medication's adverse effects and negative impact.

The value of prehospital intravenous infusions for trauma patients is being debated. Early consensus seems to indicate that a minimal infusion, one that maintains end-organ perfusion (i.e., a minimal systolic pressure of approximately 80 to 90 mmHg), should be established.[37,38] A runaway infusion during trauma resuscitation can adversely affect the patient in multiple ways, including increasing intracranial pressure, diluting coagulation factors, and increasing hemorrhagic losses.[39] A runaway infusion can be just as devastating for the medical patient as well. A runaway infusion can quickly volume overload the patient with kidney or heart failure. Subsequently, the patient can experience hypertension, pulmonary edema, or cerebral swelling.

Mechanical Flow Control Device

Paramedics use mechanical flow control devices to more accurately control intravenous flow of any drug infusions which are caustic, viscous, or have vasoactive medications. Several types of flow control devices are available on the market. Some work by a venturi effect, controlling the flow by adjusting an aperture, described as dial-a-flow devices. Others work by placing pressure on the tubing, either through a rotary piston or a linear compression (such as massaging fingers), and "milking" the tubing at a precise rate. Smaller syringe pumps apply pressure to the plunger in precise pulsations to inject the drug into the fluid stream.

The advantage of all of these devices is that they can more accurately control flow (Figure 27-23). Many are also equipped with air-in-line alarms, indicating a break in the

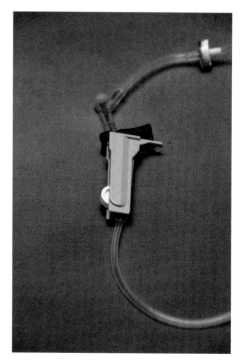

Figure 27-23 Flow control device.

closed intravenous system, and fluid empty alarms as well as obstruction alarms. The greatest advantage of these flow control devices may be the margin of safety that they bring to the less-controlled environment of out-of-hospital emergency medicine. While not impossible, the risk of a runaway infusion is virtually eliminated by these devices. On the downside, the costs of flow control devices, including the costs of training Paramedics in their proper use, may be prohibitive.

Secondary Intravenous Infusions

If a continuous infusion is running and an intermittent infusion of a medicated solution is needed, the Paramedic can establish a secondary infusion, or **piggyback infusion**, to the primary infusion. This practice has several advantages, including the ability to immediately terminate the intermittent infusion (e.g., if the patient had an allergic reaction) and permit a bolus and/or drug to counteract any ill effects, such as anaphylaxis-induced hypotension. Use of a secondary intravenous infusion also eliminates the need for a second IV access and the accompanying difficulty, and time, of preparing and establishing an intermittent infusion device (saline lock) which would normally be necessary.

After assessing to ensure that the primary infusion is running and that the IV access is patent, the Paramedic would prepare the secondary IV. Special secondary administration sets which have a shorter length are available (Figure 27-24). The secondary set would be run out as per the procedure described previously for a continuous infusion administration set. The secondary intravenous set would be connected to the continuous intravenous set, now called the **primary infusion**, via a medication port. If a needle is used to attach the two sets, it will be necessary to first cleanse the port with an alcohol prep pad.

With the two administration sets now attached, the primary set is placed lower than the secondary set. This is usually accomplished by using a plastic or metal hanger that comes with the secondary administration set. The secondary administration set will now take dominance over the primary administration as its fluid column is higher and thus there is more pressure. When the column of fluid in the secondary administration set equals the level of the fluid in the primary administration set's drip chamber, then the primary drip will resume flow at its previous adjusted rate.

Intravenous Injection

Paramedics frequently use IV access as a means for the rapid injection of IV medications during an emergency. Early insertion of an intravenous access device during patient care provides Paramedics a nearly instant ability to administer drugs directly into the circulation and to target organs.

If the IV access site has an intermittent infusion device attached, then the Paramedic would attach a syringe and withdraw about 10 mL of fluid from the device and discard the waste into an approved sharps container. The Paramedic would then attach another syringe, either filled or prefilled with the medication, to the infusion device and inject the medication. This process is called **IV push**. Note that if a needle is used then the self-sealing membrane of the injection port must be cleansed. Immediately after injecting the medication, the device is flushed with 10 to 20 mL of NSS to clear the medication from the device and assure that all of the medication goes into the circulation (Figure 27-25).

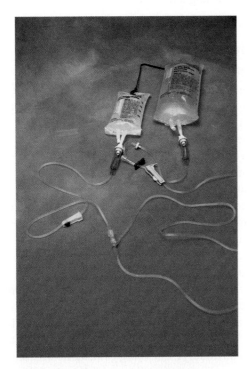

Figure 27-24 Secondary intravenous administration set.

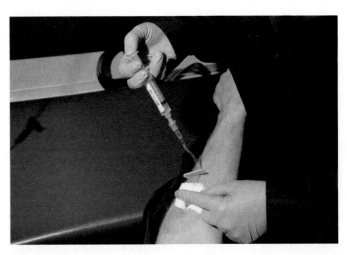

Figure 27-25 Saline flush with prefilled syringe.

If the IV access site has a continuous infusion in place, then the Paramedic would first clamp the tubing, using the roller clamp or slide clamp, and then attach the syringe or prefilled ampoule, as just described. Once the IV push is completed, the Paramedic may elect to flush the tubing with 20 mL of NSS and then unclamp the line. He may also choose to unclamp the line and allow a free flow of fluid to flush the IV line for approximately one minute, then re-adjust the flow rate.

If the patient is in cardiovascular collapse, then the patient's arm should be raised to help the medication drain out of the limb. Similarly, if the patient is in cardiac arrest, then the limb should be raised and a minimum of one minute of external chest compressions performed to ensure that the drug is circulated.

In every case it is important that the Paramedic observe the IV access site for swelling, pain, and other signs of infiltration while injecting the medication. Some Paramedics purposefully place the medication port proximal to the IV access site so that the IV insertion site can be observed. If an infiltration is suspected, then the IV push is stopped and measures taken to counteract the effects of any medication that has leaked into the subcutaneous tissue. It is important to report any intravenous infiltration. If unchecked, some medications (for example, 50% dextrose) can cause severe local tissue necrosis with the potential for subsequent tendon, muscle, and nerve damage.

Obstruction of Intravenous Flow

The flow of an IV may slow, or even stop, for a number of reasons. Before removing the IV catheter, the Paramedic should assess the situation for correctable errors. Starting at the solution bag, the Paramedic would methodically inspect the entire intravenous apparatus. For example, flow will stop if the solution bag is empty, a clamp has slipped, or the tubing is kinked. After assessing the administration set and determining that it is clear of mechanical obstructions, the Paramedic would then turn his attention to the IV access site.

An infiltrated IV access site will eventually slow or stop an infusion. If the IV access site is infiltrated, then the IV catheter must be removed immediately (this process is discussed later in the chapter). Finding no visible obstructions or infiltration, the Paramedic may elect to see if there is a return of blood, called a **flashback**, when the solution bag is lowered below the level of the patient's heart. A flashback (Figure 27-26) indicates that the IV access remains patent.

Some IV catheters are positional, meaning that the catheter lodged up against the wall of a vein or a valve and the IV flow has been obstructed. To correct a positional IV catheter, the Paramedic may elect to withdraw the needle slightly. This process includes breaking the dressing down or raising the hub of the IV catheter off the skin with a gauze pad. If the IV access is in a joint, it is advisable to place the joint onto a padded splint. If a padded splint is used, then distal circulation, sensation, and movement should be assessed before and after the splint's application to ensure that the splint is not

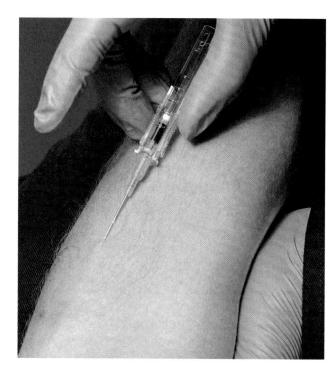

Figure 27-26 Flashback of blood verifies venous competency.

constrictive. The distal circulation, sensation, and movement should be checked periodically thereafter.

An obstructed IV catheter should never be forcibly injected with solution (IV flush) to remove any obstructions. The risk of forcing a thrombus into the circulation is not equal to the benefit of having an intravenous access. The Paramedic should consider removing the suspect IV catheter and re-establishing a new IV access.

Complications of Intravenous Infusions

Despite the best efforts of Paramedics, local or systemic complications can occur as a direct result of an IV access or infusion. An attentive Paramedic can usually detect these complications and mitigate the circumstances in order to reduce the harm to the patient.

Arteries and nerves tend to be bundled with veins, particularly deep veins. Therefore, they are at risk for accidental needle puncture. An unintentional arterial puncture would be recognized if the Paramedic noticed a pulsating column of blood within the fluid column. However, recognition of an arterial puncture is more difficult in zero flow states, such as cardiac arrest. Careful attention to anatomy, noting the location of proximal arteries by their pulse points, can help decrease the incidence of accidental arterial puncture.

A nerve can also be accidentally punctured during an IV insertion attempt. Patients usually alert the Paramedic immediately following an accidental nerve puncture. The patient will complain loudly of shooting pain, numbness, and tingling in the affected limb. Immediate withdrawal of the offending needle should provide the patient with immediate relief.

Immediately following successful cannulation of a vein by an IV catheter, and frequently thereafter, the Paramedic should assess the IV access for signs of infiltration or infection. Infiltration can occur by several mechanisms puncture of the posterior wall, enlargement of the initial incision site, or displacement of the catheter. Regardless of the mechanism, the IV solution seeps into the interstitial fluid compartment (ICF) (i.e., the third space). The resultant swelling can create increased pressure within a compartment, which can lead to impingement of nerves, muscle damage, and compression of blood vessels (compartment syndrome).

One of the earliest signs of infiltration can be a slow infusion. Other signs of infiltration include local edema, complaints of pain at the site, and localized cooling of the skin (Figure 27-27). An infiltration of an unmedicated solution should be treated by immediate removal of the catheter and application of a warm compress to the site. Any infiltration of medicated solutions should be reported and treated immediately.

Occasionally IV sites become infected. While a Paramedic would not see an infection of an IV site from a recently placed IV, patients receiving at-home intermittent intravenous infusions with temporary indwelling intravenous catheters and those who are discharged home after a short hospital stay may have signs of an infection at the insertion site. An infection at the insertion site is called a **thrombophlebitis**. An IV access site is essentially a puncture wound, and the body responds to an IV cannulation as it would any wound. A thrombus is formed at the wound and the injury healing process begins. However, the catheter keeps the wound open. Bacteria tends to track into the wound, by capillary action, and the area becomes inflamed.[40–42]

Signs of thrombophlebitis include warmth in the area, pain upon palpation, and reddened and swollen tissues. As the infection progresses, the infection can advance up the vein, creating a visible red trail along the course of the vein and pain along the vein's length.

While a Paramedic may rarely see a thrombophlebitis related to a fresh IV, Paramedics may be witness to a **pyrogenic reaction**, a devastating systemic complication of intravenous therapy. A pyrogenic reaction occurs when a contaminated fluid, or fluid run through a contaminated administration set, is infused and leads to nearly immediate sepsis. Symptoms of a pyrogenic reaction usually occur within 30 minutes of the initiation of the infusion and include complaints of headache, chills, and backache. Signs that will accompany a pyrogenic reaction include fever, tachycardia, and, in severe cases, cardiovascular collapse. Examination of the solution for contaminants as well as verification of the expiration date can help reduce the incidence of pyrogenic reaction (Figure 27-28).

If a pyrogenic reaction is suspected, the Paramedic should immediately discontinue the infusion. The administration set and intravenous solution should be retained for microbiological examination and the lot numbers of the solution recorded on the patient care report. Fortunately, with the advent of disposable single-use administration sets and tightly controlled manufacturing processes, the number of pyrogenic reactions is very low.

Another potentially devastating complication of intravenous infusions is **volume overload**. A volume overload occurs when a positional IV access is inadvertently adjusted and the infusion flow is unrestricted. It can also occur when a clamp is released (e.g., to administer a fluid bolus) and the infusion rate is not re-adjusted.

The symptoms of a volume overload include a nonproductive cough, wheezing, and complaints of shortness of breath or headache. Accompanying signs of volume overload include hypertension, marked jugular venous distention, and crackles in the lung fields that are indicative of pulmonary

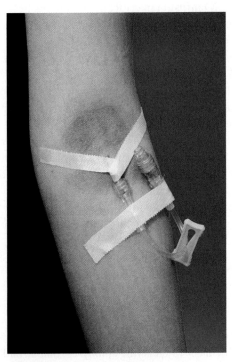

Figure 27-27 Infiltration of medication at intravenous site.

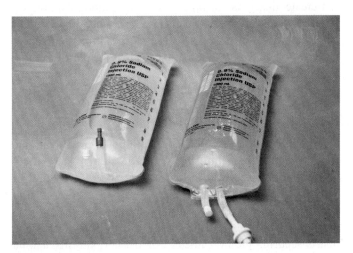

Figure 27-28 Grossly contaminated solution (on the right), as compared with clean solution (on the left).

edema. Initially, the Paramedic should reduce the infusion to KVO/TKO or consider using an intermittent infusion device (a saline well). Prehospital care of the patient with a suspected volume overload centers on symptomatic relief and supportive care.

Another serious complication of intravenous infusions is an air embolism. An air embolism can occur when the Paramedic fails to run fluid through an intravenous administration set to **flush the line** prior to use. Symptoms of air embolism include chest pain and lightheadedness. Signs of air embolism include cyanosis, as well as hypotension which can, in severe cases, lead to cardiovascular collapse. If an air embolism is suspected, the infusion should be stopped. The patient should then be placed in the left lateral recumbent position, with the right lung superior and the feet elevated above the level of the heart. The Paramedic should provide supportive care and contact medical control for further instructions.

Infusion-Induced Hypothermia

An all too common complication of intravenous infusions is hypothermia. The infusion of large quantities of room-temperature solutions will rapidly cool the body and lead to hypothermia.[43,44] If it is necessary to infuse large quantities of solutions, then consideration should be given to providing a warming blanket (hypothermia blanket) or other similar device. Some Paramedics use commercially available blood warmers, special heated compartments or thermal sleeves to warm the intravenous fluids prior to administration. Abbott Corporation, a major supplier of intravenous solutions, recommends the use of a "conventional warm air oven" which warms the fluids before administration. Once the fluids are removed from the oven, they should be used within 24 hours and not re-warmed again.

The use of microwave ovens to warm intravenous solutions is commonly practiced in emergency departments and operating rooms. Caution should be used when microwave ovens are used to warm intravenous solutions because microwave ovens can create "hotspots" of fluid within the solution that, during infusion, could scald the epithelial (inner) lining of the vein.

The use of warm water baths is also not recommended. Water from the warm water bath may cross the plastic flexible container wall and contaminate the solution. Such contamination could lead to a potential pyrogenic reaction.

Removing Intravenous Access

Paramedics may be called upon to remove, or discontinue (DC), an intravenous infusion. A careful step-by-step procedure will minimize pain for the patient and the potential of contamination to the Paramedic. The first step is to clamp the administration set and stop the infusion. With the infusion stopped, the Paramedic should gently loosen any tape that is securing the IV catheter. An alcohol prep pad can be used to undermine the tape's adhesive. With the tape loose, the Paramedic would then place a small gauze pad over the insertion site and apply gentle downward pressure with the

gloved nondominant hand. With the gloved dominant hand, the Paramedic would gently apply traction to the catheter's hub in the opposite direction of the insertion. With the entire length of the catheter out of the vein, the Paramedic would continue to apply direct pressure to the wound and elevate the limb. If the IV access was in the antecubital fossa, the patient should be encouraged to keep the limb straight and elevate it. Bending the elbow will widen the opening created by the IV catheter and thus increase bleeding. The catheter and administration set should be discarded safely in a biohazard bag and a notation made of the removal of the IV access, including the exact location of the access site.

Intraosseous Access

Before the invention of the plastic IV catheter, venous access was obtained using large metal needles, needles that would be resharpened, sterilized, and reused again and again. These large gauge needles often made venous access in the elderly or the vasculopathic patient difficult to obtain and alternatives were sought to peripheral venous access.

In 1922, Dr. C.K. Drinker, of Harvard University, demonstrated that the use of metal needles inserted into the bone marrow of the sternum (**intraosseous (IO)**) could provide venous access to the circulation. Dr. Drinker confirmed that these intraosseous infusions rapidly infused into the bone marrow and then later into the central venous circulation.

Later, Dr. Tocantins and Dr. O'Neill expanded on sternal intraosseous access sites and included the long bones (tibia and femur). With multiple sites readily available, and the invention of the bone needle for intraosseous access, IO access became practical and convenient. During the 1940s and 1950s, IO infusion in critically ill patients became somewhat commonplace and was used by military medics in World War II in over 4,000 documented cases.

However, with the advent of plastic catheters and improved venous catheter technology, IO use saw a decline after World War II and remained an historic relic of past medical practice until 1984. In 1984, Dr. Orlowski, after witnessing IO use in children afflicted with cholera in India, wrote an article in the *American Journal of Diseases in Children* citing the advantages of IO in pediatrics. IO infusion was reborn for pediatrics and is now commonplace. Pediatric IO is discussed in detail at the end of the chapter.

More recently, due to a growing population of aged patients, vasculopathic patients, and emerging new medical technologies that hold promise for use in the field, the need for venous access has grown more acute. Therefore, the interest in IO infusion for adults has been revisited.

Anatomy and Physiology of the Long Bones

A long bone has two ends (the epiphyses) and a shaft (the diaphysis). Within the shaft of the bone or the medullary cavity is the bone marrow. At the ends of the bones, within the epiphysis, is the soft, sponge-like cancellous bone. Together the medullary space and the cancellous bone make up the intraosseous space.

The IO space contains a complex network of blood vessels that connect to the major veins of the central circulation via a series of longitudinal Haversian canals that exit the bone and connect directly into the major veins. Infusing fluids into the intraosseous space ultimately infuses fluids into the central veins via these Haversian canals.

Intraosseous Devices

A number of IO devices are presently on the market. These devices range from manually inserted IO needles, the type used primarily in children, to medical drills that create a precise opening for insertion of an IO needle. Because of the large number of IO devices on the market, Paramedics are advised to read the accompanying medical literature that comes with each device and to familiarize themselves with the device by practicing on a manikin or model before trying to utilize the IO in the field.

Indications and Contraindications

There are several indications for adult IO placement. One indication is cardiac arrest.[45,46] During cardiac arrest, the cardiovascular system is in collapse and venous access can be a challenge. Intravenous access can be difficult to obtain or is obtained at a cost of prolonged scene times. The rigid container of the IO, the bone, provides a ready access even during zero blood flow states. Other indications include any time there is a need for an immediate access for medication administration for the patient in extremis.

Advantages of IO access are also several-fold. IO access is rapid, quicker than IV access in many cases, and generally requires less skill and training to master. In one study, IO access was able to be obtained in the field within 20 seconds or less with a 97% success rate.[47–50]

However, IO insertion is not without its risks. IO insertion can be painful in conscious patients, although that is not always the case. Some patients have compared the pain of an IO insertion to the discomfort of a large bore IV. IO infusions can also be painful, but with a bolus of lidocaine can further reduce the pain of infusion. Finally, the IO has a potentially higher risk of osteomyelitis. However, the incidence of osteomyelitis is uncommon. It has been reported that the osteomyelitis rate for IO infusions is about one in 200 cases. Other attendant risks include fat embolism, fracture, extravasation, and compartment syndrome. It should be noted that these complications are rare and can usually be prevented by careful insertion and monitoring.

The single largest drawback to IO may be the inability to infuse large bolus of fluids. The IO infusion is generally similar to that of a 20 gauge IV catheter.[51] The addition of a pressure infusion bag enhances flow rates to more acceptable levels.

Intraosseous Placement

Preparation of the IO site is similar to preparation for an IV insertion. First the Paramedic needs to select a site. Depending on the device and the manufacturer's recommendations, an IO needle can be placed in the sternum, the tibia, the femur, or the humerus. Next, the exact point of placement must be identified, often using adjunct landmarks, and properly prepared with povidone-iodine or similar antiseptic (Skill 27-3).

For a step-by-step demonstration of Intraosseous Access, please refer to Skill 27-3 on pages 589–590.

After inserting the needle, following the manufacturer's recommendations, the needle should be flushed with 5 to 10 cc of sterile saline to ensure patency. If the patient is conscious, an additional bolus of lidocaine (approximately 10 cc) can help to reduce the pain of infusion.

STREET SMART

Improper placement of an IO needle in an obese patient can be avoided if the Paramedic monitors the insertion. If bone resistance cannot be felt once the needle has been placed to a depth of approximately 5 cm, indicated by a black band on some IO needles, then the needle should be withdrawn and an alternative site prepared.

Medication Administration

The majority of prehospital medications can be administered via the IO route (Table 27-1). The exceptions to IO administration include 9% saline, also known as super saline, and adenosine.

This list includes medications typically used during a cardiac arrest. Considering the speed of attaining therapeutic levels of these drugs via the IO route, IO is considered by most authorities to be preferable over endotracheal administration.

Phlebotomy

A sample of the patient's blood, for laboratory analysis, may be drawn at the time that the IV access is obtained. However,

Table 27-1 List of IO Medications

• Amiodarone	• Furosemide
• Atropine	• Lidocaine
• Dextrose 50%	• Naxolone
• Diazepam	• Rocuronium
• Dopamine	• Succinylcholine
• Epinephrine	• Vasopressin
• Etomidate	• Vecoronium
• Fentanyl	• Versed

there are times when a blood sample is required but IV access is not necessary. In this case, a Paramedic would perform a phlebotomy, drawing blood through a straight needle, to obtain the sample.

Prior to performing the venipuncture, the Paramedic needs to assemble the necessary equipment, including blood sample tubes. There are a number of blood sample tubes and each has a specific purpose. The color of the stopper indicates a blood tube's use. The patient's condition usually dictates which blood tubes will be used and is based upon the expectation that a certain battery of diagnostic laboratory tests will be performed to help discern the pathology and guide the treatment.

The red top tubes are sometimes called **clot tubes** because the tube contains no additives or preservatives to prevent blood clotting. Without additives, such as an anticoagulant, the blood clots and the serum rise to the top. The percentage difference between the amount of space filled by the clot (formed elements such as red blood cells) and the total volume is the **hematocrit**. The patient's hematocrit is an important indicator, particularly for trauma patients.

Samples of the serum are used to test the **blood chemistry** (i.e., the electrolytes, etc.) in the blood. The clot is used to identify the variety of blood (**blood-typing**) and to **crossmatch** it to blood that is available in the blood bank. It is important that the serum separates from the formed elements in the blood; therefore, it is counterproductive to invert or shake the blood tube.

The light blue and lavender-topped tubes have anticoagulants (3.2% sodium citrate and sodium EDTA, respectively) added to them to prevent the blood from clotting. These anticoagulant tubes are used for special clotting studies, such as the partial prothrombin time (PPT), as well as red blood cell studies, including hematocrit and hemoglobin (H&H). The laboratory results from these studies are important if the patient is destined for the operating room or may receive fibrinolytics.

A number of other blood tubes are available—gray, green, royal blue, and yellow—and each has a specific indication. For example, tan-topped tubes have sodium heparin, another anticoagulant, and are used for tests of lead.

When in doubt, or when no orders exist, a standard blood sample usually includes drawing a red-topped tube, a blue-topped tube, and a lavender-topped tube. The order of the blood draw is also important. To prevent potential contamination from additives, the tubes without additives (red-topped tubes) are drawn first and the "wet" tubes (those with additives) are drawn last.

To perform a phlebotomy, the Paramedic could prepare the site as if an IV access was going to be attempted. Frequently, the preferred site for a phlebotomy is the antecubital fossa, although any peripheral vein is acceptable.

Commonly, a straight hollow-bore needle attached to a vacuum tube apparatus is used for phlebotomy. With the vein prepared, the needle shield is removed from the needle and the gloved dominant hand stabilizes the vein. The needle is then advanced, bevel up, into the skin and then the vein, at about a 15 to 20 degree angle. Once the Paramedic is confident that the needle is in the vein, then the blood tube is joined with the sheaved needle inside the barrel and blood is automatically drawn up.

After the first flash of blood occurs, confirming placement, the tourniquet is released and the blood tube allowed to fill completely. Red-topped tubes should be placed aside while other colored-topped tubes are generally gently inverted approximately 10 times, but not shaken, before being set aside. Multiple blood tubes can be filled in this manner.

Once the phlebotomy is completed, a cotton gauze pad is placed over the needle insertion site and the needle quickly withdrawn in the direction opposite of insertion. Cotton balls should not be used as they tend to adhere to and pull out platelet plugs at the insertion site. With the bleeding controlled, the Paramedic can proceed with marking the blood tubes with the name of the patient, the date and time of the phlebotomy, and the Paramedic's initials.

After placing the blood tubes in a clear plastic bag, the Paramedic should ensure the blood tube's safe transportation to the receiving hospital. Some Paramedics tape the blood tubes to the outside of the intravenous solution bag. This practice is acceptable provided the contents are clearly visible. The use of a nonsterile glove is discouraged, as the contents inside the glove are not visible. All **potentially infectious materials (PIM)** must be clearly marked with the biohazard symbol or some other warning that indicates the presence of PIM. A cut sustained from the broken glass of a blood tube is an exposure to blood-contaminated sharps and may be a reportable incident.

Pediatric Phlebotomy

Drawing blood from a child can be a challenge. By applying the principles of pediatric venous access (discussed later in the chapter), along with the principles of phlebotomy (just discussed), the Paramedic can expect to have success.

A heel stick is performed to obtain a blood sample from an infant. A **heel stick**—puncturing the infant's heel with a lancet then drawing the blood off with a capillary tube—is performed on newborns. Practice while under the careful supervision of a practiced provider is the best means for Paramedics to master this technique.

For older children, phlebotomy is performed as it is on adults, with a few exceptions. Children have smaller veins; therefore, smaller needles (25 g to 27 g) are used to draw blood. Children's veins also tend to collapse under the pressure that a vacuum tube system produces. Venous collapse can be averted by either using a pediatric vacuum tube system or using a 5 mL or 10 mL syringe attached to a butterfly needle. Gentle intermittent traction on the syringe's plunger will gradually draw the sample from the vein. With a little patience, the application of age-specific therapeutic interventions, and the right equipment, the Paramedic can expect to be successful with a phlebotomy on a child.

Blood Cultures

When a patient has a fever or the Paramedic suspects that the patient may have septicemia (an infection in the blood), then a blood culture could be drawn. The blood culture is a special laboratory analysis used to test the blood for the presence of sources of infection called pathogens. Common blood culture specimen collection units are either aerobic and anaerobic (Figure 27-29). Blood cultures usually involve obtaining enough blood to fill two broth-containing blood tubes or bottles, the broth being a medium for bacterial growth. One of the blood cultures is used to test for aerobic microorganisms and the other blood culture is used to test for anaerobic microorganisms.

It is important that medical asepsis be practiced whenever a blood culture is drawn. The venous access site must be cleansed with a povidone-iodine-based solution, such as Betadine®, or similar antigermicidal solution and the solution allowed to dry. While the solution is drying on the skin, the Paramedic should take a new swab and cleanse the top of the blood culture tube/bottle. The remainder of the phlebotomy would proceed as usual. Although practices vary from hospital to hospital, in every case medical asepsis is practiced the prevention of accidental contamination of the specimen is important.

Pediatric Intravenous Access

Pediatric intravenous access can be challenging to even the most experienced Paramedic. The key to success in pediatric IV access is to match the IV access site chosen to the urgency of the situation and then take a therapeutic approach to the child that is matched to the child's developmental level.

The choice for a peripheral pediatric venous access can be very age-dependent, owed to the child's changing body habitus. For example, an umbilical venous access may be appropriate in a newborn whereas a venous access in the dorsal venous arch of the hand may be more appropriate for a toddler.

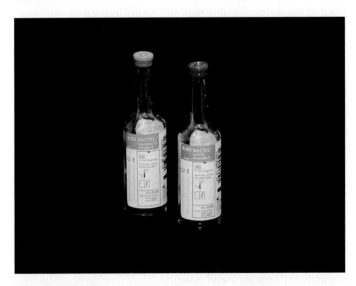

Figure 27-29 Blood culture specimen collection units.

Age-Appropriate Approaches to Pediatric Patients with IV Access

Regardless of a child's age, each child views intravenous therapy as a painful procedure that he would rather avoid. Gaining a child's trust and cooperation will tend to improve success with pediatric IV access. Trust and cooperation is earned when the Paramedic carries out the child's IV therapy with an age-appropriate therapeutic approach.

As a general rule, the Paramedic should not separate the child and parent during the IV attempt. However, practice, experience, and personal interaction with the parent is a better basis for that decision. Involving the child in the preparations and decision making may help the child feel more in control, provided the child is not given the opportunity to say no, and helps foster trust between the Paramedic and the child.

The child should never be told, by either the Paramedic or the parent, that the insertion of an IV will not hurt. Rather, the focus should be on the benefit of the IV and how quickly the IV will be over. Needless to say, this places a burden on the Paramedic to ensure that all of the necessary supplies are immediately available and prepared. Similarly, the child should not be told that only one IV attempt will be necessary. The number of IV attempts is a function of the child's condition and the importance of the IV. Finally, regardless of a child's age, he should be encouraged to cry, privately, without fear of ridicule, and to express his anger or frustration without fear of judgment. The Paramedic understands that these outbursts are not meant personally. Such expressions are healthy and an indication that the child is coping appropriately with the situation.

Developmentally speaking, infants are learning trust and have a strong child–parent bond. The infant may not trust the Paramedic but does trust the parent to protect him. A parent should be encouraged to comfort the infant before and after the venipuncture. Often a pacifier can help to sooth the infant while the procedure is going on; however, the infant should not be given a bottle-feeding, as the risk of vomiting and aspiration offsets any advantage. If the infant is fussy, and there is a risk of accidental catheter displacement, then a swaddling board (e.g., an infant blanket over a short padded board) may be used to immobilize the infant.

Toddlers exhibit their growing autonomy by attempting to assert their control. The toddler should be dealt with matter-of-factly and told (in simple, age-appropriate terms) what is about to happen. Age-appropriate distractions are often very useful at this age as the child attempts to demonstrate her self-control. However, it is not uncommon for a child at this age to regress. A parent should be available to comfort the child.

Preschoolers are capable of assisting with preparation and setup (e.g., tearing pieces of tape) and want to appear confident. However, preschoolers have a fear of the unknown, particularly about pain. Therefore, they should be told, in a straightforward manner, what is going to occur. This approach helps to eliminate some of the fear-producing fantasy the child might imagine. When the IV access has been obtained, the preschooler should be commended for her cooperation and permitted to express her emotions. Paramedics may be taken back by the articulate manner which the preschooler may express herself.

School-aged children, up to adolescence, are thoughtful and generally understand the implications behind the statements that the Paramedic makes. The Paramedic should encourage the school-aged child to ask questions and then provide answers at an age-appropriate level. Limited decision making, such as determining the arm that the IV is to be started, can help the child feel more in control and less fearful.

Adolescents can be treated like an adult, more or less. Time spent with fuller explanations and a question and answer period helps to gain both their trust and their cooperation. Adolescents are concerned about body image and peer approval. The Paramedic should be forthcoming with praise regarding positive aspects of the relationship and avoid any criticism of the adolescent's conduct. In some instances, an adolescent may be content to listen to music from a headset while the IV is being started. This is not a demonstration of contempt or aloofness, but rather an effective distraction technique.

Umbilical Venous Access (UVC)

For a newly born, with a medical emergency, it may be possible to gain venous access via the umbilical cord to administer fluids and drugs, such as epinephrine. The umbilical cord, that rope-like appendage between mother and child, has two arteries and one vein, surrounded by Wharton's jelly, and has no nerves. The two umbilical arteries carry deoxygenated blood from the fetus to the placenta, and the umbilical vein carries oxygenated blood from the mother to the fetus. Some umbilical cords, however, have only two vessels: an artery and a vein. Newborns with only two vessels often have associated congenital anomalies.

To begin, the Paramedic would loosely tie off the umbilical cord, around the base, with cloth umbilical tape. Tying the umbilical tape too tight can prevent the passage of the venous catheter. If the tie is too loose, as evidenced by bleeding, it can be re-tied tighter later. The umbilical stump is now cleansed with a povidone-iodine solution. While waiting for the povidone-iodine solution to dry, the Paramedic would prefill a 5 French umbilical catheter with NSS via a syringe attached to a three-way stopcock (Figure 27-30).

After donning sterile gloves, the Paramedic would take the sterile scalpel and perform a perpendicular transection of the umbilical cord proximal to the clamp. Examination of the cord should reveal three orifices—two arteries and one vein—with the vein typically at the 12 o'clock position. The thicker-walled arteries are usually inferior, at 4 and 8 o'clock, unless the cord is twisted, which is a common presentation.

The umbilical catheter would be advanced through the umbilical vein, the larger orifice, and toward the heart for a distance of approximately 2 to 4 cm. Once the umbilical catheter is past the orifice, there should be a flash of blood inside

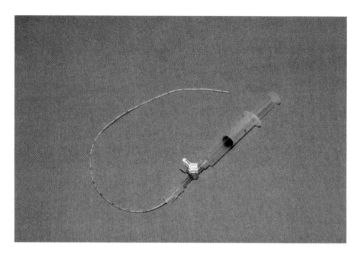

Figure 27-30 Umbilical catheter attached to a three-way stopcock.

the catheter. Opening the stopcock, the Paramedic should gently aspirate, by pulling back on the syringe's plunger, until a free flow of blood is observed.

With the catheter now in place, fluids and/or medications (such as 0.1 mg of epinephrine 1:10,000) can be rapidly administered. The Paramedic should tighten the umbilical tie to secure the umbilical catheter in place and prevent excessive bleeding from the umbilical stump.

Scalp Vein Access

The thought of inserting a needle into an infant's scalp may sound bizarre to many Paramedics. However, pediatricians and pediatric nurses have used scalp veins for venous access for decades. Scalp veins can provide a reliable venous access that is easy to obtain and even easier to maintain.

The scalp veins are generally very prominent, have no valves to interfere with cannulation, and are only thinly obscured by the fine hair of the infant. The most commonly used scalp veins are the metopic vein, located at the midforehead region, and the superficial temporal veins located bilaterally on the forehead (Figure 27-31).[52] A broad rubber band placed around the head at approximately ear level will help distend the scalp veins.

The infant should be restrained, as needed, and the area prepared. Using scissors, any negligible amount of hair should be clipped and the area cleansed with povidone-iodine or similar antiseptic solution, using care to not have the solution run into the eyes.

After flushing the intravenous catheter (either a butterfly needle or an over-the-needle device) with sterile saline, the Paramedic would pull gentle traction on the vein with the nondominant hand and proceed with inserting the needle. When a flash of blood is visible, the tourniquet can be removed and a small amount of saline solution injected to test the catheter's patency and position.

If the saline solution flushes easily, without evidence of infiltration, then the IV catheter should be secured in place.

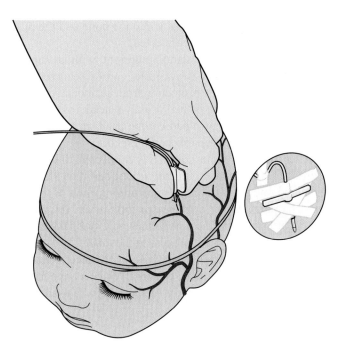

Figure 27-31 Anatomy of infant scalp veins.

Many Paramedics place a clear plastic cup-like shield over the site to protect it from incidental trauma.

Peripheral Pediatric Venous Access

The techniques for peripheral venous access are the same for children as they are for adults with just a few minor variations. However, attention to these differences will help to ensure the Paramedic is successful in obtaining venous access in a child.

Unlike adults, children cannot be expected to remain motionless while an IV needle is being inserted. Two Paramedics may be needed: one to start the IV and the other to deal with the child, including restraining the child as needed. The child should be placed supine. In an ambulance, it is common to have the parent sit at the head of the stretcher, to comfort the child, while two providers sit on each side. Use of a small blanket, used as a swaddling cloth, can help immobilize a child. With one limb exposed, the child is ready for an IV.

Next, the vein needs to be distended. Adult venous tourniquets apply too much pressure and pinch the child's tender skin. It is easier and more effective if another Paramedic encircles the limb, with a firm grasp, effectively distending the veins while stabilizing the limb.

Next, the venous access sites are chosen. The venous access sites for a child are generally the same as an adult's access sites. The Paramedic may have difficulty finding an IV access site on a pudgy infant's forearms, so the use of warm compresses can increase venous distention and improve visualization; observing caution to prevent burns.

With the IV site selected, the Paramedic should choose the appropriate IV device. Generally, Paramedics choose to use the butterfly IV needle. Butterfly needles should not be placed in freely movable joints but rather in areas, such as the scalp or dorsum of the hand, which can be immobilized.

To insert a standard IV catheter into the dorsum of the hand, the Paramedic should grasp the child's fingers with the thumb, pulling traction on the vein while immobilizing the hand. Once the hand is stabilized, the Paramedic would approach the vein with the needle almost parallel to the skin and advance the needle until a flash of blood is visible in the catheter's hub.

It is good practice to immobilize the limb with the IV catheter to a padded short board. Caution should be observed to ensure that the securing straps/tape is not acting as a venous tourniquet, creating backpressure, compromising the IV site, and possibly causing an infiltration.

Next, the IV site should be dressed. After the transparent dressing is in place and the tubing is secured, with an omega loop, a length of protective netting can also be applied lengthwise along the limb. The netting permits observation of the site while protecting the tubing, catheter, and so on. Alternatively, a small paper cup can be cut in half and placed over the site to act as a protective shield.

 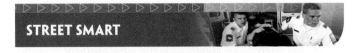
Pediatric Intraosseous Access

In high-priority situations, such as pediatric cardiac arrest, immediate venous access is imperative. In those cases, establishing an IV catheter is too time-consuming and has the attendant risk of failure. In times of high peril, an intraosseous infusion is indicated.[46, 54–57] When time is of the essence, the intraosseous route offers many advantages over traditional peripheral venous access. To begin, the intraosseous route remains available even during cardiac arrest, unlike peripheral venous access that collapses. Next, the intraosseous infusion can generally be established within a minute and a half. Then, once the needle is in place it is essentially fixed to the bone and is fast and secure. Finally, the amount of distal blood flow inside the bone's marrow quickly clears medication and circulates it directly to the central circulation and onto the heart.

Common complications of intraosseous needle (IO) placement include misplacement of the needle, inadvertent puncture of the posterior wall of the bone, and extravasation of fluids into the tissues. Other complications, such as interruption of the growth plate and osteomyelitis, are rare if the Paramedic closely follows needle insertion guidelines.

While technically there are numerous locations for an intraosseous needle placement, Paramedics concentrate on four primary sites. The first site, and the site of choice, is the proximal tibia.[58] The insertion site on the tibia is located approximately 2 centimeters, or two finger widths, distal and medial to the tibial tuberosity on the tibial plateau. Alternatively, another insertion site is available on the distal femur, 2 centimeters above the distal epicondyle and in the midline of the femur. While the distal tibia, proximate to the medial malleolus, and the anterior iliac spine are also acceptable sites, they are rarely used by Paramedics.

Intraosseous needles, like all other peripheral venous access, cannot be placed into an extremity with a fractured bone. If the limb has a painful, swollen area, secondary to trauma, then a fracture should be suspected and the area avoided for IO needle placement.

Once the desired insertion site has been identified, the Paramedic should prepare the site with a povidone-iodine swab or similar antiseptic solution. While surgical asepsis is not necessary, it is important that Paramedics practice strict medical asepsis, taking all precautions to prevent bone infection.

If the child is conscious, then it may be necessary to infiltrate the area with an anesthetic such as 2% lidocaine. However, in the field, the placement of an intraosseous needle is generally performed under emergency conditions. The patient is either unconscious or semiconscious and can feel the pain.

With the intended site properly prepped, the Paramedic grasps the limb from above with the nondominant hand to stabilize the limb. The limb should not be held in the palm of the hand. The risk of slipping with the IO needle and piercing the palm is too great. The IO needle is now placed against the skin at a 90-degree angle perpendicular to the skin or slightly caudal, away from the epiphyseal plate (growth plate) and inserted with a twisting action. As the IO advances, it will advance quickly until it meets the resistance of the bone's cortex. At this point, the Paramedic must make a forceful, but controlled, insertion into the bone with a twisting action.

After removing the IO needle's stylet, the Paramedic should attach a sterile 10 mL syringe and attempt to aspirate bone marrow. The absence of bone marrow, a common occurrence, does not indicate that the IO needle is out of the bone. If the aspirate is unsuccessful, then a 10 mL bolus of physiologic saline should be attempted. Use of a saline-filled syringe during aspiration makes it easier to visualize the flash of bone marrow and blood. The saline, blood, and bone marrow may all be injected back into the bone and the intravenous administration line connected.

The needle should be standing upright, without support. The IO needle's flanges, if available, can be secured to the limb with tape to provide protection from accidental displacement. A sterile dressing is then usually placed around the IO needle first. A split gauze pad can be used, although precut surgical sponges are available commercially.

After the intravenous solution is connected, the clamp is released. The solution should run freely, and then slowed to the desired rate of infusion. The posterior portion of the limb should be palpated for evidence of infiltration. Intravenous solution infusing into the soft tissues will swell the tissues, making them firmer in the process to the touch.

As is the case with all peripheral venous access, attempts should begin distal and move proximal. Once a bone has had one attempt made for IO access, it should not be used again.

Central Venous Access

Ideally, the best route of medication administration would be by injection directly into the central circulation where it can be quickly carried to the target organs almost instantly. Central venous access, long intravenous catheters placed into the great vessels, provides a route for central venous medication administration. An access to the central venous system would also permit the measurement of **central venous pressure (CVP)**, a measurement used to assess a patient's hemodynamic status. Finally, central venous access permits frequent blood sampling without the annoyance of repeated needlesticks.

It is estimated that five million central venous access devices (CVAD) are placed annually in the United States alone. A small fraction of those are put in place by Paramedics in the field. However, every Paramedic should know how to access a CVAD during an emergency.

Types of Central Venous Access Devices

A large number of central venous access devices are available on the market. Some CVADs are put in place during a special surgical procedure whereas others can be placed in the field during an emergency by specially trained Paramedics. The common feature of all of the central venous access devices is that they place the distal tip of a catheter proximal to the junction of the vena cava with the right atrium. Because of the high flow at the catheter's distal tip, it is possible to infuse irritating or hypertonic solutions as well as inject normally incompatible drugs consecutively.

The original central venous catheters, the Broviac® and the Hickman®, were developed during the 1970s and used extensively in the critical care areas. These skin-tunneled devices exit the body in the vicinity of the right, or left, clavicle and have a medication access port for medication infusions. A central venous access device could remain in place for five to seven days, and potentially up to two weeks in special cases, thus avoiding the trauma of repeated needlesticks.

The next generation of central venous access devices, the **percutaneous central venous catheters (PCVC)**, were inserted into the deep veins via the subclavian vein (in the chest), the internal jugular vein (in the neck), and the femoral vein (in the groin). These central venous catheters have been developed with single-, double-, and triple-lumen catheters (Figure 27-32).

Later CVAD models included an implanted port that was accessed from the outside by a special needle (described later) that could remain in place for even longer periods of time, an advantage during chemotherapy.

The most recent addition to the line of central venous access devices is the **peripherally inserted central catheter (PICC)**. The PICC is a very long catheter placed within a vein in the antecubital fossa and threaded into the vena cava while under fluoroscopy. Subsequent radiographs of the chest are taken to confirm placement of the PICC. Newer PICC devices are fiber-optic. The progress of these newer fiber-optic PICCs allows the provider to observe the progress of the catheter under the skin and into the vena cava. The ease of placement, without fluoroscopy, permits the insertion of a PICC in the physician's office, or in the field.

The PICC is rapidly becoming the CVAD of choice for patients who are at risk for hemorrhage, secondary to anticoagulants or low platelet counts (thrombocytopenia), or who are immunocompromised. The site is easily accessible and visible (for infection surveillance) and compressible (in cases of hemorrhage). The PICC line, properly maintained, can remain in place for over a year, and many patients are sent home with a PICC in place (Figure 27-33).

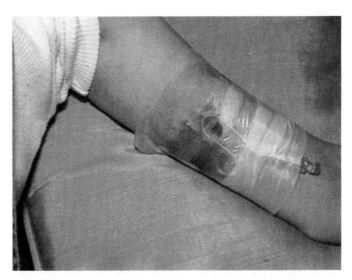

Figure 27-33 PICC line used to administer antibiotics, at home, to a 12-year-old trauma patient who subsequently had developed osteomyelitis.

Field-Placed Central Venous Access Device

The value of obtaining central venous access in the field must be weighed against the dangers of CVAD placement. While the advantages of central venous access (e.g., during cardiovascular collapse) are impressive, the disadvantages, including accidental arterial puncture with subsequent hemorrhage and permanent nerve damage, can outweigh those advantages. For those reasons, CVAD placement in the field is generally reserved for cases where a critical or cardiac arrested patient could clearly benefit and the risks are outweighed by the benefits.

The choice of the device is a function of the method of insertion. While the long catheter-over-the-needle CVAD may seem more familiar to the Paramedic, as it is similar to the regularly used peripheral intravenous access device, overinsertion of the long needle has serious implications for the patient, such as creation of a pneumothorax or accidental arterial puncture.

An alternative CVAD is the catheter-through-the-needle device, described earlier in the chapter. This CVAD is less popular among Paramedics because the opening it creates in the vein is larger than the catheter that will pass through it. Subsequently, there can be hemorrhage at the site. This CVAD is reserved almost exclusively for use in compressible sites, such as the veins within the antecubital fossa.

The preferred method of central venous access in the field is the catheter-over-the-guidewire CVAD. This device starts with a smaller intravenous needle, which is familiar to Paramedics, and progresses to a larger catheter. The technique for inserting a catheter-over-the-guidewire will be described shortly.

Although a variety of external central venous access devices are available, each with a different number and/or gauge of catheter, these catheters are generally either 20 cm

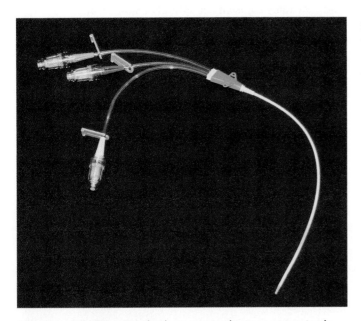

Figure 27-32 Triple-lumen catheter, a central venous access device.

long, for use in the subclavian or internal jugular vein, or 60 cm long, for femoral or basilac veins.

Placement of the Central Venous Access Device

A number of sites are available for the placement of a central venous access device, and each has its drawbacks. The internal jugular vein (JV), while readily accessible, is in the same vicinity as other resuscitative efforts, such as intubation. This makes it inconvenient. Furthermore, the proximity of the carotid arteries to the internal jugular vein makes insertion of a needle into the internal jugular vein more problematic and an "overshoot" could cause arterial puncture. However, in the hands of an experienced operator, the IJV has the highest rate of success with the lowest incidence of complications.[59]

An alternative location for a CVAD could be the subclavian vein. Located inferior to the clavicle, the subclavian vein is proximal to the apex of the lung. An all-too-common complication of a subclavian CVAD insertion is the creation of a pneumothorax.

Another complication of insertion, seen with the catheter-over-the-wire approach, is the positioning of the wire inside the heart. As the wire is literally whipped against the walls of the heart with each contraction, it can create an ectopic beat and dysrhythmia. This site, like the IJV, is in proximity to other resuscitative efforts.

The femoral vein is perhaps the safest site for the placement of a CVAD by an inexperienced operator. The topographic anatomy needed to identify the location of the femoral artery is easy to locate. Therefore, the femoral vein can be cannulated without any serious interruption to either efforts to intubate the patient or external cardiac compressions. However, because the femoral CVAD lies below the diaphragm, it is not possible to measure accurate central venous pressure (CVP). This is generally not a priority in the out-of-hospital setting, whereas immediate venous access is a priority.

The femoral vein, like most deep veins, lies in a neurovascular bundle, alongside the femoral artery and nerve. To locate the femoral vein, the Paramedic can trace its course from the saphenous opening in the thigh to its terminus at the inguinal ligament. The Paramedic should imagine a triangle, a mental triangle, in the inguinal fold, with the femoral vein lying in the middle, within the femoral sheath. The femoral artery should be found, by palpation, just lateral to the vein, and the femoral nerve lies lateral to the femoral artery (i.e., from inside to out, vein, artery, and nerve). Needle entry into the femoral vein is complicated by the presence of the superficial and deep fascia, a strong membranous sheath that protects these important structures.

Preparation and Insertion of a Femoral CVAD

To perform a femoral insertion of a catheter-over-the-wire CVAD, the Paramedic must first position the patient supine, with the legs abducted approximately 30 degrees and the thigh rotated slightly. When the insertion site for the CVAD has been identified, it must be adequately prepared before proceeding with the needle insertion. While not a sterile procedure, the insertion of devices into the central circulation (bypassing many of the body's immune defenses in the process) requires strict medical asepsis.

The immediate area surrounding the area should be swabbed with a povidone-iodine or similar antiseptic solution, starting at the intended point of insertion and moving outward in ever-expanding, overlapping circles until an adequate field has been created (usually a 6- to 8-inch circle). If the area is covered with hair, obscuring the insertion site, it may be necessary to either clip the hair with scissors (preferred) or shave the area. Excessive time should not be spent clearing the area of unwanted hair. The Paramedic would then palpate for the femoral pulse with a gloved hand. The femoral pulse should be located approximately 2 cm below the inguinal ligament at the midpoint of the mental triangle.

Using the **Seldinger technique**, a catheter-over-the-wire technique, the Paramedic will cannulate the femoral vein. With a finger on the pulse, the Paramedic inserts the long 18g intravenous needle and catheter at a 30-degree angle, approximately 1 cm medial to the femoral pulse, with the tip aimed toward the head into the femoral vein. When the Paramedic observes a blood flash, the needle is stabilized with the nondominant hand and the needle withdrawn, leaving the catheter in place. A special wire (a **J-wire**) is then inserted into the hub of the needle. The J-wire, a tightly wound spring wire, has an open hook at the end, preventing it from puncturing soft tissues.

Once the wire is in place, the needle is withdrawn. During the entire process, the Paramedic has a hold of either the needle or the J-wire. With the J-wire in place, a longer catheter is placed over the wire and slid into position. After confirmation of placement, the CVAD is secured in place and fluid flow rates adjusted accordingly (**Skill 27-4**).

On occasion, a Paramedic may inadvertently misdirect the needle and puncture the adjacent femoral artery. If this occurs, and after the needle is withdrawn, a large dressing and direct pressure (with the palm of the hand, if necessary) is applied to the area until the bleeding stops.

For a step-by-step demonstration of Obtaining a Femoral Line, please refer to Skill 27-4 on pages 591–592.

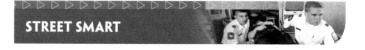

STREET SMART

If intra-abdominal or pelvic injuries are suspected, then the risk of distorted anatomy and subsequent accidental arterial puncture, as well as increased bleeding in the area, make the femoral site undesirable for central venous access.

Access of a Central Venous Access Device

Peripherally inserted central catheters (PICC), percutaneous central venous catheters, and tunneled central venous catheters all have external ports that provide easy access for Paramedics in the event of an emergency. To access these devices, the Paramedic disconnects the catheter cap, connects a syringe, draws off approximately 3 mL to 5 mL of solution (either physiologic saline or heparin), maintains the patency of the catheter, and discards the drawn off waster. Then the Paramedic connects the intravenous administration set and adjusts the flow.

If the catheter cap is a self-sealing membrane, similar to a medication port, then it will be necessary to cleanse the catheter cap with povidone-iodine solution and then introduce a needle-tipped syringe (usually a 19g needle) to withdraw the discard. Subsequently, a needle will need to be attached to the end of the intravenous administration set securely and the two mated. Many Paramedics reinforce the connection of the needle to the catheter cap with tape.

The greatest concern with accessing these devices is accidental disconnection that can result in massive hemorrhage and/or air embolism. To prevent this potentially fatal complication, most CVAD have luer lock fittings that connect together tightly and/or self-sealing membranes (similar to those on a medication port) that seal the catheter.

The insertion of a CVAD is a costly and time-consuming process and it is important to maintain the patency, and thus the viability, of a CVAD for these reasons. The patency of a CVAD can be maintained by either continuous infusion or intermittent infusions (e.g., with heparin solution). Most Paramedics prefer that, once access has been made into a CVAD, the patency of CVAD is maintained by a continuous infusion, running at KVO, until the patient arrives at the hospital.

Implanted Vascular Access Devices

For long-term venous access, a special **implanted vascular access device (IVAD)** is used. An IVAD is a central venous catheter that has the port buried in a subcutaneous pocket under the skin's surface. Implanting the entire device affords the IVAD the skin's protection, which decreases the rate of infection, as well as protect the port from physical trauma.

IVADs are generally reserved for patients who are going to receive intermittent infusions of irritating solutions for a prolonged period of time (e.g., chemotherapy). Infusion of these irritating solutions via traditional peripheral venous access would cause the veins to become inflamed (**sclerosis**) and hardened. Venous access to these hardened veins becomes increasingly difficult over time and the patient is often subjected to repeated attempts. IVADs eliminate the need to attempt, and to re-attempt, IV access on those patients who have a poverty of veins. Instead, the IVAD is accessed. The infusion is run through a plastic catheter and into the central circulation, where it can be diluted.

The subcutaneous port of an IVAD may be implanted in either the upper chest wall or the upper arm. The port consists of a reservoir, a hollow metal disk with a self-sealing membrane, and a silicone catheter.

This population of patients frequently has a medical emergency and requires EMS assistance, including medications and/or fluids. If traditional peripheral venous access cannot be obtained during an emergency, and it is imperative to gain such access, the Paramedic may elect to access the IVAD. Some Paramedics have been specially trained by oncology nurses or oncology specialists to access the IVAD during an emergency.

To access an IVAD, the Paramedic must first locate the device in either the upper chest or upper arm. Once located, the skin overlying the IVAD is prepared in the same manner as a peripheral IV site. Once the site is prepared, the Paramedic opens all necessary equipment, prefills a saline-filled syringe, and attaches it to a special non-coring needle called a **Huber needle**.

Donning sterile gloves, the Paramedic carefully picks up the Huber needle, avoiding contamination, and holds the Huber needle with the dominant hand. Taking the gloved nondominant hand, the Paramedic holds the subcutaneous port firmly, like holding a quarter on its side, and places the needle over the skin (Figure 27-34).

If the patient were a child, many Paramedics would prepare the site with EMLA cream before the procedure. In the case of adults, after repeated access, a callous commonly forms over the site, and the needle inserted is relatively painless. With the needle poised over the port and perpendicular to the skin, the needle is advanced, with authority, until the needle strikes the back plate of the port and stops. With the needle in place, the Paramedic first checks for a blood return, then flushes the IVAD.

Similar to a CVAD, once the IVAD is accessed the Paramedic has a choice between continuous infusion and intermittent infusion. Most Paramedics elect to maintain a continuous infusion and attach the intravenous administration set adaptor to the hub of the Huber needle. The entire assembly can then be secured with a transparent occlusive dressing, with or without gauze, under the arm of the Huber needle to help stabilize it.

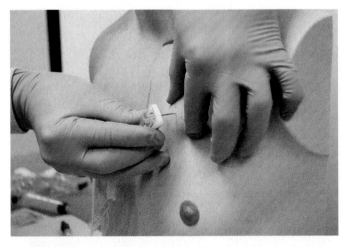

Figure 27-34 IVAD access with a Huber needle. (Courtesy of Emergency Preparedness Systems, LLC and EMS Magazine)

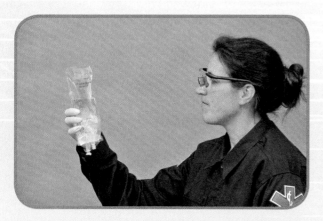

1 Select solution, checking for solution type, clarity, and expiration.

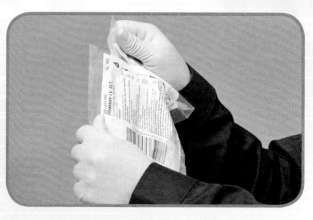

2 Select intravenous administration set, choosing between micro-drop and macro-drop.

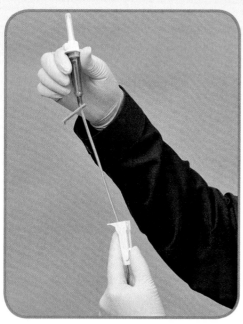

3 Place the roller clamp just proximal to drip chamber and stopped.

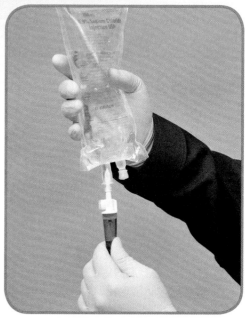

4 Squeeze drip chamber, filling drip chamber one-half full.

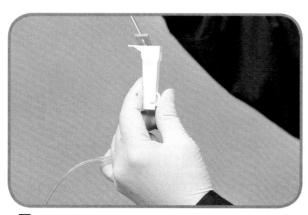

5 Run solution out while maintaining sterility of end.

Skill 27-2 Venous Cannulation Using a Catheter-Over-the-Needle Device

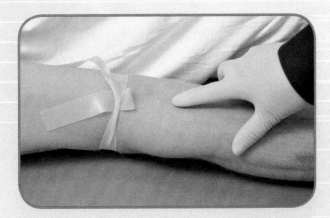

1 Apply the venous tourniquet and select the optimal site for cannulation.

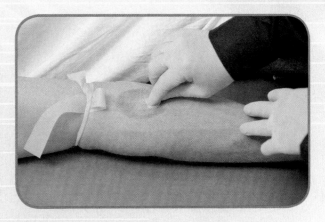

2 Cleanse the immediate area using appropriate antiseptic solution.

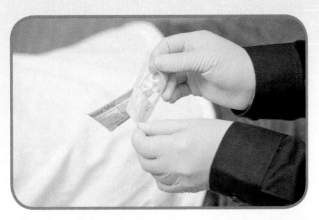

3 Select appropriate venous catheter.

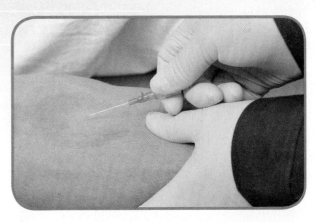

4 Visualize the insertion site (approach the site with authority).

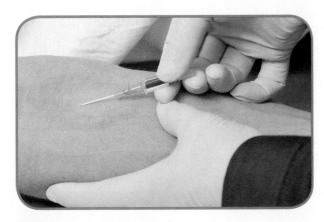

5 Confirm venous cannulation by looking for flashback in the catheter.

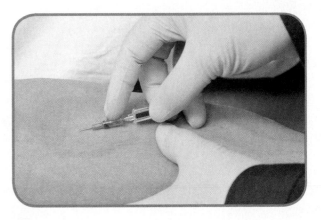

6 Slide the catheter over the needle into the vein.

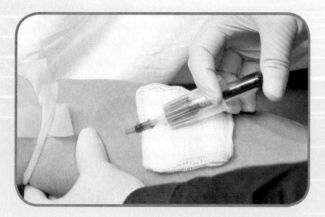

7 Draw blood as appropriate and remove tourniquet.

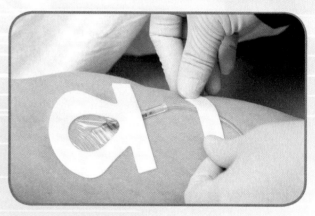

8 Secure the IV catheter using a semipermeable membrane dressing.

Skill 27-3 Intraosseous Access

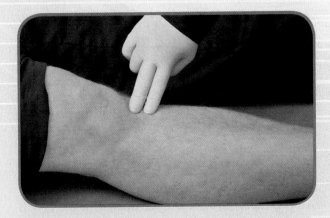

1 Identify the preferred site.

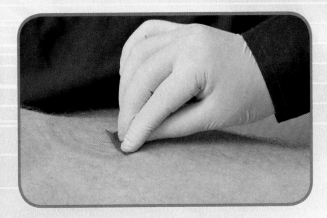

2 Prepare the site with antiseptic solution.

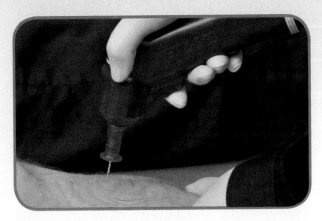

3 Approach the site with intraosseous needle, perpendicular to the bone.

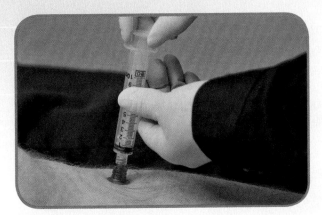

4 Aspirate to establish placement.

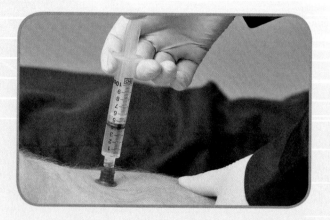

5 Flush with saline, observing for infiltration.

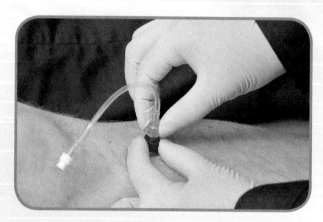

6 Attach administration set.

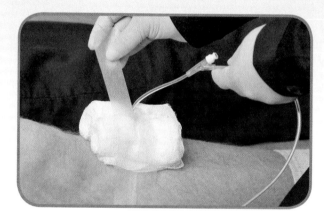

7 Secure IO access.

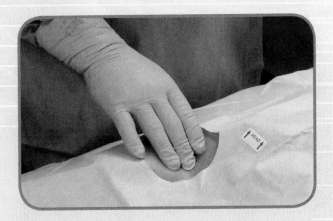

1 Identify the femoral triangle.

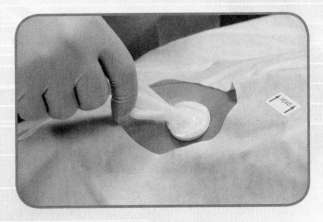

2 Prepare the area with antiseptic solution.

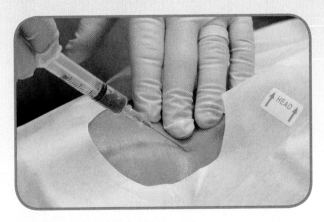

3 Insert the needle and observe flash.

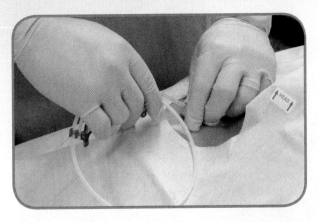

4 Thread the J-wire into the catheter.

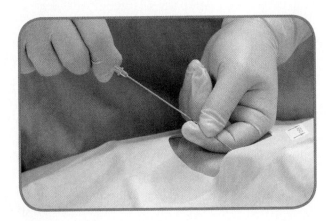

5 Remove the catheter over the wire and hold the wire.

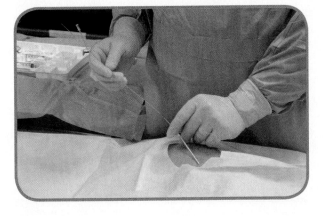

6 Introduce the dilator, then remove.

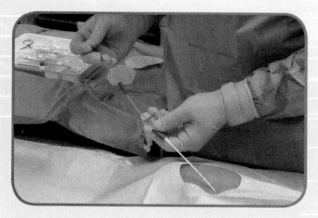

7 Thread the line over the wire, holding the line in one hand while threading with the other.

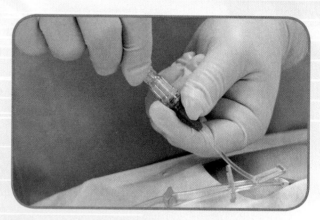

8 Attach the infusion set.

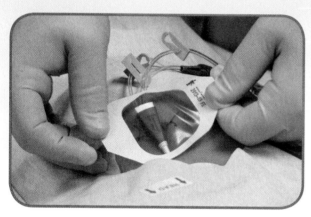

9 Dress the insertion site.

CONCLUSION

Venous access for both fluid replacement and medication administration during an emergency is critical. The Paramedic's skill in obtaining venous access is often regarded as an indicator of the Paramedic's capability. Without venous access, very little can be done to alleviate the patient's suffering and lessen the pain.

KEY POINTS:

- Body fluids are distributed across three compartments: the intravascular space, intracellular compartment (ICF), and as extracellular fluid (ECF) in the interstitial space.

- Indications for intravenous access include medication administration and the replacement of intravascular volume.

- Fluid loss may be insensible (such as perspiration and vapor on the breath) or sensible (such as urine, GI fluid loss, and wound drainage).

- Pre-existing medical conditions that can contribute to increased fluid loss include diabetes insipidus, emphysema, hyperglycemia, and the alcoholic patient. Decreased levels of responsiveness, tachypnea, tachycardia, hypotension, or postural hypotension may indicate a significant loss of intravascular volume secondary to dehydration.

- Crystalloid fluids contain electrolytes commonly found in the blood, while fluids containing proteins are called colloids.

- A balanced or isotonic solution has a percentage of solute similar to what is found in blood.

- A solution that draws water out of the cell by osmotic force, due to a greater percentage of solute than blood, is a hypertonic solution.

- A solution that has fewer solutes than blood, causing water to be drawn into the cells, is a hypotonic solution.

- Intravenous access bypasses many of the body's defenses against infection, so the Paramedic has the responsibility to take all reasonable precautions to prevent blood infection.

- After the correct solution has been chosen, the Paramedic must verify that the solution is in date, clear, and intact.

- The intravenous administration set provides a sterile pathway for the intravenous fluid to get from the container into the patient.

- A macro-drop administration set is often used when volume replacement is needed.

- A micro-drop administration set is used for fine control of the infusion stream.

- An administration set consists of a spike that pierces the fluid container and a drip chamber where a hanging drop is formed.

- A specific rate of flow may be established by adjusting the flow to the required drops per minute.

- The drip rate control device, slide clamp, and medication administration ports are located along the length of tubing, which is then connected to a catheter via an adaptor.

- Trauma tubing has a larger internal diameter, allowing the rapid administration of large volumes of solution. Other infusion sets include large-bore tubing found in blood transfusion sets and in-line burettes that are used to carefully control fluid infusion, often used with pediatric patients.

- A pressure bag will increase the flow rate by exerting direct pressure onto the solution bag.

- Connecting and priming the administration set, or running the line out, begins by clamping off the line and inserting the spike into the port of the solution. Fluid is then drawn into the drip chamber and the fluid is run through the length of tubing. Venous access is divided into peripheral access and central access.

- The smaller the gauge of an intravenous needle, the larger the needle.

- A larger gauge needle is preferred for trauma patients while a smaller gauge needle reduces the risk of thrombophlebitis and can be maintained for a longer period of time.

- The most common IV access device used is the needle-through-the-catheter variety.

- Two other IV access devices include butterfly IV catheters and needle-over-the-catheter devices, which are used almost exclusively for central venous access in the hospital setting.

- Whenever an intravenous access is attempted, a sharps container should be immediately available (i.e., within arm's reach of the Paramedic).

- A venous tourniquet should not remain in place for more than a few minutes and the distal arterial pulse should remain palpable at all times. Tamponade of a vein, or manual compression of a vein, can achieve a similar effect.

- Venous access points of the upper extremity include the dorsal arch of the hand, cephalic and basilic veins along the forearm, the cubital arch in the antecubital space, and the axillary vein in the upper arm. Access points in the lower extremity include the saphenous veins. The external jugular vein may also be accessed in an emergency.

- Venous site selection includes knowledge of hand dominance, potential future procedures, past surgical interventions, or current medical or trauma history.

- The Paramedic must assess and select a primary and secondary IV site.

- The Paramedic should clean the selected site by placing the alcohol or povidone-iodine swabs on the intended insertion site and sweep outward in expanding and ever-widening circles, creating a sterile field twice the length of the IV needle.

- The Paramedic should not re-palpate the intended IV access site once the preparation has begun.

- Venous cannulation can be performed by the direct approach by placing the IV needle atop the vein. The indirect approach involves inserting the IV needle under the skin and next to the vein, and then directing the needle into the vein. The catheter must be advanced into the vein to ensure placement.

- When the needle is completely withdrawn, it must be immediately rendered safe. Some IV needles are self-sheaving whereas others are not. Regardless of the presence of any engineered safety devices, all IV needles should be immediately placed in a sharps container.

- The entire time for insertion should be approximately two minutes, from the time the tourniquet was applied to the time the tourniquet was released. Proper preparation of supplies, preassembled as necessary, helps to improve overall efficiency.

- The IV administration set can be attached to the IV catheter and run continuously or intermittently.

- A saline lock can be used to cap off the IV catheter for later use.

- The IV catheter can be secured with tape and/or a transported membrane dressing.

- Several types of mechanical flow control devices may be used to accurately control intravenous flow.

- Complications of IV infusions include infiltration, infusion-induced hypothermia, infection that may cause thrombophlebitis and/or pyrogenic reactions, fluid volume overload, or embolisms.

- Infusing fluids into the intraosseous space ultimately infuses fluids into the central veins.

- Indications for IO access include cardiac arrest or the need for immediate access for medication administration.

- Complications of IO insertion include the risk of fat embolism, fracture, extravasation, and compartment syndrome.

- The majority of prehospital medications can be administered via the IO route except for 9% saline and adenosine.

- Phlebotomy is performed when a blood sample is required but IV access is not necessary. Phlebotomy is carried out using a straight needle and a vacuum tube apparatus.

- To prevent potential contamination from additives, the tubes without additives (red-topped tubes) are drawn first and the "wet" tubes (those with additives) are drawn last.

- When transporting samples, all potentially infectious materials (PIM) must be clearly marked with the biohazard symbol or some other warning that indicates the presence of PIM.

- Drawing blood cultures is a specialized technique that requires medical asepsis to prevent contamination of the sample.

- Specialized phlebotomy techniques are used with pediatric patients. A heel stick may be used to draw blood from infants. A smaller needle, 25g to 27g butterfly, is used along with a syringe to gradually draw the sample from the vein.

- The umbilical catheter is advanced throughout the umbilical vein, the larger orifice.

- Scalp veins may also be used for IV access on infant patients.

- Pediatric intraosseous access provides vascular access directly into the central circulation, can be established quickly, and remains available even during cardiac arrest.

- Common complications include misplacement of the needle, inadvertent puncture of the posterior wall of the bone, and extravasation of fluids into the tissues.

- The IO site of choice is the proximal tibia. Like peripheral venous access, the IO needle cannot be placed into an extremity with a fractured bone.

- Central venous access provides a route for medication administration as well as the measurement of central venous pressure (CVP).

- Central venous access devices include percutaneous central venous catheters (PCVC) that are inserted into deep veins and the peripherally inserted central catheter (PICC).

- For long-term central access, a patient may have an implanted vascular access device (IVAD). To access this device, the Paramedic needs a special non-coring needle called a Huber needle.

▷ REVIEW QUESTIONS:

1. Name the indications for venous access.
2. What is a crystalloid solution?
3. What role does the amount of solute play in the movement of water?
4. Describe insensible loss of fluid and its relationship to the disease process.
5. What clinical signs indicate dehydration?
6. What type of intravenous administration set would you select for a trauma patient? Why?
7. Name the components of an administration set.
8. What are the steps to prepare a solution and intravenous administration set?
9. Starting proximal and moving distal, identify and describe the veins that may be used to establish intravenous access.
10. State the similarities and differences between intravenous access and phlebotomy.
11. What precautions should be taken when selecting an intravenous access site?
12. Describe the procedure for performing a venipuncture.
13. Describe methods of securing the IV catheter.
14. How is a secondary intravenous infusion prepared and set up?
15. What signs and symptoms would indicate a pyrogenic reaction?

16. Name the three basic vacuum blood tubes and for which tests each is indicated.

17. Describe age-appropriate methods of establishing an IV for infants, toddlers, school-aged children, and adolescents.

18. What are the indications for placement of an implanted central access device?

19. What sites exist for an implanted central access device?

CASE STUDY QUESTIONS:

Please refer to the Case Study at the beginning of the chapter and answer the questions below:

1. Where would you look first for access on Mrs. Gorino? Explain your answer.

2. If you were unable to initiate an IV in her upper extremities, what other sites exist that you can try?

3. What other methods may be appropriate for access?

REFERENCES:

1. Reithner L. Insensible water loss from the respiratory tract in patients with fever. *Acta Chir Scand*. 1981;147(3):163–167.

2. Lamke LO, Nilsson G, Reithner L. The influence of elevated body temperature on skin perspiration. *Acta Chir Scand*. 1980;146(2):81–84.

3. David K. IV fluids: do you know what's hanging and why? *Rn*. 2007;70(10):35–40; quiz 41.

4. Soreide E, Deakin CD. Pre-hospital fluid therapy in the critically injured patient—a clinical update. *Injury*. 2005;36(9):1001–1010.

5. Roberts I, Alderson P, Bunn F, Chinnock P, Ker K, Schierhout G. Colloids versus crystalloids for fluid resuscitation in critically ill patients. *Cochrane Database Syst Rev*. 2004;4:CD000567.

6. Fan E, Stewart TE. Albumin in critical care: SAFE, but worth its salt? *Crit Care*. 2004;8(5):297–299.

7. Perel P, Roberts I. Colloids versus crystalloids for fluid resuscitation in critically ill patients. *Cochrane Database Syst Rev*. 2007;4:CD000567.

8. Fodor L, Fodor A, Ramon Y, Shoshani O, Rissin Y, Ullmann Y. Controversies in fluid resuscitation for burn management: literature review and our experience. *Injury*. 2006;37(5):374–379.

9. Hemington-Gorse SJ. Colloid or crystalloid for resuscitation of major burns. *J Wound Care*. 2005;14(6):256–258.

10. Kreimeier U, Messmer K. Small-volume resuscitation: from experimental evidence to clinical routine. Advantages and disadvantages of hypertonic solutions. *Acta Anaesthesiol Scand*. 2002;46(6):625–638.

11. Guisto JA, Iserson KV. The feasibility of 12-gauge intravenous catheter use in the prehospital setting. *J Emerg Med*. 1990;8(2):173–176.

12. Stoneham MD. Factors affecting flow through blood administration sets. *Eur J Anaesthesiol*. 1997;14(3):333–339.

13. Elad D, Zaretsky U, Heller O. Hydrodynamic evaluation of intravenous infusion systems. *Ann Emerg Med*. 1994;23(3):457–463.

14. Zamos DT, Emch TM, Patton HA, D'Amico FJ, Bansal SK. Injection rate threshold of triple-lumen central venous catheters: an in vitro study. *Acad Radiol*. 2007;14(5):574–578.

15. Dutky PA, Stevens SL, Maull KI. Factors affecting rapid fluid resuscitation with large-bore introducer catheters. *J Trauma*, 1989;29(6):856–860.

16. Krivchenia A, Knauf MA, Iserson KV. Flow characteristics of admixed erythrocytes through medex tubing with a pall filter. *J Emerg Med*. 1988;6(4):269–271.

17. Merrer J, De Jonghe B, Golliot F, Lefrant JY, Raffy B, Barre E, et al. Complications of femoral and subclavian venous catheterization in critically ill patients: a randomized controlled trial. *Jama*. 2001;286(6):700–707.

18. Hagley MT, Martin B, Gast P, Traeger SM. Infectious and mechanical complications of central venous catheters placed by percutaneous venipuncture and over guidewires. *Crit Care Med*. 1992;20(10):1426–1430.

19. Karapinar B, Cura A. Complications of central venous catheterization in critically ill children. *Pediatr Int*. 2007;49(5):593–599.

20. Rivera AM, Strauss KW, van Zundert AA, Mortier EP. Matching the peripheral intravenous catheter to the individual patient. *Acta Anaesthesiol Belg*. 2007;58(1):19–25.

21. Frelich R, Ellis MH. The effect of external pressure, catheter gauge, and storage time on hemolysis in RBC transfusion. *Transfusion*. 2001;41(6):799–802.

22. Gerberding JL. Management of occupational exposures to bloodborne viruses. *N Engl J Med*. 1998;332(7):444–451.

23. Kistner RL, Kamida CB. 1994 update on phlebography and varicography. *Dermatol Surg*. 1995;21(1):71–76.

24. Stone MB, Price DD, Anderson BS. Ultrasonographic investigation of the effect of reverse Trendelenburg on the cross-sectional area of the femoral vein. *J Emerg Med*. 2006;30(2): 211–213.

25. Parry G. Trendelenburg position, head elevation and a midline position optimize right internal jugular vein diameter. *Can J Anaesth.* 2004;51(4):379–381.

26. Goldstein AM, Weber JM, Sheridan RL. Femoral venous access is safe in burned children: an analysis of 224 catheters. *J Pediatr.* 1997;130(3):442–446.

27. Murr MM, Rosenquist MD, Lewis RW, 2nd, Heinle JA, Kealey GP. A prospective safety study of femoral vein versus nonfemoral vein catheterization in patients with burns. *J Burn Care Rehabil.* 1991;12(6):576–578.

28. Stitik TP, Foye PM, Nadler SF, Brachman GO. Phlebotomy-related lateral antebrachial cutaneous nerve injury. *Am J Phys Med Rehabil.* 2001;80(3):230–234.

29. Orme RM, McSwiney MM, Chamberlain-Webber RF. Fatal cardiac tamponade as a result of a peripherally inserted central venous catheter: a case report and review of the literature. *Br J Anaesth.* 2007;99(3):384–388.

30. Greenfield RH, Bessen HA, Henneman PL. Effect of crystalloid infusion on hematocrit and intravascular volume in healthy, nonbleeding subjects. *Ann Emerg Med.* 1989;18(1):51–55.

31. Lobo DN, Stanga Z, Simpson JA, Anderson JA, Rowlands BJ, Allison SP. Dilution and redistribution effects of rapid 2-litre infusions of 0.9% (w/v) saline and 5% (w/v) dextrose on haematological parameters and serum biochemistry in normal subjects: a double-blind crossover study. *Clin Sci (Lond).* 2001;101(2):173–179.

32. Schulze T, Mucke J, Markwardt J, Schlag PM, Bembenek A. Long-term morbidity of patients with early breast cancer after sentinel lymph node biopsy compared to axillary lymph node dissection. *J Surg Oncol.* 2006;93(2):109–119.

33. Rietman JS. Geertzen JH, Hoekstra HJ, Baas P, Dolsma WV, de Vries J, et al. Long term treatment related upper limb morbidity and quality of life after sentinel lymph node biopsy for stage I or II breast cancer. *Eur J Surg Oncol.* 2006;32(2):148–152.

34. Ververs JM, Roumen RM, Vingerhoets AJ, Vreugdenhil G, Coebergh JW, Crommelin MA, et al. Risk, severity and predictors of physical and psychological morbidity after axillary lymph node dissection for breast cancer. *Eur J Cancer.* 2001;37(8):991–999.

35. Lambert MJ, 3rd. Air embolism in central venous catheterization: diagnosis, treatment, and prevention. *South Med J.* 1982;75(10):1189–1191.

36. Kashuk JL, Penn I. Air embolism after central venous catheterization. *Surg Gynecol Obstet.* 1984;159(3):249–252.

37. Deitch EA, Dayal SD. Intensive care unit management of the trauma patient. *Crit Care Med.* 2006;34(9):2294–2301.

38. Mackinnon MA. Permissive hypotension: a change in thinking. *Air Med J.* 2005;24(2):70–72.

39. Dubick MA, Atkins JL. Small-volume fluid resuscitation for the far-forward combat environment: current concepts. *J Trauma.* 2003;54(5 Suppl):S43–S45.

40. Idvall E, Gunningberg L. Evidence for elective replacement of peripheral intravenous catheter to prevent thrombophlebitis: a systematic review. *J Adv Nurs.* 2006;55(6):715–722.

41. Katz SC, Pachter HL, Cushman JG, Roccaforte JD, Aggarwal S, Yee HT, et al. Superficial septic thrombophlebitis. *J Trauma.* 2005;59(3):750–753.

42. Tagalakis V, Kahn SR, Libman M, Blostein M. The epidemiology of peripheral vein infusion thrombophlebitis: a critical review. *Am J Med.* 2002;113(2):146–151.

43. Moore TM, Callaway CW, Hostler D. Core temperature cooling in healthy volunteers after rapid intravenous infusion of cold and room temperature saline solution. *Ann Emerg Med.* 2008;51(2):153–159.

44. Soreide E, Grande C. *Prehospital Trauma Care.* New York; Informa Health Care; 2001:357–367.

45. Iserson KV. Intraosseous infusions in adults. *J Emerg Med.* 1989;7(6):587–591.

46. Buck ML, Wiggins BS, Sesler JM. Intraosseous drug administration in children and adults during cardiopulmonary resuscitation. *Ann Pharmacother.* 2007;41(10):1679–1686.

47. Findlay J, Johnson DL, Macnab AJ, MacDonald D, Shellborn R, Susak L. Paramedic evaluation of adult intraosseous infusion system. *Prehosp Disaster Med.* 2006;21(5):329–334.

48. Miller DD, Guimond G, Hostler DP, Platt T, Wang HE. Feasibility of sternal intraosseous access by emergency medical technician students. *Prehosp Emerg Care.* 2005;9(1):73–78.

49. Suyama J. Knutsen CC, Northington WE, Hahn M, Hostler D. IO versus IV access while wearing personal protective equipment in a HazMat scenario. *Prehosp Emerg Care.* 2007;11(4):467–472.

50. Fowler R, Gallagher JV, Isaacs SM, Ossman E, Pepe P, Wayne M. The role of intraosseous vascular access in the out-of-hospital environment (resource document to NAEMSP position statement). *Prehosp Emerg Care.* 2007;11(1):63–66.

51. LaSpada J, Kissoon N, Melker R, Murphy S, Miller G, Peterson R. Extravasation rates and complications of intraosseous needles during gravity and pressure infusion. *Crit Care Med.* 1995;23(12):2023–2028.

52. Soong WJ, Jeng MJ, Hwang B. The evaluation of percutaneous central venous catheters—A convenient technique in pediatric patients. *Intensive Care Med.* 1995;21(9):759–765.

53. Zempsky WT, Cravero JP. Relief of pain and anxiety in pediatric patients in emergency medical systems. *Pediatrics.* 2004;114(5):1348–1356.

54. Hurren JS, Dunn KW. Intraosseous infusion for burns resuscitation. *Burns.* 1995;21(4):285–287.

55. Curran A, Sen A. Best evidence topic report. Bone injection gun placement of intraosseous needles. *Emerg Med J.* 2005;22(5):366.

56. Skippen P, Kissoon N. Ultrasound guidance for central vascular access in the pediatric emergency department. *Pediatr Emerg Care.* 2007;23(3):203–207.

57. DeBoer S, Seaver M, Morissette C. Intraosseous infusion: not just for kids anymore. *Emerg Med Serv.* 2005;34(3):54, 56–63; quiz 119.

58. Driggers DA, Johnson R, Steiner JF, Jewell GS, Swedberg JA, Goller V. Emergency resuscitation in children. The role of intraosseous infusion. *Postgrad Med.* 1991;89(4):129–132.

59. Sneff M. Central venous catheters. In: Rippe JM, Irwin RS, eds. *Intensive Care Medicine* (2nd ed.). Boston: Little Brown; 1991:17–37.

CHAPTER 28

BLOOD PRODUCTS AND TRANSFUSION

KEY CONCEPTS:

Upon completion of this chapter, it is expected that the reader will understand these following concepts:

- Components and production of blood
- Blood groups, compatibility, and cross-matching
- Identification and treatment of transfusion reactions
- Specific transfusion procedures before, during, and after transfer

▶ CASE STUDY:

The Paramedics were called to the local community hospital for a trauma patient who needed to be transferred to the trauma center. The patient had a serious motorcycle crash and his friends dropped him off at the hospital rather than calling for an ambulance. Now it was storming and the helicopter was grounded due to bad weather.

The local hospital had placed a chest tube to drain blood from the patient's thoracic cavity and he was receiving multiple blood transfusions. He would need more during the transport.

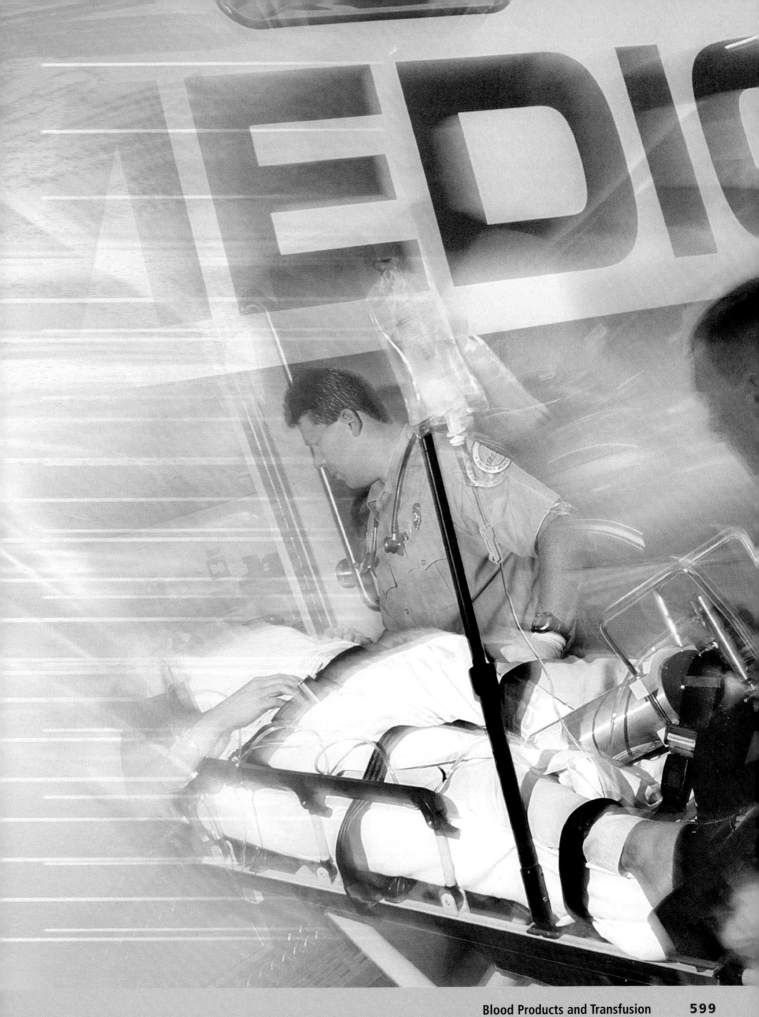

OVERVIEW

Blood product transfusion can be a life-saving therapy for patients who are critically ill or injured. In certain situations, the Paramedic may be asked to transfer patients who are undergoing a transfusion during an interfacility transfer. The Paramedic may also be asked to transfuse additional blood products during the transfer. These types of situations are often heavily regulated by each state's oversight body and regulations differ from state to state. It is important for the Paramedic to follow the regulations and protocols for her state and agency. This chapter will discuss the different blood products and the indications for transfusing those blood products.

History of Transfusions

The first recorded transfusion took place in 1665, when English physician Richard Lower started transfusing blood between dogs in his experiments. In 1667, French physician Jean-Baptist Denis transfused approximately 9 ounces or 260 mL of blood from a sheep to a young male patient. This patient survived but was described as having urine "as black as soot" after the transfusion. Dr. Denis continued animal to human transfusions over the following six months. Late in the same year, animal to human transfusion was outlawed in France and several other countries after several deaths were attributed to reactions to the animal blood. Around this same time, early microscopists were examining blood under the early microscopes and describing the different components of blood. While Anthony van Leeuwenhoek (1632–1723) is often credited with discovering red blood cells, scientist Jan Swammerdam actually discovered blood cells in the late 1650s.

The first human-to-human transfusion was performed in 1795 by Dr. Philip Physick, a surgeon in Philadelphia, Pennsylvania. The case was not publicized and little information is available about it. A little more than 20 years later, British obstetrician James Blundell performed the first known blood transfusion to treat severe postpartum hemorrhage by transfusing the blood from a husband to his wife after delivery.

In 1901, Austrian physician Karl Landsteiner discovered the existence of different proteins on red blood cells and was the first to describe blood groups. The safety of blood transfusion improved as physicians began to match the patient's blood group with the donor's blood group. In addition, around the time of World War I methods were discovered to prevent blood from clotting during storage. Researchers also discovered that blood could be stored at cooler temperatures, allowing its use for a longer period of time after it had been collected from a donor. The first **blood bank** was created in anticipation of heavy casualties by U.S. Army physician Oswald Robertson when he collected and stored blood before the Battle of Cambrai in World War I. Within 20 years, civilian blood banks began to develop in the United States and Europe.

In the 1940s and 1950s, scientists developed methods to separate whole blood into components that could be transfused separately, thus improving storage capability and longevity as well as allowing more directed treatment of a patient's deficiencies. Plastic bags were developed that were safe to use in storing blood. These replaced the cumbersome and breakable glass bottles that were used at the time.

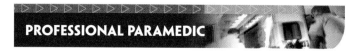

PROFESSIONAL PARAMEDIC

Carl Walter and W. P. Murphy, Jr., introduced the plastic bag for blood collection in 1950.

During the 1960s and 1970s, important advancements were made in the development and identification of specific components that could be used to prevent antibody formation, treat hemophilia, and detect infections that could be transmitted by blood product transfusion. The issue of transfusion safety moved to the forefront during the mid to late 1980s after discovering the HIV virus was transmitted through blood transfusion. This led to widespread testing. Currently, donated blood is tested for several infectious diseases (Table 28-1). Due to widespread testing and donation procedures designed to minimize risk of disease transmission, the risk of contracting HIV from a blood donation ranges from 1 in 493,000 to 1 in two million.[1]

Table 28-1 Infectious Diseases Tested for in Donated Blood

- HIV-1
- HIV-2
- Human T-lymphotropic virus (HTLV-1 and HTLV-2)
- Hepatitis B virus
- Hepatitis C virus
- West Nile virus
- Treponema pallidum (causative agent of syphilis)

Blood Components

As the early microscopists discovered, whole blood is made up of several components bathed in plasma (the liquid portion of blood). Scientists and physicians have studied blood over the last 400 years and have discovered the origin, structure, and function of these components. Each component has a unique function to carry out within the body.

Hematopoiesis is the manufacturing process the body uses to create the three main solid components of blood: red blood cells (**erythrocytes**), white blood cells (**leukocytes** and **lymphocytes**), and platelets (**thrombocytes**). All three of these major types of blood cells develop from the same **hemocytoblast** (Figure 28-1), which is the generic stem cell for blood cells. Blood cells are manufactured within the bone marrow of the long bones, pelvis, cranium, sternum, and

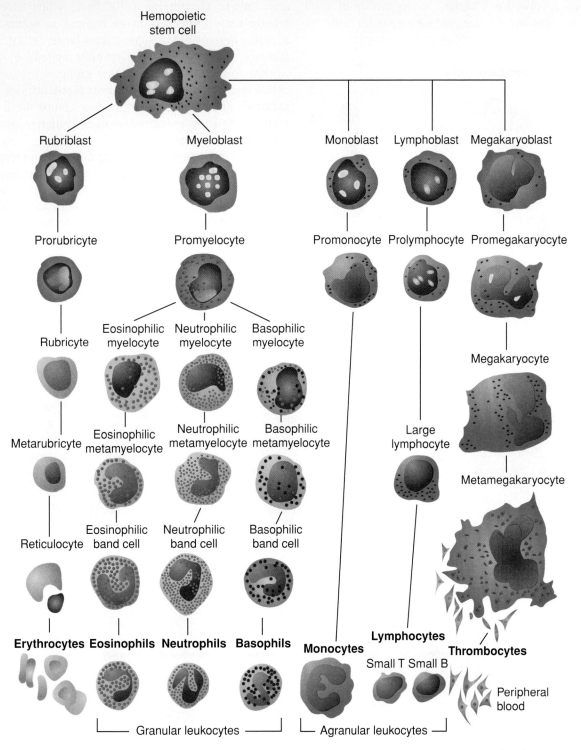

Figure 28-1 Hematopoiesis is the production of the major blood cell types from the hemopoietic stem cell.

vertebrae. The spleen, thymus, and lymph nodes are responsible for maturing certain white blood cells after production in the bone marrow.

Red blood cells, also known as erythrocytes, are small doughnut-shaped cells which act to transport oxygen from the lungs to the cells (Figure 28-2). Hemoglobin, the component of the red blood cell that binds to oxygen, is manufactured from iron. Each molecule of hemoglobin can bind up to four molecules of oxygen. The physiology of oxygen delivery was discussed in Chapter 25. The surface of a red blood cell contains proteins that produce antibodies to the red

Red blood cells

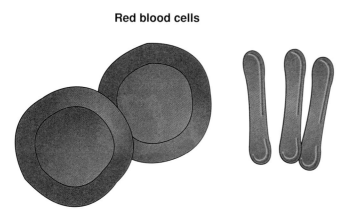

Figure 28-2 The erythrocyte.

blood cell if transfused into another person with a different blood type. Blood compatibility is discussed more fully later in this chapter.

White blood cells, or leukocytes (Figure 28-3), function as part of the immune system to react to foreign challenges. There are three different subtypes of leukocytes—basophils, neutrophils, and eosinophils—which react against, and attach themselves to, certain types of infectious organisms, whether bacterial, viral, or fungal. After attaching to the foreign cells, these white blood cells release toxic chemicals in an attempt to neutralize the invading organism. Macrophages are larger cells that attack and destroy the foreign invaders after the leukocytes identify the foreign material. Another group of immune cells, called lymphocytes, are responsible for identifying foreign materials and developing antibodies against those foreign materials to allow enhanced immune system response during future infections.

Platelets, or thrombocytes (Figure 28-4), are responsible for blood clotting. Platelets are attracted to a damaged blood vessel's endothelium, the innermost layer of the blood vessel. Coagulation factors and other proteins attract other circulating platelets to the damaged area to build a plug that achieves **hemostasis** and stops bleeding from the damaged blood vessel.

Coagulation factors are proteins which act to attract platelets to each other to build platelet plugs. Additionally,

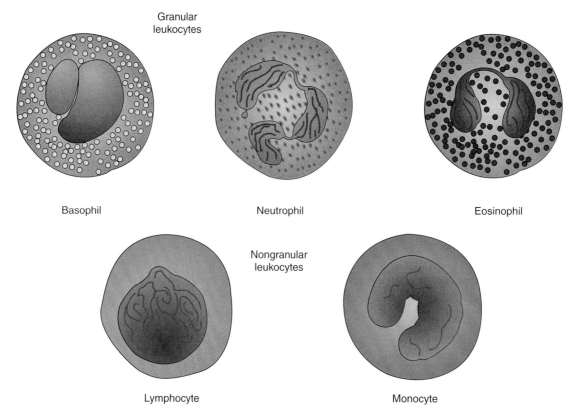

Granular
leukocytes

Basophil   Neutrophil   Eosinophil

Nongranular
leukocytes

Lymphocyte   Monocyte

Figure 28-3 Leukocytes.

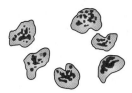

Platelets

Figure 28-4 Platelets.

coagulation factors are key to the production of fibrin and fibrinogen, two materials that serve to solidify and stabilize the platelet plug, making it impermeable to liquid. The **coagulation cascade** (Figure 28-5) outlines the process the body uses to manufacture fibrin and fibrinogen. Most of the coagulation factors are made in the liver, some of which depend on vitamin K during the manufacturing process. Both congenital and acquired deficiencies of coagulation factors can cause difficulty in clotting or spontaneous bleeding.

Blood also has many other proteins that circulate throughout the system which serve multiple different functions. Some of these circulating proteins are the antibodies that help protect against infection, albumen that helps regulate blood volume, and hormones that act in a variety of ways on the body's organs. The blood also transports nutrients and other building block materials to the cells.

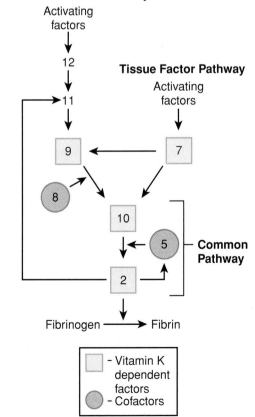

Contact Activation Pathway

Figure 28-5 The coagulation cascade.

Table 28-2 Normal Serum Blood Values Found in a Complete Blood Count (CBC)

Component	Normal Range
Red blood cells	4.5–5.5 million per mL
White blood cells	4,000–10,000 cells/mL
Hemoglobin	13–16 g/dL (male)
	12–15 g/dL (female)
Hematocrit	41%–50% (male)
	36%–44% (female)
Platelets	100,000–450,000 platelets/mL

Many of the blood components discussed are measured as part of a **complete blood count (CBC)** that is often performed in the ED or physician's office (Table 28-2). The amount of **hemoglobin** differs between males and females largely due to the females' blood loss during normal menstrual cycles. The **hematocrit** measures the ratio between the volume of the solid components of blood compared against both its solid and liquid components, listed as a percentage (solid/total).

Blood Products

Since the technique of fractionating blood into its individual components was perfected in the 1950s and 1960s, transfusion of whole blood in civilian medicine has become uncommon. However, transfusion of whole blood is more frequent in the combat environment when large quantities of blood are required.[2] The advantage of fractionating blood into its components is more directed transfusion based on the patient's specific needs as well as longer storage life for the components as opposed to whole blood. The four blood components most frequently transfused include **packed red blood cells (PRBC)**, **fresh frozen plasma**, **cryoprecipitate**, and **platelets**.

Packed Red Blood Cells

PRBCs are formed by removing nearly all of the plasma from a unit of blood and adding a small volume of preservative to the unit. PRBCs are often stored at near freezing temperatures but can be frozen for longer-term storage. Each unit of blood is approximately 250 mL in volume, which includes both the solid and liquid component of the unit. Assuming bleeding is controlled and does not continue during the transfusion, each unit of blood is expected to raise the patient's hemoglobin by 1 gm/dL.[3]

PRBCs are transfused primarily in the situation of acute blood loss (e.g., in bleeding from trauma or from gastrointestinal bleeding). PRBCs are also transfused to patients who are anemic, those with a significantly decreased hemoglobin level, and those who have signs and symptoms of impaired oxygen delivery (e.g., dyspnea, lightheadedness, or chest pain). Anemic patients with known cardiac disease may also be transfused to ensure sufficient oxygen delivery and prevent cardiac events due to each patient's anemia. Each unit of PRBCs can be transfused in as little as several minutes in critically ill, hypotensive patients with acute blood loss, and up to two to four hours for patients who have poor cardiac function. Most often, PRBCs are transfused at a rate of approximately one unit per hour to two hours. However, in severely hypotensive patients, a unit of PRBCs can be transfused in a matter of minutes.

At times, the patient requires so much blood that additional blood components are required. The term "massive transfusion" is used to describe a situation in which a patient has significant ongoing blood loss to the point where one to two body volumes of blood are required. For the average weight person, this translates to a transfusion of 10–20 units of PRBCs. In situations in which the total blood volume needs replacement, other components which are absent in PRBCs—including platelets and coagulation factors—will also need to be replaced in order to prevent continued bleeding due to loss of the blood's clot-forming ability.

Fresh Frozen Plasma

Fresh frozen plasma (FFP) is formed by removing the red blood cells and platelets from whole blood. The remaining liquid component of the blood is still rich in several of the clotting factors needed as part of the coagulation system. Two of these key coagulation factors are factors V and VIII. One unit of FFP has a volume of approximately 200 mL and is transfused in 30 to 60 minutes.

FFP is most often used to treat clotting disorders which accompany several diseases that include decreased clotting factor production (e.g., liver disease). FFP is also used to treat patients who have taken an overdose of the anticoagulant warfarin because of its action in inhibiting the production of clotting factors. FFP is also used to treat a condition called disseminated intravascular coagulation, in which the clotting factors are rapidly used up and the patient develops bleeding because of the clotting factor deficiency.

Cryoprecipitate

Cryoprecipitate is the protein portion of plasma made up of concentrated clotting factors in a much smaller volume than FFP. One unit of cryoprecipitate has a volume of between 25 and 50 mL, much less than one unit of FFP. Cryoprecipitate is transfused between 15 and 30 minutes per unit. Cryoprecipitate contains factors V, VIII, and XIII. Additionally, cryoprecipitate contains fibrinogen and fibronectin, proteins that help solidify a clot, and von Willebrand factor, which helps to initiate clot formation.

Cryoprecipitate is indicated in overanticoagulation or disseminated intravascular coagulation. It is also indicated in patients who have hemophilia A or von Willebrand's disease who are bleeding, as it quickly replaces the deficient factor. Cryoprecipitate is also used when patients are receiving a massive transfusion to replace coagulation factors that are lost and not present in PRBC units.

Platelets

Platelets are separated from plasma in the blood bank by one of two methods. In order to raise the patient's platelet count by 50,000 platelets, the patient needs to receive approximately six units of platelets, which can be a significant amount of volume. Each unit of platelets should be transfused over a 30 to 60 minute time period. The indications for platelet transfusion vary based upon the patient's platelet count, presence of bleeding, or risk of bleeding with a planned procedure. Platelets are often transfused in patients undergoing massive transfusions as they are usually deficient in platelets. Platelet transfusions may not be effective in conditions where platelet function is decreased (e.g., in renal disease).[4]

Blood Groups and Compatibility

Early transfusions caused reactions in an inconsistent manner. Some transfusions occurred without problems. In others, the recipient had severe and sometimes fatal reactions. It was not until the early 1900s that a physician researcher, Dr. Karl Landsteiner, discovered that red blood cells have proteins on the cell's surface that are responsible for producing some transfusion reactions. This section will discuss the concept of blood grouping and matching donor blood to the recipient.

Blood Grouping

The proteins that exist on the surface of the red blood cells help the body identify which cells are its own cells as opposed to foreign invaders. If a donor has different proteins on the surface of donated blood products, the recipient's immune system will identify those components as foreign material, and set off an immunological chain reaction that will lead to the clumping together of red blood cells, called **agglutination**. The clumping causes the red blood cells to break apart, a process called **hemolysis** (Figure 28-6).

Dr. Landsteiner identified the existence of two proteins—an A protein and a B protein—on the surface of red blood cells. Red blood cells that have the A protein on the surface are called Type A blood. If the B protein is present on the surface of the red blood cell, the blood is Type B blood. He also noticed that some red blood cells do not have either an A or a B protein on the surface. Cells without these proteins were called Type O blood. The A-B-O designations formed the first system of determining blood type. At a later time, it was observed that some red blood cells have both an A and a B protein on their surface, and thus the blood type is called Type AB blood, the fourth major blood group in the A-B-O typing scheme (Figure 28-7).

These surface proteins are also antigens, meaning that they can produce an immune system response. Patients with Type A blood have antibodies against Type B blood in their plasma. Conversely, patients with Type B blood have antibodies to Type A blood in their plasma. Patients who have Type O blood have antibodies to both Type A and B blood in their system and patients with Type AB blood do not have any of these antibodies in their system. As previously described,

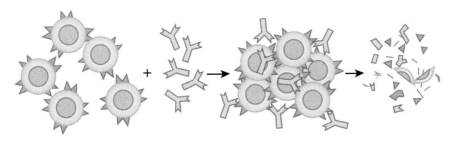

Figure 28-6 Agglutination and hemolysis occur when cells of incompatible blood types are mixed together.

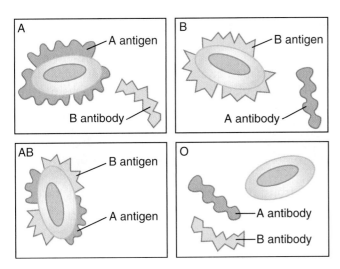

Figure 28-7 The major red blood cell types.

Table 28-3 The Frequency of Blood Type in the United States Based on the A-B-O and Rh Systems[5]

A-B-O and Rh	Frequency
O+	37.4%
O−	6.6%
A+	35.7%
A−	6.3%
B+	8.5%
B−	1.5%
AB+	3.4%
AB−	0.6%

Table 28-4 Examples of the 29 Different Blood Grouping Systems Recognized by the ISBT

- A-B-O
- Rh
- MNS
- Lewis
- Duffy
- Kidd
- Diego
- Cartwright

these antibodies are responsible for the agglutination and hemolysis of foreign blood cells.

Dr. Landsteiner also discovered a second protein that existed along with the A and B proteins. This protein, the Rh factor, was named after the Rhesus monkey, whose blood was used for the experiments that led to the discovery of the Rh factor. The Rh factor is either present or absent, which is denoted by adding a plus (+) or minus (−) to the A-B-O type. Patients with Rh+ blood do not have antibodies against the Rh protein; however, some patients with Rh− blood have developed antibodies against the Rh protein and can develop a transfusion reaction. Between these two typing systems, there are eight major blood types that exist (Table 28-3).

In addition to the major A-B-O and Rh blood types, the International Society of Blood Transfusion (http://www .isbt-web.org/) recognizes a total of 29 different groups used for blood typing. The 27 other typing schemas were classified by identifying other minor proteins that occur on the surface of blood cells which also cause immunological reactions when different types of blood are mixed together (Table 28-4).

Compatability

As blood grouping was discovered and testing became available, every effort was made to decrease the likelihood of a severe transfusion reaction by matching the recipient's blood with potential donor's blood. The greater the match between the recipient's and donor's blood, the more compatible they are and the less likelihood of severe transfusion reaction. As previously discussed, blood of a certain type will often have antibodies present that attack other types of blood. A recipient may be able to safely receive other types of blood if the recipient's type of blood is not available (Table 28-5). Notice that Type O blood can be given to any of the A-B-O blood types because Type O blood does not have surface proteins that incite the immune response which ends in hemolysis. Type O blood is sometimes termed the **universal donor** due to this property. In contrast, patients with Type AB blood can receive blood from any donor because the patient does not have antibodies against A or B proteins present in the plasma. Due to this property, individuals with Type AB blood are called **universal recipients**.

Table 28-5 Who Can Receive What Blood Types?

If the Recipient Has Type:	The Recipient Can Receive:
A blood	Type A and O blood
B blood	Type B and O blood
O blood	Type O blood only
AB blood	Type A, B, AB, and O blood only
Rh+ blood	Type Rh+ or Rh− blood
Rh− blood	Type Rh− blood only

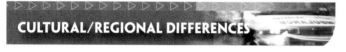

CULTURAL/REGIONAL DIFFERENCES

Some religious groups refuse blood transfusions due to their belief that it is specifically forbidden. Courts have been asked to order blood transfusions in cases of vulnerable populations such as children. Overruling a patient's or family's religious beliefs is not done lightly.

Transfusion Terms

Several terms are used to refer to the different blood products regarding their types and compatibilities. It is important for the Paramedic to understand these terms as it may impact the transfusion process.

During this process, which typically takes a half hour to accomplish, the blood bank uses a sample of the recipient's blood and identifies antibodies present in the sample. Using this information, the blood bank can find a blood match that does not have antigens which will react with the antibodies in the recipient's blood. In some cases, the recipient has numerous antibodies present in the blood and a prolonged time is required in order to identify blood for transfusion. In more complicated cases, sufficiently matched blood may need to come from another center or blood bank in order to be safe for transfusion. Donor blood that is successfully matched to recipient blood is called **type and crossed** or **type and cross-matched** blood.

In some cases, there is insufficient time to complete a cross-match of recipient and donor blood. In cases of severe shock from acute blood loss (e.g., trauma, gastrointestinal bleeding), a patient may require an immediate blood transfusion in order to sustain life. In these cases, uncross-matched blood is transfused using either O− or O+ donor blood that does not undergo the usual **cross-matching** procedure. In general, O− blood is preferred for women of childbearing age to avoid the development of antibodies to Rh+ blood that may be transfused into the recipient with an unknown blood type. This is important because during a subsequent pregnancy, the maternal antibodies can attack the fetal blood cells, potentially resulting in fetal death. In some cases, the patient's blood type is known and it is possible to administer type-specific blood that has the same A-B-O and Rh types as the recipient's blood, even though it has not been completely cross-matched. This often occurs when blood is required emergently while the blood bank is in the middle of the cross-matching process. All efforts to use cross-matched blood for subsequent units of blood products are made once the uncross-matched or type-specific blood is used on a patient. Patients receiving uncross-matched or type-specific blood must be monitored closely for transfusion reactions.

Identification and Management of Transfusion Reactions

Transfusion reactions vary from minor to life-threatening. The Paramedic must be able to confidently identify and treat the wide range of potential transfusion reactions that may occur during transfer.

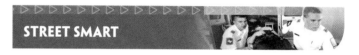

STREET SMART

Some transfusion reactions can occur with as little as 10 mL of blood transfused. However, most tend to occur by the time the first unit has fully transfused.

Transfusion-Associated Circulatory Overload

Transfusion-associated circulatory overload (TACO) occurs when the patient receives more volume of blood products than can be handled by the circulatory system. This overload essentially produces pulmonary edema and is more likely to occur in patients with impaired cardiac function, including the elderly, those with underlying CHF or coronary artery disease, or pediatric patients. It is important to note that a significant amount of volume is infused into any patient, including those who are healthy with normal heart and kidney function, and that TACO can develop. As previously discussed, each unit of PRBCs is a volume of 250 mL. Blood products are always run together with a second saline infusion running at a to-keep-open rate so the intravenous line does not clot off at the end of the transfused unit. In addition to the 250 mL in the unit of blood, up to another 100 mL of normal saline is infused per unit of blood product. As most critically ill patients requiring transfusion are given several units of blood or blood products, it is easy to provide a significant amount of volume in a short period of time. To address this issue, patients at risk of circulatory overload should be transfused at a slower rate than normal.

Allergic Reaction

Allergic reactions can occur due to MAST cell activation in the recipient's blood once exposed to the donor's blood, and are seen in up to 1% of transfusions.[6] The allergic reactions can range in severity from a mild reaction that includes itching or some hives to anaphylaxis and airway edema. Most allergic reactions of this type will resolve spontaneously. Some reactions will require administration of medications or slowing of the transfusion. Severe allergic reactions will definitely require medication treatment and may require airway management.

Febrile Non-Hemolytic Reaction

Febrile transfusion reactions are defined as an elevation of the patient's temperature of 1°C from baseline within two hours of the start of the transfusion.[6] A **febrile non-hemolytic reaction** more often begins shortly after the initiation of the transfusion or a new unit and is often secondary to minor antibodies present in the recipient's blood that cause a mild reaction when exposed to the donor's blood. In addition to fever, the patient may develop chills, rigors, headache, nausea, or vomiting. The fever may resolve spontaneously, but often an antipyretic (e.g., acetaminophen) is administered to treat the symptoms. If the fever persists or elevates, the transfusion may need to be stopped.

Acute Hemolytic Reaction

An **acute hemolytic reaction** is one of the most serious transfusion reactions and most often occurs as a result of an A-B-O incompatibility (Table 28-6). In other words, an incorrect blood type was administered to the patient; for example, Type A blood was administered to a patient who has Type B blood. This produces agglutination and hemolysis of the transfused blood. The hemolysis may involve native red blood cells. Around 10% of patients who are exposed to A-B-O incompatible blood die of the hemolytic reaction.

The administration of the wrong type of blood to a patient can occur for several reasons, and an entire system of checks and balances has been developed in order to minimize these errors. It is of the utmost importance that the Paramedic take on a personal responsibility to ensure that any units of blood products that are transported with the patient are correctly labeled. The procedure will be discussed further in a later section of this chapter. Ultimately, if the transfusion continues, the patient can develop shock, renal failure, disseminated intravascular coagulation, and death.

Bacterial Contamination

Bacterial contamination of blood products is estimated to occur at a rate of 1 in every 15,000 units of platelets and 1 in every 500,000 units of PRBCs.[7] The higher incidence of bacterial contamination of platelets is due to the higher temperature at which platelets are stored. Contamination is rarely due to an illness in the donor. More often, it is due to contamination which occurred during the collection or storage process. The patient may become septic due to the contamination, though most often the patient exhibits signs of an infection, including fever, chills, and rigors. Patients may also develop dyspnea, hypotension, nausea, vomiting, or diarrhea.

Transfusion-Related Acute Lung Injury

Transfusion-related acute lung injury (TRALI) is defined as a new acute lung injury that occurs within six hours of a transfusion and is directly related to the transfusion.[8] The patient develops hypoxemia, dyspnea, and bilateral infiltrates that can be best seen on a chest x-ray in the ED but may produce bilateral rales (crackles) on auscultation by the Paramedic. TRALI occurs as a result of pulmonary capillary leakage of plasma into the tissues surrounding the alveoli in the lung. It is believed that TRALI is set off by antibodies against white blood cells present in the donor's blood that react with the recipient's white blood cells. Less frequently, the recipient's blood contains the antibodies that attack white blood cells that may be present in the donor unit of blood. The antibodies set off an inflammatory reaction that produces compounds with the end result of leakage of plasma from the pulmonary capillaries. Alternatively, other inflammatory proteins may be present in the donor's blood that causes the inflammatory reaction in the recipient's lungs (Table 28-7). While TACO and TRALI may be difficult to differentiate in the field, TACO tends to produce a more frank pulmonary edema, whereas TRALI produces finer rales (crackles) without a significant fluid overload.

Treatment of Transfusion Reactions

Regardless of the transfusion reaction identified by the Paramedic, the first key step is to stop the transfusion, change the tubing, and flush the line with normal saline. These actions will prevent a continued reaction to the blood product. The unit of blood product and the line must be saved and given to the blood bank at the receiving hospital for testing. Draw a red or pink top tube from the patient for testing by the blood bank at the receiving hospital. The blood bank at the receiving hospital will retest both the donor unit and the sample

Table 28-6 Signs and Symptoms of an Acute Hemolytic Transfusion Reaction

- Fever > 2°C above the patient's baseline temperature
- Hypotension
- Dyspnea
- Pain at the site of the transfusion, back, and chest
- Hemorrhage and/or hemoglobinuria (dark-colored urine)
- Nausea and vomiting
- Jaundice and icterus

Table 28-7 Signs and Symptoms of TRALI

- Dyspnea
- Tachypnea
- Cyanosis
- Fever
- Tachycardia
- Froth in the endotracheal tube

from the recipient to ensure there is a match and identify any cross-matching errors. Contact on-line medical control to discuss the specific patient and develop a treatment plan as well as to decide whether to continue the transfusion.

Administer supplemental high-flow oxygen if the patient is not already on supplemental oxygen. For the patient who develops an allergic reaction, administer diphenhydramine and methylprednisolone intravenously to treat the allergic reaction. For anaphylactic reactions with hypotension, severe dyspnea, or throat edema, administer epinephrine intramuscularly to treat the anaphylaxis. TACO is treated by administering furosemide intravenously and applying CPAP to support ventilation and off-loading of fluid from the lungs. Patients who develop TRALI will often require CPAP or intubation. Care is supportive and does not require medications.

Transfusion Procedure and Documentation

Having reviewed the different types of blood products and the indications for transfusion and transfusion reactions, the next section discusses the procedure for blood product transfusion. These steps must be followed with every unit transfused. Remember, there is a mortality rate of 10% for patients who receive mismatched blood products regardless of treatment. This is a very serious complication of blood product transfusion.

STREET SMART

Hyperkalemia may occur due to infusions with irradiated red blood cells. Hypocalcemia may result from multiple transfusions due to the citrate preservative binding serum calcium and is indicated by circumoral tingling and tremors.

Prior to Transfer

During the patient report received from the RN in the sending facility, the Paramedic needs to confirm several items before receiving the patient and blood products (Table 28-8). These steps are important to ensure that the blood products match the patient's A-B-O and Rh factor and that only blood products intended for that specific patient are transfused. Ideally, the transfusion will have been initiated in the sending emergency department and the patient monitored for 15 to 30 minutes in order to identify major transfusion reactions before transport. Review the pre-transfusion set of vitals, including a temperature, as some of the transfusion reactions rely on a change from baseline temperature in identifying the reaction.

Table 28-8 Items to Confirm Prior to Transport

- Verify patient identity
- Verify consent for transfusion or indication of reason for implied consent
- Verify the patient's blood type (A-B-O and Rh)
- Verify transfusion orders:
  ○ Type of blood product
  ○ Rate of administration
  ○ Order of administration (if multiple products)
- For each unit hanging or carrying during transport, verify with another Paramedic, RN, physician, or mid-level provider:
  ○ Blood type of unit
  ○ Rh factor of unit
  ○ Patient ID label
  ○ Unit expiration date
  ○ Donor unit number and patient information match

STREET SMART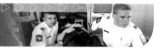

The Paramedic should document what items were verified and with whom on the regular patient care record in addition to completing the blood bank record.

During the Transfer

Blood is transfused through one of two types of administration sets. The blood transfusion set is preferred over the piggyback set (both described in Chapter 27) because the blood administration set has a larger lumen, providing less resistance to flow than a piggyback setup. The second advantage of blood tubing is that both ports of the "Y" shaped tubing flow into the same drip chamber, allowing less resistance to flow for the normal saline that is administered with the blood. Normal saline should be set to run at "to-keep-open rate" so it flushes the line with saline after the unit of blood product is finished.

During transport, blood products must be stored in an appropriate transport cooler that is certified by the blood bank (Figure 28-8). This is essential as most blood products should be stored at a temperature between 1°C and 6°C. The shelf life of a unit of blood at room temperature is approximately 30 minutes. Warmer temperatures increase the risk of bacterial contamination as well as developing proteins in the donor blood that can initiate transfusion reactions.

The Paramedic should record vital signs, including temperature, at 15-minute intervals during transfer. Vital signs should also be recorded after completing each unit. The Paramedic should auscultate the patient's lungs between units to identify signs of fluid overload. This is especially

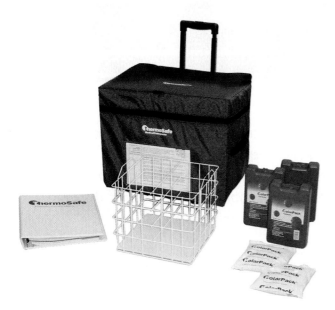

Figure 28-8 A transport cooler certified by the blood bank. (Courtesy of Thermosafe Brands, a Strategic Business Unit of Tegrant Corporation)

important in intubated or sedated patients as they may not be able to complain of dyspnea. A final set of vital signs should be recorded on arrival to the receiving facility.

The Paramedic should evaluate the patient's skin each time vital signs are obtained for indications of an allergic reaction.

After the Transfer

The Paramedic must document at a minimum vitals, times, reactions, and information about the blood products administered to that patient during transfer. This information may be documented on a usual patient care report or a specific special form may be required. The Paramedic should use the specific form required by her agency. One copy of the transfusion record should be left at the receiving hospital and another copy kept with the prehospital documentation.

Any unused blood products should be given to the blood bank at the receiving hospital. The blood is then retested and either used for the transferred patient or made available for others who match that donor's blood. In the event of a transfusion reaction, the unit of blood that was hanging at the time of the reaction, the blood tubing, and the patient's blood sample should be brought to the blood bank for testing.

CONCLUSION

The transfusion of blood products during critical care transport by the Paramedic can provide a life-saving therapy to the critically ill patient who requires blood products. It is important for the Paramedic to approach blood transfusions methodically and systematically in order to ensure patient safety during the transfusion. It is also critical to continuously monitor the patient during transfer so as to identify and treat transfusion reactions early.

KEY POINTS:

- Refinements in the process of giving blood from one animal to another, and ultimately from one human to another, has been ongoing for over 400 years.

- Blood groups are identified by specific antigens located on the red blood cell.

- Other proteins also affect blood compatibility.

- Donated blood is tested for multiple infectious diseases.

- Whole blood consists of solid components (red and white blood cells plus platelets) and plasma.

- Hematopoiesis is the process that the body uses for the development of solid blood components.

- All blood cells develop from a hemocytoblast.

- Blood cells are manufactured within the bone marrow of the long bones, pelvis, cranium, sternum, and vertebrae.

- Red cells transport oxygen.

- White cells are part of the immune system.

- Platelets are a part of the blood clotting process.

- The coagulation cascade, using multiple factors, leads to the development of fibrin, a blood clot.

- Normal hemoglobin amounts vary from males to females.

- Hematocrit compares the ratio of solid components of blood to the volume of blood.

- The four blood components most frequently transfused include packed red blood cells (PRBC), fresh frozen plasma, cryoprecipitate, and platelets.

- When no further blood loss occurs, a unit of packed red cells will increase the hemoglobin levels by 1 gm/dL.

- Fresh frozen plasma (FFP) is formed by removing cells from whole blood and is rich in several of the clotting factors needed as part of the coagulation system.

- Cryoprecipitate is the protein portion of plasma made up of concentrated clotting factors.

- Platelets may be transfused in patients undergoing massive transfusions.

- There are eight major blood types:
  - Type O positive or negative
  - Type A positive or negative
  - Type B positive or negative
  - Type AB positive or negative

- Type O blood is called the universal donor as it does not have surface proteins that trigger an immune response.

- Type AB is called the universal recipient as there are no circulating antibodies capable of attacking A or B red cells.

- The process of determining blood compatibility between the recipient and donor blood is called cross-matching.

- Transfusion reactions vary from minor to life-threatening.

- Treatment depends on the type of reaction.

- Prior to transfer, verify pertinent details regarding the patient and the blood products.

- Blood may be transfused via a "Y" shaped blood administration set or a piggy back system. The blood administration is the preferred method.

- Blood must be kept cool to reduce the risk of reactions.

- The patient should have vital signs taken every 15 minutes during transfusion.

- The transfusion record must be completed after each unit of blood product.

- Any blood product and tubing involved in a transfusion reaction should be brought to the blood bank at the receiving hospital.

REVIEW QUESTIONS:

1. What determines a blood group?
2. Name the blood groups.
3. What is a universal donor? Universal recipient? How are antigens and antibodies involved in these designations?
4. What are the solid components of the blood?
5. What is the process by which the solid components of blood are formed? Where are they formed?
6. What is the liquid portion of blood called?
7. What four blood products are routinely transfused (not necessarily to the same patient)? How do they differ from each other?
8. Define hemoglobin. Define hematocrit.
9. Name each transfusion reaction and list its prehospital treatment.
10. What items should be verified before transport?
11. How often should the patient be assessed (minimally)?
12. Describe the process of completing a blood transfusion including its documentation.

CASE STUDY QUESTIONS:

Please refer to the Case Study at the beginning of the chapter and answer the questions below:

1. How are blood transfusions managed?
2. What complications can occur during transfusion?
3. What blood components is this patient likely receiving? Explain your answer.

REFERENCES

1. Schreiber GB, Busch MP, Kleinman SH, Korelitz JJ. Risk of transfusion-transmitted viral infections. *N Engl J Med.* June 27, 1996;334(26):1685–1690.
2. Kauvar DS, Holcomb JB, Norris GC, Hess JR. Fresh whole blood transfusion: a controversial military practice. *Journal of Trauma.* 2006;61(1):181–184.
3. Department of Medicine, Washington University School of Medicine. Chapter 19: Anemia and transfusion therapy. *Washington Manual of Medical Therapeutics.* 2007.
4. Wittler MA, Hemphill RR. Acquired bleeding disorders. In: Tintinalli JE, Kelen GD, Stapczynski JS, eds. *Emergency Medicine: A Complete Study Guide* (6th ed.). New York: McGraw Hill; 2004:1324–1329.
5. Stanford School of Medicine Blood Center. Blood types in the U.S. Available at: **http://bloodcenter.stanford.edu/about_blood/blood_types.html.** Accessed October 31, 2008.
6. Santen SA. Transfusion therapy. In: Tintinalli JE, Kelen GD, Stapczynski JS, eds. *Emergency Medicine: A Complete Study Guide* (6th ed.). New York: McGraw Hill; 2004:1348–1353.
7. Nester T, Lopez-Plaza I. Bacterial contamination of cellular blood products. Transfusion Medicine Update. Epub February 2001. Available at: **http://www.itxm.org/TMU2001/tmu3-2001.htm.** Accessed October 28, 2008.
8. Toy P, Popovsky MA, Abraham E, et al. Transfusion-related acute lung injury: definition and review. *Critical Care Medicine.* 2005;33(4):721–726.

CHAPTER 29

INTRODUCTION TO PHARMACOLOGY

KEY CONCEPTS:

Upon completion of this chapter, it is expected that the reader will understand these following concepts:

- Pharmacology as a study of drug treatments
- Regulation, classification, and referencing of drugs
- New drug development and public safety
- Mechanisms of action
- Special considerations of the pregnant, pediatric, and geriatric patients

▶ CASE STUDY:

Katie O'Rielly had fallen from her bike while trying some tricks on her brother's homemade skateboard ramp. While the junior Paramedic partner completed the assessment and obtained vital signs, his senior partner called for medication orders. After reporting that Katie was 7 years old, had significant deformity to her left wrist and forearm, and had no allergies (according to her dad), the Paramedics relayed Katie's vital signs, weight, and pain scale. After completing Katie's care, which included some IV pain medication and medication to prevent nausea, the Paramedics transferred her to the hospital and began completing their paperwork. "Have you administered narcotics with this agency as yet?" asked the senior Paramedic. "There are very specific procedures and paperwork to complete."

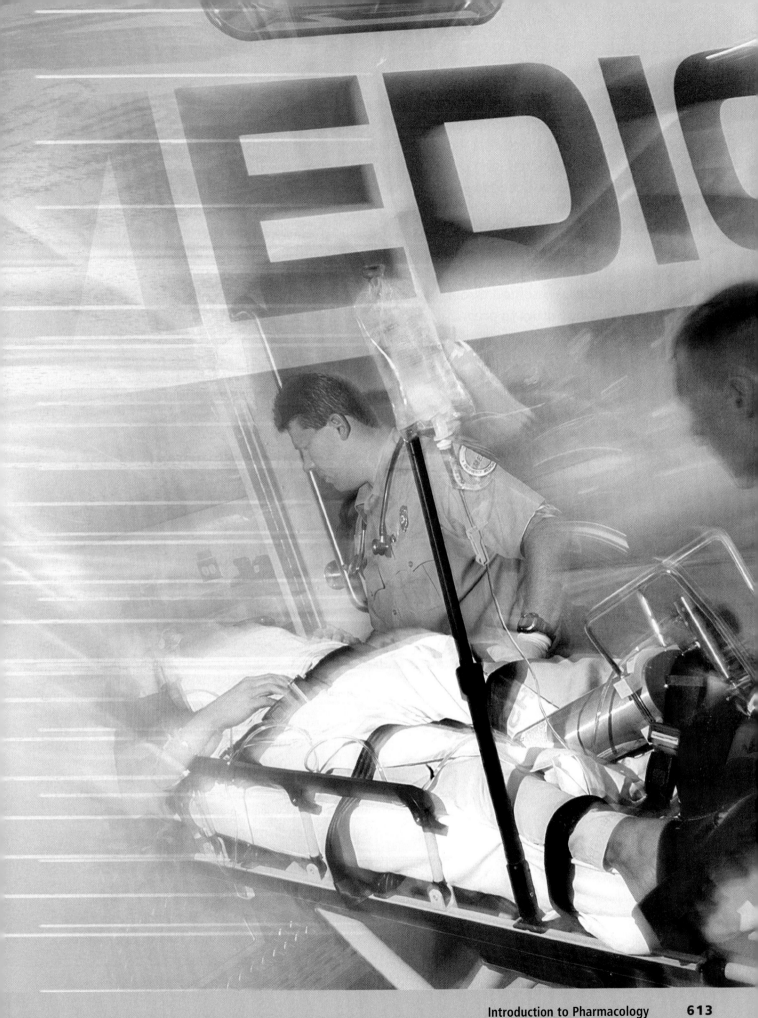

OVERVIEW

Pharmacology has its origins in medicinal treatments used to restore humoral balance to the body. As experience and experimentation pushed forward, the paradigm shifted from humoral imbalance to the idea that illness is caused by disease. This chapter will outline how drugs are classified, regulated, and developed as well as how the Paramedic may reference an unfamiliar medication. Becoming familiar with pharmacology also requires the Paramedic to understand basic pharmacokinetics and how drugs are absorbed, distributed, detoxified, and eliminated from the body. Just as important as understanding how a drug moves through the body is how a drug specifically works upon a cell. Pharmacodynamics helps to explain how drugs create their therapeutic effect and helps the Paramedic to understand a drug's mechanism of action. Presented throughout the chapter are the special considerations that apply to administering drugs to pregnant, pediatric, and geriatric patients.

Paramedic Pharmacology

Drugs have had, and continue to have, a dramatic impact on life. In 1901, the average American could expect to live to be about 49 years old. One hundred years later, the average American can expect to live to be at least 78 years of age.[1] A number of factors, such as safer working conditions, improved nutrition, cleaner water, better sanitation, and the advent of potent medications, have led to this dramatic increase in life expectancy. In addition, great medical breakthroughs have dramatically improved the quality and duration of life (Table 29-1).

Advances in safety and ease of administration of pharmacological agents, as well as the advantage of early intervention in acute medical emergencies, has prompted emergency physicians to promote the use of these medications by Paramedics. Today, Paramedics carry some of the most powerful drugs available in medicine. These medicines are capable of saving a life when used appropriately. However, these drugs are equally capable of causing death if given without due regard to their mechanism of action and possible side effects. The

term "pharmacy" comes from the Greek word "pharmakos," which can be translated to mean either "to remedy" or "to poison." It is imperative that all Paramedics understand the actions of these medications and their potential for harm before administering them.

Historical Development of Pharmacology

In 1889, Sir Petri discovered an Egyptian papyrus written in 1900 B.C. that described the treatment of a "falling womb" with a gruel made of cool milk and grain. Believed to be the oldest written prescription, it represented the timeless effort of people to rid themselves of disease. Throughout world history, continuous discoveries and advancements in the use and creation of medications have taken place. Many medications have revolutionized the practice of medicine.

Some of the earliest accounts of medication use came from the work of priests in the temple of Asclepius (the Greek God of healing). Here priests would instruct patients on a variety of treatments, ranging from the application of poultices made of herbs to the use of charms to frighten evil spirits. Each attempt to use medications was met with varying degrees of success, with the outcome more likely to be poor than good. Most people felt that illness was created by the gods or was the result of evil spirits. Therefore, it was believed that illness was inevitable and, more importantly, immutable to physician interventions.

Table 29-1 Major Medical Breakthroughs

1796	Vaccines
1865	Antiseptic
1895	X-ray
1897	Aspirin
1905	Vitamins
1922	Insulin
1929	Antibiotics
1933	CPR
1953	Polio
1960	Pacemaker
1967	Heart transplant
1972	Medical filming
1980	Smallpox
1982	Artificial heart
1990	Human genome
1997	Cloning
1998	Stem cell research

STREET SMART

Asclepius, the Greek God of healing, was thought to hold the serpent as sacred. His symbol, a staff with a coiled snake around the shaft (known as a caduceus), is now used as a symbol of medicine.

Hippocrates (460–560 B.C.), a member of the healing guild Asclepiadae named after the god Asclepius, is considered the "father" of western medicine. Hippocrates advanced the idea that disease was not caused by evil spirits but rather by natural causes, i.e., an imbalance in the body. Imbalances in the "humours" contained within the body was a revolutionary idea in its time.[2,3]

These humours were red blood, white phlegm, yellow bile, and black bile, each representing the fundamental elements of air, water, fire, and earth. Hippocrates also believed in the recuperative powers of the human body and felt that medicine could help to support the body's efforts at bringing itself into balance from "humoral pathology."

Some of the most important advances in medical practice during that time are credited to Galen, a physician to the gladiators and later court physician to Commodus, the son of Marcus Aurelius. Galen wrote volumes about medicine and established a system of medicinal practice that remained intact until after the Dark Ages. He wrote of the nature of pulses and described certain "ores" and potions of medicinal value, including the "balm of Gilead," a juice-balsam.

After the time of Hippocrates and Galen, the science of medicine developed along several different paths. Although the contributions early Chinese and Indian practitioners made to the science of medicine were significant, the focus of medicine in the western world lay along the paths created by Hippocrates and followed by Galen. However, the Arab world was to have a great influence on western medicine as well. Arabic medicine, practiced from the fertile crescent of Persia to the south of Spain, made significant advances, particularly in pharmacy. This was due in part to the introduction of arithmetic, which allowed addition and subtraction in measurements of raw materials and substances.

Early Arabic influence in medicine was seen in the writings of Ibn Sina (Avicenna), physician-in-chief in Baghdad. He wrote volumes about medicine, 290 manuscripts in total, including his treatise on medicine entitled *Kitah al-Qanun* (translated *The Medical Code*). He was second only to Galen in his influence on western medical thought. Ibn Sina's five-volume *Kitah al-Qanun* arranged medical knowledge by subject, described some 760 drugs alphabetically, and described diseases and their treatment.[4]

Later, in the sixteenth century, pharmacy was to be further advanced by a German botanist named Valerius Cordus who wrote the first authoritative collection of formulas of drugs called a "pharmacopeia."[5] A pharmacopeia, also called a compendium, is a comprehensive list of drugs which not only includes formulas but usual strengths, standards of purity, and ranges of doses that are available in a certain country or region. By creating "drug standards"—specifications for the mixture of minerals, chemicals, and biological materials—a large number of deaths secondary to accidental overdose were avoided and the effects of specific ingredients upon the body were better understood.

At about the same time, a physician named Paracelsus (1493–1541) denounced Hippocrates' "humoral pathology"

theory, publicly burned copies of Galen's writings and Avicenna's "materia medica," and suggested instead that illness was caused by disease. He believed that disease could be treated with mineral baths of mercury, arsenic, lead, or copper and alcoholic extracts, formulas of which he added to the pharmacopeia.[4] This idea, that illness was caused by disease, was a radical departure from the theory of humoral imbalances. It suggested that, with experience and experimentation, medications could lead to the cure of disease. Paracelsus was credited with establishing the scientific method in his study of medicine, a practice that continues even today.

In the centuries that followed, medicine made great strides toward relieving suffering and curing disease through the use of drugs and herbal remedies. Widespread experimentation with these new formulas in order to create new remedies heralded the dawn of **pharmacology**, the study of drugs.

In the early 1600s, the first London pharmacopeia was compiled. This was followed in 1618 by creation of the first national pharmacopeia, the French Codex. Thereafter, many national pharmacopeias were compiled. Drugs, as a commodity, were then traded from city to city and country to country since these national pharmacopeias allowed free trade of similar drugs. With the widespread availability of the drug information contained within these national pharmacopeias, pharmacies began to appear in marketplaces all over Europe. Exact formularies also allowed industries to be developed for the mass production of medicine. Thus, medications began to become more widely available to the public. Examples of these early medications include tincture of opium, used to treat diarrhea (a common malady in a time when dysentery was rampant), and syrup of ipecac, used in presumed poisonings to prevent illness.[5]

Sources of Drugs

When pharmacy was in its infancy, most medications came from plants. Advances in pharmacy and chemistry resulted in the development of new sources for drugs, including drugs from animal by-products, minerals, synthetic medicines, and, most recently, genetic engineering.

Plants

Early pharmacists would take the roots, flowers, and seeds of a plant; crush them; mix them together in different amounts, or formulas; and create crude drugs. While many of these herbal concoctions were impure and impotent, some had active ingredients which had an intended or therapeutic effect. The bark of the willow tree, for example, was used as a cure for a number of ailments including headaches. It contains the active ingredient salicylate, which is still used in aspirin today.

While most medications are chemically manufactured today, plants are still an important source of many medicines. Many of the essential plant elements of crude drugs are more highly refined, making them more potent, and they are manufactured in mass quantities. Plant derivatives used to make drugs can be grouped together according to common physical or chemical properties. These organic-based groups are alkaloids (glycosides), oils, and gums.

The Alkaloids

The **alkaloids**, as the name suggests, are nitrogenous chemicals which are alkaline in nature and often chemically combined with acids to create water-soluble salts, such as morphine sulfate or atropine sulfate. When these alkaloids are absorbed into the body they dissolve easily. The acid and alkaline components dissociate and the alkaloid drug can be transported in the bloodstream and eventually deposited at the target organ, where it can produce its intended therapeutic effect.

One of the earliest drugs obtained from a plant was digitalis. Digitalis, a cardiac stimulant found in the nightshade plant, was used to treat a cardiac condition referred to then as dropsy, which is now known to be congestive heart failure.[6] The active ingredient in plant-based drugs like digitalis is side-linked to a simple sugar, a glucose molecule, in the plant. Thus, it is called a **glycoside**. Glycosides are easily absorbed into the bloodstream and the active ingredient is taken up by the target organ when the sugar is absorbed.

The Oils

Oils are substances that have been extracted from plants for centuries for their use as food additives as well as medications. An example is olive oil. Some plant-based oils have medicinal properties. For example, caster oil is used as a laxative. Oils that give off an odor are called aromatic oils. The aroma is caused by volatile chemicals that evaporate, or off-gas, into the atmosphere. These aromatic oils are often used as flavoring essences for medicine (e.g., oil of peppermint) or as soothing topical astringents, such as oil of spearmint.

The Gums

The **gum** of a plant, sometimes called its resin, is actually a complex sugar, a polysaccharide, that when moistened becomes a gelatinous material. Complex sugars are also called colloids because they are too large to pass through a semipermeable membrane. When a gum is swallowed, it swells because of osmosis, forming a gelatinous bulk. This property is useful when a laxative effect is desired. Applied externally, certain gums help to soothe irritated skin.

Minerals, Chemicals, and Salts

Natural salts and minerals have also been used for centuries for their medicinal qualities. For example, magnesium citrate, contained within a lemon-flavored carbonated beverage, is used as a laxative to relieve constipation and cleanse the bowel before certain medical procedures.

The chemical mercury and a large number of mercury-based compounds were used to halt the epidemic spread of the blood-borne disease syphilis. Syphilis is the only disease thought to have been transmitted from the New World to the Old World.[5]

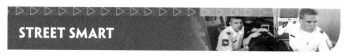

STREET SMART

The antibacterial action of common household bleach solution (Sodium hypochlorite 5%), used in EMS to clean surfaces contaminated with blood, is due to the off-gassing of hypochlorous acid from chlorine in water. The resulting chlorine gas is toxic to most bacteria.

Animal

Many drugs have their origins, in whole or in part, from animal tissues. The discovery of insulin is a case in point. Diabetes mellitus is a disease that causes the patient to excrete massive amounts of thick syrup-like urine. The resulting diabetes-induced dehydration can lead to severe shock. In the summer of 1921, Fred Banting noted that an injection of extract from the pancreas of animals, specifically the islets of Langerhans, reversed the ill effects of the diabetes and allowed the patient to return to a near-normal life. That extract was first called isletin and then later insulin. Sir Frederick G. Banting, MD, won the Nobel Prize for his discovery of insulin. Shortly thereafter, the Eli Lilly Drug Company began to mass-produce insulin, which it extracted from the pancreas of cows (beef insulin) and pigs (pork insulin). This resulted in improved lives for many diabetic patients. Many other drugs, such as epinephrine (adrenaline), were discovered in similar fashion and the study of "organotherapy" flourished in the late 1800s.[5]

Synthetic

One of the difficulties of manufacturing animal-based drugs was the pure volume of animal tissue that was sometimes needed to create them. For example, only one-half ounce of corticoid steroid could be distilled out of one ton of cows' adrenal glands.[7] Drug manufacturers had a tremendous hurdle to overcome to produce these drugs profitably.

In the 1940s, a basic building block of human hormones was discovered as naturally occurring in wild Mexican yams. These yams could be transformed, with chemical processing, into the female hormone progesterone. That discovery (using select plant stuffs and chemically processing them to produce drugs) led to an explosion of research into plant-based synthetic drugs. Today, this research continues as roots and tubers from newly discovered species of plants from the Amazon basin are being tested for possible medicinal use.[5]

Genetic Engineering

The future of drug manufacturing may be in genetic engineering. Genes are the architects of cell construction and contain the blueprint for protein production—the proteins that regulate cell function. Some diseases (e.g., hemophilia and cystic fibrosis) are thought to be caused by a failure of a gene to produce a certain protein. Genetically engineered medicine involves inserting a therapeutic gene into the malfunctioning cell via a benign viral vector and allowing the cell to produce the correct protein again. This process could eradicate the disease.

This approach to treating disease is still experimental but holds a great deal of promise. **Pharmacogenomics**, a combination of pharmaceutical research with the study of the human genome, promises to find other new ways to treat disease. With the human genome map completed in February 2001, scientists have started to look at individual gene variations, called "single nucleotide polymorphisms" or snipes, that cause or lead to disease or adverse drug reactions.

For example, a liver enzyme called CYP2C6 eliminates at least 30 different drugs from the body including beta-blockers, tricyclic antidepressants, antidysrhythmics, and opiate derivatives. By affecting this liver enzyme, it is possible to give smaller but still effective doses of medicine. The efficiency of drugs in the future may be vastly improved if scientists can make cells produce enzymes which assist the transportation of drugs into the cell.[7]

Currently, some drugs are genetically engineered proteins that replace missing proteins in the body. For example, Humulin™ is a genetically engineered form of human insulin.

Drug Terminology

By definition, a **drug** is any material which, when injected, ingested, inhaled, or absorbed into the body, is used for the diagnosis, treatment, or cure of a disease or condition. Some drugs may have more than one purpose. For example, the drug naloxone is often given to patients who are unconscious for an unknown reason but who are suspected of having over-dosed on opiates. Naloxone reverses the physiologic effects of the opiate. If the unconscious patient does not respond to the naloxone, then an opiate overdose is less likely to be the cause of unconsciousness. In this situation, naloxone is used as both a diagnostic drug and a treatment for opiate overdose.

Every drug is assigned three names, each with a specific meaning to a different group of people (Figure 29-1). As chemists and pharmacists develop new drugs they normally assign each a **chemical name**. A chemical name is a description of the drug according to its elemental chemical makeup and molecular structure. By utilizing a chemical name,

chemists are able to group drugs into classifications according to their common chemical makeups and thus understand the specific chemical nature of a drug.

After further development, manufacturers will assign a simpler to pronounce **generic name** to the drug. The generic name is often the drug name listed by the manufacturer in the United States Pharmacopeia (USP). The U.S. Pharmacopeia is a listing of all of the drugs legally manufactured or for sale in the United States. The letters USP follow the generic name after it is listed in the U.S. Pharmacopeia.

After sufficient research has been done and a drug is approved for distribution by a company, that company often will patent the drug to prevent other manufacturers from producing the same drug. To distinguish a patented drug, manufacturers will assign a unique third name, called the **trade name**.

Drug Classification

Drugs are divided into two classifications: prescription and nonprescription. Drugs that cannot be dispensed by a pharmacist without the written or verbal order of a physician or a mid-level healthcare provider, such as a physician's assistant, are called **prescription drugs**. The amount, or dose, of drug in a prescription drug can have serious side effects. Therefore, their administration requires careful patient monitoring by a healthcare provider.

> **STREET SMART**
>
> All prescription medications are federally mandated to display the legend "Caution: Federal law prohibits dispensing without prescription" and therefore are called legend drugs.

Although Paramedics are seldom asked to read a prescription from a physician, the pharmacist often directly transcribes the physician's written prescription onto the prescription label. Paramedics frequently read, review, and document what is on a patient's prescription label. Therefore, Paramedics should understand abbreviations that are routinely found on prescription labels (Table 29-2). There is an increasing practice of using plain English in a prescription, especially because of electronic prescriptions.

As the name implies, nonprescription medications can be purchased by the public without a prescription. Nonprescription drugs are generally sold by pharmacists **over-the-counter (OTC)** so patients can self-treat minor illnesses. The Health Care Financing Administration (HCFA) estimates that 6 out of 10 medications purchased in the United States are OTC. Presently, there are over 300,000 OTC medications on the market.[5,8]

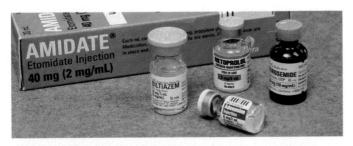

Figure 29-1 An example of a drug's names.

Table 29-2 Common Prescription Notations

a	before	kg, Kilo	kilogram	PRN, prn	whenever necessary
ac	before meals	KVO	keep vein open	pt	pint, patient
ad lib	as desired	L	liter	qh	every hour
AM, am	morning	LA	long acting	q2h	every 2 hours
amp	ampule	lb	pound	q3h	every 3 hours
bid	twice a day	mcg	microgram	q4h	every 4 hours
C̄	with	mEq	milliequivalent	QNS	quantity not sufficient
cap	capsule	mg	milligram	qs	quantity sufficient
Cl	chloride	ml, mL	milliliter (equivalent to cc)	qt	quart
cm	centimeter	mm	millimeter	R	rectal
DC	discontinue	Na	sodium	RL, R/L	Ringer's lactate
DS	double strength	NaCl	sodium chloride	S̄	without
DW	distilled water	NEB	nebulizer	SubQ, subq	subcutaneous
D5W	dextrose, 5% in water	NG	nasogastric	SL	sublingual
EC	enteric coated	noc	night	sol	solution
elix	elixir	NPO, npo	nothing by mouth	SR	sustained release
ER	extended release	NS, N/S	normal saline (sodium	stat	immediately and once only
Fe	iron		chloride, 0.9%)	supp	suppository
fl	fluid	Ø	none	tab	tablet
Gm,g	gram	OTC	over the counter	tbsp, T, tbs	tablespoon
gr	grain	oz	ounce	tid	three times a day
gtt	drop	p	after	TO	telephone order
h, hr	hour	pc	after meals	tsp, t	teaspoon
IM	intramuscular	PCA	patient controlled	vag	vaginal
IV	intravenous		analgesia	Vit	vitamin
IVPB	intravenous piggyback	PM, pm	afternoon	VO	verbal order
K	potassium	po, PO	by mouth, orally		
KCL	potassium chloride				

Note: Abbreviations should be written without periods.

STREET SMART

Seasoned Paramedics know that the patient's prescriptions can often lend a great deal of insight into the patient's past medical history. Patients frequently store prescription medications in medicine cabinets in the bathroom, in the bedside stand, or in the kitchen next to the water glasses. In some cases, patients may have already listed the prescriptions for emergency responders and placed the list in a "vial of life." These vials are often stored in the refrigerator and a "vial of life" sticker placed on the outside of the refrigerator door.

The public, in an effort to lower healthcare costs, have increasingly been self-diagnosing, self-prescribing, and self-administering OTC medicine. This practice is not without its dangers. Serious symptoms can be masked by OTC medications. Subsequent errors in medical judgment can occur, resulting in a life-threatening medical condition that may remain undiagnosed until the illness reaches crisis proportions. Furthermore, citizens who are attracted to an OTC drug's purported action, as advertised by means of the popular press or the Internet, may not read the FDA mandated warnings on the drug's label. Complicating matters, it is estimated that 20% of the American public are functionally illiterate and cannot read the label's warnings.[9] As an overall result, OTC drugs can be unsafe or, when improperly used, can cause unexpected side effects.

For these reasons, Paramedics should recognize that OTC medications are potentially dangerous, can have undesirable interactions with other drugs, and that OTC drugs are a part of the patient's medical history. The Paramedic should consider including a list of the OTC drugs that the patient is taking in the patient care report.

The difference between prescription and OTC drugs can sometimes be just the strength of the preparation (i.e., its potency). In smaller doses, the drug may be relatively safe for patient self-administration, whereas at higher doses there is a greater potential for harm to the patient if the OTC drug is misused. For this reason, the higher dose medication requires a prescription. Ibuprofen is an example. Ibuprofen comes in 200 mg, 400 mg, and 800 mg strengths. The public can buy the 200 mg dose of Ibuprofen over-the-counter, whereas the higher strength tablets require a physician's prescription and a pharmacist to dispense it. This prescription guarantees a licensed healthcare provider has determined the medication is safe for the patient to use at that strength and that a licensed healthcare provider is monitoring the patient's health while taking the drug.

Herbal Remedies

The medicinal use of herbs, also called botanicals, is also increasing across the United States. This increased use of herbal remedies may possibly be as a result of disenchantment with traditional western medicine on the part of some. However, the use of botanicals can create new problems for the patient and the Paramedic. Many patients who are taking herbal remedies are confounding their medical treatment with the addition of untested herbal preparations which can cause unpredictable consequences. Therefore, Paramedics should know the effects of some of the more common botanicals and their potential interaction with the drugs that the Paramedic would be administering (Table 29-3). It is important that the Paramedic list all herbal products along with over-the-counter and prescription medicines on the patient care report.

Observant Paramedics may note the presence of teapots, pots and pans, and the like and ask the patient questions about herbal remedies. Methods of botanical administration include **potable infusions** (boiling water over the top of the herbs and immediately drawing off the solution), **decoction** (bringing water to a boil then steeping the herbs like one would a teabag and drinking the resulting solution) and **cold maceration** (letting herbs steep in cold water).

Sources of Drug Information

A pharmacopeia is a list of the drugs commonly used in a country. The first U.S. Pharmacopeia was published in 1820 as a guide to apothecaries who collected plants and flowers and for physicians who compounded their own remedies.[10] Typically, a group of physicians, pharmacists, and other professionals, create a pharmacopeia.

The **United States Pharmacopeia (USP)** drug reference is created by an independent nongovernmental science-based public health organization called the United States Pharmacopeia. The United States Pharmacopeia is made up of over 1,000 scientists, practitioners, and representatives from various colleges of medicine and pharmacy who set the standards for medication manufacturing in the United States. This group of physicians, pharmacists, and scientists meets every five years, at the United States Pharmacopeial Convention, to discuss and adopt recommendations presented from the internal Council of Experts (COE) regarding new drugs to be added to the United States Pharmacopeia listing. The **National Formulary (NF)**, another drug reference, is a manual that lists medications which are approved for prescription. It contains specific chemical information that is more helpful to the pharmacist and manufacturer than the physician. Today, the U.S. Pharmacopeia (USP)—as well as the National Formulary (NF), which is part of the USP—is recognized by the Federal Drug Administration and contains the standards of purity, dose, formula, and other information for drugs. The USP is, per the Federal Food, Drug, and Cosmetic Act (2 U.S.C.321), the authority for drug manufacturing in the United States. The USP is a two-volume text. The first volume includes all prescription medications and the second volume includes all over-the-counter medications.

Another reputable source of information about prescription and over-the-counter medications is the **Physician's Desk Reference (PDR)**. The PDR is a compendium of manufacturer drug-prescribing information which is usually found in a package insert required by law to accompany all medications. These Food and Drug Administration (FDA)-mandated inserts contain information, including common side effects, obtained during drug testing trials.

It is sometimes difficult for a Paramedic to obtain information quickly and in useful form from the USP, the NF, or the PDR. Quick reference books, such as *Delmar's Drug Reference for the EMS Provider* by Richard Beck, are fast and convenient ways to obtain that information in a user-friendly manner. These references typically group medications

Table 29-3 Partial List of Common Botanicals

Name	Use	Side Effect/Precaution
Aloe vera	Heal wounds; Laxative	Potassium loss
Cascara sagrada bark	Laxative	Intestinal obstruction; Potassium loss
Chamomile	Anti-inflammatory	Anaphylaxis; Cross allergy—Ragweed
Cranberry	Urinary deodorizer	Diarrhea
Echinacea	Infections	Cross allergy—Sunflower seeds
Garlic	Lower blood pressure	Reduces platelet aggregation; Interacts with blood thinners
Ginger	Morning sickness	Reduces platelet aggregation; Affects calcium channel blockers (pregnancy-induced hypertension)
Ginkgo biloba	Depression; Alzheimer's disease	Reduces platelet aggregation; Cross allergy—Poison ivy
Ginseng root	Improve concentration	Interferes with digoxin; Hypoglycemia
Kava kava	Sedative	Worsens Parkinson symptoms
Licorice	Upper respiratory infection	Use with thiazides—increased potassium loss
St. John's wort	Herpes simplex; Depression	Hypertensive crisis—if taken with tyramine-containing foods

together in classification by body system or by clinical indication. These reference manuals provide further information on a drug's action, dose, use, risk during pregnancy, common side effects, and treatment of overdose. Every Paramedic should have a drug reference available to identify unfamiliar patient medications. Knowledge of a patient's medication history can lend insight into the patient's condition. Many Paramedics also create their own drug cards, handy pocket references that contain a partial listing of pertinent information (Figure 29-2).

MANNITOL
Osmitrol
CLASSIFICATIONS
Pharmacologic: Osmotic diuretic
Therapeutic: Diuretic

MECHANISM OF ACTION: Mannitol increases osmotic pressure in the **glomerular filtrate.** This inhibits the reabsorption of water and electrolytes, which causes their excretion in the urine.

THERAPEUTIC BENEFIT: The diuretic action of mannitol causes a dehydrating effect on the brain.

INDICATION FOR PREHOSPITAL USE: Mannitol is used to relieve excessive intracranial pressure.

CONTRAINDICATIONS: ■ Do not administer mannitol to patients with: ■ Hypersensitivity to the drug. ■ Preexisting dehydration. ■ Active intracranial bleeding.

PRECAUTIONS: Use caution in administering mannitol to patients who show a tendency to congestive heart failure, because mannitol may cause a sudden expansion of extracellular fluid, which could bring on congestive heart failure.

ROUTE AND DOSAGE

Adult: 1.5–2 g/kg of a 20% solution by IV infusion, using an in-line IV filter. Mannitol comes in a 5, 10, 15, or 20% 500-mL solution.

Pediatric: Not recommended for prehospital use.

ADVERSE REACTIONS AND SIDE EFFECTS

* *CNS:* Headache, confusion.
* *Cardiovascular:* Tachycardia, chest pain, congestive heart failure, pulmonary edema.
* *Eyes:* Blurred vision.
* *Fluids and electrolytes:* Dehydration.
* *Gastrointestinal:* Nausea, vomiting, thirst.

PARAMEDIC IMPLICATIONS: ■ Monitor the patients closely for any signs of dehydration, which include: ■ Fever. ■ Thirst. ■ Decreased skin turgor. ■ Dry skin and mucous membranes. ■ Mannitol has a tendency to crystalize at temperatures below 45°F. Use an in-line filer when administering mannitol to filter any crystals out of the solution.

DRUG INTERACTIONS: ■ Additive CNS depression can result if mannitol is administered with other CNS depressants. ■ Mannitol can also cause additive adrenergic effects and anticholinergic effects when used with CNS depressants.

Figure 29-2 An example of a drug card.

Historical Legal Developments in Pharmacology

The image of a medicine man in a top hat leaning over the side of a painted wagon, extolling the virtues of a snake oil remedy, is all part of the lore of the American West. It is also the genesis of many modern drug laws. These medicine men, as well as catalog mail order houses and self-anointed doctors, sold a variety of concoctions which promised to cure everything from arthritis to the common cold. Many of these cures did not work and, worse yet, many of them contained dangerous drugs such as opium and chloral hydrate.[11]

In an effort to protect the public from false advertising and adulterated medicine, Congress enacted the **Pure Food and Drug Act of 1906**. The law prohibited the use of false or misleading claims. The law further stipulated that if a medicine contained any of the 11 "dangerous" drugs, then the drug(s) had to be listed on the label. Additionally, the Pure Food and Drug Act of 1906 recognized the National Formulary and the United States Pharmacopeia (USP) as the official drug standards for the United States.

Unfortunately, there were many loopholes in the law. For example, the federal law did not apply to drugs produced in a state and then sold only within that state. The addition of the Durham-Humphrey amendment in 1952, which included new regulations regarding labeling and the refill of prescription medications, closed some of these loopholes. The amendment also required the addition of a written warning, called a legend, for drugs that are injected, that are investigational, or that are potentially habit-forming (Figure 29-3). Perhaps more importantly, the amendment described a new class of drugs for which a prescription was not required, the over-the-counter (OTC) drugs.

Controlled Substances Legislation

The use of opium, with its long and undistinguished history as a drug of abuse, ultimately led to many of the modern narcotic drug laws. Opium, a product obtained from the poppy plant (Papaver somniferum), was freely available over the counter

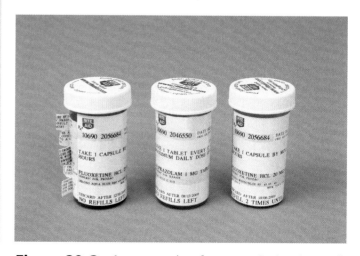

Figure 29-3 An example of a prescription legend.

in the 1700s. Mothers used tincture of opium to control diarrhea, brought on by cholera or dysentery, because opium has a powerful constipating effect. Unfortunately, these early opium preparations, including laudanum and paregoric, were very crude and the effects often unpredictable. Occasionally, these drugs would harm the patient as a result.

In 1820, a German pharmacist, Friedrich Serturner, attempted to refine opium into its active ingredient, ridding it of its impurities. He named the resulting drug "morphia," after the Greek god Morpheus, the god of dreams.[12] The combination of the increased availability of morphine and the invention of the hypodermic needle in 1850 led to the widespread use of morphine as an pain reliever (analgesic).

In a continuing effort to improve on opium, other derivatives of opium were also produced. In 1898, the German pharmaceutical company Bayer produced the semi-synthetic opium derivative diacetylmorphine and branded it "hero-in," the hero drug which had the same ability to relieve pain as morphine but was safer. Unfortunately, heroin did not live up to its promise and the medical community largely abandoned its use in favor of morphine.

Opium and morphine use in the United States reached its pinnacle in the late 1800s and opium was readily available to the public. As opium dens and pharmacies started to dispense larger and larger amounts of opiates, correspondingly larger numbers of people were becoming addicted to opium.

In response to the growing drug problem, the United States Congress passed the **Harrison Act** of 1914.[13] The Harrison Act made it illegal to obtain "narcotics" (e.g., morphine) without a prescription. The list of narcotics included drugs such as cocaine, which is a stimulant. (Marijuana would later be added to the list.)

However, the problem of opiate addiction was largely unaffected by the Harrison Act because physicians continued to prescribe the opiates. In a challenge to the Harrison Act, the Supreme Court ruled that the act of supplying addicts, even when the narcotics were obtained under physician's prescription, was illegal. In 1930, the Federal Bureau of Narcotics,

made up of mainly out-of-work prohibition officers, was formed to enforce the Harrison Act. Newly deputized federal narcotic agents immediately arrested some 3,000 doctors for illegally prescribing opiates to addicts. The Federal Bureau of Narcotics was later reorganized and became the Drug Enforcement Administration (DEA) in 1973.[5]

In furtherance of the intent of the Harrison Act, and as a part of his "war on drugs" campaign, President Nixon signed the **Comprehensive Drug Abuse Prevention and Control Act of 1970 (Controlled Substance Act)** into law. This expanded the authority of the DEA. Contained within the Controlled Substance Act were schedules of potentially dangerous and addictive drugs which had special restrictions (Table 29-4).

STREET SMART

It is important to remember that the federal schedule of narcotics includes non-opiate substances, such as marijuana and cocaine. The term "narcotic" should not be used interchangeably with opiates. The Paramedic should specifically refer to opiates by name.

Drug Misuse versus Drug Abuse

The difference between drug misuse and drug abuse is an important distinction. Drug misuse implies that the drug is not being used as prescribed and can lead to problems of toxicity. Drug abuse implies concerns about dependency and intentional improper use of a drug. Drug misuse is a complex issue which includes unintended drug interactions as a result of polypharmacology (multiple drug actions).

Drug abuse involves the intentional misuse of drugs, prescription as well as illicit, for a purpose other than the diagnosis, treatment, or cure of a disease or condition. Drug abuse

Table 29-4 Schedule of Drugs and Examples of Controlled Substances

Class	Definition	Examples	Restrictions
I	High abuse, No medical use	Opium, Marijuana, LSD	Special protocol
II	High abuse, Limited use, Severe dependence	Fentanyl, Codeine	Triple prescription, No refill, See *Note*
III	Lower abuse, Medical use, Moderate dependence	Small amounts of codeine combined with aspirin or acetaminophen paregoric	Limit six months, No more than five refills, See *Note*
IV	Minor abuse, Medical use, Minor dependence	Barbiturates, Benzodiazepines	Limit six months, No more than five refills, See *Note*
V	Low abuse Medical use Limited physical or psychological dependence	Cold remedy	May require prescription

Note: Federal law prohibits the transfer of this drug to any person other than the patient to whom it was prescribed.

Source: DEA pharmacist's manual—an informational outline of the Controlled Substance Act of 1970. U.S. Department of Justice, Washington D.C. Red Book, 1996.

often leads to dependency, a craving for the drug that can lead to socially unacceptable behaviors and/or the person's inability to perform activities of daily living (ADL).

Dependence on a drug occurs when a person has a compulsive desire to have a drug, and the drug becomes the sole source of satisfaction for that person. Dependence also can be physical, a biochemical change in the body as a result of taking the drug, or it can be psychological, the compulsive desire to have the drug. Habituation is the mildest form of psychological dependence. Cigarette smokers, dependent upon the stimulant effects of the nicotine in the cigarette, have a "smoking habit." In some cases, the habit can be stopped without any harm to the individual. Psychological dependence becomes pathological when the person insists that the drug is needed in order to survive, despite scientific evidence to the contrary, and takes antisocial action in order to obtain it.[14]

Physical Dependence

Physical dependence is more than severe psychological dependence. Physical dependence occurs when the body adapts, biochemically speaking, to the constant presence of the drug and integrates the drug into the body's metabolism. In short, the body needs the drug in order to maintain homeostasis. The following example is illustrative of physical dependence.

Coffee drinkers enjoy coffee because it contains the stimulant caffeine. Caffeine interferes with adenosine receptors by means of a competitive blockade. Adenosine, a neuromodulator in the peripheral and central nervous systems, normally attaches to adenosine receptors and reduces cyclic AMP levels. Cyclic AMP is important to neurotransmission. After a time, the body adapts to the high caffeine levels and greater amounts of caffeine are needed to produce the same effect. Subsequently, when a coffee drinker suddenly stops drinking coffee he can experience irritability, headache, and weakness as a result of the unbalancing of the nervous system. These withdrawal symptoms indicate a physical dependence upon the drug.

New Drug Development

After the death of over 100 people in 1937, following an ingestion of a new drug called "elixir of sulfanilamide," Congress enacted the **Food, Drug, and Cosmetic Act**, which prohibited the sale of new drugs before thorough safety testing. While the federal government had previously required that a drug be properly labeled and safe to use, there was no guarantee that the drug was even effective against the condition for which it was prescribed.

The passage of the **Kefauver-Harris Act** in 1962 went beyond the Food, Drug, and Cosmetic Act of 1937 by adding a new condition to the sale of drugs within the United States. The law required that all drugs undergo an extensive review that not only ensured the public's safety, but also reassured the public that a drug would do what it claimed to do.[15,16] The

FDA immediately established a drug approval process that reflected these regulations.

Now, when a pharmaceutical company manufactures a new drug, or has an old drug that is being used for a new purpose or at a new strength, it has to apply to the FDA to make the drug an "investigational new drug" (IND). Before a drug can be IND certified, the manufacturer is required to submit animal studies to the FDA that identify the drug's therapeutic dosage, its lethal toxicity, its therapeutic range, and its therapeutic index.

The therapeutic range of a drug starts at the minimally effective dose (the dose that elicits the desired therapeutic response) and concludes with a maximum dose (the dose after which any more drug does not produce any more of the desired therapeutic effect). Somewhere between the maximum and minimum dosage, within the therapeutic range, is the therapeutic dose (the amount of drug that effectively creates the therapeutic effect in a majority of patients). The therapeutic dose can also be thought of as the median effective dose, the **ED50**.

At the other extreme is the lethal dose of the drug, or LD50. The **LD50** is shorthand for lethal dose 50%, where 50% of the test animals given a certain dose of medicine died. LD50 is the median lethal dose. It should be recognized that patients can still succumb to doses far less than the LD50 and caution should always be practiced whenever giving a drug. Manufacturers also have to describe the modes of absorption, distribution, metabolism, and excretion of the drug (i.e., its pharmacokinetics) before the FDA can approve the drug as an IND.

A drug's **therapeutic index** is the ratio of the difference between the median effective dose (the ED50) and the median lethal dose (the LD50) of a drug. Drugs with less than a two-fold difference between the ED50 and the LD50 are defined as having a narrow therapeutic index, as defined in the FDA regulations (320.33(c)CFR 21). A drug with a narrow therapeutic index has a greater chance of causing toxicity in a patient (Table 29-5). Therapeutic index represents a calculated safety margin used when prescribing a drug. The prescribing healthcare provider has to carefully monitor the patient for toxicity.

Table 29-5 Drugs with a Narrow Therapeutic Index

- Aminophylline
- Digoxin
- Isoproterenol
- Lithium
- Phenytoin
- Procainamide
- Quinidine
- Valproate
- Valproic acid
- Warfarin

FDA IND Status

Once designated as an IND, further studies of the drug are required. In Phase I, an initial pharmacologic evaluation has to be performed on the drug to determine modes of absorption, distribution, metabolism, and excretion in normal healthy human volunteers. These trials are intended to prove the safety of the IND in human use, not necessarily the effectiveness of the IND.

In Phase II, a limited controlled evaluation of the drug is performed upon target populations who have the disease for which the drug was developed. Modes of absorption, distribution, metabolism, and excretion then are established for this special population of patients.

Assuming no difficulties, the IND would next undergo the final phase, or phase III, an extended clinical evaluation among the target population under selected conditions. Study "protocols" would be published and then a determination of clinical effectiveness would be established. Issues such as drug dosage range and patient drug tolerance are clarified. During phase III, common side effects are usually described and ranked according to prevalence in the study's participants. After the thalidomide tragedy of the late 1950s, special attention has been given to the effects and potential risks to an unborn fetus. The FDA establishes a drug's safety for a pregnant woman and places the drug into one of five categories (Table 29-6).

After completion of the IND process, the FDA either permits the drug to be marketed and places it in a "new drug" category or returns the drug for further testing (a "one, two, three, and out" approach). If a drug is designated a new drug, then the pharmaceutical companies monitor for post-marketing drug interactions and adverse reactions as part of ongoing surveillance.

It can take over 12 to 15 years for each new drug to complete the FDA process and may cost as much as $500 million in research.[17] Only one in 5,000 potential drug compounds makes it through the process. Seven out of ten new drugs do not make enough profit to cover the costs of initial research and subsequent development costs. These factors have led to increased drug costs for the consumer but have also ensured that safer and more effective drugs are being manufactured.

Table 29-6 Pregnancy Safety Categories

A	Adequate, well-controlled studies in pregnant women	No risk to human fetus
B	Animal studies	No risk but no studies to substantiate human risk
C	Animal studies	Adverse risk but no studies to substantiate human risk; question of risk/benefit analysis
D	Adequate, well-controlled studies or observational studies in pregnant women	Positive human fetal risk; question of maternal versus fetal life
X	Adequate, well-controlled studies or observational studies in animals or pregnant women	Known fetal anomalies; risks outweigh benefits

Drug companies willingly undertake this expense, in part because it lowers their **product liability**. A manufacturer can be held responsible (liable) if the product is defective (not fit for its suggested use or results in harm to the consumer). The FDA process helps to ensure that risks are revealed, that the manufacturer knows the effect of the product, and that a reasonable amount of research was performed to protect the public. The remaining jeopardy for the manufacturer exists during the drug's processing. Major drug manufacturers have vigorous quality assurance programs to ensure that the drug is pure throughout the manufacturing process, from production to packaging.

Patented Drugs

New drugs are typically patented, ensuring the manufacturer exclusive dominion over the drug for a specified period of time. This allows for a profit to be made as the manufacturer markets the new drug against older drugs. However, patents are time-limited. In many cases, another drug manufacturer is waiting to produce the same (or a similar) drug, without the expense of research and development, in hopes of making a profit. To extend the patent, some pharmaceutical companies will expand the drug's use to include children, a new use of an existing drug. Eventually, however, the patent expires on all drugs and the drug profitability declines. This fact of business is factored into the decision to develop a new drug.

Off-Label Use

In some cases, a physician may elect to use a drug for other than its FDA-approved use. While there is some risk involved for the physician in prescribing a drug to be used for other than its FDA-approved use, such an action is permitted and is considered to be part of the practice of medicine.

Off-label use often occurs when a generic drug, which is no longer protected by patent, is used for a new indication. In some instances, it is not cost effective for the pharmaceutical companies to research the new indication of these older drugs. Fortunately, this does not preclude the physician from prescribing that drug if, in the physician's professional opinion, the benefits outweigh the risks.

Orphan Drugs

Drug therapies for rare or uncommon diseases are generally nonprofitable. Development and research for drugs designed for these special conditions, called **orphan drugs**, are often underfunded at best. To provide this population of patients with viable treatment alternatives, Congress passed the Orphan Drug Act of 1983.

The Orphan Drug Act provides grants to manufacturers and research centers to investigate drug therapies for rare diseases such as Von Willebrand's disease or Raynaud's disease and create these orphan drugs.[17] The FDA classifies these orphan drugs as "V."

Medicine Errors

Despite all of the precautions that are taken during the research, manufacture, distribution, and preparation of drugs, mistakes can occur. In 1993, the FDA launched its drug watchdog program called MedWatch.[18,19] MedWatch is a voluntary program utilized by healthcare professionals to report adverse or unusual drug reactions and errors. MedWatch identifies those drugs and medical devices that have, or could have, resulted in death or risk of death, hospitalization, disability, or birth defects. The problems are then reported to the drug manufacturers for corrective action.

Despite this effort, in 1999 the Institute of Medicine—in its report, "To Err Is Human"—reported that there were 44,000 to 98,000 preventable deaths and 500,000 preventable injuries due to medical errors.[20,21] A subset of those medical errors is medication error. The Institute of Medicine estimated that over 7,000 deaths occur annually as a result of medication administration errors.

Alarmed by these statistics, and the attendant implications, professional pharmacists began their own program of medication administration error reporting through the United States Pharmacopeia (USP) called MedMARx.[22] While pharmacists had a program for medication error reporting (MER) since 1991, the new program sought to understand medication administration errors, not just medication labeling and packaging errors.

The MedMARx program of the USP is a self-reporting Internet program. The focus of these anonymous and voluntary reports is problems with the process by which medications are given rather than medication side effects and reactions. During 2000 alone, over 184 medical facilities reported over 41,296 medication errors.[23] Medication errors were classified as causing harm, no harm, or having a potential for harm. Fortunately, 97% of the errors caused no harm. However, 5% of reported medication administration errors did cause harm and affected about 1,200 patients.

Principles of Pharmacology

Well over a half million medications—both prescription and OTC—are available on the market, each asserting that it is the most effective medication for a specific condition or disease. The basis of these claims lies in the drug's **intended biological effect**. The intended biological effect of a drug, also called its **therapeutic effect**, is to modify a tissue or an organ's function. Drugs can enhance a bodily function by increasing or replacing a chemical in the organ. They can also preclude or prevent a chemical from having an effect on the organ by blocking or competing with the body's own chemicals. However, a drug does not add a new function; rather, it affects the organ's functions.

While a drug may have a desired therapeutic effect, it often has additional unintended effects as well. These unintended effects, called **side effects**, may be so noxious that the person stops taking the medicine. Frequently the goal of drug research is to eliminate these unwanted side effects. For example, early asthma treatments effectively reversed bronchospasm, but a frequent side effect was tachycardia, a problem for patients with a cardiac condition. Continuing pharmaceutical research aimed at reducing or eliminating these bothersome side effects resulted in a more refined drug. The next **generation** of asthma drugs caused less nervousness, palpitations, and tachycardia.

Pharmacokinetics

A drug's therapeutic value is influenced by several factors including the speed of onset of the drug's effect, the intensity of the drug's effect, and the duration of the drug's effect. These factors are largely the result of the drug's time and ease of absorption, its distribution from the plasma into the tissue of the target organ, and its eventual retention or elimination from the body. **Pharmacokinetics** is the study of how these factors—drug absorption, distribution, detoxification, and elimination—affect a drug's therapeutic value.

Absorption

In a sequential fashion, the first phase of a drug's "life" is absorption. For a systemic drug to be effective, it must get into the bloodstream and be transported to the target organ. The drug's movement from its site of administration into the plasma in the blood is a function of the route of administration. In the case of drugs given intravenously (IV), the drug is instantly available in the blood plasma. However, most medications are not given IV; most are given PO ("per os" or Latin for "by mouth"). In that case, the absorption goes through a complicated process which will be discussed shortly. Specifics of the methods of drug administration are discussed in Chapter 26. However, it is important to understand the impact of medication administration of the various drug administration techniques as they relate to drug absorption and distribution. For purposes of this discussion, medication administration can be grossly categorized as either enteral (via the gastrointestinal system) or parenteral (other than the gastrointestinal system).

Enteral Drug Administration

Enteral administration of medication, via the GI tract, is the most common form of medication administration. While easy to administer, multiple intervening factors make enteral medication absorption less predictable and therefore less desirable during an emergency.

To begin, once a PO medication is swallowed, the first impediment to drug absorption is the stomach. While the stomach has a rich network of blood vessels for ready absorption, stomach acid, with a pH as high as 1.4, can destroy the drug before it can be absorbed. The stomach acid will break down most substances, whether food or drugs, into their elemental components and therefore neutralize many medications in the process.

If the drug is either unaffected by the stomach acid, or is protected from stomach acid, it passes through the stomach into the intestines. In some cases, the drug is transferred from the lining of the intestine and moves into the plasma by a simple process of passive diffusion. The mechanics of passive diffusion assume that there is more of the drug, often in the form of a salt, on the inside of the gut's membranous lining than in the blood stream, establishing a **concentration gradient** across that membrane. Whenever a concentration gradient exists, the higher concentration will diffuse across the intestinal wall to an area of lower concentration until a balance of concentrations (equilibrium) is met (Figure 29-4).

In some cases, a drug molecule is too large to pass across the intestinal wall into the blood via passive diffusion. In those cases, a protein carrier will convey the drug across the intestinal wall and into the plasma, a process called **active transport**. This form of transport requires energy, in the form of adenosine triphosphate (ATP).

However, many physical factors—including shock states, which slow absorption, and decreased surface contact time secondary to diarrhea—can affect the absorption of drugs from the gut into the blood, making the absorption unpredictable (Figure 29-5).

Once the drug has crossed over the intestinal wall, it is in the hepatic portal system. The hepatic portal system is a subsystem of the systemic circulation. The blood volume in the entire gut is in the hepatic portal system and drains through the liver before rejoining the systemic circulation. This passage through the portal vein permits the liver to detoxify any foreign substance including drugs. The liver's actions upon the drugs, called **first pass metabolism**, can markedly reduce the amount of active drug available for the target organ when it reaches the systemic circulation. These drugs are immediately affected by the C450 system and the majority of the drug is inactivated.[24-27] To overcome this loss, healthcare providers must administer 10 to 100 times the dose that would be given intravenously (IV). For example, propranolol, a popular antihypertensive, is usually given 1 to 3 mg IV, whereas the oral dose is 80 to 100 mg. Lidocaine cannot be given orally because it is completely deactivated by the cytochrome P-450 system. To eliminate the effects of first pass metabolism, many drugs (such as lidocaine) are administered directly into the systemic circulation.

Parenteral Drug Administration

When a drug is injected directly into the bloodstream, without going through the gastrointestinal tract (the enteral route), then that drug has been given via a parenteral route. Examples of parenteral routes include intramuscular injection and intravenous injection. There are 10 parenteral routes for drug administration. The need for numerous parenteral routes underscores the significance of first pass metabolism upon drugs.

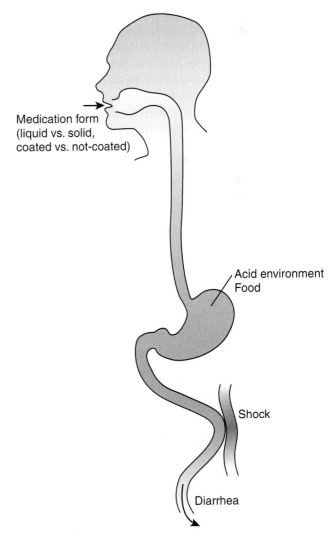

Medication form (liquid vs. solid, coated vs. not-coated)

Acid environment Food

Shock

Diarrhea

Figure 29-5 Factors that influence drug absorption in the gut.

Figure 29-4 Drugs diffusing into the cell.

Passive diffusion of a water-soluble drug through an aqueous channel or pore.

Passive diffusion of a lipid-soluble drug dissolved in a membrane.

ATP

ADP

Drug

Carrier-mediated active transport of drug

Of the 10 parenteral routes, intravenous (IV) drug infusions are generally preferred during an emergency. This is due to the fact that drug levels in the blood are obtained more rapidly and drug levels can be maintained at more of a steady state. The steady-state level of drug results from a combination of two factors. On the one hand is the amount of drug being infused and on the other, the speed or rate of the infusion. If a Paramedic starts at the zero state (with no drug in the blood) and constantly runs an infusion in, without being affected by other influences, then the amount of drug in the blood will increase at an arithmetic rate until it reaches a steady state (Figure 29-6).

However, attaining a drug's steady state is not that easy. Once a drug is in the bloodstream a number of factors begin to act upon it. First, and perhaps most importantly, the liver starts to detoxify the drug (a process called biotransformation) as the blood passes through the liver. Thus, while a drug is being infused it is also being continuously eliminated. The **drug decline** is largely a function of the liver's health and capabilities. Even with a healthy liver, there is a limited capacity to neutralize a drug. Eventually the drug infusion can overwhelm the liver's capabilities to neutralize the drug and the level of drug in the bloodstream will climb. These two factors—infusion rate and drug decline—slow the climb of the drug concentration toward a steady state. Instead of a straight linear rise in drug levels, a curved exponential rise is observed. When the drug levels attain the targeted value, as manifested by observation of the therapeutic effect, then the drug is at the **therapeutic level (t)**. When the decline of drug in the bloodstream reaches 50%, this is equivalent to the drug's **half-life (t½)**.

On occasion, it is inconvenient to wait for a therapeutic level to be attained by a slow and constant infusion of drug. In those cases a single fixed dose, called a **bolus**, is given to rapidly boost the drug to the therapeutic level. Thereafter, an infusion is started to maintain the drug at that t-level.

In some other cases, it is impractical to continuously infuse a drug intravenously. Instead, repeated boluses of drug are given until a steady state of drug is reached in the blood. While the drug level is constantly climbing and then falling, if the repeat bolus is given before the drug's half-life (t½), then the sum of the levels will always be at or above the therapeutic level (Figure 29-7).

An example may help clarify this concept. Lidocaine has been used to treat ventricular ectopy, irregular beats of the heart. A constant infusion of lidocaine would take the better part of an hour to attain a therapeutic level. To speed the process, the Paramedic would start with a bolus of lidocaine to boost the level of lidocaine to the therapeutic range and then start an infusion, an IV lidocaine drip, to maintain that level. Because of the relatively short half-life of lidocaine, the drug level drops below the therapeutic level before the infusion has assumed dominance. This lapse in drug level is called the **chemical hiatus**. Logically, if the chemical hiatus is

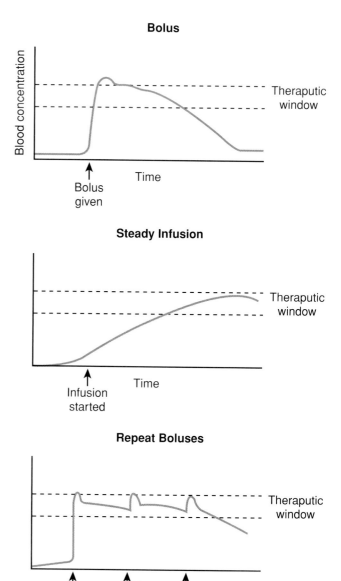

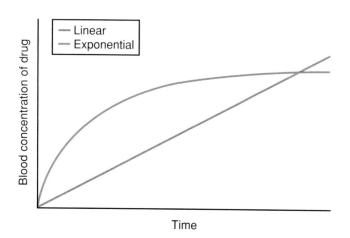

Figure 29-6 Linear and exponential drug infusion rate.

Figure 29-7 Effects of bolus, steady infusion, and repeat bolus on serum drug levels.

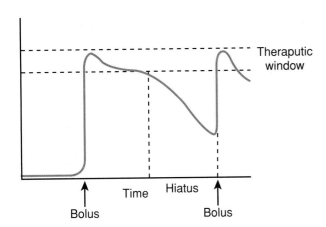

Figure 29-8 Chemical hiatus and lidocaine administration.

left untreated, a potentially life-threatening return ventricular ectopy could occur. To prevent this occurrence, a repeat bolus of one-half the initial dose is given to boost the drug back up to a therapeutic level. This practice illustrates all three injection techniques: bolus, infusion, and repeat bolus (Figure 29-8).

Distribution

Once the drug is in the bloodstream it is carried to all the body's tissues and organs. This distribution is affected by several factors including blood volume, blood flow within the tissues, and permeability of the capillary walls.

Blood volume can have a dramatic impact on drug distribution. If a patient is hemorrhaging, then the physical amount of blood which can carry the drug is diminished. The body, as a part of its compensatory mechanisms, redistributes blood to core organs. However, key organs may not get the medication needed. Even under normal conditions, certain tissues get higher blood flow rates than others; for example, the heart, lungs, liver, and kidneys get more blood than does adipose (fat) tissue. The fact that muscle and fat receive less perfusion than other organs during a resting state can be used to advantage. Injection of medication into deep muscles is more likely to be slowly absorbed into the bloodstream than medications injected into a vein.

Capillary Diffusion

Once the drug gets into an organ's capillary beds, it must pass through the interstitial fluid and into the cells directly in order for the drug to have its therapeutic effect. Capillary walls have selective permeability to drugs. Slit junctions, physical breaks in the integrity of the capillary wall, allow the drug to pass into the interstitial space. Capillary beds in specific organs, such as the liver, have large slit junctions. These larger-than-normal slit junctions facilitate large molecules, including drugs, to pass easily from the bloodstream into the interstitial fluid and then into the hepatic cells. The drug can then be chemically altered by special enzymes within the hepatic cell into an inert or non-active chemical called a **metabolite**.

Alternatively, the capillaries of the brain have tight slit junctions, preventing toxins and chemicals, including drugs, from easily passing into the brain. This obstacle is referred to as the **blood-brain barrier**. For drugs to enter the brain, the drug must be **lipid-soluble** (i.e., able to be dissolved in lipids [fat]). Since the capillary wall membranes are partially made of lipids, the drug literally dissolves into the capillary wall, passes through to the opposite wall, and moves into interstitial fluid in the brain. These drugs are also referred to as **lipophilic**, meaning attracted to lipids.

The placenta also provides a partial barrier to toxins, such as chemicals and drugs, present in the mother's bloodstream. While certain enzymes within the placental tissue can render some chemicals inert (e.g., catecholamines such as epinephrine), many other drugs are not acted upon or blocked by the placenta and pass easily through the placenta and into the fetus (e.g., narcotics and anesthetics). Paramedics should always keep in mind that drugs which may be at the therapeutic blood level (ED50) for the mother may be at the toxic (LD50) level for the fetus. Also, the placenta offers a less-than-perfect barrier for the fetus from these drugs. The relatively nonselective transfer of drugs across the placenta, and paucity of research regarding placental drug transfer, requires the Paramedic to be extra vigilant whenever drugs are being given to a pregnant patient.

Drug Reservoirs

Drugs bind to certain substances in the body and, in doing so, form **drug reservoirs**. A drug reservoir acts as a drug depot, storing the drug until it is needed. The effect of a drug reservoir is to prolong the drug's action within the body. There are two types of drug reservoirs: plasma protein reservoirs and tissue reservoirs.

The plasma proteins of the blood serve as the first drug reservoir. The blood contains plasma proteins (e.g., albumin). As a drug enters the bloodstream, it is attracted to the plasma protein within the blood and forms a union, binding the drug to the plasma protein. The protein-bound drug is not free to interact with target organs, and the measurable level of free-drug in the bloodstream is lower. In effect, the drug is held in reserve on the plasma protein, in a circulating depository, until needed.

There is a limit to the amount of drug that can be bound to plasma proteins. Once all available blood proteins are bound with the drug, then free-drug in the bloodstream becomes available for tissues. Therefore, not all of the active drug becomes protein-bound. The difference between protein-bound and free-unbound drug which is pharmaceutically active is expressed in terms of a percentage.

For example, warfarin (a commonly prescribed anticoagulant) is 99% protein bound; that means it is 99% bound to plasma proteins and 1% active drug in the system. For this reason, warfarin stays in the patient's bloodstream for long periods of time and the patient need only take the drug occasionally.

The amount of free-drug available from the plasma protein reservoir is therefore a function of the amount of blood proteins in the blood. Albumin and other blood proteins are primarily formed in the liver. The patient who has liver failure, secondary to alcoholism, or diseases such as hepatitis is unable to produce these blood proteins. Understandably, the doses of highly protein-bound drugs, such as propranolol, must be adjusted and smaller doses administered.

An impact of aging is the decline in liver function. As a result, Paramedics tend to administer one half the normal dose of highly bound medications, such as lidocaine, to avoid toxicity in this patient population.

Drug Competition

There is a limited amount of blood protein available in the blood plasma at any one time. When two protein-binding drugs are present, each will compete for the available protein. In effect, this increases the level of free-unbound drug for both drugs. For example, both aspirin and warfarin have high protein-binding capabilities. Giving an aspirin, an anticoagulant, to a patient on warfarin, another anticoagulant, may lead to an increased chance of internal bleeding as a result of the release of plasma-bound wafarin.[28–30] Drug interaction, and subsequent increases in blood serum levels of certain drugs secondary to competition, is a common source of drug toxicity. A careful medication history from the patient and cross-reference to drug tables will reveal protein-binding capacity and potential competition.

Tissue Binding

Some drugs have an attraction to, and will bind with, certain tissues. For example, lipid-soluble drugs, the kind that can pass through the blood-brain barrier, are attracted to adipose tissue (fat). Diazepam is both highly protein-bound and lipid-soluble. After an initial dose of diazepam is bound to the plasma protein, a percentage of the drug will further accumulate in the adipose tissue. The result is a depot-like effect, with a quantity of drug being stored in the fat for a prolonged period of time. If the patient is given too large a dose, or repeated doses, then the result may be a persistent drug effect beyond the desired timeframe. For example, if diazepam is given for sedation, and the patient is obese, then it may take larger doses of the drug to attain a therapeutic level, the clinical goal of sedation. However, once the patient is sedated he will tend to remain sedated for a prolonged period of time.

Bioavailability

Once the drug is free within the blood's plasma it is said to be bioavailable (i.e., capable of creating its therapeutic effect). **Bioavailability** is the difference between the amount administered and the amount that is bound and unavailable for use. For example, if an aspirin pill with 325 mg of active ingredient is swallowed, and after various factors come into play, only 150 mg is free and unbound in the blood plasma. Thus, less than 50% of the medication is bioavailable. In the case of IV medications, almost all of the drug is usually bioavailable immediately.

Volume of Distribution

After a drug is in the bloodstream (intravascular space), it will enter into the extracellular space, via diffusion and active transport, where it will come in contact with the target organ's tissues. Subsequently it will enter the organ's cells, where it will have a therapeutic effect upon the cell. While normally the drug should be equally distributed across all three compartments—the intravascular, the extracellular, and the intracellular—in drug equilibrium, often this is not the case. Factors that prevent equal distribution of drug across all three compartments include the size of the molecule, protein-binding, and the constitution of the fluid within the compartments.

The last factor, the constitution of the fluids in the tissue, has a major impact on the distribution of drugs (Figure 29-9). Some drugs have an affinity for water. These hydrophilic drugs are attracted to the large volume of water that is contained within the extracellular space. Once a drug is in the extracellular space, outside of the central circulation, it tends to persist longer. It has a longer half-life, because it is not acted upon by the liver (biotransformation) or kidneys (elimination).

Detoxification

The body has an incredible capacity to detoxify drugs using the cytochrome P-450 enzyme system. The cytochrome P-450 system simply transforms a drug—by oxidation, hydrolysis, or reduction—into a water-soluble compound which can be excreted in the urine. This process, called **biotransformation**,

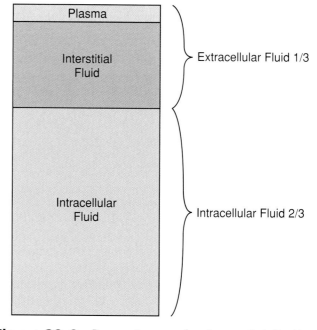

Figure 29-9 Percentages of volume distribution.

primarily occurs in the liver, though biotransformation also occurs in the lungs, intestinal lining, and the kidneys. In some instances, pharmacists have taken advantage of this process and administer inert **prodrugs** that are converted, by the liver, into their metabolically active form. For example, heroin is a prodrug that, when acted upon by the liver, metabolizes into morphine.

Rates of hepatic metabolism are affected by the health of the individual's liver. Liver cirrhosis (an obstructive disease), decreased blood flow (shock liver), and even old age all conspire to reduce the liver's ability to metabolize drugs. Outside influences can also have an impact on the liver's ability to biotransform toxins. Dyes, pesticides, CNS depressants, and xanthine derivatives, such as those found in coffee, can enhance the cytochrome P-450 system's effectiveness, and the result is reduced drug serum levels.

Prolonged exposure to certain drugs causes the liver to produce new enzymes to deactivate the drugs, resulting in a decreased blood serum level and a condition called tolerance to be created. It takes increasing doses of drug to overcome the liver's tolerance of a drug and attain a therapeutic level.

Toxicity

Every drug, in the wrong dose, has the potential to be a poison. **Toxicology**, the study of poisons, is therefore a subdiscipline of pharmacology. While some think of poisons as those drugs which, when given in a small amount, can cause death, this narrow-minded thinking precludes the possibility that an untold number of other factors could potentiate the drug's effect. This more enlightened perspective is helpful for the Paramedic who has to treat a patient for whom there is very little background information.

It is not the intention of this section to discuss toxicology in depth, but rather to bring to the Paramedic's attention that unintentional drug overdoses can be treated with the same approach as a classic overdose. Unintentional drug overdoses, and the resultant toxicity, are a common occurrence whose potential can be mitigated by the Paramedic obtaining a good history, particularly a good drug history. Also, paying careful attention to details like age, weight, sex, and so on, to arrive at a field diagnosis and then establishing a plan of treatment are important.

Elimination

The primary organ for drug excretion is the kidney. The liver's cytochrome P-450 system neutralizes toxins, including drugs, into water-soluble by-products that pass through the kidneys easily. Some drugs, particularly those with a lower molecular weight, pass through the kidney in their active form. This results in a reduced therapeutic level and the need for repeat doses of the drug.

The majority of drugs and their inactive metabolites are excreted from the kidneys by a process of passive filtration. Therefore, free-drugs, those not bound by proteins, and water-soluble drugs are excreted easily, whereas protein-bound and lipid-soluble drugs are not excreted.

Filtration, reabsorption, and eventual secretion are also greatly affected by the urine's acidity. Drugs that are weak acids, such as aspirin, are more easily excreted in a slightly alkaline urine.

While the kidneys are the primary organ of excretion, secondary organs of excretion do exist. For example, water-soluble drugs (e.g., salts) can be excreted by any exocrine gland, including sweat glands, mammary glands, and saliva glands. Certain drugs, after biotransformation in the liver, are excreted along with the bile into the intestine. These drug residuals are then passed out along with the feces. Drugs such as anesthetics and alcohol are highly volatile and literally "off-gas" into the lungs, where they are exhaled with every breath.

The sum of all drug excretion—from the kidneys, skin, lungs, and liver—is called the **total body clearance**. Hypoperfusion (shock) or diseases of the kidneys, liver, and/or lungs can markedly lower total body clearance, resulting in a potential toxic accumulation of a drug in the body.

Pharmacodynamics

Understanding how each drug specifically works upon a cell, its **mechanism of action**, helps to explain how the cell will respond, how the organ is affected, and the total systemic response. The study of how drugs come to create their therapeutic effect is called **pharmacodynamics**.

Drugs can have many effects upon a cell. A drug can cause a cell to increase or decrease its production of proteins, enzymes, and hormones or to inhibit a metabolic function. If the drug inhibits the production of a lipoprotein that is essential to cell wall production, for example, then the cell wall will be incomplete and the cell will malfunction. This tactic, called **chemotherapy**, is useful for fighting infections. If a drug cannot differentiate between foreign bacteria and normal host cells during chemotherapy, then both cells die in the process. At first this may appear to be a limitation for a drug, but even that situation can been used to a therapeutic advantage. The use of these drugs for cancer patients helps to eliminate the more rapidly dividing cancer cells while preserving a sufficient mass of host cells for survival.

While there are many different mechanisms of action, the mechanism of action for most drugs can be classified as either drug-receptor interaction, drug-enzyme interaction, or non-specific drug interaction.

Drug-Receptor Interaction

Receptor drugs have an affinity to a **receptor**, the portion of a cell which attracts a certain molecule. If activation of the receptor causes the cell to react in a specific manner, it is called a cell receptor stimulator or **agonist**. If a drug occupies the receptor but does not activate the cell or prevents other natural receptor molecules from attaching to the receptor, and the cell is therefore unable to biologically respond normally, then the drug inhibits the cell and is called an **antagonist**.

The more a drug is like a naturally occurring chemical compound within the body, the more likely that the drug will have an attraction, an **affinity**, to the receptor. In some cases (e.g., epinephrine), the affinity is extremely strong and the drug is said to be extremely **potent**.

Another influence on the drug's potency is its **efficacy**. Once a drug has interacted with a receptor, it may or may not cause the cell to react completely; in other words, it may or may not have realized its full intended therapeutic effect. The better a drug's ability to stimulate the cell to act, the better its efficacy is said to be. Often one of the goals of pharmaceutical companies is to increase a drug's efficacy.

Drug-Enzyme Interaction

Enzymes act as stimulators within the body, forcing certain chemical reactions to occur within the cell. Enzymes work by combining with a molecule, called a substrate, and acting upon the substrate. Enzyme drugs work by simulating the substrate, thereby attracting and engaging the enzyme and preventing the natural enzyme/substrate combination from working on the cell. These drugs are called **antimetabolites** because they prevent the enzymes from stimulating the cell's metabolism. Certain cancer drugs, such as methotrexate, are antimetabolites.

Enzyme drugs can also work by inhibiting the action of an enzyme directly, thereby preventing the enzyme from working. The result is that the cell continues to either produce or break down a chemical.

Nonspecific Drug Interaction

Some drugs act less specifically. For example, mineral oil physically coats the intestinal walls and blocks absorption of nutrients as well as drugs. Other nonspecific drug interactions include antacids, such as sodium bicarbonate, which mix with and neutralize stomach acids. Many of these crude drug preparations are effective because they often work at a physical level.

Biological Response

Regardless of the mechanism of action, any drug that is capable of producing the desired therapeutic effect, to affect the cell's function, is considered effective or potent. The amount of drug that it takes to be potent is called the **dose**. Dosages can vary from person to person, each according to his individual metabolism and genetic makeup.

Some individuals develop a resistance to a drug. If this happens, increasing doses of the drug are required to obtain the same therapeutic effect, a development called **tolerance**. Drug tolerance may be the result of the patient's genetic makeup, which produces a body chemistry that is less affected or unaffected by the drug. Tolerance may also occur because of the development of additional cell receptors.

The interaction between drugs can occasionally lead to unexpected or extra effects. For example, two drugs given at the same time may create a new and unexpected third effect. That third effect is called **synergism**. Synergism can be desirable. For example, when promethazine is given with meperidine, the efficacy of the combination is better than each drug when given on its own. Synergism can also be undesirable, such as when phenobarbital and diazepam are given together. The combined sedative effects can result in central nervous system depression and respiratory arrest.

When one drug increases the effectiveness of another drug, this is called **potentiation**. If the drug's effectiveness is improved, then this may be desirable. Unfortunately, the more common effect is that one drug is more potent than expected, which leads to toxicity problems.

Adverse Drug Reaction

Sometimes a drug creates an unwanted or harmful biological response. The subsequent negative impact upon the patient's health is an **adverse drug reaction**. When patients experience an adverse drug reaction, then drug administration is stopped immediately and efforts are undertaken to mitigate the negative effects of the drug.

Factors that affect if a patient will have an adverse drug reaction include extremes of age, extremes of weight, patient sex, the time of administration, the patient's physical condition, and genetic factors. Careful attention to these factors and prompt intervention can create a situation in which, instead of an intolerable adverse drug reaction, a milder side effect is experienced and the patient continues to take the medicine.

Side effects are other unwanted biological responses to a drug, which are not harmful, adverse drug effects. Whether a patient takes a medication is often a function of the patient's tolerance to these side effects. Common side effects of many drugs include nausea, dizziness, dry mouth, or diarrhea. Some side effects are short-lived. Simple interventions, such as dividing the dose or slowing the infusion, can make the side effect tolerable. For example, a common side effect of nitroglycerin, a drug given for chest pain, is dizziness and temporary postural hypotension. Therefore, to prevent this side effect, the patient should always be forewarned about dizziness and cautioned about standing quickly after using nitroglycerin.

Other side effects, usually long-term side effects, can sometimes be mitigated by use of other medications. For example, diarrhea is common with antibiotic therapy.

Therefore, the patient might be instructed to take an antidiarrheal medication.

The relationship of the patient's weight to drug dose is becoming more important in North America as the population tends toward obesity. Several factors come into play when calculating an appropriate dose of medicine for the obese patient, such as a greater volume of blood for drug distribution, altered blood flow (hemodynamics), increased adipose tissue for lipid-binding drugs, and alterations in metabolism in general. This subpopulation of patients is at great risk for receiving subtherapeutic doses of medication.[31-33]

Allergic Reaction

Allergic reactions can be the most problematic of the adverse drug reactions, with complications ranging from a contact dermatitis to anaphylactic shock and death. Formerly, terms such as "hypersensitivity," "drug allergy," and "anaphylaxis" were used to describe this adverse drug reaction. These three different syndromes (hypersensitivity, drug allergy, and anaphylaxis) have a similar mechanism. Whenever a foreign substance, such as a drug, enters the body, it can potentially stimulate the immune response and cause the creation of antibodies. These antibody generators (antigens) react with antibodies within the body to form an antigen/antibody complex. The antigen/antibody complex, in turn, causes the release of certain substances, such as histamine, which then produce the classic symptom pattern of an allergic reaction. Currently, allergic reactions are designated as types I, II, III, and IV.

Type I allergic reactions are often the most severe and can occur within minutes of exposure.[34, 35] Also called an anaphylactic reaction, a type I reaction is mediated by the IgE antibody found attached to mast cells and basophils. Drugs most accountable for type I reactions are the penicillins and other antibiotics that have a similar structure, including the cephalosporins.

Type II allergic reactions involve the IgG and IgM antibodies and lead to an autoimmune response. An autoimmune response is an unfortunate condition where the body literally attacks itself. Methyldopa, a drug used to treat hypertension, has been implicated for drug-induced hemolytic anemia, for example.

Type III allergic reactions are delayed drug reactions that are caused by the IgG antibodies in the blood. Formerly called serum sickness, the patient experiences symptoms between one and three weeks after taking the medicine. Certain antibiotics, such as sulfonamides and the anticonvulsant phenytoin, have been identified as higher risk for type III drug reactions.

A type IV allergic reaction is an inflammatory reaction secondary to T-lymphocytes and macrophages, such as a contact dermatitis from poison ivy, that may result from cross-contamination of topical ointments or crèmes.[36]

Idiosyncratic Reaction

When a drug produces an unpredictable reaction that is not allergic in nature or due to overdose and resultant toxicity, it is called an **idiosyncratic reaction**. An idiosyncratic reaction can be described as a highly unusual or abnormal reaction, within a small subpopulation of patients, to a drug that the rest of the population can normally tolerate. The basis for these rare idiosyncratic reactions is most likely based in the individual's genetic makeup. Malignant hyperthermia (e.g., an increased core body temperature caused by exposure to certain anesthetics) is thought to be a genetically linked idiosyncratic reaction.

CONCLUSION

An understanding of the basic principles of pharmacology, pharmacokinetics, and pharmacodynamics provides a foundation for the Paramedic when learning new drugs.

KEY POINTS:

- Paramedics must understand the actions of any medications that are to be administered.

- Drugs originally came from plant, animal, and mineral sources. Many are now synthetically produced or genetically engineered.

- A drug is any material which, when injected, ingested, inhaled, or absorbed into the body, is used for the diagnosis, treatment, or cure of a disease or condition.

- Every drug is assigned three names:
    - The chemical name is a description of a drug according to its elemental chemical makeup and molecular structure.
    - The generic name is the drug name listed by the manufacturer; if officially listed in the U.S. Pharmacopeia, it is followed by the initials USP.
    - The trade name is a unique one given to a drug by its manufacturer.

- Prescription drugs require a pharmacist to have a written or verbal order from a physician or mid-level provider to dispense the medication.

- Over-the-counter (OTC) medications are available to self-treat minor illness. This type of medication does not require a prescription.

- Herbal preparations are a form of OTC medications.

- The Paramedic should inquire about prescription medications as well as any herbal products and OTC medications the patient may have taken.

- Information about drugs that are recognized by the Federal Drug Administration can be found using the United States Pharmacopeia (USP) and National Formulary (NF) drug references.

- Healthcare providers use the Physician's Desk Reference (PDR) as a source of drug information in the clinical setting.

- The Pure Food and Drug Act of 1906 and later amendments worked to regulate medicine sold to the public by establishing drug standards and classifications.

- The Harrison Act of 1914 made it illegal to obtain "narcotics" without a prescription.

- The Controlled Substance Act expanded drug enforcement and placed special restrictions on potentially dangerous and addictive drugs.

- Misuse is defined as a drug not being used as prescribed.

- Drug abuse involves the intentional misuse of drugs, whether prescription or illicit.

- The ratio of effective dose for 50% of the population to lethal dose for 50% of the population is defined as the therapeutic index.

- Physicians may choose to use a drug for something other than its intended use, called off-label use.

- A drug can enhance a bodily function by either increasing or replacing a chemical in an organ or by blocking the body's own chemicals.

- Pharmacokinetics is the study of how drug absorption, distribution, detoxification, and elimination impact a drug's therapeutic value.

- Enteral drug administration involves the absorption of a drug via the GI tract by either passive or active transport.

- Parenteral drug administration does not use the GI tract. Examples include IM or SQ injections and IV administration.

- Distribution of medication is affected by blood volume, blood flow within the tissues, and permeability of the capillary walls.

- Only lipid-soluble drugs pass the blood-brain barrier.

- The placenta provides a barrier to some medications.

- Drugs bind to substances, forming plasma protein reservoirs and tissue reservoirs.

- Pharmacodynamics examines a drug's mechanism of action.

- Receptor drugs have an affinity for a receptor on a cell. A drug is called an agonist if the receptor is activated by the drug, which in turn causes the cell to react in a specific manner. An antagonist drug occupies the receptor side but does not activate the cell.

- Medication dosages are based on the amount of drug necessary for potency.

- Tolerance is the physical need for additional amounts of a drug to accomplish the same effect.

- Synergism occurs when two drugs, given at the same time, create an unexpected third effect.

- The unwanted or harmful biological response to a drug that has a negative impact upon the patient's health is an adverse drug reaction.

- An allergic reaction is an adverse drug reaction. It is caused by the body's response to a foreign substance which produces the classic symptom pattern of an allergic reaction. Hypersensitivity, drug allergy, and anaphylaxis are syndromes that each have this common response mechanism and can be designated as types I, II, III, and IV.

- An unpredictable reaction that is not allergic in nature and that is not due to overdose and resultant toxicity is called an idiosyncratic reaction.

- Biotransformation, which primarily occurs in the liver, detoxifies drugs by using enzymes to transform the drug into a water-soluble compound that can be excreted in the urine.

- Toxicology is considered a subdiscipline of pharmacology.

- Elimination of drugs is primarily carried out by the kidneys. The total body clearance is the sum of all drug excretion carried out by the kidneys, skin, lungs, and liver.

REVIEW QUESTIONS:

1. Name five sources of drugs.
2. Differentiate between prescription medications and over-the-counter medications.
3. Differentiate a drug's chemical, generic, and trade names and give an example of each.
4. Name at least three drug references.
5. Explain how drug misuse is different than drug abuse.
6. Describe the steps in the development of a new drug.
7. What is the intended biological effect of any drug?
8. What factors impact a drug's therapeutic value?
9. What is first pass metabolism? How does it affect drug development?
10. How does impaired liver function lead to high or toxic levels of protein-bound drugs?
11. Differentiate between an agonist and antagonist drug-receptor interaction.
12. What is an adverse drug reaction?
13. Differentiate between the three syndromes of an allergic reaction.

CASE STUDY QUESTIONS:

Please refer to the Case Study at the beginning of the chapter and answer the questions below:

1. Which drug laws affect the Paramedic's administration of a narcotic analgesic?
2. What does the Controlled Substance Act of 1970 require of a Paramedic:
   - At shift change?
   - When only a partial volume of a prefilled amount of narcotic is given?
   - During documentation?
3. Which drug effect is illustrated by giving Katie a pain medication along with a drug to control nausea?

REFERENCES:

1. Centers for Disease Control and Prevention. Life expectancy data: United States. Available at: **http://www.cdc.gov/nchs/fastats/lifexpec.htm.** Accessed at May 27, 2009.
2. Goldberg H. *Hippocrates: Father of Medicine*. New York: Authors Choice Press; 2006.
3. Hippocrates, Francis Adams, Translator. *The Genuine Works of Hippocrates*. New York: Kessinger Publishing, LLC; 2007.
4. Logan, Clendening C. *Source Book of Medical History*. New York: Hoeber; 1942.
5. Porter R. *Greatest Benefit to Mankind: A Medical History of Humanity*. London: HarperCollins; 1997.
6. Berndt L.*William Withering. Journal of Interventional Cardiology*. Netherlands: Springer; 2005.
7. Asimov I. *Human Brain: Its Capacities and Functions*. New York: Mentor Book; 1965.
8. Phillips KA, et al. Potential role of pharmacogenomics in reducing drug reactions: a systematic review. *JAMA*. 2001;286(18):270–279.
9. Rodman M, Smith D. *Pharmacology and Drug Therapy in Nursing* (2nd ed.). Philadelphia: Lippincott; 1979:17.
10. United States Pharmacopeial. *United States Pharmacopeia: National Formulary 2005 (United States Pharmacopeia/National Formulary)*. Washington, DC. United States Pharmacopeial; 2004.
11. Salerno E. *Pharmacology for Health Professionals*. St. Louis, MO: Mosby; 1999.
12. Somogyi AA, Barratt DT, Coller JK. Pharmacogenetics of opioids. *Clin Pharmacol Ther*. 2007;81(3):429–444.
13. Inciardi J, ed. *Handbook of Drug Control in the United States*. New York: Greenwood Press; 1990.
14. Forrest G. *Chemical Dependency and Antisocial Personality Disorder: Psychotherapy and Assessment Strategies*. New York: Haworth Press; 1994.
15. Krantz JC, Jr. New drugs and the Kefauver-Harris amendment. *J New Drugs*. 1966;6(2):77–79.
16. Barron BA, Bukantz SC. The evaluation of new drugs. Current Food and Drug Administration regulations and statistical aspects of clinical trials. *Arch Intern Med*. 1967;119(6):547–556.
17. Welling, P, ed. *Drug Development Process: Increasing Efficiency & Cost Effectiveness (Drugs and the Pharmaceutical Sciences)*. Stockholm: Informa Healthcare; 1996.
18. White GG, Love L. The MedWatch program. *J Toxicol Clin Toxicol*. 1998;36(6):645–648.
19. Meadows M. MedWatch: managing risks at the FDA. *FDA Consum*. 2003;37(5):10–11.
20. Kaldjian LC, Jones EW, Wu BJ, Forman-Hoffman VL, Levi BH, Rosenthal GE. Disclosing medical errors to patients: attitudes and practices of physicians and trainees. *J Gen Intern Med*. 2007;22(7):988–996.
21. Kaldjian LC, Jones EW, Wu BJ, Forman-Hoffman VL, Levi BH, Rosenthal GE. Reporting medical errors to improve patient safety: a survey of physicians in teaching hospitals. *Arch Intern Med*. 2008;168(1):40–46.
22. Hicks RW, Becker SC. An overview of intravenous-related medication administration errors as reported to MEDMARX, a national medication error-reporting program. *J Infus Nurs*. 2006;29(1):20–27.
23. Savage SW, Schneider PJ, Pedersen CA. Utility of an online medication-error-reporting system. *Am J Health Syst Pharm*. 2005;62(21):2265–2270.
24. Jacquot C. Bioavailability and "first pass" effect of a drug. *Therapie*. 1978;33(6):683–697.
25. Pond SM, Tozer TN. First-pass elimination. Basic concepts and clinical consequences. *Clin Pharmacokinet*. 1984;9(1):1–25.
26. Lalka D, Griffith RK, Cronenberger CL. The hepatic first-pass metabolism of problematic drugs. *J Clin Pharmacol*. 1993;33(7):657–669.
27. Kwan KC. Oral bioavailability and first-pass effects. *Drug Metab Dispos*. 1997;25(12):1329–1336.

28. Andreotti F, Testa L, Biondi-Zoccai GG, Crea F. Aspirin plus warfarin compared to aspirin alone after acute coronary syndromes: an updated and comprehensive meta-analysis of 25,307 patients. *Eur Heart J.* 2006;27(5):519–526.

29. Larson RJ, Fisher ES. Should aspirin be continued in patients started on warfarin? *J Gen Intern Med.* 2004;19(8):879–886.

30. Jeddy AS, Gleason BL. Aspirin and warfarin versus aspirin monotherapy after myocardial infarction. *Ann Pharmacother.* 2003;37(10):1502–1505.

31. Nieman CT, Manacci CF, Super DM, Mancuso C, Fallon WF, Jr. Use of the Broselow tape may result in the underresuscitation of children. *Acad Emerg Med.* 2006;13(10):1011–1019.

32. Lee JB, Winstead PS, Cook AM. Pharmacokinetic alterations in obesity. *Orthopedics.* 2006;29(11):984–988.

33. Erstad BL. Dosing of medications in morbidly obese patients in the intensive care unit setting. *Intensive Care Med.* 2004;30(1):18–32.

34. Untersmayr E, Jensen-Jarolim E. Mechanisms of type I food allergy. *Pharmacol Ther.* 2006;112(3):787–798.

35. Romano A, Demoly P. Recent advances in the diagnosis of drug allergy. *Curr Opin Allergy Clin Immunol.* 2007;7(4):299–303.

36. Brunton L, Lazo J, Parker K. *Goodman & Gilman's the Pharmacological Basis of Therapeutics.* New York: McGraw-Hill Professional; 2005.

PHARMACOLOGICAL INTERVENTIONS FOR CARDIOPULMONARY EMERGENCIES

KEY CONCEPTS:

Upon completion of this chapter, it is expected that the reader will understand these following concepts:

- Maintenance of cardiac rate, rhythm, and pumping ability as support for the brain
- Autonomic nervous system control
- Mechanisms of action of drugs affecting the heart, lungs, and kidneys

▶ CASE STUDY:

Mrs. Fein called 9-1-1 because she felt faint and very fatigued. One Paramedic interviewed Mrs. Fein while her partner scanned the medication bottles. "Do you take all of these medications?" one Paramedic asked. Mrs. Fein answered, "Oh yes. I always do what my doctors tell me to do. I am so glad that I have so many fine doctors to take care of me."

There were multiple antihypertensives, antidysrhythmics, and diuretics. At least four different pharmacies had filled the prescriptions. "I see that you go to several pharmacies to have your prescriptions filled," said the Paramedic. Mrs. Fein replied, "Well, each of my daughters likes a different pharmacy and they often pick up my prescriptions for me."

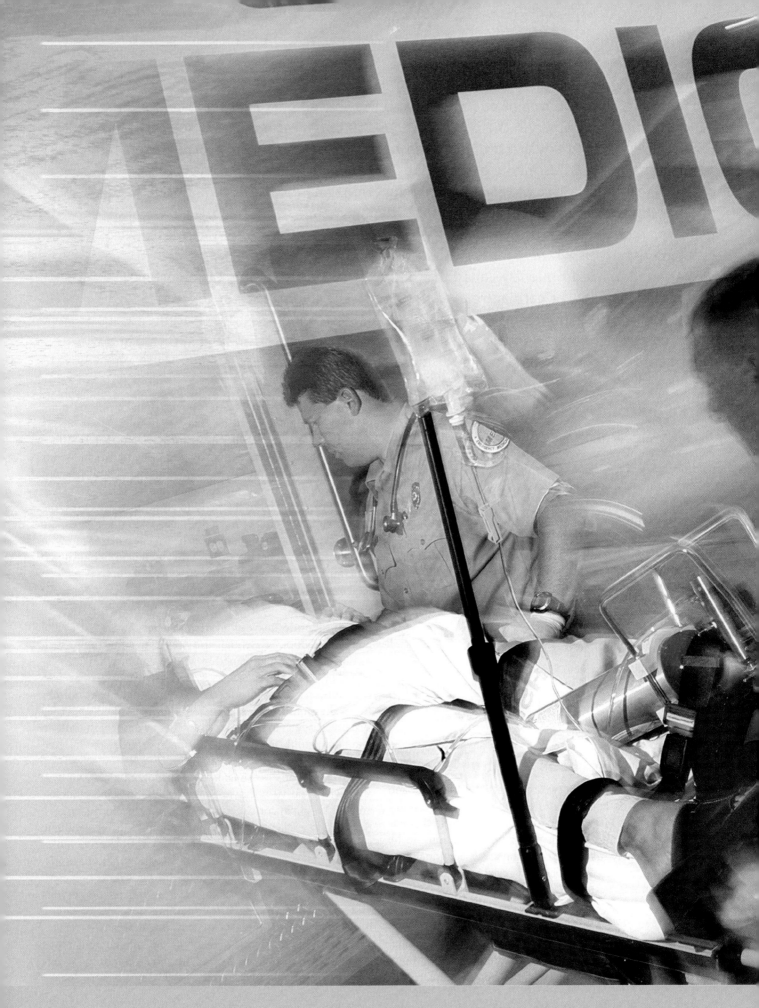

OVERVIEW

The brain, as the source of one's being and the seat of one's consciousness, is the most important organ in the body. Perhaps the two most important support systems for the brain in the body are the heart and lungs. These two organs, through constant adjustment and readjustment, ensure that the brain gets sufficient oxygen and perfusion of glucose-rich blood in order to function. Any disequilibrium between the heart and lungs results in cerebral hypoxia, hypoglycemia, or hypoperfusion. Persistent hypoxia, hypoglycemia, or hypoperfusion can lead to an alteration in mental status, loss of consciousness, and eventually death.

Paramedics are frequently called to treat a patient with loss of consciousness, shortness of breath, or cardiac-related problems. The importance of these two interconnected organ systems to the patient's health cannot be understated. Paramedics must have an intimate understanding of the heart and lung systems and the treatments which they can provide to support them.

The Nervous System

The brain controls these two vital organ systems through the autonomic nervous system. Therefore, cardiopulmonary pharmacology is focused on affecting the autonomic nervous system. To understand the effects of cardiopulmonary pharmacology, the Paramedic must have an expansive knowledge of the autonomic nervous system.

In about 200 A.D., Galen, the father of medicine, identified something "non-tendon" in the muscle. He had identified a nerve.[1] Later, anatomists would note that stimulation of these nerves caused muscle movement and they sought to discover what other functions nerves provided.

In the mid-1900s, Dr. William Cullen advanced the idea that the nervous system was responsible for maintaining the physiological balance of all organs within the body. He was correct. The nervous system is responsible for the regulation of body functions. Through an intricate system of wire-like fibers, called neurons, which are present throughout the body, messages are sent which stimulate the cells within the organs to respond.

The Central Nervous System

The central nervous system, which consists of the brain and the spinal cord, is analogous to the command and control center of an army. Information, or intelligence, from the outside world flows through the spinal cord to the brain to be processed. In many instances, the brain sends a command (a signal) to the organs to respond in a certain manner, via the peripheral nervous system.

The Peripheral Nervous System

The peripheral nervous system consists of the 12 cranial nerves and the 31 spinal nerves that extend from the brain and spinal cord to the organs of the body.[2] Similar to a two-lane highway, information flows to and from the brain along the peripheral nervous system. The afferent division is the portion of the peripheral nervous system that is stimulated by the environment (e.g., by heat or by touch) and sends a signal to the central nervous system. The central nervous system, in turn, interprets the data and sends a signal via efferent nerve fibers to the body to react. In some cases, the act is voluntary (e.g., to pat a dog's head). In other cases, the act is involuntary (e.g., a quicker heartbeat when faced with the threat of a menacing bear). This involuntary control is a function of the autonomic nervous system.

Autonomic Nervous System

The **autonomic nervous system** can be thought of as the body's autopilot.[3] Essential, life-preserving functions, such as digestion, are maintained by the autonomic nervous system. The autonomic nervous system is further divided into two divisions: the **sympathetic** division and the **parasympathetic** division. These two divisions of the autonomic nervous system compete, to some degree, with one another in order to maintain equilibrium while adjusting to external and internal stress.

The sympathetic division of the autonomic nervous system, whose nerve fibers originate in the thoracic or lumbar area of the spinal cord, serves to accelerate the body's organs. Referred to as the "fight or flight" response, the sympathetic nervous system increases heart rate, dilates the bronchioles to allow more air movement, and constricts blood vessels, causing the shunting of blood to the vital core organs.[4-7] Because of its "crisis" orientation, the sympathetic nervous system tends to create an "all or nothing" response, meaning it simultaneously stimulates all of its target organs.

The parasympathetic division of the autonomic nervous system, whose nerve fibers originate and extend from the cervical or sacral area of the spinal cord, is responsible for the more vegetative functions. Referred to as the "feed or breed" portion of the nervous system, the parasympathetic nervous system increases gastric motility as well as stimulates erections in men.

The **vagus nerve** (from the Latin word meaning "wandering") is the major parasympathetic nerve. The vagus nerve originates in the medulla, exits the skull at the base of the brain, travels down the neck (proximal to the larynx), branches into the heart and lungs, innervates the stomach, passes through the digestive tract, and ends in the anus.

Most organs have dual innervations, both sympathetic and parasympathetic. However, the parasympathetic nervous system usually dominates. For example, the upper portion of the heart, the atrium, has both sympathetic and parasympathetic nerve fibers. Yet the parasympathetic nerve, the vagus nerve, dominates, creating a "vagal tone."

Certain select organs only have sympathetic innervation. For example, the adrenal medulla (which excretes the hormone adrenaline), the kidney, and the lower portion of the heart (ventricles) are innervated by sympathetic nerve fibers only.

Neurotransmitters

The autonomic nervous system transmits its signal to the target organ (the effector organ), causing the organ to act in response to the signal. The transmission of the signal from the nerve to the organ is by means of a messenger called a **neurotransmitter**. There are many neurotransmitters in the central nervous system.

The chief neurotransmitter for the sympathetic nervous system is **norepinephrine**, which is chemically similar to the hormone adrenaline. Because of its utilization of an adrenaline-like chemical, these nerves are also called **adrenergic** nerves.

The chief neurotransmitter for the parasympathetic nervous system is **acetylcholine**. Because of its use of acetylcholine, these nerves are also called **cholinergic** nerves. These terms—"adrenergic" and "cholinergic"—are important to understanding some descriptions of drug effects.

For each neurotransmitter, there is a corresponding **neuroreceptor** that receives the neurotransmitter, chemically connecting with it in a key and lock-like fashion. The linkage of neurotransmitter to cell receptor can cause a cell to change the conductivity of an ion channel in the cell wall, thus making it more or less responsive to a stimulus.

For example, norepinephrine can cause the cell to open its potassium channels, which in turn causes a cascade of events, called depolarization.[8–10] This collectively causes the heart to contract quicker and stronger.

Alternatively, the neurotransmitter can stimulate a protein to perform a certain intracellular function. **Serotonin**, a neurotransmitter found primarily in the gastrointestinal tract, is also present in platelets and within the brain. Serotonin, released by damaged platelets, causes arterial and venous constriction; this is thought to be one of the causes of migraine headaches.[11–14] Serotonin within the brain is primarily located in the hypothalamus, where it affects sleep, temperature, pain perception, and mood. Its impact on mood is an important feature which many anti-depressant medications depend on for their effectiveness (see MAO inhibitors and selective serotonin re-uptake inhibitors).

Neurotransmission

The process of neurotransmission is a cycle (Figure 30-1). Understanding this is the key to understanding the drugs which can affect the autonomic nervous system. The phases in the cycle are preparation for action, feedback, and preparation for another action. The speed or strength of a cycle can be increased or decreased by a drug's influence during that cycle.

To review, the nerve ending makes and stores neurotransmitter in pockets called "vesicles" in the terminal end of the neuron. With stimulation, the neurotransmitter is released into the space between the nerve and the target cell, called the synapse. In the synapse, the neurotransmitter floats over to the cell and attaches to a receptor. Once the cell is stimulated to act, the neurotransmitter is released. It is either reabsorbed by the nerve, called **re-uptake**, after which it is stored in a vesicle; or it is broken down by enzymes and excreted. If the process of enzymatic degradation or re-uptake and absorption did not occur, the cell receptors would be continuously stimulated (hyperexcited) or exhausted (desensitized).

The effects of drugs on the autonomic nervous system can be one of two impacts. The drug either increases the neurotransmitter's ability to stimulate the cell's receptors (**agonist** effect) or it blocks the cell's ability to be stimulated (**antagonist** effect).

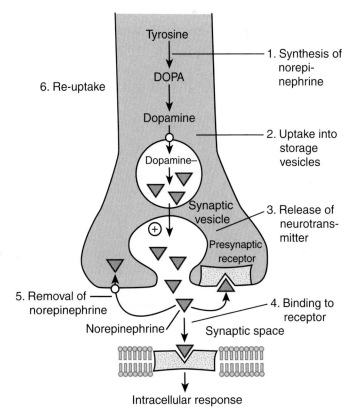

Figure 30-1 The cycle of neurotransmission.

Agonist drugs work by either increasing the amount of neurotransmitter (a direct effect) or decreasing the amount of re-uptake or enzymatic degradation, thereby indirectly increasing the amount of neurotransmitter. In both cases, these drugs would be considered an agonist.

Alternatively, a drug can act to block the neurotransmitter, and thus act as an antagonist. Drugs in this class work by either decreasing the amount of neurotransmitter, increasing enzymatic destruction of the neurotransmitter, or by competing with the neurotransmitter for the receptor, called competitive inhibition.

Cholinergic Receptors

Acetylcholine attaches to cholinergic receptors within the parasympathetic nervous system. These cholinergic receptors can be further divided into muscarinic and nicotinic receptors.

Originally, the **muscarinic** receptors were identified for their affinity for muscarine, a poison found in mushrooms. Five different muscarinic receptors (M1-M2-M3-M4-M5) have been subsequently identified.[15,16] For example, M2 receptors have been found in the cell wall of cardiac muscles.

Nicotinic receptors, the other cholinergic receptor, are located in the adrenal medulla, the central nervous system, and at many neuromuscular junctions, such as the muscles within the bronchioles. Similar to muscarinic receptors, nicotinic receptors were identified for their affinity to nicotine. Blockage of the nicotinic receptors, an antagonist effect of drugs like pancuronium, results in smooth muscle paralysis, diaphragmatic paralysis, and respiratory arrest.

The main neurotransmitter that connects with either a muscarinic or nicotinic receptor is acetylcholine. Any chemical that mimics the action of acetylcholine (e.g., nicotine) is said to be a **parasympathomimetic** agent. Poison mushrooms often contain muscarinic-like chemicals that are cholinomimetic.[17,18]

Cholinergic Agents

The action of acetylcholine on the heart is to slow its rate through direct stimulation of the vagus nerve. Any drug which has a similar action, that mimics the effects of acetylcholine, would be called a cholinergic drug. Drugs of this sort usually have a subcomponent of acetylcholine, such as an ester or alkaloid-like molecule of acetylcholine, which binds directly to the cholinergic receptor. Pilocarpine is a drug in this classification.

Using an alternative mechanism to increase the amount of naturally occurring acetylcholine available, some drugs bind with the enzyme that breaks down the acetylcholine (acetylcholinesterase), thus rendering the enzyme inert. As a result, less acetylcholine is broken down and there is more acetylcholine available in the synaptic junction. An example of a drug that uses this mechanism is physostigmine, a drug used to treat open-angle glaucoma. Papillary constriction (miosis) is controlled by the parasympathetic nervous system. Physostigmine is also used to treat overdoses of atropine (whose action is discussed later) and tricyclic

antidepressants; albeit rarely. Physostigmine is an example of a parasympathomimetic, a drug that mimics the action of the parasympathetic neurotransmitter acetylcholine.

Another anticholinesterase drug with parasympathomimetic properties is neostigmine bromide. Neostigmine is used to help reverse the effects of certain neuromuscular blocking agents, called paralytics, which are used during emergencies to facilitate intubation.[19]

Anticholinergic Agents

Cholinergic blockers, those drugs that block acetylcholine from binding to either muscarinic or nicotinic receptors, are called **anticholinergics**. Drugs in this classification would stop parasympathetic activity.

Antimuscarinic drugs inhibit parasympathetic activity at the muscarinic receptors. Their greatest impact is on the core organs, such as the eyes, the gut, and the heart, because peripheral skeletal muscle primarily has nicotinic receptors.

An example of a muscarinic blocker is atropine sulfate. Atropine sulfate is a plant alkaloid derived from the deadly nightshade plant (latin—*atropa belladonna*).[19] Its fruit, a small black cherry, is poisonous. It was used, in small quantities, by Ladies of the Court in medieval Italy to add "brilliance" (pupil dilation) to their eyes; hence the name "bella donna" or beautiful lady. The name "atropine" comes from the Greek *atropos*, one of the Fates who held the shears to cut the thread of life. This reference is interesting in light of the fact that atropine is used to treat life-threatening bradycardia. Atropine's effect is to block the vagus nerve (parasympathetic nerve) in the heart and reduce the vagal tone that slows the heart, causing the heart rate to rise.[20]

Because it is a parasympathetic blocker, atropine also decreases saliva production in the mouth, leaving the mouth dry (xerostomia). This effect is desirable prior to intubation. Atropine is also used as a pretreatment to prevent bradycardia induced by vagal stimulation of the hypopharynx, which is occasionally seen during pediatric intubation.

Atropine has received more interest lately as an antidote for certain nerve agents used as weapons of mass destruction. These nerve agents are structurally similar to the organophosphate fertilizers. This treatment works by blocking parasympathetic receptors. Atropine is now available in auto-injectors for deep IM injection during an exposure to these deadly nerve gasses.[21–24]

The alternate anticholinergic is the nicotinic blocker. Nicotinic blockers have been used for decades in the operating room as a muscle relaxer. The earliest nicotinic blocker, curare, owes its origin to tribesmen in the equatorial Amazon. These tribesmen would easily bring down large animals, without killing them, by arrows that were dipped in curare. The animal was seemingly paralyzed and died from suffocation while still awake. In the 1850s, Claude Bernard showed that the South American Indian drug curare worked primarily at the neuromuscular junction and that a substance, later identified as acetylcholine, was blocked from receptors on the muscle cell. The idea that cells had receptors which could be affected by drugs had wide ranging implications for pharmaceutical research.[20]

Curare was a crude cholinergic blocker that was specific to the nicotinic receptors found in skeletal muscle. By blocking acetylcholine from attaching to nicotinic receptors on skeletal muscle, the muscles were, in effect, paralyzed. The advantages of a drug which could paralyze are numerous. For example, a paralyzed patient is easier to intubate and mechanically ventilate.[25-27] Used together with sedatives and analgesics, these drugs have created an ideal intubation condition. Paralytics, as a class, do not cross the blood-brain barrier easily. Therefore, while the patient is paralyzed, he remains completely awake and sentient (sensing surroundings) and can experience feelings of pain. It is standard practice to co-administer a sedative and/or pain medication (analgesic) along with the paralytic agent to decrease the patient's anxiety and relieve discomfort while paralyzed.

Some paralytics, particularly the early nondepolarizing agents, release histamine, a vasodilator, from the mast cells in the blood. Therefore, the patient's blood pressure would fall. The next generation of paralytics (e.g., pancuronium) does not release histamine and therefore is more useful when treating patients at risk for hypotension, such as the trauma patient.

Depolarizing and Non-Depolarizing Neuromuscular Blockers

Neuromuscular blockers can be classified as either depolarizing or non-depolarizing. Depolarizing agents attach to the nicotinic receptor at the neuromuscular junction. In the resting state, the cell has charged sodium ions on the outside and potassium ions on the inside of the cell. This results in a difference in the electrical potential between the outside of the cell and the inside. This difference is called the **resting membrane potential**. With the nicotinic receptor stimulated by the drug, the cell opens the sodium channels in the cell wall and a rapid influx of sodium occurs. This results in depolarization and subsequently causes a cascade of events which then cause muscular contraction. These transient fine muscle contractions, seen after administration of a depolarizing neuromuscular blocker, are called **fasciculations**.

The depolarizing paralytic agent, however, remains bound to the receptor, unable to be broken down easily by the normal enzymes. This persistent action of depolarizing agents prevents the repolarization of the cell and a return of the cell to its normal resting state. Instead, the cell and the muscle remain flaccid (unable to be stimulated) and paralyzed.

As an alternative, non-depolarizing paralytic agents also bind with the nicotinic receptor but do not have the same effect on the cell. These agents simply bind to a receptor without causing depolarization. With the receptor site occupied, the cell remains in a ready resting state. However, the cell is unable to be stimulated because the receptor is blocked. This prevents the unwanted muscular fasciculations seen with depolarizing agents.

Adrenergic Neurotransmitters

Adrenergic neurotransmitters function in a manner similar to cholinergic neurotransmitters except that they act on the sympathetic nervous system. In the sympathetic nervous system norepinephrine, not acetylcholine, is the primary neurotransmitter.

Similar to the process in the parasympathetic nervous system, the sympathetic (adrenergic) nerve produces norepinephrine. To produce norepinephrine, the neuron takes the amino acid tyrosine and synthesizes it into dopamine, which is in turn converted into norepinephrine in the vesicles.

Norepinephrine is released from the vesicle, by an influx of calcium that occurs with neuronal stimulation, and floods the synapse between the nerve and the target cell. Attracted to adrenergic receptors on the cell wall membrane, the norepinephrine binds with the cell receptor and activates the enzyme adenyl cyclase, in a second messenger system, to convert adenosine triphosphate (ATP) into cyclic adenosine monophosphate (cAMP), releasing two phosphate molecules in the process. The two liberated phosphates are an energy-rich substrate which is used by many proteins within the cell to power metabolic processes (Figure 30-2).

After having caused the intended effect, the norepinephrine is released from the receptor and may either diffuse into the general circulation or be taken up again by the adrenergic neuron.

The norepinephrine, assisted by an ATPase (enzyme), re-enters the neuron where it can either be stored in a vesicle or broken down by monoamine oxidase (enzyme) into inactive by-products (metabolites).

Adrenergic Drugs

It is important for the Paramedic to understand the sympathetic response because many drugs owe their therapeutic effect to the impact of these adrenergic drugs in the process of neurotransmission. For example, cocaine prevents the uptake of norepinephrine, thereby causing a buildup of norepinephrine in the synapse, and hyperstimulation of the cell.[28,29]

Norepinephrine is an important neurotransmitter in the central nervous system (CNS). Inhibition of uptake of norepinephrine by tricyclic antidepressants, or the blockade of monoamine oxidase (MAO) breakdown of norepinephrine by MAO inhibitors, can improve clinical depression, for example.[30]

There are two adrenergic receptors in the sympathetic nervous system: the alpha-receptors and the beta-receptors. These adrenergic receptors are further divided into alpha$_1$ or alpha$_2$ according to the organs on which they predominate (Figure 30-3). For example, beta$_1$ receptors are found on cardiac muscle cells whereas beta$_2$ receptors are found on arterial smooth muscle and bronchial smooth muscle.[31-33]

Adrenergic Agents

Several drugs have been created which mimic the effects of the sympathetic neurotransmitter norepinephrine. These drugs are called **sympathomimetics**. Sympathomimetics (often either prodrugs or analogs of norepinephrine) share a

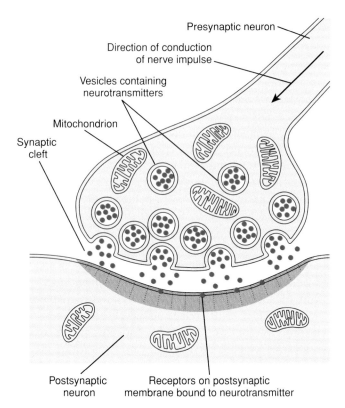

Figure 30-2 Neurotransmission.

common base molecule, a catechol ring. Thus, they share a drug classification, and are called **catecholamines**.

All catecholamines are very potent adrenergic agonists because they can cause a direct response from the adrenergic receptor. In fact, most catecholamines, such as dopamine and epinephrine, have naturally occurring counterparts in the body. Because of this, the body also has a means of breaking down the drug more rapidly; in this case, with the enzymes monoamine oxidase (MAO) and another enzyme called catechol-O-methyltransferase (COMT). In order to maintain a therapeutic effect, these drugs are continuously infused intravenously. The infusion is then slowed, a process called weaning, to the point where the body is able to sustain itself and is no longer dependent on the infusion to maintain vital functions such as blood pressure.

Realizing the limitations of catecholamines, newer non-catecholamine compounds have been created (i.e., those without catechol ring). Without the ring, the enzymes COMT and MAO have more difficulty neutralizing the drug into an inactive metabolite. Therefore, these drugs enjoy a longer duration of action. Ephedrine, a common ingredient in decongestants, is an example.

Adrenergic agonists may work by direct action or by indirect action. Direct acting adrenergic agonists couple with and excite the adrenergic receptors. The indirect agonists cause the release of norepinephrine from the terminal neuron, which in turn causes the norepinephrine to attach to the adrenergic receptors and the receptors to react.

The five direct-acting adrenergic agonists—norepinephrine, epinephrine, dopamine, dobutamine, and isoproterenol—all have similar effects on the cardiovascular system.[34] These drugs elevate blood pressure and thus are also called **vasopressors**. However, each drug has an action that is slightly different from the others, thus making one more desirable than another for different circumstances.

The indirect adrenergic agonists are stimulants that cause the release of norepinephrine. An example of an indirect adrenergic agonist is the class of drugs called amphetamines.

Systemic Pharmacologic Effect

Owing to the widespread distribution of adrenergic receptors in the major core organs, and the often dramatic effect these sympathomimetic drugs can have upon the sympathetic nervous system, a review of systems will be discussed.

The heart may be the organ system most affected by adrenergic agonists. These powerful medicines can markedly increase the heart's strength of contraction (positive inotropic effect) as well as rate (positive chronotropic effect) as a result of increased calcium influx in the myocardium. The calcium influx causes a higher action potential and quicker depolarizations. Left alone, stronger, faster contractions lead to more complete ventricular emptying and an increased cardiac output.

Catecholamines, such as epinephrine, can be potent cardiac stimulators. This is the anticipated action of epinephrine during a cardiac arrest. Epinephrine should either (1) increase the fibrillatory action of the arrested heart, coarsening the ventricular fibrillation, so that subsequent defibrillations are more likely to be successful, or (2) induce spontaneous pacemaker activity in the heart in cardiac standstill (asystole).

Conversely, catecholamines like epinephrine, when inappropriately administered, can induce spontaneous depolarizations and extra-systoles by the same mechanisms. These actions can disrupt a normal cardiac sequence and send the heart into chaos and ventricular fibrillation.

The peripheral capillary beds are largely controlled by alpha$_1$ receptors of the sympathetic nervous system as well.[35,36] During times of stress, when blood is needed in the core organs, these capillary beds can be preferentially shut down. Blood will then be directed toward the body core in a process called shunting. This shutdown of capillary beds also causes a higher total peripheral vascular resistance (PVR) to forward blood flow.

In certain abnormal perfusion states, such as anaphylactic shock or septic shock, peripheral vascular resistance is reduced. Then catecholamines, such as dopamine or norepinephrine, can help to restore a higher PVR.

Administration of catecholamines, such as dopamine, can result in a higher PVR through alpha$_1$ receptor stimulation. While dopamine is a very useful drug when used appropriately, a high PVR presents an obstacle to forward blood flow from the heart (i.e., cardiac output). This effect can create such a large demand on the heart's muscle that it cannot keep up with demand and the patient may manifest symptoms such as chest pain (angina) and possibly sustain a myocardial infarction.

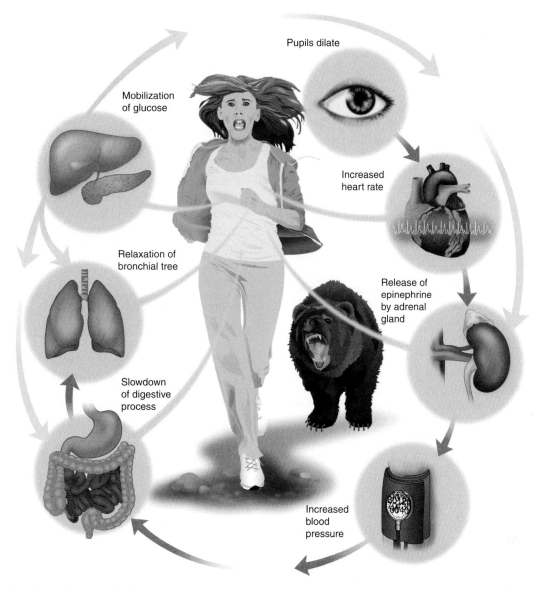

Pupils dilate

Mobilization
of glucose

Increased
heart rate

Relaxation of
bronchial tree

Release of
epinephrine
by adrenal
gland

Slowdown
of digestive
process

Increased
blood
pressure

Figure 30-3 The effects of adrenergic receptor stimulation.

The differences between the effects produced by each of the catecholamines, and even the differences between the effects of a single catecholamine at different doses, requires careful monitoring of the patient for untoward effects.

The smooth muscles of the bronchi and the bronchioles are also richly supplied with beta$_2$ receptors and are easily affected by catecholamines. When activated, these receptors cause dilation of medium-sized airways. This positive effect is so pronounced that these agents have become a mainstay in the treatment of bronchoconstriction and are discussed in more detail in the section on drugs that affect the respiratory system.

One of the notable effects of catecholamines on the endocrine system is the increase in the amount of blood glucose available to be used as energy. This is achieved through a combination of decreased insulin secretion from the pancreas and increased breakdown of glucagon in the liver and muscles. The intended effect of the elevated blood glucose

STREET SMART

Topically applied, epinephrine and epinephrine derivatives such as phenylephrine can create a localized vasoconstriction in exposed capillary beds in the mucosa. A solution sprayed into the nasal mucosa of the nostril prior to intubation can reduce the likelihood of bleeding during a nasal intubation.[37,38] The key to successful use of these agents is to apply them before other lubricating substances and in time for the medication to take the desired effect. Upon quick visualization, the mucosa should appear pale after vasoconstriction has occurred.

Alpha-Adrenergic Blockers

Most **alpha-adrenergic blockers** are competitive blockers, occupying the adrenergic receptor and preventing the catecholamine drug from attaching to the adrenergic receptor. Alpha-adrenergic blockers can be divided into either long-acting and short-acting or competitive and noncompetitive. Noncompetitive antagonists are longer acting and generally used for special conditions. For example, a pheochromocytoma, a tumor of the medulla of the adrenal gland, can induce life-threatening hypertensive crisis through secretion of high doses of epinephrine. The use of longer-acting alpha antagonists, such as phenoxybenzamine, can reduce dangerously high blood pressures.

Longer-acting alpha antagonists are also used to relieve the symptoms of benign prostate hypertrophy (BPH). BPH is a common consequence of aging for men. Alpha-adrenergic blockers relax the bladder muscles, allowing for a greater passage of urine. A patient who is under treatment for BPH with a long-acting alpha antagonist, who subsequently needs hemodynamic support from a catecholamine infusion, such as dopamine, will not respond as briskly secondary to competition from the alpha-adrenergic blocker.

Competitive short-acting alpha antagonists, such as phentolamine, are more commonly used to treat acute hypertensive crisis, especially hypertension secondary to a pheochromocytoma. Its emergency application can also prevent acute hypertension and stroke secondary to an overinfusion of a catecholamine, such as a "runaway" dopamine infusion.

Cerebral vasoconstriction is thought to be one of the causes of migraine headaches. Logically, an alpha blocker would prevent or reverse any vasoconstriction created by the sympathetic nervous system. Ergot is an alpha-adrenergic blocker used to treat both dementia and migraine headaches. A plant alkaloid, ergot is extracted from a fungus which grows on rye. Another extract of note from this extraction is lysergic acid diethylamide (LSD).

Ergot compounds are thought to depress the central nervous system's vasomotor centers and thus inhibit the pulsations, described as pounding by the patient, characteristic of a migraine.[39,40] Ergot compounds do not treat migraines, they only prevent them from occurring and thus must be taken early during the aura phase in the attack in order to be effective.

Beta-Adrenergic Blockers

Beta-adrenergic blockers, more commonly called **beta-blockers**, can be divided into two classes: selective and nonselective. Nonselective beta-blockers inhibit both beta$_1$ and beta$_2$ receptors by direct competition with norepinephrine for available receptors. This mixed effect can be problematic depending on the desired therapeutic outcome.

Beta-selective drugs specifically target either the heart, and are referred to as **cardioselective**, or target the lungs (beta$_2$ selective agents). Cardioselective drugs, such as atenolol, only affect the heart, which predominantly has beta$_1$ receptors, and prevent catecholamine-stimulated tachycardia. This effect can have a significant impact on mortality and infarction size during acute coronary syndrome.

Beta-blockers, particularly nonselective beta-blockers, are used to treat hypertension. These beta-blockers, such as propranolol, prevent peripheral vasoconstriction and subsequent increased peripheral vascular resistance with the overall result of a lower blood pressure.

Caution should be advised any time a beta-blocker is given to a diabetic patient. Beta-blockers can mask many of the classic signs of hypoglycemia. Concerns about hypoglycemia, secondary to history or physical, should be followed up with a blood glucose measurement.

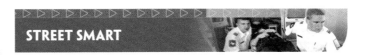

STREET SMART

Sudden withdrawal of a beta-blocker may result in symptoms of an acute coronary syndrome, including chest pain (angina), rebound hypertension, tachycardia, and bronchospasm. Patients on beta-blockers should be weaned off the medicine slowly to prevent these symptoms. Prehospital treatment may include re-instituting the beta-blocker intravenously until the patient stabilizes. Only a complete drug history would reveal that the patient's symptoms are the result of suddenly not taking his beta-blocker.

Pharmacological Interventions during a Respiratory Emergency

The pulmonary system, starting at the pharynx and ending in the capillary beds surrounding the alveoli, through mechanical ventilation and pulmonary respiration, is responsible for oxygenation, removal of wastes (including carbon dioxide), and the regulation of acid–base balance. When any one of these functions is disrupted, illness and even death can ensue. Airflow into the lungs is partially controlled by the diameter of the airway passages, the absence of obstructions, and proper air pressure gradients. Of these, the diameter of the airway may be most important. The airways within the tracheobronchial tree are surrounded by smooth muscle arranged in a double helix, like a Chinese finger-trap, which expands and contracts. This increases or decreases the airway's lumen.

All muscles within the body are controlled by the nervous system, and the muscles in the airway are no exception.

Parasympathetic nerves (from the vagus nerve) narrow the airway's lumen, called **bronchoconstriction**, while the sympathetic nerves widen the airway, called **bronchodilation**.

Overview of Pulmonary Pathophysiology

The majority of pulmonary diseases can be linked to what is referred to as the "three S's": spasm, swelling, and secretions. Bronchospasm, as manifested in the wheezing of an asthmatic patient, is a narrowing of the airway or bronchoconstriction.[41] This bronchoconstriction is the result of stimulation of the muscarinic receptors of the parasympathetic nervous system.

Any irritant, such as pollen and aerosolized medications, can stimulate this protective airway reflex. The muscarinic receptors, in turn, stimulate the production of cyclic GMP, which causes the muscle contraction and subsequent bronchoconstriction. Cyclic GMP can also cause the release of chemical mediators from mast cells, such as histamine and leukotrienes.

One common bronchospastic respiratory illness treated by Paramedics is **asthma**. Asthma is a potentially reversible airway spasm that is triggered by a stimulus. The stimulus can either be an internal or **intrinsic trigger**, such as stress or exercise, or it can be an external or **extrinsic trigger**, such as pollen, dust, and mold.

The severity of a patient's disease can be classified according to the frequency of exacerbations experienced. An occasional exacerbation or asthma attack (less than once or twice a week) is considered mild intermittent asthma and is treated with episodic medications intended to treat bronchospasm and inflammation. More frequent attacks, and particularly those which occur while asleep, are treated with routine medications on a daily basis in an attempt to prevent bronchospasm and inflammation. Persistent bronchospasm that is resistant to routine treatments, called **status asthmaticus**, can lead to suffocation and death and must be treated aggressively.[42–45]

An asthma exacerbation can be treated with an aerosolized beta-agonist, often called a "rescue drug," such as albuterol. The importance of immediately administering rescue drugs to an asthmatic patient in distress cannot be understated.

The earliest treatment for asthma, sympathomimetic epinephrine, is still used today. Whether given subcutaneously or inhaled, epinephrine proved effective in reversing bronchospasms, and every other rescue drug since has been some derivative of epinephrine.[46] Epinephrine is not without its side effects. A nonselective adrenergic stimulant, epinephrine causes tachycardia and palpitations (the feeling of one's own heart racing), peripheral vasoconstriction (which raises the PVR and the work of the heart), as well as restlessness, anxiety, and insomnia.

The next generation of asthma medications is intended to reduce these undesirable side effects. They still affect the beta$_2$ receptors. The prototypical medication in this class, a nonselective beta-adrenergic drug, is isoproterenol. Able

to be administered by inhalation, injection (sublingual), or intravenous infusion, isoproterenol does not have the alpha effects of epinephrine. However, it still causes the same cardiotoxic effects.

Beta-Selective Drugs

Improvements and refinements have led to a group of drugs that is more highly selective for beta$_2$ receptors and has little or no impact on beta$_1$ receptors. These drugs are called beta-selective adrenergics. The first beta-selective adrenergic drug (isoetharine) was still a direct-acting catecholamine derivative (i.e., sympathomimetic), but had weak beta$_1$ properties.

The next generation of beta-selective drugs was non-catecholamines. Non-catecholamine drugs had significant advantages over earlier catecholamine-based drugs. The body has enzymes, such as MAO and COMT, to break catecholamines down at the neuromuscular junction. The non-catecholamine drugs were not as strongly affected by these enzymes and thus their effects tended to last longer. The non-catecholamine drugs were also more discriminating, having primarily beta$_2$ effects and almost no beta$_1$ effects.

The model non-catecholamine beta-selective drug is albuterol. Albuterol stimulates the beta$_2$ receptor to produce the cAMP, which results in smooth relaxation without stimulating the heart to race (beta$_1$ effect) or the blood pressure to rise (alpha$_1$ effect).

Xanthine Derivatives

The active ingredient in coffee and teas is caffeine, another plant alkaloid, which is perhaps the most widely used stimulant in the world. Caffeine, a xanthine derivative, relaxes smooth muscle in the bronchial tree, stimulates the heart, and stimulates the CNS. More discussion about caffeine can be found on the section on drugs which affect the CNS.

The liver converts xanthines, as a prodrug, to theophylline, which causes bronchodilation. For a variety of reasons, most notably cigarette smoking, the conversion to theophylline can be unpredictable and toxicity is not unusual.

As a class, xanthines work by inhibiting an enzyme (phosphodiesterase), which results in an increase in cAMP and GMP, which in turn alters calcium levels in the muscle as well as blocking adenosine receptors. The end result is bronchial dilation. Methods of administration of theophylline compounds include orally in a liquid, intravenously as an infusion, and rectally as either a suppository or a retention enema.

Unfortunately, xanthine derivatives interact with several other commonly prescribed drugs. For example, phenytoin, a commonly prescribed anticonvulsant, causes an increase in xanthine metabolism, leading to subtherapeutic levels of xanthine as well as lower levels of phenytoin. Subtherapeutic levels of phenytoin for patients with a seizure disorder can result in a breakthrough seizure.

Cigarette smoking, mentioned earlier, also interferes with theophylline metabolism. The dose of theophylline for smokers has to be increased between 50% and 100% because of increased metabolism. Due to the unpredictable therapeutic level, the narrow therapeutic index, and undesirable side effects, theophylline use has markedly decreased as newer medications with more tolerable side effects have been proven equally effective.

Cholinergic Antagonists

As a class, cholinergic antagonists are not as effective as bronchodilators but rather prevent further bronchoconstriction by occupying the muscarinic receptors on the bronchial smooth muscle that cause bronchoconstriction. Treatment of bronchospasm with anticholinergic medications is most effective either immediately preceding the bronchospasm or immediately after treatment with a bronchodilator, to prevent a return of bronchospasm. Therefore, during the treatment of reactive airway diseases such as asthma, beta-selective adrenergic drugs are preferred. However, concurrent administration of cholinergic antagonists, such as ipratropium, is a common practice.[47]

Prophylactic Medications for Pulmonary Disease

The actions of prophylactic asthma medications generally revolve around decreasing inflammation (specifically, preventing the degranulation of mast cells) and subsequent releasing of histamine, prostaglandins, and leukotrienes (leukotrienes were known as slow reaction smooth muscle-stimulating substance (SRS)—the name is descriptive of the action of leukotrienes). Histamine and leukotrienes cause swelling, bronchospasm, and subsequent narrowing of the lumen of the airways.

Cromolyn, a mast cell stabilizer, inhibits the release of histamine, prostaglandins, and leukotrienes from mast cells, in part, by stabilizing the cell wall via blockage of calcium ion channels in the cell wall. Cromolyn is therapeutically equal with a maintenance dose of theophylline and has fewer side effects than theophylline. For this reason, cromolyn has largely replaced theophylline as a prophylactic agent for the treatment of asthma.

A new class of anti-inflammatory drugs, called leukotriene antagonists, are becoming available. Drugs in this class block leukotriene receptors. **Leukotriene** is the slow-acting substance of anaphylaxis that causes mucous plugs and constricts bronchial airways. Leukotriene antagonists, such as zileuton, have the distinction of affecting all three of the "S's" of pulmonary disease (swelling, secretions, and spasm). Leukotriene antagonists are indicated for the treatment of long-term or chronic asthma.

Commonly prescribed inhaled corticosteroids reduce inflammation as well, but by a slightly different action. Corticosteroids stabilize lysosomal membranes, preventing the release of hydrolytic enzymes which produce the inflammatory response in the tissues, as well as decrease the production of leukotrienes.

Inhaled corticosteroids have many systemic side effects, including cough, dizziness, and headache. Newer generations of corticosteroids have been developed which reduce some of these unwanted side effects.

Caution regarding corticosteroids is advised. Corticosteroids suppress secretion of hormones from the hypothalamus, pituitary, and adrenal glands. Sudden withdrawal from corticosteroids can precipitate a potential acute adrenal insufficiency, or Addisonian Crisis. Patients taking steroids must be gradually weaned off corticosteroids, by tapered doses, while the body readjusts.

Mucolytics

Thickened secretions in the airway obstruct the airway and serve as a breeding ground for infection. These secretions are difficult to expel (expectorate), leading to partial airway obstructions via mucous plugs, as well as acting as a foci for inflammation and infection. For these reasons, it is important to clear these secretions from the airway.

Mucus is made up of a combination of protein-like materials, and complex sugars called polysaccharides. Sputum, mucus with cellular debris such as white blood cells (leukocytes) and bacteria, is largely made up of water. By adding physiologic saline (0.9% sodium chloride in sterile water) to the airway, via aerosol or bolus flush, the thinned sputum is easier to remove by suction.

Ridding the airway of thickened secretions, called pulmonary toilet, can also be achieved through sterile endotracheal suctioning, hydration (oral or intravenous), and administration of drugs which thin the secretions, called **mucolytics**.

Mucolytics physically break down the viscosity of mucus by breaking apart the mucoprotein structure. An example of a commonly used mucolytic is acetylcysteine which is absorbed directly into the airway and exerts a local effect. Acetylcysteine begins to work within one minute and peaks in as little as 5 to 10 minutes, destroying the mucoprotein structure of mucus and allowing for easier expectoration.

Pharmacological Interventions during a Cardiac Emergency

Over 60 million Americans have cardiovascular disease and over 12 million Americans have coronary artery disease. Over 7 1/2 million of those Americans will have an acute myocardial infarction (AMI) and over one million will not survive the event. Additionally, nearly five million will have congestive heart failure.[20]

These figures serve to illustrate the prevalence of cardiovascular disease and its impact upon Americans. In fact, cardiovascular disease has been the number one killer in the United States since 1918, with the exception of the year of the great influenza outbreak.

As the major health issue in the United States for the past nine decades, great efforts have been made to reduce the number of deaths, many of them out-of-hospital, from cardiovascular disease. In fact, the genesis of EMS is owed, in part, to cardiovascular disease. Beginning with Dr. Pantridge in Belfast, Ireland, whose experiment with using coronary care

nurses out-of-hospital demonstrated the efficacy of prehospital care and ranging to today's 12-lead ECG technology, EMS has always had a focus on cardiac care.

The Paramedic's first mission was and still is to reduce dysrhythmic death. The use of cardiac medications, as an adjunct to rapid defibrillation and cardiopulmonary resuscitation, is thought to have had a significant impact on the morbidity and mortality from cardiovascular disease and continues to be the mainstay of advanced cardiac life support. Therefore Paramedics must have an understanding of the indications and mechanism of action of many cardioactive drugs in order to effectively and efficiently treat their patients and prevent sudden cardiac death.

Today, the mission of EMS is even more complex, and advances in cardiology have added new demands on Paramedics. Paramedics must not only understand the drugs which prevent or treat cardiac arrest, but also drugs that are used in the treatment of acute myocardial infarction.

In the past the diagnosis of a "heart attack" (acute myocardial infarction) was viewed as an inevitable death sentence. Today, new drugs, such as fibrinolytics, and new technologies, such as angioplasty, can literally halt the myocardial damage, but only if the patient can obtain these treatments in time.[48]

This changing focus from dysrhythmic death (mortality) to myocardial salvage (morbidity) has even changed the nomenclature. Acute myocardial infarction, an event once seen as occurring in isolation, is now looked upon as a part of the **acute coronary syndrome (ACS)**. ACS is a complex of symptoms associated with the continuum of cardiovascular disease, emphasizing its morbidity (and more importantly, its mutability) and not simply its mortality.[49–51]

Coronary Artery Disease

Coronary artery disease is primarily due to atherosclerosis. Unchecked, atherosclerosis blocks coronary arteries, which leads to hypoperfusion distal to the occlusion and death of the cardiac muscle tissue, **acute myocardial infarction (AMI)**. The series of events that leads up to and includes the myocardial infarction is referred to as **coronary artery disease (CAD)**.

Atherosclerosis, the underlying pathology of coronary artery disease, starts as a streak of fat (cholesterol) on the walls of an artery, any artery. This includes the cerebral arteries as well as the coronary arteries. The fat infiltrates into the wall of the artery, below the tunica intima, and forms a fatty lesion referred to as **plaque**. The plaque has a thin fibrous covering, created by the tunica intima, called the cap. This bulges into the lumen of the artery, partially obstructing blood flow.

The presence of **nitric oxide (NO)**, created in endothelium of the walls of the blood vessel, which prevents vasoconstriction; and **heparin sulfate**, an anticoagulant released from the endothelium of the walls of the arteries, temporarily prevents blood clot formation in the narrowed coronary arteries.

As time progresses, macrophages and T-lymphocytes, defender cells in the circulation, enter the plaque and begin the process of phagocytosis, literally enveloping the cholesterols and fats (lipids) in an effort to destroy the invaders. The now engorged macrophages swell and become foam cells. Foam cells are filled with dead and dying muscle cells and lipids. Proteins entrapped within the toothpaste-like liquid lipid core also begin to form collagens and von Willebrand's factor, two elements in clotting.

Plaques, especially newer, less mature plaques, are softer, have a thinner cap, and are prone to rupture. Any hemodynamic stress (e.g., a sudden increase in blood pressure) can cause a plaque to rupture (Figure 30-4).[52–55]

When a plaque ruptures and the thin cap is torn, the uplifted plaque now exposes the collagen in the basement layer underneath the endothelial lining. Blood clotting factors in the plasma, attracted to the exposed collagen, react as if the blood vessel had been ruptured, or cut, and attempt to plug the breach.

The response to the rupture begins with the attachment of von Willebrand's factor and ADP released from inside the plaque to glycoprotien (Gp)IIB/IIIA receptors found on passing platelets. The now "activated" platelets change from a disc shape to a sphere shape and attach to the exposed collagen and to each other. The eventual mass of platelets forms a **platelet plug**. Platelet plugs are the short-term solution to the problem.

For a more stable blockade, the platelet plug needs to be reinforced. The entire process, from platelet plug production to the reinforcement of the thrombus, is called **coagulation**. Coagulation starts when coagulation factors—adenosine diphosphate (ADP), serotonin, and thromboxane (TxA2)—are released from the damaged endothelial wall, which triggers a series of events, called the **coagulation cascade**.

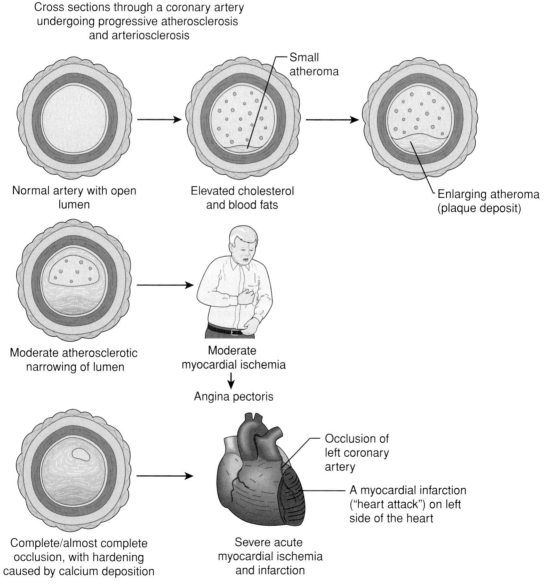

Cross sections through a coronary artery undergoing progressive atherosclerosis and arteriosclerosis

Small atheroma

Normal artery with open lumen

Elevated cholesterol and blood fats

Enlarging atheroma (plaque deposit)

Moderate atherosclerotic narrowing of lumen

Moderate myocardial ischemia

Angina pectoris

Complete/almost complete occlusion, with hardening caused by calcium deposition

Occlusion of left coronary artery

A myocardial infarction ("heart attack") on left side of the heart

Severe acute myocardial ischemia and infarction

Figure 30-4 The development of plaque. Plaque rupture occludes the narrowed lumen causing a myocardial infarction.

First, a fibrous soluble protein called **fibrinogen**, which is found floating in the blood, becomes activated. Normally fibrinogen is coated with amino acids that have an outward facing negative charge. As like-charges repel, these negatively charged amino acids keep the fibrinogen molecules separated.

When clotting factors are released, a protein-cutting enzyme (protease) called **thrombin** literally clips off the negatively charged amino acids. Without the negative charge repelling the fibrinogen molecules, the fibrinogen clumps together, becomes strand-like, and forms **fibrin**.

What follows are two processes, one intrinsic and the other extrinsic, which result in a mature clot made of platelets cross-linked with fibrin and other blood cells in a firm meshwork called a **thrombus**. With the thrombus in place, the lumen of the blood vessel is blocked.

Decreasing the incidence of cardiovascular disease, and subsequent acute coronary syndrome, revolves around interfering with one or more of the processes previously described. Starting with chemotherapeutic agents which eliminate the fatty streak on the inner lumen of the artery that signals the start of atherosclerosis, cardioprotective agents will be discussed individually.

Antihyperlipidemic Drugs

The easiest means to prevent thrombus-induced coronary artery disease is to reduce unwanted lipids which form plaques at the onset. Despite dietary control, some individuals continue to have elevated lipid levels in the blood (**hyperlipidemia**), possibly due to genetic influences. Hyperlipidemia is an abnormally high level of triglycerides and cholesterol which, when uncontrolled, can lead to atherosclerosis.

Normally, lipids are bound to protein, forming lipoproteins (a protein shell around a lipid core), and are found floating in the blood. There are three varieties of lipoproteins: very-low density lipoproteins (VLDL), low-density lipoproteins (LDL), and high-density lipoproteins (HDL). Of the three types of lipoproteins, LDL is considered the most dangerous because of its high cholesterol content, about 50% cholesterol by weight.[56-58]

Some lipid-lowering agents lower cholesterol, thus eliminating it for conversion to LDL, by sequestering the cholesterol in the bile. The bile is then excreted into the gallbladder and, in turn, into the small intestine. Cholesterol is a precursor to bile; therefore, increasing bile elimination indirectly helps to rid the body of cholesterol. An example of a bile sequestering agent is cholestyramine.

Niacin, a water-soluble vitamin, is also occasionally prescribed as a lipid-lowering agent. Niacin inhibits the lipolysis (division of fats) in adipose tissue, which would liberate free fatty acids.[59-61] These free fatty acids would normally be used by the liver to create new triglycerides and then cholesterol. In the case of the patient with hyperlipidemia, the added cholesterol would also boost the process of atherosclerosis.

Niacin in high dosages, or in persons sensitive to niacin (e.g., diabetic patients and those with liver disease), may also cause an anaphylactoid (anaphylactic-like) reaction, including pruritus, diffuse skin flushing, as well as dysrhythmias.

The reductase inhibitors, a group of drugs referred to as "statins" because of the common ending, have grown increasingly popular as a treatment for hyperlipidemia. This class of drugs inhibits an enzyme, 3-hydroxy-3-methylglutaryl coenzyme A reductase (HMG-CoA), which is essential for the liver to make cholesterol. Without the enzyme HMG-CoA, the liver cannot make cholesterol and the process of atherosclerosis is slowed.

Patients with liver disease, particularly alcoholics, are at risk for severe side effects from the statin class of lipid-lowering drugs, including rhabdomyolysis (a necrosis of skeletal muscle) which may lead to kidney failure. Examples of reductase inhibitors are fluvastatin, lovastatin, and atorvastatin.

Anticoagulants

Unchecked, the process of atherosclerosis will eventually culminate in plaque formation, plaque rupture, and thrombus formation via the coagulation cascade. Anticoagulants are intended to prevent the formation of a thrombus, which is the culmination of the coagulation cascade.

Anticoagulants include those agents that prevent platelet adhesion, fibrin collection, thrombus formation, and other thromboembolic events. While anticoagulants are discussed under the acute coronary syndrome, these drugs are used under the larger umbrella of conditions caused by thrombus formation including pulmonary embolism, deep vein thrombus, and thromboembolic ischemic stroke.

One of the earliest anticoagulants was salicylate. Extract of willow bark, salicylate, had long been known for its analgesic qualities as "Oil of Wintergreen" (methyl salicylate). However, until Felix Hoffmann eliminated the painful side effect of stomach irritation by reformulating salicylate, it was not widely used. Following the reformulation to acetylsalicylic acid (ASA), the German pharmaceutical company Bayer™ took out a patent and renamed the drug aspirin. Over 80 billion tablets of aspirin are used annually in the United States as a pain reliever and fever reducer.[62] Thanks in part to Bayer™ Company aspirin television commercials, aspirin is also widely known for its ability to prevent heart attacks. A study of 90,000 patients showed that aspirin alone prevented the reocclusion of coronary arteries in 23% of patients who had a prior AMI, especially if given within four hours.[63]

As a class, platelet inhibitors prevent platelet aggregation by preventing a critical enzyme, cyclooxygenase, from creating thromboxane A2 (TxA2). TxA2 promotes platelet aggregation and vasoconstriction. Without TxA2, platelets remain "slippery" and cannot form the initial platelet plug needed for thrombus formation.

Prior to administration of aspirin or an aspirin-like product, the provider should inquire if the patient has a history of asthma. Aspirin-induced asthma (AIA) is present in about 10% to 15% of the patient population with asthma. AIA is an idiosyncratic type of reaction which presents with allergy-like symptoms and is akin to the reaction seen to CT contrast dyes. Treatment with ASA is acceptable for patients with asthma, although the patient must be carefully monitored. Symptomatic relief should be immediately available if symptoms should occur. There are several other platelet inhibitors, such as dipyridamole, for those who absolutely cannot tolerate aspirin side effects.

The body also naturally produces anticoagulants, such as heparin, in the liver, lungs, and lining of the intestine which prevent clotting. Circulating heparin helps prevent spurious blood clots from forming in the body by preventing the formation of fibrinogen from fibrin.

The addition of intravenous heparin to the body is commonly used to help prevent new thrombus formation. It is used as a prophylactic measure post-surgery, to prevent deep vein thrombus-induced pulmonary embolism, to prevent clot formation during blood transfusion, and to prevent clots from forming on the wall of the heart during atrial fibrillation (mural thrombi).

It is important to note that heparin does not dissolve pre-existing clots and therefore cannot be used as the sole therapeutic agent during a thromboembolic emergency. Other fibrinolytic agents, discussed shortly, are used during a thromboembolic emergency to actually dissolve a blood clot. Heparin is often used in conjunction with these fibrinolytic agents to prevent fresh clots from occurring or to prevent the current clot from enlarging.

Most of the heparin used in-hospital is low-molecular weight (LMWH) heparin. LMW heparin has a longer half-life (t1/2) than standard heparin, permitting daily or twice daily administration, by subcutaneous injection, as compared to standard heparin, which must be continuously infused intravenously. This quality makes it desirable for outpatient use.

An intravenous infusion of unfractionated (standard) heparin is indicated for use in patients with ST-elevated AMI, in conjunction with aspirin. LMWH shows promise in the treatment of the patient with a ST-elevated AMI, but its use has not been definitively supported in the large scale studies. That said, LMWH is well supported by research for unstable AMI, non-ST elevated AMI and angina.[64]

Heparin and its oral counterpart, warfarin, can lead to bleeding complications. Once anticoagulants have been administered, the patient must be monitored for signs of occult hemorrhage, such as tachycardia and hypotension.

Fibrinolytics

Fibrinolytics dissolve blood clots, which can cause heart attacks (acute myocardial infarction/AMI), brain attacks (stroke/CVA), and pulmonary emboli (PE). If successful, the artery is re-opened (a process called **recanalization**) and the blood flow is restored to distal ischemic tissue in the affected organ.

The first generation of fibrinolytics included urokinase and streptokinase. Initially used to dissolve blood clots from long-term, indwelling central venous catheters, they were eventually used for the treatment of heart attacks and other thromboembolic events. An unfortunate consequence of the use of these early fibrinolytics was systemic bleeding. Intracerebral hemorrhage, for example, occurred with enough frequency that criteria for use of these drugs was tightened in an attempt to limit this sometimes fatal complication.

The second generation of "clot-busters" were more specific to a newly forming thrombus. These new fibrinolytics used the naturally occurring tissue plasminogen activator (tPA) to convert plasminogen into plasmin. Plasmin, a fibrinolytic enzyme, dissolves fibrin within the platelet plug. The net effect is that tPA disassembles the platelet plug.

Administered intravenously, tPA was an effective and rapid treatment for AMI. It was also relatively inexpensive when compared to the costs of interventional cardiology, such as angioplasty or open heart surgery.

Administration of fibrinolytics is not without its dangers. Caution must be observed before administering fibrinolytics to patients with a history of cerebrovascular disease, such as active ulcer disease and recent trauma. Some use a checklist when administering fibrinolytics (Figure 30-5).

FIBRINOLYTIC CHECKLIST

Rev. 5/07

Central Shenandoah EMS Council, 2312 W. Beverley St., Staunton, VA 24401 • 540-886-3676 • www.csems.vaems.org

INCIDENT DATA

Date ☐☐☐☐☐☐☐☐ Agency ☐ Unit # ☐☐☐☐

Patient Name ☐ Age ☐☐☐ DOB ☐☐☐☐☐☐☐☐

INDICATIONS FOR USE OF CHECKLIST

Patient experiencing chest discomfort for greater than 15 minutes and less than 12 hours, **AND...**
12-lead ECG shows STEMI or presumably new LBBB.

Are there any contraindications to fibrinolysis?

Systolic BP greater than 180 mm Hg	☐ YES	☐ NO
Diastolic BP greater than 110 mm Hg	☐ YES	☐ NO
Right vs. left arm systolic BP difference greater than 15 mm Hg	☐ YES	☐ NO
History of structural central nervous system disease	☐ YES	☐ NO
Significant closed head/facial trauma within the previous 3 months	☐ YES	☐ NO
Recent (within 6 weeks) major trauma, surgery (including laser eye surgery), GI/GU bleed	☐ YES	☐ NO
Bleeding or clotting problem or on blood thinners	☐ YES	☐ NO
CPR greater than 10 minutes	☐ YES	☐ NO
Pregnant female	☐ YES	☐ NO
Serious systemic disease (eg, advanced/terminal cancer, severe liver or kidney disease)	☐ YES	☐ NO

Is patient at high risk?

Heart rate greater than or equal to 100 bpm AND systolic BP less than 100 mm Hg	☐ YES	☐ NO
Pulmonary edema (rales)	☐ YES	☐ NO
Signs of shock (cool, clammy)	☐ YES	☐ NO
Contraindications to fibrinolytic therapy	☐ YES	☐ NO

Comments

Figure 30-5 Fibrinolytic checklist.

Prehospital fibrinolytics have been shown to improve survival in a few studies and should be considered when transport times exceed 30 to 60 minutes. Studies continue to investigate which groups of patients would benefit the most from field fibrinolytics.[65]

A growing body of evidence indicates that certain subsets of patients benefit more from mechanical revascularization (angioplasty) than standard fibrinolytics. Rapid transportation, with appropriate stabilization, to a cardiac care center may become the standard of care. Consideration should be given to incorporate criterion-based triage into EMS protocols for the treatment of the suspected AMI.[66]

Glycoprotein IIB-IIIA Receptor Blockers

Activation of glycoprotein receptors on platelets and the formation of fibrin represent the final common pathway in platelet plug formation. Blocking these receptors prevents the binding of fibrinogen and thereby prevents platelet aggregation and plug formation.

The intravenous administration of medications called glycoprotein IIB-IIIA receptor blockers, like tirofiban and eptifibatide, is useful in preventing the re-formation of platelet plugs and arterial re-occlusion immediately following fibrinolysis or angioplasty.

The combination of aspirin (ASA), heparin, and a glycoprotein IIB-IIIA receptor blocker can reduce the risk of sudden cardiac death substantially.[67]

Acute Coronary Syndrome

Atherosclerotic coronary plaque growth narrows the blood vessel's lumen. The narrowing, called a stenosis, causes a reduction in blood flow to the portion of the myocardium distal to the stenosis. Decreased distal coronary artery blood flow can lead to chest pain, or angina pectoris. Unchecked, these plaques rupture and can lead to complete coronary artery occlusion and an infarction of myocardium distal to the occlusion.

The entire process leading up to and including angina and AMI is called the acute coronary syndrome (ACS). This change in perspective, from treating a heart attack as an isolated event to one of treating atherosclerosis as a part of the continuum in a common process, reflects a more considered approach to coronary care and reflects the growing knowledge about atherosclerosis and coronary artery disease as a result of practice experience (Table 30-1).

Syndromes are, according to *Taber's Medical Dictionary*, "the sum of signs associated with any pathological process." In this case, the pathological process is atherosclerosis. Acute

Table 30-1 Inclusion Criteria for Acute Coronary Syndromes

- Unstable angina
- Non ST-segment myocardial infarction
- ST-segment elevation myocardial infarction (STEMI)

coronary syndrome is a process which has many stages, from intermittent angina to cardiac ischemia to acute myocardial infarction.

In most cases, the Paramedic's job is the early recognition of acute coronary syndrome; stabilization of the patient's hemodynamics and any other complications, such as dysrhythmia; and the provision of expeditious transfer of the patient to a cardiac care center for further treatment. In some cases, Paramedics are starting the process of treatment of the coronary artery syndrome in the field through use of fibrinolytics. In every case, whether it is the use of prehospital fibrinolytics or expeditious transportation following initial stabilization to a cardiac care center, re-establishing blood flow to ischemic myocardial tissue is a top priority. Use of nitrates can improve myocardial blood flow, reduce pain, and potentially avert sudden cardiac death.

Nitrates

One of the oldest treatments for cardiac-related angina has been nitroglycerin. For centuries, amyl nitrate (a volatile organic nitrate when in alcohol) had been used to relieve angina. In 1867, the Scotsman Lauder Brunton thought the positive effects of amyl nitrate were from hypotension. In 1933, Sir Thomas Lewis more correctly postulated that the effect of amyl nitrate was due to dilation of the blood vessels.[20]

However, nitrate's exact mechanism of action was still unknown until recently. Previously, it was known that some substance, labeled endothelial-derived relaxing factor (EDRF), relaxed the smooth muscle in the walls of blood vessels, which in turn led to vasodilation. The involvement of nitrates in this process was largely unsuspected.

In 1998, Furchgott, Ignarro, and Murad were awarded the Nobel Prize in medicine for their discovery of the role of nitric oxide in human physiology. Nitric oxide (NO), a short-lived gas, is released from endothelial cells within the inner lining of the blood vessel where it acts as an intercellular chemical messenger, signaling an increase in cGMP within muscle cells. This increase in cGMP, in turn, relaxes the smooth muscle in the blood vessel, leading to vasodilation.

It is now known that acetylcholine, the chief neurotransmitter in the parasympathetic nervous system, acts by stimulating the production of nitric oxide and thereby results in vasodilation through this mechanism.

In many cases, coronary artery vasodilation can offer symptomatic relief from the cardiac patient's angina by increasing the diameter of a chronically narrowed, stenotic vessel. Ironically, Alfred Nobel, inventor of nitroglycerin-based dynamite and originator of the Nobel Prizes, suffered from angina and was prescribed nitroglycerin for his pain. So as to not alarm the pharmacist, the physician labeled the nitroglycerin "trinitrin" (TNT).

Nitrates administered to a patient provide an exogenous (external) source of NO. Nitrates have their greatest impact on the venous circulation and reduce venous return, or preload, to the heart. Reduced preload into the heart means less work for the heart's muscles.

Nitrates' secondary vasoactive effect, particularly at higher doses, is arterial dilation. Arterial vasodilation creates reduced peripheral vascular resistance (PVR), or afterload. Afterload can be thought of as the resistance which the heart pump must overcome in order to achieve forward blood flow. It is grossly measured as the diastolic blood pressure.

There is some debate whether nitrates create a coronary artery-specific vasodilation. Coronary vasodilation would increase blood flow to oxygen-starved myocardium and lessen the angina.[68,69] What is not disputed is nitrates' ability to reduce preload and lessen afterload, which culminates in a total reduced workload for the heart. This effect may have the greatest impact on relieving the angina.[70,71]

Regardless of the primary mechanism, decreased workload, or coronary artery vasodilation, nitrates have become standard therapy for the patient with angina. In either tablet or spray form, sublingual nitrates have an onset of action of less than one minute and peak in the bloodstream within two minutes. With a half-life of only five to seven minutes, any hypotensive effects created by the venous dilation will subside quickly and usually are treated conservatively, at least initially, by placing the patient supine for a few minutes.

Nitroglycerin loses its potency when exposed to light, heat, and moisture. Therefore, it is usually carried in a sealed glass bottle with cotton wadding. A commonly noted side effect of nitroglycerin is a transient headache for between 5 to 15 minutes. Other side effects include transient hypotension, bradycardia or tachycardia, or dizziness.[72,73]

Nitrate pastes provide a more sustained release of the medication over four to six hours. In contrast, newer time-released patches are formulated with nitrates to create a reservoir of medication which can last 1 1/2 to 24 hours.

Nitroglycerin is also available in an intravenous form that allows precise titration of the level of drug needed in order to obtain relief from chest pain without the risk of common side effects, such as hypotension. Intravenous nitroglycerin is administered in micrograms of drug using an intravenous pump, a biomechanical device that carefully controls the rate of administration. Intravenous nitroglycerin is readily absorbed into plastic; therefore, special polyvinyl chloride (PVC) administration sets are used with nitroglycerin infusion.

Nitrate Tolerance

Nitrates, an essential ingredient in smokeless gunpowder, have long been used in munitions production. Workers at the munitions factory in places like Springfield, Massachusetts, often experienced a headache when returning to work after the weekend. Workers learned that if they took a bag of nitrate-laced gunpowder home and rubbed it on their hands they would not experience a headache when returning to work after the weekend.

What these workers had developed was a classic example of tolerance to a drug, in this case nitrate. After continuous exposure they developed a resistance to its effects and/or its side effects, such as a headache. Whenever these workers went home for the weekend, they essentially went on a "drug holiday," a period without the drug. They then lost their tolerance to the drug. By continuing their exposure to the nitrate-laced gunpowder during the weekend, they ensured that their tolerance for nitrates continued. Patients who are prescribed nitrates regularly can also develop a tolerance to nitrates and will not respond as well to routine doses of nitrates in the field. In some cases, it may be advisable to consider an alternative therapeutic approach, such as the use of morphine sulfate.

Indications for Nitrate Use

The chief use of nitrates is for the relief of cardiac-related chest pain called angina pectoris, or simply angina. Angina is brought about by a mismatch between the work required of the heart (workload) and the heart's ability to do that work. This limitation is a function of the coronary blood flow to the heart.

Nitrates are also used to treat pre-infarction angina, formerly known as unstable angina, in an effort to prevent some of the damage of coronary artery occlusion. By increasing collateral blood flow to the affected area, distal to the obstruction, as well as decreasing the heart's overall work, the damage can potentially be lessened.

Frequently, physicians and Paramedics assumed that if nitroglycerin relieved the chest pain, then the chest pain must be suspected of being cardiac in origin and the likely diagnosis was coronary artery disease (CAD).

A study at Johns Hopkins showed that of 459 patients treated with nitroglycerin for chest pain, all of whom had relief, only 30% had coronary artery disease (CAD). The results of this study should cause Paramedics to pause and consider other potential etiologies of chest pain whenever nitroglycerin is effective in relieving chest pain. This is particularly important in light of the fact that one in five patients coming to the emergency department complains of chest pain.[74]

Nitrates have also proven themselves to be markedly effective in the treatment of acute pulmonary edema associated with **congestive heart failure (CHF)**. CHF is the result of the heart's inability to pump strongly enough to completely overcome peripheral vascular resistance (PVR) and meet the body's needs for oxygen and nutrients. Subsequently, backpressure from the left ventricle, or backward failure, is transmitted through the pulmonary circulation, creating pulmonary edema in the process, and eventually extending into the right ventricle. The right ventricle, being a weaker pump than the left, is overwhelmed by the combination of venous preload and left ventricular backpressure and fails as well.

Nitrates are starting to gain increased favor for the emergency treatment of pulmonary edema. While loop diuretics are immediately effective in reducing pulmonary edema, they can create a hormonal rebound when the kidneys sense the volume depletion and respond naturally to create further fluid retention. The patient with cardiogenic pulmonary edema may not be volume overloaded, but more correctly, volume unbalanced. Nitrates provide the heart with a respite while it regains control of hemodynamics.

Contraindications

In general, any volume-sensitive condition can be worsened by the use of nitrates. Nitrates temporarily remove a volume of blood from the central circulation by sequestering it in the venous pool. Volume-sensitive conditions can be divided into cardiac and extra-cardiac pathologies. An example of an extra-cardiac pathology that is volume sensitive is cardiac tamponade.

The heart is dependent on adequate filling pressures (preload) obtained from the venous circulation in order to overcome the compressive consequence of pericardial tamponade. Nitrates decrease preload, via venous dilation, and the cardiac output can drop precipitously. Nitrate administration to a patient with a tension pneumothorax can have the same consequence as a result of a similar mechanism.

The right ventricle is acutely sensitive to changes in filling volumes (preload). An acute inferior wall myocardial infarction which extends into the right ventricle can cause the right ventricle to lose its ability to pump a given volume of blood. That volume of blood serves as the "prime" for the left ventricle; any pump that loses its prime loses output and fails. The administration of nitrates decreases the left ventricular filling pressures (prime) by reducing preload into the right ventricle from the venous circulation. Without adequate filling pressures, the cardiac output from the left ventricle can fall to dangerously low

levels. Life-threatening hypotension then ensues (cardiogenic shock or forward failure).

Precautions

Hypotension-induced syncope, or near-syncope, is a common complication of nitrate administration.[75,76] The impact of the abrupt loss of preload secondary to venous dilation is transmitted downstream, the fallout being loss of blood pressure and possible loss of consciousness (syncope).

Fortunately, nitrates have a short half-life. Therefore, the hypotensive effects are short-lived. Laying the patient supine with feet elevated, and exhibiting some patience, are usually the only treatments needed. If the patient's blood pressure does not return within five minutes, then a volume-sensitive pathology (e.g., internal bleeding or right ventricular myocardial infarction) should be considered.

Dysrhythmia

Despite remarkable advances in medicine's understanding of cardiac pathophysiology, and particularly coronary artery disease, over 500,000 Americans will die from heart disease each year.[77] Over 60% of these deaths will be secondary to a fatal dysrhythmia called ventricular fibrillation.

Ventricular fibrillation is one of many **dysrhythmias**, an abnormality of the electrical activity in the heart. Ventricular fibrillation is a life-threatening problem because there is no cardiac output.

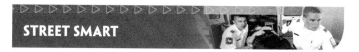

STREET SMART

Not all dysrhythmias are dangerous. A study of 1,302 professional NFL football players completed by Dr. Choo and Dr. Hutter, Jr., of Massachusetts General Hospital demonstrated that 55% had an abnormality of the electrical activity in the heart. However, after extensive testing, it was decided that the hearts of these athletes were healthy.[78]

The most common persistent dysrhythmia may be atrial fibrillation, which affects over two million Americans. Atrial fibrillation, a dysrhythmia more often seen in the elderly, is associated with an increased risk of brain attack (stroke) and associated quality of life issues. The incidence of atrial fibrillation is expected to rise as the mean age of Americans continues to climb (referred to as the "graying" of America).

Therapeutic Goal

The therapeutic goal of antidysrhythmics, drugs which prevent or abolish dysrhythmias, is to alleviate the symptoms associated with an irregular heartbeat and, in some

Technically, an arrhythmia would be defined as the absence of a rhythm (a without rhythm pattern) such as occurs in asystole. A dysrhythmia would be an abnormal pattern of electrical discharges. However, it is common practice to use the terms interchangeably.

cases, to help ensure the patient's survival. However, the mechanisms of action of many of the drugs in this class are also dysrhythmia producing or pro-dysrhythmic.

The results of the Cardiac Arrhythmia Suppression Trial (CAST) appear to indicate that there may be a significant increase in mortality associated with use of certain antidysrhythmic drugs. Therefore, the decision to administer an antidysrhythmic must be carefully considered in terms of risk versus benefit (CAST). The notable side effects of some of the dysrhythmia drugs, in addition to the creation of new dysrhythmia, have encouraged the development of alternative therapeutic approaches.

Some of the devices and techniques in use are radio-frequency ablation to disrupt alternative conductive pathways, particularly those of supraventricular origin; automated implantable cardioverter defibrillators (AICD) with an ability to terminate ventricular tachycardia and ventricular fibrillation; and a new generation of dual-chamber sensing electronic pacemakers. Use of these devices and techniques have brought about a decrease in the prophylactic use of antidysrhythmic medications.[79]

Nevertheless, antidysrhythmic drugs are still used, particularly in the setting of sudden cardiac death (SCD), and will probably continue to be used in the foreseeable future to prevent dysrhythmic death and abate symptoms associated with dysrhythmia.

Review of Action Potential

Pivotal to an understanding of the actions of most antidysrhythmic drugs is an understanding of the action potential of the heart's muscle cells (the myocardial cells, known collectively as myocardium), which these drugs affect.

Myocardial cells are essentially "charged" in a fashion similar to any conventional car battery. Ionic differences, two opposing polarities, between the inside of the cell, representing one pole, and the outside of the cell, representing the other pole, are the result of a difference in electron numbers. Typically this difference would be negated as the additional electrons are exchanged (neutralized). The cells' ability to prevent this exchange across the cell membrane is called the resting membrane potential (RMP).

The greater the electrical difference between poles, or across the membrane in this case, the greater the charge. The

resting membrane potential of a cardiac cell, measurable at approximately $+/-(-)90$ millivolts, is created by the relatively negative charge inside the cell as opposed to the positive charges outside the cell. In this resting state, the cell wall is impenetrable to charged ions such as sodium, potassium, and calcium.

A stimulus called an **action potential**, such as one produced by the normal pacemaker activity of the sinoatrial (SA) node, can change the resting membrane potential. It raises the resting membrane potential above a specific threshold. A cascade of ionic changes at the cell wall, called **depolarization**, occurs as electrolytes transfer across the cell in an attempt to balance (neutralize) the charge.

The cascade of events in depolarization can be divided into five distinct segments, each segment characterized by a different ionic event and numbered 0 to 4. These different segments represent the changes in the electrical charges from within and outside of the cell (Figure 30-6). For simplicity, the depolarization of ventricular myocardial cells is being described, although all cardiac tissues—nervous as well as muscle—respond in a similar fashion. However, nerve cells are more "excitable" (i.e., able to sustain a larger membrane resting potential).

After the action potential overcomes the resistance created by the resting potential of the cell membrane (threshold), the sodium channels in the cell wall membrane open wide, allowing an influx of sodium into the cell. This influx of sodium, via the fast sodium channels, corresponds with phase zero (0) of the action potential and completely depolarizes the membrane; an event which can be recorded on a surface electrocardiogram or ECG.

With the now abundant sodium (Na+) inside the cell, as well as native intracellular potassium (K+), the cell becomes positively charged. These ionic shifts within the cell will surpass neutrality and the cell wall will become slightly positive. This ionic overshoot, about $(+)20$ millivolts, represents phase 1.

To this point, at the end of phase 1, myocardial cells have acted in the same manner as skeletal muscle cells. The difference between skeletal muscle and cardiac muscle occurs in phases 2 and 3. In phases 2 and 3, the depolarization of myocardial cells is sustained for about 200 to 300 milliseconds during a "plateau" phase, unlike the more rapid "spike" of skeletal muscle

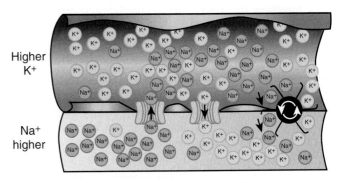

Figure 30-6 Action potential of cells.

depolarization. This permits a longer sustained contraction. The key to this sustained contraction is calcium.

In an effort to attain neutrality, calcium flows into the cell, via slow calcium channels, and potassium flows out. This is the start of the mechanical activation of the myocardium. Calcium now binds to the troponin complex, which is found within the myocardial fiber. This normally inhibits the binding of intertwined actin and myosin strands within the muscle fiber, and thus permits the sliding (contraction) of muscle fibers. The amount of calcium present partly determines the duration, and therefore the strength, of contraction. The duration of contraction is represented by the length of the plateau in phase 2.

The myosin filaments, now coupled with the actin filaments, contain quantities of an enzyme called ATPase. ATPase, in the presence of magnesium, divides the intercellular ATP, by hydrolysis, and releases the energy-rich substrate phosphate needed to sustain the contraction. Potassium within the myocardial cell now starts a rapid exodus from the cell in an attempt to regain the original resting potential but is unable to do so. Phase 3 thus ends.

The recovery of the myocardial cell (**repolarization**) occurs in phase 4. During phase 4, the sodium-potassium pump returns sodium and potassium ions to their original position, juxtaposed across the cell membrane from each other. The cell is again in a state of charged readiness, with a resting action potential of (−) 90 millivolts. The cell is now ready for another cycle of depolarization–repolarization and subsequent myocardial contraction.

Origins of Dysrhythmia

Normally, a clump of tissue in a small region near the opening where the vena cava enters the right atrium, called the sinus-atrial (SA) node, spontaneously depolarizes and thus initiates the wave of depolarization across the heart. As the SA node typically depolarizes earlier than any other tissues, it assumes dominance over the process of depolarization of the entire myocardium.

Spontaneous electrical activity in the SA node results from a loss of resting potential (ionic decay) in the cell wall membrane during diastole. When the ionic decay reaches a threshold, then the cell will spontaneously depolarize. This quality, which is exclusive to cardiac cells, is called automaticity. However, this automaticity is not solely restricted to the tissues in the SA node.

If other myocardial tissues reach the same point of decay more quickly, and become excitable earlier, then they will spontaneously discharge (i.e., self-depolarization) before the SA node. Typically, pacemaker cells such as the ones found in the SA node decay quicker than other cardiac cells and thus take dominance over the cycle. However, abnormal events at the cellular level (e.g., hypoxia, ischemia, or potassium imbalances) may cause a spontaneous depolarization from an isolated portion of myocardium, called a focus, which becomes an atypical or **ectopic** pacemaker. This mechanism, the creation of an ectopic pacemaker, is thought to be responsible for sudden cardiac death secondary to ventricular fibrillation.

Ideal Antidysrhythmic Drug

As ectopic pacemakers have been implicated in ventricular fibrillation, the ideal antidysrhythmic drug would preferentially select ectopic pacemakers (rapidly depolarizing cells) over normally functioning myocardial cells and suppress their activity.

Many of the antidysrhythmic drugs display this ectopic-specific quality. To explain this phenomenon, Hodgkin and Huxley offered the Modulated Receptor Theory (MRT). MRT suggests that ionic channels are in one of three states: resting, active, or inactive. In the polarized state (phase zero), the ionic channels (particularly the sodium channels) are resting and nonconducting. When the action potential depolarizes the cell, then (in sequence) first the sodium (Na+), then the potassium (K+), and then the calcium (Ca++) channels open and therefore are active.[80-82] Once opened, these ionic channels become inactive until repolarization occurs and the channel is returned to a resting state.

Antidysrhythmic drugs have their effect during the transitions between these states of resting: open/active and inactive. The drugs which act upon the ionic channels during the open/active state will preferentially be attracted to rapidly depolarizing ectopic pacemakers. These antidysrhythmic drugs can be said to be **use- (rate) dependent** drugs. Examples of use-dependent drugs include quinidine and procainamide.

Drugs that affect the ionic channels in myocardial cells in the inactive state would have an affinity to slower depolarizing tissues and would demonstrate a **reverse use- (rate) dependent** quality. Reverse use-dependent drugs prolong the repolarization of normal myocardial tissues, as electrographically demonstrated by a prolonged QT interval. This slowing of repolarization can lead to repolarization disturbances, such as Torsades de Pointes (twisting of the points), a form of polymorphic ventricular tachycardia that can deteriorate rapidly into ventricular fibrillation.

STREET SMART

In the past, antidysrhythmic drugs, such as lidocaine, were chosen based upon the provider's past experience or empiric evidence. Recent research has cast doubt on the efficacy of some of these drugs. Providers are now more likely to choose an antidysrhythmic drug based on research (an evidence-based approach) rather than simply upon past experience.

Vaughn-Williams Antidysrhythmic Drug Classifications

All antidysrhythmic drugs affect the action potential of the myocardial cell by altering ionic influx of sodium (Na+), potassium (K+), and calcium (Ca++) into the cell during the depolarization/repolarization cycle (Figure 30-7).

Using the schema of electrolyte changes along the myocardial cell wall as a foundation for understanding cardiac tissue function, all antidysrhythmic drugs can be divided according to their effect on a specific ion channel in the myocardial cell membrane. Drugs so grouped can be recognized for their similar therapeutic effect, even if they have slightly different actions. The Vaughn-Williams classification uses this approach, categorizing drugs according to similar electrophysiologic actions.

While the Vaughn-Williams classification system is useful in helping to predict a drug's action, it is not perfect.[83] Many drugs have effects which cross over to other classes. For example, amiodarone is predominantly a potassium channel blocker, and thus is grouped with class III drugs. However, it also has some other actions which are found in all four Vaughn-Williams classes (Table 30-2).

The common characteristic of all antidysrhythmic drugs is their ability to suppress the excitability (automaticity) of the myocardial cell. Suppression of aberrant automaticity, the principal source of ectopic pacemakers, results in the elimination of the dysrhythmia. Elimination of dysrhythmia may prevent sudden cardiac death as well as some of the symptoms associated with dysrhythmia.

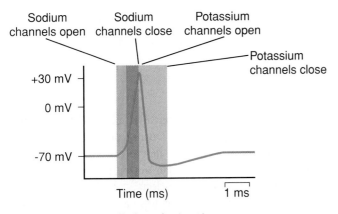

STREET SMART

Vaughn-Williams classifications (I, II, III, IV) should not be confused with the American Heart Association's classifications (I, IIa, IIb, III) of the drug's effectiveness.

Sodium channels open | Sodium channels close | Potassium channels open

Potassium channels close

+30 mV
0 mV
-70 mV

Time (ms)   1 ms

Figure 30-7 Cell depolarization.

Class I Drugs

All Vaughn-Williams Class I drugs block the sodium channels in the cell wall membrane, which normally open in phase zero. By blocking the sodium channels, Class I drugs decrease the speed of the depolarization (i.e., the conduction velocity through the myocardium). In this manner, Class I drugs decrease chronotropy during the upstroke portion of the action potential of phase zero.

This therapeutic approach is effective for treating tachyarrhythmias, particularly those that occur because of reentry phenomena. Reentry phenomenon, an error of conduction, is a common cause of arrhythmia and is the result of impaired conduction in a portion of the cardiac conduction pathway. Specific supraventricular rhythms and ventricular tachycardias utilize a reentry pathway mechanism, which creates a circus movement of rapid depolarization and repolarization around a block. The result is a tachyarrhythmia.

Class I drugs bind to sodium channels which open more frequently. This property of Class I drugs, called use- (rate) dependence, means that Class I drugs will create a total blockade at the site of the conduction defect and effectively terminate the circus movement.

On the downside, the slowed conduction caused by Class I drugs negatively affects the myocardium's contractility or V_{max}. (V_{max} is a measure of the myocardium's contractility.) A loss of contractility directly translates to a loss of force of contraction, or inotropy. Negative inotropy can cause loss of cardiac output and create hypotension or aggravate heart failure.

As a result of slowed conduction velocity, the QRS of the ECG, which is representative of ventricular depolarization, is widened and the QT interval, which represents the total time of depolarization to repolarization, is prolonged.

Patients with a prolonged QT interval, either as an inborn error of conduction or as a drug-induced complication, who are given Class I drugs are prone to life-threatening monomorphic ventricular tachycardia.[84] This is particularly true if the patient also has poor left ventricular function (ejection fraction < 40%) secondary to previous AMI.

Class I drugs are even further divided into Class A, Class B, and Class C according to their similar electrophysiologic effects on the duration of the action potential. Class IA drugs slow phase zero depolarization. Class IB drugs have a lesser effect on phase zero depolarization, but shorten the repolarization time in phase 3. Class IC drugs slowly bind to the sodium channels, and thus greatly depress the rate of rise in the action potential in phase zero.

Class IA

One of the earliest antidysrhythmic drugs was quinidine, a Class IA antidysrhythmic. Quinidine attaches to sodium channels as soon as they open during phase zero. Quinidine also creates a potassium channel blockade, which increases the duration of the action potential, and in effect, leaves sodium channels open longer so that more drug can bind with the sodium channels.

Table 30-2 Actions of Antidysrhythmic Drugs per Vaughn-Williams Classification

V-W Class	Mechanism of Action	Effect on Ionic Channels	Effect on Action Potential	Examples	Use-Dependence	Dysrhythmia*	Pro-dysrhythmia	Inotropic Effect
IA	Sodium channel blocker	Prolongs open/active state	Slows phase zero depolarization– prolonging depolarization	Quinidine Procainamide	Reverse use-dependence	Atrial fibrillation Ventricular dysrhythmia	Torsades de pointes Infranodal block	Negative inotropic effect
IB	Sodium channel blocker	Prolongs open/active state Shortens inactive state	Slows phase zero depolarization Shortens phase 3 repolarization – effectively shortening repolarization	Lidocaine Phenytoin	Use-dependence	Ventricular dysrhythmia	Infranodal block	Negative inotropic effect
IC	Sodium channel blocker	Prolongs open/active state	Greatly slows phase zero depolarization – little effect on repolarization	Encainide+	Use-dependence	AV nodal re-entry WPW-related	Torsades de pointes	
II	Beta-receptor blocker Calcium channel blocker	Prolongs open/active state	Supresses phase 4 depolarization	Propanolol Metoprolol	Reverse use-dependence	Atrial fibrillation WPW ventricular dysrhythmia	AV block	Depress left ventricle function
III	Potassium channel blocker	Prolongs inactive state	Prolongs phase 3 repolarization	Amiodarone Breytlium	Reverse use-dependence	Atrial fibrillation Ventricular dysrhythmia	Torsades de pointes	
IV	Calcium channel blocker	Shortens open/active and inactive states	Shortens entire action potential	Diltiazem Verapamil	Use-dependence	AV nodal re-entry Atrial fibrillation	AV block	Negative intropic effect

Quinidine may be most noted for its ability to create profound hypotension. Dubbed the "Quinidine effect," Class IA drugs all tend to lower blood pressure through massive vasodilatation created by an alpha-sympathetic blockade. Other Class IA drugs include procainamide and disopyramide, which both have similar drug effects to a lesser or greater degree.

Procainamide saw a great deal of use in the out-of-hospital setting for the treatment of ventricular dysrhythmias in the 1970s and 1980s. However, it has fallen out of favor as more effective drugs, with fewer side effects, have since become available.

Class IB

Lidocaine is the prototypical drug for Class IB agents. Lidocaine inhibits fast sodium channels, like Class IA drugs, but does not block the potassium channels. The result is a shorter repolarization time. Without a prolonged depolarization–repolarization cycle, represented by a prolonged QT interval, there is less opportunity for torsades de pointes to occur.

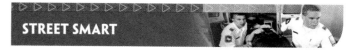

STREET SMART

The effects of Class I drugs on nervous tissues makes them useful as local anesthetics. Lidocaine and procaine (the source of procainamide) alter nerve conduction and thus change the patient's pain perception.

Lidocaine has been extensively used for the treatment of ischemia-induced ectopy. During periods of ischemia, the speed of ionic exchange in the myocardial tissues is impaired. The result is a longer action potential and occasional spontaneous depolarizations, called after-potentials, which can create ventricular ectopy and induce ventricular fibrillation.

Class IB drugs, such as lidocaine, preferentially block the sodium channels of ischemic tissues, preventing spontaneous depolarizations. Lidocaine has seen a great deal of use in the treatment of ventricular fibrillation during cardiac arrest.

Lidocaine is almost immediately metabolized by the liver, via first pass biotransformation, and therefore must be continuously infused intravenously. Understandably, patients with liver dysfunction, such as the elderly, are at greater risk for toxicity.

Class IC

Class IC agents block sodium channels, as do the other Class I agents. Class IC drugs also have the added effect of slowing conduction in all cardiac tissues, including the Purkinje fibers.

Use of Class IC drugs, particularly flecainide, presents a therapeutic quandary. On the one side, Class IC drugs are very effective in the treatment of refractory ventricular dysrhythmia. On the other side are the results of the Cardiac Arrhythmia Suppression Trial, which showed a two-fold increase in mortality for patients on the drug.[85] Class IC agents are now prescribed for very limited circumstances to patients without a history of myocardial infarction where the benefits are thought to outweigh the risk.

Class II Drugs

Class II agents block the sympathetic nervous system's stimulation of beta receptors in the heart. At first glance, inclusion of beta-blockers in the Vaughn-Williams schema would appear inconsistent with the other classes of antidysrhythmic drugs. Other antidysrhythmic drugs in the Vaughn-Williams classification depend on blocking electrolyte channels in the cell wall membrane. Beta-blockers also block electrolyte channels. Beta-blockers work indirectly on electrolyte channels in the cell wall membrane by inhibiting the chemical messenger, which opens calcium channels.

The heart has abundant beta$_1$ receptors; about 85% of the sympathetic receptors within the heart are of the beta$_1$ type. The direct effect of stimulating a beta$_1$ adrenergic receptor is to cause a series of messenger proteins, such as cyclic AMP, to stimulate calcium channel opening. Increased calcium in the myocardium increases the strength of contraction (a positive inotropic effect) and thereby improves cardiac output.

Open calcium channels also have a number of other associated electrophysiologic effects. These include increased automaticity of the SA node with accelerated conduction through the AV node, resulting in the customary tachycardia which accompanies administration of adrenergic agonists. An increase in spontaneous depolarization of ischemic tissue can be seen as well.

A blockade of the beta-adrenergic receptors in the myocardium prevents calcium channels from opening by decreasing the level of cellular cAMP available to open the calcium channels.[86–88] With fewer calcium channels open, the result is an inhibition of spontaneous depolarization during phase 4. In short, beta-blockers prevent firing of ectopic myocardial cells by blocking the beta$_1$ receptors of the sympathetic nervous system in the heart, which could have triggered earlier ectopic beats.

Administration of Class II agents, such as propranolol, blocks the beta$_1$ receptors in a lock-and-key fashion, decreasing intracellular cAMP, and thereby prevents unwanted tachycardia. The prevention of tachycardia and unwanted ectopic beats can be life-saving.

Class II agents can be used to treat hypertension, to prevent angina, as a cardioprotective agent, and to decrease mortality associated with acute coronary syndrome. Thus, beta-blockers are a useful drug for the treatment of patients with risk factors for sudden cardiac death.

Pharmaceutical Properties

The first generation of beta-blockers were relatively nonselective (i.e., blocking both the beta$_1$ receptors, which dominate the heart, as well as the beta$_2$ receptors, which dominate the lungs). Blocking beta$_2$ receptors can result in bronchoconstriction. Therefore, use of these drugs required extreme caution in patients with asthma or similar reactive airway diseases.

The next generation of beta-blockers are more cardioselective, meaning they primarily affect the heart and have a lesser impact on the lungs. Thus, they are safer to use. The newest, third generation of beta-blockers have additional vasodilatory properties which can be helpful in reducing the work of the heart.

Antihypertensive Properties

Beta-blockers exert a powerful antihypertensive effect by blocking the alpha-adrenergic receptors in the peripheral blood vessels, leading to vasodilation and a reduction in peripheral vascular resistance. This is measured crudely by the diastolic blood pressure.

STREET SMART

Sudden withdrawal from beta-blocker medication, a consequence of unpleasant side effects in many cases, can lead to rebound hypertension. Unchecked, the hypertension can increase to the level of a hypertensive crisis during which damage to the eyes, brain, heart, and kidneys can occur.

Antidysrhythmic Properties

Beta-blockers are effective antidysrhythmic agents. These medications are most effective for dysrhythmias caused by errors of automaticity (i.e., abnormal automaticity) or errors of conduction (e.g., Wolff-Parkinson-White syndrome (WPW) or Lown-Ganong-Levine (LGL)). Untreated, these errors in rhythm can lead to hypotension, syncope, and sudden cardiac death.

Beta-blockers indirectly preclude the myocardium from creating errors of impulse generation by preventing sympathetically induced tachycardia. These tachycardias can create a mismatch between the work of the heart and the coronary arteries' ability to supply oxygen-rich blood to the myocardium so the heart can do its work. This mismatch can result in myocardial cell hypoxia, which in turn leads to abnormal depolarization and the formation of ectopic pacemakers.

Extra-cardiac causes of excessive tachycardia include pheochromocytoma, an epinephrine-excreting adrenal tumor, and a thyroid storm (thyrotoxicosis), to name just a few. Regardless of the etiology, beta-blockers prevent tachycardia, which can lead to ventricular irritability.

Beta-blockers can also effectively treat errors of impulse conduction. Errors of impulse conduction are created by either a unidirectional block in the conduction pathway or the presence of an additional accessory pathway (seen in WPW). These errors in conduction create an abnormal conduction mechanism called **reentry phenomenon**.

Under normal conditions, the impulse from the SA node creates an action potential that flows down the conduction system to the base of the bundle branches where the conduction bifurcates into two branches. It is then transmitted across the ventricular myocardium in a wave.

If a segment of the pathway experiences hypoxia and ischemia, or has already been depolarized by an accessory pathway which electrically connects the atrium and the ventricle, then the cells will be unresponsive to stimulation, in effect creating a block. However, when the depolarization wave comes back around to the block from the opposite direction, it can pass this time, in effect making the block unidirectional. Both normal conduction and abnormal conduction are created by ischemia and an accessory pathway (Figure 30-8).

The myocardial cells beyond the block now have had time to recover and can be depolarized, albeit in retrograde fashion. Since the conduction path is now altered, the action potential will continue to depolarize tissue by following a reverse pathway. The consequence can be either localized depolarization and the creation of an ectopic pacemaker, or creation of a circular conduction depolarization (called a circus movement) that can lead to ventricular tachycardia and supraventricular tachycardia.

The impact of beta-blockers on this type of dysrhythmia is to slow conduction so that the SA node can retake dominance. Beta-blockers do not affect either oxygenation of the heart or block accessory pathways such as the one seen in WPW.

Acute Myocardial Infarction

Early administration of beta-blockers during an acute myocardial infarction can reduce the size of infarction, decrease the risk of re-infarction, prevent cardiac rupture, preclude episodes of ventricular tachycardia and supraventricular tachycardia, and prevent sudden cardiac death.[89–93]

Normal

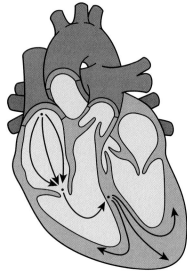

Accessory pathway

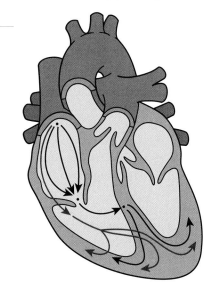

Figure 30-8 Normal conduction and abnormal conduction created an accessory pathway.

This impressive list of cardioprotective effects is owed in large part to the negative chronotropic effect of beta-blockers. By decreasing heart rate (negative chronotropy), beta-blockers create increased diastolic time. The diastolic time is that period in the cardiac cycle when the coronary arteries fill. Increased coronary artery filling directly translates to improved myocardial perfusion.

As an added bonus, beta-blockers also dilate the peripheral blood vessels, creating a reduction in the resistance against which the heart must pump (afterload) and the total work of the heart.

Early administration of beta-blockers, within the first four hours of onset of the suspected myocardial infarction, holds the greatest promise for decreasing mortality (according to one study, a decrease by 15% in the first week).[63]

When administered within the first four hours, infarction size can be reduced by as much as 30% and the risk of re-infarction of reperfused myocardium strikingly reduced. Those patients who received beta-blockers within the first two hours of symptom onset had a 61% reduction in six-week mortality in another study.[94]

These findings lend support to the concept that beta-blockers should be administered as early as possible. Some Paramedics routinely administer beta-blockers when confronted with a patient who is suspected of having an acute myocardial infarction as evidenced by history and 12-lead ECG.

Electrical Storm

Patients with a recent myocardial infarction can be prone to multiple recurrent episodes of ventricular fibrillation (V. Fib.) called an **electrical storm**. Treating patients with electrical storm conventionally (with standard Advanced Cardiac Life Support [ACLS]) has produced uniformly poor outcomes.

A trial of patients with electrical storm, for whom beta-blockers were used after successful conversion of ventricular fibrillation, has shown promise. A remarkable increase in survival in the study group was shown (5% with traditional ACLS versus 67% with a beta-blocker).[95]

Heart Failure

Traditionally, healthcare providers avoided the use of beta-blockers in the treatment of heart failure patients, fearing that the hypotension sometimes created by beta-blockers would aggravate the already failing heart.

In a recent international study which enrolled over 4,000 patients, beta-blockers have shown new promise in treating chronic heart failure. Patients with heart failure subsequent to acute myocardial infarction who are treated with carefully titrated beta-blockers evidence a slower progression in heart failure and an overall 35% decrease in mortality.[96]

However, beta-blockers are still considered potentially harmful (Class III) in acute pulmonary edema and should not be used in the field unless under direct orders of a medical control physician.[77]

Therapeutic Keystone

The benefits of decreased heart rate and blood pressure (which in turn decreases myocardial oxygen demand) and the advantage of enhanced coronary artery blood flow produced by a beta-blockade combine to improve myocardial perfusion and decrease associated mortality and morbidity.

For these reasons, the American Heart Association and the American College of Cardiology have made administration of beta-blockers in acute myocardial infarction a Class I intervention, which is defined as conditions for which there is evidence and/or general agreement that a given procedure or treatment is beneficial, useful, and effective (Table 30-3).

Table 30-3 American Heart Association and American College of Cardiology Guidelines for the Management of Patients with Acute Myocardial Infarction—Use of Beta-Blockers

Class 1
1. Acute myocardial infarction
   a. Within 12 hours of onset of infarction
   b. Without contraindication to beta-blocker therapy for example
      i. Active heart failure
      ii. Asthma/COPD
      iii. bradycardia
   c. Non ST-segment elevation (Confirmed by enzyme tests)
2. Recurrent chest pain
   a. Unstable angina
3. Tachyarrhythmia
   a. Atrial fibrillation with a rapid ventricular response

Contraindications

Beta-blockers should be administered cautiously in patients who are diabetics prone to hypoglycemia, have unstable asthma, or have chronic obstructive pulmonary disease, for the reasons that were previously described.

Beta-blockers have to be administered cautiously, if at all, in cases of cocaine-induced tachycardia, with or without chest pain.[97-99] Cocaine prevents the re-uptake of the neurotransmitter epinephrine, creating an overload of epinephrine in the synaptic junction. By blocking the beta-adrenergic receptors only, cocaine's effect on alpha-adrenergic receptors is unimpeded and profound hypertension from peripheral vasoconstriction can occur.

Toxicity

Beta-blocker toxicity can be absolute, as in the case of an overdose, or relative, as in the case of a patient with a pre-existing heart block that results in a worsening of the heart block. The immediate impact of beta-blocker toxicity is a profound bradycardia with all of its attendant complications. In many cases, the administration of atropine, a parasympathetic blocker, is effective in restoring a tolerable heart rate.

In cases where atropine is ineffective, such as in a ventricular bradycardia secondary to complete heart block, then transcutaneous external pacing may be used. To mitigate the discomfort created by external pacing, many providers premedicate the patient with an analgesic.

Frequently, hypotension is a complication of bradycardia. Added hypotension created by analgesics would only compound the situation. In those cases, glucagon may be administered. Glucagon bypasses the beta-adrenergic receptors and stimulates the formation of cyclic AMP (cAMP) directly. This in turn increases the intercellular calcium, creates stronger contractions, and improves conduction, particularly within the calcium-sensitive AV node.

In extreme cases, when none of the aforementioned treatments are effective or they are contraindicated, then high-dose dobutamine can be used to overcome the competitive blockade.

Class III Drugs

When the sodium channels are all open, at the end of phase zero, the cell is incapable of being further stimulated and is said to be refractory to stimulation. This period of time corresponds with the first one-half of the T wave of an ECG.

The exodus of potassium from the cell marks the start of the repolarization, or phase 1 of the action potential. The speed of repolarization is a function of local conditions at the cellular level (acidity, hypoxia, etc.) as well as the order of depolarization. Therefore, each cell repolarizes at a slightly different rate.

Some repolarized myocardial cells are vulnerable to reactivation. Thus, the myocardial tissue is said to be relatively refractory (the second one-half of the T wave). A strong stimulus (e.g., from a late depolarizing ectopic focus) can initiate a premature second action potential during this vulnerable period. The result can be a chaotic depolarization of myocardial cells (recorded as ventricular fibrillation on the ECG) or creation of a unidirectional block, setting the stage for a circus movement.

Class III drugs prolong the absolute refractory time of myocardial tissues by blocking the potassium channels and decrease the incidence of early depolarizations. Class III drugs are also taken up more quickly by normal cells than by ischemic cells, demonstrating a reverse use-dependence. As a result of a prolonged refractory period of normal myocardial cells secondary to reverse use-dependence, slower ischemic myocardial cells can depolarize without danger of initiating a second ectopic action potential.

The effect of Class III drugs upon the action potential can be observed by the lengthened QT interval on the ECG, the visible demonstration of the depolarization–repolarization time. In a small population, the prolonged QT produced by Class III drugs can precipitate torsades de pointes.[100,101] This complication of treatment is more common in patients with low blood potassium, possibly secondary to use of a potassium-wasting diuretic like furosemide. Torsades, as it is more commonly referred to, appears similar to ventricular tachycardia on the ECG. This similarity can lead to disastrous consequences as ventricular tachycardia erroneously treated with Class III drugs can further worsen the patient's condition.

Indications

Class III drugs can be thought of as "wide-spectrum" anti-dysrhythmics, effective in treating both atrial and ventricular dysrhythmia. Amiodarone, for example, prolongs the refractory period of all cardiac conductive tissues and therefore is effective in treating atrial fibrillation, atrial flutter, and WPW, as well as ventricular tachydysrhythmia.[102]

Amiodarone does not exhibit the reverse use-dependence that is common with other drugs in this class. Amiodarone also exhibits some Class I and II qualities as well, making its exact mechanism of action more difficult to establish. However, its predominant effect is on the duration of the action potential.

Amiodarone has received a great deal of attention for its reported effectiveness during ventricular fibrillation or ventricular tachycardia. The ARREST study (Amiodarone in the Out-of-Hospital Resuscitation of Refractory Sustained Ventricular Tachyarrhythmias), published in the *New England Journal of Medicine*, seemed to demonstrate that patients receiving amiodarone during cardiac arrest are more likely to survive until arrival at the hospital. However, the study did not have the statistical power to detect differences in survival to discharge from the hospital.[103]

Based on the power of this study, the American Heart Association (AHA) has given amiodarone a Class IIb recommendation (possibly helpful) in its Advanced Cardiac Life Support (ACLS) guidelines.

The ALIVE trial (Amiodarone vs Lidocaine in Prehospital Refractory Ventricular Fibrillation Evaluation) seems to indicate the superiority of amiodarone over lidocaine in the treatment of out-of-hospital cardiac arrest due to ventricular fibrillation or ventricular tachycardia.[104]

Class IV Drugs

Free calcium, released from within the cells via calcium channels during depolarization, binds with troponin and initiates muscular contraction (excitation-contraction coupling). There are two types of calcium channels in myocardial and smooth muscle: L-type (long-lasting) and T-type (transient). L-type calcium channels are more abundant in the heart and calcium channel blockers predominantly affect L-type calcium channels.

The different effects of calcium channel blockers upon the heart are owed to the various types of tissues within the heart and give rise to the therapeutic benefits of calcium channel blockers during coronary artery syndrome. Calcium channel blockers are also effective antihypertensive agents. These drugs inhibit the contraction of the smooth muscle found within the middle layer, the tunica media, of blood vessels. The result is widespread vasodilation in the peripheral circulation. Peripheral vasodilation reduces peripheral vascular resistance, crudely measured as diastolic pressure, and lowers the blood pressure. This reduction in afterload decreases the work of the heart as well. As a group, calcium channel blockers are well-tolerated and have fewer side effects than other antihypertensive agents, such as beta-blockers.

Calcium channel blockers are also effective anti-anginal agents. The pain of the ischemic heart (i.e., angina) is the result of a mismatch between blood supply (usually from compromised coronary arteries) and demand (from an overtaxed heart). The combination of peripheral vasodilation (reduced afterload, which in turn reduces the work of the heart) and local coronary artery vasodilation re-establishes the balance between myocardial supply and demand and eliminates angina.

Perhaps the most important use of calcium channel blockers is as an antidysrhythmic drug which decreases automaticity. The effect of calcium on the cardiac conduction is dissimilar to the effect of calcium upon muscle. In the muscle, calcium combines with troponin to create a contraction. In the cardiac conduction, calcium is part of the depolarization–repolarization cycle. Specifically, depolarization is generated by the inward flow of calcium during phase zero.

Portions of the cardiac conduction system that are especially sensitive to increased calcium are the SA node (resulting in increased automaticity) and the AV node (resulting in increased conduction).

Calcium channel blockers decrease the automaticity of the SA node, resulting in a slower heart rate (negative chronotropic effect). Calcium channel blockers also decrease the conductivity across the AV node, resulting in slower conduction in the AV node (negative dromotropic effect). The combination of a slower heart rate and slowed conduction to the ventricles creates an overall reduction in the number of contractions. These effects make class IV agents, the calcium channel blockers, the preferred antidysrhythmic agents for specific dysrhythmias such as supraventricular tachycardia.

Contraindications

Calcium channel blockers are particularly effective in the calcium-sensitive AV node. However, any calcium channel blocker can worsen a pre-existing AV heart block and therefore should be given with extreme caution to patients with pre-existing AV nodal disease or sick sinus syndrome. Calcium channel blockers can also interact with beta-blockers to create extreme bradycardias.

Digitalis, a medication prescribed for heart failure, has a similar inhibitory effect upon the AV node. The combination of a calcium channel blocker and digitalis can create profound bradycardia and subsequent syncope.

Precautions

The first generation of calcium channel blockers, starting with verapamil (which was developed in Europe in 1963), frequently created profound hypotension, secondary to widespread vasodilation. Second generation calcium channel blockers, including diltiazem (which was developed in Japan), are less likely to create hypotension and are therefore preferred for prehospital use during an emergency.

If life-threatening hypotension does occur, co-administration of calcium gluconate can provide free calcium for improved muscle contraction and a return toward a normal blood pressure. Similarly, profound bradycardia can be treated with the parasympathetic blocker atropine to restore a normal heart rate.

Unclassified Antidysrhythmic Agents

There are a certain number of antidysrhythmic agents which do not fall cleanly into one of the Vaughn-Williams classifications and are therefore presented separately. For example, adenosine, a naturally occurring purine nucleoside, does not fit into the Vaughn-Williams classification system, yet is used to treat certain tachydysrhythmias.

Adenosine affects the nervous system of the heart, yet it is not a neurotransmitter nor is it a hormone. Adenosine is a **neuromodulator**. A neuromodulator is a substance that adjusts, or modulates, the rate of a neuron's discharge. Adenosine's effect is to either increase or decrease cyclic AMP levels, which in turn adjusts calcium levels and influences the strength of contraction.

Adenosine may serve a special protective function in ischemic heart tissue. In normal heart tissue, adenosine stimulates purine receptors (which in turn reduce the inward flow of calcium) and increases the outward flow of potassium during phase 4 (repolarization) of nervous tissue. It thus increases the strength of contraction of heart muscle.

During periods of tissue hypoxia, ischemic cells release cyclic AMP (cAMP) into the interstitial space in the form of adenosine. Free serum adenosine then enters the coronary blood vessels and blocks adrenergic receptors as well as stimulating the release of nitric oxide (NO), the vasodilator thought to be at work in nitroglycerin. This combination of effects creates vasodilatation and increased coronary circulation. However, this vasodilatation is not limited to the heart. When adenosine is given intravenously, it produces a generalized flush and produces hypotension in about 20% of the patient population.

Adenosine also acts to inhibit the effects of epinephrine on the SA node (negative chronotropic effect) and generally slows the conduction (negative dromotropic effect). It is this action which makes adenosine useful as an antidysrhythmic agent.

Adenosine's inhibition of norepinephrine release is so overwhelming that often, following rapid intravenous administration, the heart is rendered momentarily asystolic. The therapeutic goal of adenosine administration in those cases is to stun the entire myocardium so as to permit the SA node to recommence its role as the dominant pacemaker.

Adenosine is particularly effective in treating aberrant conduction over accessory conductive pathways (e.g., the bypass tracts in WPW and LGL) or in preventing a unidirectional block. Unidirectional blocks can, under the right circumstances, create a circus movement within the conduction tract and cause an extreme rate supraventricular tachycardia.

Indications

Adenosine is used to treat supraventricular tachycardias associated with WPW or LGL syndromes as well as a number of other narrow-complex tachycardias. Adenosine is ineffective in treating the rapid ventricular response associated with atrial fibrillation or atrial flutter; errors of automaticity. These conditions involve ectopic pacemakers outside of the normal conductive system and thus are less affected by adenosine.

STREET SMART

A wide-complex tachycardia of unknown origin can present a diagnostic dilemma. The dysrhythmia could be a potentially lethal ventricular tachycardia or it could be an atrial fibrillation in a patient with WPW. Inappropriate treatment can produce less than desired effects. As adenosine is not an effective treatment for ventricular tachycardia, its administration can serve as a diagnostic tool for differentiating the two rhythms and help guide subsequent therapeutic interventions.

Precautions

Adenosine, as a naturally occurring nucleoside, is rapidly taken up by red blood cells and vascular endothelial cells, where it is metabolized into inosine and then uric acid. This metabolism occurs so rapidly (the half-life of adenosine is 5 to 10 seconds) that toxicity is nearly impossible. This rapid

uptake also has implications for intravenous administration. In order for therapeutic levels to be achieved in the heart (the target organ in most cases), adenosine must be given as a rapid bolus via the shortest route to the heart.

Xanthine, a prodrug of respiratory medication aminophylline, causes bronchodilation by blocking adenosine receptors. Foods that commonly contain xanthine compounds include teas and coffee. Higher than normal doses of adenosine may be needed to overcome the competitive blockade produced by the xanthine compounds.

Conversely, adenosine should be administered cautiously to patients with reactive airway diseases, such as asthma, for fear of precipitating a life-threatening bronchospasm.

Vasopressin

Vasopressin, or antidiuretic hormone (ADH), is a naturally occurring peptide created in the posterior lobe of the pituitary gland. Vasopressin was known to have potent vasoconstricting properties at higher doses and has been used to treat diabetes insipidus and bleeding esophageal varices, with varying degrees of success, in the past. However, vasopressin was primarily regarded as a hormone for maintaining water balance in the kidney. Researchers were surprised to find elevated levels of vasopressin in survivors of cardiac arrest.[105] Upon closer examination, medical researchers felt that vasopressin might have some theoretical advantages over epinephrine in cardiac arrest.

Epinephrine is traditionally considered the drug of choice in cardiac arrest because it increases the strength of contraction, or in the case of ventricular fibrillation, it coarsens the fibrillation and thereby improves the chance of success with defibrillation. Epinephrine also raises peripheral vascular resistance, thereby increasing backflow into the coronary arteries and improving cerebral circulation. On the other hand epinephrine, particularly high-dose epinephrine, increases the oxygen demand—as well as the demand for ATP—at a time when the heart is depleted.[106] Epinephrine also appears to adversely affect pulmonary function during cardiac arrest, by shunting blood away from the lungs to the heart and brain.[105]

In fact, currently no research exists which suggests that epinephrine administration increases survival. Several uncontrolled studies indicate that epinephrine administration during cardiac arrest negatively correlates with survival to discharge.[107] However, until better studies are available, epinephrine remains in the standard guidelines for management of cardiac arrest.[108]

Vasopressin increases vascular tone and perfusion pressures, like epinephrine, but does not have the associated negative catecholamine-induced effects of increased heart rate and oxygen consumption which are seen with epinephrine. Vasopressin has a relatively long half-life and therefore need only be administered once in order to achieve therapeutic levels. Early research findings seem to indicate better patient survival when vasopressin is administered along with epinephrine every three to five minutes.[109]

A large out-of-hospital clinical trial is needed before it can be definitively stated that vasopressin is of greater benefit than epinephrine in cardiac arrest.

Cholinergic Blocking Agents

Cholinergic blocking agents, as a class, were discussed earlier. However, atropine, a specific parasympathetic blocking agent commonly used to treat symptomatic bradycardia, is now revisited.

Atropine blocks the parasympathetic neurotransmitter acetylcholine at the muscarinic receptors. This effectively diminishes the influence of the primary parasympathetic nerve, the vagus nerve (vagal tone), and permits the sympathetic nervous system to re-establish dominance over the heart's rate. Excessive vagal tone is often seen in cases of AV node ischemia secondary to occlusion of the right coronary artery, as occurs during an inferior wall myocardial infarction. The ensuing bradycardia can be treated effectively with atropine. However, increasing tissue demands within the AV node at a time when the tissues are ischemic may accelerate damage and lead to an infarction of the AV node, resulting in complete heart block. The decision to use atropine in the setting of an AMI must be made with caution.

STREET SMART

Profound hypoxia produces pupillary dilation. During a cardiac arrest, providers often check pupillary response to assess the effectiveness of cardiopulmonary resuscitation. Atropine dilates pupils, thus rendering this sign inaccurate.

Heart Failure

Heart failure is the heart's inability to pump enough blood to meet the body's demands. The result is hypoperfusion of vital organs and potentially the onset of a shock syndrome. Heart failure affects over 4 million people in the United States and is the most common hospital discharge diagnosis in patients over the age of 65.[110,111]

Heart failure can be divided into two categories: systolic heart failure and diastolic heart failure. Systolic heart failure is the condition in which the heart cannot pump adequate amounts of blood into the circulation. The result can either be forward failure (a loss of cardiac output and systolic blood pressure) or backward failure (a retrograde buildup of pressure that is transmitted to the low pressure lung fields and creates pulmonary congestion and pulmonary edema). Frequently, this left-sided heart failure progresses through the right ventricle and into the systemic venous circulation.

Causes of systolic heart failure include loss of contractile strength secondary to acute myocardial infarction or an obstruction in the outflow from the heart due to valve disease.

Diastolic heart failure is that condition in which the heart has difficulty filling properly and there is subsequent loss of cardiac output. Causes of diastolic heart failure include remodeling of the ventricular chamber secondary to chronic hypertension, obesity, and systolic heart failure.

The pathophysiology of heart failure begins with a loss of cardiac output, from whatever cause, which stimulates the baroreceptors. The baroreceptors in turn increase sympathetic discharge (epinephrine) to adjust for the volume difference and maintain perfusion of vital organs.

Sympathetic stimulation has a two-fold impact. First, stimulation of alpha-adrenergic receptors preferentially vasoconstricts peripheral vascular beds, effectively shunting blood to core organs, as well as increasing the amount of blood returned to the heart (preload). With the ventricles now "overfilled," Starling's law dictates that the ventricle will contract more forcefully and the stroke volume will increase.[112]

Sympathetic stimulation also increases the heart rate (positive chronotropic effect) as well as strength of contraction (positive inotropic effect).

The combination of increased stroke volume and increased heart rate should result in improved cardiac output (SV x HR = CO). This is the body's normal response to hypovolemia. The difficulty lies not in the blood's volume but in the heart's inability to pump that volume.

Alpha-adrenergic stimulation from epinephrine excreted secondary to hypotension increases the systemic vascular resistance (the afterload) against which the heart must pump. This "afterload mismatch" causes blood to back up into the pulmonary circuit, resulting in pulmonary congestion and edema. Elevated pressure is transmitted across the pulmonary circuit and through the right ventricle back into the systemic circulation, creating peripheral edema.

The kidneys, now underperfused, activate the renin-angiotensin-aldosterone mechanism, a tri-axis of hormones which combine to preserve blood volume. This results in more fluid retention, further increasing the work of the overtaxed heart.

In an effort to compensate, the heart dilates to accept more blood and the muscle fibers thicken, a process called hypertrophy, in order to pump more forcefully. Along with a sustained tachycardia secondary to persistent sympathetic stimulation, the heart is able to compensate, sometimes for years.

The dual effect of dilation and hypertrophy upon the left ventricle slowly changes the shape of the interior chamber, called **remodeling**, into a less effective configuration. The remodeled chamber can no longer fill properly and diastolic heart failure ensues.

When the heart reaches the point where it can no longer compensate and overcome the increasing demands put upon it, the heart enters the descending limb of the Frank-Starling curve and cardiac output falls. In 1918, Frank and Starling advanced the idea that the force of the heart's contraction is proportional to the length of the muscle fibers, which are increased with increased ventricular filling. When the myocardial fibers can no longer stretch, then the muscle loses contractile strength (the backside of the curve). The pharmaceutical goals in heart failure are essentially twofold: reduce the preload and provide inotropic support to the failing heart.

Angiotensin-Converting Enzyme (ACE) Inhibitors

Baroreceptors in the kidneys, sensing a low flow state due to reduced arterial pressure caused by heart failure, release the enzyme renin. Renin is converted into angiotensin through a number of steps.

Angiotensin has a number of physiologic effects. Angiotensin stimulates the production of aldosterone in the adrenal cortex. Aldosterone, a mineralocorticoid, promotes the excretion of potassium by the kidney in exchange for retaining sodium and thus water. Angiotensin also stimulates the secretion of vasopressin, which in turn causes peripheral vasoconstriction and increased peripheral vascular resistance. Perhaps most importantly, angiotensin is a potent vasoconstrictor in itself. It is 40 times more potent than norepinephrine in causing peripheral vasoconstriction.

The conversion of renin into angiotensin depends on an enzyme called angiotensin-converting enzyme (ACE). ACE inhibitors, such as captopril, oppose the conversion of renin to angiotensin and thus upset the renin-angiotensin-aldosterone

mechanism (Figure 30-9). This is an effective treatment for hypertension in many patients.

ACE inhibitors are seeing greater use in heart failure patients as they appear to not only interrupt the renin-angiotensin-aldosterone mechanism, thereby preventing fluid retention, but they also control hypertension and thus reduce the work of the heart. They are also effective in reversing left ventricular systolic dysfunction. Long-term use of ACE inhibitors have been shown to improve survival of even severe heart failure patients by returning the heart to its original condition.[113]

Therapeutic Approaches to Heart Failure

Hippocrates advanced the idea that the four humors, including blood, had to be in balance in order to maintain good health. When the body was swollen (e.g., from heart failure), then it was thought that blood had to be released from the body to restore balance. For centuries, first monks, and then barber-surgeons, continued the practice of bloodletting to relieve "dropsy," the term used for heart failure. Leeches replaced the lancet in the 1800s, but the practice continued. In fact, the word "leech" comes from the Old English "laece" which means physician.[114] Even George Washington was bled by Dr. Benjamin Rush. Washington's leeching is thought to have been a contributing cause to his death. While this treatment may appear to be barbaric by today's standards, it nevertheless was effective for treating heart failure in some instances.

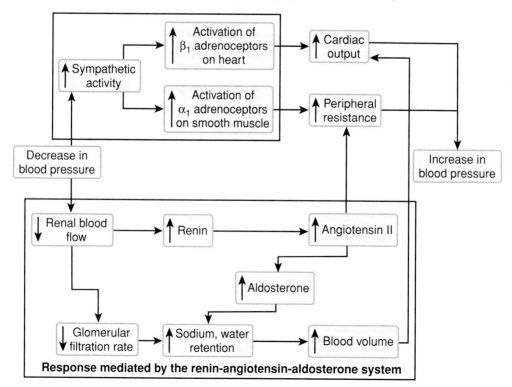

Figure 30-9 Afterload mismatch.

As primitive as these early interventions may have seemed, subsequent pharmaceutical approaches to heart failure have used the same tactic—reduce the volume of blood in order to decrease the work of the heart and allow the heart to function more efficiently.

The reduction of blood can occur in two ways: either removal of fluid from the circulation via the kidney (diuresis) or relocation of fluid into other compartments (vasodilation).

Diuresis

Approximately 20% of the blood entering the kidney's glomerular process diffuses its water and solutes (salts in solution) into the Bowman's capsule of the kidney's nephron. Only the formed elements, such as red blood cells and plasma proteins, are held back. The water and plasma solutes, now called filtrate, pass through the different portions of the nephron and are reabsorbed to go back into the circulation. In an average day the kidney will filter 180 liters of blood but only produce one to two liters of urine.

The reabsorption of water and salts occurs in various portions of the nephron. Approximately 65% of the water—as well as bicarbonate, glucose, and two-thirds of the sodium—is reabsorbed in the proximal tubule (Figure 30-10).

The proximal tubule is also the site of absorption of organic acids, such as uric acid, and metabolites of medications. The remaining filtrate passes into the loop of Henle. The cells lining the narrow ascending loop of Henle are extraordinary because they are watertight (i.e., impermeable to water). This section of the nephron actively reabsorbs chloride and sodium. To this point the exchange has been unregulated.

The remaining 15% of filtrate which remains now enters the distal convoluted tubule. The regulation of potassium and sodium reabsorption in this portion of the nephron is controlled by aldosterone.

The remaining filtrate, now called urine, is passed into the collecting duct. Vasopressin, or antidiuretic hormone (ADH), regulates the final reabsorption of water in this portion of the nephron. The process of renal filtration is complete with 99.2% of the filtrate returned to the central circulation

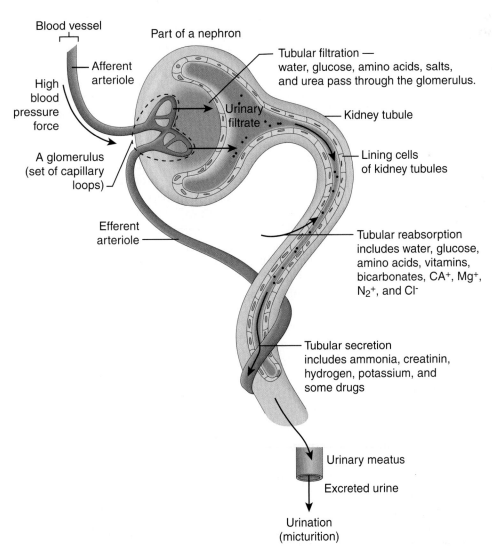

Figure 30-10 Cross-section of nephron.

and the remainder, the urine, being sent to the bladder via the ureters to be excreted.

Diuretic Agents

The creation of urine is controlled by the pressure of the blood entering the kidney, which in turn is controlled (in part) by the sympathetic nervous system, and the concentration of the salts in the blood, as well as the ADH level.

Each class of diuretics affects a different portion of the kidney's nephron and therefore has a slightly different effect on diuresis. Carbonic anhydrase inhibitors affect water reabsorption in the proximal convoluted tubule, whereas the loop diuretics and the thiazides affect the loop of Henle. Finally, the potassium-sparing diuretics affect the distal convoluted tubule.

Regardless of the affected portion of the nephron, all medications which cause the increased loss of fluid and salts from the body are called **diuretics**. This loss of fluid volume decreases the amount of circulating blood volume and ultimately decreases the work of the heart. Therefore, the universal goal of diuretic therapy is to reduce the work of the heart and permit the heart to function more efficiently.

Proximal Tubule Diuretics

The enzyme carbonic anhydrase mediates the acid and bicarbonate reaction that creates water and carbon dioxide (H+ $HCO_3 = H_2O + CO_2$) in the blood. In the sodium bicarbonate and acid reaction, carbonic anhydrase inhibitors hold onto a hydrogen ion in exchange for a sodium ion that is subsequently secreted by the kidneys. As a matter of principle, water follows salt, and water is also excreted.

Carbonic anhydrase inhibitors include acetazolamide (a sulfonamide without antibacterial properties). In comparison to loop diuretics, carbonic anhydrase inhibitors are a weak class of diuretics which are used in very limited cases. For example, mountain climbers who hike above 10,000 feet are prone to high-altitude pulmonary edema (HAPE) and high-altitude cerebral edema (HACE).[115,116] Acetazolamide is sometimes prescribed to climbers to prevent HACE and HAPE. The exact mechanism of action is unknown but is thought to be associated with the mild metabolic acidosis created by the drug and the resulting deeper respirations which occur during the mountaineer's sleep.

Loop Diuretics

Loop diuretics, as a class, inhibit the reabsorption of the electrolytes: sodium, potassium, calcium, and magnesium, as well as water in the ascending loop of Henle. This portion of the nephron is largely responsible for the concentration of urine electrolytes and subsequent volume of urine. Loop diuretics are very effective and have a rapid onset of action. For these reasons, loop diuretics are often preferred in an emergency. Furosemide is an example of a commonly used medication in this class.

Bumetanide, another loop diuretic, also blocks the reabsorption of chloride in the proximal tubule. This dual effect makes bumetanide more potent than furosemide. This second site of action makes bumetanide effective for patients who are resistant to furosemide.

Precautions

Patients without prior experience with diuretics may unpredictably experience a diuresis of large quantities of urine. The result can be severe hypovolemia, hypoperfusion, and frank shock. In those cases, gentle rehydration with intravenous solutions, such as Ringer's lactate, can re-establish lost volume and restore the blood pressure.

Overly aggressive treatment of congestive heart failure, usually manifested by pulmonary edema, can also lead to even greater problems in the care of the patient over the long term. When confronted with a patient with pulmonary edema, Paramedics may be inclined to think that the patient is fluid overloaded. More accurately, these patients are fluid misplaced. That is, the blood is being sequestered in the venous circulation (venous pool) and is putting pressure on the failing heart to pump it forward. There are two treatment pathways to relieve this condition. First, the Paramedic can cause a diuresis which will in turn reduce the blood volume returning to the heart. Alternatively, the Paramedic can increase the venous pool's capacitance, temporarily relieving the heart's burden and allowing it to recover.

The classic diuretic for the treatment of acute pulmonary edema has been furosemide. Prompt treatment with furosemide will provide the patient with immediate relief of symptoms.[117,118] This relief is due to the two-fold action of furosemide. Furosemide's immediate effect is as a vasodilator. Within five minutes of administration, furosemide reduces the heart's work by reducing the preload through vasodilation, increasing the venous pool capacitance. Following the vasodilatation, within 20 minutes of the onset of action furosemide causes diuresis. This diuresis removes fluid from the central circulation and reduces the heart's work.

Patients in acute heart failure are not suffering from being fluid-overloaded. More correctly, the blood volume is improperly distributed, leading to an input–output mismatch. Vasodilator therapy may be more beneficial to the patient in the long run. More discussion about vasodilator therapy follows.

Potassium, an important cardiac electrolyte, is closely associated with sodium. As loop diuretics cause the excretion of sodium, they also cause a loss of potassium, earning them the label "potassium wasters." Serious potentially life-threatening cardiac dysrhythmias can follow the development of low serum potassium or **hypokalemia**. For this reason, potassium supplements are often co-prescribed to patients on loop diuretics. True toxicity from loop diuretics is rare. For example, patients have been given 2,000 mg of furosemide without toxic effect. This "high ceiling" makes these diuretics relatively safe to administer.

Osmotic Diuretics

Any substance with a large molecular weight which cannot pass through a semipermeable membrane will create an osmotic effect. The presence of formed elements and blood proteins, such as albumin, in the bloodstream creates an osmotic effect. This effect, called colloidal osmotic pressure (COP), occurs because these large molecules cannot pass through the blood vessel walls.

Similarly, when chemicals with a large molecular weight (i.e., heavy molecules) pass into the filtrate via the fenestrated membranes within the kidney (a very forgiving membrane that is 100 to 400 times more permeable than ordinary capillaries) and travel to the loop of Henle to encounter a semipermeable membrane, they are entrapped. However, these heavy molecules continue to create an osmotic effect and thus draw fluids into the filtrate.

Examples of heavy molecules that are effective osmotic diuretics include mannitol (a complex sugar) and urea. Osmotic diuretics are used to reduce edema in special cases; for example, mannitol is used to treat increased intracranial pressure secondary to cerebral edema. Osmotic diuretics are also used to prevent kidney failure by forcing a continuous diuresis.

Caution must be exercised whenever osmotic diuretics are administered. Overly aggressive treatment can result in hypovolemia (leading to hypoperfusion and shock), hypokalemia (leading to ventricular dysrhythmias), and hyponatremia (leading to seizures).

Distal Tubule Diuretics

The thiazides were one of the first diuretics used in medical therapeutics for the treatment of heart failure. As sulfonamide derivatives, the thiazides also work like carbonic anhydrase inhibitors. However, they work in the distal tubule instead of the proximal tubule.

Thiazides inhibit the reabsorption of sodium and therefore increase the excretion of sodium in the urine. The urine, now hyperosmolar, collects more water as it passes through the tubules. Thiazides also increase the excretion of potassium along with the sodium.

Indications for thiazides, such as hydrochlorothiazide, include relief from mild to moderate heart failure as well as the treatment of mild to moderate hypertension. Thiazides are often preferred as a treatment for hypertension because they are inexpensive (a benefit for patients on a fixed income), easy to administer, and have fewer side effects than other diuretics.

Thiazides are also potassium wasters and have the same precautions as other potassium wasters. Potassium depletion can, for example, predispose a patient to a number of dysrhythmias.

Potassium-Sparing Diuretics

Potassium-sparing diuretics are particularly attractive for use in patients who are sensitive to hypokalemia (e.g., patients on digitalis) or patients who require a diuretic therapy but who cannot tolerate potassium supplements. Unfortunately, potassium-sparing diuretics, as a class, are weak diuretics. To improve their efficiency, as well as maintain the advantage of preserving potassium, they are often given in combination with the thiazides.

Several agents (e.g., amiloride and triamterene) work indirectly in the distal tubule, while spironolactone works by blocking the effects of aldosterone in the distal tubule. As a result of these two actions, sodium and water are excreted and potassium is retained.

Spironolactone, as an aldosterone-antagonist, also has a secondary use in the treatment of hyperaldosteronism, an adrenal disease.

Vasodilator Therapy

Certain vasodilators work on the same mechanism as nitrates, thereby creating a direct vasodilation in the blood vessels. Since a larger portion of blood and blood vessels is on the venous side of the central circulation, the venous side is more affected. This causes a drop in the venous pressure and therefore the amount of preload the heart receives.

Alternatively, other vasodilators create relaxation of the muscle within the vessel walls, resulting in dilation. Since arteries and arterioles have more muscle than veins and venules, these medications have a more pronounced effect on the arterial side of the central circulation. Arterial vasodilation directly translates to lowered diastolic pressure, reduced peripheral vascular resistance, and a reduction in cardiac afterload.[119]

Afterload Reduction

The arteriole beds are largely controlled by the alpha receptors of the sympathetic nervous system. Alpha-receptor antagonists prevent vasoconstriction and the resulting increases in peripheral vascular resistance (afterload) that occur as a result of vasoconstriction. An example of an alpha-blocker is hydralazine, a current and commonly used alpha-blocker.

The difficulty with using alpha-blockers lies in the sympathetic nervous system's response to the decrease in diastolic pressure. The baroreceptors reflexively stimulate the sympathetic nervous system to increase the blood pressure. This is achieved via peripheral vasoconstriction, now inhibited by the alpha-blockers, and tachycardia. This tachycardia can tax the already overtaxed heart and induce ischemia. To prevent this reflexive tachycardia, a beta-blocker is often given in combination with the alpha-blocker in an effort to balance the effects of each.

Other arterioles affecting antihypertensives work directly upon the smooth muscles in the arteriole walls. These agents, usually administered intravenously, are very effective in reducing peripheral vascular resistance (the diastolic blood pressure) and reduce the heart's work.

Unfortunately, the same issue exists for these agents (e.g., diazoxide) as did for the alpha-blockers. Again, beta-blockers are occasionally co-prescribed to balance the effects of each.

Preload Reduction

In the not too distant past, Paramedics used a device called a "rotating tourniquet" to mechanically sequester blood in the periphery. That technique, though fraught with complications, was effective in reducing preload. Today, medications are used to obtain a similar effect.

Nitrates are potent vasodilators, and their main impact is on the venous circulation. Dilating the venous circulation, nitrates increase the "pooling" of blood in the venous circulation and reduce the preload returning to the heart. In essence, nitrates create an "internal phlebotomy" by withholding blood from the central circulation.

A number of long-acting nitrates have been developed for this purpose. Perhaps the earliest long-acting nitrates were oral preparations, such as isosorbide. Isosorbide now comes in extended release capsules, chewable tablets, and sublingual tablets.

To further extend the vasodilator effects, nitrates are also available in transdermal systems. These "patch" systems contain nitrate in a gel-like "reservoir." After the gel melts, the drug passes through the skin and then is absorbed, by passive diffusion, into the bloodstream. There are a number of patch systems on the market and each works in a slightly different manner.

Paramedics often use nitroglycerin paste for the same effect. A ribbon of paste, measured in one-half inch increments, is placed on an impervious paper and placed against the patient's skin. The selection of a site for the paste's placement is important. The paste should be applied to a hairless area, usually on the upper anterior chest, where it is clearly visible. Avoid placing the patch below the knees or elbows. Circulation is frequently poor in these areas and absorption less predictable.

Alternative placement sites include the shoulder or the inside of the upper arm. Some Paramedics will loosely encircle the limb with a plastic wrap to prevent liquefied nitroglycerin paste from dripping.

In every case, it is important to report where the paste was applied when patient care is transferred. Nitroglycerin can induce significant hypotension, in which case the first action should be to remove the paste. Failure to notify other providers of the presence of nitroglycerin paste can lead to inappropriate treatment of the hypotension.

Nitroprusside is an effective intravenous vasodilator that has a greater impact on the venous circulation (preload) than on the arterial circulation (afterload), making it attractive for the treatment of acute heart failure, especially heart failure secondary to valvular regurgitation. Nitroprusside is also used to treat acute hypertensive crisis, an abnormal and potentially life-threatening elevation of blood pressure.

Chemically, nitroprusside contains five cyanide groups bound to nitric acid, the active ingredient in nitroglycerin, within its structure. When the nitric acid breaks off and causes vasodilation, the cyanide remains. The free cyanide is then metabolized into thiosulfate by the liver and excreted harmlessly.

When the level of cyanide exceeds the liver's capacity to detoxify it, then cyanide poisoning can occur. Fortunately, the half-life of nitroprusside is 2.7 days. Cyanide levels can be tested daily to ensure that the patient remains symptom-free.

Nitroprusside infusions are easily identified because the solution container must be protected from light. Therefore, the IV bag is always covered with aluminum foil or another similarly opaque material.

Nitroprusside infusions must be very carefully titrated, typically to the patient's blood pressure, starting at 0.3 micrograms per kilogram of patient's weight per minute (mcg/kg/min). Therefore, nitroprusside infusions are typically placed on an infusion pump.

Cardiac Glycosides

Digitalis is the quintessential cardiac glycoside. One of the few plants that make a steroid similar to animal steroids, digitalis is processed from the foxglove plant. Used for hundreds of years as the "housewife's recipe" for swelling and edema, digitalis did not enter into modern pharmacy until 1876.[120] The story is told of a patient who went to Dr. William Withering, a Scottish physician, with "dropsy" (congestive heart failure) and was diagnosed as incurable. The patient then went to a gypsy who treated him with a secret herbal remedy and he recovered. Intrigued, Dr. Withering sought out the gypsy and bartered for the remedy. The key ingredient in the concoction was the purple foxglove, digitalis purpurea (L).

Digitalis had long been known for its toxicity, having been used by the Romans as rat poison and in medieval "trials by ordeal." However, it was not thought to have many medicinal uses. Dr. Withering made his fortune on the "discovery" of the medicinal uses of digitalis after he recounted its benefits in a treatise entitled, "An Account of Foxglove." In that treatise, he strongly advised that the effects of digitalis on the patient be closely monitored and that it was imperative to individualize the dose and schedule. No wiser words could have been offered as digitalis toxicity is a common impediment to the drug's use.[20]

Mechanism of Action

Digitalis has two unique therapeutic benefits: a slowing of the cardiac conduction, resulting in increased ventricular filling, and increased strength of contraction without the use of additional oxygen. Together, these effects culminate in an overall decrease in the heart's work. This is a desirable situation for the compromised myocardium, as it allows for more efficient functioning.

Digitalis acts by binding to and disabling (blocking) Na+/K+ ATPase, the enzyme that breaks down ATP to release its energy. Without ATP breakdown there is no energy to power the Na+/K+ pump during repolarization. The accumulation of intracellular sodium, which results from the failure of the sodium-potassium pump, leads to an ionic imbalance. Calcium is then exchanged to help maintain that balance.

The slowed depolarization prolongs the cardiac cycle (a negative chronotropic and negative dromotropic effect), leading to reduced heart rate. This maximizes the diastolic potential of Starling's Law, as the slowed heart has more time for ventricular and coronary artery filling.

The heart is further slowed when digitalis inhibits the calcium-sensitive AV node from passing the action potential down the bundle branches to the ventricles. This slowing of AV node conduction can be observed by a lengthening of the PR interval.

The increased calcium also produces more excitation-coupling of actin and myosin in the ventricle's myocardial fibers and a stronger contraction of the now overfilled ventricle. This improvement in the strength of contraction, a positive inotropic effect, is done without consuming additional oxygen.

Electrocardiographically, the digitalis effect can be seen by the prolonged PR interval, the shortened QT interval, and an inverted T wave, the impact of altered repolarization opposite of the major QRS forces (Figure 30-11).

Indications

In the past, a common cause of congestive heart failure was the loss of atrial kick, which contributes approximately 25% of the cardiac output. It also accompanied new onset atrial fibrillation.[121] In this situation, digitalis slows the racing heart, which was trying to compensate for the ventricular filling pressure lost to atrial fibrillation. Slowing the heart rate allowed for more ventricular filling and thus led to an augmented cardiac output. The positive inotropic effect of digitalis can further improve cardiac output to levels that are tolerable for the patient. It should be noted that digitalis does not convert atrial fibrillation back into normal sinus rhythm, but instead merely slows the ventricular response.

Currently, digitalis has been replaced with better Class II and III agents, which slow the heart without the serious side effects and dangers of digitalis toxicity, some of which will be explained shortly. In many cases of atrial fibrillation, the etiology is identified and eliminated (if possible), sometimes by radio ablation therapy in the electrophysiology lab of a cardiac care center.

Digitalis may still have a therapeutic advantage in treating congestive heart failure from other causes. No other single chemotherapeutic agent has the same dual actions—negative chronotropy and positive inotropy—as digitalis.

Precautions

A new-onset atrial fibrillation may mask the tell-tale ECG signs of Wolff-Parkinson-White (WPW) syndrome. Digitalis mistakenly administered in those cases allows uninhibited conduction over the bypass tract, as the AV node conduction is slowed by the digitalis. The resulting antegrade conduction over the bypass tract, in concert with normal conduction down the intra-atrial pathways, can contribute to circus movement and high rate tachycardia, which may eventually deteriorate into ventricular tachycardia/fibrillation.

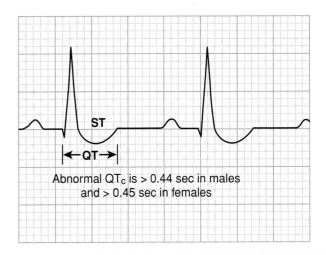

Abnormal QT$_c$ is > 0.44 sec in males and > 0.45 sec in females

Shortened QT interval
Characteristic down-sloping ST depression
Classic scooped-out ST segment

Figure 30-11 The digitalis effect demonstrated on ECG.

Digitalis also has a relative contraindication during heart block. The impact of digitalis upon the calcium-sensitive AV node can further slow conduction through the AV node and aggravate a pre-existing heart block, causing profound bradycardia and hypotension.

Digitalis Toxicity

Digitalis has a narrow therapeutic range. As a result, the incidence of toxicity is fairly high, so much so that between 10% and 20% of nursing home patients receiving digitalis will develop digitalis toxicity during the course of treatment. The early identification and treatment of digitalis toxicity will help to decrease the estimated 34% moderate to severe morbidity associated with digitalis toxicity.

Several conditions contribute to the problem of digitalis toxicity. For one, digitalis is primarily excreted via the kidneys. Therefore, any change in kidney function, such as can occur with heart failure, can cause an increase in digitalis to toxic levels.[122]

Digitalis also affects the sodium-potassium pump. Ordinary doses of digitalis administered to a patient with hypokalemia can result in toxicity. This toxicity is not a true toxicity, but rather a pseudo-toxicity (the relative imbalance between the regular dose and the desired therapeutic effect, which is exaggerated by the hypokalemia). This pseudo-toxicity is sometimes occasioned by the concurrent use of the potassium-wasting diuretic furosemide.

The mechanism of cardiotoxicity relates to the intracellular calcium overload, which results from high levels of digitalis. This increased calcium load has a two-fold effect. First, it increases spontaneous afterdepolarizations in the myocardium. These afterdepolarizations create ectopic beats, including junctional and ventricular extrasystoles. Unabated, the heightened reactivity of the myocardium can lead to junctional tachycardia and ventricular tachycardia/flutter.

Concurrent calcium buildup within the AV node depresses the AV node, causing bradycardia, as low as "35 beats in a minute."[120] It can even create a complete AV block. This ECG manifestation, AV blocks of varying degrees, is seen in 30% to 40% of patients with digitalis toxicity.

Extreme digitalis-induced AV dissociation sets the stage for a rare but potentially lethal phenomenon called "bidirectional tachycardia." Bidirectional tachycardia is the result of concurrent atrial and junctional/ventricular tachycardia with a complete heart block at the AV node.

Signs of Digitalis Toxicity

Initial signs of digitalis toxicity include bradycardia, as well as nausea and diarrhea. The latter symptoms of abdominal distress, visual changes, and general malaise may be misinterpreted by the patient as flu-like symptoms and ignored by the patient. The combination of the losses of potassium from both diarrhea and vomiting only serve to worsen the situation and lead to more nausea, vomiting, and diarrhea.

As the intoxication continues, the patient may experience confusion, which may be misinterpreted as dementia or depression in the elderly. The patient may also complain of seeing yellow-green halos around lights. At this point, significant cardiac manifestations typically occur, including tachycardia-induced syncope.

Overt digitalis overdose, either accidental or otherwise, may be treated emergently with digitalis-specific antibody fragments (digoxin immune fab). Otherwise, treatments focus on the cause of the toxicity: reversing hypoperfusion leading to kidney failure, withdrawal of the numerous drugs which interact negatively with digitalis, or correcting hypokalemia. If the patient is hypokalemic, then potassium replacement is provided. Phenytoin has been found useful in treating digitalis-induced dysrhythmia because of its anticholinergic effects.[123] Administration of magnesium as a competitive ion may be helpful in reducing ventricular ectopy, including ventricular tachycardia/flutter.

Acute Heart Failure

Acute heart failure is a medical emergency that, if untreated, can quickly culminate in death. Acute heart failure can present in several ways. The first syndrome is forward failure, a loss of cardiac output that results in hypotension and rapidly progresses to end-organ failure. The other syndrome is backward failure, a backup of pressures into the low-pressure lung fields which produces acute pulmonary edema. Acute pulmonary edema literally suffocates the lungs, leading to hypoxia and respiratory acidosis.

Backward Failure

The goal of treating backward failure, manifested by acute pulmonary edema, is to quickly reduce the preload. Treatment with diuretics can provide rapid symptomatic relief but can also lead to rebound edema later in the course of the patient's care. This rebound edema is the result of activation of the renin-angiotensin-aldosterone mechanism by the diuresis.

In many cases, these patients are already on diuretics and are not "fluid-overloaded." More correctly, these patients are fluid "maldistributed" and only need temporary relief from excessive preload. Patients at particular risk are those with restrictive cardiomyopathy, early phase acute myocardial infarction, and mild chronic heart failure.

Repeated doses of nitrates may be more effective in these cases. Nitrates will cause immediate venodilation, increasing the volume within the venous pool, and effectively create an internal phlebotomy. That is to say, a portion of blood volume will be temporarily warehoused in the venous circulation (which has a large capacitance) and taken out of the core circulation until the heart can recover.

Forward Failure

Acute forward failure, or cardiogenic shock, is a failure of the heart as a pump. Regardless of the underlying cause of the pump's failure, it is imperative to increase the heart's cardiac output (blood pressure).

The body's own compensatory mechanisms depend on the hormone epinephrine (a catecholamine) to increase the heart rate (positive chronotropy), speed of conduction (dromotropy), and most importantly, the strength of contraction (inotropy). Supporting the body's own compensatory mechanisms, Paramedics can infuse additional sympathomimetics classified as catecholamines: three naturally occurring catecholamines—dopamine, epinephrine, and norepinephrine—plus two synthetic catecholamines—dobutamine and isoproterenol.

These vasopressors, drugs which affect blood vessels directly, increase blood flow to vital organs. However, some are associated with significant side effects and should be used carefully in the patient with acute heart failure.

STREET SMART

Before starting any catecholamine infusion, it is important to rule out hypovolemia as a cause of hypotension. Failure to do so may compromise already ischemic tissue. "Squeezing dry pipes" with vasopressors will not improve blood pressure significantly.

Catecholamines

All catecholamines interact directly with sympathetic receptors throughout the body. Alpha-receptor stimulation will increase vasoconstriction of peripheral capillary beds, increasing blood in the core circulation while also increasing the peripheral vascular resistance the heart must overcome.

Beta-receptors in the heart will both increase the speed of the heart (positive chronotropy) as well as the strength of contraction (positive inotropy) and dilate the bronchial smooth muscle, thereby improving oxygen delivery. However, this comes at a cost of increased work of the heart.

Precautions

Catecholamines are potent medications, so potent that the dose is measured in micrograms (mcg) instead of milligrams (mg). Typically infused intravenously, catecholamines are carefully titrated to a dose of micrograms per kilogram of patient weight per minute of infusion (mcg/kg/min) and often infused via an intravenous pump which can ensure precise delivery.

The patient receiving a catecholamine infusion, in order to sustain an adequate perfusing blood pressure, may be drug-dependent. A sudden interruption in the infusion, for any reason, can result in a precipitous fall in blood pressure. For this reason, most providers ensure the presence of a second intravenous access site for use if the first intravenous access is lost.

Inadvertent infiltration of a catecholamine into subcutaneous tissue, secondary to a dislodged or misplaced catheter, can result in localized ischemia and necrosis of the tissue. Phentolamine, an alpha-adrenergic blocking agent, injected subcutaneously around the catecholamine infiltration may help prevent tissue necrosis, but special care should be taken to assure IV patency prior to and during administration of catecholamines.

STREET SMART

Commercially prepared catecholamines contain a preservative (sulfite) which helps maintain potency. Some patients are sensitive to sulfites and may have an allergic reaction to the drug, compounding the severity of the situation instead of improving it.

Epinephrine

Epinephrine, the original catecholamine, is available for injection, inhalation, and infusion. Epinephrine is a powerful direct-acting synthetic catecholamine. In small doses, epinephrine is used to treat severe asthma exacerbation and serves as an adjunct to local anesthetics to control bleeding during wound repair (sutures). In larger doses, epinephrine can reverse cardiovascular collapse secondary to anaphylaxis or coarsen ventricular fibrillation for more effective defibrillation.

Epinephrine's rapid onset of action (three to five minutes by subcutaneous injection) makes it useful in an emergency.

Occasionally, after a subcutaneous injection or intravenous bolus, it is necessary to continuously infuse epinephrine to maintain blood pressure, particularly in cases of distributive shock, such as septic shock and anaphylactic shock.

Dopamine

Dopamine, a naturally occurring catecholamine, is the precursor to epinephrine and has effects similar to epinephrine. At lower doses, one-half to two micrograms per kilogram per minute infusion (0.5 to 2 mcg/kg/min), dopamine dilates renal arteries, increasing blood flow and subsequent production of urine.

At higher doses, up to 10 micrograms per kilogram per minute infusion (10 mcg/kg/min), dopamine stimulates the beta-receptors of the heart, increasing heart rate and force of contraction. At the highest doses, 10 to 20 micrograms per kilogram per minute infusion, alpha-adrenergic receptors are increasingly stimulated.

Alpha-adrenergic receptor stimulation leads to peripheral vasoconstriction, an increase in peripheral vascular resistance (afterload), and more work for the heart, while elevating the blood pressure via increased venous return (preload). The trade-off, a perfusing blood pressure for increased work of the heart, may induce an acute myocardial infarction and renal ischemia.[124] For those reasons, high dose dopamine is reserved for severe hemodynamic imbalance.

STREET SMART

While dopamine at 4 to 20 mcg/kg/min can increase blood pressure, dopamine 3 mcg/kg/minute or less can actually lower the blood pressure. These lower, or renal, doses of dopamine also cause a vasodilation of the mesenteric vessels resulting in venous pooling. Therefore, dopamine infusions should always be started at more than 5 mcg/kg/min in the field.

Dobutamine

Dobutamine is the synthetic analog of dopamine but is more beta-selective than dopamine. This quality makes it less desirable in cases of distributive shock (e.g., septic shock), but very desirable for cardiogenic shock.

Dobutamine is a potent inotropic agent and a weak chronotropic agent. Therefore, dobutamine does not significantly increase the oxygen demands of the heart but can improve cardiac output. This makes it attractive for use in cardiogenic shock secondary to pump failure.

Dobutamine is very effective for patients in cardiogenic shock who have an elevated left ventricular filling pressure, often manifested by elevated jugular venous distention (JVD), but who are not remarkably hypotensive (systolic B/P greater than 90 mmHg). These patients, on the border of severe cardiogenic shock, often benefit from a combination of dobutamine (to maintain blood pressure) and dopamine at renal doses (for diuresis).

As an added bonus, dopamine and dobutamine are compatible and may be infused together via the same intravenous access. This approach is often preferable, especially in patients with potential for hypokalemia, because of a decreased risk of tachydysrhythmia.

Norepinephrine

Norepinephrine, in contrast to dobutamine, has a high affinity for alpha-adrenergic receptors. Norepinephrine is a powerful peripheral vasoconstrictor which is effective in treating cardiovascular collapse secondary to distributive shock (e.g., advanced septic shock).

The use of norepinephrine in patients in cardiogenic shock is questionable, as the increased peripheral vascular resistance (afterload) translates to increased work for the heart and offsets any advantage obtained by increasing the blood pressure. In fact, imprudent administration of norepinephrine can lead to acute myocardial infarction in patients with pre-existing coronary artery disease.

STREET SMART

Monoamine oxidase oxidizes catecholamines, like dopamine and norepinephrine, into inactive metabolites. Monoamine oxidase inhibitors (MAO inhibitors), a class of antidepressant medications, prevents the breakdown of these catecholamines. Routine doses of dopamine administered to a patient who has prescribed MAO inhibitors can result in serum dopamine levels that are increased ten-fold and lead to acute hypertensive crisis.

CONCLUSION

Two of the most common chief complaints of patients are chest pain and shortness of breath. By understanding the underlying cardiopulmonary physiology and pathophysiology, Paramedics can establish effective therapeutic interventions earlier in the course of the patient's illness. Early intervention can translate directly into decreased morbidity and mortality.

KEY POINTS:

- The central nervous system consists of the brain and spinal cord.

- The peripheral nervous system consists of the cranial, nervous, and spinal nerves.

- The autonomic nervous system is that portion of the peripheral system that controls involuntary functions.

- The autonomic nervous system consists of two branches: the sympathetic division, which serves to accelerate organs, and the parasympathetic division, which controls vegetative functions.

- The vagus nerve is the primary parasympathetic nerve.

- Messengers which relay signals from nerve to organ are called neurotransmitters.

- Neurotransmitters attach to a receptor.

- Agonist drugs increase the neurotransmitters' ability to stimulate the receptor.

- Antagonist drugs block stimulation of the receptor.

- Parasympathetic receptors are classified as cholinergic (responding to acetylcholine), i.e., muscarinic, or nicotinic receptors.

- Muscarinic receptors are found in organs, whereas nicotinic receptors are located in the adrenal medulla, CNS, and skeletal muscles.

- Cholinergic agents are agonists which stimulate a parasympathetic response.

- Anticholinergic agents would slow or stop parasympathetic responses.

- Blocking nicotinic receptors causes paralysis. Depolarizing agents cause fasciculations before paralysis while non-depolarizing agents lead directly to paralysis.

- Adrenergic agents directly or indirectly stimulate a sympathetic response.

- Adrenergic blockers would prevent a sympathetic response.

- Alpha-adrenergic agents or blockers primarily affect the vessels.

- Beta-adrenergic agents or blockers affect the heart or lungs.

- Drugs used to treat pulmonary diseases usually target one of the three S's: spasms, swelling, or secretions.

- Beta-adrenergic agonists, xanthine derivatives, and cholinergic antagonists prevent or reduce spasms.

- Corticosteroids, leukotriene antagonists, and mast cell inhibitors reduce swelling.

- Mucolytics liquefy mucus.

- Drugs used to treat coronary artery disease usually target vessels, platelets, coagulation cascade, or lipids.

- Antilipidemic drugs either prevent absorption of cholesterol, sequester in the bile for elimination, or prevent the liver from making cholesterol.

- Anticoagulant drugs interfere in the clotting cascade, preventing the formation of a fibrin clot.

- Antiplatelet drugs alter platelet membranes, preventing aggregation, adherence, and vasoconstriction.

- Fibrinolytics disassemble the fibrin clot.

- Nitrates dilate the venous system (reducing blood return to the heart), dilate the arterial system (reducing workload of the heart), and may dilate coronary vessels (increasing blood flow to the myocardium).

- Dysrhythmias are an alteration in the heart's rate or rhythm. Not all dysrhythmias require treatment.

- The goal of dysrhythmic treatment is to alleviate symptoms. Antidysrhythmic drugs can cause other dysrhythmias and are proarrythmic.

- Drugs used to treat dysrhythmias affect the transition of the ionic channels from resting to open/active or inactive.

- The cations of the heart's action potential are sodium, potassium, and calcium. The Vaughn-Williams classification system divides drugs according to the ion affected.

- Class I drugs affect sodium influx. Class I drugs are subcategorized as IA, IB, or IC, depending upon where in the sodium influx stage they act.

- Class II drugs are beta-blockers. They affect the chemical which opens the calcium channels. They also reduce myocardial infarct size by decreasing heart rate and thus allow a longer diastole and increased coronary blood flow. By also dilating peripheral vessels, they decrease myocardial oxygen demand.

- Class III drugs block potassium movement from the cell, lengthening the period of time in which the cell cannot respond to another stimulus.

- Class IV drugs block the movement of calcium into heart cells, reducing the rate of depolarization or the mechanical initiation of contraction.

- Class V drugs have miscellaneous effects and include the cardiac glycoside digitalis and the antiarrythmic adenosine.

- An indirectly acting drug which allows the heart rate to increase is the cholinergic blocker called atropine.

- When underperfused, the kidneys release a substance called renin. Through several steps, renin is converted to angiotensin, which affects vessel dilation and the movement of water and sodium from the kidney.

- The conversion of renin to angiotensin requires an enzyme. Inhibiting the enzyme (with an angiotensin-converting enzyme inhibitor or ACE inhibitor) prevents an increase in blood pressure through constriction and increased volume.

- Diuretics affect the release of water and other ions from the kidney. Depending upon the exact location of action, more or less water is released and potassium may be excreted or retained.

- Vasodilators usually cause dilation of the venous side and reduction of blood return to the heart. Those that cause arterial dilation decrease diastolic pressure, peripheral vascular resistance, and afterload.

- Digitalis, a cardiac glycoside, slows electrical conduction and increases the strength of contraction. It is both an antidysrhythmic and a treatment for heart failure.

- Digitalis has a narrow therapeutic range and can rapidly lead to toxicity.

- Catecholamines act with sympathetic receptors. They are indicated for vascular support.

REVIEW QUESTIONS:

1. Differentiate the central nervous system, peripheral nervous system, and autonomic nervous system from each other based on location, components, and general action in the body.

2. How are the actions of the sympathetic division different from those of the parasympathetic division?

3. Define a neurotransmitter and describe how it works.

4. Which division of the autonomic nervous system has cholinergic receptors?

5. Name the types of adrenergic receptors.

6. Which adrenergic receptors primarily affect vessels?

7. Which cholinergic receptors primarily affect skeletal muscles?

8. Define agonists and antagonists as they relate to receptors.

9. Which classes of drugs reduce spasms associated with pulmonary disease?

10. Which classes of drugs reduce swelling associated with pulmonary disease?

11. From which class of drugs do "rescue drugs" for pulmonary disease come?

12. List the five main classifications of the Vaughn-Williams system.

13. What condition(s) are treated by drugs of the Vaughn-Williams system?

14. How do ACE inhibitors work?

15. Describe the concern regarding the administration of digitalis preparations.

CASE STUDY QUESTIONS:

Please refer to the Case Study at the beginning of the chapter and answer the questions below:

1. Using the information in this chapter, describe at least five ways in which medications prescribed for Mrs. Fein's blood pressure control and dysrhythmias can cause her complaints of fatigue and nearly fainting.

2. In what ways do pharmacies try to prevent patients from taking similar medications prescribed by different physicians?

3. How do Paramedics assist in educating their patients about medication use?

REFERENCES:

1. Greenblatt S. *A History of Neurosurgery*. New York: American Association of Neurological Surgery; 1997.

2. Shields RW, Jr. Functional anatomy of the autonomic nervous system. *J Clin Neurophysiol*. 1993;10(1):2–13.

3. Hilz MJ, Dutsch M. Quantitative studies of autonomic function. *Muscle Nerve*. 2006;33(1):6–20.

4. Motzer SA, Hertig V. Stress, stress response, and health. *Nurs Clin North Am*. 2004;39(1):1–17.

5. Arun CP. Fight or flight, forbearance and fortitude: the spectrum of actions of the catecholamines and their cousins. *Ann N Y Acad Sci*, 2004;1018:137–140.

6. Wortsman J. Role of epinephrine in acute stress. *Endocrinol Metab Clin North Am*. 2002;31(1):79–106.

7. Lechin F, van der Dijs B. Central nervous system circuitry and peripheral neural sympathetic activity responsible for essential hypertension. *Curr Neurovasc Res*. 2006;3(4):307–325.

8. Moratinos J, Reverte M. Effects of catecholamines on plasma potassium: the role of alpha- and beta-adrenoceptors. *Fundam Clin Pharmacol*. 1993;7(3-4):143–153.

9. Wood EH, Geraci JE. Photoelectric determination of arterial oxygen saturation in man. *J Lab Clin Med*. 1949;34(3):387–401.

10. Waterhouse BD, Sessler FM, Liu W, Lin CS. Second messenger-mediated actions of norepinephrine on target neurons in central circuits: a new perspective on intracellular mechanisms and functional consequences. *Prog Brain Res*. 1991;88:351–362.

11. Hamel E. Serotonin and migraine: biology and clinical implications. *Cephalalgia*. 2007;27(11):1293–1300.

12. Johnson MP, Fernandez F, Colson NJ, Griffiths LR. A pharmacogenomic evaluation of migraine therapy. *Expert Opin Pharmacother*. 2007;8(12):1821–1835.

13. Agosti RM. 5HT1F- and 5HT7-receptor agonists for the treatment of migraines. *CNS Neurol Disord Drug Targets*. 2007;6(4):235–237.

14. Tfelt-Hansen P. A review of evidence-based medicine and meta-analytic reviews in migraine. *Cephalalgia*. 2006;26(11):1265–1274.

15. Racke K, Juergens UR, Matthiesen S. Control by cholinergic mechanisms. *Eur J Pharmacol*. 2006;533(1-3):57–68.

16. Felder CC. Muscarinic acetylcholine receptors: signal transduction through multiple effectors. *Faseb J*. 1995;9(8):619–625.

17. Diaz JH. Evolving global epidemiology, syndromic classification, general management, and prevention of unknown mushroom poisonings. *Crit Care Med*. 2005;33(2):419–426.

18. Blackman JR. Clinical approach to toxic mushroom ingestion. *J Am Board Fam Pract*. 1994;7(1):31–37.

19. Ulbricht C, Basch E, Hammerness P, Vora M, Wylie J, Jr., Woods J. An evidence-based systematic review of belladonna by the natural standard research collaboration. *J Herb Pharmacother*. 2004;4(4):61–90.

20. Porter R. *The Greatest Benefit to Mankind*. New York: Harper-Collins; 1999.

21. Treatment for nerve-poisoning agents. *FDA Consum*. 2006;40(6):6.

22. McCain KR, Sawyer TS, Spiller HA. Evaluation of centrally acting cholinesterase inhibitor exposures in adults. *Ann Pharmacother*. 2007;41(10):1632–1637.

23. Lawrence DT, Kirk MA. Chemical terrorism attacks: update on antidotes. *Emerg Med Clin North Am*. 2007;25(2):567–595; abstract xi.

24. Lynch M. Atropine use in children after nerve gas exposure. *J Pediatr Nurs*. 2005;20(6):477–484.

25. Doran JV, Tortella BJ, Drivet WJ, Lavery RF. Factors influencing successful intubation in the prehospital setting. *Prehosp Disaster Med*. 1995;10(4):259–264.

26. Bulger EM, Copass MK, Sabath DR, Maier RV, Jurkovich GJ. The use of neuromuscular blocking agents to facilitate prehospital intubation does not impair outcome after traumatic brain injury. *J Trauma*. 2005;58(4):718–723; discussion 723–724.

27. Perry J, Lee J, Wells G. Rocuronium versus succinylcholine for rapid sequence induction intubation. *Cochrane Database Syst Rev*. 2003;1:CD002788.

28. Weinshenker D, Schroeder JP. There and back again: a tale of norepinephrine and drug addiction. *Neuropsychopharmacology*. 2007;32(7):1433–1451.

29. Hall FS, Sora I, Drgonova J, Li XF, Goeb M, Uhl GR. Molecular mechanisms underlying the rewarding effects of cocaine. *Ann N Y Acad Sci*. 2004;1025:47–56.

30. Jayanthi LD, Ramamoorthy S. Regulation of monoamine transporters: influence of psychostimulants and therapeutic antidepressants. *Aaps J*. 2005;7(3):E728–738.

31. Insel PA. Structure and function of alpha-adrenergic receptors. *Am J Med*. 1989;87(2A):12S–18S.

32. Taylor MR. Pharmacogenetics of the human beta-adrenergic receptors. *Pharmacogenomics J*. 2007;7(1):29–37.

33. Bristow MR. Mechanistic and clinical rationales for using beta-blockers in heart failure. *J Card Fail*. 2000; 6(2 Suppl 1):8–14.

34. Andersson KE. Adrenoceptors—classification, activation and blockade by drugs. *Postgrad Med J*. 1980;56 (Suppl 2):7–16.

35. Insel PA. Adrenergic receptors. Evolving concepts on structure and function. *Am J Hypertens*. 1989;2(3 Pt 2):112S–118S.

36. Ruffolo RR, Jr., Hieble JP. Alpha-adrenoceptors. *Pharmacol Ther*. 1994;61(1-2):1–64.

37. Havell EA, Hayes TG, Vilcek J. Synthesis of two distinct interferons by human fibroblasts. *Virology*. 1978;89(1):330–334.

38. Singer AJ, Konia N. Comparison of topical anesthetics and vasoconstrictors vs lubricants prior to nasogastric intubation: a randomized, controlled trial. *Acad Emerg Med*. 1999;6(3): 184–190.

39. Muller-Schweinitzer E, Fanchamps A. Effects on arterial receptors of ergot derivatives used in migraine. *Adv Neurol*. 1982;33:343–356.

40. Schiff PL. Ergot and its alkaloids. *Am J Pharm Educ*. 2006;70(5):98.

41. Barnes PJ. Cyclic nucleotides and phosphodiesterases and airway function. *Eur Respir J*. 1995;8(3):457–462.

42. Cohen NH, Eigen H, Shaughnessy TE. Status asthmaticus. *Crit Care Clin*. 1997;13(3):459–476.

43. Restrepo RD, Peters J. Near-fatal asthma: recognition and management. *Curr Opin Pulm Med*. 2008;14(1):13–23.

44. Kaza V, Bandi V, Guntupalli KK. Acute severe asthma: recent advances. *Curr Opin Pulm Med*. 2007;13(1):1–7.

45. Higgins JC. The "crashing asthmatic." *Am Fam Physician*. 2003;67(5):997–1004.

46. Wiebe K, Rowe BH. Nebulized racemic epinephrine used in the treatment of severe asthmatic exacerbation: a case report and literature review. *Cjem*. 2007;9(4):304–308.

47. Qureshi F, Zaritsky A, et al. Efficacy of nebulized ipratropium in severely asthmatic children. *Ann Emerg Med*. 1997;29(2):205–211.

48. Quinn MJ, Brener SJ. Early invasive strategies for acute coronary syndromes. *Curr Cardiol Rep*. 2002;4(4):334–340.

49. Diop D, Aghababian RV. Definition, classification, and pathophysiology of acute coronary ischemic syndromes. *Emerg Med Clin North Am*. 2001;19(2):259–267.

50. Fesenko RI, Artemova Iu V, Virnik AD, Rogovin ZA, Iakovlev VA. Synthesis and study of the properties of water-insoluble products of the interaction of urease and cellulose derivatives. *Vopr Med Khim*. 1975;21(1):82–84.

51. Achar SA, Kundu S, Norcross WA. Diagnosis of acute coronary syndrome. *Am Fam Physician*. 2005;72(1):119–126.

52. Gronholdt ML, Dalager-Pedersen S, Falk E. Coronary atherosclerosis: determinants of plaque rupture. *Eur Heart J*. 1998;19 (Suppl C):C24–29.

53. Zhou J, Chew M, Ravn HB, Falk E. Plaque pathology and coronary thrombosis in the pathogenesis of acute coronary syndromes. *Scand J Clin Lab Invest Suppl*. 1999;230:3–11.

54. Shah PK. Pathophysiology of plaque rupture and the concept of plaque stabilization. *Cardiol Clin*. 1996;14(1):17–29.

55. Klein LW. Clinical implications and mechanisms of plaque rupture in the acute coronary syndromes. *Am Heart Hosp J*. 2005;3(4):249–255.

56. Hersberger M, von Eckardstein A. Low high-density lipoprotein cholesterol: physiological background, clinical importance and drug treatment. *Drugs*. 2003;63(18):1907–1945.

57. Meyers CD, Kashyap ML. Pharmacologic elevation of high-density lipoproteins: recent insights on mechanism of action and atherosclerosis protection. *Curr Opin Cardiol*. 2004;19(4):366–373.

58. Howard BV, Ruotolo G, Robbins DC. Obesity and dyslipidemia. *Endocrinol Metab Clin North Am*. 2003;32(4):855–867.

59. Ito MK. Niacin-based therapy for dyslipidemia: past evidence and future advances. *Am J Manag Care*. 2002;8(12 Suppl): S315–S322.

60. Morgan JM, Carey CM, Lincoff A, Capuzzi DM. The effects of niacin on lipoprotein subclass distribution. *Prev Cardiol*. 2004;7(4):182–187; quiz 188.

61. Miller M. Niacin as a component of combination therapy for dyslipidemia. *Mayo Clin Proc*. 2003;78(6):735–742.

62. Babu KS, Salvi SS. Aspirin and asthma. *Chest*. 2000;118(5):1470–1476.

63. ISIS-2 Collaborative Group. Randomized factorial trial of high-dose intravenous streptokinase, of oral aspirin and of intravenous heparin in acute myocardial infarction. ISIS (International Studies of Infarct Survival) pilot study. *Eur Heart J*. 1987;8(6):634–642.

64. Morrison LJ, Verbeek PR, et al. Mortality and prehospital thrombolysis for acute myocardial infarction: a meta-analysis. *JAMA*. 2000;283(20):2686–2692.

65. Sayah AJ, Roe MT. The role of fibrinolytics in the prehospital treatment of ST-elevation myocardial infarction (STEMI). *J Emerg Med*. 2008;34(4):405–416.

66. Anderson PD, Mitchell PM, et al. Potential diversion rates associated with prehospital acute myocardial infarction triage strategies. *J Emerg Med*. 2004;27(4):345–353.

67. Cannon CP. Acute coronary syndromes: risk stratification and initial management. *Cardiol Clin*. 2005;23(4):401–409, v.

68. Abrams J. Beneficial actions of nitrates in cardiovascular disease. *Am J Cardiol*. 1996;77(13):31C–37C.

69. Abrams J. Mechanisms of action of the organic nitrates in the treatment of myocardial ischemia. *Am J Cardiol*. 1992;70(8):30B–42B.

70. Abrams J. Hemodynamic effects of nitroglycerin and long-acting nitrates. *Am Heart J*. 1985;110(1 Pt 2):216–224.

71. Thadani U. Nitrate tolerance, rebound, and their clinical relevance in stable angina pectoris, unstable angina, and heart failure. *Cardiovasc Drugs Ther*. 1997;10(6):735–742.

72. Engelberg S, Singer AJ, Moldashel J, Sciammarella J, Thode HC, Henry M. Effects of prehospital nitroglycerin on hemodynamics and chest pain intensity. *Prehosp Emerg Care*. 2000;4(4): 290–293.

73. Wuerz R, Swope G, Meador S, Holliman CJ, Roth GS. Safety of prehospital nitroglycerin. *Ann Emerg Med*. 1994;23(1):31–36.

74. Henrikson CA, Howell EE, et al. Chest pain relief by nitroglycerin does not predict active coronary artery disease. *Ann Intern Med*. 2003;139(12):979–986.

75. Thadani U, Rodgers T. Side effects of using nitrates to treat angina. *Expert Opin Drug Saf*. 2006;5(5):667–674.

76. Waddell S. Vasovagal syncope. *Crit Care Nurse*. 1989;9(6):35–43.

77. Ryan TJ, Antman EM, et al. 1999 update: ACC/AHA guidelines for the management of patients with acute myocardial infarction. A report of the American College of Cardiology/American Heart Association Task Force on Practice Guidelines (Committee on Management of Acute Myocardial Infarction). *J Am Coll Cardiol*. 1999;34(3):890–911.

78. Pelliccia A. Athlete's heart and hypertrophic cardiomyopathy. *Curr Cardiol Rep*. 2000;2(2):166–171.

79. Haugh KH. Antidysrhythmic agents at the turn of the twenty-first century: a current review. *Crit Care Nurs Clin North Am*. 2002;14(1):53–69.

80. Hondeghem LM, Katzung BG. Antiarrhythmic agents: the modulated receptor mechanism of action of sodium and calcium channel-blocking drugs. *Annu Rev Pharmacol Toxicol*. 1984;24:387–423.

81. Carmeliet E. Selectivity of antiarrhythmic drugs and ionic channels: a historical overview. *Ann N Y Acad Sci*. 1984;427:1–15.

82. Hondeghem LM. Antiarrhythmic agents: modulated receptor applications. *Circulation*. 1987;75(3):514–520.

83. Chaudhry GM, Haffajee CI. Antiarrhythmic agents and proarrhythmia. *Crit Care Med*. 2000;28(10 Suppl):N158–N164.

84. Shantsila E, Watson T, Lip GY. Drug-induced QT-interval prolongation and proarrhythmic risk in the treatment of atrial arrhythmias. *Europace*. 2007;9 (Suppl 4):iv37–iv44.

85. Wyse DG. Are there alternatives to mortality as an endpoint in clinical trials of atrial fibrillation? *Heart Rhythm*. 2004;1(2 Suppl):B41–44, discussion B44.

86. Tilley DG, Rockman HA. Role of beta-adrenergic receptor signaling and desensitization in heart failure: new concepts and prospects for treatment. *Expert Rev Cardiovasc Ther*. 2006;4(3):417–432.

87. Sucharov CC. Beta-adrenergic pathways in human heart failure. *Expert Rev Cardiovasc Ther*. 2007;5(1):119–124.

88. Lohse MJ, Engelhardt S, Eschenhagen T. What is the role of beta-adrenergic signaling in heart failure? *Circ Res.* 2003;93(10):896–906.

89. Antman EM, Hand M, Armstrong PW, Bates ER, Green LA, Halasyamani LK, et al. 2007 focused update of the ACC/AHA 2004 guidelines for the management of patients with ST-elevation myocardial infarction: a report of the American College of Cardiology/American Heart Association Task Force on Practice Guidelines: developed in collaboration with the Canadian Cardiovascular Society endorsed by the American Academy of Family Physicians: 2007 Writing Group to review new evidence and update the ACC/AHA 2004 guidelines for the management of patients with ST-elevation myocardial infarction, writing on behalf of the 2004 Writing Committee. *Circulation.* 2008;117(2):296–329.

90. Kopecky SL. Effect of beta blockers, particularly carvedilol, on reducing the risk of events after acute myocardial infarction. *Am J Cardiol.* 2006;98(8):1115–1119.

91. Senior R, Basu S, Kinsey C, Schaeffer S, Lahiri A. Carvedilol prevents remodeling in patients with left ventricular dysfunction after acute myocardial infarction. *Am Heart J.* 1999;137 (4 Pt 1):646–652.

92. Fonarow GC. Epidemiology and risk stratification in acute heart failure. *Am Heart J.* 2008;155(2):200–207.

93. Himmelmann A. New information on the role of beta-blockers in cardiac therapy. *Cardiovasc Drugs Ther.* 1999;13(6):469–477.

94. Roberts R, Rogers WJ, et al. Immediate versus deferred beta-blockade following thrombolytic therapy in patients with acute myocardial infarction. Results of the Thrombolysis in Myocardial Infarction (TIMI) II-B Study. *Circulation.* 1991;83(2):422–437.

95. Nademanee K, Taylor R, et al. Treating electrical storm: sympathetic blockade versus advanced cardiac life support-guided therapy. *Circulation.* 2000;102(7):742–747.

96. Gottlieb SS. Time to practice what we preach: the use of beta-blockers post myocardial infarction. *Eur Heart J.* 1999;20(10):701–702.

97. Page RL, 2nd, Utz KJ, Wolfel EE. Should beta-blockers be used in the treatment of cocaine-associated acute coronary syndrome? *Ann Pharmacother.* 2007;41(12):2008–2013.

98. Sen A, Fairbairn T, Levy F. Best evidence topic report. Beta-blockers in cocaine induced acute coronary syndrome. *Emerg Med J.* 2006;23(5):401–402.

99. Pitts WR, Lange RA, Cigarroa JE, Hillis LD. Cocaine-induced myocardial ischemia and infarction: pathophysiology, recognition, and management. *Prog Cardiovasc Dis.* 1997;40(1):65–76.

100. Flemenbaum A. Pavor nocturnus: a complication of single daily tricyclic or neuroleptic dosage. *Am J Psychiatry.* 1976;133(5):570–572.

101. Hohnloser SH. Proarrhythmia with Class III antiarrhythmic drugs: types, risks, and management. *Am J Cardiol.* 1997;80(8A):82G–89G.

102. Tsikouris JP, Cox CD. A review of Class III antiarrhythmic agents for atrial fibrillation: maintenance of normal sinus rhythm. *Pharmacotherapy.* 2001;21(12):1514–1529.

103. Kudenchuk PJ, Cobb LA, et al. Amiodarone for resuscitation after out-of-hospital cardiac arrest due to ventricular fibrillation. *N Engl J Med.* 1999;341(12):871–878.

104. Gonzalez ER, Kannewurf BS, et al. Intravenous amiodarone for ventricular arrhythmias: overview and clinical use. *Resuscitation.* 1998;39(1-2):33–42.

105. Mayr V, Luckner G, et al. Arginine vasopressin in advanced cardiovascular failure during the post-resuscitation phase after cardiac arrest. *Resuscitation.* 2007;72(1):35–44.

106. Ditchey RV, Lindenfeld J. Failure of epinephrine to improve the balance between myocardial oxygen supply and demand during closed-chest resuscitation in dogs. *Circulation.* 1988;78(2): 382–389.

107. Herlitz J, Estrom L, et al. Survival among patients with out-of-hospital cardiac arrest found in electromechanical dissociation. *Resuscitation.* 1995;29(2):97–106.

108. Gueugniaud PY, David JS, et al. Vasopressin and epinephrine vs. epinephrine alone in cardiopulmonary resuscitation. *N Engl J Med.* 2008;359(1):21–30.

109. Lindner KH, Ahnefeld FW, et al. Comparison of epinephrine and dopamine during cardiopulmonary resuscitation. *Intensive Care Med.* 1989;15(7):432–438.

110. Fonarow GC. The role of in-hospital initiation of cardiovascular protective therapies to improve treatment rates and clinical outcomes. *Rev Cardiovasc Med.* 2003;4 (Suppl 3):S37–S46.

111. Fonarow GC, Corday E. Overview of acutely decompensated congestive heart failure (ADHF): a report from the ADHERE registry. *Heart Fail Rev.* 2004;9(3):179–185.

112. Solaro RJ. Mechanisms of the Frank-Starling law of the heart: the beat goes on. *Biophys J.* 2007;93(12):4095–4096.

113. Stojiljkovic L, Behnia R. Role of renin angiotensin system inhibitors in cardiovascular and renal protection: a lesson from clinical trials. *Curr Pharm Des.* 2007;13(13):1335–1345.

114. Seigworth GR. Bloodletting over the centuries. *N Y State J Med.* 1980;80(13):2022–2028.

115. Metcalf KM. The helper model: nine ways to make it work. *Nurs Manage.* 1992;23(12):40–43.

116. Basnyat B, Murdoch DR. High-altitude illness. *Lancet.* 2003;361(9373):1967–1974.

117. Faris R, Flather MD, Purcell H, Poole-Wilson PA, Coats AJ. Diuretics for heart failure. *Cochrane Database Syst Rev.* 2006;1:CD003838.

118. Salvador DR, Rey NR, Ramos GC, Punzalan FE. Continuous infusion versus bolus injection of loop diuretics in congestive heart failure. *Cochrane Database Syst Rev.* 2005;3:CD003178.

119. Hollenberg SM. Vasodilators in acute heart failure. *Heart Fail Rev.* 2007;12(2):143–147.

120. Fisch C. William Withering: An account of the foxglove and some of its medical uses 1785–1985. *J Am Coll Cardiol.* 1985;5(5 Suppl A):1A–2A.

121. Alpert JS, Petersen P, Godtfredsen J. Atrial fibrillation: natural history, complications, and management. *Annu Rev Med.* 1988;39:41–52.

122. Litovitz TL, Klein-Schwartz W, Dyer KS, et al. Annual report of the American Association of Poison Control Centers toxic exposure surveillance system. *American Journal of Emergency Medicine.* 1998;16(5):443–497.

123. Roberts DM, Buckley NA. Antidotes for acute cardenolide (cardiac glycoside) poisoning. *Cochrane Database Syst Rev.* 2006;4:CD005490.

124. Schreiber W, Herkner H, Koreny M, Bur A, Hirschl MM, Glogar D, et al. Predictors of survival in unselected patients with acute myocardial infarction requiring continuous catecholamine support. *Resuscitation.* 2002;55(3):269–276.

PHARMACOLOGICAL THERAPEUTICS FOR MEDICAL EMERGENCIES

KEY CONCEPTS:

Upon completion of this chapter, it is expected that the reader will understand these following concepts:

- Mechanism of action for common medications
- Prehospital drug interventions
- Recognition of expected actions and other actions of patient and prehospital medications

▶ **CASE STUDY:**

The ambulance squad received a call for a 35-year-old man complaining of severe back pain. En route to the call, one Paramedic said to his partner that this guy was probably just a drug seeker. His partner replied, "Maybe, but we need a lot more information. Many medical conditions cause severe pain and I'd want someone to care for me and reduce my pain if possible."

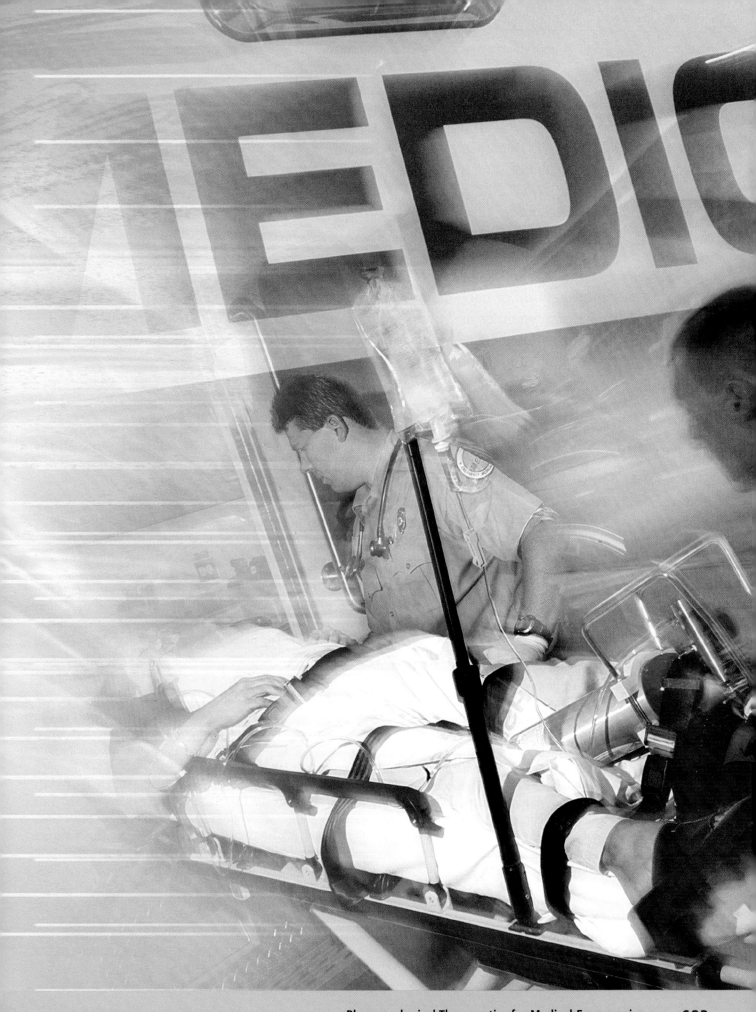

OVERVIEW

Paramedics are expected to treat an enormous variety of diseases in the field. Considering the lack of information normally known about a patient in the field, the enormity of the EMS task becomes even more daunting. Nevertheless, using a limited pharmacy, Paramedics persist in trying to accomplish their missions of care and support to the sick and injured.

The following drug review supplies the Paramedic with information about drugs that are commonly prescribed to patients, as well as those drugs that a Paramedic might use to care for that patient. The development and distribution of new drugs, and the use of old drugs/technologies for new applications, makes it impractical to discuss each drug individually. Instead, the general action of each classification of drug (i.e., its pharmacotherapeutics), including its pharmacodynamics and pharmacokinetics, is discussed. The Paramedic is well advised to consult the most recent and up-to-date drug reference regarding a specific drug before administering any medicine.

Drugs That Affect the Central Nervous System

The central nervous system consists of the brain and the spinal cord. Although the brain is considered the seat of consciousness (that uniquely human condition), it has not always been thought of that way. Aristotle viewed the brain as just an elaborate cooling apparatus for the blood. It took centuries to dispel that myth. Today, the importance of the brain is undisputed. The brain is so important that the prime directive for EMS could be "to keep the brain alive at all costs!"

The brain that controls the central nervous system is actually not one brain but three brains working together. The first brain, the so-called primitive brain, is the brainstem, which is made up of the midbrain, pons, and the medulla oblongata. Vital life functions, such as breathing and heart rate, are controlled in the brainstem.[1] The brainstem also contains the **reticular activating system (RAS)**, a complex network of interconnected reflexes that maintain wakefulness. The next brain is the cerebellum. The cerebellum is responsible for balance (equilibrium) and muscular coordination, hence its title "the athletic brain." The last brain, the cerebrum, is perhaps the most important to a person's sense of being. The cerebrum is responsible for a person's emotions, memories, and speech, as well as reasoning, judgment, and creativity. The cerebrum is actually a hollow sphere. The outside, called the cerebral cortex ("cortex" is a Latin word meaning "bark"), contains the gray matter. The inside of the cerebrum contains white matter, myelinated fibers that connect with different sections of the brain and the spinal cord.

The entire brain, as well as the spinal cord, is surrounded by the fluid-producing meninges.

Blood-Brain Barrier

Capillaries in the body have small gaps, called slit junctions that permit hormones, enzymes, and drugs to move into the interstitial space. Capillaries in the brain are distinctive in that they have nearly impenetrable tight slit junctions.[2] Reinforcing these tight junctions are cells called astrocytes. These two factors combine to make the brain nearly impassable to most drugs, permitting only lipid-soluble drugs (like diazepam) to enter the brain and preventing ionized (polar) drugs that are dissolved in solution from entering into the brain.

Central Nervous System Sedatives

A state of reduced central nervous system activity (i.e., sedation) is desirable for a number of medical reasons. Exhausted patients (e.g., insomniacs) need sleep and literally dozens of drugs can induce sleep. In another case, a fear-induced anxiety attack can lead to acute myocardial infarction (AMI) in some patients. Perhaps the earliest CNS depressant used medicinally was alcohol. While alcohol is effective as a CNS depressant, it has many undesirable qualities that limit its medical use. For this reason, and for a wide variety of clinical situations, other **central nervous system depressants** have been created.

These CNS depressants have some common effects. At low doses, many of these drugs are **sedatives**. They cause relaxation, lessened irritability, and decreased excitability. At higher doses, many of these CNS depressants induce a

hypnotic state, a sleep-producing effect. Many of these CNS depressants also are **anxiolytics**, reducing apprehension, fear, and anxiety. While anxiety is normal, and is in fact a healthy response to stress because it encourages action, excessive anxiety is unhealthy. Excessive anxiety can mentally paralyze a person and interfere with his ability to perform the activities of daily living (ADL).

Barbiturates

Barbiturates, such as phenobarbital, have been used extensively in the recent past as a CNS depressant. While barbiturates have been largely replaced by safer benzodiazepines, barbiturates are still useful in certain clinical situations. As a class, barbiturates can be divided into three groups according to the duration of action: long-acting, short-acting, and ultra-short-acting.[3]

Long-acting barbiturates, such as phenobarbital, are frequently used for seizure prophylaxis, the prevention of recurrent seizures. The intended pharmaceutical effect of long-acting barbiturates can last for as long as 10 to 12 hours, making them ideal for twice daily (BID) administration.

Short-acting barbiturates, such as pentobarbital or secobarbital, produce an onset of action within 10 to 15 minutes and can last up to four hours. This rapid onset of action makes them ideal as presurgical anxiolytics in preparation for the induction of anesthesia.

Ultra-short-acting barbiturates, such as thiopental, create a sedative/hypnotic effect, depending on the dose, within seconds. This rapid speed of onset of action makes these drugs excellent for use in emergency situations where time is of the essence and rapid induction of anesthesia is mandatory.

Mechanism of Action

The mechanism of action of all barbiturates is the same: Barbiturates interfere with the transfer of sodium and potassium across the cell membrane. Inhibition of the sodium-potassium ionic transfer blunts the action potential of muscle cells generally and of nerve cells particularly. This nonselective mechanism of action means barbiturates impact the entire central nervous system. At higher doses, barbiturates induce anesthesia by this action, in effect paralyzing the brain at the cellular level. At toxic levels, barbiturates suppress chemoreceptors that are sensing carbon dioxide and oxygen levels, inducing respiratory depression. If unresolved, toxic levels of barbiturates can lead to complete coma and respiratory arrest.

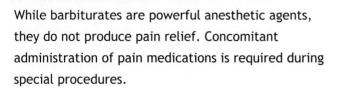

STREET SMART

While barbiturates are powerful anesthetic agents, they do not produce pain relief. Concomitant administration of pain medications is required during special procedures.

Benzodiazepines

Benzodiazepines were introduced in the 1960s and largely seen as a replacement for barbiturates. Compared to barbiturates, benzodiazepines are relatively safe, the lethal dose being one-thousand times greater than the therapeutic dose (i.e., it has a large therapeutic index). Benzodiazepines were also reported to have fewer side effects and less of an abuse potential than barbiturates.

Like barbiturates, benzodiazepines can be divided into three groups according to the duration of their action. Long-acting benzodiazepines include diazepam, the classic anticonvulsive medication. Intermediate-acting benzodiazepines (e.g., lorazepam) are useful in treating acute alcohol withdrawal (delirium tremens). Short-acting benzodiazepines (e.g., midazolam) are useful in treating neurological medical emergencies such as status epilepticus, a condition of continuous convulsions. At present, there are over 20 different benzodiazepine formulations available on the market.

Mechanism of Action

Benzodiazepines work indirectly by occupying a receptor next to a receptor. GABA receptors on cell membranes control the flow of the chloride (Cl-) ion in and out of the cell via a chloride channel. The amount inside a cell, in milliequivalents (mEq) of chloride, affects its resting membrane potential. Benzodiazepine occupies a receptor next to the GABA receptor (now called the benzodiazepine receptor). The benzodiazepine receptor, when occupied by a benzodiazepine, stimulates the GABA receptor to hold onto GABA longer when it is stimulated. The result is prolonged GABA stimulation, which in turn increases the amount of chloride (Cl-) in the cell.[2] The cell, now loaded with chloride, is hyperpolarized and therefore much more difficult to depolarize.

Indications

When benzodiazepines hyperpolarize cells, they are in effect raising the action potential of those cells. Within the central nervous system, raising the action potential also raises the seizure threshold. Seizures are the result of spontaneous depolarization of the neurons in the brain. Seizures are analogous to ventricular fibrillation in the heart, a chaotic firing of cells without purpose. Raising the action potential of the heart raises the ventricular fibrillatory threshold. The heart is thus less likely to go into ventricular fibrillation. Raising the action potential within the brain raises the seizure threshold; thus, the brain is less likely to seize. This mechanism of action makes benzodiazepines very desirable as anticonvulsive medication, especially in cases of life-threatening continuous seizures termed "status epilepticus."

Benzodiazepines also inhibit the neurons within the limbic system, the seat of human emotions. Benzodiazepine receptors are more concentrated in the limbic system than anywhere else in the brain. The inhibition of the limbic system also makes benzodiazepines effective as a tranquilizer.[4] The combination of tranquilizer effect and anxiolytic effect makes benzodiazepines desirable as a premedication before painful procedures such as elective cardioversion. However, benzodiazepines are not pain relievers. Analgesic, concomitant administration of pain medication may be indicated.

Benzodiazepines are also useful in treating muscle spasms (secondary to neuromuscular disease) and spasticity of muscles from traumatic paraplegia or cerebral palsy. By inhibiting neural control of muscles at the level of the spinal cord, spasms can be prevented and patient management made easier.

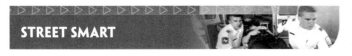

STREET SMART

All CNS depressants, including alcohol, barbiturates, and benzodiazepines, cause a loss of motor dexterity. Operation of complex machines, such as automobiles and ambulances, should be avoided while under the influence of these medications.

Benzodiazepine Toxicity

At high levels, benzodiazepines can produce drowsiness and respiratory depression. Fortunately, the therapeutic index for benzodiazepines is so high that true overdose is relatively rare. However, that is not the case when benzodiazepines are mixed with other CNS depressants, such as alcohol. These substances intensify, or potentiate, the effects of the benzodiazepines. In those cases, the incidence of respiratory depression/arrest becomes much higher. This fact is not lost on the public, some of whom use the combination of benzodiazepines and alcohol to cause a peaceful suicide.

The metabolism of benzodiazepines occurs in the liver, where even the metabolic by-products are often still pharmacologically active. The elderly, and others who have decreased liver function, may react more profoundly to the administration of benzodiazepines. For example, diazepam, which normally has a half-life of 24 hours, can remain active in the bloodstream of an elderly patient for 72 hours.

The antidote for benzodiazepine overdose is flumazenil. Flumazenil is a benzodiazepine receptor blocker. It is effective in blocking the effects of all benzodiazepines but is not effective against narcotics. Flumazenil has a half-life that is shorter than most intermediate-acting benzodiazepines. Therefore, Paramedics must be alert to the chance of rebound respiratory depression and be prepared to administer a repeat dose of flumazenil every hour.[5] Paramedics must also be cautious using flumazenil as it may induce acute benzodiazepine withdrawal (discussed shortly) and eliminate the protection from seizures created by the prophylactic administration of benzodiazepines.[6] The resultant "breakthrough" seizures can develop into life-threatening status epilepticus. For this reason, flumazenil is not recommended for use in altered mental status from unknown ingestions.

Withdrawal from Central Nervous System Depressants

Withdrawal of all CNS depressants can result in a dramatic rebound within the central nervous system. The common symptoms of depressant withdrawal include anxiety, agitation, restlessness, and symptoms of overstimulation of the sympathetic nervous system, such as tachycardia and hypertension. Onset of symptoms is usually patient and drug specific. For example, symptoms of alcohol withdrawal, called the delirium tremens, can occur in as little as 12 hours after the patient has taken his or her last drink.

Untreated depressant withdrawal can be life-threatening. Delirium tremens, for example, only occurs in about 5% of the patients in ethyl alcohol withdrawal. Yet, if left untreated, it can have up to a 35% mortality rate. Alcohol withdrawal frequently presents as a seizure, a frequent comorbid condition of alcoholism.[7] Treatment usually includes reintroduction of a CNS depressant, such as Librium, from which the patient is then carefully weaned off.

Anesthesia

While Paramedics rarely, if ever, perform general anesthesia while in the field, they are occasionally witness to anesthesia in the emergency department, critical care units, or operating room. An understanding of the fundamentals of anesthesia can potentially improve the Paramedics' experience as well as improve interdisciplinary communication between anesthetists and EMS.

Anesthesia, by definition, is the lack of sensation, painful or otherwise. Anesthetic drugs primarily induce anesthesia by interfering with or blocking nerve conduction. Local anesthesia, as the name implies, means that local nerves are incapacitated (i.e., left to feel numb). General anesthesia is much more complex. With the brain incapacitated, the patient becomes unconscious and general relaxation of muscles and loss of protective reflexes occurs.

Incremental doses of anesthetic medications can result in several levels or degrees of anesthesia, with the patient becoming deeper under the influence of the anesthetic with each successive dose or medication. The first state of anesthesia is called analgesia. **Analgesia** is a condition where the patient does not feel pain, yet remains conscious. More importantly, the patient retains his or her protective reflexes. This level of anesthesia is also referred to as **conscious sedation**. The second state of anesthesia is called excitement. At this level of anesthesia, the patient may be combative, delirious, and evidence irregular breathing. Vomiting and/or incontinence is also common in this stage. The third state of anesthesia is **surgical anesthesia**. The third state is further divided into four planes. These planes are varying levels of unconsciousness. Anesthesiologists are masters at the individualization of anesthetic doses to produce the exact plane of surgical anesthesia desired for the specific procedure being performed. By monitoring respirations, which return to normal after excitement, and reflexes, such as pupil size, the anesthesiologist can lead the patient to near-coma.

As the patient becomes more deeply anesthetized, he will lose protective reflexes in a head-to-toe (cephalocaudal) direction. The first reflex lost is the blink reflex. When the eyelashes are brushed gently, the eyelid closes (blinks); hence, the blink reflex. Level one of surgical anesthesia starts with the loss of consciousness and loss of the blink reflex. Conversely, when a patient is brought out of anesthesia, the last reflex to return before consciousness is the blink reflex.

The fourth and last state of anesthesia is medullary paralysis. With the vital life centers in the medulla oblongata paralyzed, the medication is now, by definition, toxic. Cardiopulmonary arrest ensues unless the medication is reduced or withdrawn.

STREET SMART

While the patient may appear unconscious, the last sense to be lost is the sense of hearing. Patients have reported, verbatim, statements made about them while they were assumed to be unconscious.[8–11]

Inhaled Anesthetics

General anesthetics may be either inhaled or injected intravenously. Anesthetists prefer inhaled anesthetic agents because these drugs can be precisely titrated to the exact level of anesthesia desired.

Most anesthetics are not gasses, with the exception of nitrous oxide. Inhaled anesthetics, like halothane or isoflurane, are volatile liquids that off-gas vapors, which are inhaled by the patient. The use of these volatile liquids requires complex apparatus and monitoring equipment that would make this procedure all but impossible to routinely perform in the field.

The only inhaled anesthetic used in the prehospital environment is nitrous oxide. Nitrous oxide (N_2O) received notoriety in the 1900s as a form of entertainment in the parlor and was dubbed laughing gas for its most notable side effect. Properly administered N_2O is a potent analgesic as well as an anesthetic that can be safely given in the field.[12–15] While ALS providers are concerned about the progression of anesthetics from analgesia to surgical anesthesia, with the concomitant problems that can occur, nitrous oxide cannot produce surgical anesthesia. This quality makes nitrous oxide even more desirable for the field. Add to that attribute the fact that nitrous oxide does not depress respirations nor increase cerebral blood flow in patients with potential head injuries, and nitrous oxide could be very useful in the out-of-hospital setting.

To administer nitrous oxide. the patient is usually asked to hold a mask that is flowing with a mixture of oxygen (minimum 20%) and nitrous oxide. When the patient can no longer hold the mask alone, the administration is completed.

Intravenous Anesthesia

Agents used in intravenous anesthesia include the ultra-short-acting barbiturates. Thiopental is particularly useful in cases where there is increased intracranial pressure (ICP) because it produces an actual decrease in ICP pressure (a neuroprotective benefit). The onset of action of these agents is usually between 60 and 90 seconds and the duration of the action is short.

Another class of agents used in intravenous anesthesia are the short-acting benzodiazepines. Benzodiazepines like lorazepam are lipid-soluble and readily cross the blood-brain barrier. While, as a class, benzodiazepines tend to have a slower onset of action than the barbiturates, they have an amnesic effect. This makes them the drug of choice for painful procedures, like elective cardioversion. Certain narcotic agents (e.g., fentanyl) are also used during intravenous anesthesia. A discussion of fentanyl follows in the section on narcotics.

Balanced Anesthesia

No single anesthetic agent is completely effective or even desirable for anesthesia. Individually, many anesthetic agents produce such significant side effects as hypotension, cardiac irritability, and nausea with vomiting. Therefore, a combination of anesthetic agents—some inhaled and some injected intravenously—are often used to minimize these side effects in an approach called **balanced anesthesia**.

In many cases, premedication with a CNS depressant, like barbiturates or benzodiazepines, is performed first. Use of these CNS depressants as a premedication before the introduction of anesthesia (**pre-induction agents**) can decrease the incidence of fear or panic (anxiolysis) or combativeness (sedation) in the patient.

Atropine is another frequently used pre-induction agent. Atropine, a parasympathetic blocker, dries the airways and prevents secretions, thus making intubation easier and aspiration less likely.[16,17] Another frequently used pre-induction agent is lidocaine. Lidocaine blunts sudden raises in intracranial pressure (ICP) that often accompany manipulation of the airway and intubation.[18–20]

The most common—and the most problematic—complication of anesthesia is nausea with vomiting. Major tranquilizers (**neuroleptics**) have a noteworthy side effect—they prevent nausea. Drugs like promethazine and chlorpromazine are used as both a sedative and as an antiemetic.

Procedural Sedation

Procedural sedation is a technique used by Paramedics to facilitate performance of technically difficult procedures (such as trauma intubation) or painful procedures (such as elective cardioversion). The goal of procedural sedation is to minimally depress the patient's consciousness, without loss of protective reflexes. Procedural sedation must also be performed with a minimum of alteration of vital signs. The use of procedural sedation can improve patient cooperation with painful or difficult procedures while ensuring safety and patient well-being. For these reasons, Paramedics are seeing a greater use of procedural sedation in the field.

Procedural sedation is the first state of anesthesia. As such, Paramedics must keep in mind that the patient can easily slip into the next state of anesthesia and lose their ability to protect their airway or become apneic. Therefore, all providers utilizing procedural sedation techniques must be prepared to protect the airway as well as treat any hemodynamic instability that might occur as a result of conscious sedation. It goes without saying that the patient undergoing procedural sedation must be continuously monitored. A more thorough discussion of procedural sedation is contained in Chapter 24.

Pain Management

Pain is the most common reason people call EMS. Yet, Paramedics are reluctant to administer pain medications. This is an unreasonable response, considering the large number of safe pain medications available.[21–23] Paramedics' unwillingness to use medications to ameliorate pain is, in part, due to lack of knowledge regarding the actions of these drugs.

The bombardment that the public, healthcare professionals, and Paramedics have received about the dangers of drug addiction has placed a needless fear in the minds of many. Yet, this fear continues, even though multiple studies have demonstrated that drug addiction to properly prescribed medications is rare.[24] The risks of addiction to single doses of pain medication administered in the field for obvious and necessary reasons is remote at best.

Other Paramedics are reluctant to administer pain medication for fear of inducing respiratory depression. This fear is unfounded for two reasons. First, with proper assessment, including dose adjustments based on condition, careful titration of the analgesic, and vigilant monitoring of the respiratory system, the incidence of respiratory depression is low. More importantly, if respiratory depression does occur, Paramedics are highly trained to properly respond. This fear represents a fundamental flaw in the Paramedics' understanding of pain management. While a dose of 4 milligrams of morphine, for example, administered intravenously might induce respiratory depression in 5 to 10 minutes, the same dose in a person with moderate burns, a fractured long bone, or advanced cancer would not. In fact, those patients may require 5 to 10 times or more than that amount of morphine to obtain relief from pain and still not be at risk for respiratory depression. In short, a patient who is truly in pain should and can receive pain medication for pain control. Paramedics should not be overly concerned about the risk of respiratory depression. However, this understanding does not relieve the Paramedic from needing to be prepared in case respiratory depression should occur.

Giving even more support to the argument that Paramedics can and should administer pain medications is the Paramedics' ability to administer an antagonist medication. Paramedics who can administer narcotics can also administer naloxone (the antagonist to narcotics) and thereby reverse any untoward effects. Thus, the availability of an antidote, plus the reality of pain management in these selected populations, and the ability to manage the consequences, combine to provide Paramedics an unparalleled safety margin.

The Experience of Pain

Perhaps the more central issue is the Paramedic's understanding of the concept of pain. A person's interpretation of pain is based, in part, upon cultural determinants and, in part, by a personal pain history. The interpretation of pain may be gender biased; for example, some feel men should be tough and not complain. The interpretation of pain may be age-biased, for example; the misconception that the elderly can tolerate pain better. The interpretation of pain is based in large part upon the patient's own experiences with pain. Each patient has a pain history which colors his interpretation of pain and how he perceives others' pain.

Therefore, when assessing someone else's pain, all healthcare professionals tend to look at that person's pain from their own perspective. This approach, while understandable, is flawed. Pain is a personal experience. Therefore, the effectiveness of pain management can only be interpreted by the person affected. Paramedics must develop tools to assess pain and trust the patient to be honest. That honesty will be rewarded as the patient–provider relationship is strengthened.

Concepts in Pain

Pain is both the cognitive awareness of the stimulus as well as the body's physiological response to the stimulus. Understanding the physiological response will allow Paramedics to lessen the pain by interfering with the process.

Pain can be divided into acute and chronic pain. Chronic pain is a persistent or reoccurring discomfort seen in long-term conditions (e.g., arthritis). Chronic pain, while important, is not germane to the topic of EMS. Acute pain, on the other hand, is a constant in the day-to-day provision of EMS. Acute pain occurs suddenly and is preceded by some identifiable event. Pain is a warning to the patient, the body's way of telling the patient that something has changed. The pain usually persists until the situation is corrected.

Acute pain can arise from the internal organs, such as the heart, and is usually described as a pressure-like, dull, or aching. This organ pain is termed **visceral pain**. Visceral pain is poorly localized and often is transmitted to other parts of the body, via common nerve pathways. This is called **referred pain**.

Acute pain often arises from the skin, ligaments, muscle, fascia, bones, or joints. This type of pain (**somatic pain**) is often described as sharp or burning. One important difference between visceral pain and somatic pain is that somatic pain can be localized to a specific area.

Every person has a tolerance to pain. At its lowest level, one person might perceive pain while another might not. This is the **pain threshold**, that amount of stimulus required to elicit a pain response.

If the person has multiple injuries, and therefore multiple painful experiences, she may not perceive the dull visceral pain of a heart attack, for example, over the intense pain of a fractured femur. When a pain (often dull visceral pain) is overshadowed by another more intense pain from another injury, it is called a **distracting injury**. The fractured femur in this case may be a distracting injury and takes perceptual dominance over the chest pain. The concept of perceptual dominance makes it more difficult to accurately assess a patient's condition.

Physiology of Pain

An injury to the skin will stimulate pain receptors in the dermis. These pain receptors, called **nociceptors**, respond to chemical, mechanical, or thermal stimulus and are not evenly distributed across the body. Once stimulated, the nociceptors' signal is transmitted either quickly over myelinated A fibers (sharp) to the spinal cord or more slowly over unmyelinated C fibers (dull or burning) to the thalamus. Reflex arcs occur over A fibers, the speed of which permits an automatic withdrawal from the stimulus before the brain even has a chance to interpret the painful stimuli and respond. The pain sensation is now transmitted to the brain via either the neospinothalamic tract (acute pain) or the paleospinothalamic tract (dull pain) in the spinal cord.

After arriving at the post-central gyrus in the midbrain, the signal is transferred to the cortex (acute pain) or the limbic system (dull pain) for interpretation and response. The body's response to pain is two-fold: regulation of inflammation and neuromodulation of the pain. **Inflammation** is the body's response to an injury. Activated by the pain, prostaglandins act as inflammatory regulators, affecting blood vessel tone, platelet aggregation, and muscle spasm in the injured area.

Neuromodulators are substances that inhibit the transmission of painful sensations to the brain and spinal cord. Examples of neuromodulators are **endorphins**. Endorphins attach to opiate receptors on the neuron which in turn inhibit neural activity. Naturally, opiates also occupy these opiate receptors, enhancing the activity of the endorphins. High levels of circulating neurotransmitters—such as norepinephrine and serotonin in the brain caused by stress, acupuncture, and excessive physical exertion—interfere with the effectiveness of endorphins and opiates alike.

Analgesics

The class of drugs that relieve pain are called **analgesics**. Analgesics work by inhibiting the synthesis or release of prostaglandins or stimulating opiate receptors (opiate agonists).

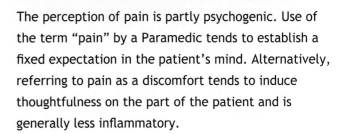

Regardless of the mechanism of action, every analgesic can mask the cause of the symptom. Simply ignoring the pain does not stop the damage that will occur. Before, during, and after pain management, Paramedics must assess and determine the underlying cause of the problem.

Opiates

Opium, isolated from the Poppy plant, may have been the first pain medication used by man. Over the span of time, physicians and laypersons alike have sought better, stronger, more effective opium. This untiring pursuit has resulted in over a dozen opiate and opiate-like medications (Table 31-1).

Mechanism of Action

All opiates work by a similar mechanism, coupling with opioid receptors in the central nervous system and the gastrointestinal system to become an opiate agonist. The stimulation of these opioid receptors decreases the cell membrane's permeability to sodium.[25] The resultant increase in intracellular sodium hyperpolarizes the cell, decreases the action potential, and slows conduction by decreasing nerve cell depolarization.

Indications

Five different opioid receptors have been identified and labeled with the Greek letters Mu, Kappa, Sigma, Delta, and Epsilon. Stimulating these opioid receptors causes a variety of effects. Stimulation of the opioid receptors in the gastrointestinal system decreases gastric motility (slowed peristalsis) as well as intestinal secretions. Disease-induced diarrhea, a common malady, can be treated very effectively with small amounts of opioids. A few drops of tincture of opium can stop diarrhea and produce constipation.[26,27] Paregoric, a camphorated tincture of opium, is an old remedy used for centuries to treat diarrhea. It is still used to treat life-threatening diarrhea in infants and neonates.

Stimulating the Mu, Kappa, and Sigma opioid receptors along the cortex–brainstem–spinal cord axis produces other desirable, as well as undesirable, effects. Some opiates, in small quantities, function as a cough suppressant (e.g., an **antitussive**). Prescription antitussive cold medications occasionally include the opiate codeine.

Table 31-1 Opiates

Drug	Method	Onset of Action	Peak Effect	Duration
Codeine	PO	10 to 31 min	31 to 60 min	4 hours
Hydrocodone	PO	10 to 31 min	31 to 60 min	4 hours
Hydromorphone	IM	15 min	31 to 60 min	4 hours
	IV	10 to 15 min	15 to 31 min	2 hours
Meperidine	IM	10 to 15 min	31 to 50 min	3 hours
	IV	1 min	5 to 7 min	3 hours
Methadone	IM	10 to 20 min	60 to 120 min	4 hours
Morphine	IM	10 to 31 min	31 to 60 min	4 hours
	IV	1 min	20 min	4 hours
Oxymorphone	IM	10 to 15 min	31 to 90 min	4 hours
	IV	5 to 10 min	15 to 31 min	4 hours
Propoxyphene	PO	15 to 60 min	120 min	4 hours

Opiates in larger doses impact the brainstem and produce constricted pinpoint pupils (*miosis*) and respiratory depression. Even moderate doses of opiates can induce some degree of respiratory depression. In some cases, this slower and deeper respiration is desirable, improving the clearance of carbon dioxide from the lungs and increasing oxygenation of the blood. In slightly higher doses, slowed respirations paradoxically result in increased carbon dioxide retention and hypoxia. The result of unattended opiate overdose can be profound respiratory depression leading to acute respiratory acidosis and cardiac arrest. Therefore, patients must be carefully monitored while receiving opiates.

The less desirable hallucinogenic effects of opiates, the **narcotic** effect, is thought to be the result of stimulation of the sigma receptors located in the limbic system. This dream-producing quality of opiates is so well known that when German pharmacist Friedrich Serturner extracted a plant alkaloid from the opium of the Poppy plant, he named it Morphium, after Morpheus, the Greek god of dreams.[28]

Perhaps the most widely known benefit of opiates is their impact on pain. A potent analgesic agent, opiates affect the Mu, Kappa, and Delta receptors in the cerebral cortex, the medial thalamus, and the spinal cord, altering the brain's perception of pain. Opiates, in effect, replace or augment the body's own neuromodulators (endophins) and lessen the sensation of pain. It should be noted that, even though the patient still perceives the pain, opiates alter the patient's perception of the pain from being an unpleasant feeling to one that is less noxious.

Such notables as Florence Nightingale used opiates for their therapeutic benefit. During one of her own illnesses she stated that the "curious little new fangled operation of putting opium under the skin" gave her relief from her discomfort. With the advent of the hypodermic needle in the 1950s, the future of opiates was ensured. Opiates have become a mainstay analgesic.[28]

Opiates, particularly morphine, are also widely used to treat the chest pain (angina pectoris) of an acute myocardial infarction (AMI). The administration of morphine not only alleviates pain—relaxing the patient and reducing circulating epinephrine levels and subsequent arterial constriction—but it also decreases the heart's work (MvO2) by creating peripheral vasodilatation. This, in turn, reduces preload. Both of these effects of morphine are accomplished without impacting heart rate significantly, making it an acceptable analgesic for acute myocardial infarction pain, though there is some controversy about the use of morphine for patients with suspected acute myocardial infarction.

Administration

Morphine is the archetypical opiate. The pain-relieving abilities of all subsequent medications are measured against it. When a dose of a new medication formulation has the same ability to produce analgesia as 10 milligrams of morphine, it is **equianalgesic** (i.e., equal to morphine). Morphine serves as the standard for comparison.

The one of the first morphine derivatives, produced by the German pharmaceutical company Bayer, was three times more potent than morphine. It was called a heroic drug, or heroin, because of its powerful pain-relieving effects.

Fentanyl, another morphine derivative, is a remarkably potent opiate agonist. It has a rapid onset of action as well as a short duration of action, and is 80 times more potent than morphine. The combination of these three qualities makes fentanyl very useful in the out-of-hospital setting.

Knowing if a drug produces an equianalgesic effect similar to morphine allows Paramedics to understand the impact of an alternative analgesic compared to morphine (Table 31-2).

Weaker derivatives of opiates (such as propoxyphene, a spinoff of methadone) are often combined with aspirin or acetaminophen for an enhanced effect. When combined, two analgesics tend to potentiate one another, allowing for smaller doses of each with the effect of giving a greater dose of one of them.

Table 31-2 Dose Equivalency of Common Opiates*

Drug	Dose
Morphine	10 mg
Methadone	10 mg
Meperidine	75 mg
Codeine	60 mg
Hydromorphone	1.5 mg
Fentanyl	25 mcg

*All medications are given IM.

Transdermal

A number of transdermal administration methods have been created to administer opioids long-term. These transdermal systems often use a gelled alcohol as a vehicle; the body's heat will melt the gel so that absorption will occur. Properly applied, the patch should be placed on smooth (hairless) and intact skin that is clear of soaps, oils, and lotions that might impede absorption. Fevers (greater than 102°F) as well as application of heating pads and electric blankets can increase the absorption of the opiate, leading to toxicity. Transdermal patches should also be removed and disposed of properly. Application of new patches without removal of used patches may result in toxicity.

Continuous Infusion

Unremitting pain from cancer, for example, requires a constant administration of opiates in order to obtain, then sustain, the analgesia. Special patient-controlled analgesia (PCA) infusion pumps provide the patient with the ability to control the amount of analgesia administered without interruption.

Precautions

While morphine has poor lipid solubility, making passage across the blood-brain barrier less likely, other opiates (such as fentanyl) rapidly pass across both the blood-brain barrier as well as the placental barrier. For this reason, caution must be advised when giving any opiate to ensure that it does not pass directly into an unborn infant, depressing the infant's respiratory drive.

Concerns related to adverse effects of opiate administration are directly related to the predictable effects of the opiates in the body. The most notorious side effect of opiates is respiratory depression. Patients who have pre-existing pulmonary disease, such as emphysema or cor pulmonale, are at risk for atypical respiratory depression and even risk respiratory arrest with standard therapeutic doses. Cases of death have been attributed to opiates given in routine doses in these patient populations.

Respiratory depression induced by opiates can also have deleterious effects upon the patient with a traumatic brain injury. Slowed respirations directly translate to carbon dioxide retention, which in turn promotes cerebral vasodilatation and subsequent increased intracranial pressure (ICP).

Opiates also complicate the neurological examination of the patient with head injuries by producing miosis (pinpoint pupils). As a general rule, opiate use is avoided in patients with potential head injuries.

Occasionally, opiates (particularly morphine) will cause the release of histamine from mast cells. The result is anaphylactoid reaction complete with urticaria (hives), pruritus (itching), and facial edema but is not a true anaphylactic reaction. Treatment usually involves symptomatic care using Benadryl.

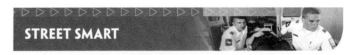

STREET SMART

Small amounts of codeine are found, along with opium, in the common Poppy. They are both plant alkaloids that are chemically related. Therefore, it is not uncommon for a patient who has an allergy to codeine to have a cross-allergy to morphine.

Synthetic Opiates

Pharmacists continue to try to create synthetic opiates that do not have morphine's undesirable effects. Methadone, a synthetic opiate, is equianalgesic to morphine and is useful in the treatment of narcotic addiction. It has many of the same effects as morphine. However, methadone's single greatest advantage may be that it can be taken orally, with the same effect, avoiding the dangers inherent in the use of needles. For this reason, and because methadone has a long half-life, methadone is used in heroin detoxification programs.

Meperidine, another synthetic opiate, is an effective analgesic but requires large oral doses to become dose-equivalent to morphine; 310 mg PO equals 75 mg IM, which is equianalgesic to 10 mg morphine. At these higher doses, meperidine has too many complications, including potentially toxic buildup of metabolites, to make it useful. Meperidine is used in smaller doses to treat moderate to mild pain.

On the positive side, Meperidine is unlikely to cause mast cells to release histamine and produce the pseudo-allergic reaction seen with morphine. Meperidine also has an atropine-like quality that causes pupil dilation, not constriction, which is unlike the other opiates.

Opiate Antagonists

Opiate antagonists can also induce acute opiate withdrawal. Opiate antagonists, like naloxone, dislodge opiates from the opiate receptors. Undesired effects of opiate administration, such as respiratory depression, are immediately reversed, as well as the euphoric feeling that some addicts crave. Unsuspecting Paramedics have been assaulted by heroin addicts because the provider "ruined the high."

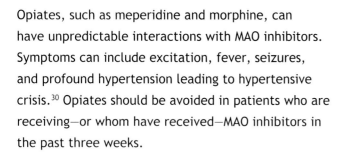
Naloxone is typically administered parenterally, either intravenously or intramuscularly. Recently, a nasal form of naloxone has been marketed, which would avoid the use of intravenous needles in this HIV-prone population.

The onset of naloxone is one to two minutes when administered intravenously and can last for up to one and one-half hours. Predictable side effects of opiate antagonists (such as naloxone) include tachycardia, hypertension, and vomiting. The half-life of most opiates is at least twice as long (four to five hours in most cases), requiring repeat doses of naloxone in order to obliterate the effects of the opiate.

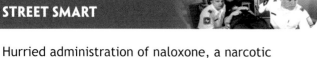
Non-Opioid Analgesics

Federal and state restrictions on opiate use, including mandatory triple prescriptions, have made acquiring opiates for pain relief difficult. Patients with minor to moderate pain often do not seek out medical assistance but rather self-treat and avoid the expense of medical care that does not include opiates. This way of thinking has led to a boom in nonprescription non-opioid analgesics sales.

This group of analgesics is also referred to as "non-narcotic," leading to the assumption that these drugs are not addictive. While strictly correct (non-opioid analgesics generally do not lead to physiological addiction), many of these analgesics are habit-forming. Unsupervised chronic use of these drugs can lead to long-term complications, including organ-specific toxicity.

Salicylates

Aspirin (ASA) is the prototypical non-opioid analgesic. Brought to the market in 1897 by the Bayer pharmaceutical company,[32] it remains the world's most popular medication. However, the central ingredient (salicylate) is found in many other over-the-counter drugs (e.g., Oil of Wintergreen). Salicylates (from the Latin *salix,* meaning willow) have three major pharmaceutical actions: analgesia, antipyretic, and antiplatelet.

In small doses (less than 1,000 mg), salicylate compounds are effective for the relief of mild to moderate pain from muscular strains, joint discomfort, headache, and the like. The pain-relieving action of salicylates is primarily at the peripheral site of inflammation, not centrally in the brain as is the case with narcotics.

Inflammatory Process

Whether caused by a break in the skin (infection), oxygen deprivation (hypoxia), chemical irritation (inhalation of gas), or trauma (mechanical injury), the body initiates an inflammatory response at the site of the injury. The inflammatory response is an exact process that begins immediately and includes nonspecific defenses, phagocytes, mast cells that release histamine (causing vasodilatation), macrophages that release lysosomal enzymes, and specific responses such as antibodies.

The activities of these various body defenses culminate in the signs of local inflammation typically manifested by redness and swelling, histamine-induced vasodilation, the accumulation of dead leukocytes and bacteria as pus, and the release of pyrogens (fever-producing chemicals) from the leukocytes.

Prostaglandins, unsaturated fatty acids, are pivotal in this response. Prostaglandins increase postcapillary venule permeability as well as smooth muscle contraction. More importantly, prostaglandins produce the pain, either visceral or somatic, that is characteristic of an inflammatory response.

Inhibition of prostaglandin production therefore reduces or eliminates the pain. Salicylates work by bonding to an enzyme called cyclooxygenase, which would normally bind with the fatty acids to produce prostaglandins.[33] Salicylates thus interrupt the production of pain-producing prostaglandins.

Without prostaglandins, prostaglandin derivatives—including thromboxane A2 (TxA2)—cannot be produced. TxA2 causes local vasoconstriction and encourages the degranulation of platelets, the first step in the coagulation cascade (sometimes called production of the platelet plug). Thus, salicylates are also anti-platelet drugs. As such, salicylates (specifically aspirin) have seen a great deal of use in preventing the formation of thrombus that can lead to acute myocardial infarction or cerebral vascular accident.

The third inflammatory response, fever, is also affected by salicylates. A febrile response is caused when pyrogens are released from the site of the inflammation and circulate to the hypothalamus. These pyrogens then affect the hypothalamus and the body's temperature is changed. Salicylates are thought to reset the body's temperature set-point back to normal by interfering with circulating pyrogens.

Salicylate Toxicity

An allergy to aspirin is a relatively common drug allergy, one whose presence is complicated by the large number of salicylate-containing compounds in drugs and over-the-counter medications. Caution is advised whenever giving any drug to determine if an allergy exists, particularly an aspirin allergy. Salicylates have also been known to induce an asthma attack in prone patients, as shown in the previous discussion of aspirin-induced asthma. Paramedics should also be particularly aware of the potential for hypoglycemia (particularly for children) that exists during a salicylate overdose.

Intentional or non-intentional overdose of salicylates creates a mixed respiratory alkalosis secondary to increased carbon dioxide production and metabolic acidosis due to the increased metabolism and increased metabolic acid production.[34] Treatment focuses on routine gut decontamination as well as reversal of the acid–base disorder.[35] If the patient experiences spasms of the muscles (titanic spasm) secondary to the acidosis, calcium gluconate is effective for offering symptomatic relief while the underlying acidosis is corrected.

While not a toxicity per se, aspirin is not given to children because of the association between aspirin given to children with a fever of unknown origin (FUO) and Reye's syndrome, an acute encephalopathy. Reye's syndrome is an abnormal degeneration of fat, especially in the viscera, that can also lead to acute encephalopathy.

STREET SMART

Aspirin in routine doses reduces fever. Aspirin in large doses can actually induce a paradoxical rise in temperature. Well-meaning parents can overdose a child on aspirin, see the child's temperature rise, and then mistakenly administer more aspirin, thinking they are treating the fever.

Nonsteroidal Anti-Inflammatory Drugs

The nonsteroidal anti-inflammatory drugs (NSAIDs), commonly referred to as aspirin substitutes, have found increasing popularity for several reasons: aspirin allergies, pediatric restrictions regarding aspirin use, and unwanted salicylate side effects (Table 31-3). The earliest non-salicylate analgesics were the para-aminophenols (short-name anilines) which included acetaminophen (APAP). Despite the difference in formulation, the mechanism of action for these NSAIDs is the same as for salicyclates (interference with the enzyme cyclooxygenase), which in turn inhibits prostaglandin production and thromboxane.

A notable difference between the two products (NSAIDs and aspirin) is that aspirin irreversibly interferes with platelet function for the life of the platelet, whereas most NSAIDs do not interfere with platelet function at all.

Acetaminophen Toxicity

The increasing popularity of any drug often results in cases of toxicity. An overdose of aspirin is usually quite evident, as the patient goes into a metabolic acidosis. His or her respirations

Table 31-3 NSAIDs

Class	Drug	Onset	Half-Life	Dose
Acetic acids	Diclofenac	31 min	2 hours	50 mg PO
	Indomethacin	31 min	4 hours	25/50 mg PO
	Ketorolac	10 min	4 hours	30 mg IV
Oxicams	Piroxicam	2 to 4 hrs	24 hours	20 to 40 mg
Propionic acids	Ibuprofen	31 min	2 hours	310 to 800 mg
	Naproxen	60 min	12 hours	250 to 500 mg

Originally, many NSAIDs were FDA approved prescription medicines. Manufacturers of these FDA prescription medicines requested (and have received) permission to sell some of these NSAIDs as over-the-counter (OTC) medications. The only difference between prescription NSAIDs and OTC NSAIDs is the dose of the drug. The assumption is that the patient using an OTC will follow the package instructions to avoid the side effects and complications associated with larger doses.

would become rapid (tachypnea) and the patient would become outwardly symptomatic.

In the case of many NSAIDs, there are no immediate outward manifestations of toxicity. Acetaminophen, for example, is highly hepatotoxic.[36] Undiscovered acetaminophen toxicity can cause permanent liver damage within three days of the overdose.

Convulsions

A generalized convulsion, the outward manifestation of a seizure, is a series of whole body contractions (**tonic**), then repetitive contractions (**clonic**), that are immediately preceded by a loss of consciousness. The underlying seizure is the result of random and disorganized neuronal discharge within the brain, particularly across the motor strip of the cerebral cortex, anterior thalamus, and basal ganglia.

The origin of the convulsion can be from an abnormal focus in the brain that is triggered by hypoxia, hypoglycemia, hyperthermia, and other stimuli. It can also be triggered by extra-cranial sources (such as toxic inhalations, electrolyte imbalances, or drugs) or iatrogenic sources, secondary to subtherapeutic anticonvulsant levels.

The chaotic brain activity during a seizure is somewhat analogous of the chaotic myocardial activity during ventricular fibrillation—purposeless and potentially life-threatening.

Regardless of the cause, the patient lapses out of consciousness and is at risk for injury secondary to falls or **status epilepticus**, a condition of unremitting convulsions.

The therapeutic goal of anticonvulsant medications is to raise the seizure threshold (by depressing the epileptic focus within the brain) without altering the patient's mental status and CNS functioning.

In every case, regardless of prior history, Paramedics should attempt to identify and treat potentially reversible causes of convulsions, such as hypoxia, hypoglycemia, or hyperthermia. Anticonvulsant medications administered in

these cases would only serve to mask the underlying pathology and put the patient at risk for more serious and potentially life-threatening complications.

For example, convulsions secondary to eclampsia (toxemia of pregnancy) can be effectively treated with either diazepam or phenytoin. However, current evidence suggests that magnesium sulfate is the drug of choice in these cases because it treats the underlying pathophysiology.[37] That said, a distinction must be made between the woman with eclampsia who is seizing and the woman with a seizure history who also has pre-eclampsia. In the first case, magnesium sulfate would be preferred, whereas in the latter case diazepam would be preferred.

While the possible teratogenic effects of seizure medication must be considered before prophylactic use is advised, a reoccurrence of a seizure can also produce fetal anoxia.

For the patient with a previous diagnosis of **epilepsy** (recurrent seizures without known cause), the most likely cause of another seizure is subtherapeutic levels of anticonvulsant medication. For whatever reason (e.g., sudden withdrawal or poor compliance), the drug level in the plasma drops below the therapeutic level and the patient experiences a **breakthrough seizure**. Regardless of this fact, other etiologies for seizure cannot be ignored and must be ruled out.

While anticonvulsant medications can help a patient return to the activities of a normal life (e.g., driving a car), these drugs do not cure epilepsy. They only control the number and severity of each seizure. However, four out of five patients with epilepsy can have their seizures controlled with medications.

Anticonvulsant Medication

Over the centuries, seizures have been variously described as the work of evil spirits, the patient's soul wrestling with the devil, and as a rabid infection, after witnessing the same frothing of the mouth as seen with patients who were infected with rabies. Not until the works of Jean-Martin Charcot, in the mid-1900s, was the *grands paroxysmes* considered a possible symptom of a greater pathology—the result of potentially curable organic lesions.[28]

In the past, treatment for epilepsy often started with a barbiturate. Phenobarbital was frequently chosen because of its margin of safety (discussed earlier). Subsequently, newer, more effective medications have largely replaced phenobarbital for the treatment of epilepsy. However, phenobarbital still sees use in the emergency setting, primarily where respiratory depression can be managed expertly and for the few cases of uncertain eclampsia and status epilepticus.

Mechanism of Action

Most anticonvulsants, including phenobarbital, negatively influence the action potential of the neuron and thus inhibit spurious discharges. The majority of anticonvulsants act as sodium channel-blockers, a mechanism that is similar to the mechanism of a Class IB antidysrhythmic medication.

Barbiturates

Barbiturates, including phenobarbital, are a class of CNS depressants that have seen second service as anticonvulsants. One advantage of barbiturates is the wide variety of delivery methods (PO, IV, IM) as well as the various duration of actions.

Primidone, whose active metabolite is phenobarbital, is seeing greater use for control of seizures and is often used in combination with carbamazepine and phenytoin. By being used together, these drugs permit lower doses of each.

Hydantoins

One of the oldest and most widely used anticonvulsants, phenytoin, belongs to the class of hydantoins. As a class, these drugs are chemically related to barbiturates and act to decrease the influx of sodium (i.e., sodium channel-blockers), thereby decreasing neuronal excitability.

Fosphenytoin, another hydantoin, is the prodrug to phenytoin. Fosphenytoin has a rapid onset of action (peaking in less than six minutes), can be administered intravenously at a rate three times faster than phenytoin (without cardiac complications), and causes less burning at the IV site.[38] Cumulatively, these advantages make fosphenytoin desirable as an emergency medication.

Hydantoin Toxicity

Maintaining a serum plasma level of hydantoins that is therapeutic—and not toxic—is complicated by the distribution and biotransformation of the drug. Hydantoins quickly become protein-bound (primarily to blood albumin) while in circulation. Thus, a large percentage of the drug is pharmacologically unavailable. Only when all available albumin becomes saturated are sufficient plasma levels of free drug available for its intended therapeutic effect.

Compounding this difficulty is the drug's biotransformation. The liver's enzymatic system, the cytochrome P-450 system, is very effective in reducing hydantoins to inactive metabolites. However, hepatic metabolism has limits. Once these limits are reached, then more free drug is available. Therefore, to reach desired therapeutic levels of hydantoin, dosing must take into account both the volume of blood proteins as well as hepatic biotransformation. Overcoming these two impediments, even with small incremental increases in hydantoin dose, can result in marked, or near-toxic, elevations in serum drug levels.

The patient who is toxic on hydantoin will present with an **ataxia** (a disequilibrium in walk that resembles a drunkard's stagger) and a **nystagamus** (a fine tremble of the eye when holding a lateral gaze).[39] Unsuspecting Paramedics may incorrectly deduce that the patient is intoxicated on alcohol. Hydantoins, in toxic doses, have significant cardiac effects, similar to Class IB antidysrhythmic drugs. Left untreated, these cardiotoxic effects can lead to cardiovascular collapse and death.

Hydantoins and Pregnancy

Women with a history of epilepsy who become pregnant are often taken off of hydantoins to eliminate the risk of **fetal hydantoin syndrome (FHS)**. Hydantoin use during pregnancy can generate birth defects such as cleft lip, cleft palate, and congenital heart anomalies.[40,41]

If left untreated, approximately 50% of pregnant women with a prior seizure history will experience at least one seizure during their pregnancy.[42] Seizure during a pregnancy can induce fetal anoxia, which can result in congenital birth defects including mental retardation.

The quandary lies in whether to prophylactically treat the seizure disorder, and potentially risk FHS, or risk a seizure and fetal anoxia. In most instances, alternative medications are explored. If these are ineffective, then the lowest possible dose of hydantoin is prescribed.

Carbamazepine

Carbamazepine has a mechanism of action that is similar to hydantoins but is chemically similar to the tricyclic antidepressants. Carbamazepine is used, with good effect, to control a large variety of seizures including partial seizures with complex symptoms, as well as generalized tonic-clonic seizures.

Carbamazepine is slow to absorb. It is not unusual for the drug to take a month or more to obtain therapeutic levels in the blood. Despite this obstacle, carbamazepine is the drug of choice for many pediatric patients because of its low incidence of side effects. Concurrent administration of erythromycin, an antibiotic occasionally prescribed to children, can lower circulating plasma levels of carbamazepine in the child with epilepsy and result in breakthrough seizures.

Carbamazepine Toxicity

Simultaneous administration of isoniazid (another antibiotic used to treat tuberculosis) and propoxyphene (an analgesic) can cause an increase in blood serum levels of carbamazepine to the point of near-lethal toxicity.

Co-administration of carbamazepine with an MAO inhibitor (an antidepressant) can also cause elevated temperature (hyperpyrexia), elevated blood pressure (to hypertensive crisis levels), and, paradoxically, seizures leading to status epilepticus.

Succinimides

Succinimides, as a class of anticonvulsant medication, raise the seizure threshold and suppress nerve conduction in the motor cortex, resulting in good seizure control. Ethosuximide, an example of a succinimide, is used to treat pediatric absence seizures.

Valproic Acid

Valproic acid and divalproex have similar actions (increasing levels of the inhibitory neurotransmitter GABA within the brain) and are used alone or in combination with other anticonvulsants to treat absence seizures.

Valproic acid is also useful in the emergent treatment of status epilepticus that is unresponsive to standard treatments.

Benzodiazepines

Benzodiazepines, discussed earlier, are also useful as anticonvulsants. Paramedics, when confronted with a patient in status epilepticus, can administer a benzodiazepine (such as diazepam or the short-acting midazolam) for control of the seizure. In those cases, Paramedics must be prepared to manage respiratory depression secondary to the benzodiazepine.

Parkinson's Disease

Parkinson's disease has an insidious onset, starting with barely perceptible rhythmic tremors and progressing to gross motor dysfunction. In an advanced stage, the patient with Parkinson's disease exhibits extremely slow (**bradykinesia**) or difficult (**dyskinesia**) movement. For example, if a patient with Parkinson's disease is gently pushed, the patient's muscles may not be able to respond quickly enough to stop a fall.

The combination of loss of airway control, manifested by drooling and slurred speech, as well as a blank mask-like stare, makes the patient with Parkinson's disease appear dull and dimwitted. Yet, Parkinson's disease affects the intellectual capacity of only 40% of the patient population afflicted with Parkinson's disease. However, the combination of events just described can often produce severe depression in this patient population, leaving an appearance of dwindling intellectual capacity.

Approximately 150 in 100,000 people over age 65 will develop Parkinson's disease, making it the fourth most common neurological disorder.[43] The onset of Parkinson's disease can start as early as 40 years of age and is slightly more prevalent in males. While Parkinson's disease itself is not a medical emergency, the effects of the disease (like falls, which often result from dyskinesia) create emergency situations.

Pathophysiology

As a person develops Parkinson's disease, the number of dopaminergic receptors in the brain is reduced (Figure 31-1). The gradual loss of these receptors results in a progressive deterioration of brain function. Dopaminergic receptors are abundant in the substantia nigra, a portion of the central nervous system's extrapyramidal motor system responsible for muscle coordination and movement.

Normally, the dopaminergic receptors produce an inhibitory effect upon the extrapyramidal motor system. In the absence of dopaminergic receptors, the cholinergic receptors take dominance by stimulating the extrapyramidal motor. The clinical manifestations of Parkinson's disease are the result of this imbalance between dopaminergic stimulation and cholinergic stimulation. Classic symptoms of Parkinson's disease include muscle rigidity, resting tremors, a forward leaning posture, and a shuffling gait.

Drugs That Are Used to Treat Parkinson's Disease

Treatment of Parkinson's disease focuses on either blocking the cholinergic receptors (suppressing the effects of acetylcholine) or increasing the level of dopamine receptor stimulation.

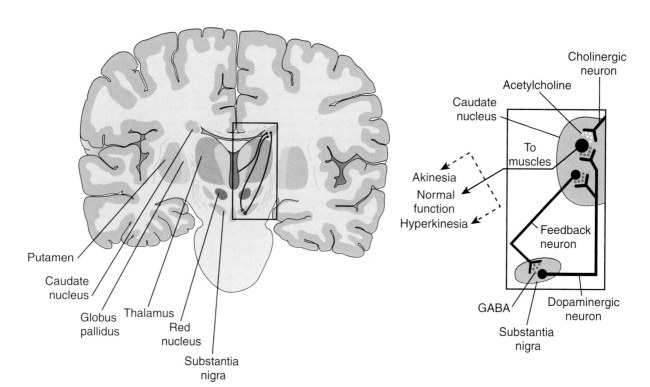

Figure 31-1 Parkinson's disease.

The quintessential cholinergic blocker is atropine, the bella donna alkaloid extracted from the nightshade plant. Atropine was used for years to treat Parkinson's disease.

More recently, newer synthetic cholinergic blockers, such as benztropine, have been used with better effect. These cholinergic antagonists decrease dyskinesia in nearly 50% of patients suffering from Parkinson's disease.

Currently, treatment of Parkinson's disease is focusing more on how to increase dopaminergic receptor stimulation than on blocking cholinergic receptors. Means to achieve this goal include administering drugs that increase dopamine levels (such as levodopa) or stimulating release of dopamine from neuronal storage vesicles (e.g., amantadine).

Alternatively, levels of dopaminergic receptor activity can be increased, not by inducing the body to produce or release more dopamine, but by using dopamine agonists. Examples of dopamine agonists include bromocriptine, a plant alkaloid, and pramipexole.

Finally, dopamine levels in the neurosynapse can be increased by decreasing dopamine destruction by monoamine oxidase during uptake. A monoamine oxidase inhibitor, such as selegiline, is often given together with levodopa. The combination of drugs permits lower doses of each, thereby decreasing undesirable side effects while still achieving the same therapeutic goal.

Precautions

Two types of monoamine oxidase exist in the body: type A and type B. MAO inhibitors used to treat Parkinson's disease primarily affect monoamine oxidase B. Inappropriate administration of other MAO inhibitors, along with levodopa, can precipitate profound hypertension or hypertensive crisis.

STREET SMART

Administration of meperidine to patients on MAO inhibitors can cause severe reactions, including profound hypertension, respiratory depression, hyperpyrexia, and seizures. Alternatively, administration of morphine is less likely to produce these unwanted side effects.

Drugs That Affect the Endocrine System

The association of the endocrine system and the nervous system is somewhat analogous to the relationship between the parasympathetic and the sympathetic nervous system. The parasympathetic nervous system, via its vagus nerve, maintains those mundane vegetative functions of life, while the sympathetic nervous system stands by, ready to react at a moment's notice to any threat to that life. Similarly, the endocrine system, via its arrangement of chemical messengers, helps to maintain an optimal internal environment for metabolism while the nervous system is ready to respond to the ever changing external conditions. The goal in both cases is identical—to maintain a balance (i.e., **homeostasis**) within the body and life.

The chemical messengers that stimulate the body's organs and help to maintain the body's internal environment (its milieu) are called **hormones** (from the Greek meaning "to arouse"). Hormones are produced and excreted from endocrine glands located in various locations within the body. The amount of hormone in the bloodstream is a function of a feedback mechanism, a mechanism that monitors and alters the amount of hormone released.

The most common feedback mechanism is the negative feedback loop. A negative feedback loop occurs when increasing levels of a hormone stop the secretion of more hormone. An exception to hormonal control by feedback mechanism is seen when the sympathetic nervous system stimulates the release of epinephrine from the adrenal medulla (an endocrine gland) during stress. This action would be classified as neuronal control.

Once a hormone is released into the blood, it circulates until it is attracted to a target cell with the correct receptor (a "key in lock" concept). When linked together, the hormone can either enhance the cell's function (a direct effect) or it can facilitate an aspect of the cell's function. For example, insulin (a hormone) attaches to insulin receptors, which then permit the passage of glucose into the cell.

Hormones and Pharmacy

The hormone's impact, at the cellular level, is a function of the amount of hormone in the bloodstream and/or the number of receptors on a cell. In the first case, if there is a hormone deficit, as is the case in diabetes mellitus, then supplemental hormone (e.g., insulin) can be administered.

When a larger than physiological dose of hormone is administered, there can also be a new or different effect, a **pharmacological effect**. An example of this pharmacological effect is when antidiuretic hormone (ADH), also called vasopressin, is given in larger than physiologic doses. When that happens, it induces a potent vasoconstrictor effect upon the blood vessels.[44]

Alternatively, there can be an increase in the number of receptors on the cell, as a result of low hormone levels, making the cell more sensitive to the available hormone. The converse is also true (i.e., there can be fewer receptors). The change in the number of cell receptors can either increase (called **upregulation**) or decrease (called **downregulation**) according to hormone levels. In certain pathological conditions it may be necessary to block these hormone receptors to moderate the hormone's effect upon the cell.

Diabetes

Type 1 diabetes is characterized by a total loss of insulin production, making necessary life-long subcutaneous injections of insulin. However, the vast majority of patients with diabetes, more than 80%, continue to produce some insulin. These patients produce insufficient quantities of insulin or have an increased resistance to the insulin, and thus are termed type 2 diabetics. The most common cause of type 2 diabetes is obesity; the hallmark of obesity-induced diabetes is insulin resistance (a case of either downgrading insulin receptors or having an ineffective insulin/receptor effect).

The first level treatment for many of these patients with type 2, or non-insulin dependent diabetes mellitus (NIDDM) is weight control through diet and exercise. Failing this, the patient must then resort to an alternative therapeutic strategy—either insulin injections or the use of hypoglycemic agents.

Drugs That Are Used to Treat Diabetes

Diabetes mellitus is not a single disease. More correctly, diabetes is a group of syndromes of varying etiologies that have a similar presentation: increased blood glucose. Even seemingly minor alterations in blood glucose can have a dramatic impact on some patients. These changes in blood glucose levels are the source of many EMS calls for assistance.

Blood glucose levels are maintained within a physiologic range by two hormones produced in the pancreas. The first hormone, insulin, is produced in the beta cells within the islets of Langerhans of the pancreas. It lowers blood glucose by facilitating passage of blood glucose into the surrounding cells and tissues. When the level of blood glucose rises, then the pancreas produces more insulin. When the level of blood glucose drops, then the alpha cells within the islets of Langerhans release glucagon (a hormone that increases blood glucose levels). Together, these two hormones help to maintain a blood glucose level within a physiological range sufficient for the body's metabolic needs.

Drugs That Are Used to Treat Diabetic Emergencies

Diabetic emergencies can be neatly divided into problems of low blood sugar (hypoglycemia) and high blood sugar (hyperglycemia). Hypoglycemia often has a more dramatic presentation, such as sudden unconsciousness or convulsions. For this reason, it is a common source of calls for EMS.

Diabetic hypoglycemia can be the result of either increased insulin levels, via self-administration or pancreatic production, or insufficient food intake in relation to insulin levels. To understand the etiology of these hypoglycemic periods, it is necessary to understand the action of the hormone insulin.

Insulin

Insulin combines with receptors in the cell wall to permit the passage of glucose into the cell. This in effect lowers the blood sugar in the bloodstream. Insulin also stimulates the storage of excess glucose in the liver in the form of glycogen.

Simultaneously, insulin inhibits the release of free fatty acids. These fatty acids would normally be excreted whenever glucagon is present. (Glucagon stimulates the use of fat for energy in a process called lipolysis.)

Since insulin is a protein, it cannot be taken orally as stomach acids would immediately break it down into inert materials. Thus, insulin must be given parenterally, usually via subcutaneous injection, into the peripheral capillary bed where it can be absorbed into the central circulation. It can also be given intravenously.

Early insulin was obtained from animals, such as pigs and cows. In some cases, patients developed an allergy to the pork or beef insulin. Currently, insulin is bio-engineered and is identical to human insulin, thereby preventing any allergy to insulin.

Insulin's onset and duration of action can be altered by mixing the insulin with other materials such as zinc. Paramedics should be aware of these other insulin preparations, especially the time of onset and peak effect, to be able to anticipate periods of hypoglycemia following an insulin overdose.

The most rapid-acting insulin is synthetically prepared insulin that is part of a zinc salt. Rapid-acting regular insulin lowers blood sugar within minutes when given intravenously.

The intermediate-acting insulin preparations use protamine to prolong their duration of action. Protamine, a peptide, makes insulin a less soluble complex, slowing absorption and increasing its duration of action. Intermediate-acting insulin, or neutral protamine Hagedorn (NPH), is never given intravenously.

Long-acting insulin preparations are the result of various processing techniques and result in insulin that has a delayed onset of action as well as a prolonged duration of action (Figure 31-2).

For most patients, a relatively stable blood glucose level would be desirable and the option of mixing various insulins (rapid, intermediate, and long-acting) to attain a near constant blood glucose level would be reasonable. With this thought in mind, Lente insulin, a mixture of 30% semilente insulin (a rapid-acting form of regular insulin) and 70% ultralente insulin (an extended-insulin zinc suspension that is poorly soluble) was created. Lente insulin helps to avoid some of the tendency toward hypoglycemia experienced by some diabetic patients.

As noted earlier, Paramedics should be aware of the peak effect of the various insulins. In cases where the patient has mixed insulin and subsequently has a period of hypoglycemia, the patient can expect to have another episode of hypoglycemia.

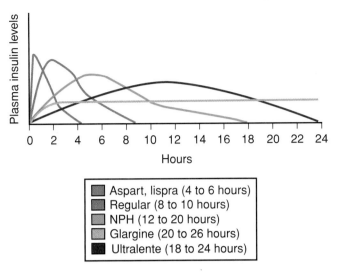

Profiles of Human Insulins and Analogues

Legend:
- Aspart, lispra (4 to 6 hours)
- Regular (8 to 10 hours)
- NPH (12 to 20 hours)
- Glargine (20 to 26 hours)
- Ultralente (18 to 24 hours)

Figure 31-2 Onset of action of insulin preparations.

Insulin and Hyperkalemia

Insulin is a negatively charged amino acid. As such, insulin binds to positively charged electrolytes, such as potassium. Elevated potassium levels (hyperkalemia) lead to significant dysrhythmias and can be life-threatening. Intravenous administration of insulin can be used to treat hyperkalemia because it binds the potassium to the insulin. When the insulin attaches to the cell, it drives the potassium into the cell with it and out of the circulation.[45-47] This technique is very effective for lowering serum potassium levels, but caution must be exercised to prevent inadvertent hypoglycemia. Typically a glucose-containing solution is concomitantly administered along with the insulin.

Diabetes is a leading cause of blindness, which occurs because of diabetic retinopathy. Patients with diabetes, who are unable to see or unable to see clearly, may unintentionally overdose themselves with insulin. Aids for the blind (e.g., guide dogs) should raise the Paramedic's index of suspicion that the cause of the medical emergency may be visual impairment that may be diabetes related.

Hypoglycemia

Untreated hypoglycemia, sometimes referred to as insulin shock, can lead to coma and even death. A number of factors—such as the stress of surgery; infections, especially when accompanied by fever; and trauma—can lead the diabetic patient to have an unexpected episode of hypoglycemia. Alternatively, changes in eating habits or activity patterns—or new medications such as MAO inhibitors, sulfonamides, salicylates, beta-blockers, and ethanol (EtOH)—can cause inadvertent hypoglycemia.[48] The clear majority of hypoglycemia cases in patients with type 1 diabetes are related to changes in insulin regime.

When the patient becomes hypoglycemic, another hormone (epinephrine) is released. Epinephrine normally inhibits insulin secretion, thereby increasing blood glucose levels in an emergency. Released by sympathetic stimulation of the adrenal medulla, epinephrine is responsible for the majority of the symptoms present during a hypoglycemic episode, such as tachycardia, tremors, diaphoresis, headache, and hypertension.

Treatment of Hypoglycemia

Treatment of hypoglycemia is simple: Replace the glucose until adequate levels of blood glucose are available to resume normal metabolism. Methods of glucose administration include oral paste as well as intravenous administration. Typically, 25 grams of dextrose is administered intravenously, either as 500 cc of 5% dextrose in sterile water (D5W) or 50 cc of 50% dextrose solution.

The effects of intravenous administration of 50% dextrose upon hypoglycemia is immediate but not without its complications. Concentrated dextrose is hypertonic. Therefore, administration through a misplaced intravenous line and subsequent subcutaneous infiltration can lead to severe tissue necrosis.

A hypoglycemic patient can present in the field with facial droop, confusion, and slurring of words. This presentation may be mistaken for a stroke and grave complications may occur subsequent to this misdiagnosis.[49] Similarly, a patient with stroke symptoms should not be assumed to have hypoglycemia. Inappropriate administration of concentrated dextrose to a stroke patient with a normal blood sugar level can induce changes secondary to the osmotic effect of the concentrated dextrose. Dextrose should only be administered to those patients with evidence of hypoglycemia (e.g., a low glucose meter reading).

An alternative treatment for hypoglycemia, when intravenous administration of glucose is not possible, is intramuscular injection of glucagon. Glucagon, which is naturally secreted by the alpha cells in the pancreas, raises the blood glucose level by liberating glucose from glycogen stores in the liver. By definition, for glucagon to work there must be adequate stores of glycogen in the liver. Patients with liver disease or those who are chronically malnourished may not have glycogen stores, thereby rendering glucagon useless.

Glucagon's onset of action is dependent upon its route of administration (15 minutes via IM injection and 31 minutes by subcutaneous injection). The delay in onset of action makes intravenous dextrose administration more desirable.

Oral Hypoglycemia Agents

The three therapeutic strategies that could potentially increase insulin levels include (1) stimulation of the beta cells in the pancreas to produce more insulin or to reduce glucagon levels, (2) suppression of the alpha cells in the pancreas, or (3) an increase in the binding of insulin to receptors on the cells.

The sulfonylureas were the first class of drugs that could produce all three of these desirable mechanisms of action. The introduction of sulfonylureas eliminated the need for some patients to inject insulin. Each successive generation of sulfonylureas, while not more effective than the previous, have as positive features a longer duration of action as well as fewer side effects.

Other oral hypoglycemia agents include (1) the alpha-glucosidase inhibitors, which delay the digestion and absorption of carbohydrates, permitting subphysiological levels of insulin production to suffice; and (2) other non-sulfonylurea agents, such as metformin, which have a similar mechanism of action.

The newest class of antihyperglycemia agents lowers insulin resistance, permitting more effective use of the patient's own endogenous insulin. These medications stimulate the release of helper proteins from the muscles and fat. These proteins enhance the cells' response to insulin by a mechanism entirely different than the sulfonylureas' mechanism of action. Currently research is on–going for medications that can lower insulin resistance, a major cause of type II diabetes, particularly in the obese patient population.

Drugs That Are Used to Treat Adrenal Disorders

The paired pyramid-shaped adrenal glands, located just above the kidneys, produce a rich supply of hormones that are essential to the body's health. All of these hormones are produced from cholesterol and have a common steroid core (hence the term "steroids").

Dividing the adrenal cortex into three zones, the outer zone (zona glomerulosa) produces the mineralocorticoids, chief among those being aldosterone. The larger middle zone

(zona fasciculata) produces the glucocorticoids, including the principal glucocorticoid cortisone. The innermost zone (zona reticularis) produces the adrenal androgens and estrogen.

The glucocorticoids help to regulate metabolism of carbohydrates, increase blood glucose by helping to convert glycogen to glucose, antagonize insulin, and help create glucose from amino acids by a process of protein catabolism (gluconeogenesis).

The glucocorticoids also inhibit both the immune system and the inflammatory response by suppressing the chemical mediators such as prostaglandins, leukotrienes, bradykinin, serotonin, and histamine.

Levels of glucocorticoids rise during periods of stress, providing needed glucose. However, they also lower resistance to infection during those times. Chief among these naturally occurring glucocorticoids is cortisol. Cortisol secretion, regulated by the hypothalamus and the anterior pituitary gland via adrenocorticotropic hormone (ACTH) stimulated by low levels of cortisol, travels throughout the body bound to blood proteins such as albumin.

Synthetic Glucocorticoids

Paramedics may be called upon to administer steroids in order to treat severe inflammatory responses that occur in severe asthma, including status asthmaticus, acute allergic reactions, and anaphylactic reactions that are unresponsive to standard treatment.

Treatment with steroids may also be indicated for gram-negative septic shock.[50] Endotoxins released from the gram-negative bacteria injure cells and alter the patient's coagulation. Glucocorticoids suppress many of the chemical mediators in the coagulation cascade, in addition to protecting cellular membranes. Glucocorticoids also potentiate catecholamines, such as dopamine, increasing their vasoconstrictive activity.

Glucocorticoids are also administered as replacement therapy for adrenocortical insufficiency (Addison's disease). Typically, a dose of hydrocortisone, the synthetic equivalent to naturally occurring cortisol, is given: two thirds in the morning and one third in the afternoon, to match the patient's circadian rhythm.

Glucocorticoids can be broken down into three subclassifications according to their duration of action. The short-acting glucocorticoids include hydrocortisone and cortisone (which is converted into hydrocortisone in the body). These short-acting agents generally have a half-life of about 8 to 12 hours in the tissues.

The intermediate-acting glucocorticoids include prednisone and methylprednisolone. They have an average half-life of 18 to 36 hours in the tissues.

Dexamethasone, an example of a long-acting steroid, is occasionally used to treat the edema seen following head injury or secondary to a brain tumor.[51] Beclomethasone dipropionate, another example of a long-acting steroid, is available in an aerosol form for long-term use in patients with severe asthma. This aerosol form permits lower doses than would be given orally and minimizes some of the undesirable systemic effects of steroids.

Precautions

Administration of glucocorticoids may cause fluctuating glucose levels, as glucocorticoids promote metabolism. Use of these steroids may cause hypoglycemia in diabetics and those prone to hypoglycemia.

Glucocorticoids also have some related mineralocorticoid activity. The result is retention of salts and water with subsequent edema and hypertension that can progress to congestive heart failure in susceptible patients. Long-term use of these steroids can result in iatrogenic Cushing's syndrome. The patient's presentation will include a puffy face (Moon face), acne (early sign), hypertension, weight gain, and an increase in body hair.

Patients on steroids become dependent on those steroids, as levels of naturally produced steroids drop off. Abrupt withdrawal of these steroids can lead to acute adrenal insufficiency.[52] Tapering doses of the steroid are required for patients who are prescribed steroids for longer than two weeks to gently re-establish a natural response from the adrenal gland.

Mineralocorticoids

The primary mineralocorticoid, aldosterone, is largely responsible for electrolyte and fluid balance and acts upon the distal tubules of the kidneys. This steroid primarily conserves sodium, while promoting potassium and hydrogen ion (acid) excretion. The production of aldosterone is controlled by the renin-angiotensin mechanism, which is activated by sodium and/or blood volume depletion.

High levels of aldosterone can induce hypokalemia, which can create cardiac irritability manifested as ventricular ectopic beats, as well as a metabolic alkalosis.

Antiadrenal Medications

Antiadrenal medications suppress adrenal cortical function, resulting in decreased production of these steroids. Used to treat Cushing's syndrome as well as adrenal tumors, these medications inhibit the enzyme that converts cholesterol into steroids.

As these medications also suppress estrogen production in the adrenals (a hormone thought to be related to breast cancer), investigational cancer studies are in progress.

Adrenal Medulla

At the core of the adrenal glands is the medulla. The adrenal medulla produces the catecholamines norepinephrine and epinephrine. Secretion of epinephrine from the medulla is largely under sympathetic nervous control (i.e., a neurohumoral regulation). Stimulation of the adrenal medulla can result from hypoglycemia, hypoxia, hypercapnia, nicotine, and angiotensin II.

While tumors of the adrenal medulla, called a pheochromocytoma, are rare (less than eight cases per million population), they can produce large amounts of epinephrine.[53] Excess epinephrine can cause paroxysms of hypertension, cause sustained hypertension, induce a hypertensive crisis, and create a "runaway" tachycardia. Occasionally, an episode of hypertension follows a meal of tyrosine-rich food, red wine, beer, or aged cheese. Tyrosine is the precursor of epinephrine.

Rupture of a pheochromocytoma can literally lead to a systemic flood of epinephrine accompanied by profound hypertension, severe abdominal pain, and a potentially fatal hemorrhage. Treatment for a hypertensive emergency includes intravenous administration of an alpha-blocking agent (e.g., phentolamine) and a beta-blocker (e.g., metoprolol) to control the runaway tachycardia.

Drugs That Are Used to Treat Ovarian Disorders

Estrogen and progesterone are the principal sex hormones produced by the ovaries. Created from cholesterol (like the steroids of the adrenal glands), estrogen and progesterone ebb and flow rhythmically, creating a woman's menstrual cycle. This continues until pregnancy interrupts the sequence.

Estrogen is primarily responsible for a woman's sexual development as well as regulation of her menstrual cycle. Besides effects upon the ovaries, estrogen also has metabolic effects. For example, estrogen helps to maintain bone density. When a woman stops producing estrogen (i.e., menopause), she is at greater risk of losing bone density (i.e., osteoporosis).

Estrogen also has a cardioprotective effect. This alters the metabolism of cholesterols, decreases serum levels of low-density lipoproteins and high-density lipoproteins, and prevents atherosclerosis.

Estrogen Therapy

Estrogen can be used to prevent pregnancy (a contraceptive effect) or during menopause at a one fifth dose. Estrogen is used during menopause to prevent atrophic vaginitis, vasomotor symptoms (i.e., hot flashes), and abnormal uterine bleeding. Post-menopausal women are at greater risk of osteoporosis. If unchecked, osteoporosis can lead to brittle bones that fracture. (Hip fractures are more common among these women.) Estrogen replacement therapy can decrease the risk of osteoporosis.

Estrogen is also an effective treatment for some estrogen-sensitive metastatic breast cancers. Paradoxically, estrogen slows tumor growth when it normally increases breast development in those cases. Conversely, some breast cancers are estrogen-dependent. These breast cancers are treated with an anti-estrogen agent, such as tamoxifen, which blocks estrogen receptors in the tumor.

High-dose estrogen, or the morning after pill, a.k.a. plan B, is sometimes used as an emergency contraceptive (e.g., following rape or contraceptive failure). If administered within 72 hours, high-dose estrogens (such as diethylstilbestrol) can induce menses, eliminating products of conception. Diethylstilbestrol, therefore, has a pregnancy class of X.

Estrogen in oral contraceptives can induce thrombophlebitis and thrombosis formation, leading to strokes and pulmonary embolism.[54] This risk is increased in women over age 35 and in women who smoke.

Drugs That Are Used to Treat Pituitary Disorders

The pituitary gland is located just inferior to the hypothalamus nestled in the base of the skull. These are connected to one another by a thin stalk of tissue called the infundibulum. This pituitary-hypothalamus axis produces a number of hormones that control other glands. Thus, the pituitary is called the master gland.

The pituitary gland can be divided into two portions: anterior and posterior. The posterior portion produces two hormones: antidiuretic hormone (vasopressin) and oxytocin. The primary effect of antidiuretic hormone is to control plasma osmolality and maintain intravascular volume. ADH achieves that goal by affecting the permeability of the distal tubules of the kidney's nephron. Oxytocin is discussed later in the section on drugs used during pregnancy.

Vasopressin

Vasopressin has received widespread attention for its potential role in cardiac arrest. The hormone's pharmacological effect (vasoconstriction) may be useful as a first-line therapy in cardiac arrest, following defibrillation.[55–58]

Vasopressin is also useful in treating diabetes insipidus. Diabetes insipidus is characterized by a lack of ADH and may be caused by basal skull fractures injuring the infundibulum, subsequently causing increased intracranial pressure. It could also be caused by a brain tumor or subdural hemorrhage that compresses the infundibulum. There are a number of reasons why the pituitary gland would fail, all culminating in a scarcity of ADH.

Without ADH, immense volumes of dilute urine are excreted (polyuria), upwards of 3 to 18 L a day, and the patient wants to drink large volumes of water (polydipsia). If unchecked, diabetes insipidus can lead to dehydration, hypovolemia, and shock.

Natural vasopressin, or synthetic derivatives such as lypressin, is prescribed to patients suffering from diabetes insipidus.

Drugs That Are Used to Treat Thyroid Disorders

The thyroid gland (from the Greek word, meaning "shield-like") straddles the thyroid cartilage, commonly known as the Adam's apple, with a thin isthmus in the middle. The follicles within the two lobes of the gland secrete the hormones responsible for metabolism.

Pathology of the thyroid gland involves either hyper- or hyposecretion of thyroxine (T4) or triiodothyronine (T3). Hyperthyroidism can be caused by Graves' disease, thyroid cancer, or a goiter. Hyperthyroidism results in tachycardia, weight loss, nervousness, and exophthalmos (a bulging of the eyes).

If left unchecked, hypersecretion of thyroid hormones can lead to thyrotoxic crisis (thyroid storm), a condition that can lead to death. Thyrotoxic storm's symptomology includes atrial tachydysrhythmia, cardiogenic shock, and hyperpyrexia secondary to a metabolism that is increased by as much as 60%.

Strong iodine solutions, such as Lugol's solution, may be administered during a thyrotoxic crisis. The iodine in the solution inhibits the formation of tyrosine, a precursor to epinephrine. Alternatively, thioamide derivatives, such as propylthiouracil, may be used. These agents inhibit thyroid hormone synthesis, preventing tyrosine production.

Hyperthyroidism is typically treated with either surgical removal of the thyroid gland or administration of radioactive iodine, which results in the destruction of the thyroid gland. The patient, like the patient with hypothyroidism, needs lifelong thyroid hormone replacement therapy.

Levothyroxine, a synthetic thyroxine, is one of the more common thyroid preparations prescribed for hypothyroidism. Poor patient compliance with the prescribed replacement therapy can result in hypothyroidism and myxedema. Myxedema is characterized by ataxia (drunken staggers), lethargy and confusion, headaches, and a non-pitting edema of the eyes, hands, and feet. Myxedema also results in edema of the tongue and laryngeal mucous membranes, making speech slurred. The combination of symptoms might lead less informed Paramedics to suspect intoxication.

Amiodarone contains large amounts of iodine, approximately 37% by weight, and can induce hyperthyroidism in a small population of susceptible individuals.[59,60] The onset of a new atrial tachydysrhythmia is often seen in these patients.

Drugs That Are Used to Treat Anaphalaxis

Inappropriate responses to allergens (i.e., allergy, autoimmunity, and alloimmunity) can be classified jointly as hypersensitivities. Hypersensitivities can further be classified as immediate or delayed.

Paramedics are most concerned about immediate hypersensitivity reactions, the most severe being anaphylaxis. Untreated anaphylaxis can progress within minutes to a life-threatening medical emergency.

A classic anaphylaxis is an IgE-mediated reaction. After exposure to a foreign protein—one that is inhaled, ingested, or injected—the body's immune system produces an antigen specific antibody (IgE). The IgE binds to special crystallizable fragment (Fc) receptors on mast cells.

When the patient is re-exposed to the allergen, it causes the Fc receptors on the mast cell surface to cross-link, one to the other, destroying the mast cell in the process and releasing the cell's contents. This process is called degranulation.

The majority of the symptoms of anaphylaxis are related to the degranulation of mast cells. Chemical mediators released during degranulation include histamine. Histamine is responsible for the majority of symptoms associated with an anaphylactic reaction: bronchoconstriction, increased vascular permeability leading to angioedema, and vasodilation-induced hypotension.[61]

Antihistamines

Antihistamines are antagonists to histamine, their mechanism of action being a competitive inhibition of naturally occurring histamines at the H1 receptors. Once H1 receptors are occupied by antihistamines, such as diphenhydramine, the development of further histamine-induced angioedema, pruritis (itching), and bronchospasm is impeded. Antihistamines do not reverse pre-existing pathology (e.g., vasodilation-induced hypotension). Furthermore, the pharmacokinetics in antihistamines are gradual, with an onset of action between 15 and 30 minutes (with a peak in one hour).

During anaphylaxis, time is of the essence and the drug of choice remains epinephrine.[62] Epinephrine, administered subcutaneously, has an immediate effect and reverses the symptoms present in anaphylaxis. Epinephrine's mechanism of action was previously discussed.

Drugs That Are Used to Treat Gastrointestinal Disorders

From ancient Greece, when Hippocrates spoke of the runny "faeces" of dysentery, to contemporary discussions of infantile diarrhea in developing countries, gastrointestinal complaints have historically plagued humanity. Many concoctions have been created to combat this malady. Oil of earthworm, listed in the Leiden pharmacopoeia in 1741, was replaced by paregoric (liquid opium) in 1788. Opium's popularity is owed, in part, to its ability to constipate, to "bind the bowel," and halt diarrhea. Subsequent mineral preparations had some degree of success and an entire pharmaceutical industry was created to treat this common disorder.[28]

Ulcer Medicines

Heartburn and the pain of peptic ulcer was formerly believed to be the result of excessive stomach acid, so medical attention was turned toward reducing or neutralizing that acid. More recently, the pathogen Helicobacter pylori has been implicated as the causative agent for peptic ulcers and a course of antibiotics as its cure. However, there are other causes of stomach inflammation. These include irritants like alcohol or aspirin, which can produce epigastric discomfort. A number of medications, many of them over-the-counter medications, are available to help with these disorders.

Antacids

Antacids chemically neutralize stomach acid and bring relief to those suffering from heartburn (i.e., gastroesophageal reflux disease (GERD)), hiatal hernia, and gastritis. The compounds calcium carbonate, sodium bicarbonate, magnesium salt, and aluminum salt are used for this purpose.

A concern with many of these medications involves some of their systemic effects. Patients with renal failure, who are on antacids, may develop toxicities and adverse reactions. Other patients may, for example, develop a metabolic alkalosis from prolonged or generous administration of sodium bicarbonate. Aluminum-containing antacids should be avoided in patients with Alzheimer's disease. Antacids will generally reduce the absorption of digoxin, possibly leading to dysrhythmia.[63]

Of greater concern is the altered absorption of many medications as a result of changed stomach acidity. For example, the pharmacokinetics of drugs that are weak bases, such as antihistamines and tricyclic antidepressants, and drugs that are weak acids, such as sulfonamides and salicylates, will be altered. Since the list of drug interactions with antacids is long, Paramedics should consider drug interaction when assessing a patient who is also taking antacids.

Histamine Antagonists

Histamine antagonists (discussed earlier), particularly the H2 receptor blockers, are effective in inhibiting all phases of stomach acid secretion. Many examples of histamine

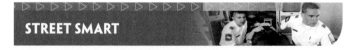

STREET SMART

Patients will dismiss epigastric discomfort as being heartburn, denying the possibility that they are having a heart attack, and will self-medicate with antacids (without relief). Paramedics should always have a high index of suspicion that heartburn has a cardiac origin (an inferior wall AMI) and treat accordingly.

antagonists, such as cimetidine and ranitidine, are now available over-the-counter.

Emetics

The quintessential emetic agent is syrup of ipecac. Used for centuries as a purgative, it stimulates vomiting by both irritating the stomach and rousing the vomiting centers in the brain. Syrup of ipecac is highly effective (greater than 80% of patients will vomit) and has a quick onset of action (within 20 minutes).[64]

Toxicity

Syrup of ipecac itself can be both neurotoxic and cardiotoxic and caution is advised anytime it is used. Emetine, the active ingredient in syrup of ipecac, is part of a mixture of alkaloids obtained from the plant Rubiaceae (Cephalus ipecacuanha). Emetine is derived from tyrosine, the intermediary of dopamine, which explains its effects upon the heart and brain.

The delay between the onset of symptoms from a poison and the onset of action of the syrup of ipecac is a concern for most Paramedics. If there is any possibility that the toxin can induce drowsiness or unconsciousness before the ipecac can take effect, then the ipecac should be withheld. For this reason, the routine use of syrup of ipecac is not recommended by the American Academy of Clinical Toxicology.[65]

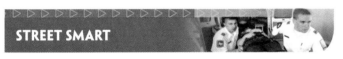

STREET SMART

The American Academy of Pediatrics no longer advocates the civilian use of syrup of ipecac and encourages that all syrup of ipecac be discarded. Syrup of ipecac should only be used, in the hospital setting, under the direct orders of a physician.

Antiemetics

Unremitting vomiting (e.g., from chemotherapy) can be debilitating and lead to potentially life-threatening dehydration and hypovolemia. The majority of antiemetics work centrally, in the brain, to control the nausea that leads to vomiting. This area, called the chemoreceptor trigger zone (CZT), contains sensory nerves that detect poisons and the like in the blood. The CTZ then triggers the emetic center in the brainstem to induce vomiting. This primitive protective mechanism is most effective with ingested toxins.

Mechanism of Action

The mechanism of action of an antiemetic generally involves blocking a receptor (an antagonist) along the neuromuscular chain that leads to vomiting. Dopamine receptors, located within the CTZ, can be blocked by dopamine antagonists.

For example, drugs in the class of phenothiazines (such as chlorpromazine) and promethazine or metoclopramide stop nausea before the process of vomiting can be started.

Anticholinergics can block acetylcholine receptors located within the emetic center, thereby preventing vomiting. This is the mechanism of action for scopolamine. Similarly, histamine receptors in the emetic center can be blocked by antihistamines such as diphenhydramine or dimenhydrate.

Another anti-emetic is odansetron, (Zofran®). Odansetron, selective serotonin receptor antagonist, is especially effective as a pretreatment for nausea and vomiting, Some providers have reported transient ECG changes, particularly QT prolongation, with intravenous odansetron administration. As ondansetron treats the symptom, not the cause of nausea, assessment and treatment of the underlying cause is imperative.

Cannabinoids (synthetically produced THC, such as the type found in marijuana) have two therapeutic advantages. First, cannabinoids are antiemetic. Second, cannabinoids stimulate appetite and reduce anorexia. This advantage can be critical when treating patients who are cachetic secondary to acquired immunodeficiency syndrome or chemotherapy.[66]

Antidiarrheal

To be medically accurate, diarrhea is not loose watery stool, but rather a frequent passage of loose watery stool. Certain populations, such as the very old and very young, are at risk for dehydration from diarrhea. Chronic diarrhea (diarrhea that lasts for more than one week) can be indicative of intestinal infections such as amebic dysentery. Acute diarrhea can be indicative of toxin ingestion and bacterial infection, such as salmonella or escherichia coli.

In many cases, resolution of the underlying cause will alleviate the symptom. In cases where more immediate relief is sought or where the patient expects a short course of illness, then antidiarrhea agents are available.

Absorbents

Absorbents essentially coat the bowel wall, preventing interaction of the intestine and bacteria or toxin, thereby stopping intestinal irritation and subsequent diarrhea. An example of an absorbent antidiarrheal agent is bismuth subsalicylate. This bismuth preparation also contains salicylate, the active ingredient in aspirin, and can increase bleeding times.

Another example of an absorbent agent commonly used by Paramedics is activated charcoal. Activated charcoal, a finely pulverized form of charcoal, absorbs the toxins until passage out of the intestine. To aid excretion, an indigestible osmotic agent such as sorbitol is added.

Opioids

Paregoric and tinctures of opium have been used as antidiarrhea agents for centuries. However, recent concern about the addictive quality of these medicines has brought about a decrease in their use. Nevertheless, these opioids remain highly effective in the control of diarrhea.

Loperamide, a synthetic opioid, decreases the peristalsis associated with diarrhea and permits reabsorption of water. This prescription medication has a duration of action of over 24 hours, making it effective when traveling in remote or frontier areas.

Laxatives

Older patients are frequently plagued by constipation as their gastrointestinal tracts slow. In some cases, constipation can lead to life-threatening small bowel obstruction. There are numerous causes of obstruction, but the effect is the same: blockage of the intestinal tract.

There are as many treatments for constipation as there are causes of constipation. Treatments for constipation can be organized into broad classifications based upon the mechanism of action.

Saline Laxatives

As soluble salts, these laxatives dry the water in the intestinal tract via osmosis. The result is an increased fecal mass and stimulation for evacuation. Many of these saline laxatives contain other minerals that may have added side effects. An example of a commonly used saline laxative is magnesium hydroxide, otherwise known as milk of magnesia. It can have a toxic effect on the kidneys. Others high in sodium complicate the management of a patient's heart failure or hypertensive control.

Stool Softeners

Stool softeners act as a wetting agent, softening the fecal mass until it can be passed. An example of a commonly prescribed stool softener is docusate. Docusate is often given to post-MI patients to prevent straining during bowel movements and the subsequent vasovagal stimulation that occurs.

Bulking Agents

Bulking agents, such as psyllium, absorb water from the fecal flow, increasing the volume of the feces and distending the bowel. The distended bowel is now encouraged to empty reflexively.

Stimulants

Stimulants act directly upon the nervous control of the bowel, increasing peristalsis and bowel emptying. Stimulants, such as senna, can also produce abdominal cramping and pain. Senna tea, an old world remedy, is made from an infusion of leaves of the Cassia plant into a tea.

Lubricants

Lubricants aid the naturally occurring mucus to coat the feces for an easier bowel movement. Many of these oil-based lubricants can also block absorption of fat-soluble vitamins, such as vitamins A, D, E, and K.

Precautions

Laxatives should not be routinely used to treat abdominal pain thought to be due to constipation. Undiagnosed abdominal pain can be the presenting symptom for appendicitis, enteritis, and mesenteric infarction.

Drugs That Are Used to Treat Bleeding Disorders

The origins of bleeding disorders can be genetic (e.g., hemophilia), disease-induced (e.g., disseminated intravascular coagulation), or iatrogenic (e.g., heparin infusion). Regardless of the etiology the result is the same: a coagulopathy (defect in blood clotting). Consequently, the patient either clots too much or bleeds too much.

Drugs that affect blood clots (antithrombolytics and antifibrinolytics) were discussed in Chapter 30. Treatment of bleeding disorders revolves around either use of antagonists that interfere with anticoagulant medication or replacement of missing coagulation factors.

Anticoagulants (such as warfarin) antagonize the fat-soluble vitamin K, an essential cofactor in the coagulation cascade. In some instances, the administration of vitamin K overcomes the warfarin dose and re-establishes normal clotting. Unfortunately, vitamin K is slow acting and can take up to 24 hours to be effective.[67] This single quality makes vitamin K less useful in an emergency.

Other anticoagulant antagonists work in direct opposition to the action of the fibrinolytics. Fibrinolytics act by encouraging plasminogen activators to degrade fibrin. These anticoagulant antagonists (such as aminocaproic acid) inhibit plasminogen activators.

Heparin, a commonly prescribed anticoagulant, is formed in the liver, lungs, and intestinal lining. It produces its anticoagulant effect by binding with naturally occurring antithrombin III and inactivating several factors in the coagulation cascade.

The heparin antidote, protamine sulfate, is a protein obtained from the sperm of salmon that has an ability to interfere with the heparin-antithrombin III complex and thereby prevents anticoagulation.

Antihemophilic Drugs

Uncontrollable bleeding secondary to a minor injury can be life-threatening to a patient with hemophilia. Born with an inability to produce one of the protein-clotting factors in the blood, these patients may have excessive bleeding into the joints, bladder, and brain.[68]

The most common hemophilia (hemophilia A) is a deficiency of factor VIII or the antihemophiliac factor (AHF). Administration of cryoprecipitated AHF, prepared by rapid freezing and thawing of fresh plasma, is useful during an emergency. As a glycoprotein, AHF is needed to transform prothrombin into thrombin.

Following AHF administration, it is common to administer anti-inhibitor coagulant complex. Anti-inhibitor coagulant complex is also obtained from plasma and is often used preoperatively for those with factor VIII deficiency.

Similarly, factor IX complex is administered to patients with hemophilia B (Christmas disease) to prevent or control bleeding.

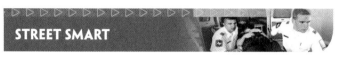

STREET SMART

Absorbable gelatin sponges, film, powder, and oxidized cellulose gauze are moving out of the operating room and into the street. These topical hemostatic agents are capable of absorbing blood in large quantities and encouraging clot formation at the bleeding site.

Anemia

Anemia is not a disease. More accurately, anemia is a symptom of other diseases that involves the body's inability to form adequate red blood cells. In most instances, anemia is the result of either a dietary deficiency of needed nutrients or poor absorption of those needed nutrients.

In some instances, the anemia is a quasi-anemia (i.e., one induced by a temporary state such as pregnancy). In other instances, chronic blood loss, infection, cancer, or drug-induced bone marrow depression can produce anemia. Regardless of the cause, the patient has a less than normal hemoglobin (Hb) concentration from either fewer circulating red blood cells or a low hemoglobin content in those red blood cells.

Treatment of anemia is usually geared toward providing supplementary nutrition while eliminating or treating the root cause of the anemia. A common anemia, iron-deficiency anemia, can occur from chronic blood loss, including menses. Iron, which is essential for the red blood cell to carry oxygen, is prescribed to those patients suffering from a deficiency. Iron stored in the intestinal mucosa can also be lost in gastrointestinal disease.

If children accidentally ingest iron supplements, it can turn into a medical emergency.[69] As the iron is absorbed, the child can become toxic and will have diffuse abdominal signs, such as cramps.[70] Unfortunately, the symptoms subside within 24 hours and the patient appears fine, which may prompt them not to seek further treatment. Subsequently, about 48 to 72 hours later, an acidosis occurs that can lead to pulmonary edema, convulsions, and hyperthermia.

If ferritin intoxication is suspected, the Paramedic may induce vomiting using syrup of ipecac and/or lavage with sodium bicarbonate solution, which converts the ferritin into poorly absorbable ferrous carbonate. Other nutrient supplements used to treat various types of anemia include folic acid and cyanocobalamin (vitamin B12). Vitamin deficiencies can occur as a result of poor diet and are often seen in patients with alcoholism.

Drugs That Are Used to Treat Psychiatric Disorders

In the past, the diagnosis of a psychiatric illness would bring out images of raving mad lunatics locked in an insane asylum forced to undergo bizarre medical treatments, such as frontal lobotomy and straitjackets. Historically, mentally ill patients were warehoused in public mental hospitals with deplorable health and sanitation conditions. Documentaries, such as the one on Millbrook, brought these appalling conditions to light and efforts were made to change conditions and the therapeutic approach. Psychiatrists, encouraged by the effectiveness of antibiotics, turned their attention to medications. They were not disappointed.

The impact of the first tranquilizer (chlorpromazine) in the 1950s cannot be overstated.[71] Patients, who were previously labeled dangerous and uncontrollable, could be tranquilized, treated, and, in some cases, allowed to lead a normal public life.

The development and widespread use of these psychiatric medications led to the widespread deinstitutionalization of hundreds of psychiatric patients, It also prompted a complete change in the focus of mental health medicine away from institutionalization and toward community-based treatment centers.

Psychosis

A large number of mental illnesses can be grossly categorized under the label of schizophrenia, anxiety disorders, and depression. Medications to treat patients who suffer from each of these mental illnesses are described further.

The patient with a diagnosis of schizophrenia has demonstrated disturbances in thought. Hallucinations, particularly audible hallucinations and delusions, plague the patient. The outcome of this deranged thinking, and what usually brings the patient to the Paramedics' attention, is an inability to perform the routine activities of daily living (ADL) such as bathing and clothing oneself.

Drugs That Are Used to Treat Psychosis

Antipsychotic medications help provide the patient with symptomatic relief from the frightening hallucinations and deranged thoughts caused by schizophrenia. While these medications induce a tranquil state in the patient, allowing the patient to cope with the illness, they are not a cure for schizophrenia. Therefore, in order to maintain control of the disease patients must remain on the drug for long periods of time. Setbacks for these patients are frequently the result of poor compliance with prescribed medications and subsequent breakthrough psychosis that is often manifested in aggressive or combative behaviors.

The phenothiazines, the major class of antipsychotic medications, are thought to block dopamine receptors within the limbic portion of the brain. (The limbic system is the seat of emotions.) This blockade results in a reduction in hallucinations and subsequent agitation. However, it should be noted that the phenothiazines do not depress the patient's intellectual function or native intelligence.

Phenothiazines can be further broken down, according to chemical makeup, into three subcategories. The first phenothiazines were all aliphatic phenothiazine derivatives (e.g., chlorpromazine). The next subcategory of phenothiazines includes the piperidine derivatives, such as thioridazine. The last subcategory of phenothiazines are the piperazine derivatives (e.g., prochlorperazine).

Most phenothiazines have a strong antiemetic effect, which blocks the chemoreceptor trigger zone (CTZ) within the medulla. The most famous of these is scopolamine, which is used to treat motion sickness. Many patients who are receiving chemotherapy for cancer are prescribed a phenothiazine, such as chlorpromazine, for nausea control.

Precautions

Phenothiazines also exert an antagonistic influence on other receptors. The majority of side effects attributed to the phenothiazines can be traced to this broad blockade of other receptors. For example, phenothiazines block alpha-adrenergic receptors in the peripheral circulation. As a direct consequence of this blockade, when a patient stands up the cardiovascular system cannot compensate and the patient may experience syncope.[72]

More troubling may be the antimuscarinic effects of phenothiazines. Through its inhibition of smooth muscle, phenothiazines cause the patient to experience blurred vision (papillary muscle), dry mouth, constipation, and urinary retention.

Extrapyramidal System

Coordination of muscles is owed, in part, to the extrapyramidal system that connects the motor coordination from the cerebral cortex with the spinal nerves. There are abundant cholinergic and dopaminergic receptors within this system. A naturally occurring imbalance between these two receptors is the pathogenesis of Parkinson's disease. Phenothiazines can produce a drug-induced Parkinsonian syndrome.

Characteristics of the extrapyramidal symptoms (EPS) of drug-induced Parkinsonian syndrome include a shuffling gait, resting tremors, muscle rigidity with resultant slurred speech, drooling, and a gross motor restlessness called akathisia.[73]

If left untreated, drug-induced Parkinsonian syndrome can lead to involuntary movements of the extremities (a **tardive dyskinesia**). These include fly-catching motions of the tongue and a spasm of the neck muscles, called torticollis, that tilts the head to one side (formerly called wryneck).

Fortunately, most of these symptoms are self-limited and diminish with the termination of the medication.

Anxiety

As a class, sedatives affect the limbic system and thus emotions. Sedatives effectively reduce anxiety (i.e., anxiolytic) as well as induce sleep (i.e., hypnotic). Some of the most commonly known sedatives are the barbiturates and the benzodiazepines. When used early, the barbiturates can create an anxiolysis, even in small doses (doses too low to induce respiratory depression). The use of barbiturates for anxiolysis has declined in favor of benzodiazepines. This is, in part, due to the greater safety margin of benzodiazepines over barbiturates. The lethal dose of barbiturates is only some 50 times greater than the therapeutic dose, whereas the lethal dose of benzodiazepines is one-thousand times greater than the therapeutic dose.

Benzodiazepines

Benzodiazepines are effective for treating such anxiety-related disorders as panic attacks, as well as seizure activity, by attaching to benzodiazepine receptors located in the Limbic system of the central nervous system. These benzodiazepine receptors are thought to enhance the attraction of gamma-aminobutyric acid (GABA) to the GABA receptor, which in turn opens chloride channels in the neuron. Increased chloride (Cl-) within the cell hyperpolarizes the neuron, making it more difficult to depolarize.

Benzodiazepines are also used for a number of other therapeutic effects including treatment of sleep disorders (hypnotic effect), seizures (see earlier discussion), and muscle spasms. However, the majority of benzodiazepines are prescribed for their anxiolytic effect. Short-acting benzodiazepines, such as lorazepam, are effective in ending panic attacks. Long-acting benzodiazepines are effective in treating the agitation and anxiety patients experience when they go through alcohol withdrawal. It should be noted that ethanol (ethyl alcohol) is also a sedative. The therapeutic goal in alcohol detoxification is to first replace the alcohol with a benzodiazepine, then to slowly wean the patient off of the benzodiazepine.

Antidepressant Medication

Depression is a disturbance in a patient's mood, not thought, and is characterized by feelings of hopelessness, helplessness, and despair. Some psychiatrists attribute these maladjusted emotions to a lack of a certain neurotransmitter in the brain, specifically the monoamines. Monoamines include norepinephrine and serotonin. Antidepressant medications that have had a positive effect are medications that either increase the amount of monoamines in the synaptic junction or decrease the destruction of monoamines by enzymes, indirectly increasing the amount of monoamines in the synaptic junction.

Tricyclic Antidepressants

The class of antidepressants that block the uptake of serotonin, norepinephrine, and dopamine into the neuron are called the tricyclic antidepressants. The first generation of tricyclic antidepressants (TCA), including imipramine and amitriptyline, are chemically related to the phenothiazines and have similar mood-altering effects. The second generation of TCA also has the same action but slightly different pharmacokinetics, with different side effects and a longer duration of action.

The primary action of TCA is to increase the monoamines serotonin, norepinephrine, and epinephrine in the brain's neuronal synapse. At issue is whether the antidepressant effect is due to increased monoamines or the observed subsequent increase in monoamine receptors in the brain. Regardless, TCA administration results in mood elevation, improved mental alertness, and increased physical activity. The TCA, as a class, are effective in between 50% and 70% of patients taking the medication.

Precautions

Tricyclic antidepressants also affect a number of other peripheral neural receptors including serotonin, alpha-adrenergic receptors, and muscarinic receptors. TCA can block muscarinic receptors in the parasympathetic nervous system, resulting in dry mouth (xerostomia), blurred vision, and urinary retention.[74]

Tricyclic antidepressants also increase catecholamine activity in the heart while blocking alpha-adrenergic receptors in the peripheral capillary beds. Subsequently, when a patient stands suddenly the central nervous system cannot reflexively adjust to the sudden change in blood distribution and the patient experiences orthostatic syncope.

Toxicity

The depressed patient may elect to attempt suicide by ingestion of the TCA prescription. A TCA overdose can be dangerous at many levels. Alone, TCA blocks sodium channels in the heart, leading to complex cardiac conduction abnormalities including AV block, reentry ventricular dysrhythmia, and ventricular tachycardia, including polymorphic ventricular tachycardia (specifically torsades de pointes).[75,76]

Co-ingestion of depressants, such as alcohol, along with the TCA can lead to a toxic sedation. Similarly, if the patient ingested MAO inhibitors (another antidepressant) along with the TCA, the two drugs can produce a significant sympathetic overstimulation that manifests as high fever (hyperpyrexia) that mimics heat stroke, marked hypertension, and convulsions.

Treatment of a TCA overdose is aimed at reversing these negative cardiovascular effects and protecting the airway. After controlling the airway, alkalinization of the blood with sodium bicarbonate (0.5 mg/kg) may be the initial treatment.[77] The sodium bicarbonate bolus is usually followed by an intravenous infusion of sodium bicarbonate.

Selective Serotonin Re-Uptake Inhibitors

Selective serotonin re-uptake inhibitors (SSRI) preferentially block the re-uptake of serotonin into the neuron and thus, indirectly, increase the amount of neurotransmitter in the synaptic cleft. The SSRI drugs are thought to have less impact on the parasympathetic nervous system as well as fewer cardiovascular side effects such as orthostatic hypotension.

Monoamine Oxidase Inhibitors

Monoamine oxidase is an enzyme that metabolizes excess catecholamines, through a process of oxidation, into inactive metabolites that can be harmlessly excreted. MAO inhibitors prevent the deactivation of catecholamines from the synaptic gap and therefore indirectly increase the amount of neurotransmitter in the synaptic junction. The MAO inhibitors are similar to TCA in effect, but different in their pharmacodynamics, as they elevate the patient's mood.

Tyramine, the fundamental substance for monoamines such as norepinephrine, is found in such foodstuffs as aged cheeses, fermented sausages (such as bologna, pepperoni, salami, and summer sausage), sauerkraut, smoked or pickled meats, beer, and red wines.

Typically, tyramine is metabolized in the intestines by MAO. When the patient has been placed on an MAO inhibitor, tyramine-rich foods are absorbed unaltered into the circulation. Tyramine taken up by the neurons displaces the monoamines in the neuron's vesicles, liberating large quantities of catecholamines.

The resulting increase of catecholamines in the neuronal synapse leads to profound sympathetic stimulation. Subsequently, tachycardia and hypertension ensues and can lead to a potentially life-threatening hypertensive crisis.

Mania

Psychotic depression is discernible by extremes of mood. One moment the patient is depressed, voicing hopelessness, and the next moment the patient is elated and demonstrates self-confidence beyond reason. Patients exhibiting these behaviors are said to be bipolar (i.e., manic–depressives) and must be treated for both extremes in emotion.

Lithium Salts

The prototypical anti-mania drug is lithium. While lithium salts are very effective, the therapeutic index for lithium is very low. Effects of lithium intoxication include ataxia (drunken staggers), confusion, and convulsions.[78]

Drugs That Are Used to Treat Childbirth Emergencies

Traditionally, medications are used sparingly during pregnancy for fear of possible teratogenic effects. However, under certain special circumstances it may be necessary to use medication. In those instances, the Paramedic should review the drug's pregnancy classification as well as contact medical control.

Eclampsia

Eclampsia, also known as toxemia of pregnancy, is the culmination of a syndrome called pre-eclampsia. It is dramatically revealed by the pregnant woman's convulsion between her third trimester (twentieth week) and immediately postpartum. Pre-eclampsia produces hypertension (rise in the baseline systolic pressure by 31 mmHg), protein in the urine (albuminuria), and peripheral edema.

Treatment of eclampsia has two objectives: stop the convulsion and preserve the life of the fetus. If left untreated, the mother's eclampsia-induced convulsion can lead to coma and stress the unborn infant. A higher incidence of placenta abruptio has also been noted following eclampsia-induced convulsions.

While diazepam is effective in treating the convulsion, evidence suggests that magnesium sulfate remains superior for the treatment of eclampsia.[79] Whenever magnesium sulfate is administered, careful monitoring of blood pressure, pulse, respirations, and fetal heart sounds (when possible) should occur at least every 15 minutes.

It is important that Paramedics make the distinction between the mother who is experiencing an eclampsia-induced convulsion and one with a pre-existing seizure disorder. This distinction is important when selecting preferred agents for emergency treatment. If uncontrolled, a convulsion can lead to fetal anoxia and brain damage. Therefore, it must be treated immediately with the most effective anticonvulsant agent.

Labor

Complications of pregnancy, such as premature labor, preterm delivery, and breech deliveries, make the field delivery of an infant more dangerous. In certain situations, it is desirable to inhibit the labor of a pregnant woman in favor of effecting an immediate transfer of the mother to a better equipped birthing center.

Another serious complication of pregnancy is postpartum hemorrhage. When the products of conception are incompletely removed from the uterus following labor, such as incomplete placental detachment, then the mother may hemorrhage uncontrollably. In those cases, Paramedics may institute a life-saving infusion of medication to force uterine contraction.

Tocolysis

Medications that cause uterine relaxation, and thus inhibit labor, are called tocolytics. Some tocolytics, such as ethyl alcohol (inhibits oxytocin) and aspirin (inhibits prostaglandin-induced labor), are impractical in the field. In some cases, a simple bolus of intravenous solution can be temporarily effective. The bolus of intravenous solution activates antidiuretic hormone from the posterior pituitary gland and also inhibits oxytocin secretion from the posterior pituitary as well.

Hypothetically, any smooth muscle relaxant should also inhibit labor, as few drugs work exclusively in one organ or even on one organ system. Terbutaline, a smooth muscle relaxant (beta-adrenergic agonist), has been given intravenously (0.025 mg/min IV drip) with some success. However, significant side effects limit its use to emergencies only.

Oxytocics

Labor, the forceful contraction of the uterine smooth muscles, is induced by the hormone oxytocin which is secreted from the posterior pituitary gland. Oxytocin, which translated literally means "rapid birth," is made synthetically and can be intravenously administered by Paramedics during a pregnancy-related emergency.

The onset of action of synthetic oxytocin, such as ergonovine or oxytocin itself, is almost immediate (one to six minutes) and causes uterine contractions to gradually increase over one hour. The strong contractions of the uterus tend to compress blood vessels and slow intrauterine bleeding.

STREET SMART

Stimulation of the mother's nipple stimulates milk discharge from the breast via release of oxytocin. This cause and effect is called the letdown reflex. Therapeutically, stimulation of the mother's nipple, by the suckling infant, can also release oxytocin that will cause uterine contractions and help control hemorrhage.

Drugs That Are Used to Combat Infection

An infection occurs whenever any microorganism, such as a virus, bacteria, parasite, fungus, or worm (helminth), invades the body and overcomes the host's native defenses. Without medical intervention, these infections can lead to generalized sepsis, septic shock, and even death.

The best defense against infection is prevention. Paramedics can utilize a variety of techniques to try and prevent infection. The first assumption of infection control is that pathogens (microorganisms capable of producing infection) are omnipresent in the community and within the work environment. To limit their transmission (i.e., prevention), Paramedics use a variety of barrier devices (gloves, goggles, mask, and gown) as well as aseptic techniques.

Hypothetically, a complete lack of all microorganisms (surgical asepsis) would be the most desirable situation for EMS. However, surgical asepsis is only possible via sterilization and is therefore impractical in the field. More realistically, the Paramedics' goal should be to attain medical asepsis (an absence of pathogenic microorganisms) in the field. Medical asepsis is obtained through a combination of hygienic measures, such as hand washing, barrier devices, antiseptics, and disinfectants.

Disinfectants are solutions and compounds, such as the phenols and chlorine compounds, which effectively remove pathogens from inanimate objects, such as work surfaces and assessment tools. However, they are generally toxic when they come in contact with living tissue. Therefore, disinfectants cannot be used in the treatment of patients unless their potency is reduced (e.g., through dilution). Weakened, these solutions tend to inhibit, rather than destroy, pathogens and are thus called antiseptics.

Antiseptics, as well as disinfectants, can be further categorized as either bacteriostatic (solutions that slow the growth of pathogens) or bactericidal (solutions that kill off the pathogens). Some solutions are effective against a broad spectrum of pathogens (i.e., fungi, virus, and bacteria) and are called germicides. An effective disinfectant must be able to kill off all bacteria (not spores), fungi, parasites, and most viruses within 10 minutes of application.

Antimicrobials

Despite meticulous medical asepsis, infections do still occur. Medical intervention is necessary to prevent the spread of infection. Treatments for infection can be broken down into surgical treatments and medical treatments. Surgical treatments include the debridement of dead and necrotic tissue, incision and drainage of infection, and excision of infected organs. A discussion of surgical treatment is beyond the scope of this text.

Medical treatments for infection include the use of chemicals (i.e., drugs) for their therapeutic benefit. Organization of these chemotherapeutic agents can be arranged according to the pathogen that the drug is most effective against. For example, antibiotics are drugs that are effective against bacteria and antivirals are most effective against viruses.

Antivirals

Viruses, the smallest pathogen, are incapable of independent reproduction and, as parasites, require a host cell for replication. Understanding how important this simple process is to a virus's infectivity, antiviral treatment is focused on preventing the virus from injecting (i.e., uncoating) its RNA into the host cell or inhibiting the synthesis of DNA once the virus is inside.

Unfortunately, due to the close relationship of the virus to the host cell, it is difficult to kill one without eliminating the other.

Antibiotics

The sheer number of antibiotics available on the market is staggering. To lend order to this collection, antibiotics can be further classified according to their action. Minimally, antibiotics should suppress bacterial infections, allowing the host's defenses to overcome the infection (e.g., tetracycline or erythromycin) or even destroy the invading pathogen (e.g., aminoglycosides, cephalosporins, and penicillins).

Some antibiotics are effective against a large number of bacteria (i.e., the antibiotic is nonspecific) and thus are classified as broad-spectrum antibiotics. Other antibiotics are very effective for only a specific bacteria. For example, isoniazid is only effective against mycobacterium tuberculosis, and thus is classified as a narrow-spectrum antibiotic.

In many cases, a patient will be placed on a broad-spectrum antibiotic while awaiting laboratory results of cultures obtained from the patient. With the results in hand, more specific, or narrow-spectrum, antibiotic therapy would be prescribed.

Antibiotics can bring about their antimicrobial effect by several means, including inhibiting cell wall synthesis, inhibiting protein synthesis, or as an antimetabolite.

Antibiotics That Inhibit Cell Wall Synthesis

Bacteria, unlike native cells, are not isotonic in the interstitial fluid. The resulting osmotic pressure places a great strain upon the bacteria's cell walls. Any antibiotic that weakens that cell wall (e.g., by inhibiting the synthesis of portions of the cell wall) will cause the cell wall to structurally fail and the cell to burst (i.e., lysis).

The pharmacodynamics of the first antibiotic (penicillin) works by this mechanism. Subsequent generations of antibiotics, such as the cephalosporins, also depend on this mechanism.[80]

Allergies to penicillin are common, occurring in about 5% of the U.S. population.[81] Not surprisingly, patients who develop an allergy to penicillin drugs often have a cross-allergy to the cephalosporins as well, since the two are chemically related. Newer broad-spectrum penicillins, such as piperacillin, are among some of the most widely used antibiotics because of their wide safety margin. Unfortunately, overuse and poor patient compliance has led to the development of penicillin-resistant bacteria, the creation of super-infections, and subsequently limited the usefulness of these inexpensive antibiotics.

Antibiotics That Inhibit Protein Synthesis

Inhibition of protein synthesis within the bacteria's cytoplasmic ribosome by these antibiotics causes the bacteria to misread the genetic code. Unable to properly synthesize the necessary proteins for cell reproduction, the bacterium dies. Tetracyclines, aminoglycosides, erythromycin, chloramphenicol, and clindamycin are all antibiotics that work by this mechanism.

Antibiotics That Are Antimetabolites

Bacteria, like the host, require certain substrates for the production of proteins and the like. For example, one of those substrates is folate. Folate, which is produced by the bacteria from PABA, is converted into folic acid, an essential cofactor in amino acid synthesis. The sulfonamide class of antibiotics competes with bacteria for the enzymes necessary for this conversion, thus inhibiting the bacteria's ability to produce amino acids and proteins. Isoniazid (IND), a potent antituberculosis agent, works by a similar mechanism, inhibiting the synthesis of mycolic acids. This, in turn, weakens the mycobacterium's cell wall.

Antifungals

Of the over one million varieties of fungus, over 400 are known to cause disease in humans. So many varieties of fungus exist that fungus is categorized as one of the five kingdoms of life. Fungus is identifiable by its rigid cell walls, among other characteristics, which makes it particularly resistant to most antibiotics. Fungal infections, called mycoses, are generally treated with antibiotics that disrupt the cell wall of the fungus, making it more permeable. The cell walls are now "leaky," essential substrates (such as potassium) leak out, and the cell dies.

Antiprotozoal

Protozoa, a one-celled organism, may be the most abundant life form on Earth, creating more "biomass" than any other life form. Of particular concern to Paramedics are the protozoa that cause malaria and the protozoa that cause amebic dysentery.

Malaria, carried in mosquito saliva, is a blood-borne infection.

Roughly 40% of the world's population is at risk for malaria. In fact, it is estimated that one African child dies every 30 seconds from malaria.[82]

Acute dysentery, characterized by large amounts of mucus-laden diarrhea and severe abdominal pain, is the consequence of intestinal amebic infection. If left untreated, dysentery can lead to profound hypovolemia and shock.

While improved sanitary conditions have decreased the incidence of these two diseases in the United States, immigrants from other countries and tourists traveling abroad can bring the disease back in the Americas.

Pregnancy and Protozoa

A particular concern of pregnant women is the possibility of contracting toxoplasmosis. The causative agent in toxoplasmosis is toxoplasma gondii, a protozoa that is carried in the feces of cats as an oocyst (encapsulated protozoa). Absorbed systemically, the protozoa are transferred to the fetus and can cause blindness, loss of hearing, and mental retardation. For this reason, women who are pregnant are advised to not empty cat litter boxes.

Antihelmintics

The helminthes (worms) include blood flukes, flatworms, and tapeworms. (Ringworm is a fungal infection.) These worms can be present in undercooked beef or pork, or transmitted by common vectors, such as the mosquito, horse fly, or black fly.

Treatment of worms is aimed at the specific helminth that has been identified. Interestingly, a number of the treatments paralyze the worm. When co-administered with laxative, the body then can purge the infestation.

Drugs Used to Treat Cancer

Cancer is the second leading cause of death in the United States. One in four patients will have a diagnosis of cancer in his or her lifetime. The goal of cancer treatment is to eliminate the cancer from the body.

Chemotherapy is one of the three mainstays of cancer treatment, the other two being radiation and surgery. Chemotherapy is aimed at eliminating the cancer at the cellular level. In some instances, the chemotherapy is calculated to reduce a tumor's mass for surgical removal later. In other cases, the chemotherapy is intended to eliminate any remaining cancer cells (micrometastases) after surgery and/or radiation.

Drugs that eradicate cancer cells are called antineoplastics. These antineoplastic drugs depend upon the rapid division of the dysfunctional cells within a tumor to be effective. To proliferate, cancer cells depend on amino acids and nucleic acids in order to build DNA and RNA. By understanding this concept, chemotherapies are designed that deprive the cancer cell of these essential substrates (i.e., antimetabolites), block the transcription of RNA to new DNA (called mitotic inhibitors), or prevent cell division entirely (such as the alkylating agents).

All antineoplastic agents are also effective against cell division among normal healthy cells, particularly the rapidly dividing epithelial cells of the mucus lining in the intestine, the dermis of the skin, and the hair. Thus, the margin between the therapeutic and toxic margins of antineoplastic agents is extremely narrow and serious side effects frequently occur.

A common side effect is a decline in the number of white blood cells. At the peak (nadir) of the chemotherapy's effectiveness, the patient's white blood cell count will be at its lowest (leukopenia) and the patient will be seriously immunocompromised. With a limited immunity, opportunistic infections can obtain a foothold and the patient can become septic. Often the first sign of infection is a fever of unknown origin.[83]

Similarly, at the nadir of the chemotherapy the patient's platelet count will also drop. The resulting thrombocytopenia will leave the patient at greater risk for spontaneous hemorrhage (e.g., cerebral hemorrhage) and bruising.

STREET SMART

The nadir of chemotherapy usually occurs in the middle of the cycle (e.g., on the seventh day of a 14-day cycle). At this time, the patient is at greatest risk for acquiring infection. Paramedics should practice reverse isolation when caring for this patient.

Palliative Care

In many instances, all a Paramedic can do is offer support and palliative measures to patients with cancer. Palliative measures are those treatments that are intended to alleviate the unpleasant symptoms of chemotherapy with antineoplastic agents.

Common symptoms associated with chemotherapy include nausea, vomiting, anorexia, and diarrhea. Use of antiemetics—such as promethazines, phenothiazines, and antihistamines—may bring the patient much needed relief and comfort.

CONCLUSION

Paramedics have a limited arsenal of effective chemotherapeutic agents with which to fight disease. Despite this apparent disability, thoughtful Paramedics can intervene early in an emergency with this limited number of medications and reduce the morbidity and mortality associated with these diseases.

KEY POINTS:

- The brain consists of the brainstem (the primitive brain), the cerebellum, and the cerebrum.

- Only lipid-soluble drugs are capable of passing into brain tissue. This blood-brain barrier is the result of tight slit junctions, gaps in capillaries that allow some substances to pass.

- CNS depressants reduce anxiety, decrease excitability, and (at higher doses) produce sleep. Depressants include barbiturates, benzodiazepines, and alcohol.

- Depressants work by interfering with ion movement across the membrane or occupying receptor sites.

- Anesthesia is lack of sensation.

- Analgesia, the first stage of anesthesia, is the lack of pain.

- Anesthetic agents can be inhaled or intravenously administered.

- Nitrous oxide is an inhaled field anesthetic.

- IV anesthetics include short-acting benzodiazepines and short-acting barbiturates.

- Conscious sedation is a technique used to depress a patient's level of consciousness without loss of protective reflexes. In the field setting, it enables the Paramedic to perform difficult or painful procedures.

- Pain is the most common reason to call EMS.

- The pain threshold, the level of stimulus that will elicit a pain response, varies from person to person.

- Nociceptors (pain receptors) send messages over myelinated A fibers (sharp pain) or via unmyelinated C fibers (dull or burning pain). A fibers connect to

reflex arcs in the spinal cord, causing an immediate withdrawal from the stimulus.

- Neuromodulators are substances that affect the transmission of pain sensations to the brain. Endorphins are natural neuromodulators and attach to opiate receptors. Sodium movement across the membrane is slowed, thus slowing nerve conduction and pain interpretation.

- Opiate analgesics act in the same manner as endorphins.

- Opiate analgesics include morphine, fentanyl, codeine, and hydromorphone. Side effects include respiratory depression, altered mental status, and vasodilation.

- Synthetic opiates, including meperidine and methadone, have less undesirable side effects.

- Opiate antagonists, such as naloxone, reverse the effects but do not affect an allergic reaction.

- Non-opioid analgesics act at the level of the injury, reducing the effects of inflammation.

- Salicylate (aspirin) toxicity results in a metabolic acidosis.

- Acetaminophen toxicity can lead to permanent liver damage.

- Anticonvulsant medications affect the sodium channels in the nerve's action potential or affect the neurotransmitter GABA, reducing rapid electrical discharges. Barbiturates, hydantoins, benzodiazepines, succinimides, and valproic acid prevent or treat seizure activity.

- Anti-Parkinson's medications block acetylcholine or increase dopamine reception in the brain.

- The endocrine system utilizes hormones to relay chemical messages. Hormones can be given to treat some endocrine diseases.

- Diabetes mellitus can cause the medical emergencies of hypoglycemia or hyperglycemia with or without acidosis.

- Insulin is a protein that must be injected. Various insulin preparations have different onset and duration of effect.

- Oral hypoglycemic agents act in one or more of the following ways:
  - Stimulate beta cells in the pancreas to produce more insulin
  - Reduce glucagon levels
  - Increase insulin binding to cell receptors
  - Delay absorption of carbohydrates
  - Lower insulin resistance

- Hypoglycemia is treated with sugar replacement by mouth or intravenously. Glucagon can be given intramuscularly to stimulate the release of glycogen and its subsequent metabolism to glucose.

- The cortex of the adrenal glands produces mineralocorticoids (which affect water and sodium balance), glucocorticoids (which affect inflammation), androgenous steroids, and estrogen. The medulla produces epinephrine and norepinephrine.

- The ovaries are the primary site of estrogen production. Altering the amount and timing of estrogen production has a contraceptive effect. Estrogen also inhibits or enhances the growth of tumors, has a cardioprotective effect, and limits bone density loss in post-menopausal women.

- The pituitary gland produces different hormones in its anterior portion compared to its posterior portion. Antidiuretic hormone from the posterior portion is given as vasopressin to cause vasoconstriction and limit water loss. Oxytocin is also a posterior pituitary hormone.

- The thyroid gland is responsible for the rate of metabolism. Drugs used to treat thyroid disorders include medications to stimulate the production of triiodothyronine (T3) or thyroxine (T4).

- Anaphylaxis is the most severe inappropriate response to an allergen. The chemical mediator (histamine) can cause bronchoconstriction, angioedema, and airway swelling, plus hypotension secondary to vasodilation. Antihistamines are antagonists and compete for the H1 receptors. They prevent further effects but do not reverse the effects already present. Epinephrine reverses the effects.

- Gastrointestinal medications include over-the-counter antacids designed to buffer stomach acids, emetics that induce vomiting, antiemetics that prevent vomiting by affecting the vomiting center in the brain, antidiarrheal medications, and laxatives that stimulate release of rectal contents, soften the stool by increased water absorption, or bulk up the stool with insoluble fibers.

- Medications that treat bleeding disorders either interfere with anticoagulant drugs or replace missing coagulation factors.

- Ineffective or decreased red blood cells may be treated with replacement substances such as iron or vitamins.

- Antipsychotic medications include those that block dopamine receptors, those that reduce anxiety, and those that enhance the neurotransmitters, called monoamines.

- Medications that slow labor are called tocolytics. Many work by beta agonism relaxing the smooth muscle of the uterus. Medications that enhance labor (oxytocics) work by stimulating or imitating the effect of oxytocin from the posterior pituitary.

- Drugs used to combat infection are directed toward the specific agent.
  - Antibiotics affect bacterial invasions through inhibiting cell wall synthesis, inhibiting protein synthesis, or as an antimetabolite.
  - Antivirals try to prevent viruses from invading host cells.
  - Antifungals affect the integrity of the rigid cell wall.
  - Antiprotozoans and antihelmintics help the body purge the invading organisms.

- Drugs used to treat cancer are antineoplastics. These affect the metabolism of the rapidly dividing cancer cell but also affect other rapidly dividing cells such as hair follicles.

REVIEW QUESTIONS:

1. Describe the mechanism of action of opiate pain relievers.

2. How does the opiate antagonist naloxone work? Does it affect an allergic reaction to an opiate drug?

3. List at least two non-opiate pain relievers, state their mechanism of action, and state their toxic effects.

4. Name two ways in which anticonvulsant medications prevent or treat seizures.

5. What is the mechanism of action of anti-Parkinson's drugs?

6. What protein is given to reduce glucose levels in the blood? Can it be taken orally?

7. List the mechanisms used by oral hypoglycemic agents to lower blood glucose levels.

8. Name two medications given to treat hypoglycemia.

9. What is the mechanism of action of antihistamines? Do these medications reverse the presenting signs?

10. Name two mechanisms of action for antipsychotic medications. What is a potentially reversible side effect of the major antipsychotic agents?

11. What is the classification of drugs that slow or stop labor? Stimulate labor?

12. Describe three mechanisms by which antibiotics work.

CASE STUDY QUESTIONS:

Please refer to the Case Study at the beginning of the chapter and answer the questions below:

1. What classifications of drugs relieve pain? Alter sensation? Modify metabolism?

2. Name at least six questions the Paramedic should ask regarding the history of the present illness (complaint).

3. Name at least five questions that the Paramedic should ask regarding the patient's past medical history.

REFERENCES:

1. Burt A. *Textbook of Neuroanatomy.* Philadelphia: W.B. Saunders Company; 1993.

2. Seigel G, ed., et al. *Basic Neurochemistry: Molecular, Cellular and Medical Aspects (Periodicals).* Philadelphia: Lippincott Williams & Wilkins; 1998.

3. Lopez-Munoz F, Ucha-Udabe R, et al. The history of barbiturates a century after their clinical introduction. *Neuropsychiatr Dis Treat.* 2005;1(4):329–343.

4. Lader M, Petursson H. Rational use of anxiolytic/sedative drugs. *Drugs.* 1983;25(5):514–528.

5. Whitwam JG, Amrein R. Pharmacology of flumazenil. *Acta Anaesthesiol Scand Suppl.* 1995;108:3–14.

6. Ngo AS, Anthony CR, et al. Should a benzodiazepine antagonist be used in unconscious patients presenting to the emergency department? *Resuscitation.* 2007;74(1):27–37.

7. Hamilton M. Researching harm reduction—care and contradictions. *Subst Use Misuse.* 1999;34(1):119–141.

8. Wobst AH. Hypnosis and surgery: past, present, and future. *Anesth Analg.* 2007;104(5):1199–1208.

9. Andrade J, Deeprose C. Unconscious memory formation during anaesthesia. *Best Pract Res Clin Anaesthesiol.* 2007;21(3): 385–401.

10. Punjasawadwong Y, Boonjeungmonkol N, et al. Bispectral index for improving anaesthetic delivery and postoperative recovery. *Cochrane Database Syst Rev.* 2007;4:CD003843.

11. Szmuk P, Aroyo N, et al. Listening to music during anesthesia does not reduce the sevoflurane concentration needed to maintain a constant bispectral index. *Anesth Analg.* 2008;107(1):77–80.

12. Jaslow D, Lemecha D. Prehospital pharmacology: nitrous oxide. *Emerg Med Serv.* 2007;36(2):71–73.

13. Faddy SC, Garlick SR. A systematic review of the safety of analgesia with 50% nitrous oxide: can lay responders use analgesic gases in the prehospital setting? *Emerg Med J.* 2005;22(12):901–908.

14. Bledsoe BE, Myers JW. Future trends in prehospital pain management. *JEMS.* 2003;28(6):68–71.

15. Schrading W, Kaplan R, et al. Effect of scavenging on ambient levels of nitrous oxide in ambulances. *Ann Emerg Med.* 1990;19(8):910–913.

16. Zelicof-Paul A, Smith-Lockridge A, et al. Controversies in rapid sequence intubation in children. *Curr Opin Pediatr.* 2005;17(3):355–362.

17. Bean A, Jones J. Atropine: re-evaluating its use during paediatric RSI. *Emerg Med J.* 2007;24(5):361–362.

18. Butler, J, Jackson R. Best evidence topic report. Lignocaine as a pretreatment to rapid sequence intubation in patients with status asthmaticus. *Emerg Med J.* 2005;22(10):732.

19. Butler J, Jackson R. Towards evidence based emergency medicine: best BETs from Manchester Royal Infirmary. Lignocaine premedication before rapid sequence induction in head injuries. *Emerg Med J.* 2002;19(6):554.

20. Robinson N, Clancy M. In patients with head injury undergoing rapid sequence intubation, does pretreatment with intravenous lignocaine/lidocaine lead to an improved neurological outcome? A review of the literature. *Emerg Med J.* 2001;18(6):453–457.

21. Lee C, Porter KM. Prehospital management of lower limb fractures. *Emerg Med J.* 2005;22(9):660–663.

22. McManus JG, Jr., Sallee DR, Jr. Pain management in the prehospital environment. *Emerg Med Clin North Am.* 2005;23(2):415–431.

23. Thomas SH, Shewakramani S. Prehospital trauma analgesia. *J Emerg Med.* 2008;35(1):47–57.

24. Salerno E. Race, culture, and medications. *J Emerg Nurs.* 1995;21(6):560–562.

25. Gordon DB. Love G. Pharmacologic management of neuropathic pain. *Pain Manag Nurs.* 2004;5(4 Suppl 1):19–33.

26. Sellin JH. A practical approach to treating patients with chronic diarrhea. *Rev Gastroenterol Disord.* 2007;7(Suppl 3):S19–S26.

27. Shah SB, Hanauer SB. Treatment of diarrhea in patients with inflammatory bowel disease: concepts and cautions. *Rev Gastroenterol Disord.* 2007;7(Suppl 3):S3–10.

28. Porter R. *The Greatest Benefit to Mankind: A Medical History of Humanity.* New York: W. W. Norton & Company; 1999.

29. Ghoneim MM, Dhanaraj J, et al. Comparison of four opioid analgesics as supplements to nitrous oxide anesthesia. *Anesth Analg.* 1984;63(4):405–412.

30. Gillman PK. Monoamine oxidase inhibitors, opioid analgesics and serotonin toxicity. *Br J Anaesth.* 2005;95(4):434–441.

31. McGuire W, Fowlie PW. Naloxone for narcotic-exposed newborn infants. *Cochrane Database Syst Rev.* 2002;4:CD003483.

32. History of aspirin. Available at: http://www.bayeraspirin.com/pain/asp_history.htm. Accessed December 9, 2008.

33. Vane JR, Botting RM. The mechanism of action of aspirin. *Thromb Res.* 2003;110(5-6):255–258.

34. Temple AR. Pathophysiology of aspirin overdosage toxicity, with implications for management. *Pediatrics.* 1978;62(5 Pt 2 Suppl):873–876.

35. Proudfoot AT. Toxicity of salicylates. *Am J Med.* 1983;75(5A):99–103.

36. Bailey BO. Acetaminophen hepatotoxicity and overdose. *Am Fam Physician.* 1980;22(1):83–87.

37. Karumanchi SA, Lindheimer MD. Advances in the understanding of eclampsia. *Curr Hypertens Rep.* 2008;10(4):305–312.

38. Craig S. Phenytoin poisoning. *Neurocrit Care.* 2005;3(2):161–170.

39. Tomsick RS. The phenytoin syndrome. *Cutis.* 1983;32(6):535–541.

40. Brewer JM, Waltman PA. Epilepsy and pregnancy: maternal and fetal effects of phenytoin. *Crit Care Nurse.* 2003;23(2):93–98.

41. Gladstone DJ, Bologa M, et al. Course of pregnancy and fetal outcome following maternal exposure to carbamazepine and phenytoin: a prospective study. *Reprod Toxicol.* 1992;6(3):257–261.

42. Karceski S. Patient page. Epilepsy and pregnancy: are seizure medications safe? *Neurology.* 2008;71(14):e32–33.

43. Ferrara JM, Stacy N. Impulse-control disorders in Parkinson's disease. *CNS Spectr.* 2008;13(8):690–698.

44. Penson PE, Ford WR, et al. Vasopressors for cardiopulmonary resuscitation. Does pharmacological evidence support clinical practice? *Pharmacol Ther.* 2007;115(1):37–55.

45. Putcha N, Allon M. Management of hyperkalemia in dialysis patients. *Semin Dial.* 2007;20(5):431–439.

46. Kim HJ. Combined effect of bicarbonate and insulin with glucose in acute therapy of hyperkalemia in end-stage renal disease patients. *Nephron.* 1996;72(3):476–482.

47. Allon M, Takeshian A, et al. Effect of insulin-plus-glucose infusion with or without epinephrine on fasting hyperkalemia. *Kidney Int.* 1993;43(1):212–217.

48. Marks V, Teale JD. Drug-induced hypoglycemia. *Endocrinol Metab Clin North Am.* 1999;28(3):555–577.

49. Cryer PE. Symptoms of hypoglycemia, thresholds for their occurrence, and hypoglycemia unawareness. *Endocrinol Metab Clin North Am.* 1999;28(3):495–500, v–vi.

50. Brindley PG, Simmonds M, et al. Best evidence in critical care medicine. Steroids in sepsis: bulking up the evidence. *Can J Anaesth.* 2008;55(9):648–650.

51. Du Plessis JJ. High-dose dexamethasone therapy in head injury: a patient group that may benefit from therapy. *Br J Neurosurg.* 1992;6(2):145–147.

52. Reimondo G, Bovio S, et al. Secondary hypoadrenalism. *Pituitary.* 2008;11(2):147–154.

53. Karagiannis A, Mikhailidis DP, et al. Pheochromocytoma: an update on genetics and management. *Endocr Relat Cancer.* 2007;14(4):935–956.

54. Jick S, Kaye JA, et al. Further results on the risk of nonfatal venous thromboembolism in users of the contraceptive transdermal patch compared to users of oral contraceptives containing norgestimate and 35 microg of ethinyl estradiol. *Contraception.* 2007;76(1):4–7.

55. Spohr FA, Teschendorf P, et al. Vasopressors in cardiopulmonary resuscitation. *N Engl J Med.* 2008;359(15):1624–1625; author reply 1625.

56. Sillberg VA, Perry JJ, et al. Is the combination of vasopressin and epinephrine superior to repeated doses of epinephrine alone in the treatment of cardiac arrest—a systematic review. *Resuscitation.* 2008;79(3):380–386.

57. Ong ME, Lim SH, et al. Intravenous adrenaline or vasopressin in sudden cardiac arrest: a literature review. *Ann Acad Med Singapore.* 2002;31(6):785–792.

58. Choong K, Kissoon N. Vasopressin in pediatric shock and cardiac arrest. *Pediatr Crit Care Med.* 2008;9(4):372–379.

59. Vassallo P, Trohman RG. Prescribing amiodarone: an evidence-based review of clinical indications. *JAMA.* 2007;298(11):1312–1322.

60. Ursella S, Testa A, et al. Amiodarone-induced thyroid dysfunction in clinical practice. *Eur Rev Med Pharmacol Sci.* 2006;10(5):269–278.

61. Fisher MM. Severe histamine mediated reactions to intravenous drugs used in anaesthesia. *Anaesth Intensive Care.* 1975;3(3):180–197.

62. Sheikh A, Shehata YA, et al. Adrenaline (epinephrine) for the treatment of anaphylaxis with and without shock. *Cochrane Database Syst Rev.* 2008;4:CD006312.

63. Allen MD, Greenblatt DJ, et al. Effect of magnesium–aluminum hydroxide and kaolin–pectin on absorption of digoxin from tablets and capsules. *J Clin Pharmacol. 1981;21*(1):26–30.

64. Scharman EJ, Hutzler JM, et al. Single dose pharmacokinetics of syrup of ipecac. *Ther Drug Monit.* 2000;22(5):566–573.

65. Krenzelok EP, McGuigan M, et al. Position statement: ipecac syrup. American Academy of Clinical Toxicology; European Association of Poisons Centres and Clinical Toxicologists. *J Toxicol Clin Toxicol.* 1997;35(7):699–709.

66. Corey S. Recent developments in the therapeutic potential of cannabinoids. *P R Health Sci J.* 2005;24(1):19–26.

67. Au N, Rettie AE. Pharmacogenomics of 4-hydroxycoumarin anticoagulants. *Drug Metab Rev.* 2008;40(2):355–375.

68. Agaliotis DP.Hemophilia overview. 2008. Available at: http://www.emedicine.com/med/TOPIC3528.HTM. Accessed November 22, 2008.

69. Dayalu P, Chou KL. Antipsychotic-induced extrapyramidal symptoms and their management. *Expert Opin Pharmacother.* 2008;9(9):1451–1462.

70. Henretig FM. Special considerations in the poisoned pediatric patient. *Emerg Med Clin North Am.* 1994;12(2):549–567.

71. Thornley B, Rathbone J, et al. Chlorpromazine versus placebo for schizophrenia. *Cochrane Database Syst Rev.* 2003;2:CD000284.

72. Schoenberger JA. Drug-induced orthostatic hypotension. *Drug Saf.* 1991;6(6):402–407.

73. Mehta M, Gharpure V, et al. Acute iron poisoning. *Indian J Pediatr.* 1997;64(4):485–493.

74. Flanagan RJ. Fatal toxicity of drugs used in psychiatry. *Hum Psychopharmacol.* 2008;23(Suppl 1):43–51.

75. Rosenbaum TG, Kou M. Are one or two dangerous? Tricyclic antidepressant exposure in toddlers. *J Emerg Med.* 2005;28(2):169–174.

76. Groleau G, Jotte R, et al. The electrocardiographic manifestations of cyclic antidepressant therapy and overdose: a review. *J Emerg Med.* 1990;8(5):597–605.

77. Bradberry SM, Thanacoody HK, et al. Management of the cardiovascular complications of tricyclic antidepressant poisoning: role of sodium bicarbonate. *Toxicol Rev.* 2005;24(3):195–204.

78. Nguyen L. Lithium I: the basics. *J Emerg Nurs.* 2008;34(3):268–269.

79. Duley L, Gulmezoglu AM, et al. Magnesium sulphate and other anticonvulsants for women with pre-eclampsia. *Cochrane Database Syst Rev.* 2003;2:CD000025.

80. Tipper DJ. Mode of action of beta-lactam antibiotics. *Pharmacol Ther.* 1985;27(1):1–35.

81. Prescott WA, Jr., DePestel DD, et al. Incidence of carbapenem-associated allergic-type reactions among patients with versus patients without a reported penicillin allergy. *Clin Infect Dis.* 2004;38(8):1102–1107.

82. Jerrard DA, Broder JS, et al. Malaria: a rising incidence in the United States. *J Emerg Med.* 2002;23(1):23–33.

83. Gaeta GB, Fusco FM, et al. Fever of unknown origin: a systematic review of the literature for 1995–2004. *Nucl Med Commun.* 2006;27(3):205–211.

CHAPTER 32

PRINCIPLES OF ELECTRO-CARDIOGRAPHY

KEY CONCEPTS:

Upon completion of this chapter, it is expected that the reader will understand these following concepts:

- Phases of the cardiac cycle
- The coronary blood supply to the major portions of the cardiac conduction system compared and contrasted with the regions of the heart.
- The heart's pacemaking control, rate, and rhythm
- The purpose of ECG monitoring
- The electrophysical and hemodynamic events occurring throughout the entire cardiac cycle correlated with the various ECG waveforms, segments, and intervals

▶ CASE STUDY:

"Something just happened to Mrs. Fitzpatrick," said the intern Paramedic. "Her ECG complexes were upright and now they are negative." His preceptor (teaching Paramedic) asked if he changed leads, but the intern Paramedic denied doing anything to the monitor. After they had checked the patient, the preceptor began reviewing the waveforms on the ECG tracing.

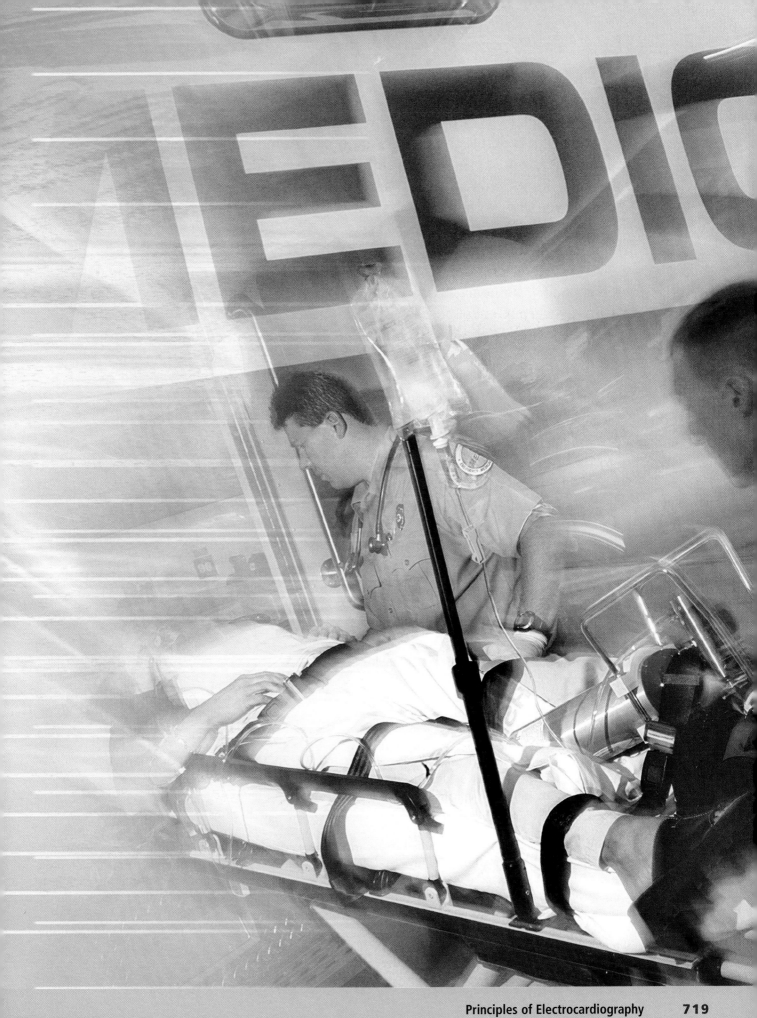

OVERVIEW:

From the toes to the nose, the heart pumps blood throughout the entire body. Similar to the fire engine's water pump, the heart has two components. It has an electrical system that controls the pump's action and a mechanical system that produces the pump's output. In the heart, both must work efficiently and in sequence in order to maintain the rhythmic pumping action that causes the 2 to 3 billion heart beats which occur over the average person's lifespan.

The electricity to run the heart's electrical system results from an electrochemical process. That electrochemical process occurs in specialized nervous cells in the heart's conduction system. This conduction system rhythmically stimulates the heart's muscles, thereby pacing the heart. Since the heart is essential to life, the heart's muscle cells (the myocardial cells) possess a special property called automaticity. That is, they can also generate electricity but at a much slower rate. This myocardial-induced pacing is a backup system that, although generally less efficient, can be life-saving.

The mechanical process, which creates the movement of blood and generates a pulse, is secondary to the electrical process and is dependent upon the electrical system for rate and rhythm. Damage and disruption to the electrical system can be catastrophic to the individual. Therefore, it is important for Paramedics to constantly assess the heart's electrical activity. Technology has given Paramedics the tools to observe the heart's electrical activity and to visually display it on an ECG monitor.

Anatomy

The heart lies within the thoracic cavity, an area in the center of the chest. This space, known as the mediastinum, also contains the great vessels (the aorta and the trachea). The heart is situated directly behind the sternum and extends slightly farther to the left of sternum than to the right. The base of the heart, where the great vessels enter, is located at the 2nd intercostal space. The apex of the heart is located at approximately the 5th intercostal space on the left midclavicular line.

The heart is composed of three layers of tissues (Figure 32-1). From outside inward, the first layer of the heart is the two-part **pericardium**. It has one part which envelops the heart and roots of the great vessels, plus another part that is closely adherent to the heart called the **epicardium**. The epicardium is considered the heart's outermost part. Between these two parts is a lubricant called pericardial fluid which decreases friction as the heart beats within the pericardial sac.

The next layer is the thicker **myocardium**. The myocardium is a muscular layer that actually performs the heart's work by contracting forcefully and ejecting blood from within the heart's chambers. Controlling this ejection are valves. Valves serve to direct blood in one direction from one chamber to another through the heart. These valves are assisted by muscles (such as the papillary muscles) and thick connective

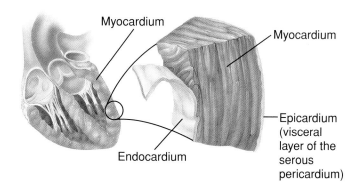

Figure 32-1 Cross-section of the myocardium.

cords (such as the chordae tendinae or, as in the case of the aorta, a thick supportive ring).

The muscle fibers of the myocardium are specially arranged in vertical bundles and figure 8 shapes called whorls. This arrangement allows maximum efficiency in both pushing and squeezing blood out of the heart during each heart beat. The muscles, valves, and rings all attach to a fibrous matrix called the **cardiac skeleton**.

The innermost layer of the heart is the **endocardium**. The endocardium is a single-layer thick sheet of epithelial cells that act as a lining, like the sleeve inside a fire hose.

Unlike the rest of the heart, this layer gets its nutrition (oxygen and glucose) directly from the circulating blood volume. Unfortunately, because of its direct contact with circulating blood, this layer is prone to infection from any pathogen circulating in the blood (e.g., an infection such as syphilis). This infected condition is called endocarditis.

Although cardiac muscle fibers function similarly to skeletal muscle fibers, there are several important differences. A specialized cell membrane in the myocardial cell reduces electrical resistance and allows an electrical stimulus to move rapidly from cell to cell. The myocardial cells are found in strands, or myofibrils, which form an extensive interrelated network. This network further enhances the rapid movement of the electrical stimulus from cell to cell and myofibril to myofibril, as well as to the myocardial mass as a whole. This networking of cells and myofibrils allows simultaneous stimulation of the whole structure so that it functionally acts as a single unit. A mass of cells that act as a unit is termed a **functional syncytium**. The atria act as one syncytium and the ventricles as another. The cardiac skeleton, made up of fibrous connective tissues, serves to isolate one syncytium from the other. As a result of electrical stimulation, muscles in the atria will contract as a unit (a functional syncytium), pushing blood from the base of the heart to the apex of the heart and the ventricles. The muscular ventricles will, in turn, function as another functional syncytium, pushing and squeezing blood from the apex of the heart and out the great vessels.

Cardiac Cycle

During a single contraction (one heart beat), blood flows through all four chambers of the heart. This contraction, including an entire sequence of events from atrial filling through ventricular filling and ejection, is called a **cardiac cycle**. The cardiac cycle is highly dependent upon pressure changes that occur within the heart's chambers to create forward blood flow. When the atria are at rest (**atrial diastole**) blood flows into the atria from the body and lungs. The blood then continues into the ventricles through the open atrioventricular valves. Approximately 70% of the blood returning to the heart passively enters the ventricles at this time. As pressure increases in the atria, the atria become stretched. The stretched atria will then contract (**atrial systole**), forcing approximately 32% more blood into the ventricles than would normally be there because of passive ventricular filling. The active contribution of blood to the ventricle by the atria is called the **atrial kick**. This atrial kick ultimately increases the amount of blood in the ventricles (the end diastolic volume (EDV) or the **preload**). The greater the preload, the greater the cardiac output.

With the ventricles maximally filled, the backpressure from the blood in the ventricles causes the atrioventricular valves to close and bulge upward toward the atria. The **chordae tendinae** (Figure 32-2), strong cords attached to **papillary muscles**, which emanate from the inferior wall, prevent the valves from inverting into the atria, which would allow a backflow of blood into the atria (**regurgitation**). With the atrioventricular valves closed, the atria begins diastole again while the ventricles prepare for systole.

As a result of the atrial kick, and because the atrioventricular valves are closed, the pressure within the ventricles rises sharply, distending the ventricular walls. This distention of the ventricles, and the resulting tension, causes the myocardium to contract more forcibly—a phenomenon predicted in **Starling's law**.

With the pressure elevated in the ventricles, the ventricular muscle fibers contract forcefully and generate sufficient

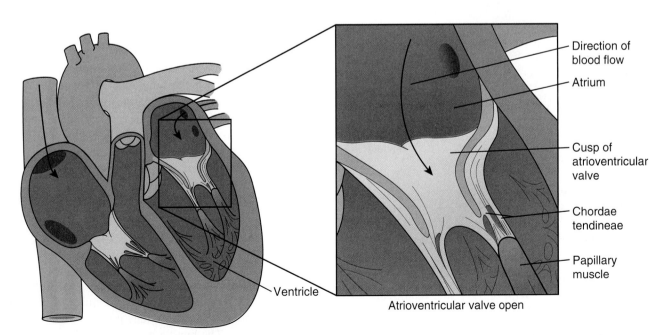

Direction of blood flow

Atrium

Cusp of atrioventricular valve

Chordae tendineae

Papillary muscle

Ventricle

Atrioventricular valve open

Figure 32-2 The chordae tendinae prevent inversion of the valves during ventricular systole.

pressure to force open the aortic and pulmonary valves and eject blood out of the heart. This process is called **ventricular systole**. The cardiac output (the volume of blood ejected out of the ventricles) flows via the aorta to the body or to the lungs. After the contraction, the ventricles relax and begin a period of **ventricular diastole**.

The arrangement of the muscle fibers efficiently ejects blood from the ventricles. However, even under optimal conditions, the ventricles cannot eject 100% of the blood from the ventricles. The percentage of blood pushed and squeezed out of the heart is called the **ejection fraction**. Normal ejection fraction of blood in a healthy heart is 60% to 75% of the end diastolic volume (the preload).[1]

Conduction System

The heart requires a taskmaster in order to perform its rhythmical work. Although this taskmaster can be influenced by other parts of the body, the heart's primary control is its own specialized cardiac cells. These cells are designed to carry on the heart's electrical rhythm. These specialized cells are collectively called the **conduction system** (Figure 32-3).

The initial portion of the conduction system is the **sinoatrial node (SA)**. This node is located just beneath the epicardium on the posterior wall of the right atrium near to the end of the vena cava and at the junction of the sinus of Valsalva and the atria. The SA node has fibers which connect it to the heart's right atrial cells. A special pathway exists for the SA node to communicate with the left atrium. This path is called **Bachmann's Bundle**.

The SA cells have the ability to initiate an electrical impulse without needing stimulation from an outside source. The SA node initiates an impulse between 60 to 100 times per minute. This rate is normally faster than in any other portion of the conduction system. The SA node assumes dominance as the pacemaker and is termed the primary or physiologic pacemaker of the heart. The SA node also has innervations from the sympathetic and the parasympathetic nervous systems. The sympathetic nervous system increases automaticity and subsequently the rate of discharge. The sympathetic nervous system can therefore cause the heart to race. Conversely, the cardiac branch of the vagus nerve, the 10th cranial nerve and a part of the parasympathetic nervous system, dampens automaticity of the cardiac conduction system. Therefore, stimulation of the vagus nerve can cause the heart to slow down. The parasympathetic nerve (the vagus nerve) ends at the AV node but the sympathetic nerves run the entire length of the conduction system from the SA node to the Purkinje fibers. This is an important fact to remember when discussing treatments for heart blocks.

Once the impulse is initiated at the SA node, it spreads across the heart like a wavefront, depolarizing the myocardium along the way. The result of this electrical stimulation of the myocardium is that the right and left atria contract immediately and nearly simultaneously (syncyctium) after the impulse leaves or exits the SA node. The impulse is then conducted toward the ventricles via the internodal pathways. The electrical signal then passes to the **atrioventricular node (AV)** located in between the atria and the ventricles.

The electrical impulse cannot normally enter the ventricles except by passing through the AV node. The cardiac skeleton, which serves as a framework for the heart's valves, also electrically separates the atria from the ventricles.

The signal next enters the AV node. The cells of the AV node are designed to conduct the impulse slowly. This electrical delay permits the atria to contract, thereby permitting maximal filling of the ventricles. This also allows the ventricle to receive the "atrial kick" that occurs when the atria contract. When atrial contraction is complete, the signal moves down the long strip of tissue below the AV node connecting the atria and the ventricles, called the **junctional tissues**. The junctional tissues are capable of independently initiating a stimulus if the SA nodal impulse should fail to depolarize them first. The intrinsic rate of the junctional tissue is approximately 40 to 60 bpm. Therefore, if the SA node fails to fire, then junction tissue at the AV node is the heart's secondary pacemaker. Often junctional rhythms produce less cardiac output because of the loss of the atrial kick that would normally occur if the SA node was the pacemaker.[2]

When the impulse reaches the ventricle, it is conducted through a wide, thick group of fibers called the **bundle of His**. The bundle of His conducts the impulse to the interventricular septum where it divides into the **right** and **left bundle branches**. The bundle branches lie deep within the myocardium just above the endocardium. The left bundle

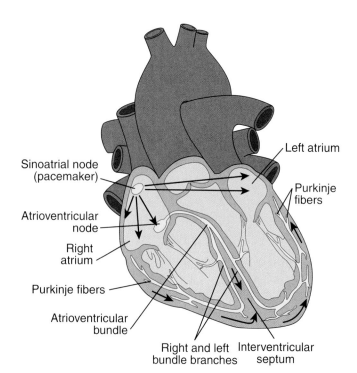

Sinoatrial node (pacemaker)

Atrioventricular node

Right atrium

Purkinje fibers

Atrioventricular bundle

Left atrium

Purkinje fibers

Right and left bundle branches

Interventricular septum

Figure 32-3 The electrical conduction system.

branch will further divide into an anterior branch and a posterior branch to adequately serve the larger, thicker left ventricle (Figure 32-4).

At the level of the ventricular cells, the bundle branches further divide to carry the impulse along the **Purkinje fibers**. Purkinje fibers, named after Jan E. Purkyne, connect directly with the ventricular myocardium, allowing the ventricles to contract nearly simultaneously as a functional syncytium.

Impulse Formation

Each part of the conduction system, from the SA node to the Purkinje fibers, is capable of initiating an electrical impulse via automaticity. Such capability serves as a backup plan for the heart in the event one pacemaker fails. Should this occur, there is another pacemaker available to take its place. The normal rate of the SA node is 60 to 100 impulses per minute. Its next closest neighbor, the AV node, can initiate impulses at a rate of 40 to 60 impulses per minute, while the bundle of His initiates impulses at only 20 to 40 times per minute. The slowest rate is that initiated in the Purkinje fibers, which has a rate of an agonizing 20 beats per minute or less.

The conduction is arranged to complement the heart's muscular action. The atrial aspect of the conduction system moves the impulse from superior to inferior just like the contraction of the atria, which is from superior to inferior. Therefore, the upper portion of the conduction system can be called the supraventricular (above the ventricles) portion. Once the impulse enters the ventricles, the conduction system takes it inferiorly to the apex and then (via the Purkinje fibers) immediately back upward, resulting in an inferior to superior route. This mimics the ventricular contraction of inferior to superior. The lower portion of the conduction system can be referred to as the ventricular portion.

Coronary Circulation and Its Relationship to Conduction

With the exception of the endocardium, the heart does not utilize the blood flowing through it for its metabolic needs. The heart is served by a special set of arteries and veins called the **coronary circulation**. These blood vessels are called the coronaries because they resemble a crown of thorns positioned on top of the heart. The coronary arteries arise from the aorta in an area adjacent to the aortic valve, an area called the **sinus of Valsalva**. They are the first arteries to arise from the aorta but they receive their blood flow last. This is because the aortic valve leaflets occlude the coronary arteries during systole. The result is that the coronary arteries fill only after the aorta valve has closed during diastole.

Because of the particular importance of the left ventricle, when the term "wall" is used it describes the portions of the left ventricle. The walls of the left ventricle are broken down into the following: the inferior wall (that portion that lies next to the diaphragm) and the anterior wall (that part of the left ventricle which faces forward). The anterior wall is the largest part of the left ventricle and contains the greatest mass of muscle in the heart (Figure 32-5).

The anterior wall of the left ventricle gets its blood from the left coronary artery. The left main coronary artery almost immediately divides and gives rise to the **left anterior descending coronary artery (LAD)** and the left **circumflex (Cx)**. The LAD provides blood to the SA node, in 45% of the population, and to the majority of the muscle mass in the left ventricle. Perhaps more importantly, the LAD provides the blood supply to the lower portion of the conduction system, the bundle of His, and the three bundle branches.

However, the most important function of the LAD is to provide blood flow to the largest part of the left ventricle, its anterior wall. In fact, 60% to 70% of the blood that travels to the coronary arteries is provided to the LAD and subsequently to the anterior wall.

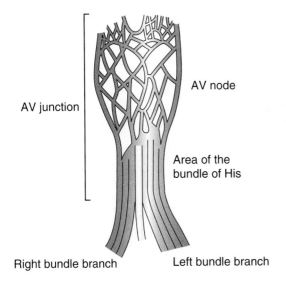

Figure 32-4 The atrioventricular node provides a pause in electrical conduction for the impulse traveling from the atria to the ventricles.

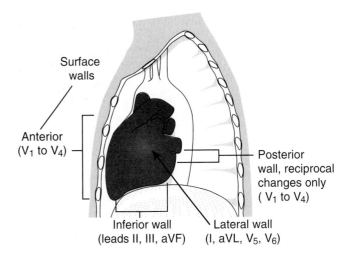

Figure 32-5 The anterior, lateral, and inferior walls of the heart.

The circumflex coronary artery, a minor branch of the left coronary artery, bends around to the left side of the heart and provides blood to the lateral wall of the left ventricle. The circumflex provides about 40% to 50% of the blood flow to the anterior wall, with the remainder supplied by the left anterior descending coronary artery.

The **right coronary artery (RCA)** serves the right atrium and ventricle and the inferior portion or wall of the left ventricle, which lies on the diaphragm. In 55% of the population, the RCA provides blood to the sinus node, and in 90% of the population it provides blood to the atrioventricular junction, both located in the upper portion of the conduction system. The sinus node and atrioventricular junction are important portions of the conduction system as they control the atria and therefore are part of the atrial kick.

The coronary veins follow the general pattern of the arteries except on the posterior wall, where an enlarged vein called the coronary sinus drains blood. The coronary sinus drains into the vena cava at its juncture with the right atrium. Other veins, called Thebesian's veins, drain directly through the heart muscle into the heart chambers (Figure 32-6).

Electrophysiology

The heart creates an impulse via an electrochemical reaction. Electrophysiology describes how the heart actually initiates the impulse by describing the electrochemical reactions that occur at the cellular level. Key to cardiac electrophysiology is the action potential of each and every myocardial cell. The term **cardiac action potential** is defined as the electrochemical activity of the heart's individual cells. This activity occurs somewhat differently in those cells designed for the work of muscular contraction and those designed to initiate and carry impulses. In both circumstances, the activity is based on the movement of ions and the electrical changes that the ions cause as they move.

The events are broken down into phases numbered from 0 to 4. In a typical cardiac working cell, which is not part of the specialized conduction system, the process will begin at phase 0. A resting cardiac cell is normally negatively charged on its inside. An electrical stimulus will change the permeability of the cell's membrane by opening special channels, allowing for the movement of sodium into the cell. The influx of sodium is very rapid, and the process of allowing the sodium in is called fast channel response. Sodium is a cation (+) so a large amount of sodium moving into the cell will cause the inside to become positive.

Phase 1 begins when the fast sodium channels close. Chloride, an anion (−), also moves into the cell during phase 1. With sodium no longer adding its positive charge to the inside of the cell, and chloride with its negative charge moving in, the cell again becomes negative.

Phase 2 is the plateau phase of the action potential. In phase 2 calcium, which is another cation (+), leaks in slowly. Calcium movement is termed "slow channel response" because of the difference in speed of movement from that of the sodium channels. At the same time calcium is coming in, potassium (+), another cation, is leaking out. The net change in electrical charge is zero and the cell remains somewhat negative inside, but does not yet return to its resting state.

In phase 3 the slow channels (i.e., calcium movement) shut down but potassium continues to move out of the cell very quickly. As a result, the cell becomes negatively charged.

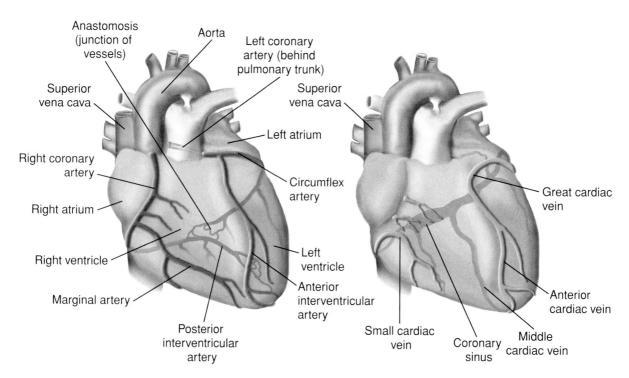

Figure 32-6 The coronary circulation.

However, it does not have the same chemical makeup as it did when everything began at phase 0. There is too much sodium but not enough potassium inside the cell. While the electrical charges are back to normal, the chemical makeup is not. During this phase, another stimulus could trigger the cell to depolarize. However, that depolarization would be out of sync with the rest of the cell's repolarization–depolarization cycle.

Phase 4 begins with the cell actively pulling potassium back into the cell while forcefully expelling sodium. The movement of these two ions is against their concentration gradients. Therefore, the cell must use energy to move these chemicals in order to achieve normalcy again. The process is termed "active transport." In this case, the movement is caused by the sodium–potassium pump powered by adenosine triphosphate (ATP). In phase 4 the cell's chemical and electrical composition is back at its baseline. This state is called the **resting membrane potential**. The charge inside of the cell at this point is approximately −90 mV and is ready to be discharged or depolarized.

When a cell initially changes its charges, it is said to depolarize. The process of returning to its resting state is called repolarization. Phase 0 is the rapid depolarization of the cell. Phases 1 to 4 describe the various stages of repolarization.

A pacemaker cell undergoes the same phases of the action potential (Figure 32-7), but the process differs slightly. The activities of phase 4 vary depending on time. Early in the phase, the sodium potassium pump is actively returning the cell to its predepolarization chemical state. Later in phase 4, a new process begins.

Pacemaker cells allow a slow movement of sodium and calcium into the cell at the same time potassium is leaking out. These ion movements cause the cell to gradually become less negative. At a certain point (or threshold) approximately −60 mV, the cell spontaneously begins phase 0, the rapid depolarization period. The inside charge of the pacemaker cell is not as negative as that of a working cell when phase 0 began. This difference causes phase 0 to occur more slowly in the pacemaker cell. It also changes the timing of phases 1 to 3.

There is variation in how quickly a pacemaker cell allows the leakage of sodium and calcium in and potassium out at phase 4. The faster the leak, the sooner the cell begins phase 0 (spontaneous depolarization). This translates into more depolarizations per minute or a faster rate. Leakage at phase 4

occurs fastest in cells of the SA node and slowest in cells of the Purkinje fibers. The SA pacemaker cells generally depolarize more times per minute and thus have a faster pacing rate, called the **intrinsic rate**. For SA cells, the intrinsic rate is 60 to 100 times per minute.

The AV node cells would spontaneously depolarize at 40 to 60 times per minute except that the SA node is faster (a concept called **dominance**). Impulses are being conducted to the AV node and cause depolarizations. The AV node is said to be **refractory**, or unable to respond to a new stimulus. It is not chemically or electrically ready to depolarize again and thus cannot spontaneously depolarize at its own intrinsic rate.

If the SA node were to stop sending impulses to the AV node, the AV node would be electrically and chemically ready to begin its own spontaneous depolarizations. Thus, the heart would still receive regular impulses from a pacemaker cell but at a slower rate. This mechanism is called an **escape mechanism**.

These impulses of the slower pacemaker site (so-called escape impulses) then become the heart's dominant pacemaker. The escape mechanism is the backup plan of the heart. If a faster pacemaker site fails, there is another slower one ready to take its place; a concept expanded on shortly.

Properties of Cardiac Cells

All muscle cells have the qualities of excitability and contractibility. Cardiac muscle cells possess additional properties that specifically govern the heart's activity. The first of these special qualities is **automaticity**. This is the cell's ability to generate its own action potential. Cardiac cells do not need an outside stimulus to depolarize. Enhanced automaticity is normally a property of the pacemaker cardiac cells which generate the stimulus in a predictable and reliable way.

The next special property of cardiac muscle is conductivity. **Conductivity** is the transmission of the electrical stimulus from cell to cell. The myocardium's ability to do this is owed to special intercellular junctions. The rate at which the stimulus is conducted varies from atrial cells to ventricular cells. This rate can be further modified by damage to cells, age changes, and drugs.

As is true with other muscles, the myocardium has the ability to respond to a stimulus, a property called **excitability**. Healthy cardiac cells respond to the stimulus generated from the pacemaker cells. When cells have been damaged by a lack of oxygen, they may respond to a much lower stimulus, causing **enhanced excitability**. In some cases, the hypoxic injured myocardial cell, for example, may even compete with the pacemaker cells by generating spontaneous impulses via **abnormal automaticity**.[3–6] The resultant aberrant beats are called **ectopic beats** (*ectopic* is Greek for "out of place").

The final special property is the cardiac cells's ability to contract. **Contractility** is the cardiac muscle fibers' ability to shorten or contract. This is the mechanical response to the electrochemical properties of automaticity, excitability,

Action Potential of Myocardial Working Cell

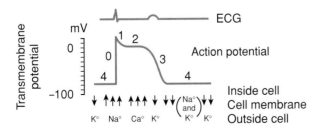

Figure 32-7 Cardiac cell action potentials.

and conductivity. In order to have a heart beat as opposed to electrical activity, the cardiac cells must be able to contract. Without the contraction, a state of electromechanical dissociation occurs.

Electrocardiographic Principles

Assessment of the heart's electrical activity forms a basis for cardiac physical assessment. The tools to assess the electrical activity have been developed over the past 200 years. However, it is only within the last 50 years that portable equipment has been developed allowing for the out-of-hospital monitoring of cardiac electrical activity.

Electrical current in a resting heart was first measured in 1843, DuBois-Raymond then coined the term "action potential" based on these measurements. Electrical changes associated with a beating heart were first recorded in 1887. Willem Einthoven developed methods of standardizing and calibrating recordings of the electrical activity in 1911 and built the first functional ECG machine. Willem Einthoven was awarded the Nobel Prize in medicine in 1924 for his contributions.[7]

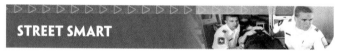

STREET SMART

Willem Einthoven's invention was originally called the "elektrokardiogramm" or EKG. The anglicized version of the same term is electrocardiogram or ECG. However, the two terms are often used interchangeably.

By understanding the concept of syncytium and with knowledge of anatomy, the Paramedic knows that electricity propagates (flows) down the heart in an activation wavefront. It moves from inside to outside (endocardium to epicardium) and from base to apex to base. The resulting voltage changes within the heart are transmitted to the skin. Einthoven's ECG machine is used to detect the voltage changes that occur between two points on the skin's surface. These changes are created by the propagating activation front of the heart's depolarization.

The ECG machine, or monitor, records the ECG on a type of graph paper to plot the amount of change or amplitude on the vertical axis of the graph and time on the horizontal axis. These recordings are explained more fully in Chapter 33. Observation and research has shown the norms for the amplitude/time of the surface ECG.

A Paramedic with knowledge of the standard ECG tracings can perform a comparative analysis with abnormal ECG tracings and relate those findings to the patient's clinical condition. It is important to remember that while the ECG

can indicate a number of abnormal cardiac and extra-cardiac conditions, it may also be normal while the patient is in jeopardy. The first rule of patient care is: *Treat the patient, not the monitor.*

Leads

The ECG machine creates leads. A lead is a view of the heart's electrical activity from a specific vantage point. The lead relies on an electrical difference between two electrodes to create a view of the passage of electricity down the heart's conduction system *over a period of time*; understanding this last statement is critical for an understanding of electrocardiology.

A lead is made up of two electrodes—one electrode is negative and the other is positive. Electricity travels from a negative electrode toward a positive electrode. As a result of having two electrical polarities—positive and negative—with a distance between the two poles, a dipole is established. Because it takes some time, even though it is a fraction of a second, for the electricity to flow between one pole to the other, Paramedics are able to determine its direction (vector). Any electrical activity which flows toward the positive electrode will be seen as upright or positive deflection on the ECG monitor screen or recording paper. Any activity traveling away from the positive electrode will be seen as downward or negative deflection (Figure 32-8).

Standard Leads

Einthoven developed recordings of the heart's electrical activity, using both arms and the left leg as electrode placement

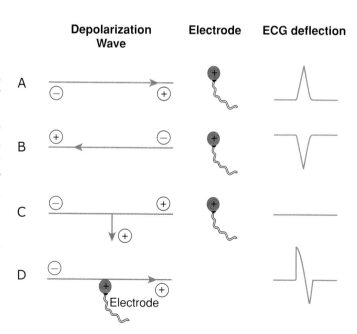

Figure 32-8 A positive deflection is recorded when current is moving toward the unipolar lead and negative when current is moving away from the unipolar lead.

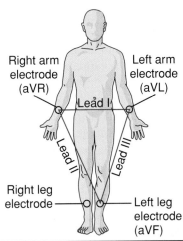

Lead	Right arm	Right leg	Left leg	Left arm
I	−			+
II	−		+	
III			+	−
aVR	+	−	−	−
aVL	−	−	−	+
aVF	−	−	+	−

Figure 32-9 Einthoven's Triangle derived from the standard limb ECG leads.

points (Figure 32-9). Using a human silhouette as background, draw a triangle extending from the left arm at the wrist, right arm at the wrist, and left leg at the ankle. This is Einthoven's Triangle. Einthoven's Triangle visually describes the relationship of any two electrode points to any other two electrode points in the triangle. While not quite an equilateral triangle, anatomically the two leads are in an equilateral triangular arrangement electrically. Einthoven called these **standard leads** and identified them with the Roman numbers of I, II, and III.

Lead I measures the voltage change between the right arm and the left arm. The negative electrode is on the right arm. The positive electrode is on the left arm. The axis of Lead I is across the chest wall and somewhat corresponds to that of the conduction which occurs leftward and downward. Under normal conditions, the electrical movement is toward the positive electrode. Deflections from baseline in Lead I are generally upright or positive but small.

Lead II notes the change between the right arm and left leg. The positive electrode is located on the left leg. This arrangement mimics the conduction system alignment of left and downward. This arrangement is almost in-line with the heart's natural conductive pathway. As a result, the deflections from baseline in Lead II are upright and much larger than in Lead I.

Lead III measures change between the left arm and left leg. The positive electrode is on the left leg. The axis is also similar to that of Lead II and the heart's natural conduction

pathway. Deflections from baseline are upright—larger than in Lead I but not as large as those in Lead II.

Under normal conditions, the largest and clearest picture of the electrical signal is seen in Lead II. For this reason, Lead II is the single best lead to monitor the conduction pathway of the heart for errors.

Waves

In order for Paramedics to interpret, describe, and discuss the tracings that occur on the ECG machine due to the heart's electrical activity, a common language is needed. If the Paramedic understands that during diastole the heart's resting membrane potential is negative (approximately (−) 90 mV) and accepts that as a baseline, and at the moment of depolarization the transmembrane potential becomes positive behind the wavefront, then the Paramedic is able to trace the path of the electricity cascading over the heart. Einthoven described these deflections away from the even baseline, or flatline, and termed them "waves." If the depolarization front is moving toward the positive electrode, then its wave will be upright or positive. If it is moving away from the positive electrode, then its wave will be downward or negative. Einthoven documented the expected changes in voltage and assigned the waves letter titles beginning with P-Q-R-S-T-U (Table 32-1). In a healthy heart, these waves are directed toward or away from the positive electrode in a predictable manner as they pass along the heart's conductive pathway.

To establish a baseline, the ECG tracing starts when the heart is at rest (diastole) and the transmembrane potential is negative. The flat line seen during this period, called the isoelectric line, indicates that the line is not a voltage change occurring.

When the SA node spontaneously depolarizes, it propagates a wavefront across the atria that takes approximately 0.08 to 0.1 seconds. This is represented on the surface ECG in Lead II as a rounded positive deflection in the normal heart. The wavefront now enters the AV node where it is slowed. The period of time when the wavefront is retarded, in the electrical sense, in the AV node is seen as a brief isoelectric line on the ECG.

Exiting the AV node, the depolarization wave continues to propagate across the entire ventricular mass in a predictable fashion, The first area to be depolarized, from right to left, is the septal wall. This momentary swing in the vector of the electrical flow away from the positive electrode in Lead II causes a small negative deflection in the ECG called a Q wave. Not every depolarization of septal wall results in a Q wave in every lead; sometimes the energy is too small to be recorded.

Having transversed the septum, and the bundle of His within, to the apex of the heart, the activation front begins to depolarize the myocardium in the apex of the heart toward the base of the heart and from the inner endocardium to the outer epicardium. This causes a contraction of the left ventricular myocardial whorl and starts the ejection of blood from the

Table 32-1 Waves on ECG with a Sinus Rhythm in Lead II 0

Name	Description
Isoelectric line	Straight line
	Represents diastole
	No voltage difference noted
	Neither (1) nor (−) deflections
P wave	First deflection from isoelectric line
	Represents atrial depolarization
	Occurs just prior to atrial contraction
	Positive upright and rounded
pT wave	Normally obscured by the QRS
	Represents atrial repolarization
	If seen, positive and upright
Q wave	First deflection of the QRS complex
	Represents septal depolarization
	Downward or negative deflection
	Less than one third of the total QRS height
	May not occur in healthy heart
R wave	Initial or second wave of the QRS complex
	Represents depolarization of bundle of His
	Upright or positive deflection
	Is the initial wave if there is no Q wave
S wave	Final wave of QRS complex
	Represents depolarization of the bundle branches
	Negative or downward deflection
T wave	Deflection from baseline ventricular
	Represents repolarization of the ventricle
	Positive or upright in deflection
U wave	Small deflection following after the T wave
	Represents after-polarizations
	Positive or upright in deflection
	Not typically seen

ventricles. The vector of this electrical wavefront down the bundle branches is parallel to the positive lead in Lead II and results in a large positive deflection on the ECG called the R wave.

Following from the bundle branches along the Purkinje fibers, the wavefront continues to propagate to its terminus in the remaining ventricular myocardium upwards toward the base of the heart. This abrupt change in the vector of the wavefront away from the positive lead in Lead II creates a negative deflection that is represented by the S wave.

Following the depolarization of the ventricular myocardium, the heart immediately begins the process of repolarization. Interestingly, while it would seem the repolarization would occur in a retrograde fashion, and thus be represented

by a mirror image of the QRS, it does not occur in this manner. The epicardium repolarizes more rapidly than the inner bundles of the endocardium, resulting in a near simultaneous repolarization. This is represented on the ECG as a T wave.

For the sake of completeness, it is necessary to discuss the repolarization of the atria as well. Like the ventricles, the atria's repolarization is represented by a small positive rounded wave called the tP wave. Under normal circumstances, the tP wave is obscured on the ECG by the QRS. However, the tP may be visible during periods of ventricular standstill. Practically, differentiating the P wave from the tP wave under those conditions is difficult. However, it is assumed that the first wave after the longer period of diastole is the P wave and therefore the wave immediately following the P wave is the tP wave.

On rare occasion there may be another small positive rounded wave that occurs immediately after the T wave and before the next cardiac cycle. Originally thought to be caused by a late repolarization of the Purkinje fibers, it is now thought to be "after-depolarizations." After-depolarizations are late depolarizations in the myocardium that occur as a result of altered chemistry (e.g., secondary to drugs) at the cellular level that changes the myocardial cell's automaticity. These errors in automaticity can lead to abnormal or ectopic beats as a result of stimulating the rest of the myocardium during phase 3 or phase 4 of repolarization. These premature depolarizations of the rest of the myocardium can lead to triggered activity such as atrial or ventricular tachycardia.

ECG waves combine in predictable ways to describe other cardiac events and are the basis for ECG interpretation, discussed in further detail in Chapter 33.

QRS complexes are a combination of two or more waves. When a wave repeats itself (e.g., there are two upward deflections in the QRS, due to errors of condution), then the first wave is considered the **prime wave** and is represented by a capital letter and the second wave is represented by a lowercase letter. For example, a proper notation of a QRS might read RSr.

Intervals and Spaces

In some instances, the activity between the waves (i.e., the timing) is more representative of cardiac pathology than the waves themselves. The space between waves is called a **segment** and a segment and a wave together are called an **interval**. Intervals and segments represent electrophysiological events as well as mechanical events within the heart.

The first interval on the standard ECG is the PR interval. The PR interval represents the retardation of the propagation of the depolarization in the atrioventricular node. Normally this interval is a fraction of a second, between 0.12 and 0.20 seconds, and is measured from the beginning of the P wave to the first deflection in the QRS. During this fraction of a second, atrial kick occurs and maximal ventricular filling occurs.

If the PR interval is shortened, it may be indicative of an accessory pathway and may lead to pre-excitation syndrome. Alternatively, a prolonged PR interval (greater than 0.20 seconds) may represent the initial electrophysiologic change of an ischemic AV node that can progress to heart block. However, some prolonged PR intervals are a function of the natural changes of aging or a drug effect. In every case, the patient's medical condition must be taken into account when there is a finding of an abnormal PR interval.

The other interval in the ECG is the QT interval. Whereas the PR interval is indicative of the atrial depolarization and repolarization, the QT interval is indicative of the ventricular depolarization–repolarization cycle. The QT interval can also be thought of as indicative of systole. The QT interval is measured from the first deflection of the QRS to the end of the T wave and is normally about 0.40 seconds. However, QT intervals vary according to the heart's rate. The faster a heart races, the shorter the QT interval becomes. To ascertain if a QT interval is abnormal, the heart rate must be taken into account. Using Bazett's formula, the measurement is corrected to account for the increased automaticity. The result is referred to as the QT corrected or QTc. Any QT interval greater than 0.44 seconds is considered abnormal and labeled a "prolonged QT interval."

Medications, such as Vaughn-Williams Class I drugs, can cause a prolonged QT interval as well as a congenital condition called prolonged QT syndrome (LQTS). Patients with LQTS are prone to ventricular tachycardias—particularly one dysrhythmia called polymorphic ventricular tachycardia or torsades de pointes.[8-10] Conversely, some patients may be born with short QT syndrome. Short QT syndrome (less than 0.32 seconds) is the cause of syncope and sudden cardiac death as well.

Perhaps the most important segment or interval is the ST segment. The ST segment, that period from the end of the QRS to the beginning of the T wave, represents an isoelectric period in the normal heart; a time when the heart is neither depolarizing or repolarizing In the ischemic heart, where there is altered electrophysiology, late depolarization may cause either a depression or an elevation in the ST segment. In some cases, the ST segment elevation may represent myocardial infarction in progress, known as an ST elevation myocardial infarction (STEMI); more discussions of this very important ECG finding are contained in the following chapters.

The ST segment starts at the J point, the point immediately following the QRS where the ECG returns to baseline and continues to the T wave. The typical ST segment is approximately the same length as the QRS (0.08 to 0.12 seconds) and corresponds with the plateau phase of the action potential. Therefore, any alteration of the action potential (e.g., ischemia or drugs such as digitalis) can result in changes in the ST segment.

The last segment, the TP segment, represents the time when phase 4 of the action potential has occurred and the heart has achieved its resting membrane potential. Normally this results in no electrical movement and is represented by an isoelectric line (Table 32-2 and Figure 32-10).

Table 32-2 Intervals and Segments

Name	Description	Significance
PR interval	P wave plus PR segment	Period of time for stimulus to travel across the atria and delay at AV node
ST segment	Point from J wave to T wave	Beginning of ventricular repolarization
QT interval	Beginning of QRS complex to end of T wave	Represents ventricular depolarization and repolarization
TP segment	Point from end of T wave to start of next depolarization	Represents the isoelectric line

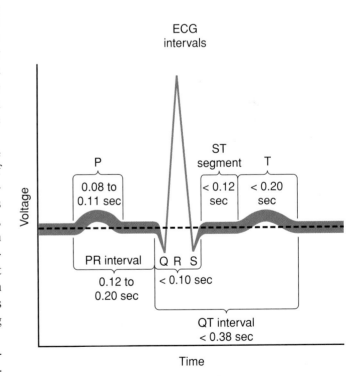

Figure 32-10 ECG complex intervals.

CONCLUSION

The measurement of the heart's electrical activity is a key objective assessment tool for the Paramedic. This chapter has provided a basis for the heart's electrophysiology and lays the foundation for the following two chapters that discuss monitoring of the cardiac rhythm and 12-lead ECG.

▶ KEY POINTS:

- The heart lies within the thoracic cavity. The base of the heart is located at the 2nd intercostal space and the apex is located at approximately the 5th intercostal space on the left midclavicular line. The heart is composed of three layers. First is the two-part pericardium which envelops the heart and roots of the great vessels plus continues on as the epicardium, or outermost layer of the heart. The next layer, closer to the center of the organ, is the myocardium. This is the muscular layer. The innermost layer is the endocardium, which lines the chambers of the heart. Valves serve to direct blood in one direction through the heart.

- An entire sequence of events from atrial filling and ejection through ventricular filling and ejection is called the cardiac cycle. The cycle consists of atrial diastole and systole plus ventricular diastole and systole.

- The heart is served by a special set of arteries and veins called the coronary circulation. The major coronary arteries are the right coronary artery (RCA) and the left coronary artery (LCA, also called the left main) which divides into the left anterior descending artery (LAD) and the left circumflex artery (LCx).

- In 55% of the population, the RCA provides blood to the sinus node. In 90% of the population, it provides blood to the atrioventricular junction. The LAD provides blood to the SA node in the remaining 45% of the population, to the AV junction in the remaining 10% of the population, and to the remainder of the conduction system in nearly 100% of people.

- The initial portion of the conduction system is the sinoatrial node (SA). The SA node has fibers which connect it to the heart's atrial cells. A special pathway exists to communicate with the left atrium. This path is called Bachmann's Bundle. The impulse is also conducted toward the ventricles via the internodal pathways to the atrioventricular node (AV). When the impulse reaches the ventricular side of the AV node, it is conducted through a wide, thick group of fibers called the bundle of His, which divides into the right and left bundle branches. The left bundle branch will further divide into an anterior branch and a posterior branch to adequately serve the larger, thicker left ventricle. At the level of the ventricular cells, the impulse is carried by the Purkinje fibers.

- The heart's rate and rhythm are initiated and controlled by an electrochemical process. Altering the ion content inside of a pacemaking cell triggers an electrical stimulus. The SA node completes this process more quickly than any part of a healthy conduction system and is therefore considered the heart's pacemaker. The number of times per minute that the SA node completes this process is termed its intrinsic rate. Should the SA node fail, the AV node has a slower intrinsic rate and will act as the backup plan or escape pacemaker. Should the AV node fail, the bundle of His or Purkinje fibers can function as an escape pacemaker, although at a much slower rate.

- The action potential has five phases numbered 0 to 4.
  - In phase 0, a resting cardiac cell is normally negatively charged on its inside. A rapid influx of sodium occurs, causing the inside to become positive.

- Phase 1 begins when the fast sodium channels close. Chloride, an anion (−), moves into the cell. With its negative charge, the cell again becomes negative.
- Phase 2 is a plateau phase. Calcium (another cation) leaks in slowly. At the same time calcium is coming in, potassium (another cation) is leaking out. The net change in electrical charge is zero and the cell remains somewhat negative inside, but does not yet return to its resting state.
- Phase 3 has the slow channels or calcium movement shut down, although potassium moves out of the cell very quickly. The cell becomes very negative but does not have the same chemical makeup as it did when everything began at phase 0.
- Phase 4 begins with the cell actively pulling potassium back into the cell while forcefully expelling sodium.

- Cardiac muscle fibers have a specialized cell membrane that reduces electrical resistance and allows an electrical stimulus to move rapidly from cell to cell. The cells also form an extensive network that further enhances the rapid movement of the electrical stimulus. This allows the whole structure to act as a unit. The atria will contract as a unit from superior to inferior. The ventricles will function as a unit, pushing and squeezing blood from inferior to superior.

- The electrical impulse cannot normally enter the ventricles except by passing through the AV node. The cells of the AV node are designed to conduct the impulse slowly, which allows the ventricles to receive the "atrial kick" that occurs when the atria contract.

- The functional properties of cardiac muscle tissue are automaticity, excitability, conductivity, and contractility.

- Using electrodes, the ECG records the voltage changes that occur between two points and are transmitted to the skin.

- Electricity travels from a negative point toward a positive one. The positive electrode is the viewing electrode. Any electrical activity that points toward the positive electrode will be seen as upright or positive on the screen or paper. Any activity traveling away from the positive electrode will be seen as downward or negative.

- The waves evident on the ECG correspond to electrical events in the body.

REVIEW QUESTIONS:

1. If a papillary muscle in the right ventricle was damaged and did not function, what could happen to forward blood flow?
2. Name two ways in which a very rapid heart rate may interfere with coronary blood flow.
3. Describe what may occur if a person had an accessory pathway around the AV node.
4. When heart cells die, they are replaced by scar tissue. The scar tissue does not possess the properties of automaticity, conductivity, excitability, or contractility. Using each of these properties, describe how the heart's normal processes can be disrupted.
5. Would it be possible for the properties of automaticity, excitability, and conductivity to function but not the property of contractility? Why or why not? What assessment would give you the answer?
6. If you could design a substance that would slow the movement of calcium into the cell at phase 2 of the cardiac action potential, what would happen to the heart rate?

CASE STUDY QUESTIONS:

Please refer to the Case Study at the beginning of the chapter and answer the questions below:

1. Why did the Paramedics check the patient before analyzing the monitoring strip?

2. What is happening at the cellular level when each of the following waves, intervals, segments, or complexes is occurring?
   a. P wave
   b. PR interval
   c. QRS complex
   d. ST segment
   e. T wave

3. Where is the electrical stimulus when each of the following waves, intervals, segments, or complexes is occurring?
   a. P wave
   b. PR interval
   c. QRS complex
   d. ST segment
   e. T wave

4. What is happening mechanically during
   a. the P wave?
   b. the QRS complex?
   c. the T wave?

REFERENCES:

1. Wayne- Alexander R, Fuster V, King SB, Nash I, O'Rourke RA, Prystowsky EN, Roberts R. *Hurst's the Heart*, Vol. 2 (11th ed.). New York: McGraw-Hill Professional; 2005.

2. Brunekreeft JA, Graauw M, de Milliano PA, Keijer JT. Influence of left bundle branch block on left ventricular volumes, ejection fraction and regional wall motion. *Neth Heart J.* 2007;15(3):89–94.

3. Sarre A, Maury P, Kucera P, Kappenberger L, Raddatz E. Arrhythmogenesis in the developing heart during anoxia-reoxygenation and hypothermia-rewarming: an in vitro model. *J Cardiovasc Electrophysiol.* 2006;17(12):1350–1359.

4. Kutala VK, Khan M, Angelos MG, Kuppusamy P. Role of oxygen in postischemic myocardial injury. *Antioxid Redox Signal.* 2007;9(8):1193–1206.

5. Hoffman JW, Jr., Gilbert TB, Poston RS, Silldorff EP. Myocardial reperfusion injury: etiology, mechanisms, and therapies. *J Extra Corpor Technol.* 2004;36(4):391–411.

6. Kaminski KA, Bonda TA, Korecki J, Musial WJ. Oxidative stress and neutrophil activation—the two keystones of ischemia/reperfusion injury. *Int J Cardiol.* 2002;86(1):41–59.

7. Cajavilca C, Varon J. Willem Einthoven: the development of the human electrocardiogram. *Resuscitation.* 2007;76(3):325–328.

8. Roden DM. Clinical practice. Long-QT syndrome. *N Engl J Med.* 2008;358(2):169–176.

9. Janeira LF. Torsades de pointes and long QT syndromes. *Am Fam Physician.* 1995;52(5):1447–1453.

10. Kannankeril PJ, Roden DM. Drug-induced long QT and torsade de pointes: recent advances. *Curr Opin Cardiol.* 2007;22(1): 39–43.

CHAPTER 33

THE MONITORING ECG

KEY CONCEPTS:

Upon completion of this chapter, it is expected that the reader will understand these following concepts:

- Use of ECG as a tool
- Correct application of electrodes
- Troubleshooting the equipment
- Interpretation of rhythms

▶ CASE STUDY:

Jane Sheehan had called EMS because she felt faint and her heart seemed to be beating too fast. The first response unit had started her on oxygen, obtained vital signs, and was asking questions about the event when the Paramedic unit arrived. The Paramedic received report while placing Ms. Sheehan on a cardiac monitor. The Paramedic quickly interpreted the rhythm, verified that Ms. Sheehan did not have any drug allergies, and then outlined a plan of care for her.

The EMTs wondered aloud what the lines on the monitor meant and what part they played in determining a diagnosis and treatment.

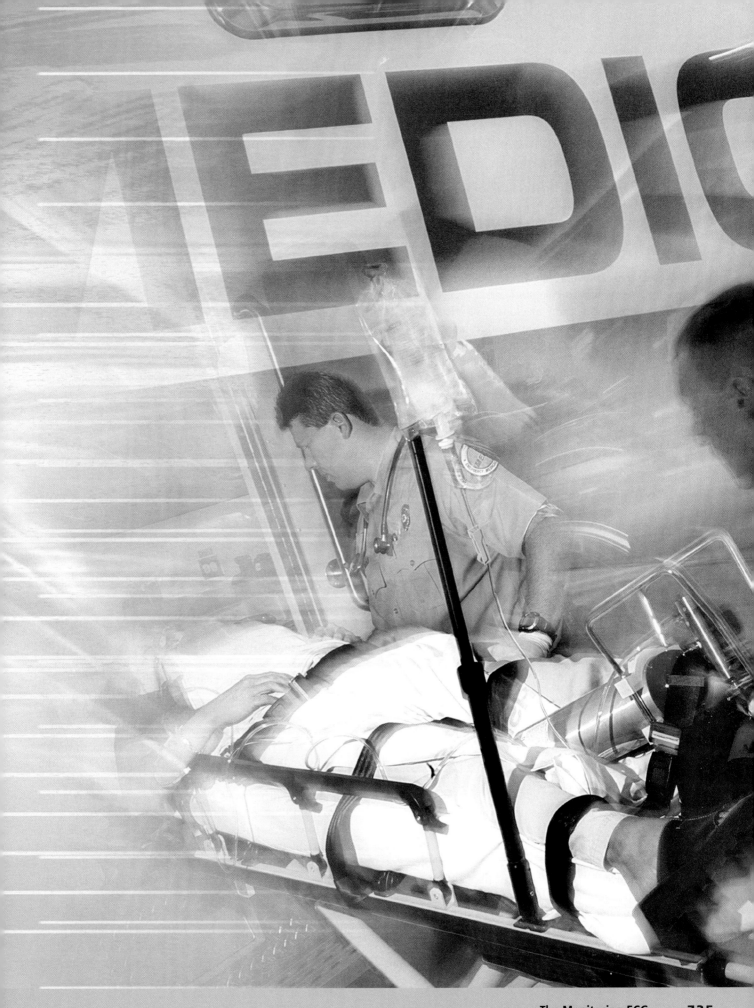

OVERVIEW:

Paramedics use an electrocardiogram each day to monitor the cardiac rhythm in a significant proportion of their patients. Most cardiac monitors today have developed into comprehensive monitoring tools that measure other parameters including blood pressure, pulse oximetry, and capnography. In this chapter, we will examine the use of the basic cardiac monitor to observe the patient's cardiac rhythm.

The Monitoring ECG

In the eyes of the public and many healthcare providers, the distinction between basic life support and advanced life support is the electrocardiogram machine. The electrocardiogram (ECG) provides Paramedics with information about the electrical activity of the patient's heart (i.e., the depolarization and repolarization of the heart through the cardiac cycle of systole and diastole). Armed with this additional data, the Paramedic can make better clinical decisions regarding treatment and transport.

By interpreting the ECG's rhythm for disorder, the Paramedic can come to suspect electrolyte disturbances that can cause errors of automaticity (conduction abnormalities) or errors of conduction, as well as signs of is-chemic heart disease. Any of these can indicate a potential life-threatening emergency. Furthermore, changes in a rhythm strip may be indicative of other medical conditions such as head injury, toxic exposure, electrolyte imbalance or other more fundamental disorders such as hypoxia and hypothermia.[1]

Continuous monitoring of the patient's heart rhythm allows the Paramedic to note changes in the patient's condition, as well as the patient's response to treatments, and thus continue or alter treatment plans accordingly. The goal of prehospital ECG monitoring is to obtain a clear and accurate view of the heart's electrical activity quickly and dependably.

When using an ECG, the Paramedic's first priority should be to monitor the heart for the presence of any life-threatening dysrhythmia. The utilization of a diagnostic 12-lead ECG always comes after the patient's initial rhythm has been confirmed.

Portable ECG Equipment

Portable ECG equipment consists of an **oscilloscope** and a printer needed to review and record ECG. The original oscilloscopes on an ECG machine operated similar to the first television sets. A beam of electrons struck a phosphorescent screen and produced a point of light. Slight differences in voltages cause movement of the beam, which is displayed on the screen as fluctuations in the point of light. The point of light could be seen to move either as an upward spike (a positive deflection) or in a downward deflection (a negative spike). The ECG oscilloscope is also called a **cardiac**

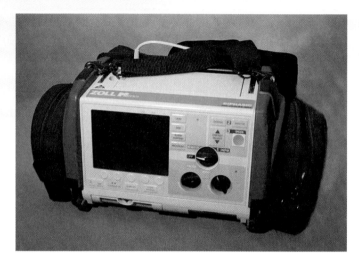

Figure 33-1 A Paramedic's cardiac monitor–defibrillator.

monitor (Figure 33-1). The monitor is analogous to a computer's visual display of the machine's output.

ECG Tracing

Like the original silver string galvanometer used in the first experiments by Willem Einthoven, the modern ECG machine senses the current changes, or fluctuations, between two electrodes—one negative and one positive—as a wave of depolarization cascades down the heart and displays that information on a screen.[2,3] A downward deflection indicates that the electricity is flowing away from a positive, or monitoring, electrode. An upward deflection indicates that the depolarization wave is flowing toward a positive monitoring electrode. If the differences in the flow of electricity resulted in a zero net difference in direction (i.e., electricity was flowing both toward and away from the positive electrode (perpendicular) at the same time), then the resulting signal is **equiphasic** or flatline.

Using this technology, the movement of electricity within the body could be observed, by the bounce of a point of light, at any given moment. However, the flow of electricity within the heart as it travels down a conductive pathway takes time. Therefore, the dimension of time must be included if the meter is to illustrate the passage of electricity down the conduction pathway. Oscilloscopes can add the dimension of time by moving the point of light across the screen from left to right at a precise rate of speed. Speed is distance over time and is measured in fractions of a second in the heart.

Compared against a static grid placed over the oscilloscope, this horizontal left-to-right movement (manifested on the screen as a **trace**) can be measured and fluctuations expressed in terms of time (seconds or milliseconds). Any vertical fluctuations seen on the monitor can also be measured. Vertical fluctuations represent the voltage change from zero, either positive or negative. The change from zero can also be measured on a grid and is expressed in terms of millivolts (mV). The larger the voltage difference, the larger the fluctuation.

Current ECG monitors not only measure the energy and the speed of conduction, but they also have many other features that are valuable to the Paramedic.

Monitor Features

The standard ECG monitor typically features a sensitivity and sweep speed control, output printer, lead selector, rate counter, monitor brightness control, and alarms. Many ECG monitors also have telemetry capabilities. Telemetry is the ability to broadcast the ECG via telephone or radio to a distant receiver, typically located at a hospital.[4-6]

To make the ECG readable, the ECG monitor must have both a sweep speed control and a sensitivity control. The sweep speed control regulates the speed of the tracing on the monitor, and subsequently on the printout. The sensitivity control alters the size of the ECG tracing. Adjusting these functions on the ECG monitor provides the Paramedic with some advantages in certain clinical situations.

To facilitate analysis, and documentation, a printer was added to print out the ECG seen on the screen. The printer provides a printed hard copy of the ECG tracing visible on the ECG monitor. In many cases manufacturers have built in a 5- to 10-second delay between what is visible on the ECG monitor and what is being printed out. This momentary delay permits the Paramedic time to activate the printer if an irregularity in rhythm is seen on the ECG monitor and thus capture the dysrythmia.

In some instances one view, or lead, is better than another when trying to make an ECG interpretation. Lead selection (changing the electrical view of the heart without moving electrodes) permits the Paramedic an opportunity to observe the heart from several angles at an instant. Optional leads and lead selection are discussed shortly.

An added feature of many ECG monitors is the rate counter. The **rate counter** is a digital readout of the number of ECG complexes that pass in a minute, usually counting the tallest, or deepest, wave on the ECG. Some ECG monitors also have a flashing light, or other visible signal, that indicates when an ECG complex has passed across a point on the monitor. Some rate counters have an audible signal which indicates the passage of an ECG complex across the monitor. The volume of these counters can be adjusted, or shut off, to reduce noise pollution on scene.

The purpose of an ECG monitor is to alert the Paramedic to potentially life-threatening dysrhythmias. To that end, some ECG monitors have **alarms** that will indicate, via visible and/or audible signal, that a patient's heart rate is above or below a certain rate. The Paramedic often has the option of choosing the rate values (called the alarm limits) according to the patient circumstances. Some EMS agencies do not permit Paramedics to alter alarm limits or to disable alarms. This fail-safe device offers another level of security to permit early detection of potentially life-threatening dysrhythmias.

Finally, an additional feature on some ECG monitors is an ability to adjust the brilliance of the ECG monitor. Depending on ambient light conditions, it may be desirable to turn up the brilliance of the ECG monitor or to dampen it in order to improve the quality of the ECG.

Monitor Adjustments

Many monitors permit the Paramedic to adjust certain variables in order to improve the ECG tracing's usefulness. For example, most monitors available to the Paramedic allow a change in speed and amplitude of a tracing. The Paramedic may want to change the speed of the rhythm passing by on the screen. An alteration in the speed of the tracing is an alteration in **sweep speed**. Standard sweep speed is 25 mm/second. Increasing the sweep speed to 50 mm/second will stretch out the trace and make the trace appear slower than it actually is. However, slowing sweep speed will also allow for closer examination of key features on the ECG, such as changes in the segments or minor deflections in the QRS.

The Paramedic may need to also enlarge the tracing shown on the monitor. This is called increasing the **gain**. The gain increases the size of the tracing shown on the monitor screen. Occasionally key features of the ECG are too small for clear examination without increasing the gain. By adjusting the gain, the Paramedic can get a clearer picture. Conditions which can cause low amplitude include a variety of medical conditions (Table 33-1).

Calibration

The ECG monitor is a medical device. As such, Paramedics should regularly ensure that the ECG monitor is accurate. Any number of medical interventions may be performed, including defibrillation and medication administration, based in large part upon the ECG tracing. A faulty ECG monitor could lead to an error of treatment. For this reason an ECG monitor should regularly serviced by a biomedical engineer who will re-calibrate the ECG monitor to factory specifications.

On a daily basis, and to assess accuracy of the ECG monitor, the Paramedic compares the ECG machine's operation against standard settings (i.e., industry standards). Making

Table 33-1 Conditions That May Cause
a Low-Amplitude ECG

- Amyloidosis—deposits of proteinaceous mass in muscle fibers
- Hypothyroidism (a.k.a. myxedema)
- Restrictive cardiomyopathy
  - Endomyocardial fibrosis
- Pericardial effusions
  - Hemopericardium
  - Infectious transudate
- Pericardial tamponade
- Tension pneumothorax
- Obesity
- Hypothermia

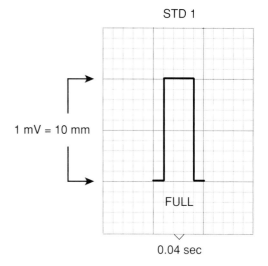

ECG standardization

Figure 33-2 Normal standardized
calibration mark.

sure that sweep speed and gain is up to standard is called **calibration**. Most ECG monitors self-calibrate, internally setting standard sweep speeds and gain, when initially switched on. However, many ECG monitors also provide an internal user test that allows the paramedic to check calibration and operational readiness at the beginning of the shift; many Paramedic services require that the Paramedic document that calibration test

The calibration mark (Figure 33-2), visible at the beginning of the ECG printout, is a square wave that is 10 mm high, or 1 mV, and 10 mm wide. Each box measures 0.1 mV vertically and 0.4 mm horizontally. The calibration mark is created by a calibration impulse, an electric impulse, by the ECG machine. The resulting wave should be sharply delineated (i.e., quick corners that make a squared wave).

ECG Paper

Reading an ECG on the monitor can be difficult at times. Therefore, a hard copy can improve the accuracy of the analysis. For this reason, most Paramedics print out a copy of the ECG, called an **ECG rhythm strip**. The paper used for ECG recordings is imprinted on heat-sensitive paper via heated stylus or is printed by a laser. It is lined in a manner similar to graph paper to enable a Paramedic to accurately measure and compare ECG waves.

In order to determine regularity, rate, timing, and amplitude of the ECG features, the Paramedic must understand the grid structure of ECG paper. The paper is lined vertically and horizontally (Figure 33-3). On the vertical axis, a line occurs every 1 mm and a darker line occurs every 5 mm. For the horizontal axis, a line occurs every 0.04 seconds and a darker line every 0.20 seconds. The amplitude markings are correct assuming there is a standard gain of 10 mm/mV, and the time markings are correct assuming a standard sweep speed of 25 mm/second.

When assessing the rate of a rhythm or the time frame of a feature on the ECG, the Paramedic will use the horizontal markings. The horizontal axis equals time (0.20 seconds per large square). When measuring the amplitude of a feature, the Paramedic will use the vertical axis. The vertical axis equals

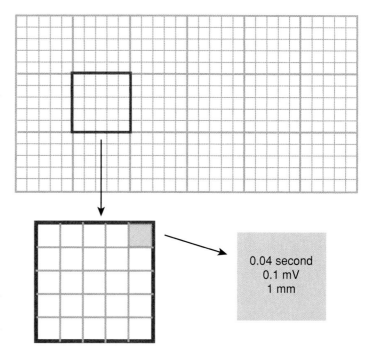

0.04 second
0.1 mV
1 mm

Figure 33-3 The standard ECG graph.

amplitude, which can be roughly equated to the strength of the electrical signal.

Wire Systems

The wiring harness, also called the ECG cable, connects the electrodes to the ECG monitor and is a single thick cable that separates into three, four, or five thinner wires. (Some harnesses will have an additional port that will accept a six-wire plug to enable the acquisition of a 12-lead ECG.)

The machine end of the harness has a pin connector that must be set firmly into its socket in order to avoid a poor connection, which will create an unreadable signal. The thinner wires are connected to electrodes at the distal end. These, in turn, are placed on the patient.

Electrodes

For a surface ECG, the electricity must pass from the heart and up through the skin in order for the ECG to detect the current. The stratum corneum, the outermost layer of the skin, does not conduct electricity well because it contains dead and dried out cells. These dead cells cause the skin to act as a resistor; resistance to the passage of electricity.[7] To permit the passage of the electrical current through the skin to the surface, the electrode must have an intermediate substance, a conductive medium which bridges the stratum corneum and connects the inside of the body with the electrode.

Typically an ECG electrode is used for that purpose. An electrode consists of a gel-like substance that conducts electricity well, such as silver chloride, with an adhesive on a foam or paper backing to help maintain contact (Figure 33-4). The conductive gel is designed to melt with body warmth and soak through the skin. This will enable it to overcome skin resistance to the electrical signal and create an electrical bridge from the inside of the body to the electrode. A sticky piece of foam or paper surrounds the gel. This serves to isolate the electrode from the surrounding environment and enables the electrode to adhere closely to the skin.

Warmth is necessary for the electrode to function. Without warmth the conductive gel does not melt, the electrical pathway is ineffective, and the signal quality will be poor or lost entirely. When the gel only partially melts, due to cold skin or poor adherence of the electrode, then the quality of signal will also be poor (degraded) and the tracing will be unreadable (**noisy**).

There are many reasons why an electrode will not function. If the gel on the electrode has dried, it will no longer serve as an electrical pathway. Electrodes should be inspected regularly to ensure new and moist electrodes.

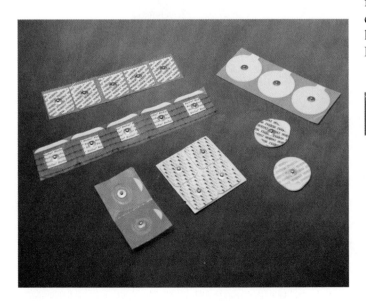

Figure 33-4 Examples of ECG electrodes.

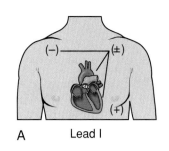

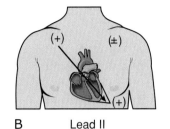
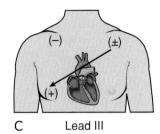

Figure 33-5 Electrode position affects the electrical view of the heart.

Electrode Placement

The primary objective of monitoring the electrical activity of a patient's heart is to discern abnormalities of conduction or automaticity that produce potentially life-threatening dysrhythmias. An ECG **lead** is a view of the heart from one particular vantage point that helps to ascertain the dysrhythmia (Figure 33-5). For example, Lead II (a commonly used monitoring lead) views the inferior portion of the heart and would help identify dysrhythmia arising from the inferior wall. Most dysrhythmias can be ascertained using one or two leads. It is important for the Paramedic to choose the lead that provides the best chance of identifying the dysrhythmia.

For Lead II, one electrode is placed on the right wrist, one electrode on the left wrist, and one electrode on the left foot (to recreate Einthoven's Triangle) (Figure 33-6). In many cases, it is inconvenient to place the electrodes out onto the limbs where the wires may become tangled. Therefore, the Paramedic may choose to place electrodes on the right and

STREET SMART

Many Paramedics use the same electrodes for the monitoring ECG as for a 12-lead ECG. Key to an accurate 12-lead ECG is the re-creation of Einthoven's Triangle. Jowett and associates suggested that placing the limb leads on the torso can lead to inaccurate interpretation of the 12-lead by producing false patterns of ischemia.[9]

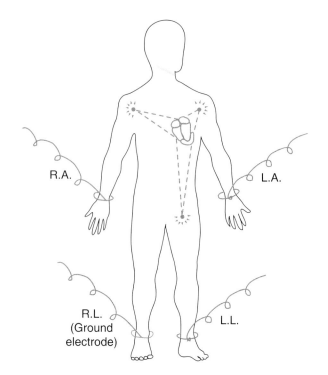

Figure 33-6 Electrode placement for limb leads.

left upper arms at the deltoids. Lower electrodes are then placed on the right and left thighs. The third alternative strategy, suggested by Takuma and associates, is to place the electrodes in the subclavicular space (the deltopectoral fossae) on the right and left and then on the right and left lower rib cage.[8] The important concept is to try to maintain Einthoven's Triangle.

Best results are obtained from placing the electrode over muscle and not over bony prominences. The Paramedic should also avoid placing an electrode over any jewelry, implanted devices such as pacemakers (automated internal defibrillator/cardioverters), or medication patches.

To ensure patient comfort, connect or clip the wires to the electrodes before attaching the electrodes to the skin. Pressing the snap connection to an electrode that is already on the skin is uncomfortable for the patient. Perhaps more importantly, it squeezes the gel out from under the electrode, potentially causing loss of signal.

Standard Lead II Configuration

If the negative lead is on the right shoulder and the positive lead is on the left leg, then the ECG machine is monitoring **Lead II**. Lead II provides a view of the inferior wall of the heart.[10–12] The upper portion of the conduction system resides within the inferior wall, from the SA node to the AV node. This portion of the left ventricle also receives its blood supply from the right coronary artery.

Whenever there is suspicion of an acute occlusion of the right coronary artery, and therefore doubt about performance of the upper portion of the conduction system (a conduction abnormality as manifest by changes in the PR interval), then the patient should be observed in Lead II. Because Lead II provides an excellent view of the inferior wall/upper portion of the conduction system, it produces the clearest P waves.

Modified Chest Lead I

While it may be easier to distinguish P waves in Lead II, the placement of the electrodes may be more difficult in the field. Also, the electrodes in Lead II may interfere with important procedures such as defibrillation. For these and other reasons, many Paramedics choose **modified chest Lead 1 (MCL1)** to monitor patients instead of/in addition to Lead II (Figure 33-7). MCL1 simulates the precordial lead V1, one of the six precordial leads of a 12-lead.

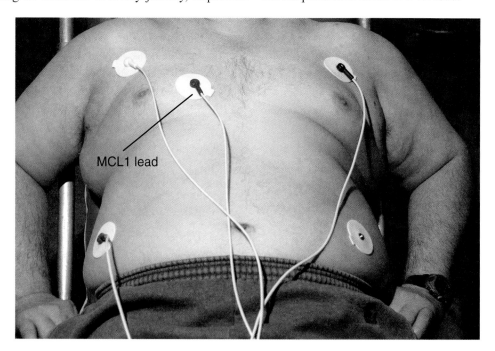

Figure 33-7 Lead placement for MCL1.

By placing the positive monitoring electrode at the right sternal border at the fourth intercostal space, between the fourth and fifth ribs, and looking across the chest from the left shoulder, the Paramedic obtains a view of the anterior wall of the left ventricle.

The MCL1 lead not only permits differentiation of ectopic complexes (ventricular from supraventricular with aberrancy), but MCL1 keeps the defibrillation platform open for defibrillation pads or paddles. MCL1 also helps the Paramedic distinguish between right and left bundle branch blocks. A new onset left bundle branch block as a sign of an acute coronary event will be discussed later.

Perhaps the most pressing reason to use MCL1 as a monitoring lead is that it views the anterior wall. The left coronary artery (LCA), including the left anterior descending coronary artery (LAD), are commonly occluded during an acute coronary event and these arteries provide blood to the anterior wall of the left ventricle. MCL1 provides a vantage point from which to monitor the anterior wall and quickly identify lethal threatening dysrhythmias such as ventricular fibrillation.

Preparation of Skin

Electrodes are designed to adhere to and transmit electrical signals from a warm, dry, flat skin surface. In order to obtain these conditions, the Paramedic must take several steps to prepare the skin before applying the electrode.[13]

First, the skin should be relatively free of hair. The Paramedic can clip some hair to ensure electrode contact. Some Paramedics use single-blade razors to clear unwanted chest hair. However, if the patient receives anticoagulants later, then microlacerations created by the razor may bleed. Some Paramedics prefer to use disposable hair clippers specifically designed for this purpose. However, handheld bandage scissors, the type with the blunted tips, are adequate to trim chest hair.

Next, skin oils must be removed. Skin oils reduce the adhesion of the electrode and hinder penetration of electrode gel. An alcohol-soaked pad applied to the area and then pressed against the skin in an outward-circling motion will remove dirt, oil, and other particulates which could prevent proper adhesion of the electrode. Visible perspiration also can prevent proper adhesion of the electrode. The alcohol pad also helps to evaporate perspiration. The skin in the target area should then be dried with gauze or a towel prior to placement of the electrodes in order to remove debris and remaining alcohol.

If the patient is grossly diaphoretic, it may be helpful to apply tincture of benzoin. Tincture of benzoin is a topical lotion that, when dried, is tacky to touch and helps electrodes adhere to the skin. It is important to not apply tincture of benzoin directly over the electrode site as it does not conduct electricity well. Properly applied, the tincture of benzoin should leave a bull's eye-appearing ring in which the middle is clear of the benzoin.

Finally, the best ECG signal is obtained when the area is gently abraded to remove dead skin cells and to improve circulation (i.e., increase warmth) to the area. The use of fine grit sandpaper (commercially available for this purpose) or even a gauze pad to abrade the skin can markedly improve the quality of the ECG signal.

Systematic Approach to ECG Rhythm Interpretation

A rapid and accurate interpretation of a patient's ECG rhythm is important and potentially life-saving. To attain speed and accuracy, the Paramedic must take a disciplined approach to ECG interpretation. Faithful adherence to a systematic approach analysis of the ECG rhythm strip, a process called **ECG interpretation**, promises the best results in the shortest amount of time.

There are a number of ECG interpretation schemas available. Some take a simple left to right approach to reading an ECG, similar to reading a book. The method originally described by Dr. Henry J. L. Marriott works well in the out-of-hospital environment as it focuses on rapid identification of high-risk patients.[14] Dr. Marriott's systematic approach to ECG interpretation also can be easily integrated with the algorithmic approach to advanced cardiac life support advanced by the American Heart Association. Regardless of the method of ECG interpretation chosen, the Paramedic should master that technique and resolve to use that systematic approach with each ECG tracing.

Descriptive Analysis

Some Paramedics have a tendency to quickly label an ECG rhythm because it looks like another ECG rhythm the Paramedic has seen before. This practice relies on **pattern recognition**. The use of pattern recognition is poor practice. Errors in ECG interpretation can be made when Paramedics fail to note the fine nuances that differentiate one rhythm from another (e.g., the difference between a bradycardia with U waves versus a sinus bradycardia with a heart block).

A **descriptive analysis** provides the building blocks to an ECG interpretation. Using the Marriott method of analysis, the elements of the descriptive analysis would consist of the rhythm, rate, width of the QRS complex, and atrial activity.

Armed with a descriptive analysis, the Paramedic assembles the information and, using an understanding of cardiac anatomy (specifically electrophysiology), generates a rhythm interpretation.

On occasion, an ECG rhythm strip baffles a Paramedic. The practice of using descriptive analysis allows the Paramedic to accurately describe the ECG rhythm strip to a physician or another colleague who, in turn, may be able to interpret the rhythm even without benefit of seeing the rhythm strip.

Emergency Decision Making

Some medical emergencies are time-sensitive. Unfortunately, there may not be time to come to a comprehensive interpretation about an ECG rhythm before definitive action must be taken. This fact is best evidenced by the advanced cardiac life support algorithms. Many of these algorithms intend that the Paramedic establish a gross analysis of the ECG rhythm strip (e.g., "wide complex tachycardia") in order to use the algorithm. This permits quick action to resolve the dysrhythmia. A descriptive analysis, as suggested by the Marriott method, lends itself to this type of swift decision making.

Determining the Isoelectric Line

The first step in an ECG interpretation is to determine the isoelectric line. The **isoelectric line** indicates that period of time when the myocardium, particularly the ventricular mass, has been repolarized and awaits depolarization. The isoelectric line extends from the end of the T wave to the start of the ventricular depolarization represented by the QRS complex. An isoelectric line on the monitor and on the rhythm strip should appear as a flat line between ECG complexes.

Artifact

In some cases, it may be difficult to distinguish the isoelectric line because of artifact. **Artifact**, a disturbance in the isoelectric line, is the result of outside interference with the signal. Some artifact may resemble ventricular fibrillation, possibly causing inexperienced EMS providers to react inappropriately. More commonly, artifact makes rhythm interpretation difficult (if not impossible). Therefore, it is important to find the source of the artifact and try to resolve it.

Artifact can result from many causes including patient movement, problems with the cable, electromagnetic interference, or vehicle motion. A systematic problem-solving approach, starting at the patient and moving to the machine, often uncovers the cause of the artifact.

Patient-Induced Artifact

There are many easily understood reasons why the patient may be the source of the artifact. For example, if a patient experiences a seizure while on the cardiac monitor the ECG strip will show artifact. In some cases, one of the first warnings that a Paramedic has that the patient is seizing is the sudden appearance of artifact on the monitor and the accompanying rate alarms. Seizures can occur for many reasons (e.g., hypoxia, hypoglycemia, and the sudden hypotension that results from ventricular fibrillation).

Cardiac compressions performed during resuscitation can also create artifact, as can placing an electrode directly over the top of an internal electronic pacemaker. One of the most common reasons for patient-related artifact is poor preparation of the patient's skin prior to printing the ECG rhythm strip. Loose electrodes—undermined by sweat, dirt, or hair—or dried electrode conductive gel can interfere with the signal and cause artifact.

Patient movement can also cause artifact (Figure 33-8). The patient should be made to be as comfortable as possible, preferably lying supine or semi-reclined and with arms to the side or on a flat surface. If artifact is still observed, check for subtle movements such as nervous finger tapping or grasping the side rails. Try to discourage the patient from raising her head in an attempt to observe the ECG monitor. Any muscle tension can cause artifact.

Shivering can also cause artifact. After placing the electrodes, the patient should be covered to prevent hypothermia and any subsequent shivering. Finally, fine tremulous body movements may be observed on the ECG monitor as artifact when the Paramedic administers defasciculating doses of paralytic drugs.

Cable-Induced Artifact

ECG cables carry the signal from the body to the ECG machine. At the start of every tour of duty, the cables should be visually inspected for cracks in the insulation and loose connections to the connectors at both ends. Extraneous movement of the ECG harness (cable) can cause artifact. Starting

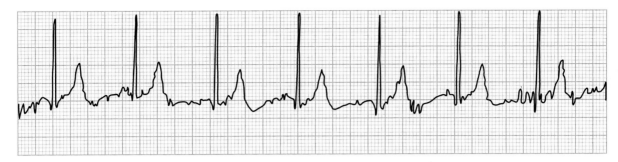

Figure 33-8 Artifact from patient movement caused the noisy baseline in this ECG tracing.

at the patient, the wires should be inspected to ensure that they are securely fastened to the electrodes.

Wires that are running over the top of electrodes can create interference. Therefore, wires should be placed in such a fashion that they run parallel to one another but not on top of one another. The Paramedic should also permit some slack in the cable running from the patient to the ECG monitor. This slack removes the tension from the electrode wires and helps prevent the electrode from being pulled off the patient.

Electromagnetic Interference

The flow of electricity through an electric device can naturally generate an electromagnetic field. In most cases, electronic devices are shielded to prevent this type of "radiation leak." If, for example, the shielding failed, then an electromagnetic field might be created. ECG machines, designed to detect changes in electricity, would logically be expected to pick up these fields and record them. **Electromagnetic interference (EMI)** of an ECG is seen as artifact.

Common sources of EMI include radios, cellular telephones, televisions—in fact, any electronic or radio device.[15-17] The first step in eliminating EMI is to turn off electronic devices in the proximity of the patient and see if the artifact resolves. Another common source of EMI is overhead fluorescent lighting. These lights, common in commercial establishments and increasingly more common in homes, create a steady electrical signal from the 60-cycle alternating current (AC). The resulting artifact distorts the ECG tracing, making it difficult to read (Figure 33-9).

If it is difficult to identify the exact source of the electrical interference (i.e., the "noise"), then the patient should be moved away from the environment. For example, perhaps the patient can be moved to the rear of the ambulance.

Vehicle Motion Artifact

Little can be done to prevent vehicle motion artifact created by rough roads. Paramedics will frequently obtain a "clean" (artifact-free) tracing before and after transport for analysis and interpretation or while stopped at traffic control devices.

Identify the QRS Complex

The next step in the ECG interpretation is to identify the QRS complex. The QRS complex shows the greatest degree of variation in **duration** (length), **polarity** (direction), and **morphology** (shape). The QRS complex, representing ventricular depolarization, is usually the largest wave visible. The QRS complex can take on a number of combinations of the waves Q, R, or S. At this juncture it is not important to describe the significance of these wave groupings, but rather to simply identify the presence or absence of a QRS complex. The purpose of identifying the QRS complex first is so that the rhythm can be described and then the rate can be calculated accurately.

Absence of a QRS Complex

If there is no artifact and no QRS complexes are discernable, then the rhythm will appear flatline and the heart may be in asystole (no ventricular activity is detected on the surface ECG). The Paramedic's first reaction should be to confirm that the patient is without pulse and has no signs of life. If the patient is indeed unresponsive, apneic, and pulseless, then it

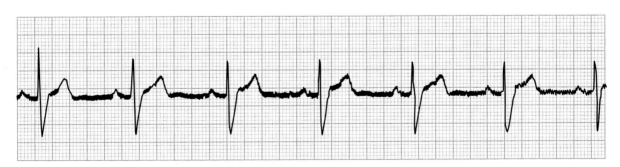

Figure 33-9 Artifact from 60-cycle interference.

may be necessary to confirm asystole in a minimum of two leads. It is recommended that asystole be confirmed in more than one lead.

If there are no QRS complexes in either lead and the monitor shows what appears to be artifact, then the Paramedic should immediately palpate for a pulse and signs of life. Again, if the patient is lacking a pulse and signs of life, the Paramedic should assume the chaotic rhythm is ventricular fibrillation and proceed accordingly. It is beyond the scope of the present discussion to talk about the treatment of life-threatening dysrhythmias.

STREET SMART

The ECG rhythm may not be visible on the surface ECG of morbidly obese patients. The heart lacks the energy to get a strong enough signal to the surface to be sensed. However, the patient may be awake and alert. This finding adds support to the Paramedic axiom, "Treat the patient, not the monitor!"

Determine Rhythm

The regularity of the rhythm is assessed by measuring from a point on the QRS complex to the same point on the next QRS complex. Typically, the tallest or deepest wave is used—the R wave in Lead II or the S wave in MCL1. By then visually inspecting the next waves in sequence and moving from left to right across the horizontal axis, the Paramedic can determine if events are occurring regularly, irregularly but with a pattern, or irregularly irregular.

Calipers make this task easy. However, care must be taken not to open or close the calipers inadvertently while moving from R to R. Many Paramedics use a flat edge or piece of paper to mark the interval between two R to R points and then assess subsequent R points. Some minor irregularity is expected in a normal rhythm. In very slow rhythms, an alteration of one to two small boxes, representing 0.04 to 0.08 seconds difference, is normal and is still considered regular.

Calculate Heart Rate

Armed with information about rhythm regularity, the Paramedic can choose the best method for determining the heart rate from among the several methods available.

If the rhythm is *regular*, then the quickest method to calculate the rate is to count the number of large boxes between any two QRS complexes and divide the result into 300. This method gives an accurate result. An understanding of this method will allow the Paramedic to substitute a

memorization trick to help in making calculations (Table 33-2 and Figure 33-10).

The most accurate method of calculating the rate of a regular rhythm is to count the number of small boxes between any two complexes and divide the result into 1,500. This method will give a very accurate result. Most Paramedics use a calculator when using this method.

If the rhythm is *irregular*, an acceptable method is to count the number of QRS complexes in a six-second strip and multiply that number by 10 to get a number per minute or a rate. Many ECG printouts have "tic" marks, a line or label, every three seconds either the top or the bottom of the ECG paper. These tic marks help the Paramedic to quickly determine a six-second strip. Therefore, between three tic marks is six seconds. The number of QRS complexes within that length of strip, times 10, equals the heart rate in beats per minute.

Since the rhythm is irregular, the choice of rhythm strip is only a snapshot in time. The rate only represents the rate at that moment. However, the rate can be altered by the choice of a different six-second rhythm strip. Therefore this method is the most inaccurate method of rate calculation.

Clinical Significance of Rate

Generally speaking, all rates are normal, fast or slow. Heart rates between 50 and 100 are considered to be normal or **normocardiac** and further clinical correlation is needed to ascertain the patient's condition.

The fast heart rate, greater than 100 beats per minute, is called a **tachycardia** and may have clinical significance to the patient's condition as well. If the patient is exercising, it is expected that the heart rate will be tachycardia. However, if the patient is lying in bed it would not be anticipated that the patient's heart rate would be tachycardia.

There are many causes of tachycardia including consumption of caffeine, cocaine, or other intoxicants that mimic adrenaline (sympathomimetics). Other causes include fever,

Table 33-2 Large Box Method of Rate Calculation

If there is one large box between two QRS complexes, then the ventricular rate is 300.

Continuing the sequence:

2 large boxes = ventricular rate of 150

3 large boxes = ventricular rate of 100

4 large boxes = ventricular rate of 75

5 large boxes = ventricular rate of 60

6 large boxes = ventricular rate of 50

7 large boxes = ventricular rate of 43

8 large boxes = ventricular rate of 37

9 large boxes = ventricular rate of 33

10 large boxes = ventricular rate of 30

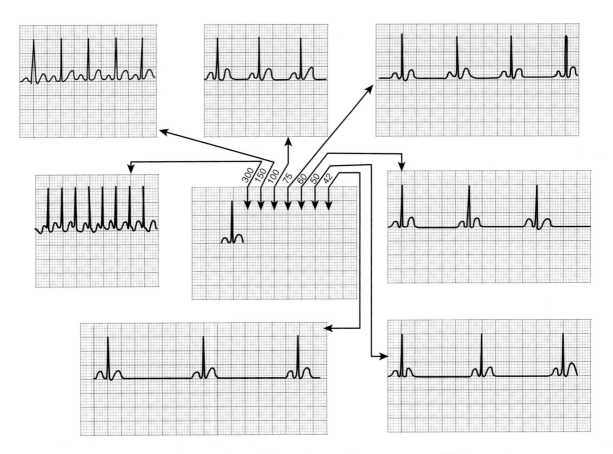

Figure 33-10 Rate based on the number of large boxes between two QRS complexes.

shock, acute coronary events, and endocrine disorders such as hyperthyroidism.

In some cases, the patient may experience a sensation of his or her heart racing, a phenomena called **palpitations**. The presence of palpitations should alert the Paramedic to the possibility of tachycardia. Typically heart rates of less than 150 beats per minute are well tolerated by the patient and the patient may not feel a palpitation.

A slow heart rate, called a **bradycardia**, may also be clinically significant but is usually not life threatening unless the rate falls below 50. In that case, the patient may be light-headed secondary to hypotension.

STREET SMART

It is important to note that the presence of a QRS complex does not always equate with the presence of a pulse. A patient can have an electrical rhythm without a pulse, a condition called **pulseless electrical activity (PEA)**. This phenomenon reinforces the Paramedic axiom of "Treat the patient, not the monitor."

QRS Width

After having determined the rhythm and rate, the Paramedic should examine the QRS more closely. The pressing concern is whether the QRS is wide, suggesting a ventricular origin, or it is narrow, suggesting either a sinus or supraventricular origin. **Ventricular rhythms** are usually, but not always, dangerous because the origin of the rhythm is in the last pacemaker in the ventricles. While a **supraventricular rhythm**, a complex originating above the ventricles, can be dangerous, it is generally better tolerated by the patient.[18] A sinus rhythm is a supraventricular rhythm and is considered the best situation.

In monitoring Lead II, the QRS is normally positive. It generally consists of a small initial Q wave (negative wave measuring less than 2 mm) followed by the positive R wave. Normal duration is from 0.04 to 0.12 second in the adult. For monitoring Lead MCL1, the complex normally begins with a small, narrow R wave followed by an S wave. The QRS duration is the same. If the QRS in any lead is greater than 0.12, then it is considered to be wide and therefore possibly of a ventricular origin.

Ectopy

It is essential to determine if every complex is wide or if only an occasional complex is wide. If there is an occasionally wide QRS, then this suggests a competing lower pacemaker

At this point in the ECG interpretation, there is sufficient information in many cases to start treatment of the patient. The Paramedic has determined if the underlying rhythm is regular, as well as the rate and the width of the QRS complex. Advanced cardiac life support algorithms include wide complex tachycardia, narrow complex tachycardia (both regular and irregular), and symptomatic bradycardia.

site, called an **ectopic focus**. Any complex that occurs outside of the sinus is considered an ectopic complex.

An ectopic focus can compete with the sinus node for **dominance** (the fastest cell) in terms of automaticity (creates the depolarization). If the ectopic focus is ventricular, and the ventricular pacemaker becomes dominant, the patient may experience a rhythm called **ventricular tachycardia**. With ventricular tachycardia, the rhythm is regular, the rate is fast, and every complex is wide.

If only the occasional complex is wide (i.e., possibly of ventricular origin), then the Paramedic should concentrate on determining the underlying **primary rhythm**. In many cases, the ectopic complexes are a result of hypoxia, rate-related myocardial ischemia, or a basic electrolyte disturbance. Correction of the ectopic rhythm is best accomplished by correction of the underlying abnormality.

In many cases, the ectopic complex appears earlier than would be expected in the course of a regular cardiac cycle. Increased automaticity of the ectopic focus leads to premature discharge, and therefore dominance, during depolarization. Therefore, these ectopic complexes could be described as wide premature complexes.

When an ectopic complex occurs at every other complex, it is called **bigeminy**. Bigeminy should not be confused with the situation in which two ectopic complexes occur together. These ectopic complexes are called **couplets**. Ectopic complexes can also occur every third beat (**trigeminy**) or every fourth complex (**quadrageminy**). Like bigeminy, ectopic complexes that occur three or four at a time are considered to be a **salvo** or a **run of ventricular tachycardia**.

P Waves

Following determination of rhythm, rate, and QRS width, the next step is to identify the P wave. The normal morphology and polarity of the P wave is upright (positive) and rounded in monitoring Lead II. It may be upright, flat, or negative in monitoring MCL1.

While the P can be **biphasic**, beginning as a positive deflection then becoming a negative wave or vice versa, it

Some Paramedics have a tendency to refer to a rhythm by its ectopy. This is analogous to referring to a friend by a nickname. However, it is more descriptive to refer to the rhythm by first describing the underlying primary rhythm and then the ectopy (e.g., sinus rhythm with a bigeminy of wide premature complexes).

is abnormal for the P to be notched or peaked. The upper limit of normal for the duration of the P wave (which reflects atrial depolarization) is 0.12 seconds.

The normal height of the P wave is less than 3 mm, or three small boxes, rounded and upright in Lead II. This is due to the size and arrangement of the atrial fibers. Any P wave larger than 3 mm suggests that the atrium may be enlarged due to an increased workload. Causes of increased atrial work include tricuspid valve disease, pulmonary hypertension, cor pulmonale, or congenital heart disease.

Lead II is the best *single* lead to view atrial activity as a rule. The P wave should be upright and rounded in Lead II.[19,20]

AV Relationships

Normally, the sinoatrial node (SA node) discharges, setting off a cascade of depolarizations down the conductive pathway in the heart. When this occurs, the surface ECG will register a P wave followed by a momentary pause, as the signal reaches the atrioventricular node (AV node) and then ventricular depolarization occurs, as represented by the QRS complex.

In a normal sinus rhythm, there should be a P wave immediately preceding the QRS. If a P wave is absent, then the pacemaker may be down further in the conduction system, either at the level of the AV node or at the level of the ventricles.

If there are more P waves than there are QRS complexes, then the complex is being blocked at some point along the conductive pathway. An interruption of AV conduction (an **AV block**) can be indicative of disease or ischemia at the level of the AV node. While AV blocks can be troubling, the resultant bradycardia is of greater concern.

Intervals

After having established rhythm, rate, QRS width, and AV relationships, the Paramedic should proceed to examine intervals. Intervals are periods of time when a certain event—in this case, a depolarization of the heart—is expected to occur. Prolonged or shortened intervals can be indicative of underlying abnormalities.

PR Interval

The time for conduction down the intra-atrial pathways is rapid. In order to allow time for the blood (a viscous fluid) to match the speed of electrical conduction, the impulse is held in the AV node. The AV delay is between 0.12 and 0.20 seconds and is measured from the beginning of the P wave to the start of the QRS complex, the **PR interval**.

If the PR interval is greater than 0.20 seconds, then the impulse is delayed. There are many causes (including ischemia) of a delayed PR interval. In some cases, the PR interval becomes progressively longer until the AV node no longer conducts the electrical impulse. This is another indication of disease.

Conversely, if the PR interval (PRI) is shorter than 0.12 seconds, then the likelihood is that an ectopic pacemaker in the atrium has assumed dominance or that a congenital abnormal pathway, called an **accessory pathway**, has become engaged in the conduction of the impulse.[21]

If there is no relationship between P waves and the QRS complex (AV dissociation), there may be a **complete heart block**. When a complete heart block occurs, pacemakers lower in the heart at the level of the bundle of His, bundle branches, or even the ventricular myocardium will take over as the pacemaker. These secondary pacemakers serve as a fail-safe for the heart but are generally not reliable for the long term.

QT Interval

Ventricular depolarization and repolarization is represented on the surface ECG tracing as the QT interval. The QT starts at the first deflection of the QRS complex, regardless of the initial wave, and stops at the end of the T wave.

While short QT intervals do exist, some patients have congenital short QT syndromes. Paramedics are generally concerned with QT widening. QT intervals are affected by sex and age. For example, men, on average, have shorter QT intervals (0.39 second) than women (0.41 second) at a heart rate of 70 bpm. However, prolonged QT intervals may represent underlying abnormal electrolyte levels, drugs, and even myocardial ischemia.

QT intervals are also affected by heart rate. When assessing a QT interval, the value obtained is corrected by using a formula. For example, Bazett's formula for corrected QT interval equals the QT interval divided by the square root of the RR interval. To accommodate the variables such as rate, QT intervals are reported as corrected (QTc). Any QTc longer than 0.40 +/− 0.06 seconds in a normal heart rate should be considered prolonged. A patient with a prolonged QT segment is at risk for unstable ventricular tachycardia, specifically torsades de pointes.[22,23] It should be noted that the QTc is of little clinical relevance in heart rates over 100 bpm.

Determination of the QT interval in the field is generally not necessary, except under certain specific circumstances (Table 33-3). It is only necessary to ascertain if the QT interval is abnormally long. A quick rule of thumb is that the QT should be less than one half of the RR interval.

Normal Sinus Rhythm

Normal sinus rhythm (Table 33-4 and Figure 33-11) is considered an optimal rhythm. The regular rhythm and rate provide for adequate filling of the ventricles and sufficient ejection of blood for perfusion.

In a regular and normocardiac rhythm, where the P wave precedes the QRS in a timely fashion and the QRS is narrow, the Paramedic may reasonably interpret the rhythm as normal sinus rhythm. The Paramedic should learn the essential parameters of the sinus rhythm, because all other rhythms that are not sinus (i.e., that do not fit into the essential parameters) are considered to be dysrhythmias.

Sinus Tachycardia

Sinus tachycardia (Table 33-5 and Figure 33-12), is a sinus rhythm with a rate greater than 100 bpm. All other measurements of the rhythm remain the same as those for a sinus rhythm. If the heart rate is greater than 150 bpm, and the rhythm is sustained, then it is less likely that the rhythm is a sinus tachycardia but another supraventricular tachycardia.

Sinus Bradycardia

A sinus rhythm becomes a **sinus bradycardia** (Table 33-6 and Figure 33-13) when the rate falls below 60 bpm, though most patients are not symptomatic until the heart rate falls below 50 bpm. Any rate below 60 is considered an **absolute bradycardia**. Alternatively, some patients can be symptomatic with a rate above 60, even though the rate does not meet the criteria for absolute bradycardia. In those cases, the patient is said to be experiencing a **relative bradycardia**, or a rate that is too slow for the patient's metabolic needs.

Table 33-3 Etiology of Prolonged QT Interval—Partial List

1. Antidysrhythmic drugs
a. Vaughn-Williams Class I
2. Tricyclic antidepressants
3. Phenothiazines
4. Electrolyte imbalance
a. Hypokalemia
b. Hypomagnesemia
5. Stroke
6. Seizures
7. Cardiomyopathy

Table 33-4 Parameters for Normal Sinus Rhythm (NSR)

Sinus rhythm originates in the sinus node, the heart's primary pacemaker. Conduction takes place along the conduction pathway, in a time frame conducive to adequate cardiac output.	
Rhythm	Regular
Rate	Ventricular
	60 to 100 bpm
QRS configuration	Same complex to complex
	Upright in Lead II
QRS duration	Less than 0.12 seconds
P wave	Rounded and upright Lead II
Atrial rate	Same as ventricular
AV conduction	P wave to QRS = 1:1
PR interval	0.12 to 0.20 seconds
QT interval	Less than 0.44 seconds

Table 33-5 Parameters for Sinus Tachycardia

Rhythm	Regular
Rate	Ventricular
	Greater than 100 bpm
QRS configuration	Same complex to complex
	Upright in Lead II
QRS duration	Less than 0.12 seconds
P wave	Rounded and upright Lead II
Atrial rate	Same as ventricular
AV conduction	P wave to QRS = 1:1
PR interval	0.12 to 0.20 seconds
QT interval	Less than 0.44 seconds

Sinus Dysrhythmia

Sinus rhythm naturally slows with exhalation and then accelerates during inspiration. During expiration, intrathoracic pressure decreases. As a result, more blood can return to the heart, thereby increasing preload. With an increase of blood in the heart, stretch receptors in the heart's atrium in turn signal the heart to contract slower. During inhalation, the opposite occurs. **Sinus dysrhythmia** (Table 33-7 and Figure 33-14) is most notable in children. The pacer site remains in the sinus node and conduction follows the usual pathways.

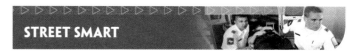

STREET SMART

Sinus dysrhythmia is a normal variant for most people. It is extremely common in children and young adults. For this reason, some Paramedics never refer to a sinus rhythm as "normal" sinus rhythm as this implies the rhythm is regular and since many people have a slight variation in rhythm which is completely natural.

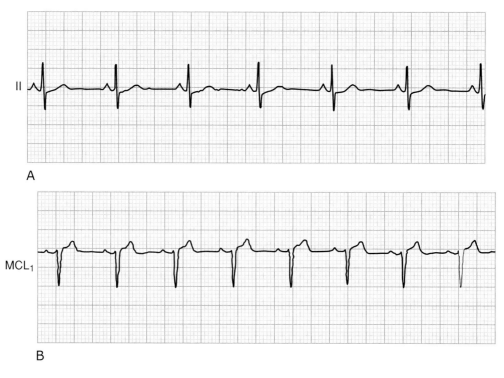

A

B

Figure 33-11 Normal sinus rhythm.

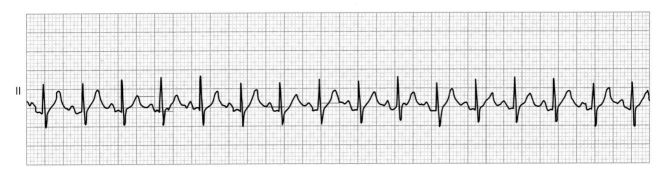

Figure 33-12 Sinus tachycardia.

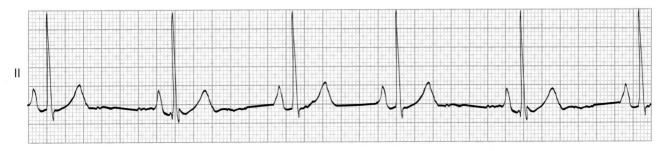

Figure 33-13 Sinus bradycardia.

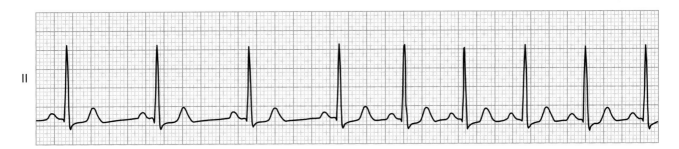

Figure 33-14 Sinus dysrhythmia.

Table 33-6 Parameters for Sinus Bradycardia

Rhythm	Regular
Rate	Ventricular
	Less than 60 bpm
QRS configuration	Same complex to complex
QRS duration	Less than 0.12 seconds
	Upright in Lead II
P wave	Rounded and upright Lead II
Atrial rate	Same as ventricular
AV conduction	P wave to QRS = 1:1
PR interval	0.12 to 0.20 seconds
QT interval	Less than 0.44 seconds

Table 33-7 Parameters for Sinus Dysrhythmia

Rhythm	Regularly Irregular
Rate	Ventricular
	60 to 100 bpm
QRS configuration	Same complex to complex
	Upright in Lead II
QRS duration	Less than 0.12 seconds
P wave	Rounded and upright Lead II
Atrial rate	Same as ventricular
AV conduction	P wave to QRS = 1:1
PR interval	0.12 to 0.20 seconds
QT interval	Less than 0.44 seconds

Out-of-Hospital ECG Monitoring Equipment

During transport within a hospital and during the patient's hospital stay, the cardiac patient will have electrodes connecting him directly to the ECG device which is both displaying and storing the ECG tracings. This type of equipment, which may be anchored above the patient's bed or may be portable, is called **hard wire monitoring**. Its limitation is that it limits the patient's ability to move around.

To allow a patient to begin walking in his hospital room or out in the hallway, some places use **telemetry** monitors. These devices are connected to the patient by two or three wires. They collect the data and send it via radio waves to an antenna. The data is then transmitted by wires to the main console. The Paramedic should be aware that the radio waves transmitted by cellular phones can interfere with both hard-wire and telemetry systems.[24–26] Care should be taken to turn off cell phones when transporting the patient within the hospital setting.

At-Home ECG Monitoring

In many cases, the problematic dysrhythmia is sporadic in nature. It is economically impossible to keep a patient in the hospital for continuous monitoring for days or weeks in order to pick up the dysrhythmia. For this reason, a continuous type of ECG monitor called **Holter monitoring** was invented. Holter monitoring allows the patient to go about his routine work and play activities while the Holter monitoring device records the ECG activity. At the conclusion of the desired monitoring period (usually 48 to 72 hours), the device is returned to the cardiologist who, in turn, downloads the information to a console or computer for analysis.

Even Holter monitoring may miss abnormal ECG activity that tends to occur very irregularly (as in days or weeks apart). This patient may possess an **event monitor**, a device that is a little larger than a credit card. When the patient senses the abnormal activity, the monitor is placed on the chest for the preset period of time. The patient can then telephone the cardiologist's office and transmit the data from the card via telephone.

If the Paramedic needs to provide care to a patient with a Holter monitor, the monitor poses no problem. While the Holter monitor may have hard wires or electrodes connected to the patient's chest, the electrode placement for the Holter monitor is different than the placement recommended for prehospital monitoring. Therefore, both may be used simultaneously without interference with the other device.

Keep in mind that some cardiac treatments, such as defibrillation and pacing, may require access to the patient's chest. If the Holter monitor needs to be removed, simply remove it and the electrodes. Turn off the Holter monitor if the device has an ON/OFF switch. Bring the Holter monitor to the hospital with the patient or give the device to a person designated by the patient. The Paramedic should document the disposition of the device including the name of the person to whom it was given.

CONCLUSION

While seemingly daunting at first appearance, ECG interpretation can be learned provided the Paramedic practices ECG analysis and remembers the fundamental rules of the monitoring ECG. To improve the quality and accuracy of ECG interpretation, the Paramedic should take a disciplined and logical approach to ECG interpretation. While an ECG is important to the overall clinical picture, a stand-alone ECG is of little clinical value. It is important to correlate the patient's clinical picture with the ECG in order to have a meaningful interpretation.

KEY POINTS:

- Monitoring equipment varies according to the specific monitoring need, the location of the patient, and the type of event being assessed.

- The Paramedic must make a judgment as to whether preexisting monitoring equipment must be removed to permit appropriate patient care.

- The speed at which the screen or paper moves is called sweep speed. A change may allow better examination of key features.

- The size of the picture on the screen or paper is called gain.

- The Paramedic must follow the agency's policy for documenting sweep speed and gain, which is called calibration.

- ECG paper is standardized to allow Paramedics to measure the timing of events and the intensity of the events.

- The horizontal axis equals time. Each light line equals a time of 0.04 seconds; each heavy line equals a time of 0.2 seconds.

- The vertical axis equals amplitude. Each light line equals 0.1 mm or 0.1 mV. Each dark line equals 0.5 mm or 0.5 mV.

- To obtain an ECG, there must be an electrical signal, an electrode to reduce skin resistance to the signal, and a wire to conduct the signal to the machine.

- Wire systems vary. The important point is to place the electrodes and attach the wires in such a way as to mimic Einthoven's Triangle.

- Measurements of duration, amplitude, and polarity are made of each ECG feature.

- Apply a consistent method of assessment and treatment. First, assess the patient for the presence of pulses. Next, assess the width of the QRS complex. Determine treatment timeliness.

- In determining the name of the rhythm:
  - Know the causes of dysrhythmias
  - Assess the QRS complex
  - Assess the P waves
  - Do not mistake blips for P waves or miss the P wave due to size
  - Determine which P wave is related to which QRS
  - Pinpoint the primary diagnosis

- Normal sinus rhythm (NSR) is considered the optimal rhythm for most people. All other rhythms are compared to NSR.

- The presence of NSR does not eliminate the presence of patient problems.

REVIEW QUESTIONS:

1. What steps should be taken before placing the electrodes?
2. What are the two standard ECG monitoring leads?
3. How does one place the ECG electrodes for these monitoring leads?
4. What are some causes of low-amplitude ECG?
5. What are some common causes of artifact?
6. What can be done to resolve artifact?
7. Why is it important to determine rhythm before rate?
8. What are the three methods of determining heart rate?
9. What are normal and abnormal heart rates?
10. What are the normal parameters of the QRS?

CASE STUDY QUESTIONS:

Please refer to the Case Study at the beginning of the chapter and answer the question below:

1. Explain why analyzing and naming the rhythm could impact the treatment provided to Ms. Sheehan.

REFERENCES:

1. Ferguson JD, Brady WJ, Perron AD, Kielar ND, Benner JP, Currance SB, et al. The prehospital 12-lead electrocardiogram: impact on management of the out-of-hospital acute coronary syndrome patient. *Am J Emerg Med.* 2003;21(2):136–142.
2. Hurst JW. Naming of the waves in the ECG, with a brief account of their genesis. *Circulation.* 1998;98(18):1937–1942.
3. Wellens HJ. Bishop lecture. The electrocardiogram 80 years after Einthoven. *J Am Coll Cardiol.* 1986;7(3):484–491.
4. Campbell PT, Patterson J, Cromer D, Wall K, Adams GL, Albano A, et al. Prehospital triage of acute myocardial infarction: wireless transmission of electrocardiograms to the on-call cardiologist via a handheld computer. *J Electrocardiol.* 2005;38(4):300–309.
5. Chen EH, Hollander JE. When do patients need admission to a telemetry bed? *J Emerg Med.* 2007;33(1):53–60.
6. Mischke K, Zarse M, Perkuhn M, Knackstedt C, Markus K, Koos R, et al. Telephonic transmission of 12-lead electrocardiograms during acute myocardial infarction. *J Telemed Telecare.* 2005;11(4):185–190.
7. Faes TJ, van der Meij HA, de Munck JC, Heethaar RM. The electric resistivity of human tissues (100 Hz-10 MHz): a meta-analysis of review studies. *Physiol Meas.* 1999;20(4):R1–10.
8. Takuma K, Hori S, Sasaki J, Shinozawa Y, Yoshikawa T, Handa S, et al. An alternative limb lead system for electrocardiographs in emergency patients. *Am J Emerg Med.* 1995;13(5):514–517.
9. Jowett NI, Turner AM, Cole A, Jones PA. Modified electrode placement must be recorded when performing 12-lead electrocardiograms. *Postgrad Med J.* 2005;81(952):122–125.
10. Bayram E, Atalay C. Identification of the culprit artery involved in inferior wall acute myocardial infarction using electrocardiographic criteria. *J Int Med Res.* 2004;33(1):39–44.
11. McManus JG, Convertino VA, Cooke WH, Ludwig DA, Holcomb JB. R-wave amplitude in Lead II of an electrocardiograph correlates with central hypovolemia in human beings. *Acad Emerg Med.* 2006;13(10):1003–1010.
12. Kataoka H, Kanzaki K, Mikuriya Y. Massive ST-segment elevation in precordial and inferior leads in right ventricular myocardial infarction. *J Electrocardiol.* 1988;21(2):115–120.
13. Learning D. *EKG Tech Video.* Utica, New York: Delmar Thomson Learning; 1998.
14. Upshaw CB, Jr., Silverman ME, Henry JL. Marriott: Lucid teacher of electrocardiography. *Clin Cardiol.* 2007; 30(4):207–208.

15. Schlimp CJ, Breiteneder M, Seifert J, Lederer W. Interference of 16.7-Hz electromagnetic fields on measured electrocardiogram. *Bioelectromagnetics*. 2007;28(5):402–405.

16. Kolb C, Zrenner B, Schmitt C. Incidence of electromagnetic interference in implantable cardioverter defibrillators. *Pacing Clin Electrophysiol*. 2001;24(4 Pt 1):465–468.

17. Fleischhackl R, Singer F, Nitsche W, Gamperl G, Roessler B, Arrich J, et al. Influence of electromagnetic fields on function of automated external defibrillators. *Acad Emerg Med*. 2006;13(1):1–6.

18. Mulroy JF, Thayer JJ, King JE. How do I manage stable narrow-complex SVT? *Nursing*. 2005;35(10):14.

19. Gorenek B, Birdane A, Kudaiberdieva G, Goktekin O, Cavusoglu Y, Unalir A, et al. P wave amplitude and duration may predict immediate recurrence of atrial fibrillation after internal cardioversion. *Ann Noninvasive Electrocardiol*. 2003;8(3):215–218.

20. Zeng C, Wei T, Zhao R, Wang C, Chen L, Wang L. Electrocardiographic diagnosis of left atrial enlargement in patients with mitral stenosis: the value of the P-wave area. *Acta Cardiol*. 2003;58(2):139–141.

21. MacKenzie R. Short PR interval. *J Insur Med*. 2005;37(2):145–152.

22. Shantsila E, Watson T, Lip GY. Drug-induced QT-interval prolongation and proarrhythmic risk in the treatment of atrial arrhythmias. *Europace*. 2007;9(4):37–44.

23. Roden DM. Clinical practice. Long-QT syndrome. *N Engl J Med*. 2008;358(2):169–176.

24. Brodlie M, Robertson D, Wyllie J. Interference of electrocardiographic recordings by a mobile telephone. *Cardiol Young*. 2007;17(3):338–339.

25. Tri JL, Severson RP, Firl AR, Hayes DL, Abenstein JP. Cellular telephone interference with medical equipment. *Mayo Clin Proc*. 2005;80(10):1286–1290.

26. Tri JL, Hayes DL, Smith TT, Severson RP. Cellular phone interference with external cardiopulmonary monitoring devices. *Mayo Clin Proc*. 2001;76(1):11–15.

CHAPTER 34

DIAGONOSTIC ECG—THE 12-LEAD

KEY CONCEPTS:

Upon completion of this chapter, it is expected that the reader will understand these following concepts:

- Paramedic use of 12-lead ECG as the first step in a critical care pathway for patients with acute coronary syndrome
- Accurate acquisition of the 12-lead ECG
- Analysis of the 12-lead ECG to make a patient prognosis, determine treatment, and plan for an appropriate destination

▶ CASE STUDY:

The Paramedics were called to the home of Jennie Swinter. Mrs. Swinter is an 82-year-old widow, living alone on a small farm that she still farms for vegetables. She called EMS because she became exhausted and out of breath after walking to the bathroom. The inexperienced Paramedic commented that at her age, Mrs. Swinter should be tired and out of breath. The more experienced Paramedic suggested that many acute processes could account for Mrs. Swinter's complaints.

The Paramedics obtained an ECG right after placing Mrs. Swinter on oxygen. It showed ST elevation and hyperacute T waves in Leads II, III, and aVF. Mrs. Swinter complained of feeling very lightheaded and afraid. Repeat vital signs were obtained. Rather than the 118/66 found earlier, she had a pressure of 80/48. She also had jugular venous distention while semi-sitting and clear lung sounds.

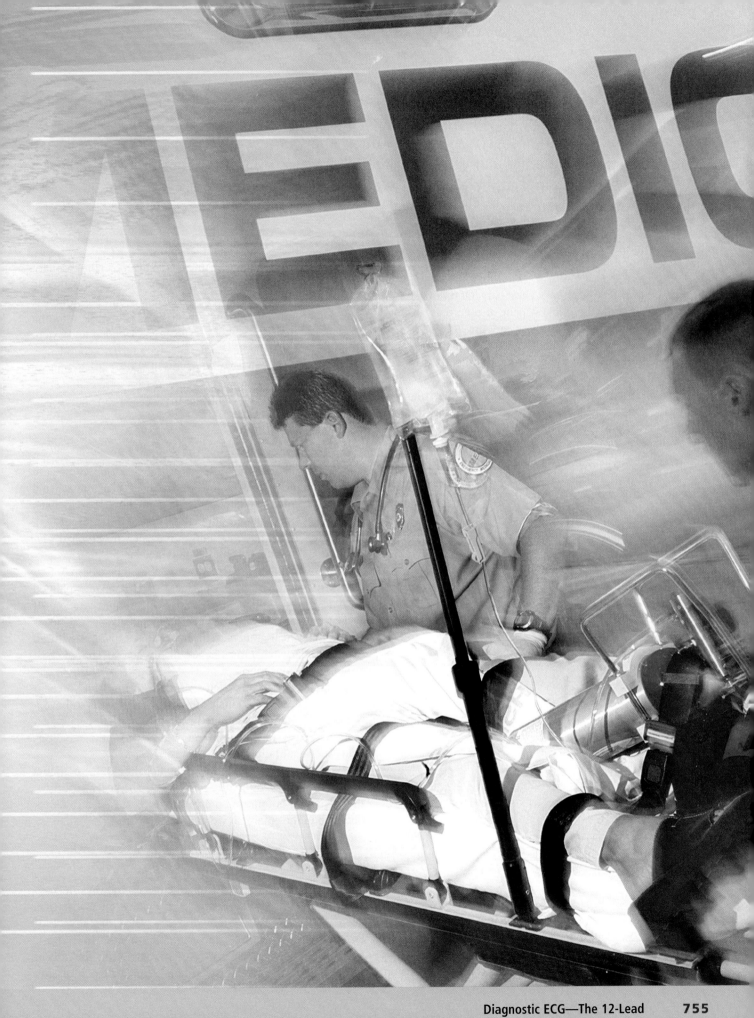

Diagnostic ECG—The 12-Lead

OVERVIEW

Death from acute myocardial infarction remains a leading reason for mortality in the United States despite advances in medicine. It has been estimated that 50% of patients with acute coronary syndrome (which, if left untreated, leads to AMI) are transported by EMS and the majority of cardiac arrests occur in the prehospital setting. It is therefore important that Paramedics be able to identify and aggressively treat these patients.

Chief Concern

There are a number of causes of chest pain. Of particular concern for the Paramedic is chest pain of a cardiac etiology. Patients with cardiac-related chest pain are at high risk for acute myocardial infarction and sudden cardiac death.

The identification of the patient with potential for acute myocardial infarction is predicated on a clinical history which is suggestive of acute coronary syndrome and electrocardiographic findings. The latter, electrocardiographic findings, are not always present in patients who are at the beginning of the event (i.e., early in the evolution of the acute myocardial infarction). The maxim "Treat the patient, not the monitor" holds true for these patients. Treatment for suspected acute myocardial infarction—specifically morphine, oxygen, nitrates, and aspirin—should not be withheld because of a lack of electrocardiographic findings. It has been estimated that upward of 50% of patients who will develop an acute myocardial infarction had no confirmatory electrocardiographic (ECG) findings upon the initial ECG.[1-4]

STREET SMART

One study suggested that serial 12-lead ECGs identified acute myocardial infarctions in 75% of patients upon whom the initial 12-lead ECG exhibited nonspecific ECG changes. The importance of an early baseline 12-lead ECG was supported by that study. Therefore, it is advisable for all Paramedics to obtain an initial baseline 12-lead ECG as soon as possible. Thereafter, serial 12-lead ECGs should be performed every 15 to 30 minutes for the first 2 hours of patient contact.

However, that is not to dismiss the importance of obtaining a 12-lead ECG as soon as possible on a patient with suspected acute coronary syndrome. A 12-lead ECG can also help the Paramedic estimate the location of the coronary occlusion, ascertain the ventricular wall involved, and predict the coronary artery that is affected. Not only is this information valuable downstream, to the emergency physicians and cardiologists who will eventually treat the patient, but it is important for the Paramedic. By being able to estimate the location and extent of injury, the Paramedic can predict, with relative confidence, the clinical course that the patient will take. This prognostic ability permits the Paramedic to prepare for predictable complications related to the acute coronary event.

Atypical Presentations of ACS

While it is obvious that patients with substernal chest pain (SSCP) should have a 12-lead ECG, other occasions when a 12-lead ECG may be necessary are sometimes less obvious. For example, middle-aged females often do not present with chest pain. These patients tend to present with atypical presentations for acute coronary syndrome.[5,6]

These atypical presentations can include sharp rather than crushing chest pain, shortness of breath, unexplained weakness, and sudden diaphoresis. Unfortunately, some of these symptoms can be mistaken for menopausal signs, leading to delayed treatment. The belief that a patient with an acute coronary event must have concomitant substernal chest pain is a misconception.

Another group of patients who have an atypical presentation are the elderly. This group of patients tends to have a higher frequency of acute myocardial infarction, even when identified early in the evolution, and complications such as heart and renal failure.

For these reasons the Paramedic should have a low threshold for 12-lead ECG acquisitions. The best support for this argument is found in the frequency that 12-lead ECG is obtained in the emergency department.

Rhythm Strip

The primary mission of all Paramedics has always been to prevent sudden cardiac death from dysrhythmia. This has been the essence of Paramedic care since the advent of Dr. Pantridge's "mobile coronary care units" in Belfast, Ireland, over half a century ago. However, with the advent of fibrinolytics and invasive cardiology, the original mission has been expanded to include rapid acquisition and interpretation of 12-lead ECGs.

The 12-lead ECG stands at the center of the decision pathway when managing patients with ischemic chest pain. Delays in obtaining the 12-lead ECG must be eliminated whenever possible. The most effective means of obtaining a 12-lead ECG at the earliest point in time is to have a Paramedic obtain one.[7]

The importance of obtaining a rapid and accurate 12-lead ECG is underscored by the American Heart Association's (AHA) statements. The AHA states that upon recognition of acute coronary syndrome and a suspected acute coronary event, a 12-lead ECG should be obtained as soon as possible but no later than ten (10) minutes upon arrival at the hospital.[8,9] This rapid 12-lead ECG acquisition and interpretation will facilitate the patient's transfer to cardiac centers for interventional cardiology. This time frame has been demonstrated to decrease both morbidity and mortality.

The efficiency of this process can be substantially improved with 12-lead ECGs being obtained by Paramedics and the diversion of ambulances to cardiac centers. The American College of Emergency Physicians (ACEP) supports this process in their position paper entitled "Out-of-Hospital 12-Lead ECG."

While ACEP acknowledges that 12-lead ECG acquisition will prolong scene times, many Paramedics have become very adept at obtaining 12-lead ECGs in minimal time. Studies have shown that Paramedics can obtain 12-lead ECGs at the point of care in the field in approximately 5 minutes.

The advent of Paramedic 12-lead ECGs has greatly affected physicians' opinions of Paramedics regarding the treatmet of acute coronary syndromes. Paramedics are viewed as a part of the continuum of care that starts in the field and ends in the interventional cardiologist suite. It is recognized that aggressive Paramedic care can substantially impact cardiac patient morbidity and mortality.

Origins of the Electrocardiogram

The electrocardiogram has a long history that may have started with Italian physicist Carlo Matteucci. Matteucci, interested in the works of the noted physicist Luigi Galvani, continued Galvani's work on bioelectricity and started to investigate the role of electricity in the human body. Matteucci observed that with every heartbeat there was a passage of electrical current in the body. What Matteucci did not realize when he made that observation was that he was actually witnessing the birth of electrocardiography.

Following Matteucci's early lead, noted British physiologist Augustus Waller, of St. Mary's Medical School in London, created the first tracing of the heart's electrical activity using his lab assistant Thomas Goswell as a patient in 1887. Subsequently, British physiologists William Bayliss and Edward Starling from the University College of London, following Waller's direction, attached a terminal to the right hand of a patient and to the skin overlying the apex of the heart. They observed a triphasic pattern to the electricity's flow.

Continuing the work of Bayliss and Starling, Willem Einthoven, who had also witnessed Waller demonstrate an ECG in 1889, used a silver string galvanometer to reproduce the triphasic waves that Bayliss and Starling had observed. Willem Einthoven named the deflections of these waves P, Q, R, S, and T, a convention that lasts to this day.

Continuing his work with the "electrokardiogram" (EKG) in 1905, Einthoven transmitted his first EKG over 1.5 kilometers to another lab using a telephone cable. This was the first recorded experience with telemetry.[10] Einthoven also went on to standardize the electrocardiogram by referencing the body and using the designators Leads I, II, and III. These first leads formed an equilateral triangle which is now referred to as "Einthoven's Triangle." From this platform, Einthoven was able to distinguish normal "EKG" from abnormal, noting premature ventricular contractions, heart blocks, atrial flutter, and other dysrhythmia. For this and other work, Einthoven was awarded the Nobel Prize in medicine in 1924 for "inventing the electrocardiogram." He is commonly referred to as the "father of electrocardiology."

Standard Limb Leads

Einthoven's limb leads used two electrodes, one negative and one positive, and measured the electrical potential between these electrodes as it flowed from negative to positive. Because the limb leads required two leads which measured the current difference between the leads' electrodes, they were—and still are—referred to as **bipolar leads**. Einthoven's original bipolar limb leads provided electrical information relating to the heart's electrical activity along the frontal plane of the body (Figure 34-1).

Perhaps the most useful of these bipolar leads was Lead II in that its orientation, from right shoulder to the left foot, was more or less in alignment with the heart's electrical conduction system. For this reason, Lead II provides the best view of error of conduction. It is often used to monitor patients for an irregular heart rhythm, a disturbance in conduction along the heart's electrical pathway, called a dysrhythmia.

Unfortunately, because of its orientation along the frontal plane, Lead II only permits a view of the heart's inferior wall. However, the bulk of the ventricular mass is in the anterior wall.[11]

Even with the use of three limb leads, the ECG only viewed the frontal plane and the inferior and lateral wall of the heart (Figure 34-2). However, the majority of the ventricular mass lies along the transverse plane in the anterior wall. Thus, even with these additional leads, the electrical activity of the anterior wall was still not being captured by the ECG.

Precordial Leads

In an effort to obtain a more comprehensive view of the heart, researchers sought to create new leads. In 1931, researchers Wilson, MacLeod, and Barker devised a method for recording

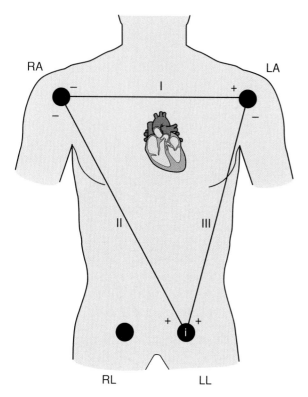

Figure 34-1 Standard limb leads.

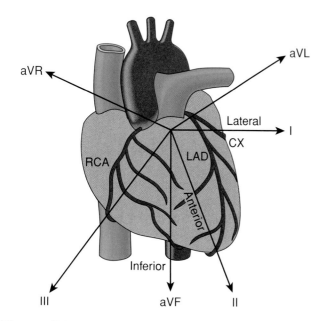

Figure 34-2 Frontal plane's relationship to the heart.

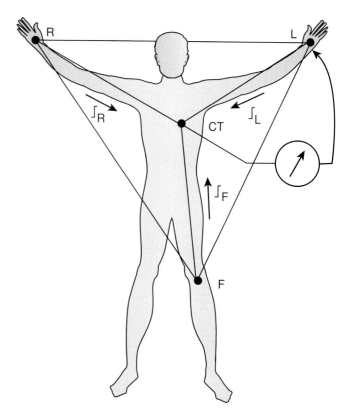

Figure 34-3 Wilson's central terminal (i.e., the virtual negative electrode) and the creation of the unipolar lead.

the electrical activity of the heart along any of its surfaces. They continued to use the three limb leads. However, through the use of electrical resistors, they were able to move the negative electrode to the center of the body, proximal to the right atria and the SA node, to form a central point called Wilson's central terminal (CT).

Because the negative electrode is a "virtual" electrode, not an actual electrode, in the center of the body, the positive electrode is now available to become an "exploring" lead which can be placed anywhere on the thorax to view any angle of the heart. The use of a single positive electrode, using Wilson's central terminal, created the **unipolar lead** (Figure 34-3).

Using the central terminal concept, Wilson placed electrodes in a semicircle around the precordium, that portion of skin that overlies the heart. Wilson's unipolar precordial **chest leads** encircled the anterior ventricular wall from the septal wall on the right to the lateral wall on the left. This permitted a complete view of the anterior myocardium.

These leads were originally called the V leads (V for voltage). In 1938, the American Heart Association standardized the precordial leads and called them V1, V2, V3, V4, V5, and V6. Adding these precordial (chest) leads to the standard limb leads gave nine views of the heart along both the frontal plane and the transverse plane.

Augmented Leads— A More Complete Picture

While six precordial chest leads gave physicians a better view of the anterior wall, the three bipolar limb leads did not give physicians the same view of the inferior wall. Einthoven's Triangle (the origin of the standard limb leads) is an equilateral triangle and has, by definition, angles of 60 degrees. Use of these angles left wide gaps with the potential for much of the heart's electrical activity to be unrecorded by these standard limb leads.

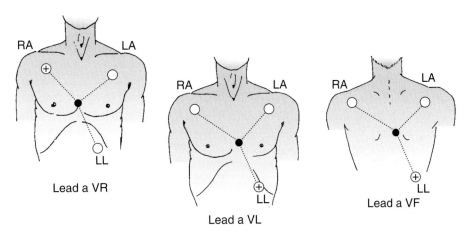

Figure 34-4 Augmented lead placement and the relationship of augmented limb leads to the standard limb leads.

Using Wilson's central terminal theory, Goldberger recorded the activity between each of the limb leads' positive electrodes and the central terminal, adding three additional limb leads. Unfortunately, when the signals were recorded, they were too small to be properly examined and required a boosting of the signal in order to identify any characteristics. In 1942, Goldberger devised a method to boost, or augment, the signal (hence the title "augmented" leads) (Figure 34-4).

Combining the lead type and the positive electrode location gave rise to the names of Goldberger's **augmented leads** (i.e., augmented voltage right or aVR, then augmented voltage left or aVL, and augmented voltage foot now called aVF).

Acquisition of the 12-Lead ECG

The importance of acquiring a high-quality 12-lead ECG, as explained earlier, cannot be overstated. Clinical decisions regarding the patient's treatment and transportation are based, in part, on the 12-lead ECG. Therefore, it is imperative that the Paramedic know how to obtain a clear and concise 12-lead ECG.

Diagnostic 12-Lead ECG versus Rhythm Monitoring

Tracings of early ECGs were often plagued with artifact and distortions that made reading the ECG difficult. These early ECG machines were intended to monitor the rhythm only. To solve these problems, electrical engineers resorted to adjusting the frequency range, that area of the electric signal that is being recorded. They also used electronic filters such as common mode rejection.

In order to capture subtle changes in amplitude and duration which are necessary for the interpretation of a diagnostic 12-lead, the 12-lead ECG monitors require a wider frequency range than simple three-lead ECG rhythm monitors. In the

simple ECG rhythm monitor, a narrower frequency range between 0.5 Hz and 30 to 50 Hz removes distortions which interfere with the rhythm's correct analysis. However, it does so at the cost of accuracy when measuring segments of the ECG complex. In the simple ECG rhythm monitor, an ST segment may appear far above (elevated) or below (depressed) the baseline, indicating potential ischemia or acute injury/infarct. Paramedics are generally directed to take patients with an ST segment above baseline to an interventional cardiology center as opposed to the local hospital.[12–15] A false positive in this regard is not only an inconvenience to the patient and to the patient's family, but misuses critical cardiac services needed for more acutely ill patients.

To obtain a proper diagnostic 12-lead ECG that correctly shows all segments, the American Heart Association recommends that a frequency range of 0.05 Hz to 150 Hz be used. However, switching from monitoring mode to diagnostic mode raises the problems of artifact which were previously eradicated. Therefore, the Paramedic must take other measures to reduce artifact.

12-Lead ECG Artifact

The common sources of ECG artifact can be broadly classified as physiologic and nonphysiologic. Physiologic artifact includes muscle artifact and skin artifact. The first, muscle artifact, is the result of muscle movement or muscle tension. Muscle tension is the result of agonist and antagonist muscles competing to maintain a limb in one position. Any time a muscle contracts, it produces an electrical current which will be detected as an **electromyographic signal (EMG)** by the ECG. An EMG is seen as narrow rapid spikes on the ECG monitor.[16]

To prevent EMG on the ECG, the patient should be positioned comfortably, in an effortless position, with arms and legs supported by the stretcher. In some cases, it may be more prudent for the Paramedic to perform the ECG on the patient's bed or couch rather than the stretcher because the patient's arms hang off the stretcher. Folding of the arms across the chest only creates muscle tension and resultant EMG.

The other source of physiologic artifact is skin movement. Whenever the skin is stretched under an electrode, it will create an epidermal signal. For example, when a patient inhales and exhales, the movement of the skin will create baseline shifts (wandering baseline) as the electrodes move along with the chest wall. To prevent epidermal signal interference, it is important to properly place the electrodes on the patient's chest away from the thoracic cage.

An example of a nonphysiologic source of ECG artifact is **electromagnetic interference (EMI)**. Whenever alternating current (AC) electricity passes through a wire, it produces an electromagnetic field. Therefore, whenever a 12-lead ECG monitor is in the vicinity of a wire carrying AC electricity, the monitor will pick up the electromagnetic field as 60-cycle interference. An example of common sources of 60-cycle EMI are florescent lights, particularly those with a malfunctioning ballast, and poorly shielded ambulance convertors. Visually, 60-cycle EMI will present on the 12-lead ECG as a fuzzy baseline.

Static electricity can also produce artifact on the ECG. The patient may build up an electrical charge (static electricity). When the patient, as the charged body, is in proximity of an uncharged body, such as the ECG monitor, then electricity will pass between the two and be recorded on the ECG. This occurs frequently in dry climates.

One of the more common sources of artifact is electrode failure. Since the outer layer of skin is electrically "dead," an electrical signal cannot be transmitted across the skin without a conductive medium to act as a bridge between the inner body and the electrode. The typical ECG electrode uses silver chloride as the conductive medium. When a metal, such as silver chloride, is placed next to an electrolyte solution (i.e., the interstitial fluid), then an electromagnetic force is created and an electromagnetic "signal" is sent to the ECG monitor.

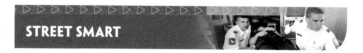

STREET SMART

Most 12-lead ECG cables are covered, or shielded, to prevent the monitor from picking up extraneous 60-cycle EMI. The presence of 60-cycle EMI on the monitor is a sign of either a defective cable or a broken lead.

If the skin is not properly prepared, then the skin can create an impedance to this signal of approximately 100,000 to 200,000 ohms. Simple site preparation can reduce the skin's impedance to less than 10,000 ohms in 90% of patients and thereby markedly improve the quality of the ECG signal.

Patient Preparation

To prevent EMG interference, the Paramedic should first place the patient in a comfortable position. Preferably, the patient should be supine with arms at the sides and the entire body supported. If the patient is not relaxed, because of a painful condition such as arthritis, then the Paramedic might consider using analgesia or sedatives.

The Paramedic should then prepare the skin before applying the electrodes. If the patient's chest hair interferes with the Paramedic's attempts to closely adhere the electrodes to the skin, then the chest hair needs to be removed. While it might be expeditious to use a straight razor to remove the hair, shaving the chest can create microlacerations that can bleed if the patient is given fibrinolytics later. Also, the hair follicles can become infected (folliculitis). The patient's chest hair should be carefully trimmed using either a commercially available clipper or a pair of blunt tipped bandage scissors.

STREET SMART

If the patient is grossly diaphoretic, some Paramedics have used antiperspirants to dry the area. These antiperspirants often contain aluminum oxide as an active agent. Aluminum oxide interferes with the electrical signal and will reduce the quality of the 12-lead ECG.

While wiping the contact surface with a gauze pad will reduce the pickup of 60 Hz EMI and motion artifact, it will only reduce the skin's resistance by 1,000 to 5,000 ohms. It is important to not only remove the dead cells of the stratum corneum but to also scratch the lower stratum granulosum.[17]

Scratching the stratum granulosum improves the ECG signal by allowing the electrode gel to permeate the skin and contact the electrolyte solution (i.e., interstitial fluid). Typically, either fine weight sandpaper (220 to 3,400 grit) or a commercially available gritty ECG preparation gel is used. Five to ten strokes of either a gel-soaked gauze pad or sandpaper is sufficient. The skin should be slightly reddened but not abraded.

The area immediately surrounding the electrode contact should be cleansed with an alcohol-soaked preparation pad. The alcohol helps to remove surface fats which can undermine the electrode's adhesive and prevent close skin contact with the electrode's gel.

It is important that the gel on the electrode be moist. Most electrodes come prepackaged and have an expiration date. The Paramedic should first confirm that the electrodes are not expired before proceeding. Next, the Paramedic should remove the electrode from the package and remove the plastic protective cover over the gel. With one finger, the Paramedic should gently compress the gel. Moist electrode gel should have a little spring when gently compressed. Dried electrode gel will be stiff and unyielding. Dried electrodes should be discarded immediately as they are of no practical use.

After confirming that the gel on the electrode is still moist, the lead wire should be attached to the electrode. The gel under the electrode is formed into a pod so that the gel stays concentrated in an area when the electrode is then placed on the skin. If the electrode is placed on the skin first and then the lead wire is attached, the pressure from attaching the lead wire can crush the pod, disperse the gel, and diminish the signal quality.

Electrode Placement

Accurate electrode placement is important. In some cases, the prehospital 12-lead ECG may not display ischemic changes. However, when serial ECGs obtained later are compared against the initial 12-lead ECG, the differences become apparent. These comparisons are only valid if the electrodes have been placed in the same position.

The American Heart Association emphasized proper lead placement in 1938 when it first standardized the placement of precordial leads. It continues to establish the standard for electrode placement in order to obtain a clinically relevant 12-lead ECG.[18]

Standard Limb Leads

Limb leads are traditionally placed where Einthoven placed them—on the end of the extremities. One electrode should be placed on the ventral surface of the right and the left wrist and another placed on the ankle proximal to the medial malleolus.

The electrode should be placed on the properly prepared skin overlying muscle, not bone. The resulting leads—Lead I, Lead II, and Lead III—are therefore a function of the polarity ascribed to them by the ECG monitor. Often these electrode wires are labeled for ease of application.

While technically correct, the placement of electrodes on the ankles and wrists of the patient is often mechanically inconvenient. Problems with resting tremors and clothing prevent the Paramedic from obtaining an accurate 12-lead ECG. This distortion can be minimized if the electrodes are moved more centrally. In 1966, Mason and Likar suggested moving the electrodes to the shoulders and the hip. To properly place the limb electrodes in the **Mason–Likar modification**, the right arm electrode is moved to the right infraclavicular fossa, approximately 2 cm below the clavicle. The left arm electrode is similarly placed in the left infraclavicular fossa, and the left leg electrode is moved next to the left iliac crest in the iliac fossa. This placement of the limb leads maintains the integrity of Einthoven's Triangle without the inconvenience of distal limb lead electrodes.

Because the ECG machine electrically converts the bipolar limb leads into unipolar augmented leads using the same leads and electrodes, it is unnecessary to add additional electrodes for the augmented leads.

Precordial Leads

Wilson's precordial leads measure the ECG potentials across the anterior wall of the left ventricle. Precordial leads are to be placed according to specific landmarks. Variation in the placement of precordial electrodes can sometimes produce diagnostically significant changes in the 12-lead ECG.

The first electrodes, V1 and V2, are placed within the 4th intercostal space at the right and left sternal border, respectively. Mistakenly, Paramedics may palpate the space just below the clavicle, assume it is the 1st intercostal space, and start counting down three more spaces. This placement is incorrect and will cause V1 and V2 to be placed too high.

The Paramedic should first identify the suprasternal notch above the sternum and palpate inferiorly until a ridge is felt. The ridge on the bone is the connection of the manubrium to the body of the sternum (the angle of Louis). Moving laterally to the right, the Paramedic should palpate the second intercostal space along the sternal border and then palpate the spaces downward until the 4th intercostal space is palpated.

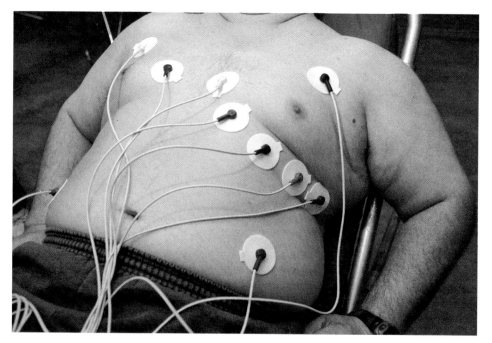

Figure 34-5 Precordial electrode placement.

The first precordial electrode, V1, is placed on the right sternal border and V2 is placed across from V1 at the same level on the left sternal border.

From the V2 position, the Paramedic should palpate the 5th intercostal space and move laterally to the midclavicular line to place the V4, the third electrode. The fourth electrode placed is V3, which is placed midpoint along an imaginary line that runs between V2 and V4.

Continuing to palpate along the 5th intercostal space, the Paramedic should place V5 at the left anterior axillary line, in line with the iliac crest, and V6 at the 5th intercostal space along the left midaxillary line (Figure 34-5 and Table 34-1).

If the patient has large breasts, male or female, place V4 under the breast and V3 over the breast. The V4 electrode should be placed flat against the chest and not partially on the breast and the chest. This position would cause the electrode to fold over on itself and will not sense the electrical activity. If the patient is small or thin, then place the electrodes between the ribs, avoiding the bony prominences, if possible.

Table 34-1 Lead Names with Correct Electrode Placement

LA	Left arm over muscle or flesh
RA	Right arm over muscle or flesh
LL	Left leg over muscle or flesh
RL	Right leg over muscle or flesh
V1	4th ICS RSB, 4th right intercostal space at the sternal border
V2	4th ICS LSB, 4th left intercostal space at the sternal border
V3	Between V2 and V4
V4	5th ICS MCL, 5th left intercostal space at the midclavicular line
V5	5th ICS LAAL, 5th left intercostal space at the anterior axillary line
V6	5th ICS LMAL, 5th left intercostal space at the midaxillary line

The Paramedic should document if it is necessary to perform the 12-lead ECG on a patient in a semirecumbent position, such as in a wheelchair or recliner. The patient's change in position from Fowler's position, at a 45-degree angle, causes the heart to swing anterior and closer to the chest wall.

Dextrocardia

Some patients have a congenital condition in which the body's organs are mirror opposite of normal. **Situs inversus**, which is a complete reversal of all thoracoabdominal organs, occurs in less than 1 in 10,000 patients but has been a documented medical phenomenon since 1643. If the heart and lungs are opposite and the abdominal organs are in their usual position, this is referred to as **dextrocardia**.[19]

When the Paramedic initially places the patient on the monitor to determine a rhythm, it will be noted that Lead I is inverted. An inversion in Lead I is suggestive of dextrocardia. A standard 12-lead ECG will support the diagnosis. The patient with dextrocardia will have a P wave axis greater than 90 degrees and a poor R wave progression, both discussed shortly.[20]

If dextrocardia is suspected, or the patient confirms dextrocardia, then the Paramedic should proceed by placing the electrodes on the right side of the thorax. The Paramedic should make a note on the 12-lead ECG printout that dextrocardia is suspected and right-sided chest leads were placed.

12-Lead ECG Tracing

Before reading a 12-lead ECG the Paramedic must understand the standard layout of the printout. Like a rhythm, a 12-lead ECG is never read off the monitor screen but instead is printed out for careful analysis.

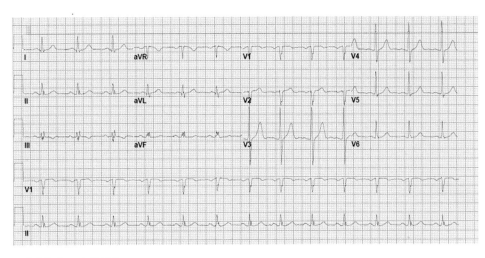

Figure 34-6 Normal 12-lead ECG.

A 12-lead ECG is printed in a standard four-column format. The 12-lead ECG machine reads three leads simultaneously for 2.5 to 3 seconds until all 12 leads are obtained and then prints out the 12-lead ECG.

Beginning on the far left column, the printout contains the standard limb leads I, II, and III. The 12-lead ECG machine then uses the limb leads and, with the creation of Wilson's central terminal, creates the augmented leads, aVR, aVL, and aVF.

Moving from the limb leads to the precordial leads, the 12-lead ECG machine reads and records the precordial leads, starting with V1, V2, and V3, then reads and records V4, V5, and V6 (Figure 34-6).

In some instances, the 12-lead ECG machine will simultaneously record both the 12-lead ECG and the monitor lead and a single monitoring strip may be printed across the bottom. Although most machines will default to Lead II for the monitoring strip, the Paramedic may choose to record a different lead depending upon the patient's condition.

> **STREET SMART**
>
> Some older 12-lead ECG machines can only print a single lead at a time. These machines, called single-channel machines, print the 12-lead ECG in the same sequence but in one very long ECG strip.

Electrocardiographic Assessment of Left Ventricular Function

The left ventricle is essential for cardiac output to the body (in general) and to the brain (in particular). All other portions of the heart (the atriums and the right ventricle) could be considered auxiliary to the left ventricle. In fact, loss of any one of these auxiliary portions of the heart is survivable, whereas loss of the left ventricle is usually fatal. For this reason, the 12-lead ECG focuses on the left ventricle.

For ease of conceptualization, the left ventricle is said to have four walls. It is actually a cone-like shape with artificially contrived sides. The lower portion of the left ventricle, next to the epigastrium, is called the inferior wall. The portion of the left ventricle that is shared with the right ventricle (the septum) is called the septal wall. That foremost portion of the left ventricle, where the bulk of the myocardium exists, is called the anterior wall. The last wall, the lateral wall, is actually an extension of the left ventricle's anterior wall.

Contiguous Leads

An ECG lead gives the Paramedic a view of a particular portion of the left ventricle. The 12-lead ECG allows the Paramedic to have several views of the heart in an effort to try and capture evidence of myocardial injury. When two or more leads look at the same wall of the left ventricle, they are said to be **contiguous leads**.

ECG leads are related to each other by the position of the positive electrode which, in turn, affords a specific view of a particular portion of the ventricle. In the standard 12-lead ECG, the limb leads II, III, and the augmented lead, aVF, the positive electrode is located on the lower extremity and looks up toward the bottom of the heart. The bottom of the heart is a portion of the left ventricle called the inferior wall. Thus, these leads (II and aVG) are called inferior leads and can be said to be contiguous.

Leads I, aVL, V5, and V6 have the positive electrode located on or beneath the left arm. These leads look at the heart's lateral wall and are called lateral leads. Similarly, leads V1 through V4 have the positive electrode on the front of the chest. These leads look at the front portion or anterior wall of the left ventricle. The front of the chest is a large area. Thus, these leads are broken into subcategories. V1 and V2 have the positive electrode over the interventricular septum and are also referred to as septal leads. V3 and V4 continue to be known as true anterior leads.

In some cases, the evidence of myocardial damage spreads across two walls of the left ventricle. In those cases, both walls are used in the description. For example, injury

Table 34-2 Contiguous Leads

- Pure changes
  - II, III, aVF   = Inferior
  - V1, V2   = Septal
  - V3, V4, V5   = Anterior
  - I, aVL, V5, V6   = Lateral
- Mixed changes
  - V1, V2, V3, V4   = Anteroseptal
  - I, II, III, aVL, aVF, V5, V6 = Inferolateral
  - I, aVL, V3, V4, V5, V6 = Anterolateral
  - II, III, aVF, V1, V2   = Inferoseptal
- Global changes
  - V1, V2, V3, V4, V5, V6 = Global anterior
  - I, II, III, aVL, aVF, aVR,
  - V1, V2, V3, V4, V5, V6 = Global

to both the anterior wall and the septal wall, as evidenced by ECG changes in the contiguous leads V1, V2, V3, and V4, would be referred to as anteroseptal. Similarly, myocardial damage to both the inferior and the lateral wall, as evidenced by ECG changes in Leads I, II, III, aVL, aVF, V5, and V6 would be called inferolateral. If there are changes suggestive of damage to the entire myocardium (i.e., ECG changes in all leads), then the term "global" is used. ECG changes in only two contiguous leads are necessary to make a presumption of myocardial injury (Table 34-2).

STREET SMART

When a Paramedic sees global changes across all of the 12-leads, consideration should first be given to extra-cardiac causes (i.e., those conditions, such as hypoxia, that could lead to damage to the entire heart).[21–23] The likelihood that all of the coronary arteries could have a catastrophic event simultaneously is extremely unlikely.

Relationship to Coronary Arteries

The main coronary arteries perfuse specific areas of the heart and, in particular, the left ventricle. By evaluating the 12-lead ECG for evidence of myocardial injury in the contiguous leads, the Paramedic can infer that ECG changes in those contiguous leads raises a suspicion of involvement of specific coronary arteries.

The coronary arteries originate at the sinus of Valsalva and proximal to the aortic valve, with which they have a symbiotic relationship. There are two coronary arteries which are simply called the right coronary artery and the left coronary

artery. The right coronary artery (RCA) runs the length of the heart and has a minor branch, called the marginal branch, towards its terminus. Conversely, the left coronary artery (LCA) divides almost immediately at its mainstem into the left anterior descending coronary artery (LAD) and the circumflex (Cx).

The right coronary artery (RCA) provides blood to the inferior wall of the left ventricle and to the AV node in the majority of patients. Thus, ECG changes in the inferior leads of II, III, and/or aVF would suggest that the RCA may be involved.

The left main coronary artery serves the entire anterior wall including the septum. Occlusions of the left main stem, referred to as "widow makers" (thus emphasizing the importance of the LCA), can cause global anterior wall damage. ECG changes in the anterior leads of V1 to V4 and the lateral leads of I, aVL, V5, and V6 suggest that the LCA is affected.

The LCA almost immediately bifurcates, giving rise to the left anterior descending (LAD) coronary artery and the circumflex coronary artery (Cx). The LAD artery serves the central portion of the anterior wall of the left ventricle. Therefore, anterior wall ECG changes would be expected (V3 and V4).

Lesser branches off the LAD, called the septal perforators (SP), provide the septum with blood, including the bundle branches. Atherosclerotic involvement of the SP will injure the septum and may cause ECG changes in leads V1 and V2 and possible bundle branch blocks.

The LAD then continues to run along the anterior interventricular (AIV) groove which separates the right and left ventricles toward the apex of the heart. Along its path another minor branch of the LAD, which cuts diagonally away from the AIV and toward the anterolateral wall and the apex of the heart, is the diagonal (Dx). Distal occlusions of the Dx can give rise to ECG changes in leads I, aVL, V5, and V6 as well as V4 and V5.

The circumflex coronary artery (Cx) was the second artery at the bifurcation of the left coronary artery. The Cx follows the atrioventricular groove to the lateral wall of the left ventricle. In most cases (approximately 85% of patients), the Cx stops at the left lateral wall. In 15% of patients, the Cx continues and provides perfusion to the AV node. Normally blood for the AV node comes from the right coronary artery. In those cases, the patient is said to be "left dominant," indicating an alternative blood supply to the AV node as opposed to the normal blood supply. The difficulty for the patient who is left dominant arises when an occlusion of the left coronary artery occurs and almost the total of the left ventricle's myocardium is hypoperfused (Figure 34-7 and Table 34-3).

Interpretation

The primary value of a Paramedic-obtained 12-lead ECG in the field is the identification of myocardial injury and the patient's transportation to the definitive care center. However, the value in a 12-lead ECG is not only in the identification of myocardial injury but also in the Paramedic's ability to make a prognosis based on that information. By

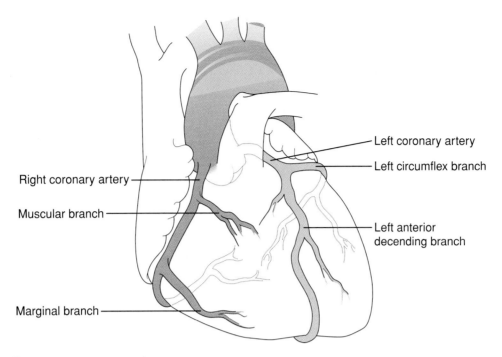

Figure 34-7 Coronary artery anatomy.

Table 34-3 Relationship of Leads to Walls to Coronary Arteries

• II, III, aVF	= Inferior	Right coronary artery (RCA)
• V1, V2	= Anteroseptal	Left anterior descending (LAD)/(SP)
• V3, V4	= Anterior	Left anterior descending (LAD)
• V3, V4, V5, V6	= Anterolateral	Diagonal (Dx)
• I , aVL, V5, V6	= Lateral	Circumflex (Cx)
• V1, V2, V3, V4, V5, V6	= Global anterior	Left mainstem (LCA)

having information about the location of the myocardial injury, the Paramedic can prepare for complications associated with that injury.

12-Lead ECG Identification of Myocardial Injury

The era of the ECG identification of acute myocardial infarction may have started with Harold Pardee when he published the first ECG of an acute myocardial infarction, describing the T wave as "tall" and "starts from a point well up in the descent of the R wave." From that point, physicians have had a keen interest in using the 12-lead ECG to identify the patient with acute coronary syndrome who is at risk for an acute myocardial infarction.

Normal Depolarization and Repolarization

Normal ventricular depolarization begins with the onset of the QRS complex. The first negative deflection, called a Q wave, represents the depolarization of the septum.

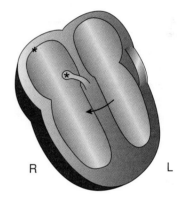

Septal activation from left to right

Figure 34-8 Septal depolarization.

A Q wave is not always visible in every patient, nor is it seen in every lead (Figure 34-8). The presence of a small Q wave, called a physiologic Q wave, is normal.[24]

Following the depolarization of the septum, ventricular depolarization occurs. Normally, ventricular depolarization proceeds from the endocardium outward to the epicardium (Figure 34-9). The specific wave pattern (i.e., rS, Rs, etc.) is a function of the electrode's placement. For example, since the energy is going away from V1, the QRS deflection should be negative. The energy is going toward V6 and the QRS deflection in V6 should be primarily positive.

Normally the segment between the QRS and the T wave, called the ST segment, is isoelectric as the Purkinje fibers start to repolarize (Figure 34-10).

Ventricular repolarization is represented by the T wave. In a reverse process, normal repolarization begins at the epicardial surface and progresses through the ventricular walls to the endocardium. The process of repolarization involves

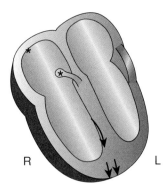

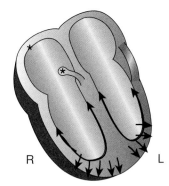

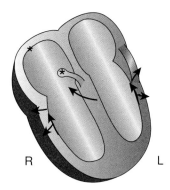

Activation of anteroseptal region of the ventricular myocardium

Activation of major portion of ventricular myocardium from endocardial to epicardial surfaces

Late activation of posterobasal portion of the left ventricle, the pulmonary conus, and the uppermost portion of the interventricular septum

Figure 34-9 Ventricular depolarization.

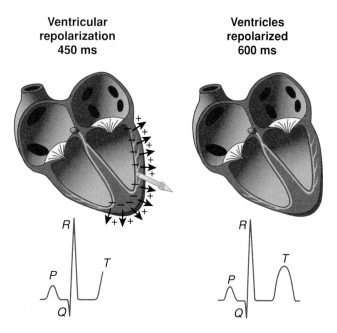

Figure 34-10 Ventricular repolarization.

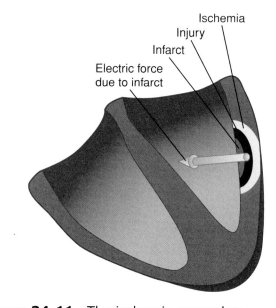

Figure 34-11 The ischemic penumbra.

resuming a negative interior of the cell compared to the outside. The combination of the interior of the cell becoming more negative while moving away from the positive electrode results in a positive deflection on the screen. The T wave representing ventricular repolarization is positive or upright in all leads except aVR.

Ischemic Patterns

A healthy myocardial cell requires oxygen, glucose, and a balance of electrolytes in order to function (i.e., to depolarize, then repolarize). Abnormal depolarization/repolarization occurs whenever the myocardial cells lack these essential conditions. The most common cause of myocardial dysfunction is acute occlusion of the coronary arteries.

As a result of this occlusion, and subsequent hypoxia, the myocardial cells go through a predictable pathway to

cell necrosis and myocardial infarction called **penumbra** (Figure 34-11). The cellular changes that occur during penumbra can be witnessed by the Paramedic as changes in the ECG. These **ischemic patterns** are the result of abnormal repolarization.

There are three successive stages before myocardial cell death: ischemia, injury, and infarction. These stages are evolutionary and affect tissues incrementally, spreading out from a central point in a bull's eye fashion. They can be described as the three "I's" of acute coronary syndrome (ACS).

Ischemia

The first change is **myocardial ischemia**. During the ischemic phase, myocardial cells are deprived of oxygen and hypoxia ensues. During this phase, the myocardial cells convert to anaerobic metabolism to conserve energy. This

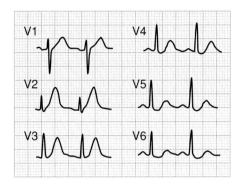

Figure 34-12 Hyperacute T waves.

decreased cellular activity slows myocardial repolarization. As coronary perfusion occurs from the surface (or epicardium) inwardly, the deeper myocardial tissues become ischemic first. This limited ischemic involvement is called **subendocardial ischemia**. This slowing of repolarization does not alter the direction of repolarization; therefore, the ECG will appear normal, but it does lengthen the time for repolarization. Accordingly, the first manifestation of myocardial ischemia can be a lengthening QT interval.

As the cell's sodium–potassium pump starts to falter, due to insufficient ATP, potassium leaks from the cell. The leaking potassium causes an increase in the amplitude of the T waves, called a **hyperacute T wave**, in the leads facing the damage (Figure 34-12).

Transmural ischemia occurs as the ischemia reaches the point where it affects the entire thickness of the myocardium, from the endocardium to the epicardium. Then, the deeper myocardial cells begin to malfunction.

Normally, when repolarization occurs, the polarity changes as potassium is pumped back into the cell. This reverses the current. Repolarization results in an upright T wave on the ECG.

However, when the ischemic endocardial cells deeper in the myocardium fail to repolarize, the result is a loss of the change in direction of polarity which normally occurs during repolarization. This failure to change in direction causes a negative deflection in the T wave. Without repolarization and the subsequent negative polarity of the myocardium, the normally upright T waves become inverted in the ECG leads that overlay the ischemic area. In some cases, **inverted T waves** will be one of the first electrocardiographic changes that the Paramedic will observe.

Injury

The persistent hypoxia causes the myocardial cells to change from ischemia to injury. The faltering sodium–potassium pump of the injured myocardial cells can no longer maintain polarization and the cell becomes electrically inert. At first the injured endocardial cells tend to draw the ST segment downward (**ST-segment depression**). An ST segment, by definition, is a >1 mm depression below the J point from iso-electric baseline. To decide if the ST segment is depressed, the Paramedic must first ascertain the J point.

J Point

To decide if an ST segment is depressed or elevated, the Paramedic starts by identifying the **J point**. The J point is the start of the ST segment and is found at the juncture of the QRS and the ST segment, the point where the angle from the QRS changes. To find the J point, the Paramedic starts at the beginning of the P wave and draws a straight line across to where it crosses the T wave. If any portion of the ST segment is below that line, then there is ST-segment depression. If any portion of the ST segment is above this line, there is an ST-segment elevation. If the Paramedic is unable to find the beginning of the P wave, then the line is drawn from the bottom of the calibration wave straight across.

ST-Segment Elevation

As the injury continues and becomes full thickness (transmural), the ST segment starts to rise (**ST-segment elevation**). Myocardial injury, as manifested by ST-segment elevation in the ECG leads overlying the area, generally occurs after 20 to 40 minutes of ischemia.[25] Some examples of ST-segment elevations in the anterior leads include some "tombstone" elevations in V2, V3, and V4 (Figure 34-13).

Patterns of Ischemia and Penumbra

At this point, the Paramedic may see a complex picture of T wave inversions, ST-segment depressions, as well as ST elevations. These markings represent the process of ischemia and are manifestations of penumbra. The key is to focus on those leads that indicate the greatest degree of damage. The other ECG changes should radiate away from the location of the primary event.

Infarction

Without oxygen, the myocardial cells eventually die (**myocardial infarction**), and the area begins **necrosis**, a physiologic process in which dead cells are removed and new cell growth may occur. The ECG hallmark of this change is the development of pathologic **Q waves**. Pathologic Q waves indicate electrical silence (i.e., no depolarization)

STREET SMART

It is estimated that in some 50% of initial ECGs taken on patient's with cardiac related chest pain, the Paramedic may not see ST-segment elevations with the initial 12-lead ECG because the event has not evolved to that level. Nevertheless, it is important to obtain a baseline ECG for later analysis, particularly for QT intervals and T wave changes.

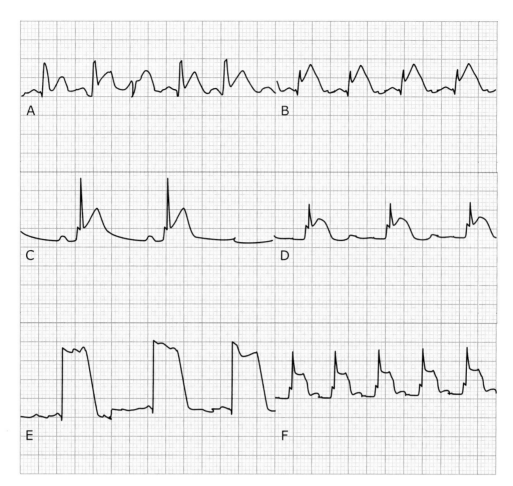

Figure 34-13 ST-segment elevation due to acute MI tracings. A and B show oblique straightening; C and D show a concave upward appearance; E and F show a more horizontal or flattened ST appearance.

in that portion of the ventricular wall. Because that portion of the ventricular wall is electrically silent, the depolarization in the opposite wall, going away from the electrodes in that lead, is the only signal present. It is recorded as a negative deflection on the ECG.

Q waves can also represent the depolarization of the intraventricular septum. As the septum depolarizes from left to right, any leads that are looking from the left (i.e., the lateral leads I, V5, and V6) will show a negative deflection. These physiologic or septal Q waves are normal (Figure 34-14).

While some Q waves are normal (physiologic), the Q waves associated with infarction (pathologic Q waves) are deep (greater than 25% of the R wave) and wide (typically 0.04 seconds). These characteristics, and the presence of Q waves in contiguous leads, suggests pathology and infarction.[26]

The presence of a Q wave in a 12-lead ECG is confirmation that the patient has had a transmural myocardial infarction. Q waves can remain for years, alerting the Paramedic to the presence of an acute myocardial infarction (AMI) in the past. In up to 30% of 12-lead ECGs with Q waves,

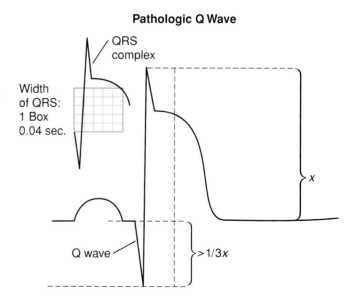

Pathologic Q Wave

A significant Q wave should be:
1. One-third height of QRS complex
2. 0.04 second (one small box wide) in duration

Figure 34-14 Q waves.

An isolated pathologic Q wave in Lead III may be a normal finding and is not indicative of an inferior wall AMI unless it is accompanied by other ECG changes in the contiguous leads II and aVF.

the Q waves resolve, especially in the inferior wall, within one year.[27]

Electrocardiographic Diagnosis of Acute Myocardial Infarction

To make an electrocardiographic diagnosis of acute myocardial infarction, the Paramedic looks for hyperacute T waves, T wave inversions, ST-segment depressions, and ST-segment elevations as well as Q waves in all leads. When a pattern of ischemia is noted (ECG changes in contiguous leads), then the Paramedic may have a high index of suspicion that the artery which perfuses the corresponding wall is occluded.[28]

The presence of Q waves in the face of concomitant ST elevation speaks to the evolution of the infarction and may indicate that this MI has been in progress for several hours (Figure 34-15). However, the presence of ST elevations indicates that there may be myocardium that can be salvaged with thrombolytic therapy or interventional cardiology.

Reciprocal Changes

Supporting evidence of an acute myocardial infarction in progress are reciprocal changes. **Reciprocal changes** are ST-segment depressions seen on the 12-lead ECG in leads that face the wall opposite of those with ST-segment elevations. Reciprocal changes are more commonly seen in inferior wall AMI (approximately 70%) versus anterior wall AMI (about 30%).[29,30] The presence of reciprocal changes is an excellent marker of acute myocardial infarction in progress and has a positive predictive value of 90%.

The ST-segment depression of reciprocal changes is thought to be due to "mirror reflections" of the electrical signal from the affected wall. The ST-segment depression seen in a reciprocal change is more downsloping than those caused early in an AMI and is typically seen when the AMI is large.

As an example of the predictive value of reciprocal changes, ST depression in leads V1, V2, V3, and V4 (all anterior leads) suggests an acute myocardial infarction in evolution in the posterior wall and an occlusion of the circumflex artery (Cx) (Table 34-4).

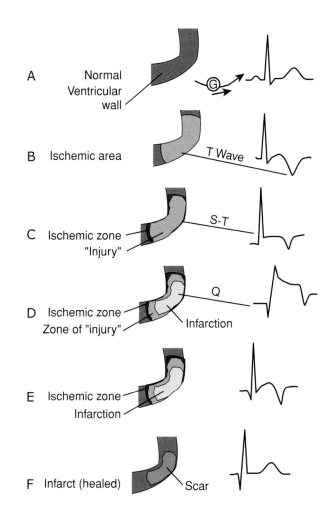

Figure 34-15 Wave changes during evolution of myocardial damage.

Table 34-4 Reciprocal Changes

Wall	Artery Lead	Reciprocal Wall	Reciprocal Leads
Inferior	RCA II, II, aVF	Lateral	I, aVL
Anterior	LAD V3, V4	Inferior	II, III, aVF
Lateral	Cx I, aVL, V5, V6	Inferior	II, III, aVF

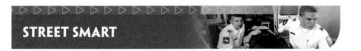

ST depressions seen in reciprocal changes can be helpful in distinguishing infarction from the normal variants in African American males who have ST elevations.

R Wave Progression

In a normal 12-lead ECG, there is a series of changes in the primary deflection of the QRS from negative in V1 to positive in V6, called an **R wave progression**, in the precordial leads. Starting with the deep S wave in V1, the deflection in the precordial leads gradually changes direction, with a transition at approximately V3 or V4, until V6, where there is a tall R wave.

Whenever there is an electrical disturbance in the anterior wall, secondary to ischemia, then the R wave progression is disturbed (specifically when there is a loss of R waves in the anterior precordial leads). The loss of an R wave progression, sometimes called a **reverse R wave progression**, is suggestive of an anterior wall AMI.

If the transition occurs early (i.e., before V3), it may be indicative of a posterior wall AMI. The Paramedic may then want to consider obtaining leads V7, V8, and V9 (discussed later). If the transient occurs later, after V4, it can be suggestive of an anterior wall AMI. However, a late transition can also occur if the patient has a thick chest or has respiratory disease, particularly if there are small R waves in the right precordial leads, or may be a normal variant in some women.

STREET SMART

Some Paramedics may use the term "poor R wave progression." The American Heart Association prefers the term "reverse R wave progression" instead. It should be noted that improper lead placement can cause a reverse R wave progression.

The isolated appearance of a reverse R wave progression (RRWP) should not be taken to mean that the patient is having an anterior wall AMI. There are other causes of RRWP which include a pre-existing left bundle branch block, dextrocardia, and Wolff–Parkinson–White (WPW) syndrome. Nevertheless, the presence of a reverse R wave progression, coupled with a good history for ACS and other 12-lead ECG changes in the anterior leads, is helpful in diagnosing an anterior wall AMI.

New Onset Left Bundle Branch Block

A left bundle branch block (LBBB) (Figure 34-16) is a partial heart block (when the impulse fails to be conducted) which involves one or both the left fascicles of the left bundle. As a result, the ventricular wall of the affected side must be depolarized by a wave front from the opposite side. This delay in depolarization prolongs the QRS to greater than 0.14 seconds for a left bundle branch and a small narrow R wave (less than 0.04 seconds) in all leads. The Paramedic

may also observe that the T wave is opposite in deflection to the QRS in all precordial leads, as well as a notching in the anterolateral leads.

The characteristic appearance of a notched QRS in V6 (i.e., RsR') is the result of the electrical impulse crossing the right bundle branch, depolarizing the right ventricle, then crossing the interventricular septum to depolarize the left ventricle.

A common cause of an LBBB is occlusion of either the left anterior descending (LAD) coronary artery or one of the septal perforators which branch from the LAD. These coronary arteries perfuse the septum and the bundle branches that lie within.

Because of the delayed repolarization, the ST segment of the septal leads will be elevated and the 12-lead ECG will have the appearance of an anterior wall AMI (AWMI). However, there are a number of benign conditions, including advanced age and hypertension, that can also cause an LBBB.[31]

In some cases, because of advanced atherosclerotic disease, the patient may experience a rate-related bundle branch block. These blocks occur because the bundle branches are incapable of repolarizing, secondary to decreased perfusion, at faster rates. Because of slower conduction, there is reduced strength of contraction and the patient may experience heart failure.

STREET SMART

Whenever an LBBB occurs, the patient is at risk of heart failure. Therefore, the administration of any Vaughn-Williams Class 1 drugs (i.e., lidocaine or procainamide) can slow conduction even further, leading to worsened heart failure and even to drug-induced complete heart block.

Typically, the altered electrical pathway associated with LBBB makes the ECG diagnosis of AMI complicated. Therefore, if a Paramedic observes an LBBB on initial 12-lead ECG, no further interpretation is possible because a diagnosis of AMI by ECG cannot be made with confidence. However, the presence of a new onset LBBB during the course of patient care is an ECG finding highly suggestive of an AMI.

The Paramedic should report the appearance of a new onset LBBB and, coupled with a patient history suggestive of ACS, have a high index of suspicion that the patient is having an AMI.[32–34] Patients with a new onset LBBB have a worse prognosis for their AMI compared to those without the conduction delay. Because of the prolonged conduction, and the resultant decreased inotropy, a patient with an LBBB may experience as much as a 25% loss of cardiac output. Paramedics should treat new onset LBBB more aggressively, with a keen eye on the development of heart failure.

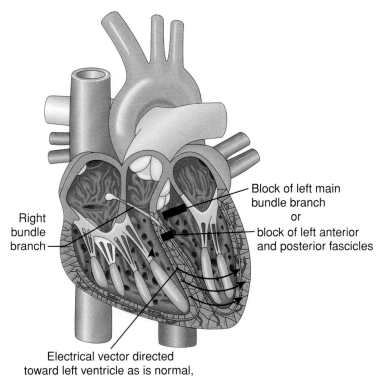

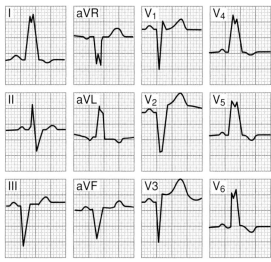

Wide QRS complex prolonged (≥ 0.12 second). with ST depressions and inverted T waves, particularly in leads I, aVL, V₅ and V₆

Figure 34-16 Left bundle branch block.

Right Bundle Branch Block

A right bundle branch block (RBBB) is a type of heart block in which the impulse fails to be conducted down the right bundle of the bundle of His. In a RBBB, the impulse travels rapidly to depolarize the interventricular septum and down the left bundle branch to activate the left ventricle. Since the right bundle branch is blocked, the impulse must cross the interventricular septum to activate the right ventricle. Because it takes more time to depolarize the entire ventricle, the QRS is greater than 0.12 seconds in width.

The ECG diagnosis of RBBB is also supported by a small terminal R wave in V1 and a slurring of the S wave in the lateral leads (i.e., Lead I and V6). The T wave in V1 will also be in the opposite deflection of the QRS.

A RBBB is one of the most common defects in ventricular conduction (Figure 34-17). RBBB occurs often, and without apparent cause, in normal hearts. Treatment is directed at the cause of the conduction defect, which can include myocardial infarction (MI) or ischemia, heart failure, pulmonary embolism, or valvular disease.

Nondiagnostic ECG

In some cases, the patient may have a benign 12-lead ECG. The absence of patterns of ischemia on a 12-lead ECG does not preclude the diagnosis of an AMI. When the 12-lead ECG is nondiagnostic, the Paramedic should maintain a high index of suspicion based on the patient's clinical presentation and, more specifically, the history of present illness.

In some cases, the diagnosis of AMI on 12-lead ECG is missed because of the low amplitude of the QRS. When the amplitude of the QRS is less than 5 mm in the standard limb leads (i.e., low amplitude QRS), an assessment of ST-segment change is nearly impossible. Causes of low voltage, resulting in a low amplitude QRS, include pericardial effusions leading to constructive pericarditis, pleural effusions, and obesity.[35–37]

Electrical Alternans

When every other ECG complex has alternating amplitude (i.e., the one QRS complex is smaller when compared to the next), then the patient may have **electrical alternans**. Electrical alternans is more frequently seen in the precordial leads and is a sign of pericardial effusion.

The alternating amplitude of the QRS is thought to be the result of the heart swinging, in a pendulum fashion, from the wave created in the pericardium as the heart beats within the accumulation of fluid.

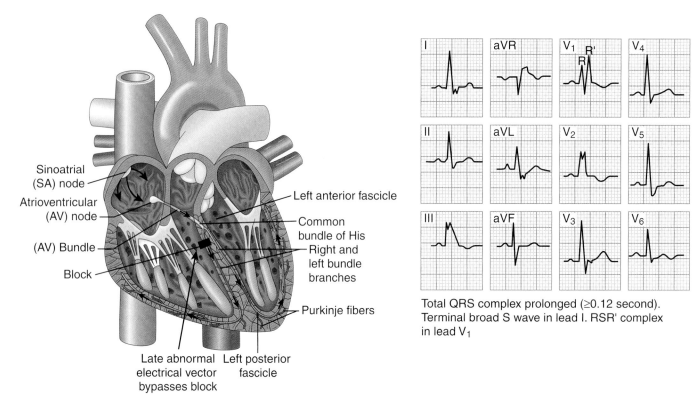

Total QRS complex prolonged (≥0.12 second).
Terminal broad S wave in lead I. RSR' complex
in lead V_1

Figure 34-17 Right bundle branch block.

Alternative Etiologies for ECG Abnormalities

The Paramedic should keep an open mind when reading a 12-lead ECG for alternative causes of prolonged QT intervals, T wave abnormalities, and ST-segment elevations. Although these aberrant changes do not typically mimic the pattern of ischemia, a quick glance could mislead a Paramedic into thinking that there is a pattern of ischemia. Careful attention to the ECG for patterns of ischemia and a disciplined approach to interpretation will yield the best results.

Prolonged QT Intervals

One of the first ECG changes which can occur as a result of anterior wall myocardial ischemia (AWMI) can be a prolonged QT interval. However, there are a host of other etiologies for prolonged QT intervals.[38,39] The majority of causes of acquired prolonged QT intervals involve electrolyte abnormalities (e.g., hypokalemia) and medications. Vaughn-Williams Class I and III drugs are the leading offenders and have been repeatedly implicated as the cause of prolonged QT intervals. Other potential offenders include psychotropic medications (particularly tricyclic antidepressants and phenothiazines), antibiotics (such as erythromycin), and toxins (such as organophosphates).[40]

In some cases, the cause of the prolonged QT interval is congenital. These patients may have presented in their youth with unexplained syncopal episodes. For this reason, any patient, regardless of age, who has an unexplained syncope should be a candidate for a 12-lead ECG.

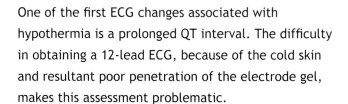

STREET SMART

One of the first ECG changes associated with hypothermia is a prolonged QT interval. The difficulty in obtaining a 12-lead ECG, because of the cold skin and resultant poor penetration of the electrode gel, makes this assessment problematic.

The length of the QT interval is inversely related to the patient's heart rate. Therefore, when calculating a patient's QT interval, it must be corrected with the heart rate. Typically, Paramedics and physicians use Bazett's formula to obtain the correct QT interval. Under emergency conditions, the QTc (corrected QT) can be derived from information on the 12-lead ECG. Alternatively, the Paramedic can take the heart rate and, for every ten (10) beats above 70, subtract 0.02 seconds from 0.40 seconds, and for every ten (10) beats below 70 add 0.02 seconds.

T Wave Abnormalities

Generally, the T wave in a normal ECG is in the same deflection as the preceding QRS in the limb leads. The normal T wave is slightly asymmetrical, with the upstroke of the leading edge of the T wave being gentle compared to the downstroke. Any deviation from those conditions would be abnormal.

T wave abnormalities can include T wave inversion, flattened or low-amplitude T waves, and peaked or hyperacute T waves. There are numerous causes for the T wave abnormalities that can be suggestive of a number of disorders (Table 34-5). With the exception of hyperkalemia, the isolated presence of a T wave abnormality is not diagnostic of any condition and requires further investigation.

Hyperacute T Waves

Hyperacute T waves are defined as T waves greater than 5 mm in the limb leads and greater than 10 mm in the precordial leads. While a peaked T wave in contiguous leads is suggestive of ischemia, hyperacute T waves in all leads is highly suggestive of hyperkalemia.[41,42] Hyperkalemia can be the result of renal failure or crush injury, or seen in cases of diabetic ketoacidosis (DKA). Conversely, flattened T waves are suggestive of hypokalemia, a deficit in serum potassium that can be the result of potassium-wasting diuretics (e.g., furosemide).

ST-Segment Abnormalities

While an ST-segment depression is suggestive of ischemia when seen in select contiguous leads, a global ST-segment depression, affecting all of the precordial leads, suggests the etiology is likely extra-cardiac (Table 34-6).

Table 34-5 Potential Causes of T Wave Abnormalities

- CNS disorders
  - Cerebrovascular accident (CVA)
  - Subarachnoid hemorrhage
- Cardiac disease
  - Mitral valve prolapse
  - Myocarditis
  - Pericarditis
  - Ventricular hypertrophy
  - Conduction disorders
    - Bundle branch block
    - Ventricular preexcitation
    - Post ventricular tachycardia
- Electrolyte disorders
  - Hyperventilation
- Pulmonary conditions
  - Pulmonary embolism
  - Pneumothorax
- Gastrointestinal conditions
  - Acute pancreatitis
  - Acute cholecystitis
- Pharmacology
  - Digitalis
  - Antidysrhythmic agents
  - Alcohol
  - Cocaine

Table 34-6 Causes of ST-Segment Depression

- Hypokalemia
- Hypothermia
- Hypertrophy–Ventricular

Medications, for example, can cause alterations in the ST segment. A classic cause of ST-segment depression is digitalis. Digitalis alters ventricular depolarization, resulting in a "ladle" appearance of the ST segment (Figure 34-18).

Other causes of ST-segment depression include subarachnoid hemorrhage and hypokalemia. Hypokalemia (serum potassium less than 2.8) will produce ST-segment depression in 80% of patients, along with flattened T waves (Figure 34-19).

Similarly, ST-segment elevation can be a normal variant, with some patients demonstrating a 1 to 2 mm ST segment rise, particularly if the ST segment has an upward concavity and/or a notch at the J point (Table 34-7). This finding is particularly common among African Americans and leaves the ST segment with a fishhook appearance.

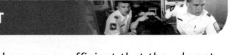

STREET SMART

Current pacemakers are so efficient that they do not leave a "foot print" (a pacer spike) on the rhythm strip. The only evidence of a pacemaker may be the slow and wide QRS as well as a slight ST-segment elevation noted in the precordial leads.

Special Case of Pericarditis

Pericarditis is an inflammation of the pericardial sac. As the pericardium surrounds the entire heart and is closely adherent to the heart's surface, inflammation of the pericardium will cause diffuse and widespread ST-segment elevation in practically all leads of a 12-lead ECG.[43]

When the ST-segment elevations appear unrelated to the pattern of ischemia seen with any specific coronary arteries, there should be a suspicion of pericarditis. Further assessment, including auscultation for a pericardial rub and an assessment of the chest pain while lying and seated, are in order.

Table 34-7 Etiologies of Normal ST-Segment Elevation

- Therapeutic digoxin
- Pre-excitation syndromes
  - WPW
  - LGL
- Early repolarization syndromes (Congenital)
  - Brugada syndrome

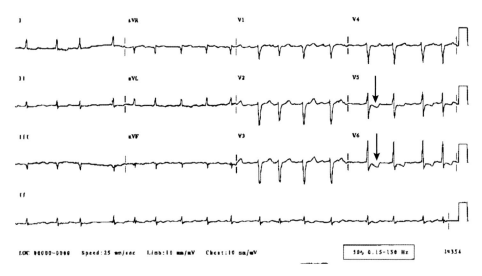

Figure 34-18 Digitalis effect on the ST segment.

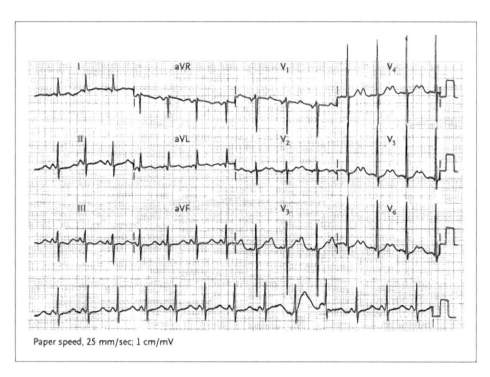

Paper speed, 25 mm/sec; 1 cm/mV

Figure 34-19 Hypokalemia.

Nonspecific ST Changes

In some instances, the ST segment changes do not fit a pattern of ischemia, nor are they contributory toward another diagnosis. In some cases, the ST changes are transitory but not evolutionary. In those cases, the Paramedic merely notes that the 12-lead ECG has **nonspecific ST changes**.

There are a number of causes of nonspecific ST changes including improper lead contacts, electrolyte abnormalities, drug-induced changes, and hyperventilation. Even a drink of cold water can cause nonspecific ST changes.

Vasospastic Angina

One of the causes of transient patterns of myocardial ischemia is vasospasm. This vasospasm may be the result of many etiologies, including hyperventilation. These patients may present with symptoms consistent with acute coronary syndrome. 12-lead ECGs taken during this time will demonstrate ST-segment elevations that seemingly disappear spontaneously. This condition is called variant or Prinzmetal's angina.

Approach to 12-Lead ECG Interpretation

There are several published approaches to the analysis and interpretation of the 12-lead ECG and each of these methods has one common characteristic. Success in accurate 12-lead interpretations requires a disciplined approach to the analysis as well as the avoidance of any presumptions. Most Paramedics read a 12-lead ECG from left to right, starting at the left corner. The left corner provides information about calibration, speed, and diagnostic quality.

Calibration

The 12-lead ECG machine is a scientific instrument. As such, it needs to be calibrated to ensure its accuracy. Unlike the past, when Paramedics had to physically calibrate the ECG machine, current machines are self-calibrating. To demonstrate this internal calibration, the ECG machine marks the calibration as a squared off calibration mark at the beginning of the recording (Figure 34-20). Standard gain is 1 mV to 10 mm (10 small boxes) of amplitude.

Speed

The paper speed (Figure 34-21) is critical for the analysis of the 12-lead ECG. The correct paper speed should be 25 mm/second. In some instances, the Paramedic may have slowed the paper speed to better analyze slope characteristics. (The delta wave of WPW is sometimes difficult to discern when the paper speed is 25 mm/second.) However, a slower, or faster, paper speed will impact on the measurement of intervals (i.e., PRI, QRS, and QT), leading to errors in interpretation.

Diagnostic Quality

The last information in the left lower corner of the 12-lead ECG is related to frequency response (Figure 34-22). When the ECG is used as a monitor for dysrhythmia, the machine reduces the frequency response (i.e., the sample from the signal) to 0.5 Hz and 20 to 50 Hz. This helps eliminate some of the artifact but also diminishes the quality of the ECG.

The 12-lead ECG must have a frequency response of 0.05 (not 0.5) Hz to 150 Hz. By "opening" the range, minor changes in the ECG are observable. In this way, the 12-lead ECG can be diagnostic. Unfortunately, the artifact and noise eliminated by the narrow sample supports the importance of proper skin preparation and proper electrode placement.

12-Lead ECG Analysis

Having confirmed that the 12-lead is accurate (calibrated) and that the 12-lead ECG is diagnostic, the Paramedic can then proceed to analysis. There are several systems of analysis. The P, Q, R, S, T method helps to ensure that no change or abnormality is left undetected. Regardless of the methodology of analysis, the Paramedic should always maintain a detailed approach to analysis and never rush to judgment over what appears to be obvious signs of ECG changes. The decision to label a 12-lead ECG as indicative of acute coronary syndrome must be coupled with the patient's clinical picture and the whole picture taken into consideration.

The start of every 12-lead ECG analysis is to confirm that the patient is not experiencing a dysrhythmia. The first mission of a Paramedic and emergency physician remains the treatment of dysrhythmia. This point is emphasized by the placement of a rhythm strip on the bottom of some 12-lead

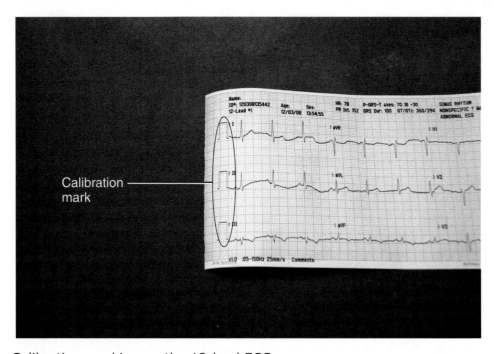

Figure 34-20 Calibration marking on the 12-lead ECG.

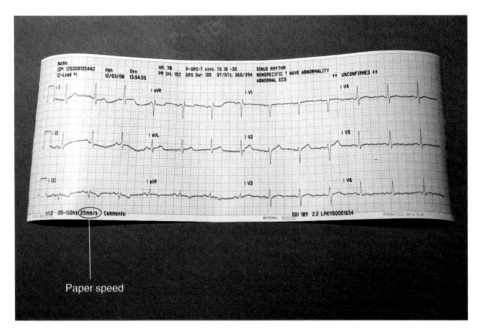

Figure 34-21 The paper speed is indicated on the 12-lead ECG.

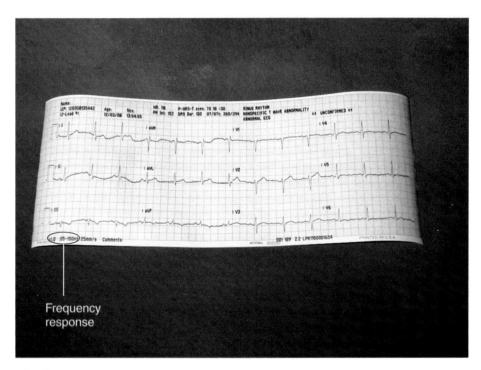

Figure 34-22 The frequency response is indicated on the 12-lead ECG.

ECGs. Once the Paramedic has confirmed that the patient rhythm is normal (i.e., there is a P wave associated with a QRS) and sinus in origin, then the Paramedic can proceed to the rest of the analysis.

Some Paramedics analyze the 12-lead ECG by proceeding in a left-to-right and top-to-bottom fashion. Other Paramedics, with a trained eye, look for Q waves in the leads that are associated with specific coronary arteries (e.g., Leads II, III, and aVF) overlying the right coronary artery located in the inferior wall. Paramedics look for pathologic Q waves

that are indicative of either an old myocardial infarction or a new myocardial infarction that is late in its evolution. The latter finding, Q waves in a late evolving MI, have some implications for further complications.

Following a search for Q waves, the Paramedic should take a moment and look at the R wave progression. A reverse R wave progression (RRWP) is suggestive of anterior ischemia. A RRWP can be likened to an early warning system, alerting the Paramedic to the possibility of sudden cardiac death before other ECG changes, such as ST-segment elevation, occur. Anterior wall MI (AWMI) can rapidly progress to either heart failure or sudden cardiac death.

Next, the Paramedic should look for ST-segment elevations and ST-segment depressions, which are indicative of reciprocal changes. The importance of delaying to find ST-segment elevations, suggestive of an ST elevation myocardial infarction (STEMI), is to reinforce the importance of a disciplined approach and to prevent the Paramedic from leaping to conclusions.

Finally, the Paramedic would turn to analysis of the T waves. While T waves are supportive of an argument for ACS, isolated T wave abnormalities may have no significance at all. Therefore, T wave changes should only be considered in the context of other ECG changes and the patient's history.

12-Lead ECG Interpretation

Like the approach to a 12-lead ECG analysis, the approach to the 12-lead ECG interpretation must likewise be disciplined. First, the Paramedic should assemble the list of abnormalities (i.e., presence and location of Q waves, R wave progression, ST changes, and T wave abnormalities). Reflecting on these changes, the Paramedic should assess for lead groupings. Lead groupings are ECG changes in contiguous leads that are suggestive of involvement of a specific ventricular wall.

Armed with this information, the Paramedic can attempt to identify the culprit artery that is involved. Understanding coronary artery involvement can help the Paramedic predict the progression of the acute coronary event and prepare for these predictable events. For example, the right coronary artery (RCA) supplies the AV node in the vast majority of patients.[44] ECG changes suggestive of an inferior wall myocardial infarction (IWMI) implicate the right coronary artery (RCA) and vis-á-vis the AV node ischemia. This AV node ischemia can manifest as type I heart block. The first indication of a type I heart block is a prolonged PR interval (PRI). Therefore, a Paramedic confronted with a possible IWMI would monitor the PRI in an IWMI for a possible heart block.

Finally, the Paramedic should consider the 12-lead ECG as a whole. ECG changes in adjoining walls may be suggestive of the extent and the evolution of the AMI. For example, ST changes and T wave abnormalities across all of the precordial leads, from V1 to V6, are suggestive of an extensive AMI. Such a pattern of ischemia could be suggestive of a left main coronary artery occlusion.[45] The implications of left main coronary artery occlusion include acute pulmonary edema (backward failure), cardiogenic shock (forward failure), and sudden cardiac death (cardiac arrest).

A combination of Q waves, ST changes, and T wave abnormalities across one or more ventricular walls may be suggestive of an AMI later in its evolution. While every STEMI has the potential for reversal, the prognosis in a late evolution AMI is poorer and the morbidity higher.

Paramedic Prognosis

If the AV node is suffering from a lack of oxygenated blood, it will malfunction. As noted in previous chapters, the AV node is responsible for delaying the impulse and allowing the atria to contract and push blood into the ventricles. The node is also the electrical connection between the atria and the ventricles. The artery that serves the AV node is the right coronary artery. If ischemic or injury patterns in the ECG leads which look at the area served by the RCA occur, the Paramedic can anticipate conduction abnormalities in the monitoring strip. The conduction abnormalities may lead to a decrease in coronary output sufficient to decrease preload and drop the blood pressure. Concurrently, blood may back up into the venous system, leading to distention in the neck veins. Also associated with RCA occlusions are bradycardias.

With LAD occlusions, the conduction is affected at the bundle of His, making for more serious conduction abnormalities and unreliable escape mechanisms. The anterior wall is the largest portion of the left ventricle and is responsible for ejecting blood into the high pressure system. Damage to the anterior wall may lead to the inability to eject the blood delivered to it and the backup of blood to the lungs. Anterior wall damage caused by occlusion of the LAD may lead to pump failure. Treatment options for anterior wall damage include anticipation of cardiogenic shock, gross irritability of the muscle cells leading to ventricular fibrillation, and reduction of heart rate and workload, leading to a reduction in myocardial oxygen demand.

Further 12-Lead ECG Interpretation

As the heart's muscle depolarizes, the energy moves down the electrical pathway from the sinoatrial node (SA node) to the atrioventricular node (AV node) as a wave front. The electrical wave front then moves across the septum in a left-to-right fashion, then to the bundle branches, and finally the wave front radiates outward across the ventricular mass. Each of these electrical events can be recorded, over time, on an ECG. The graphic representation of these events is the traditional PQRS complexes seen on an ECG.

There is another way to look at the electrical event. Instead of looking at depolarization in fragments of P, Q, R, and S, the Paramedic could look at the sum of these events. The sum of these electrical events would be the common direction of the electrical wave front called the mean electrical **vector** (Figure 34-23).

To explain vectorography in another way, these electrical events could be likened to a battle front during a war. While an army may send out many patrols, some going in different directions, the main objective of the army is to move the front forward. This common direction would be the army's vector. Similarly, while there may be minor deflections on the ECG, the major direction of the energy during depolarization is toward the apex of the heart. This common direction, or vector, of the energy of depolarization is called the heart's

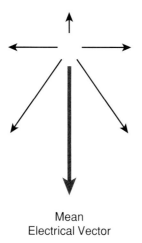

Figure 34-23 Electrical vector.

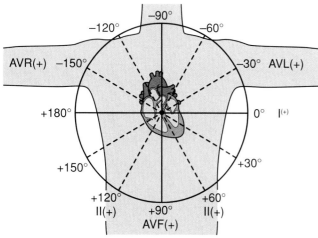

Figure 34-24 Hexaxial reference system.

electrical **axis**. Any aberration from a normal electrical axis could be indicative of disease (which is explained in more detail shortly).

To help conceptualize the heart's normal axis, and to help determine if there is any axis deviation, an artificial construct called the **hexaxial reference system** was created. To create the hexaxial system, the limb leads were drawn around the heart and Lead I, the lead that is horizontal and on the right side, was assigned zero degrees and the left side 180 degrees. As the limb leads are part of Einthoven's Triangle (an equilateral triangle), then Lead II would be at 60 degrees and negative 120 degrees and Lead III would be at 120 degrees and negative. The three axes are then all drawn into the middle of the heart and the three augmented leads overlaid with aVF at 90 degrees, aVL at negative 30 degrees, and aVR at 30 degrees and negative 150 degrees. The resulting construct shows the heart divided into equal 30-degree segments (Figure 34-24).

The traditional method of calculating the mean electrical axis was to find the most equiphasic lead of the frontal leads (I, II, III, aVR, aVL, and aVF). An equiphasic lead is an QRS complex with an R wave that is equal in height to

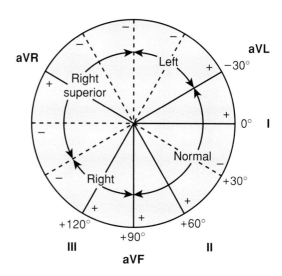

Figure 34-25 Axis determination using the hexaxial reference system.

the depth of the S wave. An equiphasic wave would be neither going toward the vector nor away from it, but would be perpendicular to it. Using that lead, the Paramedic would plot it on the hexaxial reference system (Figure 34-25). The lead represented on the perpendicular spoke would be the heart's mean electrical axis in degrees. For example, if the equiphasic QRS was Lead I, then the perpendicular axis would be 90 degrees.

This method of axis determination, while very accurate, is cumbersome in the field. An acceptable alternative is the Grant method. With the Grant method, the Paramedic would refer to Lead I and Lead II only (Figure 34-26). If both leads are upright, then there is a normal axis deviation. If Lead I is upright but Lead II is primarily downward in deflection,

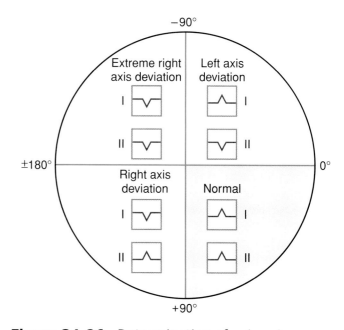

Figure 34-26 Determination of axis using Lead I and Lead II.

then a left axis deviation is assumed. Alternatively, if Lead I is primarily downward but the QRS in Lead II is upright, then it can be assumed it is a right axis deviation. If the QRS for both Lead I and Lead II is negatively deflected, then the axis is called an extreme left axis deviation; nicknamed "no man's land" because it represents extreme abnormal depolarization.

STREET SMART

Many 12-lead ECGs provide a reading of the axis, listed as P-R-T axes. The Paramedic need only read the R axis and compare it to the hexaxial reference to determine the axis.

STREET SMART

To reduce confusion, some Paramedics use their thumbs to represent the QRS deflection—Lead I on the right hand and Lead II on the left hand. If Lead I is upright (i.e., the right thumb is up and the left thumb is down), then there is a left axis deviation. If both Lead I and Lead II are negative, then both thumbs are down.

Axis Deviation

Axis deviation is any time the heart's axis is not normal. Determining axis deviation is another means of observing many pathological conditions. Coupled with other physical findings, axis determination can help the Paramedic establish a diagnosis. For example, a right axis deviation which is abnormal can often suggest pulmonary pathologies such as pulmonary embolism and chronic obstructive pulmonary disease.[46]

A slight left axis deviation, from 0 to (-) 30 degrees, may be physiologic and seen in obese patients or women who are in their third trimester of pregnancy. A larger left axis deviation, from (-) 30 to (-) 90 degrees, is often associated with left ventricular hypertrophy, secondary to heart failure, inferior wall MI, or (in some cases) Wolff Parkinson White syndrome.[47]

Of greater concern to the Paramedic is an extreme left axis deviation (>180 degrees) into "no man's land." While conditions such as congenital transposition of the great vessels and dextrocardia can produce this, extreme left axis deviation in the normal heart is suggestive of ventricular tachycardia. During ventricular tachycardia, the electrical source is in the ventricle and the wave front runs backward through the conduction system.

Differentiating VT from SVT with Aberrant Conduction

Paramedics (and other practitioners) often have difficulty determining whether a fast rhythm with a wide QRS complex is ventricular tachycardia or supraventricular tachycardia with aberrant conduction. Some patients can tolerate a sustained monomorphic ventricular tachycardia for a prolonged period of time, despite opinion that patients cannot tolerate ventricular tachycardia (VT). Because the patient is tolerating what appears to be a wide complex tachycardia of unknown etiology, the assumption is it must be supraventricular tachycardia (SVT) with aberrant conduction. Some patients do develop a rate-related bundle branch block.

The determination is important as treatments for SVT, such as calcium channel blockers, can lead to rapid patient deterioration if the rhythm is actually VT. Instead of trialing a medication to "see if it works," at the risk of patient discomfort and wasted time, a 12-lead ECG can provide the necessary information.

Ventricular tachycardia occurs most often in patients with acute cardiac ischemia or those with a cardiac history. The Paramedic should first obtain a quick patient history, paying attention to antiarrythmic medications that indicate a previous history of cardiac dysrhythmia or medications that may predispose the patient to arrhythmias (proarrhythmic medications).

Alternatively, supraventricular tachycardias often occur in otherwise healthy individuals. Some of these patients may have a history of SVT or a diagnosis of WPW or LGL syndromes.

Next, the Paramedic should obtain a 12-lead ECG, paying particular attention to axis deviation and R wave progression. The first step is to determine if the rhythm is regular. Ventricular tachycardia is usually very regular. SVT with aberrancy is also usually regular unless the underlying cause is an atrial fibrillation with a rapid ventricular response. If the rhythm is atrial fibrillation, then the ventricular response will be irregularly irregular. While regularity will not help differentiate an interpretation of either VT or SVT, an irregularly irregular rhythm is suggestive of atrial fibrillation.[48]

Next, the Paramedic should examine the QRS morphology in V1. In ventricular tachycardia, the V1 lead will be an R wave, where typically there is no R wave. Looking across the chest leads, the Paramedic may also observe an S wave where typically there is no S wave.

In fact, if all of the QRS complexes in the chest Leads V1 through V6 are in the same direction (a phenomena called concordance), the ECG interpretation favors VT. The direction of the QRS (the polarity) can be either positive or negative but should be in the same direction.

Next, the Paramedic should look at Lead I and Lead II. If both leads are negative, or the R vector on the 12-lead ECG reads between (-) 90 degrees and (-) 180 degrees (i.e., extreme left axis deviation), then the interpretation of VT is supported.

Table 34-8 Comparison of VT vs. SVT with Aberrancy

Ventricular Tachycardia	Supraventricular Tachycardia
• History of ischemia	• Healthy individual
• Proarrythmic medications	• History of SVT
• Regular or irregular rhythm	• Regular or irregular rhythm
• Dissociated P wave activity	• P waves before each QRS
• Concordance in the chest leads	• R wave progression
• In V1 (MCL1), R wave, Rr', QR, RS	• In V1 (MCL1), rSR'
• In V6 (MCL6), rS, QS, QR	• In V6 (MCL6), qRs
• QRS duration of 0.16 sec or more	• QRS duration > 0.12 but < 0.16 sec
• Initial notching or slurring of QRS	• Absent or ending slurring of QRS
• Axis of −90 to −180 degrees	• Axis of −90 to +180

Finally, the Paramedic should observe the 12-lead ECG for the presence of P waves. Atrial depolarization still occurs in VT, independent of the ectopic ventricular pacemaker. Because of the independent atrial and ventricular activity (i.e., atrial–ventricular dissociation), P waves will randomly appear throughout the 12-lead ECG. P waves that appear regularly in front of a QRS suggest a supraventricular ectopic pacemaker (Table 34-8).

Miscellaneous Effects on the ECG

Electrolyte abnormalities, particularly potassium, can cause changes in the appearance of the 12-lead ECG. While the Paramedic does not usually have access to lab results, the patient's history may suggest the potential for electrolyte disturbances. For example, patients in end-stage renal disease may experience elevation of potassium levels while those patients receiving diuretics may have a decreased level of potassium unless they receive potassium supplementation.

A normal potassium level, between 3.5 mEq/L and 4.5 mEq/L, is important for optimum cardiac cell function. If the patient is hypokalemic (i.e., serum potassium less than 3.5 mEq/L), then the patient may be prone to decreased inotropy. This can lead to generalized weakness or malaise, and/or dysrhythmias such as atrial flutter and bradycardia.

Causes of hypokalemia are numerous and include vomiting, aggressive gastric suctioning, diarrhea (secondary to infectious diseases), or abuse of potassium-wasting diuretics such as furosemide. With hypokalemia, the 12-lead ECG may show T wave flattening, ST-segment depression, and/or U wave development.[49,50]

Hypokalemia is often associated with low magnesium levels or hypomagnesemia (Figure 34-27). Hypomagnesemia may predispose the patient to a form of polymorphic ventricular tachycardia called torsades de pointes.[51]

Albuterol is a bronchodilator but also drives potassium into the cells. Aggressive use of albuterol (i.e., stacked treatments) may cause changes in cellular uptake of potassium, putting the patient at risk for low potassium levels and dysrhythmias.

Perhaps more problematic for the Paramedic may be hyperkalemia. A serum potassium level above 4.5 mEq/L is considered hyperkalemia. One of the most common causes of hyperkalemia is kidney failure. Patients who are on kidney

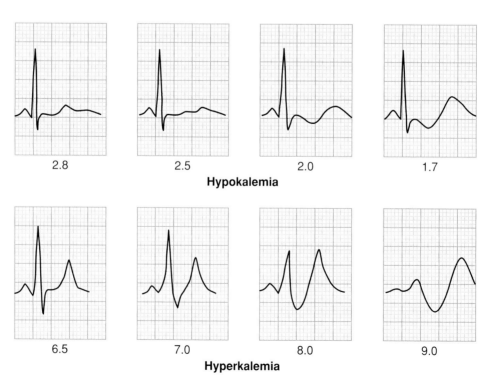

2.8   2.5   2.0   1.7

Hypokalemia

6.5   7.0   8.0   9.0

Hyperkalemia

Figure 34-27 ECG changes associated with hypokalemia and hyperkalemia.

dialysis are at obvious risk of hyperkalemia prior to dialysis. Other at-risk patients include patients with diabetes who are experiencing diabetic ketoacidosis, patients with severe burns, patients with crush injury, and those patients with acute tubular necrosis secondary to shock.

The common ECG alterations seen in hyperkalemia are changes in the T wave. At potassium levels greater than 4.5 mEq/L but less than 6.5 mEq/L, the T wave appears tall and peaked and is best seen in inferior leads (Lead II and Lead III). As the potassium level continues to climb toward 8 Eq/L, the QRS starts to widen and a left axis deviation may be appreciated. Finally, as the potassium level climbs above 8 mEq/L, the P waves all but disappear and the QRS starts to flatten into a sine wave configuration. It is at this time the patient's cardiac output has dropped precipitously and the patient is at risk for ventricular fibrillation or asystole.

Arrhythmias caused by hyperkalemia are very difficult to treat with defibrillation or the usual emergency drugs without lowering the serum potassium level. Calcium chloride, calcium gluconate, or sodium bicarbonate, all competitive electrolytes, may be used to lower potassium levels. Alternatively, serial treatments with Albuterol may help to treat mild to moderate hyperkalemia. In severe cases, it may be necessary to administer 50% dextrose with short-acting insulin.[52] The insulin helps to drive both glucose and potassium into the cells.

STREET SMART

Calcium is needed for regular cell function. Loss of calcium (serum calcium levels less than 8.5 mg/dL) or hypocalcemia is rare. Typical causes of calcium disturbances are chronic diseases. The effect of calcium is seen on the QT interval. Hypocalcemia causes a widened QT interval whereas an elevated serum calcium causes a short QT interval. To remember that calcium is related to QT, the Paramedic need only remember that QT interval is corrected for heart rate and recorded on the 12-lead ECG as such (i.e., QTc). The little c could represent calcium, to remind the Paramedic of other causes of prolonged/shortened QT intervals.

Extra-Cardiac Causes of ECG Changes

Potentially devastating extra-cardiac pathologies, such as intracranial hemorrhage, hypothermia, and pericarditis, can also cause changes on the 12-lead ECG. While not pathognomonic for these pathologies, they are another sign to be added to the symptom complex for diagnosis.

An acute rise in intracranial pressure secondary to subarachnoid hemorrhage, intracerebral bleed, or an epidural bleed may lead to wide and deeply inverted T waves in the chest leads.[53-55] The Paramedic's attention is likely focused on other more urgent matters during one of these events. However, 12-lead ECG evidence, if obtained, may be useful at the emergency department.

Hypothermia affects all cellular functions and can also cause changes in the ECG. When a patient is hypothermic, all of the interval durations (i.e., PR, QRS, and QT) lengthen and positive deflections at the J point, or point where the ventricular complex ends and the ST segment begins, become noticeable. These deflections are in the same direction (polarity) as the QRS and are termed Osborn waves (sometimes called the camel-hump sign). The Osborn wave is seen in all leads, but is more prominent in the inferior limb leads. The size of the Osborn waves correlates directly with the degree of hypothermia. Osborn waves are often difficult to discern because of artifact from muscle tremors (Figure 34-28), but are seen in 80% of patients with hypothermia (below 33°C/91.4°F).[56]

Finally, pericarditis, an inflammation between the pericardium and the epicardium, can cause chest pain and 12-lead ECG abnormalities. Initially, the Paramedic may be led to believe that the chest pain is secondary to acute coronary syndrome. However, nitrates are not useful in treating the pain of pericarditis, so it is important for the Paramedic to seek historical clues to the diagnosis of pericarditis (i.e., fevers, etc.) as well as ECG evidence.

The inflammation that occurs between the sac surrounding the heart and the epicardium leads to swelling which puts some pressure on the myocardium. The myocardium cannot repolarize as it normally does due to the swelling, so there are T wave changes. The T will become pointed and tall (similar to a hyperacute T wave found in an MI). However, the changes tend to occur in all leads rather than within contiguous leads only, leading the Paramedic to suspect other causes for the chest pain, such as pericarditis.

Evaluation

One of the advantages of the 12-lead ECG is its ability to predict the clinical progression of the patient's disease if left unchecked. For example, in the case of a patient with an anterior wall myocardial infarction (AWMI), the patient may eventually develop cardiogenic shock secondary to lost myocardial function. In this case, the patient had an IWMI that could, predictably, either extend to the mitral valve (causing

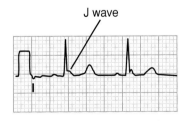

Figure 34-28 Osborn wave secondary to hypothermia.

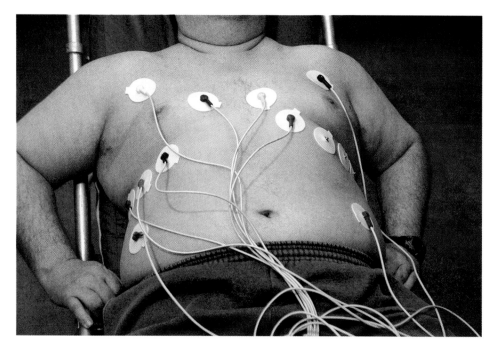

Figure 34-29 Lead placement for a 15-lead ECG, which is helpful in assessing the right ventricle.

mitral valve regurgitation) or extend into the right ventricle. It is estimated that 50% of IWMI extend into the right ventricle, with a resultant loss of preload.

15-Lead ECG

An additional diagnostic test available to the Paramedic if the Paramedic suspects right ventricular involvement is the 15-lead ECG.[57] The electrode placement for a 15-lead ECG will place positive electrodes onto the right side of the chest and view the right ventricle.

Locations for these electrodes are the 5th right intercostal space at the midclavicular line, 5th right intercostal space anterior axillary line, and 5th right intercostal space at midaxillary. The corresponding V4 to V6 wires from the left chest electrodes are switched over to the right electrodes and the ECG is rerecorded (Figure 34-29). The repeated ECG is marked **right chest leads** or V4R, V5R, and V6R.

CONCLUSION

The diagnostic 12-lead electrocardiogram is a useful tool in the Paramedic's assessment tool box with the potential to improve patient outcome by early detection of cardiac abnormalities. This is especially true in situations where the patient presents with an acute ST elevation myocardial infarction, where the patient can be triaged to the appropriate hospital, or in cases of dynamic changes in the ECG that change with treatment, uncovering underlying cardiovascular disease.

KEY POINTS:

- Death from AMI remains a national health problem.

- Aggressive prehospital treatment including obtaining and interpreting a 12-lead ECG can favorably impact patient mortality and morbidity.

- Paramedics must have a higher index of suspicion with patient populations that may present with atypical cardiac symptoms.

- A regular ECG uses standard limb leads, augmented limb leads, and precordial leads.

- The regular ECG allows for inferior, anterior, and lateral views of the left ventricle, as well as combinations.

- Accurate 12-lead ECG requires proper patient preparation including standardized electrode placement.

- A 12-lead ECG is printed in a standard configuration.

- Viewing a specific combination of leads, called contiguous leads, allows correlation to specific ventricular walls.

- Based upon coronary artery anatomy, ECG changes in contiguous leads permit Paramedics to estimate damage in specific arteries.

- Estimation of damage in specific arteries permits prognosis and planning.

- Understanding an acute myocardial infarction requires an understanding of penumbra.

- Additional ECG evidence, such as new onset left bundle branch block (LBBB) and reverse R wave progression (RRWP), are important in supporting the diagnosis of myocardial infarction.

- Some 12-lead ECGs do not show acute changes. The Paramedic should focus on treating the patient based on history.

- There are numerous extra-cardiac causes to ECG abnormalities.

- 12-lead ECG interpretation takes a disciplined approach that gathers all the pertinent information to prevent premature interpretation.

- Based on the 12-lead ECG interpretation and the patient history, the Paramedic can make a field diagnosis.

- Additional information is also available from the 12-lead ECG that can lend insight into other health conditions.

- The 12-lead ECG can help differentiate ventricular tachycardia (VT) from supraventricular tachycardia.

- The addition of three right-sided leads can help identify right ventricular AMI.

- Early detection of MI, via 12-lead ECG, and rapid transportation to an interventional cardiac care center can lead to better patient outcomes.

REVIEW QUESTIONS:

1. Why is Paramedic use of 12-lead ECG the first step in a critical pathway for patients with acute coronary syndrome?
2. What are the key elements necessary for an accurate acquisition of a 12-lead ECG?
3. List the ECG abnormalities associated with an inferior wall MI, anterior wall MI, and lateral wall MI.
4. Which leads are affected on an ECG of a patient experiencing an inferolateral MI? An anterolateral MI?
5. Where are leads placed for a right-sided ECG?
6. What are some atypical presentations of acute coronary syndrome that might require the Paramedic to obtain a 12-lead ECG?
7. List the ECG changes that occur as an acute myocardial infarction evolves.
8. What is penumbra?
9. What is the significance of a new onset left bundle branch block?
10. List potential causes of T wave abnormalities.

CASE STUDY QUESTIONS:

Please refer to the Case Study at the beginning of the chapter and answer the questions below:

1. What is the benefit of a baseline ECG?
2. How can an early ECG assist the Paramedic in determining appropriate patient destination?

REFERENCES:

1. Pope JH, Selker HP. Diagnosis of acute cardiac ischemia. *Emerg Med Clin North Am*. 2003;21(1):27–59.
2. Lau J, Ioannidis JP, et al. Diagnosing acute cardiac ischemia in the emergency department: a systematic review of the accuracy and clinical effect of current technologies. *Ann Emerg Med*. 2001;37(5):453–460.
3. Schweitzer P. The electrocardiographic diagnosis of acute myocardial infarction in the thrombolytic era. *Am Heart J*. 1990;119(3 Pt 1):642–654.
4. Spiers CM. Using the 12-lead ECG to diagnose acute myocardial infarction in the presence of left bundle branch block. *Accid Emerg Nurs*. 2007;15(1):56–61.
5. Stephen SA, Darney BG, et al. Symptoms of acute coronary syndrome in women with diabetes: an integrative review of the literature. *Heart Lung*. 2008;37(3):179–189.
6. Canto JG, Goldberg RJ, et al. Symptom presentation of women with acute coronary syndromes: myth vs reality. *Arch Intern Med*. 2007;167(22):2405–2413.
7. Myers RB. Prehospital management of acute myocardial infarction: electrocardiogram acquisition and interpretation, and thrombolysis by prehospital care providers. *Can J Cardiol*. 1998;14(10):1231–1240.
8. Antman EM, Hand M, et al. 2007 focused update of the ACC/AHA 2004 guidelines for the management of patients with ST-elevation myocardial infarction: a report of the American College of Cardiology/American Heart Association Task Force on Practice Guidelines. *J Am Coll Cardiol*. 2008;51(2):210–247.
9. Cahoon W, Jr., Flattery MP. ACC/AHA non-ST elevation myocardial infarction guidelines' revision 2007: implications for nursing practice. *Prog Cardiovasc Nurs*. 2008;23(1):53–56.
10. Moukabary T. Willem Einthoven (1860–1927): father of electrocardiography. *Cardiol J*. 2007;14(3):316–317.
11. Spodick DH. Electrocardiology teacher analysis and review. Deceptiveness of Lead II as a rhythm strip. *Am J Geriatr Cardiol*. 2003;12(1):59.
12. Zanini R, Aroldi M, et al. Impact of prehospital diagnosis in the management of ST elevation myocardial infarction in the era of primary percutaneous coronary intervention: reduction of treatment delay and mortality. *J Cardiovasc Med (Hagerstown)*. 2008;9(6):570–575.

13. Sejersten M, Sillesen M, et al. Effect on treatment delay of prehospital teletransmission of 12-lead electrocardiogram to a cardiologist for immediate triage and direct referral of patients with ST-segment elevation acute myocardial infarction to primary percutaneous coronary intervention. *Am J Cardiol.* 2008;101(7):941–946.

14. Brown JP, Mahmud E, et al. Effect of prehospital 12-lead electrocardiogram on activation of the cardiac catheterization laboratory and door-to-balloon time in ST-segment elevation acute myocardial infarction. *Am J Cardiol.* 2008;101(2):158–161.

15. Nallamothu BK, Bates ER, et al. Driving times and distances to hospitals with percutaneous coronary intervention in the United States: implications for prehospital triage of patients with ST-elevation myocardial infarction. *Circulation.* 2006;113(9):1189–1195.

16. Drake JD, Callaghan JP. Elimination of electrocardiogram contamination from electromyogram signals: an evaluation of currently used removal techniques. *J Electromyogr Kinesiol.* 2006;16(2):175–187.

17. Davis-Smith C. Skin preparation to reduce ECG artifact. *Biomed Instrum Technol.* 2000, 34(4):246.

18. Hubbell K, Massey D, Novak A. *Emergency Care Technician Curriculum.* Boston: Jones & Bartlett Publishers; 2002.

19. Rao PS. Dextrocardia: systematic approach to differential diagnosis. *Am Heart J.* 1981;102(3 Pt 1):389–403.

20. Momma K, Linde LM. Cardiac rhythms in dextrocardia. *Am J Cardiol.* 1970;25(4):420–427.

21. Riera AR, Uchida AH, et al. Early repolarization variant: epidemiological aspects, mechanism, and differential diagnosis. *Cardiol J.* 2008;15(1):4–16.

22. Tingle LE, Molina D, et al. Acute pericarditis. *Am Fam Physician.* 2007;76(10):1509–1514.

23. Pelter MM, Adams MG. Nonischemic ST-segment elevation. *Am J Crit Care.* 2004;13(2):167–168.

24. Goldberg RK, Fenster PE. Significance of the Q wave in acute myocardial infarction. *Clin Cardiol.* 1985;8(1):40–46.

25. White HD, Chew DP. Acute myocardial infarction. *Lancet.* 2008;372(9638):570–584.

26. Lilly L. *Pathophysiology of Heart Disease: A Collaborative Project of Medical Students and Faculty.* Philadelphia: Lippincott Williams & Wilkins; 1997.

27. O'Brien TX, Ross J, Jr. Non-Q-wave myocardial infarction: incidence, pathophysiology, and clinical course compared with Q-wave infarction. *Clin Cardiol.* 1989;12(7 Suppl 3):III3–III9.

28. Eskola MJ, Nikus KC, et al. Value of the 12-lead electrocardiogram to define the level of obstruction in acute anterior wall myocardial infarction: correlation to coronary angiography and clinical outcome in the DANAMI-2 trial. *Int J Cardiol.* 2008;131(3):378–383.

29. Parle GP, Kulkarni PM, et al. Importance of reciprocal leads in acute myocardial infarction. *J Assoc Physicians India.* 2004;52:376–379.

30. Hayes DD. Picturing reciprocal changes in an MI. *Nursing.* 2003;33(5):53.

31. Upshaw CB, Jr. Seeing through the maze of complete left bundle branch block. *J Med Assoc Ga.* 1993;82(11):593–599.

32. Reuben AD, Mann CJ. Simplifying thrombolysis decisions in patients with left bundle branch block. *Emerg Med J.* 2005;22(9):617–620.

33. Klimczak A, Wranicz JK, et al. Electrocardiographic diagnosis of acute coronary syndromes in patients with left bundle branch block or paced rhythm. *Cardiol J.* 2007;14(2):207–213.

34. Sgarbossa EB. Value of the ECG in suspected acute myocardial infarction with left bundle branch block. *J Electrocardiol.* 2000;33 (Suppl):87–92.

35. Chinitz JS, Cooper JM, et al. Electrocardiogram voltage discordance: interpretation of low QRS voltage only in the limb leads. *J Electrocardiol.* 2008;41(4):281–286.

36. Cuculi F, Jamshidi P, et al. Precordial low voltage in patients with ascites. *Europace.* 2008;10(1):96–98.

37. Sweetwood HM. The clinical significance of low QRS voltage. *Crit Care Nurse.* 1997;17(3):73–78.

38. Vohra J. The long QT syndrome. *Heart Lung Circ.* 2007;16 (Suppl 3):S5–S12.

39. Sauer AJ, Moss AJ, et al. Long QT syndrome in adults. *J Am Coll Cardiol.* 2007;49(3):329–337.

40. Gupta A, Lawrence AT, et al. Current concepts in the mechanisms and management of drug-induced QT prolongation and torsade de pointes. *Am Heart J.* 2007;153(6):891–899.

41. Somers MP, Brady WJ, et al. The prominant T wave: electrocardiographic differential diagnosis. *Am J Emerg Med.* 2002;20(3):243–251.

42. Fuller F. Hyperacute T waves: "The eye cannot see what the mind does not know."—Anonymous. *JEMS.* 2007;32(5):36–38.

43. Sternbach GL. Pericarditis. *Ann Emerg Med.* 1988;17(3):214–220.

44. Yesil M, Arikan E, et al. Locations of coronary artery lesions in patients with severe conduction disturbance. *Int Heart J.* 2008;49(5):525–531.

45. Nikus KC. Acute total occlusion of the left main coronary artery with emphasis on electrocardiographic manifestations. *Timely Top Med Cardiovasc Dis.* 2007;11(8):E22.

46. Baydur A. Pulmonary physiology in interstitial lung disease: recent developments in diagnostic and prognostic implications. *Curr Opin Pulm Med.* 1996;2(5):370–375.

47. Klein RC, Vera Z, et al. Electrocardiographic diagnosis of left ventricular hypertrophy in the presence of left bundle branch block. *Am Heart J.* 1984;108(3 Pt 1):502–506.

48. Rawles JM, Rowland E. Is the pulse in atrial fibrillation irregularly irregular? *Br Heart J.* 1986;56(1):4–11.

49. Martin ML, Hamilton R, et al. Potassium. *Emerg Med Clin North Am.* 1986;4(1):131–144.

50. VanderArk CR, Ballantyne F, 3rd, et al. Electrolytes and the electrocardiogram. *Cardiovasc Clin.* 1973;5(3):269–294.

51. Janeira LF. Torsades de pointes and long QT syndromes. *Am Fam Physician*. 1995;52(5):1447–1453.

52. Weisberg LS. Management of severe hyperkalemia. *Crit Care Med*. 2008;36(12):3246–3251.

53. Salvati M, Cosentino F, et al. Electrocardiographic changes in subarachnoid hemorrhage secondary to cerebral aneurysm. Report of 70 cases. *Ital J Neurol Sci*. 1992;13(5):409–413.

54. Mayer SA, LiMandri G, et al. Electrocardiographic markers of abnormal left ventricular wall motion in acute subarachnoid hemorrhage. *J Neurosurg*. 1995;83(5):889–896.

55. Stober T, Kunze K. Electrocardiographic alterations in subarachnoid haemorrhage. Correlation between spasm of the arteries of the left side on the brain and T inversion and QT prolongation. *J Neurol*. 1982;227(2):99–113.

56. Ortak J, Bonnemeier H. Cool waves: resolution of Osborn waves after prolonged hypothermia. *Resuscitation*. 2007;75(1):5–6.

57. Somers MP, Brady WJ, et al. Additional electrocardiographic leads in the ED chest pain patient: right ventricular and posterior leads. *Am J Emerg Med*. 2003;21(7):563–573.

ACRONYMS

A&O Alert and oriented
ABC Airway, breathing, circulation
ABF American Burn Foundation
ABG Arterial blood gas
AC Alternating current
AC Antecubital
ACE Angiotensin-converting enzyme
ACEP American College of Emergency Physicians
ACLS Advanced cardiac life support
ACS Acute coronary syndrome
ACTH Adrenocorticotropic hormone
ADA Americans with Disabilities Act
ADEA Age Discrimination in Employment Act
ADH Antidiuretic hormone
ADL Activities of daily living
ADP Adenosine diphosphate
AED Automated external defibrillator
AEIOU-TIPS Alcohol, epilepsy, insulin, overdose, uremia, trauma, infection, psychiatric, stroke
AEMT Advanced emergency medical technician
AHA American Heart Association
AHF Antihemophiliac factor
AICD Automated implantable cardioverter defibrillators
AIDS Acquired immune deficiency syndrome
AIA Aspirin-induced asthma
AIR Allergies, intended effect, reasonable risks
AIV Anterior interventricular
ALJ Administrative law judge
ALS Advanced life support
AM Amplitude modulation
AMA Against medical advice
AMA American Medical Association
AMI Acute myocardial infarction
AMPLE Allergies, medications, past medical history, last meal, events
ANI Automatic number identification
ANSI American National Standards Institute
APA American Psychiatric Association
APAP Acetaminophen
APCO Association of Public Safety Communications Officials
APHA American Public Health Association
ARC American Red Cross
ARDS Adult respiratory distress syndrome
ARF Acute renal failure
ASA Acetylsalicylic acid
ASTM American Society of Testing and Materials
AT&T American Telegraph and Telephone
ATLS Advanced trauma life support

ATP Adenosine triphosphate
ATSDR Agency for Toxic Substances and Disease Registry
ATV Automatic transport ventilator
AV Atrioventricular node
avdp *Avoir de pois*
AVPU Alert, voice, pain, unresponsive
AWMI Anterior wall acute myocardial infarction
BAAM Beck airway airflow monitor
BARNACLE Benefits, alternatives, risks, nature, answers, consents, lacks treatment, explanations
BIAD Blind insertion airway devices
BiPAP Bilevel positive airway pressure
BLS Basic life support
BOLO Be on the lookout
BP Blood pressure
BPG Blood pressure gas
BPH Benign prostate hypertrophy
BPM Beats per minute
BSA Body surface area
BSI Body substance isolation
BTE Behind the ear
BURP Backward, upward, rightward pressure
BVM Bag-valve mask
CAAHEP Commission on the Accreditation of Allied Health Education Programs
CAAS Commission on the Accreditation of Ambulance Services
CABG Coronary artery bypass graft
CAD Computer-assisted dispatch
CAD Coronary artery disease
CAMP Cyclic adenosine monophosphate
CAST Cardiac arrhythmia suppression trial
CBC Complete blood count
CBF Cerebral blood flow
CC Chief concern
cc Cubic centimeter
CCU Coronary care unit
CDC Centers for Disease Control and Prevention
CFR Code of Federal Regulations
CHART Chief complaint, history, assessment, Rx [prescription], treatment
CHARTIE Chief complaint, history, assessment, Rx [prescription], treatment, intervention, evaluation
CHB Complete heart block
CHEATED Chief concern/complaint, history, examination, assessment, treatment, evaluation, disposition
CHF Congestive heart failure

CINAHL Cumulative Index to Nursing and Allied Health
CIRT Critical incident response team
CISD Critical incident stress debriefing
CMS Centers for Medicaid and Medicare Services
CNS Central nervous system
CoAEMSP Committee on Accreditation of Educational Programs for the EMS Professions
COE Council of Experts
COHgb Carboxyhemoglobin
COMSPEC Communications specialists
COMT Catechol-O-methyltransferase
COP Colloidal osmotic pressure
COPD Chronic obstructive pulmonary disease
CO$_2$ Carbon dioxide
CPAP Continuous positive airway pressure
CPP Cerebral perfusion pressure
CPR Cardiopulmonary resuscitation
CPS Cycles per second
CQI Continuous quality improvement
CRF Corticotrophin-releasing factor
CSF Cerebrospinal fluid
CT Central terminal
CTZ Chemoreceptor trigger zone
CVA Cerebrovascular accident
CVAD Central venous access devices
CVP Central venous pressure
Cx Circumflex
DARE Data, action, response, evaluation
DC Direct current
DEA Drug Enforcement Administration
DEEDS Data Elements for Emergency Departments
DG Dorsogluteal
DHHS Department of Health and Human Services
DIC Disseminated intravascular coagulation
DKA Diabetic ketoacidosis
DNAR Do-not-attempt-resuscitation
DNR Do-not-resuscitate
DO Designated officer
DO Doctor of Osteopathic Medicine
DOPE Displacement, obstruction, pneumothorax, equipment
DOT Department of Transportation
DP Dorsalis pedis
DPAHC Durable power of attorney for health care
DPI Dry powder inhalers
DRG Diagnosis-related group
DSD Dry sterile dressing
DSMB Data and Safety Monitoring Board
DSM-IV *Diagnostic and Statistical Manual*, fourth edition
DTR Deep tendon reflex
D$_x$ Diagonal
EAS Emergency alert system

ECF-A Eosinophil chemotactic factor of anaphylaxis
ECF Extracellular fluid
ECG Electrocardiogram
ED Emergency department
EDD Esophageal detection devices
EDD Expected date of delivery
EDRF Endothelial-derived relaxing factor
EDV End diastolic volume
EGTA Esophageal gastric tube airway
EHF Extremely high frequency
EJV External jugular vein
ELF Extremely low frequency
EMD Emergency medical dispatch
EMG Electromyographic signal
EMI Electromagnetic interference
EMLA Eutectic mixture of local anesthetics
EMR Emergency medical responder
EMS Emergency Medical Services
EMSC EMS for children
EMT Emergency medical technician
ENA Emergency Nurses Association
ENS Emergency notification system
EOA Esophageal obturator airway
EOM Extraocular movements
EOMI EOM intact
EPIC Eliminate preventable injuries of children
EPS Extrapyramidal symptoms
ER Emergency room
ERIC Educational Resources Information Center
ERV Emergency response vehicle
ET Endotracheal
ETA Estimated time of arrival
ETC Esophageal tracheal Combitube
EtCO$_2$ End-tidal carbon dioxide levels
EtOH Ethanol
ETT Endotracheal tube
EVO Emergency vehicle operator
FAX Facsimile
FCC Federal Communications Commission
FDA Food and Drug Administration
FDNY Fire Department of New York
FEMA Federal Emergency Management Agency
FF Firefighters
FFP Fresh frozen plasma
FHS Fetal hydantoin syndrome
FLSA Fair Labor Standards Act
FM Frequency modulation
FMLA Family and Medical Leave Act
FUO Fever of unknown origin
GABA Gamma aminobutyric acid
GCS Glasgow Coma Scale
GERD Gastroesophageal reflux disease
GTT Drops

HACE High-altitude cerebral edema

H&H Hematocrit and hemoglobin

HAPE High-altitude pulmonary edema

HAPI-SOCS History, activity, pain, infection, smoker, orthopnea, cough, sputum

Hb Hemoglobin

HBV Hepatitis B

HCFA Health Care Finance Administration

HCV Hepatitis C

HDL High-density lipoproteins

HELP Head elevated laryngoscopic position

HF High frequency

HFNC High-flow nasal cannula

HIPAA Health Insurance Portability and Accountability Act

HIV Human immunodeficiency virus

HMO Health maintenance organization

HOH Hard of hearing

HPI History of present illness

HPV Human papillomavirus

HSV Herpes simplex virus

HTLV Human T-lymphotropic virus

IAFC International Association of Fire Chiefs

IAFF International Association of Firefighters

I&D Incision and drainage

ICD-10 International Classification of Diseases, 10th Revision

ICF Intracellular fluid

ICP Intracranial pressure

ID Internal diameter

ILMA Intubating LMA

ILO International Labor Organization

IM Intramuscular

IN SAD CAGES Interest, sleep disorder, appetite, depression, concentration, activity, guilt, energy, suicidal ideation

IND Investigational new drug

IO Intraosseous

IOM Institute of Medicine

IRB Institutional Review Board

ITE In the ear

IU International unit

IV Intravenous

IVAD Implanted vascular access device

IWMI Inferior wall myocardial infarction

JV Jugular vein

JVP Jugular venous pressure

KVO Keep vein open

LAD Left anterior descending coronary artery

LBBB Left bundle branch block

LCA Left coronary artery

LDL Low-density lipoproteins

LEMON Look, evaluate, Mallampati, obstruction, neck mobility

LEO Law enforcement officer

LEO Low Earth orbit

LES Lower esophageal sphincter

LF Low frequency

LGL Lown-Ganong-Levine

LMA Laryngeal mask airway

LMP Last menstrual period

LMR Land mobile radio

LMWH Low-molecular weight

LOS Line of sight

LOX Liquid oxygen

LPM Liters per minute

LQTS Prolonged QT syndrome

LR Lactated Ringer's

LSD Lysergic acid diethylamide

MAC Membrane attack complex

MAO Monoamine oxidase

MAP Mean arterial pressure

MCI Multiple casualty incident

MCL1 Modified chest Lead 1

MDI Metered dose inhaler

MDT Mobile data terminals

MER Medication error reporting

MeSH Medical subject headings

MetHgb Methemoglobin

MF Medium frequency

MFI Medication-facilitated intubation

MHS Marine Hospital Service

MI Myocardial infarction

MMR Measles, mumps, rubella

MMWR *Morbidity and Mortality Weekly Report*

MODS Multiple organ dysfunction syndrome

MOI Mechanism of injury

MRT Modulated receptor theory

MSU Mobile subscriber units

MVC Motor vehicle collision

NAD No apparent distress

NAEMSE National Association of EMS Educators

NAEMSP National Association of Emergency Medical Services Physicians

NAEMT National Association of Emergency Medical Technicians

NAP Narrative, assessment, plan of treatment

NASEMSO National Association of State EMS Officials

NEMSES National EMS Education Standards

NEMSIS National EMS Information System

NEMSSOP National EMS Scope of Practice

NF National formulary

NG Nasogastric

NHANES National Health and Nutrition Examination Survey

NHR Natural hormone replacements

NHTSA National Highway Traffic Safety Administration

NIDDM Non-insulin dependent diabetes mellitus
NIH National Institute of Health
NKDA No known drug allergies
NMBA Neuromuscular blocking agent
NO Nitric oxide
NP Nasopharyngeal
NPH Neutral protamine Hagedorn
NPO Nothing by mouth
NRB Nonrebreather
NREMT National Registry of Emergency Medical Technicians
NRFM Nonrebreather face mask
NRHA National Rural Health Association
NS Normal saline
NSAID Nonsteroidal anti-inflammatory drugs
NSC National Standard Curriculum
NSR Normal sinus rhythm
NSTEMI Non-ST-segment elevation myocardial infarction
OG Orogastric
OJT On the job
OPA Oropharyngeal Airway
OPQRST AS/PN Onset, provocation, quality, radiation, severity, timing, associated symptoms, pertinent negatives
OSHA Occupational Safety and Health Administration
OTC Over the counter
PaCO$_2$ Arterial pressure of carbon dioxide
PAD Public access defibrillation
P&S Physicians and surgeons
PCA Patient-controlled analgesia
PCP Primary care provider
PCR Patient care report
PCS Personal cellular service
PCVC Percutaneous central venous catheters
PDA Personal digital assistant
PDCA Plan-do-check-act
PDR Physician's Desk Reference
PE Physical examination
PE Pulmonary embolism
PEA Pulseless electrical activity
PEARLS Partnership, empathy, apology, respect, legitimization, support
PEEP Positive end expiratory pressure
pH Potential hydrogen
PHI Personal (or protected) health information
PHS Public health service
PICC Peripherally inserted central catheter
PIER Public information, education, relations
PIM Potentially infectious materials
PIO Public information officer
PL Private line
PM Preventative maintenance
PMH Past medical history

PMI Point of maximal intensity
PO "Per os" or by mouth
POLST Physician's order of life-sustaining treatment
POMR Problem-oriented medical recordkeeping
POS Point of service
PPE Personal protective equipment
PPO Preferred provider organization
PRBC Packed red blood cells
PRI PR interval
PSAP Public safety access point
PSDA Patient Self-Determination Act
PSI Pounds per square inch
PT Prothrombin times
PTL Pharyngeal-tracheal lumen
PTSD Post-traumatic stress disorder
PTT Partial prothrombin time
PVC Polyvinyl chloride
PVC Premature ventricular contractions
PVR Peripheral vascular resistance
PVS Persistent vegetative state
QA Quality assurance
QI Quality improvement
QRS Quick response system
RAS Reticular activating system
RBBB Right bundle branch block
RCA Right coronary artery
RCT Randomized clinical trial
REM Rapid eye movement
RF Radio frequency
RFR Radio frequency radiation
RIC Rapid infusion catheter
RMA Refusal of medical assistance
RMP Resting membrane potential
ROSC Return of spontaneous circulation
RR Respiratory rate
RRWP Reverse R wave progression
RSI Rapid sequence intubation
SA Sinoatrial
SAFE-R Stimulation reduction, acknowledgement, facilitate, explain, restore
SAMPLED Signs, allergies, medications, past medical history, last of something, events, directives
SARS Severe acute respiratory syndrome
SCD Sudden cardiac death
SCT Specialty care transport
SHF Super high frequency
SI *Le Systeme Internationale d'unites*
SIR Special incident report
SIRS Systemic inflammatory response syndrome
SLF Super low frequency
SLUDGEM Salivation, lacrimation (tearing of the eyes), urination, defecation, gastrointestinal pain, emesis, miosis
SMS Slow muscle stimulating

SOAP Subjective, objective, assessment, plan
SP Septal perforators
SRS-A Slow acting substances of anaphylaxis
SSCP Substernal chest pain
SSM System status management
SSRI Selective serotonin re-uptake inhibitors
STD Sexually transmitted disease
STEMI ST-segment elevation myocardial infarction
SVN Small volume nebulizer
SVT Supraventricular tachycardia
SWAT Special weapons and tactics
TACO Transfusion-associated circulatory overload
TBI Traumatic brain injury
TBW Total body weight
TCA Tricyclic antidepressants
TEMS Tactical EMS
TKO To keep open
TNT Trinitrin
TOT Turned over to
TPA Tissue plasminogen activator

TRALI Transfusion-related acute lung injury
TROPO Tropospheric
TTJV Transtracheal jet ventilation
TV Tidal volume
UCLA University of California at Los Angeles
UHF Ultra high frequency
ULF Ultra low frequency
USP United States Pharmacopeia
UVC Umbilical venous access
VHF Very high frequency
VL Vastus lateralis
VLDL Very-low density lipoproteins
VLF Very low frequency
VT Ventricular tachycardia
WEMT Wilderness EMT
WFPHA World Federation of Public Health Associations
WHO World Health Organization
WO Wide open
WPW Wolff-Parkinson-White syndrome

GLOSSARY

Abandonment Situation in which a Paramedic walks away from or discontinues care for a patient without turning over care to another provider who has the same or higher level of training.

Abnormal automaticity Spontaneous impulses generated in cardiac muscle that may interfere with the SA node's contraction-regulating impulses.

Abrasions An irritated area on the skin caused by wearing or rubbing away by friction.

Abscess A localized collection of pus surrounded by inflamed tissue.

Absolute bradycardia A sinus rhythm with a rate below 60 bpm.

Abstract An abbreviated summary that hits a research study's highlights.

Accessory muscles Muscles recruited to assist with body functions when the normal muscles used for that task are inadequate. For example, in respiratory distress, accessory muscles may be used to help expand the rib cage, allowing the patient to inhale.

Accessory pathway A congenital abnormal cardiac electrical pathway that may be indicated by a short PR interval.

Acetylcholine The chief neurotransmitter released into the synapse from the nerve's presynaptic membrane during neurotransmission.

Acetylcholinesterase A chemical that breaks down acetylcholine.

Acid A substance with a pH value less than 7; a molecule that has a proton that is not orbited by a paired electron.

Acid load Excessive amounts of acid in the tissues to the point that tissues are acidotic.

Acidemia Condition in which the amount of hydrogen atoms in an arterial blood gas sample is below 7.35.

Acidosis Excessive acid in a body system that can have a profound effect upon the body's uptake, distribution, and the effectiveness of medications administered.

Acknowledging Responding to a patient's answer to a question with a positive reply, either verbal or nonverbal, that encourages further dialogue.

Actionable Determination if a claim can be the basis for a lawsuit. To be actionable , a claim must generally have the four elements of a tort.

Action potential A stimulus that raises the resting membrane potential above a specific threshold.

Active transport The movement of a chemical substance through a gradient of concentration in the opposite direction to that used for normal diffusion, which requires an expenditure of energy.

Activities of daily living (ADL) The everyday events people perform in the course of their life, such as eating, dressing, driving, performing personal hygiene, and generally caring for themselves.

Act-utilitarianism An approach to ethical decision making in which the Paramedic weighs the outcomes or consequences of performing the act against not performing the act and then makes a decision that maximizes the intrinsic good.

Acute coronary syndrome (ACS) A complex of symptoms associated with the continuum of cardiovascular disease, emphasizing its morbidity (and more importantly, its mutability) and not simply its mortality.

Acute hemolytic reaction A serious bodily response to a transfusion that most often occurs as a result of an A-B-O blood type incompatibility, which leads to agglutination and hemolysis of the transfused blood.

Acute myocardial infarction (AMI) Death of cardiac muscle tissue.

Acute renal failure (ARF) The net effect of prolonged hypoperfusion, leading to a reduction in the kidneys' ability to function.

Acute respiratory distress syndrome (ARDS) A serious reaction to various injuries that involve the lungs.

Acute respiratory failure Dysfunction within the lungs that impairs respiration.

Acute traumatic stress An unexpected and sudden stressful event which is unlike the stress of day-to-day EMS and understandably requires a different approach to relieve.

Adenosine triphosphate (ATP) The chemical energy source in a cell used to power the rest of the cell's functions.

Administrative law judge (ALJ) One who decides cases involving violations of a department's regulations.

Adrenergic transmission The transmission of a nervous system signal using adrenaline as the neurotransmitter.

Advanced directives Written declarations of patient intent during specific circumstances, which are designed to provide guidance when a patient is threatened with living in a persistent vegetative state or being afflicted with a terminal illness.

Advanced emergency medical technician (AEMT) An EMS professional trained to administer a limited number of drugs and perform skills that have been shown to positively impact patient survival.

Advanced life support (ALS) Additional skills and equipment offered by Paramedics over and above basic life support, such as intubation and ventilation.

Adverse drug reaction An unwanted or harmful biological response to a drug that creates a subsequent negative impact upon the patient's health.

Aerobic metabolism The step in the metabolism process in which the cell uses oxygen to create ATP from glucose.

Affidavit A sworn written statement which attests to facts that pertain to a legal case.

Affinity An attraction to or liking of something.

Against medical advice (AMA) Situation in which patients refuse medical care in opposition to all logic when confronted with a clear and immediate danger to their health.

Ageism A stereotypical view of the elderly as frail or feeble.

Age of majority The legal age a person must be in order to consent to a medical procedure; 18 years of age in most states.

Agglutination Clumping together of red blood cells.

Agonist A drug or other chemical that can combine with a receptor on a cell to produce a physiologic reaction typical of a naturally occurring substance.

Airlock A technique in which the Paramedic injects a small bubble of air into the injection, essentially sealing off the drug below from leaking out to the subcutaneous tissues above.

Akinetic State of being without motion.

Alarm A signal on an ECG machine that indicates, via visible and/or audible signal, that a patient's heart rate is above or below a certain rate.

Alarm stage The first stage of the general adaptation syndrome, during which the body responds to the stressor via the central nervous system.

Alert report A notification sent to the receiving medical facility about an incoming patient arrival. The information in the alert report is brief and concise: age, sex, chief complaint, mental status, vital signs, treatments in progress, and an estimated time of arrival (ETA).

Algorithm A logic tree in flowchart format that simply states: if this, then do that; if not this, then do this other thing. Algorithms can be useful during an emergency when time is of the essence.

Algor mortis The body's natural cooling. As the body's metabolic processes cease, so does the production of heat.

Alkalemia Condition in which the amount of hydrogen atoms in an arterial blood gas sample is above 7.45.

Alkaloids Nitrogenous chemicals which are alkaline in nature and often chemically combined with acids to create water-soluble salts, such as morphine sulfate or atropine sulfate.

Allergic reactions A bodily response that occurs when exposed to a certain substance, ranging from sneezing and rashes to severe complications.

Alpha-adrenergic blockers Competitive blockers occupying the adrenergic receptor and preventing the catecholamine drug from attaching to the adrenergic receptor. Alpha-adrenergic blockers can be divided as either long-acting and short-acting or competitive and noncompetitive.

Alpha$_1$ adrenergic receptors Sympathetic neuroreceptors primarily involved with excitation. They are located in the peripheral vascular beds, on the arteriole side, and control the sphincters (round muscles) of the bladder, intestine, and the iris of the pupil.

Alpha$_2$ adrenergic receptors Sympathetic neuroreceptors found in the gastrointestinal tract where they decrease bowel motility, via relaxation of the smooth muscles within the intestinal walls.

Alternative hypothesis A result in a research study indicating the treatment is a plausible explanation for a change.

Alternative medicine Techniques other than traditional western medicine people may attempt for a more natural treatment, such as use of mega-vitamins, therapeutic massages, chiropractic medicine, and acupuncture.

Alveoli A large collection of small sacs in the lung that provides a larger surface area for gas exchange than if the lung were made up of a single large sac; singular is alveolus.

Ambulatory Able to walk.

Americans with Disabilities Act (ADA) A law that prohibits discrimination based on disability in hiring, promoting, training, and retiring.

AMPLE A mnemonic used to determine a patient's past medical history, consisting of questions about allergies, medications, past medical problems, last oral intake, and events preceding the incident.

Amplitude modulation (AM) When modulating an audio signal, changing the wave's height.

Anaerobic metabolism The phase of glucose metabolism that does not utilize oxygen, in which the cell changes glucose into pyruvate acid, which is in turn converted into lactic acid.

Analgesia A condition where the patient does not feel pain, yet remains conscious. More importantly, the patient retains his or her protective reflexes.

Analgesics Medications that relieve pain by inhibiting the synthesis or release of prostaglandins or stimulating opiate receptors (opiate agonists).

Anaphylactic response An exaggerated immune response that can lead to severe airway compromise and/or cardiovascular collapse secondary to relative hypovolemia.

Anaphylatoxins Substances that increase the degranulation of mast cells and attract other white blood cells (leukocytes) to the site.

Anasarca Total body edema.

Anemia Condition in which the blood is lacking red blood cells, hemoglobin, or volume.

Anemic hypoxia A low hematocrit, or other red blood cell abnormality, that can lead to oxygen deprivation at the cellular level.

Anesthesia A lack of sensation, painful or otherwise. Anesthetic drugs primarily induce anesthesia by interfering with or blocking nerve conduction.

Angulated Describes an extremity where the bone is obviously fractured and displaced at an abnormal angle.

Anorexia nervosa A psychiatric illness involving problems with self-image characterized by self-starvation and bulimia.

Antagonist A drug or other chemical that interferes with the physiological action of another substance, especially by combining with and blocking its nerve receptor.

Antecubital fossa (AC) A triangular cavity of the elbow joint that contains a tendon of the biceps, the median nerve, and the brachial artery.

Anticholinergics Drugs that block acetylcholine from binding to either muscarinic or nicotinic receptors and stop parasympathetic activity.

Antigens Foreign proteins found in bacteria.

Antimetabolites Drugs that prevent enzymes from stimulating a cell's metabolism.

Antitussive A cough suppressant.

Anoxia Hypoxia of such severity that permanent damage results.

Anxiolytics CNS depressants that reduce apprehension, fear, and anxiety.

Aortic stenosis A condition in which the leaflets of the aortic valve become scarred over time and the pathway through the valve narrows.

Apical pulse The pulse rate at the chest.

Apologize An admission of fault or error accompanied by a request for acceptance of that admission.

Apoptosis A normal physiological process in which old or damaged cells are destroyed so new ones can take their place.

Appeal A request for an appellate court to change the decision issued by a trial level court.

Artifact A disturbance in the isoelectric line of an ECG as a result of outside interference with the signal.

Arytenoid One of three separate cartilaginous structures in the aryepiglottic folds that are attached to each other and other structures by ligaments as well as the intrinsic and extrinsic muscles of the larynx.

Ascites Accumulation of fluid in the peritoneal cavity.

Assault An intentional tort involving a threat of violence, either physical or verbal.

Asthma A chronic lung disorder marked by recurrent airway obstruction and labored breathing.

Ataxia A disequilibrium in one's walk that resembles a drunkard's stagger.

Atherosclerosis The underlying pathology of coronary artery disease, which starts as a streak of fat (cholesterol) on the walls of an artery. The fat infiltrates into the wall of the artery and forms a fatty lesion.

Atrial diastole State during the cardiac cycle in which the atria are at rest.

Atrial kick The active contribution of blood to the ventricle by the atria during the cardiac cycle.

Atrial systole State in which the atria contract during the cardiac cycle.

Atrioventricular (AV) node A small mass of specialized cardiac muscle fibers, located in the wall of the right atrium of the heart, that receives heartbeat impulses from the sinoatrial node and directs them to the walls of the ventricles.

Atropine A parasympathetic blocker that decreases vagal response.

Augmented leads A modified unipolar limb type made from combining the lead type and the positive electrode location (i.e., augmented voltage right or aVR, augmented voltage left or aVL, and augmented voltage foot now called aVF).

Auscultation An assessment performed by listening, typically using a stethoscope.

Autoimmune response An immune response triggered by some infections that causes damage to the host.

Automatic answers Short, single-word responses such as "yes" or "no" given in reply to closed-ended questions.

Automaticity A cell's ability to generate its own action potential.

Automatic transport ventilators (ATV) Mechanical devices that deliver a specified volume of respiratory gas.

Autonomic nervous system The body system that maintains the involuntary, yet essential, life-preserving functions such as digestion.

AV block An interruption of AV conduction that can be indicative of disease or ischemia at the level of the AV node.

AVPU A technique used to report the patient's general level of consciousness. A stands for alert, V stands for responsive to voice, P stands for responsive to pain, and U stands for unresponsive.

Axis The major direction, or vector, of the energy of depolarization in the heart.

Axis deviation Any situation in which the heart's axis is not normal.

Bachmann's Bundle A special pathway the SA node uses to communicate with the left atrium.

Bacterial contamination Infection of blood products often due to contamination during the blood collection process, which can lead to septic patients following transfusions.

Balanced anesthesia Process of using a combination of anesthetic agents—some inhaled and some injected intravenously—to minimize the side effects that occur with using only one particular anesthetic agent.

Barotrauma Physical damage to tissues, or an injury caused by an imbalance between pressures in the environment and those within the body.

Barrel The shaft of a syringe.

Base Atoms that lack a proton and therefore want to accept protons from an acid in order to become electrically balanced; a substance with a pH value greater than 7.

Baseline vital signs An initial set of vital signs taken from the patient against which all subsequent vital signs are compared to check for changes.

Basic life support (BLS) The early assistance given to patients in the field, such as CPR, oxygen, and suction.

Battery An intentional tort involving unwanted touching.

Behavioral emergency Abnormal or bizarre behavior that may include violence or threats of violence.

Beneficence A belief that the physician's actions are acts of mercy and charity, a good act performed for people at a time of need.

Benign Something that will not harm or threaten health.

Benzodiazepines Medicines that help relieve nervousness, tension, and other symptoms by slowing the central nervous system. These drugs are short acting, share the characteristics of the other benzodiazepines, and have been studied in the prehospital environment as a sole agent to facilitate intubation.

Best practices Those actions which have led to the most desirable outcomes in the past.

Beta$_1$ adrenergic receptors Sympathetic neuroreceptors that cause the muscle of the heart, the myocardium, to beat harder and stimulate the heart to beat faster. Beta$_1$ adrenergic receptors are also found in the kidneys where they cause the secretion of renin.

Beta$_2$ adrenergic receptors Sympathetic neuroreceptors that act upon the smooth muscles found in the bronchial walls, the level of the terminal bronchioles, and cause bronchodilation.

Beta-blockers Medicines that block the sympathetic nervous system action at the Beta receptors.

Beta-selective Drugs that preferentially targets either Beta$_1$ or Beta$_2$ receptors.

Bevel An angled surface of a needle point designed to quickly pierce the skin with a minimum of pain.

Bigeminy Condition in which an ectopic complex occurs at every other complex.

Bilateral Relating to both the left and right sides.

Bioavailability The difference between the amount of a drug administered and the amount that is bound and unavailable for use. For example, imagine an aspirin pill with 325 mg of active ingredient is swallowed, and then after various factors come into play, only 150 mg is free and unbound in the blood plasma. Thus, less than 50% of the medication is bioavailable.

Bioethics A form of applied ethics—that is, ethics applied to the medical situation—which creates a set of guiding principles for the medical practitioner.

Biological death Death associated with irreversibility, meaning that any efforts to prolong life would be futile.

Biotransformation A detoxification process in the body that simply transforms a drug—by oxidation, hydrolysis, or reduction—into a water-soluble compound which can be excreted in the urine.

Bipolar leads Use of two electrodes—one negative and one positive—to measure the electrical potential between the leads' electrodes.

Blastocyst A hollow, fluid-filled ball formed by the zygote. The cells inside of the blastocyst will form the human, whereas the cells on the outside will form a protective covering that eventually develops into the placenta.

Blebs A small blister created when injecting medication, which is about the size of a mosquito bite; a change in the cell wall membrane.

Blind insertion airway device (BIAD) An airway management tool that is placed blindly and provides an airway that is superior to face-mask ventilation, yet is not as protective as an endotracheal tube.

Blocking behaviors Self-protective behaviors that inhibit free dialogue with the Paramedic. Many of these blocking behaviors are manifestations of psychological defense mechanisms.

Blood bank Location where donated blood and blood products are evaluated and stored for future transfusions.

Blood-brain barrier Tight slit junctions in the capillaries of the brain which prevent toxins and chemicals, including drugs, from easily passing into the brain.

Blood chemistry A study of the blood's chemical composition, such as its level of electrolytes.

Blood pressure A measure of the pressure within the blood vessels that make up the circulatory system. The pressure will vary depending upon the type of vessel and the phase of heart contraction.

Blood-typing Classifying blood as A, B, AB, or O based on antibodies.

Body armor A form of personal protective equipment used to protect the Paramedic from thrown objects or projectiles like bullets.

Body habitus One's physique or body build.

Body language The transmission of a message by nonverbal visual cues. Experts suggest that 70% of any spoken message is conveyed by body language.

Body substance isolation Protection worn to keep a patient's body fluids from coming in contact with the Paramedic, such as latex gloves.

Bolus A concentrated volume of fluid infused rapidly over several seconds or minutes.

Borrowed servant doctrine Situation in which the Paramedic in charge of an emergency is responsible for the actions of those Paramedics working in a subordinate role.

Bounce A radio wave phenomenon that occurs whenever a short wave strikes a reflective surface and is redirected in another direction.

Bradycardia A heart rate that is under 60 beats per minute for an adult or below the lower limit of normal for a child.

Bradykinesia Extremely slow movement.

Brain dead A state in which an electroencephalogram shows zero brain activity, indicating brain death.

Breach of duty Situation in which a Paramedic fails to perform patient care in conformance with the standard of care.

Breakthrough seizure An unexpected epileptic seizure in a person who has had good seizure control, which occurs when the drug level in the plasma drops below the therapeutic level.

Bronchial sounds Lung sounds auscultated over the larger airways that are louder and sound like air rushing through a hollow tube.

Bronchoconstriction Narrowing of the airway's lumen.

Bronchodilation Widening of the airway's lumen.

Bronchospasm Temporary narrowing of the smaller air passages of the bronchi due to violent, involuntary contraction of the smooth muscle of the bronchi that sometimes accompanies a respiratory infection.

Bronchus Either of the two primary divisions of the trachea that lead into the right or left lung; plural is bronchi.

Buffered Actions taken to render an atom neutral (not to have an electrical charge).

Bulimia Eating disorder characterized by binge-eating and then purging via laxatives or vomiting.

Bundle of His A wide, thick group of cardiac muscle fibers that conducts an electrical impulse to the interventricular septum.

BURP technique A method to improve laryngoscopic view through backward, upward, and rightward pressure.

Butterfly IV catheters A throwback to the days of steel needles, in which short steel needles are embedded into a plastic anchor device that has wings, like a butterfly.

Calibration Process used to assess the accuracy of the ECG monitor, in which the Paramedic compares the ECG machine's operation against standard settings.

Capacity The mental ability to understand what one is being told.

Capillary refill A measure of the patient's ability to perfuse the extremities with oxygenated blood.

Capnography The process of tracking the carbon dioxide in a patient's exhaled breath, which enables Paramedics to objectively evaluate a patient's ventilatory status.

Capnometry The determination of the end-tidal partial pressure of carbon dioxide.

Capsule Medicinal powder placed within a gelatin casing that generally makes it easy to swallow and keeps it from easily dissolving in the water-based saliva of the mouth.

Cardiac action potential The electrochemical activity of the heart's individual cells.

Cardiac cycle A single contraction (one heartbeat), during which blood flows through all four chambers of the heart. This contraction includes an entire sequence of events from atrial filling through ventricular filling and ejection.

Cardiac monitor A device that shows the electrical and pressure waveforms of the cardiovascular system; the ECG oscilloscope.

Cardiac output The volume of blood pumped out of the left ventricle with each contraction.

Cardiac skeleton A fibrous matrix to which the muscles, valves, and rings of the myocardium are attached and that separates the atria from the ventricles.

Cardiogenic shock Problems with the heart that lead to its failure to pump.

Cardioselective Beta-selective drugs that only affect the heart.

Carina Level of the 5th thoracic vertebrae; an anatomical part, ridge, or process.

Carotid bruit A whooshing sound heard in a carotid artery that has plaque buildup on the artery walls.

Carotid pulse A measure of the beats produced by blood flow taken in the anterior neck.

Carrier squelch A type of squelch control that eliminates background static during pauses in a radio transmission, essentially muting the radio between transmissions and thereby improving the message's overall quality.

Case law Law established by previous judicial decisions.

Case report An example of a descriptive study Paramedics use to report interesting or unique cases, which allow other Paramedics to gain insight into a problem.

Case-control study An observational study method in which the Paramedic compares cases—those patients with the disease—to controls—those patients without the disease—and then examines the procedures performed on both to see if there was an association between outcomes.

Catecholamines A classification of very potent adrenergic agonists that cause a direct response from the adrenergic receptor.

Cell An area that a mobile radio transmission tower services for cell phone calls.

Cell-mediated immunity Immunity that results from the activity of T lymphocytes

Cellular telephones Low-powered wireless transmitters (radios) that work within close proximity to a radio tower.

Cellulitis A skin infection.

Cell wall membrane A porous semipermeable dual layer lipid-protein matrix that makes up the outside of a cell.

Celsius scale A method of measuring temperature based on a system of 10 in which water freezes at 0°C and water boils at 100°C.

Central nervous system depressants Drugs that produce a state of reduced central nervous system activity.

Central venous pressure (CVP) A measurement used to assess a patient's hemodynamic status.

Cerebellum The portion of the brain responsible for coordination of muscles and balance.

Channel crowding Situation in which several agencies share the same radio frequencies.

Chart audit A system of quality review performed retrospectively in which the Paramedics reviews the chart against care standards.

CHEATED A mnemonic for an EMS-specific, user-friendly documentation method highlighting chief concern/complaint, history, examination, assessment, treatment, evaluation, and disposition.

Chemical hiatus Situation in which the drug level in the body drops below the therapeutic level before the infusion has assumed dominance. If left untreated, a potentially life-threatening return ventricular ectopy could occur.

Chemical name A description of a drug according to its elemental chemical makeup and molecular structure.

Chemotactic factors Chemical messengers released by mast cells that attract specific leukocytes (white blood cells) to the injury site.

Chemotherapy Use of drugs to combat infections and diseases, most notably cancer.

Chest leads Leads in which the exploring electrode is placed on the chest and the other is connected to one or more limbs.

Chevron Method for securing a catheter hub that involves slipping the inverted tape, sticky side up, under the hub until it adheres to the hub, then crossing it over the hub.

Chief concern or complaint (CC) The main reason for which the patient is seeking medical care.

Cholinergic transmission The transmission of a nervous system signal using acetylcholine as the neurotransmitter at the motor endplate.

Chordae tendinae Strong cords of connective tissue that connect the mitral valve to the papillary muscle of the heart's left ventricle.

Choreography The ability to organize a team's efforts in order to deliver appropriate interventions in a timely manner.

Chromosomes A double helix of DNA that carries genetic information.

Chronotropy To make the heart beat faster.

Circumflex (Cx) A minor branch of the left coronary artery that bends around to the left side of the heart and provides blood to the lateral wall of the left ventricle.

Civil law The legal system designed to handle cases not of a criminal nature, often involving business transactions, such as contracts, torts, estates, trusts, wills, real estate matters, commercial matters, and grievances against the government.

Clarification Communication technique in which a Paramedic asks the patient to restate the message in other words.

Climacteric An age-related decrease in sex hormone production that occurs in both men and women.

Clinical death The absence of vital signs. Clinical death is characterized by unresponsiveness to loud verbal and painful stimuli, absence of breathing, and an absence of a central pulse.

Clinical decision making The process of systematic analysis and critical thinking the Paramedic uses to make clinical decisions that will be incorporated into a patient's treatment plan.

Clinical trial Experimental medical research process in which subjects are assigned at random to either the treatment group or to the non-treatment group (i.e., those receiving standard care [control group]).

Clock method Procedure used to determine the infusion rate in which the Paramedic mentally visualizes a clock with a sweep hand pointing out the drug infusion rate. When the sweep hand is at the 15 second point, it represents 1 milligram of drug at 15 drops per minute or 15 milliliters an hour. When the sweep hand is at the 30 second position, it represents 2 milligrams of the drug infusing at 30 drops per minute, and so forth.

Clonic Repetitive muscle contractions during a convulsion.

Closed-ended questions Questions that generally start with words like "do," "is," or "are" and require the answer to be a short, direct reply—usually just "yes" or "no." Closed-ended questions are used when specific information is needed quickly.

Clot tubes A red top blood sample tube that contains no additives or preservatives to prevent blood clotting.

Coagulation The thickening process through which the blood makes clots.

Coagulation cascade The process the body uses to manufacture fibrin and fibrinogen.

Coagulation factors Proteins which act to attract platelets to each other to build platelet plugs. Additionally, coagulation factors are key to the production of fibrin and fibrinogen, two materials that serve to solidify and stabilize the platelet plug, making it impermeable to liquid.

Coagulative necrosis Condition in which muscle cells die, such as in myocardial infarction, the skeleton of the cell remains, and the tissue remains firm.

Coded (or tone) squelch Sometimes called private line, a type of squelch control that permits the radio to receive only the intended signal by eliminating reception of nearby broadcast messages and only accepting signals with the correct code.

Cognitive restructuring Action taken to reframe the brain's interpretation of a stimulus so that it is non-threatening.

Cohort study An observational study method that examines patients who have been exposed to a treatment and compares them to a group that was not exposed to the same treatment. The patients are followed to determine outcomes.

Cold maceration Process of letting medicinal herbs steep in cold water.

Colloid Blood substitutes that contain proteins and are capable of both pulling fluids from within the interstitial space into the circulation (to help augment the circulating volume) and remaining within the bloodstream for a prolonged period of time (to help maintain the circulating volume).

Colorimetric device Encapsulated pieces of litmus paper over which an exhaled breath flows. When carbon dioxide is in the presence of water, it forms carbonic acid; the pH sensitive litmus paper in the colorimetric device detects this acid and changes color.

Combining forms Creating a word by placing two or more roots together, separated by a vowel, to explain a complex process. For example, the term "cardiomyopathy", meaning disease of the muscle of the heart, is made up of "cardia-" (meaning heart), "my" (meaning muscle), and "patho" (meaning disease), with the letter "O" separating the roots "cardia", "my", and "patho."

Command presence The ability to present oneself as the person of authority.

Commercial ambulance services For-profit EMS services that provide interfacility medical transportation as well as emergency medical services to patients. Many of these commercial ambulance services originated from the funeral homes that previously provided the service.

Communications Act of 1934 A resolution which states that the President of the United States has control over all government radios and that the Federal Communications Commission (FCC) has control over the civilian use of radios.

Communications specialists (COMSPEC) Enhanced 9-1-1 staff that dispatch emergency responders to people who are unable to speak or who have lapsed into unconsciousness.

Community-based EMS Volunteer (nonprofit) EMS squads that operate independently of local fire departments or hospitals.

Competency assurance The necessity of the Paramedic not only to maintain minimal skills and an adequate knowledge base, but to continue to remain current with updates to EMS.

Complementary medicine See Alternative medicine.

Complete blood count (CBC) The quantity of each type of blood cell in a given sample of blood, often including the amount of hemoglobin, the hematocrit, and the proportions of various white cells.

Complete heart block Obstruction of electrical signals through the AV node or at the bundle of His, in which case pacemakers lower in the heart at the level of the bundle of His, bundle branches, or even the ventricular myocardium will take over as the pacemaker.

Comprehensive Drug Abuse Prevention and Control Act of 1970 (Controlled Substance Act) A law that expanded the Drug Enforcement Administration's authority to include schedules of potentially dangerous and addictive drugs that had special restrictions.

Concealment Any object that blocks the pursuer's vision of the Paramedic, although it does not offer physical protection.

Concentration gradient The difference in concentration between two solutions in different areas (i.e., on two sides of a membrane). When a concentration gradient exists, the higher concentration will diffuse across the membrane to the lower-concentration solution until a balance is reached.

Concept formation The inductive logic process of forming ideas about what is causing a patient's condition based on the patient's history and the Paramedic's knowledge base.

Conduction system Specialized cardiac cells designed to carry on the heart's electrical rhythm.

Conductivity The ability of an electrical stimulus to be transmitted from cell to cell.

Congestive heart failure (CHF) The heart's inability to pump strongly enough to completely meet the body's needs for oxygen and nutrients.

Conjunctiva The mucous membrane that lines the inner surface of the eyelids.

Conscious sedation The first stage of anesthesia where the patient does not feel pain but is awake enough to maintain protective airway reflexes.

Constitutional examination An evaluation that assesses the patient's general appearance.

Constitutional signs/symptoms General nonspecific findings, such as fevers, unexplained weight loss, night sweats, chills, headaches, nausea, and vomiting, that are often common to all sick patients.

Contiguous leads Situation in which two or more leads look at the same wall of the left ventricle.

Continuous infusion A volume of fluid evenly administered over the course of a period of time (i.e., an hour).

Continuous quality improvement (CQI) An ongoing process of review and re-engineering, in order trying to refine a process and improve its delivery.

Contractility The cardiac muscle fibers' ability to shorten or contract.

Contributory negligence A legal assertion that an action, although not directly causing an injury or problem, nonetheless made it worse.

Cormack-Lehane grading system A quantitative measure system that grades the view of the glottic opening by how much is occluded by the tongue—Grade I is a clear view of the entire glottic opening whereas IV is visualization of the tongue or soft palate only. Proper patient position and external laryngeal manipulation can improve the view by one to two grades.

Coronary artery disease (CAD) The series of events that leads up to and includes myocardial infarction.

Coronary circulation A special set of arteries and veins that supplies blood to the muscles of the heart.

Cortisol A glucocorticoid hormone that stimulates the production of glucogen from amino acids and fatty acids contained in lipids.

Cost–benefit ratio A classic economic analysis that asks the question of whether it is advantageous (i.e., cost-effective) to take a particular action or make a change in a procedure.

Costal margin The lower edge of the chest (thorax) formed by the bottom edge of the rib cage.

Costovertebral angle Area located over the lower ribs just medial to the posterior axillary line.

Countermeasures Steps that could be effective in reducing injury.

Couplets Situation in which two ectopic complexes occur together.

Cover Any object that cannot be penetrated by a projectile, from bullets to frying pans. Examples of cover include telephone poles and even fire hydrants.

Crenate Dehydration and collapse of a cell.

Crepitus Crackling or popping sounds under the skin or near joints.

Cricoid pressure Also called the Sellick's maneuver, a procedure that involves identifying the cricoid ring and gently applying approximately 10 pounds of pressure in a posterior direction throughout airway management; from the onset of ventilation until completion of intubation.

Criminal law Laws dealing with violations of a person's duties to the community and for which the written law requires the person to provide satisfaction.

Critical incident response team (CIRT) Individuals called in during an acute stress situation to meet with the affected personnel, typically front-line responders.

Critical incident stress debriefing (CISD) An intervention to defuse stressors in an acute stress situation, such as a line-of-duty death, serious injury of a coworker while on-the-job, and post-event suicide of a fellow responder.

Cross-match Comparing a donor's blood to a patient's blood to determine compatibility of antibodies and type.

Cross-sectional survey A snapshot of a certain aspect of a population at a given moment in time that the researcher is interested in, obtained by means of observation.

Crowning Part of the childbirth process in which the infant's head begins the passage into the birth canal, indicating delivery will occur within several minutes.

Cryoprecipitate The protein portion of plasma made up of concentrated clotting factors.

Crystalloids Electrolyte-containing fluids Paramedics use during trauma resuscitation that, when dehydrated, create crystals.

Cultural competence A Paramedic's ability to function effectively within the diverse populations that she serves.

Culture The culmination of life experiences in a locality or region that affects the way a person thinks and behaves.

Cyanosis A bluish hue that develops when the patient develops a decreased oxygen level in the blood.

Cytopathic Manifestations of disease at the cellular level.

Cytoplasm A fluid mixture inside a cell, primarily made up of water and organelles, which has a specific cellular function(s).

Dangerous instruments Any object that could be used, under the right circumstances, to produce serious injury or even death, such as a broken bottle or box cutter.

Data and Safety Monitoring Board (DSMB) A group of individuals who are not directly involved in a research study but who can nonetheless make an objective decision about the research based on the merits of the data.

Data dredging Sometimes called data mining, it means conducting research by searching through a database without a predefined scientific question in mind (i.e., without a predefined hypothesis).

Dead airtime A period in which no radio transmissions are made on a particular channel.

Deadly weapons Objects that are, by design, intended to inflict death or disability (e.g., a gun or a knife).

Decoction Process of bringing water to a boil then steeping medicinal herbs in the water (like one would steep a teabag), then drinking the resulting solution.

Decode To interpret and understand a message.

Decubitus ulcers Also known as pressure ulcers, tender or inflamed patches that develop when skin covering a weight-bearing part of the body is squeezed between bone and another body part, or a bed, chair, splint, or other hard object, creating pressure or friction.

Deep tendon reflexes (DTRs) Involuntary muscle contraction in the muscle associated with a tendon.

Defasciculating dose A small dose of a non-depolarizing paralytic which, when administered before administering a certain drug, prevents the fasciculations associated with that drug.

Defensive medicine The practice of a Paramedic performing a wide variety of random tests to limit liability or criticism from the medical director, rather than performing just those tests that benefit the patient.

Defusing An immediate intervention intended to avert acute stress reactions among the emergency responders.

Degranulate The process of breaking down or losing granules.

Delirium A sudden change in mental function, usually associated with reversible metabolic derangements (e.g., hypoxia, or the toxic effects of medications).

Deltoid An intramuscular injection site in the muscle that overlays the shoulder and extends downward toward the elbow, forming an inverted triangle in the process.

Demobilization An opportunity to mitigate the effects of the acute stressors and to decrease the incidence of acute traumatic stress reactions.

Denature To break down a protein's complex folded structure.

Deontology Duty-based ethics in which the decision as to whether an action is right or wrong is based on principles and not upon the consequences.

Depolarization A cascade of ionic changes at a cell wall that occurs as electrolytes transfer across the cell in an attempt to balance (neutralize) the charge.

Depolarizing neuromuscular blocker One of the two major classes of neuromuscular blockers; binds to the acetylcholine receptor and causes the muscle to depolarize or contract.

Deposition Out-of-court testimony made under oath and recorded by an authorized officer for later use in court.

Descriptive analysis Based on the Marriott method of analysis, a way to gather information for a thorough ECG interpretation consisting of review of the rhythm, rate, width of the QRS complex, and atrial activity.

Descriptive study Documentation that simply states that a condition or situation exists without trying to offer an explanation.

Detailed physical examination A more thorough evaluation given to low-priority patients with whom the Paramedic has more time.

Developmental milestones The skills and abilities a child achieves at certain ages in his or her life, measured against the norms of other children.

Dextrocardia Condition in which the heart and lungs in a body are opposite their normal position while the abdominal organs are in their usual position.

Diagnosis Identification of a disease or disorder based on available symptoms and testing.

Diagnosis-related groups (DRG) Groups of patient populations with the same or similar diagnosis, who may benefit from similar treatments.

Diaphoretic To be profusely sweaty.

Diaphragm A large, thin, dome-shaped muscle that divides the abdomen from the thorax.

Diastolic blood pressure The minimum blood pressure measured during diastole when the heart relaxes and fills.

Digital intubation An endotracheal intubation technique that uses the Paramedic's hand to identify laryngeal structures and to guide tube placement.

Diminished autonomy Standard that states any person who is mentally incapable of making an informed decision (e.g., by virtue of age or infirmity) cannot willingly consent to participate in research.

Diphasic A wave that begins as a positive deflection then becomes a negative wave or vice versa; having two phases.

Diplomacy To calmly and thoughtfully resolve issues without angering the parties in the dispute.

Direct questioning An interviewing technique in which a Paramedic asks simple, unambiguous questions of the affected party about the situation at hand.

Disclosure An open dialogue between patient and provider in which the provider tells the patient about the procedure, including its attendant risks, and recommends the procedure.

Disease An abnormal change in the function of cells, tissues, or organs. An example of each is cancer in cells, emphysema in tissues, and acute myocardial infarction in organs.

Disorder A physiological deviation from a normal homeostasis.

Disseminated intravascular coagulation (DIC) A condition in which, after initial blood clotting factors are partially consumed by massive coagulation throughout the body, the remaining clotting factors are insufficient to protect the body.

Distention An abnormal expansion, such as in a vein or the abdomen.

Distracting injury Situation in which a pain (often dull visceral pain) is overshadowed by another more intense pain from another injury; for example, a fractured femur taking attention away from chest pain.

Distress A negative response to stimuli that overcomes the body's innate defenses and serves as the body's maladaptive reaction to stress.

Distributive shock The third category of the Hinshaw-Cox shock classification, which is descriptive of the problem of poor blood distribution. Distributive shock includes shock caused by the widespread vasodilatation seen with severe infections and during anaphylactic reactions, to name a few causes.

Diuretics Medications that cause the increased loss of fluid and salts from the body.

Divine command ethics Extrinsic ethics based upon a higher authority, such as the Bible's Ten Commandments or Buddha's Four Noble Truths and Eight Paths to Righteousness, in which that higher authority has predetermined what qualities a virtuous person would have and calls upon the person to display those virtues through correct action.

Dominance A condition of superiority, as in when the actions of one bodily function are faster than or overpower the actions of another.

Do-Not-Resuscitate (DNR) order Sometimes called a Do-Not-Attempt-Resuscitation (DNAR) order, a directive from the patient that artificial means of life support should not be used, generally in cases when a condition is terminal and artificial life support will just delay the inevitable.

DOPE A mnemonic Paramedics use to help remember the causes of problem intubations. The D in dope stands for displaced endotracheal tube; the O stands for obstructions of the endotracheal tube, such as a mucous plug; the P suggests the possibility of a pneumothorax; and the last letter, E, indicates equipment failure.

Dormant A state of biological rest a disease may stay in until favorable conditions exist for it to reanimate.

Dorsalis pedis (DP) pulse A measure of the beat created by blood flow measured over the dorsum of the foot.

Dorsiflex The ability to raise toes above the horizontal toward the tibia.

Dorsogluteal (DG) The most common intramuscular injection site, located in the gluteus medius.

Dose The amount of drug needed to produce the desired effect.

Double-blinded randomized clinical trial (RCT) A prospective scientific study that controls known and unknown variables, leaving only one variable to be manipulated. Subjects are then chosen at random to be included in either the experimental treatment group or in the control group.

Double-blind study A research study in which both the researcher and the participants are unaware of which group the subject is in.

Downregulation A decrease in the number of cell receptors in a cell due to changes in hormone levels.

Dress-up philosophy Technique in which Paramedics add barrier devices for protection as the situation warrants.

Drug Any material which, when injected, ingested, inhaled, or absorbed into the body, is used for the diagnosis, treatment, or cure of a disease or condition.

Drug decline The idea that while a drug moves through the body various forces and organs are weakening it, reducing its effectiveness.

Drug reservoir A type of drug depot in the body, created when drugs bind to certain substances, that stores the drug until it is needed. The effect of a drug reservoir is to prolong the drug's action within the body.

Dry powder inhalers (DPI) Respiratory device that uses a solid drug pulverized into micro-fine particles for inhalation.

Duplex A radio that uses two frequencies—one to transmit and one to receive—so that an operator can talk and listen at the same time, permitting more rapid communications.

Duration The length of a QRS complex wave.

Duty to act An element of a tort that implies a Paramedic must act whenever called upon to perform patient care (i.e., the Paramedic is "on duty").

Dyskinesia Lack of ability to control body movements.

Dysplasia Situation in which there are too many new, or immature, cells being produced that are not functional.

Dysrhythmias An abnormality of the electrical activity in the heart.

Ecchymosis Blood from ruptured vessels moving into other tissues; bruising.

ECG interpretation A systematic approach used to rapidly and accurately analyze an ECG rhythm strip.

ECG rhythm strip A printed hard copy from an ECG machine of at least one lead that shows the ECG complexes over a long period of time allowing Paramedics to analyze the rhythm.

Echo technique Communication method in which the physician gives an order and the Paramedic, in order to ensure it's been interpreted correctly, repeats the order back to the physician exactly as received.

Ecological study Sometimes called a correlational study, this type of research design serves to provide information about trends and rates of disease within a population, often cited as X number of cases of Y disease per 1,000 or per 100,000 of Z population.

Ectopic To occur in an abnormal or atypical position.

Ectopic beats Aberrant cardiac beats resulting from abnormal automaticity.

Ectopic focus Any complex that occurs outside of the sinus of the heart's cavity.

ED50 The dose of a drug that effectively creates the therapeutic effect in a majority of patients.

Edema A dramatic fluid buildup in the body's tissues.

Edentulous A state of having no teeth.

Efficacy The power to produce an effect; the ability of a drug to realize its full intended therapeutic effect.

Ejection fraction The percentage of blood pushed and squeezed out of the heart, typically 60% to 75% of the end diastolic volume.

Elastic gum bougie A device made entirely of wound gum rubber, with a hard, smooth, and round plastic tip, that resembles a very long stylet. The device is directed through the vocal cords and into the trachea to serve as a guide for an endotracheal tube.

Electrical alternans Situation in which every other ECG complex has alternating amplitude (i.e., the one QRS complex is smaller when compared to the next).

Electrical storm Multiple recurrent episodes of ventricular fibrillation.

Electrocardiogram A device used to monitor cardiac rhythm.

Electromagnetic interference (EMI) Disruptions of an ECG signal caused by the flow of electricity through an electric device, such as a radio, cellular telephone, or television, which creates an electromagnetic field.

Electromyographic signal (EMG) An electrical current recorded by the ECG any time a muscle contracts, appearing as narrow rapid spikes on the ECG monitor.

Electroporation The effect of electrical current passing through the tissue.

Elixir A sweetened tincture used for medicinal purposes.

Emancipated minors A special class of youths who are below the age of majority but are permitted to give informed consent, provided they are capable of understanding the consequences of their decisions and that they are not impaired by alcohol or drugs. These include married persons, single parents, the military, and youth living on their own.

Embryo An unborn child at any stage of development between conception and birth.

Emergency doctrine Policy invoked when family members or guardians are not present that states if a parent was present the parent would want the child treated and transported to the hospital. The emergency doctrine is usually invoked only in cases of life- or limb-threatening emergencies.

Emergency exception A situation in which a care provider performs a procedure without fully explaining it to the patient because the delay created by a lengthy explanation might compromise the patient's health.

Emergency medical dispatch (EMD) A dispatch algorithm in which the communications specialist interrogates the caller, gives prearrival instructions, and uses preset criteria to make a response determination before dispatching the appropriate EMS responder units.

Emergency medical responder (EMR) An EMS provider who is expected to render life-saving care with minimal equipment; for example, a police officer or fire fighter providing rapid response.

Emergency Medical Services (EMS) The field of medicine that involves transporting the sick or wounded to medical care and providing treatment to patients prior to their arrival at the hospital.

Emergency Medical Technician-Ambulance A national standard curriculum established in 1969 for the training of ambulance drivers/attendants in new skills and life-saving techniques.

Emergency Medical Technician (EMT)–Basic Part of a team that responds to the emergency scene, typically aboard an ambulance, and is trained to provide initial care on scene as well as medical care to the patient while in transit to the hospital.

Emergency vehicle operator (EVO) Any individual who operates a vehicle en route to a response call.

Emergent An assessment classification in which the patient's condition unexpectedly developed and is in need of immediate medical attention.

Empathy An emotional understanding of the patient's feelings; to be able to understand what it is like to walk in the other person's shoes.

Empiric therapy Treatment based on initial observations obtained during the primary assessment.

EMS Act of 1973 Federal legislation that delineated the 15 aspects of an EMS system that needed improvement including education (both public as well as provider), improved communications (including public access), and system evaluation, but offered little money to help make those improvements.

EMS Agenda for the Future Overall framework which suggests that EMS will be more intimately intertwined with public health, as well as public safety, over time and continue to evolve along with health care.

EMS Education Agenda for the Future The plans that emerged from the 1996 meeting of over 30 EMS organizations held with the intent of implementing the educational portions of the EMS Agenda for the Future.

Emulsions Finely pulverized particles placed into oils, such as cod liver oil.

Endocardium A single-layer thick sheet of epithelial cells that act as a lining in the heart; the heart's innermost layer.

Endocrine shock A fifth classification of shock, which recognizes the importance of hormones in maintaining homeostasis. The classic endocrine shock is hypoglycemic shock.

Endogenous Originating within the body.

Endorphins Neuromodulators that reduce the sensation of pain and affect emotions by attaching to opiate receptors on the neuron, which in turn inhibit neural activity.

Endotoxins Poisons produced by bacteria during an infection that stimulate chemical mediators to affect the hypothalamus.

Endotracheal tube The basic tool of endotracheal intubation which provides a conduit for oxygenation and ventilation between the patient's lungs and the ventilator (person or machine).

End-tidal carbon dioxide (ETCO$_2$) A standard method of measurement and monitoring carbon dioxide levels used for both confirming endotracheal tube placement and monitoring patient status, ventilation, and continuing tube placement.

Enhanced excitability The ability to respond to a much weaker stimulus.

Enteral Administration of drugs through the gastrointestinal tract, either through pills taken orally or through suppositories.

Enteric coating A protective coating on a tablet that permits the tablet to travel, unaltered, through the stomach and into the intestine for absorption.

Environmental risk Modifiable risk factors that are a function of one's lifestyle or occupational choice, such as farmers developing respiratory issues from their exposure to dust.

Epicardium The heart's outermost part; a part of the pericardium that is closely adherent to the heart.

Epidemiology The study of the causes, distribution, and control of disease in populations.

Epiglottis A "U" shaped structure in the upper airway attached to the anterior pharynx between the base of the tongue and the larynx that protects the lower airway from foreign body aspiration.

Epilepsy A neurological disorder characterized by recurrent seizures that occur without known cause.

Epistaxis Nosebleed.

Equianalgesic Drug characteristic in which a dose of a new medication formulation has the same ability to produce analgesia as 10 milligrams of morphine.

Equiphasic A flatline pattern on an ECG machine that occurs if the differences in the flow of electricity result in a zero net difference in direction.

Equity A concept of fairness or evenhandedness. To be accepted, any change must appear to be equitable to all parties concerned.

Erythema Abnormal redness of the skin caused by capillary congestion.

Erythrocytes Red blood cells that transport oxygen and carbon dioxide through the blood.

Escape mechanism A form of backup pacemaker in the heart that will continue to prompt contractions (at a slower rate) if the SA node stops sending impulses.

Esophageal intubation detection devices (EDD) Devices used to confirm endotracheal tube placement. Two major styles of these devices exist: self-inflating bulbs and syringe style aspirators.

Esophageal-tracheal Combitube (ETC) A rescue device placed into the esophagus that allows tracheal placement. The double-lumen design allows for endotracheal as well as esophageal intubation.

Ethical relativism When a majority of Paramedics agree to a specific conduct or course of action, determining that it does more good than harm, which suggests the act is ethical.

Ethics From the Greek "ethos" meaning character, a system of guiding principles that govern a person's conduct.

Ethics committee A group that can help individuals, including Paramedics, deal with common ethical concerns.

Ethnocentrism A view that one's own cultural practices and customs are superior.

Etiology The origin of a disease.

Etomidate A sedative that functions primarily as a hypnotic, although it also is an excellent amnestic.

Eustress A positive, manageable form of stress from daily activities.

Eutectic mixture of local anesthetics (EMLA) A cream that helps to reduce the pain of needle insertion, consisting of lidocaine 2.5% and prilocaine 2.5%.

Evaluation and Management Documentation Guidelines Standardized histories that permit the Paramedic to identify diseases, disorders, and syndromes, vis-á-vis, through symptom pattern recognition, and document the medical necessity of the therapeutic services provided to the patient.

Event monitor A credit-card sized device patients may use to record abnormal ECG activity that occurs very irregularly (as in days or weeks apart). When the patient senses the abnormal activity, the monitor is placed on the chest for a preset period of time.

Event report Documentation following a mass casualty incident that details the situation and conditions that occurred which led to the incident. Triage tags are attached to this report.

Evidence-based practice A research approach based on observed experimental results, in hopes of making the results more reliable and valid than peer reviews.

Exacerbation Periodic episodes in which a chronic disease returns, or flares up.

Excitability The ability to respond to a stimulus.

Excited delirium A physical state a restrained patient may reach if agitated and combative in which he becomes tachycardic, hypertensive, and has hyperpyrexia.

Exercise A series of physical activities, both aerobic (e.g., walking or jogging) and strength training, which is considered optimal to perform for maintaining health.

Exhaustion The final, recovery stage of the general adaptation syndrome, which occurs when the body's response is insufficient to meet the challenge of the stressor.

Exogenous Originating outside of the body.

Exotoxins Proteins produced by bacteria that are released into the interstitial fluid. They are then absorbed, because they are highly soluble, into surrounding cells.

Expanded scope of practice Assigning additional duties and responsibilities to Paramedics beyond the scope of practice to provide health care where scarce healthcare resources exist.

Exposure Situation in which blood or bodily fluids from a patient are spilled, splashed, or dripped onto or injected into a Paramedic.

Exposure report A special incident report completed after an exposure that details the circumstances that resulted in the Paramedic being exposed, in hopes that a future exposure will not occur in the same manner.

Expressed consent During an emergency situation, an assumption that if a patient does not object to receiving care, consent for the procedure has been given.

External laryngeal manipulation A technique used to improve visualization of the glottic opening in which the Paramedic performs direct laryngoscopy with his left hand while manipulating the larynx with his right hand. Once he has an improved view of the glottic opening, the Paramedic has an assistant take over the external laryngeal manipulation, holding the larynx absolutely still.

Extracellular water The water that is outside of cells.

Extrinsic trigger A stimulus prompting an airway spasm that originates outside the body, such as pollen, dust, and mold.

Exudate A collection of white blood cells and fluids; whitish discharge.

Facilitation Interviewing technique in which the Paramedic nods his head in acknowledgement and says "Go on," as well as tries to make eye contact, which may encourage the patient to continue talking about a subject.

Facsimile machine A device that, using digital technology, can transmit a high-quality copy of documentation from one location to another.

Fading Progressive weakening of a radio wave as it encounters more and more obstacles.

Fahrenheit scale A standard used to measure temperature based on freezing and boiling temperatures of a water and salt solution. In this scale, water freezes at 32°F, water boils at 212°F, and a person's body temperature is 98.6°F.

Failure to thrive Situation in which a child does not grow as expected, perhaps due to psychosocial or nutritional imbalances.

Fallout Situation that occurs in the airway whenever large particles carried in the air current settle out as airflow velocity is lost.

False imprisonment A restriction of movement or a confinement that abridges the patient's right to freedom, such as by the use of restraints.

FarMedic© An EMS course specifically directed to the rural or farm emergency.

Fasciculations Transient fine muscle contractions, seen after administration of a depolarizing neuromuscular blocker.

Febrile non-hemolytic reaction An elevation of the patient's temperature of 1°C from baseline within two hours of the start of a transfusion which begins shortly after the initiation of the transfusion or a new unit. It is often secondary to minor antibodies present in the recipient's blood that cause a mild reaction when exposed to the donor's blood.

Federal Communications Commission (FCC) The agency with rule-making and enforcement responsibility for civilian radio frequencies.

Feedback The mechanism by which the Paramedic can ensure the message sent was the message received and decoded; that is, the message heard was the message sent.

Fee for service A "pay as you go" approach to health care, with a certain amount of medical care provided gratis to the poor or uninsured.

Femoral pulse A count of the beats created by blood flow in the femoral artery that is measured at the patient's groin.

Fetal alcohol syndrome Umbrella term covering a variety of birth defects caused by a mother drinking during pregnancy.

Fetal hydantoin syndrome (FHS) Birth defects such as cleft lip, cleft palate, and congenital heart anomalies seen in children born to mothers taking hydantoins during pregnancy.

Fibrin An elastic, insoluble, whitish protein produced by the action of thrombin on fibrinogen and forming an interlacing fibrous network in the coagulation of blood.

Fibrinogen A protein in the blood plasma that is essential for the coagulation of blood and is converted to fibrin by the action of thrombin in the presence of ionized calcium.

Fick principle The process of getting oxygen to the cells, which can be summed up in five key concepts: oxygenation, ventilation, respiration, circulation, and cellular respiration.

Fidelity The physician's obligation, and therefore the Paramedic's obligation, to keep any promises made to the patient.

Field A place to enter data on a chart or form.

Field diagnosis See **Paramedical diagnosis**

Fight or flight The body's instinctive response to a potential life threat, either to resist it or avoid it. This primitive stress response may have been critical to the survival of primeval man, but can be unhealthy today.

Fire-based EMS Using the fire service, with their combination of trained personnel, life-saving equipment, emergency vehicles, and strategically located stations, as the platform for delivery of EMS; the predominant means of delivering EMS in the United States.

First-due report A brief synopsis of the scene size-up obtained by the first arriving responder.

First pass metabolism A chemical degradation of a drug by the liver that markedly reduces the drug's bioavailability.

Fixed-post staffing The method of resource allocation in which EMS is stationed in centrally located standing facilities, from which ambulances respond to emergencies.

Fixed-wing aircraft A traditional airplane, rather than a helicopter, used by flight Paramedics to transport patients.

Flail segment Condition that develops when two or more adjacent ribs are fractured in two or more places, which produces an unstable area of the chest that impedes normal respiration.

Flashback A return of blood that may be observed in the tubing when an IV solution bag is lowered below the level of the patient's heart, which indicates that the IV access remains patent.

Flight Paramedic The most highly trained level of EMS provider; this individual transports critically ill patients from emergency scenes or other facilities to definitive care.

Fluori-methane A topical refrigerant, sometimes called vapocoolant spray, that numbs the skin at the injection site in as little as 15 seconds.

Flush the line A procedure in which the Paramedic runs fluid through an intravenous administration set to remove any air bubbles in order to prevent an air embolism.

Focused/vectored physical examination (PE) A more detailed evaluation following the primary assessment in which the Paramedic looks for observations that the physician will most likely request.

Followership A willingness to follow a leader's direction and to support the mission, putting aside personal ambitions.

Food, Drug, and Cosmetic Act Law that prohibits the sale of new drugs before they go through safety testing.

Foreseeable harm Risks that can reasonably be expected as a result of a medical procedure.

Frequency modulation (FM) When modulating an audio signal, changing the wave's speed.

Fresh frozen plasma Blood component formed by removing the red blood cells and platelets from whole blood. The remaining liquid component of the blood is still rich in several of the clotting factors needed as part of the coagulation system.

Functional job description Tasks described in a job description that are needed to perform the functions of the job, excluding rare or marginal job functions.

Functional syncytium A group of myocardial cells that act as a unit.

Gain Enlargement in the size of the tracing shown on the ECG monitor screen.

Gait The way a patient walks.

Gallop The combination of the normal and extra heart sounds that occur with changes in ventricular filling. This produces a galloping rhythm, similar to hearing a horse gallop.

Garbage can diagnosis An imprecise and overgeneralized field diagnosis the Paramedic might make that lends little direction to patient care.

Gene A sequence of nucleotides in DNA on a chromosome that determines an individual's physical characteristics.

General adaptation syndrome The body's predictable pattern of response to stressors.

General impression A Paramedic's overall evaluation of the patient, in which she assesses the patient's mental status, airway, breathing, and circulation, to determine which patients require immediate transport.

Generation A span of time used to differentiate advancements (e.g., the next generation of drugs).

Generic name A simple name given to a drug, often listed by the manufacturer in the United States Pharmacopeia (USP).

Genetic make-up Those physical characteristics that make up a person, including appearance, disposition, and so on.

Genotype An individual's genetic make-up.

Gestalt A decision-making process in which the Paramedic comes to a conclusion not through a summation of symptoms but rather from patterns observed in similar situations in past practice and experience. Also referred to as the Paramedic's "gut feel."

Glottis The space between the vocal cords.

Glucagon An enzyme that breaks down glycogen into individual glucose molecules.

Glycogen A dual molecule in the liver and muscles that stores any glucose which is not needed immediately by the body.

Glycolysis An aerobic process during which the body uses eight different enzymes to divide glucose and create a chemical called pyruvate.

Glyconeogenesis The production of glucogen from amino acids and fatty acids contained in lipids.

Glycoside Any of a group of organic compounds, occurring abundantly in plants, that yield a sugar and one or more nonsugar substances on hydrolysis.

Good Samaritan statutes Laws that protect well-meaning people who, although they have no duty to provide care to an injured person, do so nonetheless.

Governmental immunity Also called sovereign immunity, a practice in which the government is exempt from liability for torts committed by its employees except to the extent that it has consented by statute to be sued.

Gross negligence Intent to willfully, or with reckless disregard for a patient, cause harm to a patient.

Ground wave High-frequency (HF) radio transmissions that are capable of being transmitted over the land.

Guidelines General rules that provide the Paramedic with direction while also permitting use of her knowledge and experience to shape clinical decisions. Whenever guidelines are in use, the Paramedic must be willing to discuss and defend the clinical decisions.

Gum Sometimes called resin, a complex sugar in plants, a polysaccharide, that when moistened becomes a gelatinous material.

Haddon matrix An easily understood concept map of injury causation and prevention. Using a model similar to the one used for disease, Haddon plotted the factors that cause injury across a horizontal *X*-axis and the stages of an injury process along the *Y*-axis. The result was an injury prevention matrix.

Half-life (t½) The point when the decline of the amount of a drug in the bloodstream due to metabolism reaches 50%.

Hands-off The process in which one mobile radio tower switches the transmission to another tower so that there is no interruption in transmission.

Hanger Hook-like device an IV bag is hung from.

Hanging the bag Process of suspending an intravenous solution for delivery to the patient.

Hard-wire Use of physical transmission lines for communication rather than radio waves, i.e., wireless.

Hard wire monitoring Devices that feature electrodes running from the device to the patient, causing limited mobility for the patient.

Harrison Act A law established in 1914 that made it illegal to obtain "narcotics" (e.g., morphine) without a prescription.

Head elevated laryngoscopic position (HELP) A patient position that places the head in extension along the atlanto-occipital joints, bringing the pharyngeal, laryngeal, and oral axes into alignment using an elevation pillow. It can also be used in patients who are unable to lay flat (i.e., CHF patients or morbidly obese patients) or to help clear secretions.

Healthcare proxy This person has a responsibility to review the medical record, consult with healthcare providers, and give consent to either initiate or to refuse care for the patient.

Health Insurance Portability and Accountability Act (HIPAA) Federal legislation that has placed conditions upon all healthcare providers that protect patient privacy during claims processing, data analysis, utilization review, quality assurance, and practice management.

Health maintenance organization (HMO) A managed care system that provides payments to healthcare providers at a negotiated annual per capita rate. These rates are based on practice history of the insured patients and helps to prevent fluctuations in payments, thus making expenses, costs, and budgets more predictable.

Heart failure Situation in which an impaired heart cannot meet the body's demands for perfusion.

Heave To cause to swell or rise. When referring to the heart, a heave indicates the heart is beating so forcibly that the chest wall is felt to move by the Paramedic assessing the patient.

Heel stick Puncturing an infant's heel with a lancet then drawing the blood off with a capillary tube to acquire a sample.

Hematocrit The volume of red blood cells in the blood expressed as a percentage.

Hematoma A mass of clotted blood that forms in a swelling as a result of a broken blood vessel.

Hematopoiesis The manufacturing process the body uses to create the three main solid components of blood: red blood cells, white blood cells, and platelets.

Hemicorporectomy Amputation at the waist.

Hemocytoblast The generic stem cell from which all other blood cells (red, white, and platelets) develop.

Hemoglobin The molecule in red blood cells that accepts oxygen in the lungs and carries it to the body's tissues to allow cellular respiration.

Hemolysis The disintegration of red blood cells, resulting in a release of hemoglobin.

Hemostasis The stoppage of blood flow through a blood vessel or body part.

Hemothorax Collection of blood in the pleural cavity which can cause lung collapse.

Heparin sulfate An anticoagulant released from the endothelium of the walls of the arteries that temporarily prevents blood clot formation in the narrowed coronary arteries.

Heparin well An intermittent infusion device filled with heparin to prevent clot formation in the device.

Hepatectomy The surgical removal of a portion of the liver.

Hepatojugular reflux An elevation of venous pressure visible in the jugular veins when firm pressure with the flat hand over the liver.

Hermeneutics The Paramedic's ability to put himself in the patient's situation, with all of the accompanying physical and cultural influences, in order to understand the patient better.

Hernia Openings in the muscle and tissue layers that allow the an organ to protrude through the opening into another cavity.

Hertz A unit of frequency measured in cycles per second.

Hexaxial reference system An artificial construct created to help conceptualize the heart's normal axis and to help determine if there is any axis deviation.

High-flow nasal cannula (HFNC) An advance in nasal cannula technology in which, by humidifying and warming the oxygen and using membrane technology, up to 40 LPM is comfortably delivered to the patient through a nasal cannula.

High priority patients Patients with the most serious, yet treatable, conditions. They are generally transported to the hospital immediately, with further assessment being performed en route.

History of present illness (HPI) A chronological description of the development of the patient's present illness, including symptoms the patient is currently displaying, which may help the Paramedic make a diagnosis. This can be determined by asking when, where, why, and how type questions about the problem.

History taking Medical questioning to determine the disorder, syndrome, or condition affecting the patient that resulted in the call for assistance.

Histoxic hypoxia The inability of the cells to accept or use oxygen, such as in cyanide poisoning.

Holter monitoring A continuous type of ECG monitor that records the ECG activity while the patient goes about his routine work and play activities, which is often used on patients with sporadic dysrhythmia problems.

Homeostasis The processes a body undertakes to try to maintain a constant state of balance or equilibrium.

Horizontal equity Injury prevention strategy in which standards are broadly applied to all individuals equally, such as the level of a legal blood alcohol content.

Horizontal leadership A leadership style that "flattens the pyramid" so Paramedic leaders work toward linking, or networking, with the members of a public safety team. Horizontal leadership emphasizes an "out and back" line of communication instead of an "up and down" line of communication and can be visualized more like a wagon wheel.

Hormones The chemical messengers that stimulate the body's organs and help to maintain the body's internal environment.

Hospice A concept of care focused on providing for the physical, emotional, and spiritual needs of a terminal patient.

Hospital-based EMS An EMS system design where a hospital provides EMS services in the form of a flycar or ambulance.

Hotline A telephone number dedicated to providing the caller with immediate assistance.

Huber needle A beveled needle intended to pierce a stopper without coring it, thereby preventing leakage of the contents within the catheter from leaking out of the stopper when the needle is withdrawn.

Human dignity The right of every person to be treated respectfully, regardless of his or her station in life.

Human rights Rights based on a commonly desired human condition (i.e., freedom from want, freedom from pain, and freedom from suffering). Human rights involve universally accepted standards of justice.

Humoral immunity The component of the immune system involving antibodies that circulate as soluble protein in blood plasma.

Hydrostatic pressure Pressure created by the force behind the volume of water in the body.

Hyoid The only bone in the body that does not directly articulate with another bone. Instead, it serves as a common point of attachment for a number of muscles and ligaments that function in swallowing and airway maintenance.

Hyperacute T wave An increase in the amplitude of T waves in the leads facing cellular damage.

Hypercapnia Condition in which the partial pressure of carbon dioxide dissolved in an arterial blood gas sample is greater than 45; increased carbon dioxide levels.

Hypercarbia Condition in which the amount of bicarbonate ions in an arterial blood gas sample is greater than 30.

Hyperlipidemia An abnormally high level of triglycerides and cholesterol which, when uncontrolled, can lead to atherosclerosis.

Hyperoxia Condition in which partial pressure of oxygen dissolved in the arterial blood gas sample is greater than 100.

Hyperplasia An abnormal increase in the number of cells due to frequent cell division/reproduction which causes the tissue or organ to increase in size.

Hyperpnea Deep breathing.

Hyperreflexive Reflexes that are significantly more brisk than normal.

Hyperresonant Percussion notes that sound similar to striking a drum, indicating an increased amount of air in the chest.

Hypertension A systolic blood pressure that is above the upper limit of normal.

Hyperthermia A condition that occurs if too much heat builds up in the body's core; a body temperature above 38°C (100.4°F).

Hypertonic Fluid that has less water and more salt (electrolytes) than the solution on the other side of a semipermeable membrane. Hypertonic fluid on the other side of a semipermeable membrane will pull fluids into itself.

Hypertrophy An increase in either the weight or functional capacity of a tissue or organ beyond what is normal.

Hyperventilation A deeper than normal respiration that may be caused by respiratory distress, a metabolic condition, or drug overdose.

Hypnotic state A sleep-like condition often induced by a large dose of CNS depressants.

Hypocapnea Condition in which the partial pressure of carbon dioxide dissolved in an arterial blood gas sample is less than 35.

Hypocarbia Condition in which the amount of bicarbonate ions in an arterial blood gas sample is less than 22.

Hypoglycemia Condition in which blood sugar (or blood glucose) concentrations fall below a level necessary to properly support the body's need for energy and stability.

Hypokalemia The development of low sodium potassium in the blood serum.

Hyporeflexive Reflexes that are significantly less brisk than normal.

Hyporesonant Percussion note that is dull in character and often indicates fluid in the lung.

Hypotension A systolic blood pressure below the lower limit of normal.

Hypothermia A condition that occurs if there is too little heat in the body's core; a body temperature less than 35°C (95°F).

Hypotonic Fluid that has more water and less salt (electrolytes) than the solution on the other side of a semipermeable membrane. In an effort to balance concentrations, the water from the hypotonic solution will cross the membrane until the two solutions are balanced.

Hypoventilation Shallow respirations that can be caused by drug overdose, head injury, or another condition.

Hypovolemic A state of decreased circulating blood volume.

Hypovolemic shock The first category of the Hinshaw—Cox shock classification, which includes shock that arises from trauma (hemorrhagic shock) but also includes other etiologies where there is a loss of circulating blood volume.

Hypoxemia A decreased oxygen level in the blood.

Hypoxia Condition in which partial pressure of oxygen dissolved in an arterial blood gas sample is less than 70; low oxygen concentration that causes cells to redirect their metabolic processes to anaerobic respiration in an effort to sustain the cell.

Hypoxic hypoxia Lack of oxygen, due to an oxygen poor environment, which can lead to hypoxia.

Iatrogenic Adverse effects or complication that results from a medical intervention.

Idiosyncratic reaction Situation in which a drug produces an unpredictable reaction that is not allergic in nature or due to overdose and resultant toxicity, but often due to the patient's genetic make-up.

Immune complex Situation in which an antibody has attached to an antigen and stimulates the complement system.

Immunocompetent Capable of providing immunity.

Immunoglobulins A type of protein globulin. Five types of immunoglobulins have been identified: IgA, IgD, IgE, IgG (gamma globulin), and IgM. Each immunoglobulin fits into the surface of an antigen in a key and lock fashion, linking them together.

Implanted vascular access device (IVAD) A central venous catheter that has the port buried in a subcutaneous pocket under the skin's surface. Implanting the entire device affords the IVAD the skin's protection, which decreases the rate of infection, as well as protects the port from physical trauma.

Implied consent An assumption that an unconscious patient in danger would consent to a life saving procedure if awake and capable of consenting.

Incidence The number of new cases of a disease per standardized group per time. An example would be 1 case per 100,000 per year of x disease.

Incision and drainage (I&D) A minor surgical procedure used to release pus or pressure from a site such as an abscess.

Indirect statement A question that asks for an explanation that is not constrained by the question. An example of an indirect statement would be, "Please tell me about your pain."

In extremis An appearance of grave illness or mortal injury.

Infarction A large area of necrosis in a tissue or organ.

Inflammation A protective reaction of tissue to irritation, injury, or infection, characterized by localized pain, redness, swelling, and sometimes loss of function.

Initial assessment See **Primary assessment.**

Initial impression A global patient assessment made on initial contact with a patient based on a myriad of factors such as patient presentation, environmental factors, gross observation, and resources on-scene.

Injury Something that damages or harms.

Injury prevention See **Prevention; Injury prevention strategies.**

Injury prevention strategies Techniques used to go about implementing Haddon's countermeasures, which include engineering safety into products or processes, educating people about the dangers, increasing or improving enforcement of laws and regulations which promote safety, and providing economic incentives for people to use safer products or processes.

Inotropy To make the heart beat harder.

Insensible loss The volume of fluid that is lost from the body in the form of perspiration off the skin (1.1 liters/daily) and the vapor in the breath.

Insight An understanding of the patient's current or chronic medical condition, as well as the consequences of inappropriate treatment; the ability to make reasonable decisions.

Inspection A physical examination technique that involves looking closely at the patient.

Inspiratory capacity The total of the tidal volume plus the inspiratory reserve volume, which is a measure of the maximum air that can be inspired.

Institutional Review Board (IRB) An independent ethics committee consisting of experts from the fields of theology, sociology, psychology, and medicine, which is responsible for reviewing all aspects of a proposed research project in terms of the potential psychosocial impact and to ensure that all human subject research is ethical.

Integrity A personal commitment to a code of moral or ethical behavior which serves as a foundation for the patient–provider relationship.

Intended biological effect The modification a drug is designed to have on the function of a tissue or an organ, such as reduce fever, eliminate pain, and so on.

Interference Extraneous electromagnetic energy heard on the radio as crackles and dead spots.

Internal locus of control The idea that one has the ability to remain in control of a given situation.

International unit (IU) A standardized measurement that reveals the quantity of a biologically active substance, such as a hormone or vitamin, required to produce a specific response.

Interpretation An interviewing technique in which the Paramedic tries to determine the meaning of a message based on what is said and the speaker's nonverbal cues.

Interstitial fluid The fluid between cells.

Interval A segment and an ECG wave together.

Intimate space In the theory of proxemics, an area about the size of a beach blanket where patients feel most vulnerable. Entry into that space is only permitted to those people whom the patient trusts.

Intracellular water The water that is within cells.

Intradermal Injections that place a small quantity of medicine just under the epidermis and in close proximity of the subcutaneous tissue.

Intramuscular injection Injection deposited between the layers of muscle, which is a common method of medication administration.

Intraosseous (IO) An injection into the bone marrow.

Intravascular fluid A type of extracellular water found in the blood, which is primarily made of plasma and constitutes about 4% of the total body weight (3 or 4 L).

Intrinsic rate The rate at which the pacemaker cells of the heart depolarize.

Intrinsic trigger A stimulus prompting an airway spasm that originates within the body, such as through stress or exercise.

Inverted T waves A negative T wave that's normally positive and upright, which may indicate coronary ischemia.

Involuntary consent Situation during a life or limb emergency in which an officer can provide consent for a person in custody (e.g., a prisoner). Involuntary consent is usually reserved for true emergencies;

the police power to provide consent is not generally invoked for minor emergencies or elective procedures.

Ions An atom that has a positive or negative charge due to a gained or lost electron.

Ischemia A deficient supply of blood going to a body part due to an obstruction of the inflow of arterial blood.

Ischemic hypoxia Problems of circulation that can lead to oxygen deprivation at the cellular level.

Ischemic patterns Changes in an ECG as the result of abnormal repolarization.

Isoelectric line A line on the ECG that extends from the end of the T wave to the start of the ventricular depolarization represented by the QRS complex. This line indicates the period of time when the myocardium, particularly the ventricular mass, has been repolarized and awaits depolarization. An isoelectric line on the monitor and on the rhythm strip should appear as a flat line between ECG complexes.

Isometric Exercise using free weights.

Isotonic In terms of exercise, resistance exercises. In terms of fluid management, a balanced solution (equal water and salt on both sides of a membrane).

IV bags Soft plastic solution containers that collapse as the solution is withdrawn, eliminating the need for venting. These create a closed system that helps to decrease the risk of outside contamination.

IV push Procedure in which a Paramedic a medication by attaching a syringe filled with the medication to an infusion device and rapidly injects the medication.

Jaundice A yellowish hue of the skin, which can indicate liver failure or obstruction of the bile duct.

Joule heat Heat caused by the buildup of thermal energy as a result of electricity overcoming resistance from the tissues.

J point The start of the ST segment found at the juncture of the QRS and the ST segment, the point where the angle from the QRS changes.

Jugular venous pressure The force at which blood flows throughout the venous system, which can help diagnose issues in the lung and heart.

Junctional tissues A long strip of tissue below the AV node connecting the atria and the ventricles that is capable of independently initiating a stimulus if the SA nodal impulse should fail to depolarize one first.

Jurisdiction The court having authority to decide a legal case, typically based on location.

Justice The application of the concept of fairness, which implies impartiality in the administration of rewards. In terms of research, the belief that one group of people should not bear all the risks of research when the benefits of said research would benefit all persons in the larger society.

J-wire A special tightly wound spring wire with an open hook at the end to prevent it from puncturing soft tissues, which is inserted into the hub of a needle during the Seldinger technique.

Kaizen Japanese concept of continual self-improvement that emphasizes process and system thinking.

Keep the vein open (KVO) A slow infusion of fluid designed to be just enough to keep the veins from occluding.

Kefauver-Harris Act A 1962 amendment to the Federal Food, Drug and Cosmetic Act that required all drugs to undergo an extensive review that not only ensured the public's safety, but also reassured the public that a drug would do what it claimed to do.

Ketamine A dissociative anesthetic that provides excellent amnesia, analgesia, and anesthesia during procedures and intubation. Most notably, however, it has minimal respiratory depression even at very high doses.

Kinematics The branch of dynamics that studies motion apart from mass and force considerations.

Kinesics The study of nonverbal behavior in interpreting communications.

Knowledge base The Paramedic's previous experiences, anecdotal information, and formal medical education.

Korotkoff sounds Sounds heard during the inflation and deflation of the cuff that are caused by the change in the nature of blood flow through the artery.

Labor Uterus contractions which signify the start of the childbirth process.

Lacerations A torn or ragged wound.

Landline A hard-wired telephone.

Laryngeal mask airway A blindly inserted airway device designed to be used in situations where face-mask ventilation was inappropriate but the invasiveness of endotracheal intubation was not necessary.

Laryngoscope The primary, compact, and self-contained device healthcare providers use to visualize the larynx.

Larynx Also known as the "voice box," the upper group of structures of the lower airway that contains the vocal cords.

LD50 Shorthand for lethal dose 50%, the drug dosage where 50% of the test animals given that dose died.

Lead Any of the conductors connected to the electrocardiograph, each comprising two or more electrodes that are attached at specific body sites and used to examine electrical activity by monitoring changes in the electrical potential between them.

Lead I An electrode point that measures the voltage change between the right arm and the left arm. The negative electrode is on the right arm. The positive electrode is on the left arm.

Lead II An electrode point that notes the change between the right arm and left leg and provides a view of the inferior wall of the heart. The positive electrode is located on the left leg.

Lead III An electrode point that measures change between the left arm and left leg. The positive electrode is on the left leg.

Leading question A question that may direct the patient toward an answer that might not necessarily have been given if asked in another manner; for example, asking "Was the pain crushing?" rather than "Tell me what the pain in your chest was like."

Left anterior descending coronary artery (LAD) A coronary artery branch that provides blood to the anterior wall of the left ventricle.

Left bundle branch A division of the bundle of His that lies within the septum and serves as a further passageway for electrical impulses into the left ventricle.

Legitimate interest A determination of which individuals need access to a patient's confidential medical information, and the extent of the information they are entitled to view.

Legitimization The process in which a Paramedic listens and seeks to understand the patient and the patient's concern, regardless of how seemingly insignificant the problem. This process supports the patient and demonstrates caring.

LEMON law A rapid mnemonic used to predict a difficult airway when evaluating a patient. The elements of the LEMON law are to:

- L—Look externally for anything that will hinder ventilation or intubation
- E—Evaluate the 3-3-2 rule to assess the airway anatomy
- M—Mallampati classification
- O—Obstruction, either new or chronic, should be evaluated
- N—Neck mobility should be determined if not contraindicated (contraindicated in suspected C-spine injury)

Les ambulance volantes Light two-wheeled carriages used by the French military in the early 1800s that carried an attendant as well as a driver, often viewed as the precursor to the modern ambulance.

Leukocytes White blood cells, which help the body fight off disease.

Leukotrienes Slow acting substances of anaphylaxis that produce chemical effects similar to histamine and help to prolong the inflammation.

Libel Situation in which a falsehood damaging to a person's reputation is written or printed and then disseminated to the public.

Lidocaine A common local anesthetic and antiarrhythmic drug.

Life-long learning The commitment made by all Paramedics when they attain their first certification to remain current with the state of the profession.

Lighted stylettes Malleable stylettes with a bright light source at the distal end and a power source at the proximal end. When placed in the trachea, a bright, well-circumscribed light is seen in the midline of the trachea.

Line of sight (LOS) The path that radio transmissions take over land, which ideally are free of obstructions that will impede the radio waves.

Line-out To place a single diagonal line across any open areas of a document in order to prevent the addition of new content to a PCR by others after the Paramedic has completed the PCR.

Lipid-soluble A substance that is able to be dissolved in lipids (fat).

Lipophilic Characteristic of being attracted to lipids.

Liquid oxygen (LOX) Concentrated oxygen in liquid form.

Liquifactive necrosis Process in which cells that are largely lipid in content, such as the neurons of the brain, simply liquefy upon death and leave a pool in their place.

Literature Published reports of research.

Livor mortis A condition caused by relaxation of the vascular bed and a pooling of blood in dependent portions of the body.

Loco parentis Legal doctrine that states if a child has been left in the custody and care of another adult (e.g., a schoolteacher) then that adult has the authority to provide consent for medical care.

Lotions Topical medications mixed in water.

Lower esophageal sphincter (LES) A functional portion of the esophagus where its walls contract inwardly, forming a physical barrier to the reflux of stomach contents up the esophagus.

Low priority patients Patients with relatively minor conditions who can typically be treated in a more focused manner on-scene.

Lozenges Medicines intended to dissolve in the mouth.

Luer lock A needle adaptor that attaches to the syringe hub by use of a twist connection, where the adaptor on the syringe is grooved and will mate with a flange on the needle hub.

Lymphangitis Inflammation of the lymphatic channels in the skin that occurs when there is spread of an infection from a site distal to the channel.

Lymphedema The swelling of tissues on a limb due to lymphatic obstruction.

Lymphocytes Almost colorless cells found in the blood, lymph, and lymphoid tissues, constituting approximately 25 percent of white blood cells and including B cells, which function in humoral immunity, and T cells, which function in cellular immunity.

Lysosomes Tiny sacs in a cell that contain enzymes which can break down proteins.

Macintosh blade A curved laryngoscope blade with common sizes from 1 to 4 with a large flange and flat surfaces to control the tongue.

Macro-drop Administration set with a short, straight line that has few obstructions, such as filters or medication portals. It is used when volume replacement is needed (e.g., during a trauma resuscitation).

Macroglossia A state of having an abnormally large tongue.

Magmas Powdered drugs with particles so large that they are visible when they are mixed, or suspended, in water.

Malfeasance Wrongdoing or misconduct; for example, if the Paramedic performed an inappropriate procedure (e.g., gave a fluid bolus to a hypertensive head-injured patient).

Malignant Cancerous; something that will cause harm or damage health.

Malignant hyperthermia A skeletal muscle disease that leads to a life-threatening reaction to succinylcholine and some other inhaled anesthetics.

Malpractice Failure to exercise an appropriate degree of professional skill during a service, resulting in injury, loss, and damage.

Managed health care A financial system where a large corporation or the government obtains health insurance for its workers via private sources, who then gather groups of healthcare providers and obtains a reduced rate in exchange for a guaranteed client base. The managed healthcare insurance plan then mandates that patients seek treatment from this preferred medical group, in essence managing the care that the patient will receive by providing medical care for the lowest price.

Mandatory reporting A situation in which one is required by law to report a crime, such as child abuse, sexual assaults, gunshot wounds, certain communicable diseases, and animal bites.

Mason–Likar modification Adjustment in the placement of electrodes to help Paramedics obtain a more accurate 12-lead ECG, which involves moving the electrodes to the shoulders and the hip rather than the ankle and wrist.

Masses A large, firm area of considerable size in the body.

Master problem list In a POMR recordkeeping system, a list of the medical conditions for which a patient had been, or currently was, receiving treatment.

Mean arterial pressure (MAP) The average blood pressure in the arterial system over time, typically about 60 to 80 mmHg.

Mechanism of action The way a drug specifically works upon a cell.

Mechanism of injury (MOI) A description of the forces applied to a patient with the potential to cause injury, such as a motor vehicle collision (MVC) or a fall.

Medical command An immediate and direct physician involvement in patient care. The physician's authority can be exercised either on-scene or over-the-air at the time of an emergency.

Medical ethics The way Paramedics behave in regard to patients.

Medical intelligence The healthcare provider's process of learning from experience and past medical practice and then coming to a decision.

Medical lines Sometimes called lifelines, a means of adding medications directly into the circulation.

Medical oversight When a physician is involved in the quality assurance/quality improvement process and provides direction, either in the form of protocols or education, to Paramedics.

Medical Priority Dispatching™ A classification system designed to ensure the right response gets to the right person at the right time.

Medical record Documentation about the patient's condition that will be used in the future by other physicians and allied healthcare professionals for patient care. As a part of the medical record, the patient care report often provides vital information to physicians about the origin of a condition or disease.

Medical restraint Any device used to immobilize a patient for both the patient's and the care provider's safety; may include straps, jackets, and so on.

Medical self-help Instructions provided to patients by 9-1-1 on self-rescue actions they can take during the time before responders arrive.

Medical utility An assumption that those with the best medical prognosis should be treated with the medical provider's limited resources.

Medication-facilitated intubation The use of adjunctive medications during intubations, either to provide sedation or cause muscular paralysis to protect patients and improve their quality of care.

Medulla oblongata The part of the brain responsible for controlling involuntary vital functions; the brainstem.

Membrane attack complex (MAC) In cases where the body does not recognize the bacteria and cannot mount an effective antigen–antibody defense, a complex created by the complement system which attaches itself to the cell's walls and forms a tube from the outside to the inside. The tube allows water to enter the cell, the cell to swell, and the cell to lysis.

Memory cells Clone cells that have a memory of the make-up of the original cell.

Meniscus A concave-curved shape liquid assumes due to tensions within a syringe.

Menopause An age-related cessation of a woman's menses for an entire year, generally indicating the end of the woman's reproductive abilities.

Mentors Experienced master Paramedics who take on graduate Paramedics as their protégés to teach them paramedicine.

Meta-analysis A technique used when it is difficult to obtain a large population of study subjects, or the event being studied is relatively rare. The results of several similar small studies are combined and a statistical hypothesis test is applied, taking into account differences in subjects and methods used before a conclusion is made.

Metabolic acids Acids formed during anaerobic metabolism and amino acids formed by the breakdown/oxidation of proteins.

Metabolism Biochemical reactions that need to occur for life processes to go on.

Metabolite A chemical produced by degradation of a medication into subcomponents that may be active or inactive.

Metaplasia Replacement of one adult cell type with another type of adult cell.

Metered dose inhaler (MDI) Portable and simple-to-operate respiratory device that delivers a specific amount of aerosolized medication to the lungs.

Micro-drop Administration set with fine control of the infusion stream, used when careful titration of medicated fluid is desired (e.g., when a medical patient needs a slow infusion of a drug).

Micrognathia A state of having a small jaw.

Milieu An environment where an action can occur.

Military emergency medicine The largest and oldest EMS service, consisting of those who provide emergency medical care to members of the armed forces.

Miller blade A straight laryngoscope blade with common sizes from 00 to 4 with a small and curved flange designed to open a conduit to the larynx on the right side of the mouth and hold the tongue in the midline to the left side of the mouth.

Minimum data sets Certain fields with requested information that must be completed on a PCR or other form.

Minute ventilation A measure of the total volume of gas that passes through the lungs in a minute. It equals the respiratory rate (RR) times the volume per breath (Tidal Volume, or TV).

Misfeasance To perform a legal action in an illegal manner; for example, if the Paramedic performs the correct procedure but does so incorrectly.

Mitochondria The largest organelle in the cell, found outside a cell's nucleus, which produces energy.

Mitosis The process of cell division.

Mobile data terminal Laptop or handheld computers inside a vehicle a Paramedic can use to create a downloadable document for transmission over a telephone line, via modem, over the Internet, or by using wireless technologies.

Mobile subscriber units (MSU) The various varieties of cellular phones for use within a cellular radio system. The three main varieties are the portable cellular telephone, the transportable cellular telephone, and the mobile telephone.

Modified chest Lead 1 (MCL1) An alternative ECG lead Paramedics may use to monitor patients instead of/in addition to Lead II. MCL1 simulates the precordial lead V1, one of the six precordial leads of a 12-lead.

Morality A personal code of conduct.

Moral obligations Certain mores that go beyond the basic human rights which every patient enjoys; for example, an off-duty Paramedic's moral obligation may be to provide care when coming in contact with an injured person.

Morbidity The incidence of disease.

Morphology The shape of a QRS complex wave.

Mortality The state of death.

Motion A request sent to a judge for some action (i.e., dismiss the case, order a party to do something, postponement, cease and desist orders, etc.). A motion can be verbal, but is most often a written request that contains pertinent points for the judge to consider.

Mucolytics Drugs that thin mucous secretions and physically break down the viscosity of mucus by breaking apart the mucoprotein structure.

Multiple organ dysfunction syndrome (MODS) A failure of two or more organ systems.

Multiplex Radios that permit the transmission of audio signals as well as data.

Municipal EMS service A government-financed and administered EMS system that may exist as an independent entity or cross-trained with the police or fire department.

Murphy's sign Right upper quadrant tenderness that worsens when the patient takes a deep breath while the quadrant is palpated. A Murphy's sign indicates gallbladder inflammation

Muscarinic receptors Parasympathetic neuroreceptors that are slower than nicotinic receptors and indirectly open ion channels that cause depolarization. Muscarinic receptors, by definition, are more sensitive to muscarine, a naturally occurring chemical found in mushrooms, than to nicotine.

Mutation A change in the DNA sequence of one gene.

Myocardial infarction The death of myocardial cells.

Myocardial ischemia A condition that occurs prior to myocardial cell death in which the heart tissue is slowly or suddenly deprived of oxygen and other nutrients.

Myocardium A muscular layer that actually performs the heart's work by contracting forcefully and ejecting blood from within the heart's chambers.

Myoglobulinuria A condition in which the protein products of muscle breakdown clog the kidneys.

Narcotic The hallucinogenic effects of opiates, thought to be the result of stimulation of the sigma receptors located in the limbic system.

Narcotics A class of drugs known for their ability to induce a profound state of sedation.

Nares The openings to the nose; nostrils.

Nasogastric tube A single-lumen tube passed through the nose into the stomach to evacuate air from the stomach.

Nasotracheal intubation The process of aiding respiration by placing an endotracheal tube through the patient's nostril and into the trachea.

National Association of EMTs (NAEMT) A professional organization, founded in 1975, whose mission is to represent the views and opinions of all prehospital care providers.

National Centers for Injury Prevention and Control A federal agency tasked with injury surveillance.

National EMS Core Content Created under the leadership of the National Association of EMS Physicians (NAEMSP) a curriculum that defines the entire universe of disorders, diseases, syndromes, and skills that an EMS provider might encounter and for which he would be expected to provide emergency care.

National EMS Education Program Accreditation A designation that assures students their EMS education will meet national standards and assures the public that graduates of those educational programs will be competent providers.

National EMS Education Standards Created under the leadership of the National Association of EMS Educators (NAEMSE), the basis for EMS instruction that provides direction for EMS educators regarding both the core content and the scope of practice.

National EMS Scope of Practice (NEMSSOP) Created under the leadership of the National Association of State EMS Officials (NASEMSO), an organizational plan that clearly defines four levels of EMS providers and identifies the knowledge and skills required for each level.

National Formulary (NF) A drug reference manual that lists medications which are approved for prescription. It contains specific chemical information that is more helpful to the pharmacist and manufacturer than the physician.

National Registry of Emergency Medical Technicians (NREMT) An organization that provides a process of practical testing and written examinations for the certification of Paramedics, providing proof that the individual being licensed is minimally competent to provide a specified level of care. The majority of states currently accept National Registry certification for state licensure.

National Standard Curriculum (NSC) A seminal document that defines the scope of practice for many EMS providers distributed by the National Highway Traffic Safety Administration (NHTSA).

Nature of illness The history of the present patient's illness, often reported by the patient himself or the patient's family.

Necrosis A physiological process in which living cells die, often due to disease, injury, or some other pathological state.

Needle cricothyroidotomy A type of surgical airway performed by piercing the cricothyroid membrane with a large bore needle and catheter, allowing rapid access to an otherwise obstructed airway.

Negative pressure ventilation A mechanical ventilation technique in which a negative pressure environment is created around the patient's chest, thus sucking air into the lungs. An iron lung is an example.

Negligence A failure to exercise the degree of care that a prudent person would exercise.

Negligence per se Situation in which a Paramedic commits a criminal act, and the patient is injured as a result of that criminal act. The assumption is that the Paramedic's negligence flows from the criminal act.

Neostigmine An acetylcholinesterase inhibitor that can be used to reverse the effects of the competitive (non-depolarizing) NMBAs.

Neuroleptics Major tranquilizers that prevent nausea.

Neuromodulator Substances that inhibit the transmission of painful sensations to the brain and spinal cord by adjusting, or modulating, the rate of a neuron's discharge.

Neuromuscular blocking agents (NMBAs) Medications that block transmission of nerve impulses to skeletal muscle at the neuromuscular junction.

Neuroreceptor A chemical receptor that receives messages from the neurotransmitters.

Neurotransmitter A chemical messenger that transmits a nervous signal across the synapse.

Nicotinic receptors Chemical receptors from the parasympathetic nervous system found in the central and peripheral nervous system as well as the neuromuscular junction with skeletal muscles. Cholinergic stimulation of nicotinic receptors is quick in onset and short in duration, causing a sodium influx and local depolarization.

Nitric oxide (NO) A colorless, poisonous gas involved in oxygen transport to the tissues, the transmission of nerve impulses, and other physiological activities.

NKDA Acronym that stands for "no known drug allergies."

No apparent distress (NAD) An appearance of not having difficulty.

Nociceptors Pain receptors in the body that respond to chemical, mechanical, or thermal stimulus.

Noisy Characteristic of an ECG signal that is of poor quality and produces an unreadable tracing.

Non-depolarizing neuromuscular blockers One of the two major classes of neuromuscular blockers; competes with acetylcholine for the receptor but does not cause the receptor to fire.

Nonfeasance A failure to perform the correct or required procedure, which would be an error of omission; for example, if a Paramedic were to arrive on-scene of a cardiac arrest and the defibrillator failed because of a dead battery, which the Paramedic should have checked during routine maintenance.

Nonjudgmental Providing services based upon human need, with respect for human dignity, unrestricted by consideration of nationality, race, creed, color or status.

Non-malfeasance A concept suggesting that no act of harm will be done during a medical treatment.

Nonrebreather face masks (NRB) Oxygen masks with an oxygen reservoir that can deliver up to 80% FiO_2; they do not deliver 100% FiO_2 because there will always be some room air mixing through the open side port.

Nonspecific ST changes Situation in which the ST segment changes do not fit a pattern of ischemia, nor are they contributory toward another diagnosis. Causes of nonspecific ST changes include improper lead contacts, electrolyte abnormalities, drug-induced changes, hyperventilation, and even a drink of cold water.

Norepinephrine The chief neurotransmitter used in the sympathetic nervous system.

Normal saline (NS) A solution of 0.9% sodium chloride in sterile water (0.9% NaCl) that contains the same amount of salt as does blood. NSS has become an EMS standard solution in many systems because it is compatible with all medications as well as blood.

Normal sinus rhythm An optimal rhythm to provide adequate filling of the ventricles and sufficient ejection of blood for perfusion.

Normocardiac A heart rate between 50 and 100, which is considered to be normal.

Nosocomial A hospital-acquired infection.

Notary public A public officer recognized by the court who can verify the Paramedic's writings to authenticate them as evidence.

Null hypothesis When considering the results of a research study, the supposition that the treatment did not create changes (i.e., any changes are purely random and coincidental). The purpose of the study is to determine if the null hypothesis is true or false.

Nutritional flow The daily process of excretion and reabsorption of approximately half the nutrient-laden fluids in the body that is essential to the body's sustenance.

Nystagmus A fine tremble of the eye when holding a lateral gaze; unequal movement or oscillating eye movements that are usually involuntary.

Obesity A growing health crisis when an individual's body mass index is 30 or greater; a common layperson definition of morbid obesity is 100 pounds over ideal weight.

Observational study In contrast to the descriptive study, a study that asks a question and poses a simple explanation or hypothesis. To have a scientifically valid result from an observational study, one must control extraneous confounding variables that could account for the desired change.

Obstructive shock The final category of the Hinshaw–Cox shock classification, which deals with the physical impairment of forward blood flow despite an effective pump, an adequate blood volume, and a normal vasculature. Examples of obstructive shock include massive pulmonary clots, embolism, and a collapsed lung (pneumothorax), which proceeds to crush the heart as well.

Ockham's razor A theory that simply states that if all things are equal, the simplest solution tends to be the best one. In other words, common things occur commonly.

Oils Substances that have been extracted from plants for centuries for their use as food additives as well as medications.

Ointments Topical medications placed in either lanolin, an oil from sheep's wool, or petroleum jelly.

Oliguria An decreased output of urine, below 20 mL per hour.

Omega loop Creation of a stress loop when securing an intravenous administration set tubing to the patient. Initially, a strip of tape is laid across the adaptor and against the skin. Then a loop of tubing is taped across

the first strip of tape, which will absorb any tension on the tubing and potentially prevent the IV catheter from being displaced.

Oncotic Caused by swelling (e.g., oncotic pressure).

On-line medical control Medical command technique in which physicians can give medical direction and exercise medical command via the base radio.

Open-ended questions Questions that allow the patient to express himself without restriction, with answers that can be used as a springboard to other questions. Open-ended questions usually begin with words like "how," "what," or "could" and ask for an explanation.

Operational competence A Paramedic knowing how the various team members interact, knowing an organization's policies and procedures, and possessing situational awareness.

Opsonization A process in which the plasma proteins mark resistant bacterium by attaching fragments of themselves to the bacterial cell wall, thus enhancing the impact of the leukocytes.

Optic Pertaining to the eyes.

Orientation A person's awareness of himself in terms of place and time.

Orogastric tube A single-lumen tube passed through the mouth into the stomach to evacuate air from the stomach.

Orotracheal intubation The most common technique used to intubate patients, in which a laryngoscope is used to visualize the larynx and the vocal cords, and an endotracheal tube is observed to pass through the vocal cords.

Orphan drugs Drug therapies for rare or uncommon diseases, which generally are unprofitable for manufacturers to produce because the drugs are so rarely used.

Orthostatic hypotension An abnormal decrease in blood pressure that occurs when someone stands up.

Orthostatic vital signs Vital signs that change with position. For example, when an individual changes position from lying down to standing, the blood pressure normally has a tendency to drop due to gravity.

Oscilloscope An electronic instrument that produces an instantaneous trace on the screen of a cathode-ray tube corresponding to oscillations of voltage and current, used in some cases to measure electrocardiograms.

Osteoporosis A loss of calcium from the bones secondary to a decrease in hormones.

Otic Pertaining to the ear.

Otitis media A middle ear infection marked by pain, fever, or hearing loss.

Outcomes evaluation A matter of comparing the level of injury or illness before and after an injury prevention program.

Over-the-counter (OTC) Nonprescription medications that can be purchased by the public without a prescription so patients can self-treat minor illnesses.

Ovum A female gamete; the egg in a female fertilized by a sperm cell to create an embryo.

Oxygenation The ability to move oxygen from the air in the lungs into the blood.

***p* value** The probability of random chance causing the changes in a clinical trial, rather than the treatment. An acceptable *p* value is arbitrarily assigned by the researcher prior to the start of the study and is symbolized as α.

Packed red blood cells (PRBC) Blood component formed by removing nearly all of the plasma from a unit of blood and adding a small volume of preservative to the unit.

Pain threshold The amount of stimulus required to elicit a pain response in a person.

Palliative care Measures used to increase comfort and reduce pain, such as medication.

Palpation Evaluation that involves the provider placing his hands or fingers on the patient's body in an effort to detect any abnormalities.

Palpitations The sensation of one's heart having an irregular and/or rapid heartbeat.

Pandemics Outbreaks of diseases that spread throughout a country or a region, which may reach disaster proportions if not prevented or controlled in an appropriate fashion.

Papillary muscle Muscles that stabilize, open, and close the valve leaflets with each myocardial contraction.

Paradigm blindness The attitude that "we have always done it this way." Paradigms can sometimes become barriers to innovation and improvement.

Paradoxical respiration A disruption in normal respiration in which, during inhalation, the flail segment is drawn inward by the negative pressure in the chest rather than expanding outward with the rest of the chest wall. During exhalation, the opposite occurs due to the increased pressure in the thorax during exhalation.

Paraglossal approach An intubation technique that involves inserting the entire length of the laryngoscope blade blindly into the esophagus and then slowly withdrawing the blade under direct visualization.

Paramedic The highest level of EMS provider, whose skill level and education includes advanced assessment and diagnosis of syndromes and disorders and the treatment thereof.

Paramedic field diagnosis See Paramedical diagnosis.

Paramedical diagnosis A broad and comprehensive identification of a syndrome, a group of signs and symptoms that suggest a disease, or a primary disorder of homeostasis, such as hypoxia, in a patient upon assessment by the Paramedic.

Paramedicine A special subset of medicine that Paramedics provide in the out-of-hospital setting.

Parasympathetic nervous system The portion of the autonomic nervous system responsible for the body's involuntary vegetative functions including digestion, heart rate, and the like, largely controlled by the vagus nerve. These functions are summarized as "feed and breed."

Parasympathomimetic A chemical agent that mimics the action of acetylcholine.

Parenteral A method of drug administration that bypasses the gastrointestinal system, such as injection, which is preferred during an emergency because of the rapidity of onset of the medication's action as well as predictability of the drug levels.

Past medical history (PMH) Significant historical information necessary to determine the nature and potential severity of the patient's illness or injury. All patients should be questioned about issues like chronic illnesses, medications taken, allergies, and use of tobacco, alcohol, or other drugs.

Pathogen An organism that causes an infectious disease.

Pathogenesis The sequence of events—at the molecular and cellular level—that leads to organ dysfunction.

Pathologic Physical changes as a result of disease.

Pathophysiology The study of the causes of suffering in the normal human condition.

Patient advocate An individual who fights for the rights and wishes of the patient in terms of health care. Whenever a Paramedic acts to help a patient obtain needed health care, he is acting in the advocacy role.

Patient autonomy The patient's ability to control her person and her personal destiny through decision making. Followed to its logical conclusion, patient autonomy implies that patients could decide to do nothing about a fatal illness, a decision that might lead to their own demise.

Patient care report (PCR) Documentation completed by the Paramedic indicating the care provided to a particular patient.

Patient concordance The process of shared decision making between the healthcare provider and patient.

Pattern recognition A tendency to quickly label an ECG rhythm because it looks like another ECG rhythm seen previously, which is poor practice because it negates nuances that differentiate one wave from another.

PCR audits A careful review of the patient care report documentation for specific data that allows healthcare managers, EMS administrators, and EMS physicians to ensure that acceptable patient care is provided to all patients equally.

Peak expiratory flow The maximum velocity of gas movement during exhalation.

Peak-load staffing EMS practice in which, during predictable hours of high demand, additional ambulances are placed in-service at strategic locations.

PEARLS A mnemonic (partnership, empathy, apology, respect, legitimization, and support) that includes the qualities needed to provide for a strong Paramedic–patient relationship.

Peer reviewed An article or research study that was critically appraised by experts in the field for validity.

Penumbra A predictable pathway of cell changes leading to cell necrosis and myocardial infarction.

Percussion The act of lightly but sharply tapping the body surface to determine the characteristics of the underlying tissue.

Percussion note The sounds that result from the act of percussion. Air-filled structures will produce a hollow, tympanic percussion note similar to that of a drum. Fluid-filled structures will produce a dull percussion note. Solid structures will provide a loud, well-defined percussion note.

Percutaneous central venous catheters (PCVC) A central venous access device inserted into the deep veins via the subclavian vein (in the chest), the internal jugular vein (in the neck), and the femoral vein (in the groin).

Percutaneous cricothyrotomy A surgical technique used to gain entry to the trachea through placement of a needle, then guidewire, then a small bore tracheostomy tube in a rapid fashion with less bleeding than a traditional surgical cricothyrotomy.

Pericarditis An inflammation of the pericardial sac that surrounds the heart.

Pericardium The membranous sac filled with serous fluid that encloses the heart as well as the roots of the aorta and other large blood vessels.

Peripherally inserted central catheter (PICC) A very long central venous access catheter placed within a vein in the antecubital fossa that is threaded into the vena cava while under fluoroscopy.

Peritoneum The inner lining of the abdomen.

Persistent vegetative state (PVS) A permanent state of unconsciousness.

Personal digital assistants (PDA) Personal palm computers Paramedics can use as they move about

the patient compartment at will, all the while transmitting and receiving critical patient information.

Personal space In the theory of proxemics, the area where a patient would engage in a one-on-one conversation. This personal space, about one and one-half feet to four feet, is the distance within which most Paramedics initially interview patients for a history.

Pertinent negatives Those symptoms which, if present in a patient, could indicate a more serious underlying problem.

pH scale A measure of the differing degrees of acidity or alkalinity in a substance. The range of pH is from 0 to 14, with 7 being neutral. Values lower than 7 are acids, values higher than 7 are bases, and pure distilled water is neutral (pH is an abbreviation for potential hydrogen).

Phagocytosis A process in which neutrophils destroy bacteria by engulfing them.

Pharmacodynamics The study of how drugs come to create their therapeutic effect.

Pharmacogenomics A combination of pharmaceutical research with the study of the human genome.

Pharmacokinetics The study of how drug absorption, distribution, detoxification, and elimination affect a drug's therapeutic value.

Pharmacological effect A new or different effect a drug generates in the body other than what was expected.

Pharmacology The study of drugs.

Pharynx The area of the airway composed of the spaces behind the nose (the nasopharynx) and the oral cavity (the oropharynx).

Phenotype The visible outward expression of the chromosome, which is the result of the genetic influences of both parents.

Phlebotomy The act of drawing or removing blood from the circulatory system in order to obtain a sample for analysis and diagnosis.

Physical examination Also called an exam, an assessment of the patient from head to toe in an effort to detect signs associated with a disease or condition.

Physician extenders Allied health professionals who work under the license granted to the physician.

Physician's Desk Reference (PDR) A reputable source of information about prescription and over-the-counter medications; a compendium of manufacturer drug-prescribing information which is usually found in a package insert required by law to accompany all medications.

Physician's Order of Life-Sustaining Treatment (POLST) A more detailed description than a DNR order of the patient's wishes, placed in the form of a physician's order. These forms are generated through a discussion between patients and their physician that addresses specific situations including utilizing artificial hydration, nutrition, intubation, antibiotics, and other medical therapies.

Physiologic A physical loss of cells as a result of the normal changes of aging or simple disuse; a natural development of cells.

Physiology The study of the body's functions, in its normal human condition, which focuses on the physical, mechanical, and biochemical processes that go on inside the body every day (i.e., how the body works).

PIER A model public education system developed by the National Highway Traffic Safety Administration (NHSTA) which stands for public information, education, and relations.

Piggyback infusion The process of administering a medication infusion by attaching the secondary intravenous line containing the medication to a primary intravenous line to eliminate the need for a second intravenous line.

Pitting edema The amount of indentation produced when the edematous limb is pressed over the tibia by the examiner's finger.

Placebos Inactive drugs used in research trials that appear similar to the actual drug in order to create blinding for the participants.

Placenta The vascular organ that connects the unborn child to the mother's uterus, providing safety and nutrition during its development.

Plain English transmissions The use of everyday speech to transmit information rather than using codes or jargon.

Plantarflexion The ability to push the toes downward and away from the tibia.

Plaque Fatty lesion formed in the artery as a result of atherosclerosis.

Plasma cells Cells that generate antibodies.

Platelet See **Thrombocytes.**

Platelet plug A concentrated mass of platelets that serve as a short-term fix to a plaque rupture.

Pleura The delicate serous membrane that lines each half of the thorax and is folded back over the surface of the lung on the same side.

Pleural effusion Excess fluid that builds up in the fluid-filled space that surrounds the lungs, which can cause difficulty breathing.

Pneumothorax Condition in which air or another gas is present in the pleural cavity as a result of disease or injury.

Point The end of a needle, often cut obliquely in such a fashion that a sharp leading edge is created.

Point of care Testing done in the field by the Paramedic, such as capillary blood draws, which enhance the Paramedic's ability to provide immediate emergency services while still in the field and to transmit critical information to the emergency department.

Point of service (POS) A managed care system with qualities of both an HMO and a PPO. The patient is allowed to choose a healthcare provider from among a list of preferred care providers (PCP) but may elect to see another "out of system" provider, without a referral, at a substantially higher copayment and/or deductible, similar to a fee-for-service arrangement.

Polarity The direction of a QRS complex wave.

Portable radios Radio devices that can be carried from place to place.

Positional asphyxia Situation in which a patient in excited delirium develops hypoxia and goes into cardiac arrest when restrained prone, particularly if hobble restrained.

Positive pressure ventilation A mechanical ventilation technique in which the pressure in the patient's airway is increased, thus forcing air into the lungs. Intubation or a bag-valve mask are examples.

Postmortem Specific changes within the body that are associated with death.

Post-traumatic stress disorder (PSTD) According to the *Diagnostic and Statistical Manual*, the development of "characteristic symptoms following exposure to an extreme traumatic stress involving direct personal experience of an event that involves actual or threatened death or serious injury, or other threat to one's physical integrity; or witnessing an event that involves death, injury or a threat to the physical integrity of another person."

Potable infusions Process of boiling water over the top of medicinal herbs and immediately drawing off the solution.

Potent Chemically or medically effective; strong.

Potentially infectious materials (PIM) Any substance with the ability to transmit bacteria to another material.

Potentiation Situation in which one drug increases the effectiveness of another drug.

Power The ability to attribute the changes in a research study to the treatment rather than chance.

Predictable injury pattern Characteristic injuries associated with a particular mechanism of injury.

Preferred provider organization (PPO) A managed care system that serves as a modified fee-for-service schedule, permitting patients to choose their healthcare provider from among a roster of approved physicians.

Prefix An affix placed at the beginning of a root word to modify that root word; for example, adding the prefix "un-" to the root word "do" makes "undo," the opposite of do.

Pre-induction agents CNS depressants administered as a premedication before the introduction of anesthesia to decrease the incidence of fear or panic (anxiolysis) or combativeness (sedation) in the patient.

Preload The volume of venous blood entering the heart during diastole.

Prescription drugs Drugs that cannot be dispensed by a pharmacist without the written or verbal order of a physician or a mid-level healthcare provider, such as a physician's assistant.

Pressured speech Condition characterized by a patient speaking so fast it appears she has an urgency or pressure to speak quickly.

Preventative maintenance (PM) A program that forestalls the incidence of failure, thereby decreasing the incidence of injury and potential litigation.

Prevention The steps taken to avoid illness or injury.

Primary assessment The Paramedic's initial evaluation performed to find and manage any life-threatening injuries or conditions the patient might have by assessing for (and correcting, if possible) any threats to airway, breathing, and circulation.

Primary infusion A continuous intravenous set to which other medications may be added as supplements.

Primary rhythm The main heartbeat.

Prime wave The first wave in a QRS complex in a situation where a wave repeats itself. The prime wave is represented by a capital letter and the second wave is represented by a lowercase letter. For example, a proper notation of a QRS might read RSr.

Primum non nocere The duty to "first, do no harm."

PR interval The distance from the beginning of the P wave to the start of the QRS complex.

Privacy officer An officer at a healthcare agency responsible for providing patient record security and recording security awareness training of all employees, as well as implementing a privacy protection plan within the agency.

Private line (PL) See Coded (or tone) squelch.

Problem-oriented medical recordkeeping (POMR) Recordkeeping system in which a master problem list records the medical conditions for which that patient had been, or currently was, receiving treatment. Indexed as such, new entries in the medical record would be placed into the patient's file under the problem listed. All healthcare professionals, from physicians to nurses to dieticians, would place their entries into the patient's record. This system provides some order to the records needed by hospitals, medical specialties, and allied healthcare providers—all of whom need the same information.

Process evaluation A measurement of the means used to carry out a program and how successful it was.

Process server A person hired by an attorney to deliver a summons and complaint to the defendant in a case.

Prodrugs A precursor of a drug that is converted into its active form in the body by normal metabolic processes. For example, heroin is a prodrug that, when acted upon by the liver, metabolizes into morphine.

Product liability The responsibility a manufacturer has to ensure a drug (or other product) is not defective (unfit for its suggested use or results in harm to the consumer).

Professional development Steps a Paramedic may take to continue advancement of his or her EMS skills, which may include attendance at state and national EMS conferences or regional workshops, consultation with medical directors for guidance and education on new technologies, and review of EMS trade journals.

Prognosis The expected outcome from a disease, determined by a culmination of modifiable risk factors, nonmodifiable risk factors, and the availability of treatments.

Progress notes In a POMR recordkeeping system, new entries in the medical record.

Pronator drift An indicator of upper motor neuron weakness that is tested for by asking the seated patient to hold her arms out with the palms facing the ceiling and then close her eyes. The test is positive if one arm drifts away from the starting position.

Prospective research The most scientifically valid research, in which an attempt is made to account for all predictable or known confounding variables, to control those variables, and then add a treatment. If change occurs, then it may be reasonable to conclude that the treatment may have caused that change.

Prostaglandin A chemical mediator released from the mast cell that creates the sensation of pain, although its primary function is to increase vascular permeability and smooth muscle contraction later in the inflammatory response.

Protected health information (PHI) Facts from a patient's medical record that are not to be dispersed to the public without authorization.

Protective custody Situation in which a law enforcement officer assumes temporary custody of a child in order for the child to receive medical care after the parent refuses to give consent.

Protocols A written set of mandatory instructions for the Paramedic to use in specific situations in the absence of the physician. Protocols, almost by definition, assume that one patient's situation is the same or similar to another patient's condition in the same situation.

Proxemics A theory based on the concept that four spaces surround a person—intimate space, personal space, social space, and public space—which provide varying levels of comfort when people move within them.

Proximate cause The immediate or direct reason why something occurred. In legal terms, the action that created an injury or reason for a claim.

Prudent layperson standard An approach to defining an emergency that simply estimates if another citizen, not a physician, who was in the same or similar circumstance would think it appropriate to call EMS.

Public Health Model A framework showing the connections between host, agent, and environment in preventing injury.

Public Health Service A federal program which makes up a key portion of the Department of Health and Human Services. With 5,700 commissioned health services officers and 51,000 civilian employees, all led by the Surgeon General, the current United States Public Health Service provides support to county and state Public Health Departments as well as health care to medically underserved areas.

Public information officer (PIO) An EMS agency employee whose responsibility is to interface with the news media and provide public information.

Public safety access point (PSAP) A centralized communications center which runs 24 hours a day, seven days a week, and contains the entire 9-1-1 operation; a place where a service callback or additional emergency information would be available.

Public space In the theory of proxemics, the area one would occupy with a stranger without fear but with an ability to flee if danger should arise.

Public trust An understanding between the patient and the Paramedic that the patient will be treated with dignity and respect in the same manner a physician would treat the patient.

Pulse oximetry A noninvasive measurement of the percentage of hemoglobin in arterial blood that is bound to oxygen molecules.

Pulse pressure The difference between the systolic and diastolic blood pressures. The pulse pressure can provide the Paramedic with an indication about the blood volume status or compensation for illness in a given patient.

Pulseless electrical activity (PEA) A situation in which the patient displays electrical activity in the heart but no signs of contraction; an electrical rhythm without a pulse.

Punitive damages Money paid to reimburse an individual for more than just the actual damages suffered that prompted a court case; a monetary fine designed to "punish" the loser of the case.

Pure Food and Drug Act of 1906 A law that prohibits the use of false or misleading claims about medicines. The law further stipulates that if a medicine contains any of the 11 "dangerous" drugs, then the drug(s) have to be listed on the label.

Purkinje fibers Cardiac muscle fibers that connect directly with the ventricular myocardium, allowing the ventricles to contract nearly simultaneously with the atrioventricular node, creating a functional syncytium.

Pursed lip breathing A sign of increased work of breathing, in which the patient puckers his or her lips while exhaling, providing some resistance to exhalation that provides pressure to keep the alveoli open.

Putrefaction A process of decomposition within the body characterized by greenish discoloration, secondary to hemolysis of blood, and slippage of the skin from the skeleton, due to breakdown of subcutaneous fat.

Pyelonephritis An infection of the upper urinary tract and kidney.

Pyrexia A fever that makes the body's environment hostile to bacteria.

Pyrogen Chemical mediator that produces fever.

Pyrogenic reaction A devastating systemic complication of intravenous therapy that occurs when a contaminated fluid, or fluid run through a contaminated administration set, is infused and leads to nearly immediate sepsis.

QRS complexes A combination of two or more ECG waves, which combine in predictable ways to describe other cardiac events and are the basis for ECG interpretation.

Quadrageminy Situation in which ectopic beats occur every fourth beat.

Quality assurance (QA) Verifying a program's compliance with established standards.

Quarantine The practice of isolating diseased individuals from the larger community.

Quickening Fetal movements during the second trimester that serve as the first signs of life.

Q waves Pathologic waves on an ECG that indicate electrical silence (i.e., no depolarization) in a certain portion of the ventricular wall.

Radial pulse A measure of the beats created by blood flow taken at the wrist over the radial artery.

Radio head A small remote radio control panel placed in the driver's and/or patient compartment of an emergency vehicle. The actual transmitter is usually placed in a different location in the vehicle.

Range A certain set of acceptable physical parameters the body uses to try maintaining a normal equilibrium.

Rate counter A digital readout on some ECG monitors that measures the number of ECG complexes that pass in a minute, usually counting the tallest, or deepest, wave on the ECG.

Reasonable accommodations Actions taken by an employer to make a workplace more accessible for a person with special needs, such as adding ramps or elevators.

Rebound tenderness Tenderness that becomes worse when the pressure is suddenly released during palpation that may indicate irritation of the peritoneum.

Recanalization The process of re-opening an artery to restore blood flow.

Reception The process of interpreting a sent message, which may be influenced by both physical and cultural factors.

Receptor The portion of a cell that attracts a certain molecule.

Reciprocal changes ST-segment depressions seen on the 12-lead ECG in leads that face the wall opposite of those with ST-segment elevations.

Recovery For cells, a return to a former functional capacity. For a person, a return to health.

Reentry phenomenon The reexcitation of a region of the heart by a single electrical impulse, which may cause ectopic beats, tachyarrhythmia, or an abnormal conduction mechanism.

Refereed A review process in which an editor will typically distribute an article to a panel of expert Paramedics, who offer input and edit the article. The article is returned to the author, who revises the article based on the edits.

Reference librarian A librarian trained in research techniques who can help researchers develop a search strategy to identify which resources, such as articles, will be most helpful in a study.

Referred pain Pain from one source transmitted to other parts of the body, via common nerve pathways.

Reflected path When using the radio wave phenomenon of bounce, using enough reflective surfaces so that the redirected radio transmission will roughly result in the intended direction of travel.

Reflection An interviewing technique in which the Paramedic repeats the patient's words, which may encourage additional responses. Reflection is helpful because it typically doesn't interrupt the patient's train of thought.

Refractory Unable to respond to a new stimulus.

Refusal of medical assistance (RMA) A situation in which a patient can consent to a medical procedure, and yet still refuses care.

Regulations Rules established by a government department to regulate the conduct of citizens.

Regurgitation A backflow of blood into the atria.

Rehabilitation Steps such as taking a rest break, eating some food, drinking fluids, and using lavatories that help EMS responders handle stress more effectively while at the scene of a prolonged incident.

Relative bradycardia A sinus rhythm with a rate that is too slow for the patient's metabolic needs.

Release of information A written authorization allowing documents to be given to an attorney.

Reliable Giving the same result on multiple trials.

Remission Situation in which the body's defenses, or medical treatment, may force the disease into a non-active state. Remission does not mean the patient has been cured, but rather means the disease has been stopped.

Remodeling To change the shape of something, such as the interior chamber of a ventricle.

Repeaters Radios that pick up, amplify, and then retransmit a radio transmission, which can extend the range of a VHF almost indefinitely.

Repolarization The restoration of a polarized state across a membrane, as in a muscle fiber following contraction or the recovery of the myocardial cell.

Rescue devices Airway management tools used when intubation is not successful, such as a blind insertion airway device.

Residual Physical or chemical changes that remain in a patient after an encounter with a disease, such as scars or hemiplegia.

Resistance The second stage of the general adaptation syndrome, during which the body attempts to reestablish homeostasis, utilizing the endocrine and/or the immune system.

Respect High regard based upon a nonjudgmental attitude toward the patient.

Respiratory acid Acid in the body formed when excess carbon dioxide reacts with water to form carbonic acid (H_2CO_3) before conversion into bicarbonate, which is the intermediary step in carbon dioxide transport.

Resting membrane potential A difference in the electrical potential between the outside of the cell and the inside of the cell while in a resting state.

Reticular activating system (RAS) A complex network of interconnected reflexes in the brainstem that maintains wakefulness.

Retrospective research Research technique in which a Paramedic looks at past practice, typically from patient care reports, to determine how to resolve a current issue or question.

Re-uptake The reabsorption of a neurotransmitter by a neuron following impulse transmission across a synapse.

Reverse R wave progression The loss of an R wave progression, which is suggestive of an anterior wall AMI.

Reverse use- (rate) dependent Drugs that prolong the repolarization of normal myocardial tissues, as electrographically demonstrated by a prolonged QT interval.

Rhabdomyolysis A breakdown of skeletal muscle releasing cell contents including myoglobin.

Rib retractions Situation in which the work of breathing increases and more effort is needed to generate the negative pressure in the thorax required for inspiration. When this happens, the skin between the ribs is pulled inward because of this negative pressure in the chest.

Right Something to which a person is entitled based on society's sense of fair play.

Right bundle branch A division of the bundle of His that lies deep within the myocardium and serves as a further passageway for electrical impulses to the right ventricle.

Right chest leads ECG recording technique in which the V4 to V6 wires from the left chest electrodes are switched over to the same relative position on the surface of the right chest and the ECG is rerecorded as V4R, V5R, and V6R.

Right coronary artery (RCA) Cardiac artery that provides blood to the right atrium and ventricle and the inferior portion or wall of the left ventricle.

Rigor mortis A stiffening of the muscles, which often occurs after death.

Risk The likelihood that a situation could lead to harm.

Risk factors Traits or practices that tend to make a person more or less vulnerable to a disease as compared to another person.

Risk management A plan that emphasizes safety and whose goal is to reduce Paramedic injury in an effort to promote a culture of safety in an organization.

Risk manager An individual in an organization who identifies known hazards and then tries to mitigate those hazards.

Root A word, often supplemented with prefixes or suffixes, that relates to the main idea and often describes the organ involved or the key symptom.

Rovsing's sign Pain in the right lower quadrant that occurs when the left lower quadrant is palpated, which is often associated with appendicitis.

Rub A low-pitched, soft scratching sound that occurs at any time during the cardiac cycle.

Rules out A deductive process in which the Paramedic eliminates all explanations for the patient's condition that don't match the symptoms, thereby leaving the correct diagnosis.

Runaway infusions An out-of-control drip infusion that results in the patient being overmedicated.

Running the line out The process of clearing intravenous administration tubing of any air and running fluid freely from the end.

Run of ventricular tachycardia Nonsustained bursts of ectopic ventricular beats that occur three or four at a time.

R wave progression A series of changes in the primary deflection of the QRS from negative in V1 to positive in V6 in a normal 12-lead ECG.

SAFE-R A crisis intervention model consisting of five steps: stimulation reduction, acknowledgement, facilitation, explanation, and return or restoration.

Safety officer In a large emergency situation, an individual assigned to maintain scene safety for the responders.

Saline locks Process of filling the intermittent infusion device with saline to seal, or lock, the device and prevent thrombus formation.

Salvo see Run of ventricular tachycardia.

Satellite phones Satellites that radio waves are sent to, in which they literally bounce off the satellite and return back to Earth, bypassing obstructions such as mountains.

Scanners Multiband radio receivers that monitor several radio frequencies, including those used by cellular telephones.

Scene safety Steps taken to ensure the Paramedic's well-being when responding to an emergency situation, such as rerouting traffic, assessing for threats, securing unstable areas, and the like.

Schizokinesis A physiological theory that suggests past painful experiences, unconsciously recalled by trigger words, can elicit an autonomic nervous system response. In some cases, this response could be harmful to the patient.

Scientific method The acquisition of knowledge through objective observation and considered reasoning.

Sclerosis An inflammation, thickening, or hardening of a body part.

Scope of practice The duties and responsibilities that fall under a particular Paramedic's experience and skill level.

Scored Adding a depression across the middle of a tablet that makes dividing the tablet in half easier.

Script An idea in the Paramedic's mind about a set of symptoms that has an associated symptom complex and an associated field diagnosis and treatment plan.

Sedative Medications used to decrease a patient's level of consciousness, lessen irritability, decrease excitability, or cause muscular relaxation.

Segment The space between ECG waves.

Seldinger technique A catheter-over-the-wire technique used to cannulate the femoral vein.

Self-awareness Possessing a conscious understanding of one's life influences and prejudices.

Semantics The meanings of words.

Senescence A breakdown in the body's ability to monitor for organ system failure and to repair those organs, which is inherent in the concept of being elderly.

Senile dementia Altered mental status caused by irreversible damage to the brain that typically is manifest over a long period of time (e.g., a series of brain attacks, such as strokes).

Sensitivity A measure of how often a medical field test gives a correct positive result.

Sepsis A toxic condition resulting from the spread of bacteria or its toxic products from a focus of infection.

Septal hematoma A form of nasal trauma that results in a bruise or bleeding.

Septic shock Condition in which the patient develops a potentially serious drop in blood pressure from a systemic infection in the blood.

Serial vital signs All vital signs taken after the baseline vital signs that are useful to illustrate trends in vital sign changes.

Serotonin A neurotransmitter found primarily in the gastrointestinal tract that causes arterial and venous constriction.

Serve In legal terms, to cause to be delivered, as in a summons or other document.

Settlement A sum of money paid to the plaintiff in order to conclude a case without going through a trial.

Shams Ineffective devices used in research trials that appear similar to the actual device in order to create blinding for the participants.

Shared decision making Collaborative medical practice in which the patient is seen as being interdependent with, rather than dependent on, the Paramedic. In a shared decision-making model, the patient is consulted about clinical decisions, empowering her with current information about her state of health.

Shared practice The knowledge that both physicians and Paramedics are responsible for the patient's care.

Shock–liver A form of liver failure.

Shunting A displacement of blood volume to the core circulation.

Side effects Unintended reactions one may have to a medication in addition to its therapeutic effect, such as drowsiness or nausea.

Sign Indication that appears during a physical examination that suggests the cause of a disease or injury.

Sign-out An authentication measure in which the Paramedic writes the time, date, and initial after the last entry. The sign-out indicates that the PCR was written and completed by the person listed "in-charge" at the time and date listed.

Simplex A radio system that only allows communication in one direction at a time, such as a walkie-talkie; the simplest radio system.

Sim's position A modified left lateral position used when administering medication rectally in which the patient is asked to bring her right knee to the chest as far as practical. This position provides optimal access to the anus while minimally compromising the patient's dignity.

Simulcast The ability to interact with several departments of an organization at once.

Single-blind study A research study in which the subjects do not know which group they are in, although the researcher does.

Sinoatrial node (SA) The initial portion of the conduction system, located just beneath the epicardium on the posterior wall of the right atrium near to the end of the vena cava and at the junction of the sinus of Valsalva and the atria.

Sinus bradycardia A sinus rhythm with a rate below 60 bpm, although most patients are not symptomatic until the heart rate falls below 50 bpm.

Sinus dysrhythmia An irregular heart rhythm characterized by alternating increases and decreases in the heart rate.

Sinus of Valsalva An area adjacent to the aortic valve that creates a space between the aortic wall and each semilunar wall.

Sinus tachycardia A sinus rhythm with a rate greater than 100 bpm.

Situs inversus A condition characterized by complete reversal of all thoracoabdominal organs, such that they are positioned the mirror opposite of normal.

Skip A radio wave transmission technique to overcome the problem of obstacles to line of sight, in which the high-frequency radio antenna is directed toward the sky. The radio signal then rises until it strikes the ionosphere, a layer of atmosphere where the sun's ultraviolet rays ionize the gasses, and the signal is reflected back to Earth.

Sky wave A radio wave transmitted into the atmosphere for a return to Earth rather than being transmitted across land.

Slander Situation in which defamatory lies about a person are told to others.

Slip-tip A syringe adaptor that simply slides inside the needle hub.

Small volume nebulizer (SVN) An alternative platform for the delivery of inhaled medications in which the medication is suspended in a stream of air which is then smashed against a round surface in the SVN, creating micro-fine particles that are ideal for inhalation.

SOAP notes One of the earliest standardized documentation formats, which contains subjective (S) information obtained from the patient or the patient's family, objective (O) information obtained during physical examination, an assessment (A) of the patient's problem, and a plan (P) for action.

Social norm A rule of conduct that regulates the interaction between people but is not specific to one individual.

Social space In the theory of proxemics, an area of relative safety where strangers can enter, with certain expectations of conduct. A dining room in a restaurant is an example of the use of social space.

Somatic pain Acute sharp, burning pain that often arises from the skin, ligaments, muscle, fascia, bones, or joints. Unlike visceral pain, somatic pain can be localized to a specific area.

Spacer A device attached to a metered dose inhaler that allows a more controlled inhalation of smaller, ideal-sized drug particles suspended in the vapor within the chamber than are possible with the metered dose inhaler alone.

Special incident reports (SIR) Documentation completed by the Paramedic that is not directly related to patient care but is instead used for administrative purposes or as a part of a court proceeding.

Specialty Care Transport (SCT) A growing subspecialty in EMS, in which Paramedics perform critical care interfacility transportation by transporting sick and injured patients from outlying clinics and critical access hospitals to tertiary care centers.

Specificity A measure of how often a patient with a negative medical field test truly does not have the condition the test is designed to detect.

Spike Sometimes called a bayonet, a very sharp point on an administration set which is used to pierce the fluid container.

Spirits Liquid medications brewed from various materials that have a volatile oil that evaporates at room temperature and leaves a distinctive odor in the air.

Spontaneous abortion Situation that occurs in about 30% of pregnancies in which the zygote fails to implant and the pregnancy prematurely ends; often referred to as a miscarriage.

Squelch control A static-reduction technique in radio transmissions that reduces the amount of signal received between transmissions, narrowing the reception of radio waves and eliminating background interference.

Standard leads The 12 leads used in a standard electrocardiogram, comprising the standard bipolar limb leads I–III, the augmented unipolar limb leads, and the standard precordial leads.

Standard of care Care and treatment that another Paramedic with the same or similar training would have rendered in the same or a similar situation.

Standing orders Preauthorized medical orders often given to Paramedics by physicians.

Star of life The symbol of EMS as represented by six points: detection, reporting, response, on-scene care, care in transit, and transfer to definitive care.

Starling's law A cardiac theory that states the heart's stroke volume increases in response to an increase in the volume of blood filling the heart (the end diastolic volume). The increased volume of blood stretches the ventricular wall, causing cardiac muscle to contract more forcefully.

Static Radio interference caused by unshielded electrical devices emitting 60 cycle interference, lightning in the atmosphere, bursts of radio waves from sunspot activity, and even the spark plugs in an automobile.

Status asthmaticus Persistent bronchospasm that is resistant to routine treatments.

Status epilepticus A condition of unremitting convulsions interspersed with brief instances of coma.

Statute A law enacted by legislation rather than previous case decisions.

Statute of limitations The time allowed from the occurrence of an incident during which a lawsuit can be filed. The statute of limitations simply states that a plaintiff (usually the patient) cannot commence a lawsuit after a certain amount of time has passed.

Sternal notch An anatomical position near the base of the neck.

Sternal retractions Situation in which the work of breathing increases and more effort is needed to generate the negative pressure in the thorax required for inspiration. When this happens, the skin at the top of the sternum is pulled inward because of this negative pressure in the chest.

Stethoscope A medical instrument used to listen inside the body, consisting of hollow flexible tubes connected to ear pieces that join to a piece placed against the area to be evaluated.

Stewardship To uphold the noble traditions of medicine while caring for patients.

Stigma A negative connotation attached to participation in a program, such as labeling and public embarrassment.

Stochastic effects Long-term complications from ionizing radiation exposure.

Stock solution A standard concentration of a solution that may be diluted to weaken its potency for certain patients.

Strain Signs of fatigue often seen when the body is repeatedly overstimulated, perhaps by constant bombardment by stress-inducing stimuli.

Stress The body's reaction to stimuli; a disruption in homeostasis.

Stress management A process of coping with chronic stress in an effort to recover from its effects.

Stress reduction Actions an individual takes to eliminate the source of stress.

Stressors Stimuli that cause stress. Modern stressors include psychosocial pressures from family, coworker complaints, and supervisors' demands, as well as such things as unrealistic expectations and noise pollution.

Strike-out A method of error correction on the patient care report in which the Paramedic crosses through the mistake with a single line, leaving the content below the strike-out legible. Next to the strike-out, the Paramedic should place the date and initial the strike-out to indicate authorship.

ST-segment depression A reduction of the ST segment, which is a >1 mm depression below the J point from isoelectric baseline.

ST-segment elevation A rise in the ST segment, which is a >1 mm depression below the J point from isoelectric baseline.

Stylet A commonly used adjunct to oral intubation that provides rigidity to the endotracheal tube.

Subcutaneous emphysema The presence of air between the layers of the skin that indicates a leak in the respiratory system.

Subcutaneous injection Injection in the layer of skin directly below the dermis and epidermis, which is the slowest and least dependable means of obtaining therapeutic drug levels in the bloodstream.

Subendocardial ischemia Condition that occurs during myocardial ischemia in which the deep myocardial tissues becomes ischemic first, since coronary perfusion occurs from the surface (or epicardium) inwardly.

Subpoena A legal command or direction issued by the court to appear at a certain place, such as the office of the plaintiff's attorney or the courthouse, at a particular time.

Substituted judgment Situation in which a surrogate decision maker has the responsibility to know the patient's preferences and must place the patients' wishes before the surrogate's wishes.

Succinylcholine A depolarizing neuromuscular blocker composed of two acetylcholine molecules hooked back to back. It offers a rapid onset of action (30 to 60 seconds) and rapid termination of effect (3 to 12 minutes) with return of sufficient ventilation to sustain life in 8 to 10 minutes. Succinylcholine produces muscle fasiculations at onset of action.

Suffix An affix placed at the end of the root word to modify that root word; for example, adding the suffix "-less" to the root word "help" makes "helpless," meaning something different than "help."

Summarization Communication technique in which the Paramedic takes the patient's own words, then paraphrases the patient's words to ensure that the message sent was correctly received.

Summary dismissal A request by the defendant's attorney to end a court action based upon the facts in the case, stating that the facts of the case are clear and without dispute.

Summary judgment Determination by a judge to dismiss or decide a case solely on the preliminary evidence without conducting a trial.

Support Assistance that promotes another's interests.

Suppositories Medication within a wax carrier that melts at body temperature and is typically given internally for a local effect; often administered in the vagina, urethra, or rectum.

Supraventricular rhythm A cardiac rhythm originating above the ventricles, indicated by a narrow QRS.

Surfactant A fluid that decreases the alveoli's surface tension and prevents the alveoli from collapsing during expiration.

Surgical anesthesia A near-coma state of sedation in which the patient loses protective reflexes in a head-to-toe (cephalocaudal) direction.

Surgical cricothyroidotomy A surgical procedure to gain entry to the trachea through the anterior neck by making an incision through the cricothyroid menbrane.

Suspension Medications that will not dissolve in a solvent and thus remain as finely pulverized particles floating in a liquid.

Sweep speed The speed of the rhythm passing by on the ECG monitor screen. Standard sweep speed is 25 mm/second, although the Paramedic may alter this speed to get a closer look at certain features of an ECG.

Sympathetic nervous system The portion of the autonomic nervous system responsible for those emergency responses that are at "stand-by," ready to provide the person with the ability to flee (flight) or fight.

Sympathomimetics Drugs that mimic the effects of the sympathetic neurotransmitter norepinephrine.

Symptom Something that indicates the presence of a physical disorder.

Symptom complex A list of abnormal conditions found by the Paramedic during the history of the present illness and the physical examination.

Symptom pattern A series of conditions associated with a known disease. The Paramedic compares the symptom complex against the symptom pattern arrive at a diagnosis.

Synapse The point at which an impulse passes from one neuron to another.

Syncope A transient loss of consciousness that spontaneously resolves.

Syndrome A collection of symptoms that characterize a condition or state.

Synergism The interaction between drugs which can occasionally lead to unexpected or extra effects.

Syntax The rules of grammar.

Syrups Medicines mixed with sugar and water.

System architecture The arrangement of radio components. Currently, two radio architectures exist in EMS: traditional land mobile radio (LMR) architecture and cellular system architecture.

Systemic Pertaining to more than one internal organ system.

Systemic inflammatory response syndrome (SIRS) Localized infection leading to systemic infection leading to sepsis, then on to septic shock and multiple organ dysfunction syndrome.

Systemic pathology Illnesses and ailments of humans related to specific organs.

Systems review A head-to-toe approach to history gathering in which the healthcare provider starts at the head, questioning about issues/concerns that may be present at the nervous system level (stroke, seizures), and moving downward to cover the cardiovascular system, respiratory system, abdomen, genitourinary system, extremities, and behavioral disorders.

System status management (SSM) A dynamic alternative to fixed-post staffing in which ambulances are "on the road" and moving to new locations to improve response times.

Systole Ventricular contraction.

Systolic blood pressure The maximum blood pressure measured during systole when the heart contracts.

Tablet A dry medicinal powder that is compressed into a pill shape.

Tachycardia A heart rate that is over 100 beats per minute for an adult or above the upper limit of normal for a child.

Tachypnea Rapid breathing.

Tactical EMS (TEMS) EMS providers working with police SWAT teams trained on how to provide care to the wounded while in hostile surroundings as well as maintain the health of the SWAT team members during prolonged operations.

Tactile fremitus Vibrations palpated on the chest wall that occur with speech.

Tamponade Compression performed to control bleeding.

Tardive dyskinesia A neurological disorder characterized by involuntary movements of the extremities often caused by long-term use of certain drugs (antipsychotic or neuroleptic).

Teachable moment The time when the patient has a heightened awareness of a problem and is receptive to information.

Telemetry The process of transmitting measurements and recordings to another location, where they are interpreted; a monitoring device connected to a patient by two or three wires that collects data and sends it via radio waves to an antenna.

Teleological A model of ethics that simply states the end justifies the means. This approach implies that, even though some harm may occur, in the end if the outcome is good then the behavior is ethical.

10-codes A system from the 1920s in which police departments that only had one radio frequency used abbreviated messages designed to minimize airtime. Plain speech is preferred over 10-codes to avoid confusion and improve interoperability.

Tenderness A soft or yielding texture; physically weak.

Tentative field diagnosis A determination of what's causing the patient's problems performed upon initial evaluation.

Teratogen Toxic substance or agent such as an illegal drug or an infection such as rubella (measles) or toxoplasmosis that could lead to fetal malformation.

Teratogenic effect Exposure to ionizing radiation that can cause birth defects and cancer in subsequent generations as a result of changes in the structure of DNA.

Tertiary care Highly specialized care provided in areas such as trauma centers and cardiac centers.

Therapeutic effect See **Intended biological effect.**

Therapeutic index The ratio of the difference between a drug's median effective dose (the ED50) and the median lethal dose (the LD50).

Therapeutic level (t) The point when the drug levels attain the targeted value, as manifested by observation of the therapeutic effect.

Therapeutic touch Intentional touching that mimics earlier comfort experiences (such as a mother stroking an infant's cheek) and telegraphs reassurance, understanding, and caring to the patient as a means to heal.

Third spacing A process that occurs when colloidal osmotic pressure is low, in which fluid leaks from the intravascular space and into the interstitial space.

3-3-2 rule A simple method for rapidly evaluating a patient's anatomy, in which a Paramedic should be able to place three fingers between the tip of the chin and the hyoid bone, place three fingers between the upper and lower teeth at the maximal mouth opening, and place two fingers between the thyroid notch and the floor of the mouth.

Thrill Vibration of the chest associated with heart contraction.

Thrombin A protease in blood that facilitates blood clotting by converting fibrinogen to fibrin.

Thrombocytes Platelets; blood cells that aid in clotting.

Thrombophlebitis An inflammation of a vein that may develop at an IV insertion site.

Thrombus A mature clot made of platelets cross-linked with fibrin and other blood cells in a firm meshwork; a blood clot.

Thyroid gland A highly vascular, "H" shaped structure that lies along the sides of the larynx and upper trachea.

Tidal volume The volume of a normal breath, approximately 5 to 7 cc/kg of ideal body weight.

Tincture Medicinal substance that is dissolved in alcohol.

Tincture of benzoin Medication often applied to skin before applying tape or another adhesive bandage, used to both prevent allergic reactions on the skin from the bandage and to help the tape or bandage adhere longer.

To keep open (TKO) The minimal infusion rate needed to keep veins from becoming occluded by a clot.

Tolerance Resistance to a drug over time, which prompts the patient to take larger doses of the drug to acquire the same effect.

Tonic A series of whole body contractions that often precede a seizure.

Tonicity A solution's ability to exert an osmotic pressure upon the membrane.

Topical Medications meant to be applied to the skin.

Tort A civil or private wrongful act, other than a breach of contract, resulting in some type of injury or harm (not necessarily physical injury).

Total body clearance The sum of all drug excretion from the kidneys, skin, lungs, and liver.

Toxicology The study of poisonous substances.

Toxin Any substance capable of causing cell injury and death, including poisons.

Trace A horizontal left-to-right movement on an ECG monitor.

Trachea A conduit for respiratory gasses to pass to and from the lungs.

Tracheobronchial suctioning Direct suctioning of the secretions in the bronchial tree.

Trade name Drug name manufacturers give a patented drug to distinguish it from other similar drugs.

Transdermal Pertaining to topical medication absorption, in which medicines are applied to the skin and absorbed into the body.

Transfusion-associated circulatory overload (TACO) Situation that occurs when the patient receives more volume of blood products than can be handled by the circulatory system.

Transfusion-related acute lung injury (TRALI) A new acute lung injury that occurs within six hours of a transfusion and is directly related to the transfusion.

Translaryngeal illumination Using a lighted stylet during endotracheal intubation to take advantage of the larynx's proximity to the anterior surface of the neck.

Translocations Gross breaks in some chromosomes with subsequent rejoinings at new locations.

Transmission The process of conveying a message, which can be either a true and accurate representation of the sender's thoughts or may be conveyed in such a way that the meaning is misconstrued by the receiver.

Transmural ischemia The stage of myocardial ischemia when the ischemia affects the entire thickness of the myocardium, from the endocardium to the epicardium.

Transtracheal jet ventilation (TTJV) Ventilation of the lungs using special high-pressure devices through a large bore catheter placed through the cricothyroid membrane, which is a commonly taught and performed emergent oxygenation technique.

Trauma Mechanical injury due to abrupt and sudden physical forces acting upon the body, such as friction, blunt force, or penetrating force.

Trauma line Intravenous access inserted into the vascular space so that intravascular volume can be replaced quickly.

Treatment pathway The continuum of patient care which starts with the primary assessment and is continued in the emergency department, critical care units, rehabilitation floors, and homecare services.

Triage tag A form of documentation tag used in mass casualty incidents to quickly prioritize patients based on how quickly they need assistance (i.e., immediate treatment vs minor injury).

Trigeminy Situation in which ectopic complexes occur every third complex.

Tripod position A position patients may assume when in respiratory distress to help with breathing, in which they place their hands on their knees or legs and lean forward in a sitting position, creating a tripod. This position allows the overworked accessory muscles to work better, although most patients begin to tire when they are in such severe respiratory distress.

Troches Lozenges that dissolve and are absorbed in the mouth through the oral mucosa.

Trunking A technique whereby, using computers, multiple users can communicate over fewer frequencies, with the computer selecting the frequency to be used based on availability.

Turgor A distended state of tension in living cells.

Turned over to A process of transferring a patient to another care provider with equal or greater skill.

Tympanic membrane Sometimes called the eardrum, a thin membrane that separates the external ear from the middle ear.

Type and crossed Donor blood that is successfully matched to recipient blood.

Type and cross-matched See **Type and crossed**

Type I error A common error made in an experiment in which the researcher rejects the null hypothesis and accepts the alternative hypothesis when in fact it is not supported.

Type II error A common error made in an experiment in which the researcher incorrectly fails to reject the null hypothesis; a failure to observe the change created by the treatment when one did occur.

Umbilical cord A connection between the mother's placenta and unborn child (at the navel) used to transfer nutrition, respiratory gasses, and wastes in the months prior to the child's birth.

Unilateral Relating to only one side.

Unipolar lead The use of a single positive electrode, using Wilson's central terminal, to record differences in electrical potential.

United States Pharmacopeia (USP) A drug reference created by an independent nongovernmental science-based public health organization called the United States Pharmacopeia. The United States Pharmacopeia is made up of over 1,000 scientists, practitioners, and representatives from various colleges of medicine and pharmacy who set the standards for medication manufacturing in the United States.

Universal donor Name given to Type O blood, since it can be given to any of the A-B-O blood types without adverse reactions. Type O blood does not have surface proteins that incite the immune response, which ends in hemolysis.

Universal law A situation that demands action by any person in that situation, as a matter of duty.

Universal recipients Name given to individuals with Type AB blood, since they can receive blood from any donor. This is because people with Type AB blood do not have antibodies against A or B proteins present in the plasma.

Upregulation An increase in the number of cell receptors in a body cell due to changes in chemical levels.

Urgent An assessment classification in which the patient's condition is not emergent, suggesting further assessment and evaluation is needed before treatment is initiated.

Use- (rate) dependent Drugs which act upon the ionic channels during the open/active state and preferentially will be attracted to rapidly depolarizing ectopic pacemakers.

Uvula A fleshy lobe that typically hangs in the midline of the pharynx.

Vagus nerve The major parasympathetic nerve which originates in the medulla, exits the skull at the base of the brain, travels down the neck (proximal to the larynx), branches into the heart and lungs, innervates the stomach, passes through the digestive tract, and ends in the anus.

Valecula The space formed between the anterior-superior surface of the epiglottis and the posterior base of the tongue.

Valid Logically correct and accurate.

Value judgment A Paramedic's decision as to which course of action is the correct course of action in terms of right or wrong.

Vapocoolant spray See **Fluori-methane.**

Vasopressor A chemical that causes vasoconstriction, particularly on the arterioles.

Vastus lateralis (VL) An intramuscular injection site on the anterior thigh. The Paramedic mentally divides the vastus lateralis muscle into three equal portions. Choosing the middle section of the VL, the Paramedic prepares the intended injection site with an alcohol-soaked pad.

Vector The sum of electrical events which makes up the common direction of the electrical wave front.

Vecuronium A non-depolarizing neuromuscular blocking agent commonly used by Paramedics in the prehospital setting.

Venous cannulation The process of threading a catheter into a vein.

Ventilation A measure of how well a patient is moving air in and out of the lungs during inhalation and exhalation.

Ventricular diastole Condition after a contraction when the ventricles of the heart are in a relaxed state.

Ventricular rhythms A heartbeat originating from the ventricle, indicated by a wide QRS. This is usually, but not always, dangerous because the origin of the beat is in the last pacemaker in the ventricles.

Ventricular systole Condition in which, with the pressure elevated in the ventricles, the ventricular muscle fibers contract forcefully and generate sufficient pressure to force open the aortic and pulmonary valves to eject blood out of the heart.

Ventricular tachycardia A rhythm experienced when the ectopic focus is ventricular and the ventricular pacemaker becomes dominant. With ventricular tachycardia, the rhythm is regular, the rate is fast, and every beat is wide.

Ventrogluteal (VG) An intramuscular injection site located on the lateral thigh proximal to the hip.

Venturi masks Special masks with a restricted intake that permits an exact percentage of oxygen. These can be used to deliver oxygen, although their use in the prehospital environment is generally limited to specialty care services.

Veracity An adherence to truthfulness. When a Paramedic practices being truthful with all of her patients, then that Paramedic can be said to have veracity.

Verbal consent A spoken request for permission to perform a procedure, accompanied by a simple explanation, which can improve patient compliance and decrease the risk of misunderstanding.

Vertical equity Injury prevention programs where the people most affected receive the major emphasis. For example, if statistics demonstrate a higher number of accidental shootings among children in low-income households, then public health programs could be justifiably organized to emphasize prevention within that population.

Vesicular sounds Lung sounds auscultated over the peripheral, smaller airways that sound like leaves rustling in the wind.

Vicarious liability Based on the legal principle *respondeat superior* ("let the master answer"), the basis that a person is accountable for the actions of others.

Virtue ethics A somewhat middle ground approach to ethics that does not depend on consequence-driven decisions or duty-driven decision making, but upon virtues. The virtue ethics approach suggests that a "right-thinking" person will make the best decision for the patient based upon a predetermined set of virtues.

Visceral pain Poorly localized pain that arises from the internal organs and is usually described as pressure-like, dull, or aching.

Vital signs Objectively measured characteristics of basic body functions, such as temperature, pulse, respirations, and blood pressure. Vital signs provide the Paramedic with an indication as to how well the patient's body is functioning or compensating for an injury or illness.

Volume overload A potentially devastating complication of intravenous infusions that occurs when a positional IV access is inadvertently adjusted and the infusion flow is unrestricted.

V/Q mismatch A mismatch between the amount of the lungs that are filled (alveolar ventilation) and the capillary circulation (pulmonary perfusion).

Walked on Suppression of a radio signal.

Wellness A state of physiologic equilibrium free of disease. More than an absence of illness, it is an active process of becoming aware of, and making choices toward, a more successful existence.

Wide open (WO) A rapid infusion of intravenous fluid.

Wilderness EMT (WEMT) An EMS provider in rural and woodland areas with special training that fosters critical thinking as well as creativity when working in an environment where supplies may be limited and patient transport to definitive care prolonged.

Witness A person who can confirm testimony or evidence presented in a case, or authenticate information provided.

Working diagnosis A presumptive conclusion the Paramedic makes based on the available signs and symptoms.

World Health Organization (WHO) The most prominent and influential international public health agency.

Z-track An injection technique in which the Paramedic holds the drug-filled syringe in the dominant hand, bevel up, and pulls gentle traction on the injection site with the nondominant hand as a means to prevent leakage.

Zygote A fertilized ovum.

INDEX

muscle relaxation, 43
muscles
    breakdown of, 160
    larynx, 357-358, 359
    rigor mortis, 194
    thoracic structures, 364-365
    thorax, 361-363
    trachea, 360
muscle wasting diseases, 167
muscular dystrophy, 167
musculoskeletal system, 285-287, 289-290, 292. *See also* bones; muscles
mushrooms, poisonous, 166, 640
myocardial infarction, 274-277
myocardial injury, 765-769
myocardial ischemia, 766-767
myocarditis, 773
myocardium, 720
myoglobulinuria, 181
myosin, 194
MyPyramid, 41
myxedema, 702, 738

N

Nadar, Ralph, 121
NAD (no apparent distress), 345
nail polish, 501
naloxone, 531, 617
names, addressing patients, 245
narcotics, 383, 479. *See also* illicit drug use; medications
nares, 293
nasal airway, 411
nasal cannula, 397, 503
nasal fossae, 354-356
nasal medications, 526
nasogastric tubes, 451, 463-464, 528
nasopharyngeal airway, 398-399, 411. *See also* airway
nasopharynx, 354-356
nasotracheal intubation, 427, 428, 444, 456-457. *See also* intubation
National Academy's Institutes of Medicine, 112
National Association of Emergency Medical Technicians (NAEMT), 6-7
National Association of EMS Educators (NAEMSE), 27
National Association of EMS Physicians (NAEMSP), 6, 25
National Association of EMS State Directors (NAEMSD), 25, 26

National Association of State EMS Officials (NASEMSO), 26
National Centers for Injury Prevention and Control, 121
National Commission for Protection of Human Subjects of Biomedical and Behavioral Research, 62
National Emergency Number Association, 28
National EMS Core Content, 26
National EMS Education Program Accreditation, 27
National EMS Education Standards (NEMSES), 6, 27
National EMS Scope of Practice (NEMSSOP), 26
National Formulary (NF), 619
National Health and Nutrition Examination Survey (NHANES), 60
national healthcare systems, 32
National Highway Safety Act, 22
National Highway Safety and Traffic Administration (NHSTA), 121
National Highway Traffic Safety Administration (NHTSA), 10, 25
National Institute for Health (NIH), 19, 111
National Institute of Medicine Report, 7
National Library of Medicine, 59
National Registry of Emergency Medical Technicians, 6
National Registry of Emergency Medical Technicians (NREMT), 6, 27
National Research Act (1974), 62
National Rural Health Association (NRHA), 7
National Standard Curriculum (NSC), 27
National Trauma Registry, 121
natural disasters, 110, 113
natural rights, defined, 74
nature of illness, 313
nebulizers, 533-534
neck, trauma, 298
necrosis, 180, 193, 767-768
needle cricothyroidotomy, 448-449
needle cricothyrotomy, 437
needles, 534-536, 562-563, 563, 576-577
negative pressure ventilation, 365
negligence, 85

negligence per se, 89
neonates, 135
neostigmine, 482
neostigmine bromide, 640
nerve agents, 640
nerves, injections, 574
nervous system
    alpha-adrenergic blockers, 644
    beta adrenergic blockers, 644
    neurotransmission, 639-640
    overview, 638-639
    respiration, 364, 365-366
    stress and, 42
    toddlers, 139
neurogenic shock, 180
neuroleptics, 687
neurological examination
    altered mental status, assessment of, 287
    chest pain, assessment of, 277
    extremity pain, assessment of, 290
    HEENT, assessment of, 293
    high blood pressure, assessment of, 292
    pregnancy, assessment of, 297
    syncope, assessment of, 282-283
neuromodulators, 689
neuromuscular blocking agents, 165, 479-482, 641
neuromuscular system, 139-140
neuropeptide neurotransmitters, 165
neuroreceptors, 164, 165-166, 639
neurotransmitters, 164-165, 639
neurovascular assessment, 279
neutrophil chemotactic factor, 186
neutrophils, 186-187, 602
new media, 11
niacin, 649
nicotine, 534
nicotinic receptors, 165, 640
nitrates, 531, 534, 652-654, 670
nitric oxide, 647-648
nitroprusside, 670
no apparent distress (NAD), 345
nociceptors, 689
nomogram, acid-base interpretation, 509-510
non-depolarizing (competitive) neuromuscular blockers, 481-482, 641
non-economic damages, 87

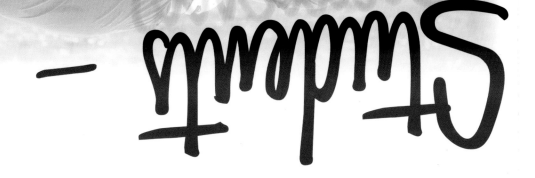

Become part of the community of more than 800,000 EMS PROVIDERS

Read what INDUSTRY LEADERS HAVE TO SAY about the EMS profession

Review NEW PRODUCTS and SERVICES you will be using in the field

Learn FROM VETERAN EMS professionals who respond to emergencies every day

Continue your EMS education BEYOND THE CLASSROOM

Receive a FREE subscription to *EMS* Magazine and:

Submit

EMS MAGAZINE
ATTN CIRCULATION DEPT
PO BOX 803
FORT ATKINSON WI 53538-9985

POSTAGE WILL BE PAID BY ADDRESSEE

BUSINESS REPLY MAIL
FIRST-CLASS MAIL   PERMIT NO. 139   FORT ATKINSON, WI 53538

NO POSTAGE
NECESSARY
IF MAILED
IN THE
UNITED STATES

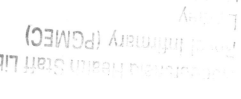

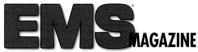MAGAZINE

PO BOX 500
FORT ATKINSON WI 53538-0500

Visit us at
www.emsresponder.com/subscribe
Priority Code: Q9STUD
or Fax to: (920) 563-1704

Please write clearly with a black pen.

1. **Please start/continue my FREE subscription to** *EMS Magazine*:
   ○ **Yes, Print**   ○ **Yes, Electronic**   ○ **No, Thanks**
   Electronic Editions may be served at the publisher's discretion

Signature (Required) _____   Date _____/_____/_____

Name (Please print) _____

Job Title _____

Company _____

Address _____

City _____

State/Province_____ Zip/Postal Code_____

Country _____

Phone (   ) _____ Fax (   )_____
By providing your fax number you are giving Cygnus Business Media permission to send you information via fax. Your fax number will not be released to any third party. Check here if you do not wish to receive subscription or industry related information via fax. ❏

Email (Required for Digital Edition) _____
Complimentary subscriptions need to be renewed annually. Check here if you do not wish to receive Product and Service information from our industry Partners via e-mail. ❏

The publisher reserves the right to serve only those individuals who meet qualification guidelines

2. **Please indicate your type of service:**
   ○ 12. Fire Department
   ○ 10. Third Service/Municipal Agency
   ○ 11. Independent EMS Service
   ○ 13. Private Service
   ○ 17. Hospital
   ○ 19. Commercial/Industrial
   ○ 14. Government/Military
   ○ 18. Manufacturer/Distributor/Dealer
   ○ Other EMS Provider
     (Please specify)_____
   ○ Other (Please specify) _____

3. **Please indicate your job title:**
   ○ N. EMS Chief
   ○ K. Fire Chief
   ○ D. Other Chief
   ○ L. EMS Director
   ○ O. Captain, Lt, Commander
   ○ M. Pres, Owner, VP, Dir, Div/Dept Head, Mgr
   ○ S. Emergency Manager, Commissioner
   ○ E. Medical Director, Physician
   ○ G. EMS Coordinator/Administrator/Supv
   ○ H. Instructor, Trainer
   ○ R. Nurse
   ○ P. Paramedic
   ○ T. EMT–Intermediate
   ○ F. EMT–Basic
   ○ J. EMS Committee Member
   ○ Other (Please specify)_____

4. **I recommend, specify or approve products or services in the following areas:**
   (Check all that apply)
   ○ 1. Firefighting   ○ 6. Hospital ED
   ○ 2. EMS   ○ 7. Emergency Mgmt
   ○ 3. Rescue
   ○ 4. Haz-Mat
   ○ 5. Other (Please specify)_____

5. **Number of stocked BLS/ALS vehicles at your location:** (check if applicable)
   ○ 1. 1-2
   ○ 2. 3-5
   ○ 3. 6-10
   ○ 4. 11-25
   ○ 5. more than 25

6. **Please also send EMS Magazine FREE to the following individuals at this location:**

   Name_____

   Title_____

   Name_____

   Title_____

*Complete this form, fold with postal side out, tape at top and mail. *DO NOT STAPLE**